SEVENTEENTH EDITION

Bailey's Textbook of
HISTOLOGY

SEVENTEENTH EDITION

Bailey's Textbook of
HISTOLOGY

Wilfred M. Copenhaver, Ph.D.

Professor Emeritus of Anatomy,
College of Physicians and Surgeons,
Columbia University
Professor of Anatomy,
University of Miami School of Medicine

Douglas E. Kelly, Ph.D.

Professor of Anatomy,
University of Southern California School of Medicine

Richard L. Wood, Ph.D.

Professor of Anatomy,
University of Southern California School of Medicine

The Williams & Wilkins Company/Baltimore

Previous editions copyrighted in 1904, 1906, 1910, 1913, 1916,
1920, 1925, 1932, 1936, 1940, 1944, 1948, 1953, 1958, 1964, 1971

Spanish translations published in 1948; 1962

Indian Edition in 1967

Made in the United States of America

Library of Congress Cataloging in Publication Data

Bailey, Frederick Randolph, 1871–1923.
    Bailey's textbook of histology.

    Bibliography: p.
    Includes index.
    1. Histology. I. Copenhaver, Wilfred Monroe, 1898– II. Kelly, Douglas E., 1932– III. Wood, Richard Lyman,
1929– IV. Title: Textbook of histology. [DNLM: 1. Histology. QS 504 B154t]
QM 551.B24 1978   611'.018   77-22879
ISBN 0-683-02078-1
Reprinted 1979

Composed and printed at the
Waverly Press, Inc.
Mt. Royal and Guilford Avenues
Baltimore, Md. 21202, U. S. A.

Preface to The Seventeenth Edition

Since the last edition of this textbook was published (1971) there have been marked advances in histology and its related fields as a result of well conceived experimental studies combined with improved techniques. A wealth of new information has been obtained by electron microscopy through improvement in technical methods, such as those for freeze-fracture replication, improvement in instrumentation, and improvement in our interpretive abilities. Results obtained by scanning electron microscopy have also provided a better understanding of structure in three dimensions. As a result, a number of the older electron micrographs used in previous editions of this textbook have been replaced and numerous additional ones that reflect some of the recent advances have been included. Numerous light micrographs of thin (1 to 2 μm) sections of plastic-embedded tissue fixed by vascular transfusion have been added to provide better light microscopic detail and to give better correlation between light and electron microscopy.

In histology, as in other disciplines, new research not only answers some questions but also raises many new questions. In this revision, as in previous ones, we have tried to make the more important points stand out somewhat from the accompanying details. We have tried to present the material in a manner that is most useful for students and we have provided selected references for those who wish to pursue particular topics in more detail.

At the University of Southern California, we have found it advantageous to teach human embryology in a closely integrated fashion with histology. Students learn the embryonic body plan and emergent organ systems as arenas in which the differentiation of the basic cells and tissues is occurring. They learn the cells and tissues as products of developmental processes and recognize thereby both essential differences and similarities among differentiated cellular populations. In this spirit, we have departed somewhat from the usual histology textbook format to include an expanded chapter on early human development and to include added embryological insight into most discussions of tissues and organs. We hope this will prove helpful to the wide variety of patterns in which courses in microscopic anatomy are taught.

This textbook has been rewritten a number of times since the first six editions by Frederick R. Bailey, M.D., between 1904 and 1926. However, the book still contains passages and illustrations incorporated by many others into subsequent editions. A resumé of these contributions before the 15th edition is given in a part of the 15th edition Preface, which is reprinted on page vii of this edition.

The present edition also contains some text material and a number of illustrations in the chapters on the cell, nervous tissue, and sense organs which were added by Drs. Richard and Mary Bunge, who participated in the 16th edition revision.

A number of illustrations included in this textbook have been obtained from colleagues at other universities and we are grateful for their generosity. Credits for those illustrations are given in the figure legends. We are also grateful to Dr. Mikel Snow for providing the brief text of the section on muscle regeneration, to Mr. Pete Mendez and some of his students, who provided new drawings, and to technicians, secretaries, and many other colleagues who have contributed immeasurably to the preparation and the content of the book.

Finally, we wish to express our appreciation to the Publishers for their cooperation and assistance in the production of this book and for their patience in awaiting its completion.

WILFRED M. COPENHAVER, PH.D
DOUGLAS E. KELLY, PH.D.
RICHARD L. WOOD, PH.D.

Excerpts from the Fifteenth Edition Preface

A brief resumé of the history of this textbook seems appropriate at this time (1964). The first edition was written by Professor Frederick R. Bailey at the College of Physicians and Surgeons and was published by William Wood and Company in 1904. Professor Bailey, with assistance from Professor Oliver Strong on the nervous system, continued the book through the sixth edition, published in 1920. Although the text has been rewritten by a number of authors since the time of Professor Bailey, it has adhered to his objective of emphasizing fundamentals.

Professors Oliver S. Strong and Adolph Elwyn revised the seventh edition (1925) and a part of the eighth edition (1932). Professors R. L. Carpenter, C. M. Goss, and A. E. Severinghaus participated with Professor Philip E. Smith and myself in completing the eighth edition (1932) and in the subsequent revisions of the ninth and tenth editions. The text retains valuable contributions made by them.

Professor Philip E. Smith served as editor of the ninth and tenth revisions and as coauthor of the eleventh, twelfth, and thirteenth editions. His contributions of material plus his sound editorial judgment had an important role in whatever success the textbook achieved during editions eight to thirteen inclusive. Professor Dorothy D. Johnson assisted with the thirteenth edition and became coauthor in the fourteenth edition. She made particularly valuable contributions to the chapters on the digestive system, respiratory system, and endocrine glands. It is regretted that unavoidable circumstances prevented Professor Johnson from participating in this edition.

I am indebted to Mr. Robert Demarest for all new drawings for this edition and for those which were added in the previous edition. I am also indebted to Mr. Carl Kellner (now retired) for the drawings which appeared first in editions nine to thirteen inclusive.

Many valuable suggestions have come from my colleagues at Columbia and from those in other schools. I am indebted particularly to Professor Thomas E. Hunt for a number of constructive suggestions.

WILFRED M. COPENHAVER, PH.D.

Introduction

All living organisms consist of minute elements which are called cells. These cells are the smallest structural units possessing those properties which we commonly associate with life. They are able to nourish themselves, to grow, to respond to stimuli, and to reproduce. Some organisms, the protozoa, consist of one cell only; the higher types, metazoa, may consist of infinite numbers of cells varying greatly in structural characteristics. Each of these multicellular organisms starts its existence as a single cell, the fertilized ovum, which by a process of proliferation and differentiation gives rise to the adult body. At first the cells of the developing embryo are similar in shape and structure. As growth continues, differentiation leads to the formation of groups of specialized cells, each group differing in structure from the others, each group adapted to subserve one or more specific functions. These specialized groups form the *tissues* of the adult body. At a very early period the cells of the embryo become separated from each other by the formation of varying amounts of intercellular substance, which may be the result of cellular secretion or actual modifications of cellular substance. In some of the tissues this intercellular material assumes enormous proportions. Thus the adult body is composed of cells and intercellular material, all elements so interrelated as to form a normally functioning machine.

Histology in a restricted sense is the study of the tissues of the body, but because the tissues are composed of cells and their products, a knowledge of the structure and activities of the cell must necessarily form the basis of histology. The first two chapters of the book are therefore given to a discussion of cells in general, the first of these these dealing with cells after fixation and the second with living cells. Each of these chapters obviously supplements the other. Succeeding these, the structure of the tissues is presented. This is followed by the microscopic anatomy of the various organs.

Over the years, histologists have tended to categorize the various cells and tissues of the body. They have classified them largely according to apparent differences, somewhat more than according to similarities. Textbooks of histology have tended to emphasize the categorizations, and students often dismiss their study of histology once they have memorized the essential differences that distinguish the categories under scrutiny. Yet we now understand ever more clearly that the similarities and common properties are as important as the differences. Nature has, in fact, not designed separate, distinct categories, but rather has evolved a spectrum of structural and functional possibilities around which the living organism is fabricated. Thus, in histology it is ultimately more important to interrelate and compare the properties of cells and tissues than it is simply to separate and name them.

Whereas histology is a structural science and complements at finer levels of resolution anatomical knowledge gained from dissection, its intimate relation to biochemistry, physiology, and pathology must be emphasized. The cell is a unit not only of structure but also of physiological activity. The formation of the specialized tissues is the structural expression of a physiological division of labor. The structures seen under the microscope assume a meaning only in the light of their functional significance. Thus the structure of muscles and glands can only be studied by constant reference to contraction and secretion. Normal physiological processes are associated with normal structure; abnormal processes are usually expressed in the altered structure and relationship of the cells and intercellular substance.

Recognition of these considerations, then, implies an awareness of increased breadth in the discipline of histology. To understand cells and tissues is to appreciate the common properties they have shared since their embryonic ancestry, the subtle and dramatic special propensities they have acquired during maturation, the minuteness of their most important parts, the delicate metabolic balance within which they normally operate, and the ease with which all of this can be altered to give conditions we define as disease. Understanding cells and tissues is not unlike understanding people and societies.

Contents

xviii   CONTENTS

CHAPTER 1

The Cell

The goal of anatomical study is not just the acquisition of an accurate, static visualization of the structural elements of living systems. Rather, such visualization must lead eventually to an appreciation of those elements as dynamic, changing entities in the flux of activity that is life. Living *structure* is the fabric upon which *function* is organized; neither can be understood without reflection upon the other. Anatomists have traditionally striven to visualize and describe as directly as possible the structural components of cells, tissues, and organs in a manner which is most representative of the living state. It is a difficult task, for important structure is often not rendered visible unless the cell or tissue is killed, and the anatomist must try somehow to assure himself that death has not rendered a distorted image of the living state. Moreover, anatomists have found repeatedly that the most challenging aspects seem to lie just beyond the resolution of the naked eye or microscopic tools at hand. Hence, the major challenge has been to develop better methods for accurate visualization of ever smaller parts.

We have recently seen an enormous expansion of histology and cytology, the youngest of the anatomical sciences. Utilizing the methods of histochemistry, light and electron microscopy, and tissue culture, cytological studies have clarified much of the structure of subcellular elements. These revelations, combined with new knowledge from biochemistry and cell physiology, have led to a firmer basic understanding of many of the ongoing processes of the living cell.

Neither the term "cell" nor the term "cell concept" will be new to readers of this text. The 19th century histologist Leydig defined a cell as "a mass of protoplasm containing a nucleus." This simple and useful description is still appropriate for animal cells today, for the minimal structural unit of protoplasm is that unit having available the genetic material (within the nucleus) which allows it to carry out, relatively independently, all of the vital functions necessary to sustain life. Although cells in higher organisms may develop considerable dependence on one another, each retains within its nucleus identical sets of genetic information necessary to carry out all cell functions. Cells which lose their nuclei may continue to function for some time because the nucleus previously made provision for the manufacture of all of the substances needed during the remaining life of the cell.

The term *protoplasm* denotes the entire living substance of the cell. This includes the cell body and its extensions and the nucleus which lies in it. The substance of the cell outside the nucleus is called *cytoplasm*; the substance of the nucleus is *karyoplasm* or *nucleoplasm*. The entire cell is circumscribed by a membrane termed the *plasma membrane* or *plasmalemma*.

Methods of Study

Our present knowledge of cell structure has been gained from an expanding variety of methods which fall logically into two groups: (1) methods employed with living cells and (2) methods involving dead cells (fixed or preserved). Some of the special methods employed in studies on the living cell are treated in the second chapter, but it should be emphasized that no single method should be used to the exclusion of all others. Studies on the living cell and those on preserved material yield supplementary data and, by their different approaches, corroborate or question the other's findings. This chapter deals with preserved cells and chapter 2 summarizes important findings from studies on living cells.

Preparation of Material

Some types of cells can be satisfactorily studied by placing them directly on slides for staining and for microscopic observation (e.g., Wright's stained blood smears). However, for most cytological work it is necessary to cut tissues into thin, translucent slices only a few microns thick. Sectioning is done on instruments called microtomes and is facilitated by freezing the tissue or by embedding it in a supporting medium such as paraffin, celloidin, or plastics. A brief outline of some of the technical procedures is given to aid the student in the interpretation of most slides prepared for his study. Those who wish more details on technique should refer to the books listed at the end of the chapter.

Most commonly, the first step in the preparation of histologic material is *fixation*. Numerous chemicals and their mixtures are used as fixatives (formalin alcohol, Bouin's fluid, Zenker's fluid, etc.), but fixation can also be achieved by rapid freezing. Fixation stabilizes tissue, preventing postmortem change, begins a hardening which facilitates sectioning, and promotes affinity of certain tissue elements for particular dyes. In the process of fixation, proteins are cross-linked or denatured and rendered insoluble; lipids and carbohydrates may or may not be preserved, depending on the nature of the fixative. For example, many fats are removed from tissues immersed in alcohols. Therefore, it has often been necessary to use different technical procedures to study the various constituents of a cell. It is significant, however, that methods for examining sectioned tissue by electron microscopy permit study of many cell constituents in a single light microscopic preparation.

For sectioning, the tissue is commonly infiltrated with paraffin. Because paraffin does not mix with water, the former will not penetrate into tissues until the latter is removed. *Dehydration* is accomplished by passing the tissues through a series of graded alcohols, up to 100%. Now, because paraffin is also insoluble in alcohol, the latter must be replaced by an agent miscible with both alcohol and paraffin, e.g., xylene or cedar wood oil. These agents also render the tissue translucent, and therefore this step in technique is known as *clearing*. The tissue is then placed in melted paraffin, which replaces the clearing agent; this step is referred to as *infiltration*. Next, the tissue is *embedded* in paraffin by allowing the latter to harden, and then the material is ready for sectioning and subsequent staining. Figure 1-1 shows photomicrographs of cells prepared by this method. Sections are usually 3 to 10 μm thick. Celloidin is an alternative embedding medium which is particularly useful for cutting large objects (e.g., brain) and for hard and brittle material (e.g., cartilage). Plastics, particularly epoxy resins, are increasingly being employed as the embedding medium for both light and electron microscopy. They produce less tissue and cellular damage than paraffin and allow the production of much thinner sections (down to 0.02 μm).

It is obvious that structures seen in sections may be altered by chemical fixation, dehydration, or the embedding process. Again and again, the description of features in the fixed cell has brought forth the objection that they are not true features of the living cell, but *artifacts* of technique. The answer to such objections must always be the consistency of the findings obtained by different technical procedures.

The *freeze drying technique* seems in some instances to cause less alteration of the living tissue than do the standard methods. In this technique, fresh tissue is pre-

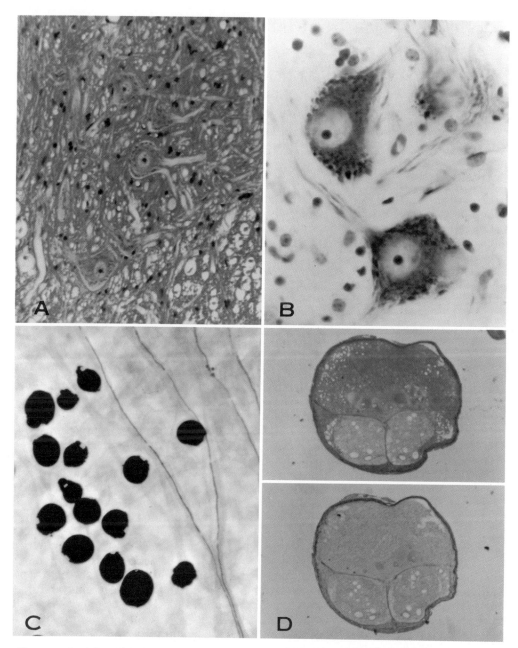

Fig. 1-1. Staining of various components. *A*, hematoxylin and eosin-stained spinal cord. Four nerve cell bodies are stained blue to purple by hematoxylin because of their high content of basophilic nucleic acid. Much of the remaining tissue is stained magenta by eosin because of the preponderance of acidophilic protein components. ×225. *B*, staining of nucleic acid by cresyl violet. In these two nerve cell bodies from spinal cord, the ribonucleic acid in the cytoplasm and in the nucleolus is heavily stained. The deoxyribonucleic acid of the nerve cell nucleus remains largely unstained because it is in a dispersed state. Smaller nuclei in which the nucleic acid is more condensed do stain with this dye. ×440. *C*, the lipid stores of these 15 fat cells are revealed by staining with Sudan black. The small indentations in some of the black deposits are the unstained nuclei. The slender strands are myelin sheaths, which also stain because of their high lipid content. Nervous tissue in culture. × 175. *D* (*upper figure*), glycogen is stained pink by the periodic acid-Schiff reaction. If the tissue is first treated with amylase, which digests glycogen, the pink staining is not seen (*lower figure*). Nonglycogen components of the sheath surrounding this lobster nerve ganglion are stained purple with or without amylase treatment. ×20.

served by placing it in a liquid such as isopentane chilled to about −170°C with liquid nitrogen. The frozen tissue is dehydrated in a vacuum and may thus be embedded without previous chemical fixation and dehydration in alcohols. This method is particularly useful for studying the localization of certain enzymes which are destroyed by the standard methods.

In the *frozen section technqiue* (not to be confused with the freeze drying method just outlined), a piece of tissue is placed directly on the stage of a special microtome equipped with an outlet for compressed carbon dioxide gas which cools the stage and freezes the tissue sufficiently for the cutting of sections. This method is widely used in clinical work for sectioning biopsy material when speed is important. In cytological work, the freezing method is particularly useful for studying the lipid content of cells because it avoids the use of fat-solvent dehydrating and clearing agents. The methods may be used for either fresh or fixed material; in the former case, it is useful for studying cell enzymes which are destroyed by chemical fixation.

The list of chemicals used for *staining* is even longer than that of those used for fixation. Most stains are classified as acids or bases. Actually, they are neutral salts having both acidic and basic radicals. When the coloring property is in the acid radical of the neutral salt, the stain is spoken of as an acid dye, and the tissues which stain with the dye are called *acidophilic*. Eosin is an acid dye with such general usage that the terms *eosinophilic* and acidophilic are often used synonymously. In some cases, it is clear that *basophilic* substances which attract basic dyes are themselves acids, as in the staining of nucleic acids with methylene blue. It has long been realized that special methods and stains are frequently necessary to demonstrate different structures, but the nature of the reaction between tissue and dye is often poorly understood.

Histochemical methods for the study of chemically recognizable substances within tissues began many years ago with the iodine test for starch. Since that time, numerous techniques have been developed for the identification and localization of chemical substances at the cellular level. Methods of particular interest include Caspersson's use of spectrophotometry for nucleic acids, Brachet's method for RNA, and Gomori's method for phosphatase. In applying spectrophotometry to cytology, ultraviolet light is useful because nucleic acids absorb light more strongly in the ultraviolet region than in other regions of the spectrum. Brachet's method uses an enzyme, ribonuclease, which selectively removes the RNA. When any material stains with a basic dye (such as pyronine or toluidine blue) in an ordinary section and then becomes unstainable after the section has been treated with pure ribonuclease, it may be concluded that the stained material was RNA. A similar principle is used in the histochemical study of glycogen. In this case, the control slides are treated with saliva; the salivary enzyme amylase removes the glycogen.

The histochemical localization of the enzyme *acid phosphatase* is widely used to identify areas of lytic (digestive) activity in the cytoplasm (see below under "Lysosomes"). The section is placed in a fluid containing a phosphate compound and lead ions. The enzyme in the tissue frees the phosphate, which combines with the lead to form an insoluble precipitate which is visible in the electron microscope (Fig. 1-31*C*). To make this visible in the light microscope, sulfide ions are added to form the coarser precipitate lead sulfide. Thus, the sites of dense reaction product may reveal the location of the enzyme. Combining histochemical procedures such as this with specific immunologic reactions, and the development of both techniques to utilize viewing by electron microscopy, improves accuracy of localization.

Radioautography is a technique whereby a radioactive precursor is supplied to living tissue and, after incorporation, its intracellular location is detected by exposure to a coating of photographic emulsion applied to the specimen. The radioactivity lodged in the tissue activates the silver halide crystals in the emulsion, and with photographic development metallic silver grains are formed. They are visible in both the light (Fig. 1-2) and electron microscopes, depending upon the preparation. Again, more precise localization of activity results from

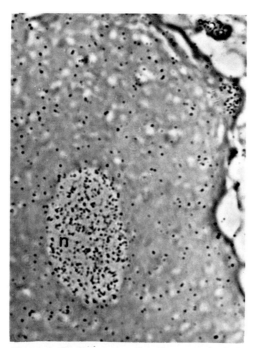

Fig. 1-2. Radioautograph photographed in the light microscope. The black dots overlying the tissue are silver grains which mark the sites of incorporation of radioactive uridine into newly formed ribonucleic acid. The silver grains are more concentrated over the nucleus (*n*) than over the cytoplasm of this large lobster nerve cell. ×500.

the combined use of radioautography and electron microscopy. Electron microscopic radioautography has proved extremely useful in tracing the path of protein synthesis in the cell cytoplasm (see "Granular Endoplasmic Reticulum"). The use of radioactive thymidine, incorporated only into replicating DNA, has been helpful in identifying dividing cells and in tracing cell migration in developing tissues.

The *preparation of sectioned tissue for examination in the electron microscope* must be done with extreme care. Fixatives are chosen to preserve structure in as lifelike a form as possible; inferior preservation is far more apparent in the electron microscope than in the light microscope. A primary aldehyde fixation (glutaraldehyde or formaldehyde) coupled with a postfixation with osmium tetroxide is most commonly employed. Buffering to slightly above neutrality is beneficial for most tissues. A highly crosslinked embedding medium (such as the epoxy resins, Araldite or Epon) is required in order to obtain the extremely thin sections that are examined in the electron microscope. Glass or diamond knives and specially designed microtomes are mandatory for such thin sectioning. Heavy metal "stains" (such as osmium, uranyl acetate, and lead citrate) are chosen for their ability to scatter electrons rather than to impart color. Because these cytological techniques yield preparations of superior quality, tissues prepared for electron microscopy are often sectioned at 1 or 2 μm, stained with a dye such as toluidine blue, and utilized for light microscopic study. Figure 1-3 is a semithin section prepared in this way.

Other methods for studying cell structure include microincineration and ultracentrifugation. By means of microincineration, microscopic sections are reduced to ash on a quartz slide. The amounts and distribution of inorganic components of the cell are demonstrated by this method. With the perfection of the ultracentrifuge, subcellular constituents can be separated. Combined with the use of solutions of varying density (density gradients), more and more precise separation has been obtained. Our present knowledge of subcellular elements was made possible by the parallel development of these separation methods and the introduction of the electron microscope for cytological analysis.

The Microscope

An understanding of the observations made with different types of microscopes requires familiarity with the units of measurement in common usage and an appreciation of the dimensions of some structures commonly studied by biologists (Table 1-1 and 1-2).

The usefulness of any type of microscope is dependent not merely upon its ability to magnify but, more importantly, also upon its ability to resolve detail. The useful magnification of an ordinary light microscope is only about 1200×. The *resolving power* of a lens is its capacity to give separate images of points close together. It is measured as the least distance between two points which can be seen as two instead of

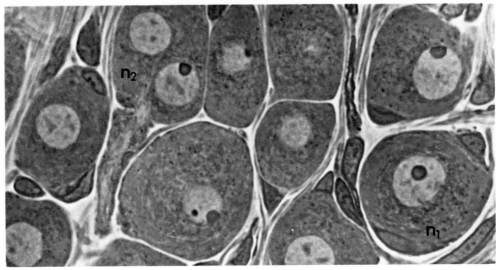

Fig. 1-3. Nerve cells fixed and embedded in plastic for electron microscopic study and then sectioned at 1 μm and stained with toluidine blue for observation in the light microscope. This type of preparation is often termed a semithin section. At *lower right,* a typical neuron (n_1) is seen to contain a large pale nucleus with a dense nucleolus. A binucleate neuron (n_2) is also shown. ×1100. (From M. B. Bunge et al.: J. Cell Biol. 32:439, 1967.)

TABLE 1-1

Measurements

Unit	Symbol and definition
Micrometer (micron)	1 μm = 0.001 mm = 10,000 Å 1 μm = 1 × 10^{-3} mm
Nanometer (millimicron)	1 nm = 0.001 μm = 10 Å 1 nm = 1 × 10^{-6} mm
Angstrom	1 Å = 0.1 nm = 0.0001 μm 1 Å = 1 × 10^{-7} mm

TABLE 1-2

Dimensions of some elements studied by biologists

Structure	Dimension
Human ovum	100 μm 1,000,000 Å
Skeletal muscle cells (cross section)	10–100 μm 100,000–1,000,000 Å
Cardiac muscle cells (cross section)	9–20 μm 90,000–200,000 Å
Lymphocytes	6–10 μm 60,000–100,000 Å
Erythrocytes	7.7 μm 77,000 Å
Bacteria	0.1–10 μm 1,000–100,000 Å
Viruses	0.05–0.5 μm 500–5,000 Å
RNP granules (ribosomes)	0.015 μm 150 Å

one. The resolving power is governed by the numerical aperture (NA) or light-gathering capacity of the objective lens and by the wavelength of light. Hence, in the light microscope, the resolution limit may be computed from the formula $R = 0.61\ \lambda/NA$, where R is the minimum distance between two resolvable points (in micrometers), λ is the wavelength of the light utilized (in micrometers), and NA is the numerical aperture of the objective lens in use. In practice, a yellow-green light with a wavelength of about 5400 Å is generally used, because the eye is more sensitive to this part of the spectrum, and with this light the limit of resolution of a 1.40-NA objective is 0.24 μm. With a 1.25-NA oil immersion objective, used on the most student microscopes,

the limit of resolution with a yellow-green light is 0.28 μm. A resolution of 0.17 μm can be achieved by using an oil immersion objective of 1.50 NA, but the refractive index of most optical material makes it impossible to increase the NA much further. It is evident that the way to increase resolving power is to use smaller wavelengths. However, glass lenses are not transparent to the wavelengths lower than 4000 Å, and it becomes necessary to use other refractive media. By using ultraviolet radiation having a wavelength of 2000 to 3000 Å and quartz lenses, resolving power can be increased to about 0.1 μm (1000 Å), but the main value of the ultraviolet microscope is for absorption spectrophotometry in histochemical studies.

The chief advance in increasing resolving power has been made with the transmission *electron microscope,* which uses electrons in place of light, and electromagnetic fields as lenses (Figs. 1-4 and 1-5). The final image is visualized on a fluorescent screen and recorded on a photographic plate. The wavelength of a stream of high velocity electrons is so short that the resolving power of an electron microscope can be less than 5 Å (0.0005 μm) with test specimens and 8 to 15 Å with biological specimens. With this amount of resolution, the electron microscope can be used profitably at very high magnifications. In common practice, the image is recorded at 1,000 to 100,000× and the photographic negative is enlarged 2 to 6 × when the positive print is made, thus giving final magnifications to about 600,000 ×. With the best equipment and with careful attention to all technical procedures, it is possible to use even greater magnifications. The appearance of a typical cell by transmission electron microscopy is shown in Figure 1-6A.

One of the limitations in transmission electron microscope work is the necessity of having extremely thin preparations (0.1 μm or less) because of the low penetration of the electrons. Another disadvantage stems from the fact that the tissues must be viewed in a high vacuum. Thus the study of living cells has not been possible with conventional specimens and instrumentation. Current experimentation with ultrahigh voltage instruments (1,000,000 to 2,000,000 V) and special wet specimen chambers show promise of alleviating this limitation. Currently, the greatest advantage in using ultrahigh voltage instruments is not the greater theoretical resolution but the ability to view thicker specimens. High voltage microscopy provides increased potential for preparing stereo pictures and visualizing intracellular components in three dimensions at high resolution.

Other types of electron microscopes are also coming into use. The *scanning electron microscope* offers less resolution, but its great depth of field allows direct visualization and three-dimensional rendition of the surfaces of fixed and dehydrated cells, organs, or small organisms. The specimen, usually coated with a conductor such as gold, emits secondary electrons when struck by a focused scanning primary electron beam. The intensity of secondary electron emission for each point of the scanned specimen surface is analyzed and displayed on a cathode ray tube, thus providing an electronic image such as is seen in Figure 1-6B.

The desire to view cells and tissues without chemical fixation and without dehydration has led to another approach for preparing material for electron microscopy, called *freeze fracturing* or *freeze etching.* After rapid freezing of the tissue, a break is made directly through the frozen cells, and a delicate metal shadow cast is made of the fractured surface. This metal cast, called a replica, is then observed in the transmission electron microscope. The technique is especially used in the study of membranes, for the fracture frequently occurs in such a manner that it splits the leaflets of the membranes of cells and organelles. Thus, not only are the contours of membranous components revealed in the replica, but the technique also provides the first fairly direct method of visualizing the interiors of individual membranes. Figure 1-7 is an electron micrograph from a freeze-fractured specimen.

The *phase microscope* is a modification of the light microscope particularly useful for the study of unstained cells, either living or fixed. Cellular components of unstained cells usually appear indistinct with the ordinary microscope because they are fairly transparent and produce very little change in the intensity of transmitted light (Fig. 1-8A). On the other hand, the different protoplasmic constituents produce phase changes because they vary in thickness and refractive index. The phase microscope converts phase variations into intensity variations and thereby enables the eye to detect more contrast between different structures (Fig. 1-8B).

The *interference microscope* utilizes the

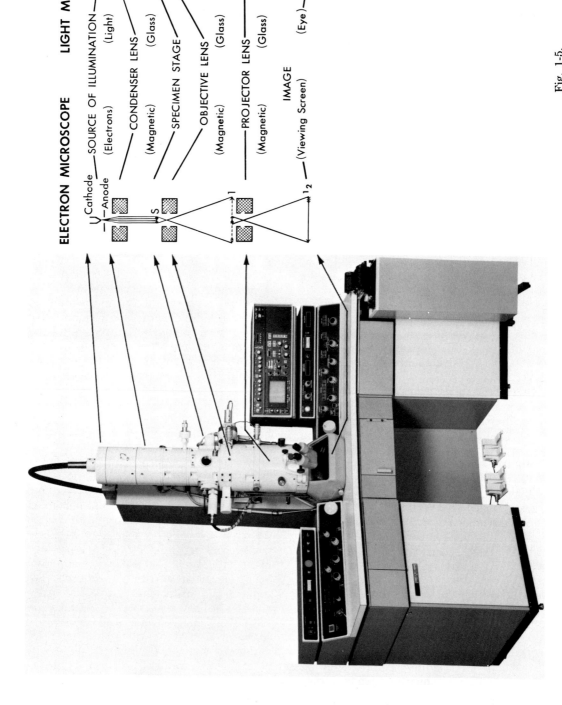

Fig. 1-5.

Fig. 1-4.

principles of the phase microscope more precisely. A light beam passing through the tissue is recombined with a separate light beam which has passed through the same optical apparatus without passing through the tissue. The manner in which these beams interfere with one another gives an index of the mass of the specimen, and it is thus possible to obtain precise information on the density of cellular regions, even in the living state. Differential interference (*Nomarski*) optics uses similar principles and provides remarkable three-dimensional images of living cells and cell components (Fig. 1-8C).

The *fluorescence microscope* has recently come into common use. Selected wavelengths of light are used to illuminate the biological specimen. Specific molecules within the tissue absorb this light and emit light at other wavelengths. The exciting wavelength is absorbed with filters, and the emitted wavelength is viewed in the microscope objective. Because it is possible to label antibodies with molecules (such as fluorescein) that fluoresce under these conditions, it becomes possible to localize antigen-antibody complexes within tissues. This can be a most precise method of localizing specific proteins within tissues.

The resolution of these phase, interference, and fluorescence optics is, of course, limited to that of all light microscopes.

Chemical and Physical Properties of Protoplasm

The basic medium in which the protoplasmic constituents are dispersed is water. In combination with soluble organic molecules and salts, this "ground cytoplasm" forms a hydrosol or a hydrogel, with the physical properties of a colloidal mass. Protoplasm is a semifluid or viscid substance whose consistency varies in different cells or in the same cell under different conditions of physiological activity. It may change from a condition of greater fluidity, a state of sol, to a more viscous gel state.

The nuclear protoplasm is ordinarily more viscous than the cytoplasm.

The chief ion of positive charge (cation) in solution in cell cytoplasm is K^+. The chief cation outside cells, in the general body fluids, is Na^+. Extracellular fluids contain about 120 meq/l of Na^+ but less than 5 meq/l of K^+; inside the cell a typical value is 10 meq/l Na^+ and 140 meq/l K^+. The tendency for Na^+ to leak into the cell and for K^+ to diffuse out to regions of lower concentration is counteracted by special properties of the cell membrane. The chief extracellular ion of negative charge (anion) is Cl^-; intracellularly, the important negatively charged molecules are HCO_3^-, HPO_4^{2-}, SO_4^{2-}, and certain proteins. The cell membrane is quite impermeable to certain of these intracellular anions (which are osmotically active), and when membrane properties are altered and metabolic processes cease after death, the intracellular molecules tend to attract water and the cell may swell.

The difficulties in understanding the life processes occurring within the cell derive in large part from their profound complexity and their remarkable miniaturization. The nucleus of human cells, which may be only a few micrometers in diameter, contains information (according to one estimate) for the manufacture of approximately 30,000 different proteins. A single cell may utilize 1000 or more different enzymes in the course of its day to day activities.

Early chemical analyses of protoplasm were primarily concerned with the types and amounts of small molecules present. Such analyses showed that the cell contains a high percentage of water and a host of small molecules, both organic and inorganic. The most characteristic components of the living cell, however, are the macromolecules: nucleic acids, proteins, complex carbohydrates, and lipids. These macromolecules are, in fact, polymers of certain of the smaller molecules, as is discussed below.

Fig. 1-4. Photograph of a modern electron microscope. The instrument shown may be used as a conventional transmission microscope (for viewing sections) or as a scanning electron microscope. Separate instruments of both types are also available. (Courtesy of JEOL (USA), Inc.).

Fig. 1-5. Comparison of optical paths in an electron microscope (*left*) and a light microscope (*right*). The light microscope diagram is inverted to facilitate comparison. (Courtesy of RCA).

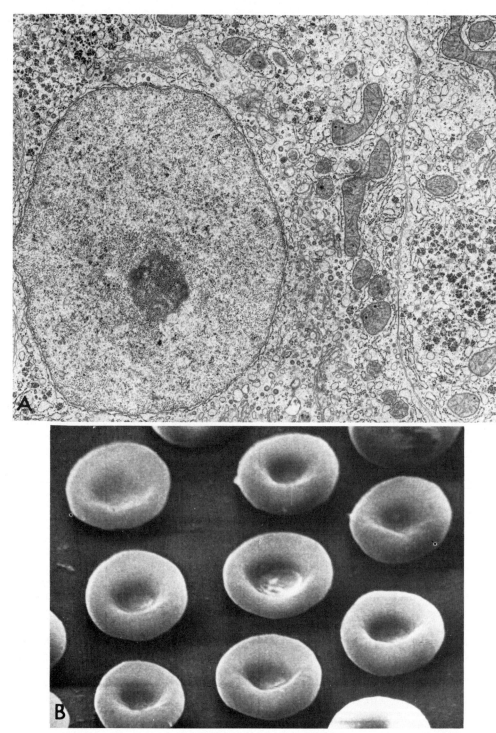

Fig. 1-6. *A*, transmission electron micrograph of a developing liver cell. Note the clarity of detail as compared to that of even the best light microscope preparations (as in Fig. 1-3). The cytoplasm contains organelles and inclusions that are considered in detail later in this chapter. ×9950. *B*, human red blood cells as they appear in the scanning electron microscope. As illustrated here, this instrument allows unsectioned objects to be visualized in three dimensions. ×3700. (Courtesy of Dr. Sarah Luse.)

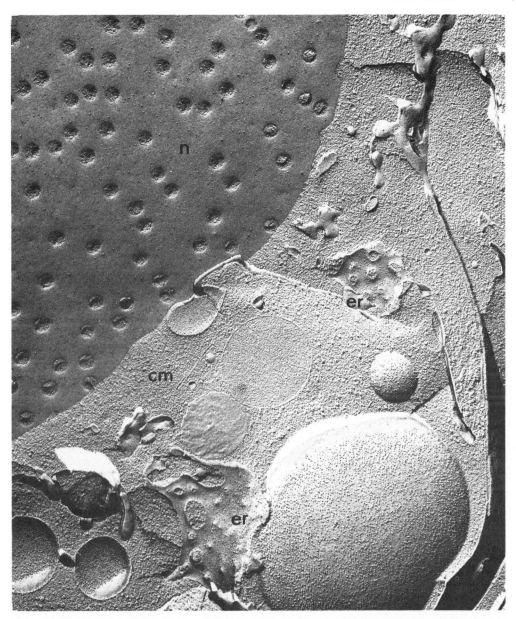

Fig. 1-7. Electron micrograph of a platinum replica of a cell which was frozen without fixation and then fractured to enable visualization of the cell interior, especially membrane faces. After freeze fracturing pores in the otherwise smooth nuclear envelope (*n*), sheets of fenestrated endoplasmic reticulum (*er*), the cytoplasmic matrix (*em*), and a variety of cytoplasmic vacuoles are all clearly visible. Onion root tip. × 36,000. (From D. Branton: Proc. Natl. Acad. Sci. U.S.A. 55:1048, 1966.)

More recently, the biochemist, by separating various cell components in a still viable state, has been able to study the dynamic relationships between various cell compounds. Such analyses indicate that many metabolic processes within the cell do not occur between constituents free in the ground cytoplasm. They occur instead within the framework of macromolecular aggregates called cell *organelles*. Many of these organelles are complex combinations of nucleic acids, proteins, and lipids. The organelles compartmentalize the cytoplasm and provide regions where specific metabolic processes occur, as is discussed below. *Protoplasm, in other words, is not a bio-*

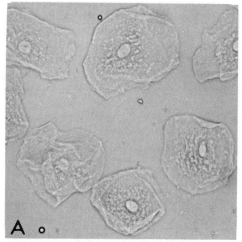

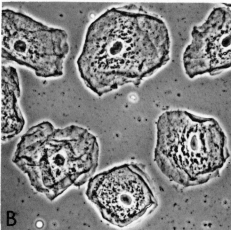

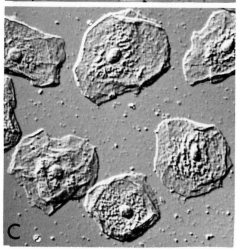

Fig. 1-8. Epithelial cells from human oral mucosa as they appear in *A*, the bright field light microscope, *B*, the phase contrast microscope, and *C*, the Nomarski optical system. ×250. (Courtesy of Carl Zeiss, Inc., New York.)

logical broth but a collection of highly organized components dispersed within the cell in a pattern suitable for their functional activities.

Despite the fact that many cell components are a combination of materials, it nevertheless is useful for the histologist to stain for specific components, because such staining can indicate regions of exceptional concentration. For example, a lipid stain will clearly delineate the nerve myelin sheath (Fig. 1-1C). Myelin also contains protein and carbohydrate, but the exceptional concentration of lipids in myelin allows its differential staining. Thus, it is useful to discuss the major macromolecular components of cells in relation to methods for their histological demonstration. The student is referred to biochemical texts for details of the structure of macromolecules.

Nucleic Acids

Nucleic acids are considered the basis of life, containing the genetic information available within the cell. They provide the blueprint for the most important products of the cell, the proteins, and the kinds and proportions of protein present give each cell its individuality.

Nucleic acids are complex compounds consisting of polymers of *nucleotides*. Each nucleotide contains a pentose sugar combined with phosphoric acid and with a nitrogen-containing base, either a purine (adenine, guanine) or a pyrimidine (thymine, uracil, cytosine). The phosphoric acid component gives the nucleic acids their marked affinity for basic dyes in stained preparations, and pyrimidines and purines absorb characteristic wavelengths of ultraviolet light. On the basis of the type of pentose sugar, the nucleic acids fall into two groups: (1) deoxyribonucleic acid (DNA, containing the sugar deoxyribose) and (2) ribonucleic acid (RNA, containing the sugar ribose). The nucleic acids combine with the basic proteins, protamine and histone, to form nucleoproteins. According to the Watson and Crick model (proposed in 1953), the DNA molecule is composed of two long polynucleotide chains coiled around each other in the form of a double helix. Certain forms of viral RNA are known to be double-stranded, as is DNA; the conformation of native RNA molecules in animal cells is presently under active investigation.

The DNA is found chiefly in the nucleus, confined to chromosomes which contain the genetic units called genes. The DNA is the chief informational macromolecule of heredity. In the cytoplasm, small amounts of DNA are present within mitochondria (see below). The quantity of DNA in the nuclei of different cells of any given species is relatively constant, with the exceptions of mature germ cells, which have a reduced (haploid) number of chromosomes, and certain other cells, which may have a multiple (polyploid) number of chromosomes (some liver cells, for example). Naturally, there must be an increase in chromosomal DNA before chromosome division at mitosis; otherwise the DNA of the daughter cells would soon be depleted. Although the amount of DNA in the chromosomes of different cells is relatively constant, the amount of DNA-associated protein varies greatly. The latter is usually high in cells which have high metabolic activity in their cytoplasm (e.g., liver and kidney cells).

Ribonucleic acids are found both in the nucleus and in the cytoplasm, particularly in the latter. The RNA carries the information stored in the DNA of the gene to the sites of actual protein synthesis in the cell. The total amount of RNA per cell varies for different tissues and for the same cell type at different times. It is usually abundant in the nucleoli and in the cytoplasm of cells, which are most active in synthesizing proteins.

Recent studies have revealed the presence of different types of RNA in the cell, with differences in function. *Messenger* RNA is formed in the nucleus and then travels out into the cytoplasm, where its linear sequence of bases provides the template for *transfer* RNA. The amino acids attached to transfer RNA are then combined in a specific sequence into a linear chain, the polypeptide chain, for the formation of proteins (Fig. 1-18). Messenger and transfer RNAs are relatively small molecules and probably contribute little to the staining of RNA in cells. Staining instead depends mostly on the presence of *ribosomal* RNA, which, in combination with protein, constitutes ribosomes (see below).

Thus, nucleic acid staining of cytoplasm depends primarily on the presence of ribosomal RNA (Fig. 1-1B). Ribosomal RNA is synthesized as two subunits of different sizes that join together to form definitive ribosomes. Ribosomes nearly always occur in clusters called *polyribosomes* or *polysomes*. Polysomes either lie free in the cytoplasm or may be attached to membranes of the endoplasmic reticulum. Ribosomes and endoplasmic reticulum are discussed further under the heading "The Cytoplasm" later in this chapter.

The Feulgen staining reaction is particularly useful for distinguishing DNA from RNA and from other basophilic substances. This cytochemical reaction is specific for DNA because, after mild acid hydrolysis, only the aldehyde group of deoxyribose is available to change the colorless leuco fuchsin (Schiff reagent) to the characteristic magenta color. Reference has already been made to the fact that the identity of RNA can be confirmed by the use of a specific enzyme, ribonuclease. Although basophilia in itself is not a specific test for nucleic acids (other acids in the protoplasm attract basic dyes), it is true that many basophilic structures contain nucleic acids. It may be pointed out again that the nucleic acids occur in combination with proteins as nucleoproteins. The nucleoprotein reaction seen in sections stained with both basic and acidic dyes varies with the proportion of the different substances present. For example, the chromatin of the nucleus is very basophilic by reason of its high proportion of nucleic acid, whereas the nucleoprotein of the nucleolus is often acidophilic by reason of its proportion of certain basic proteins.

Amino Acids and Proteins

Proteins are indispensable for the metabolic processes of the cell, and they are also important in the structural organization of protoplasm. All enzymes, the vital catalysts of the chemical reactions in the cell, are proteins. Each type of protein is made up of a particular number and variety of amino acids joined in a precise sequence. Living systems contain about 20 different amino acids, each a single letter in the alphabet of protein structure. They have a characteristic capacity for combining with each other to form long chains. This property results from the presence of a carboxyl group (—COOH) and an amino group (—NH₂) in each molecule. Condensation occurs when the acid group of one amino acid molecule combines with the basic group of another, with the loss of one molecule of water. This is known as a peptide linkage, or a *peptide bond*. Chains of amino acids connected by peptide bonds are known as polypeptides. The sequence of amino acids in the peptide chain is very important. For instance, the hemoglobin of patients with sickle cell anemia differs from normal hemoglobin only in the substitution of a molecule of valine in the place of a molecule of glutamic acid.

Protein molecules consist of one or more peptide chains, and they have molecular weights ranging from 10,000 to 1,000,000 or more. These large molecules are generally described as having three levels of organization. The *primary structure* is provided by the amino acid sequence. The primary structure of a substantial number of protein molecules is known. Insulin, for example, is known to be composed of two polypeptide chains (with a total of 51 amino acids) bound together at two points by disulfide bonds between sulfur-containing amino acids within the chain. The *secondary structure* of proteins is formed when peptide chains spontaneously coil as a result of secondary bonding (such as hydrogen bonding) between their constituent amino acids. This secondary coiling produces the helical arrangement of the protein molecules in hair and wool and in other fibrous proteins. Sometimes these helical arrangements involve a number of polypeptide chains coiled together, as in collagen (discussed in chapter 5).

A *tertiary structure* of proteins may be formed when relatively straight sections of the polypeptide chain are sharply bent at a number of points to fold the molecule up into a globular configuration. The more biologically active proteins in the cell (such as enzymes and hormones) are globular in overall configuration, and are often soluble in the cell cytoplasm and in general body fluids. These globular proteins become partly unfolded in the presence of heat; this

denaturation accounts for egg albumin's turning white upon heating. Histological fixatives are often selected to stabilize the structural components of tissue while causing as little protein denaturation as possible.

Many proteins contain chemical entities in addition to amino acids; this forms the basis for another method of protein classification. The *simple proteins* yield only amino acids on hydrolysis. This group includes albumins, globulins, protamines, and histones. *Conjugated proteins* consist of a simple protein combined with another organic substance called the prosthetic group. The conjugated proteins yield amino acids plus the prosthetic group on hydrolysis. The conjugated proteins include nucleoproteins (proteins combined with nucleic acid), glycoproteins or mucoproteins (proteins combined with a carbohydrate), lipoproteins (proteins with fatty acids), and chromoproteins (e.g., hemoglobin).

The amino acids which form proteins contain groupings which ionize to form acids in some cases and bases in others. Thus, proteins may be predominantly acidic or basic and take up dyes which bind either to acid groups (basic or cationic dyes, such as methylene blue) or to basic groups (acid or anionic dyes, such as eosin). Eosin colors acidophilic material (primarily basic proteins) pink or red (Fig. 1-1*A*). A commonly used counterstain, hematoxylin, contains components which together stain basophilic material (nucleic acids and acid proteins) blue.

Lipids

Lipids form a diverse group of compounds (including fats, phospholipids, glycolipids, and sterols) which are generally insoluble in water. Three examples of their functional role within the cell are as follows. First, they provide the most concentrated energy reserves of the cell. Fats, which contain fatty acids linked to glycerol, are generally stored within cells in droplets of varying size. These fats can be hydrolyzed to fatty acids and glycerol, and the fatty acids can then be oxidized for energy production. Further energy is derived as the 2-carbon fragments resulting from oxidation are used to fuel the citric acid cycle (see below). Second, certain lipids, particularly phospholipids and cholesterol, form important components of cell membranes. The phospholipids are key compounds, for they have the important property of having a hydrophobic end, which repels water, and a hydrophilic end, which attracts water; this property contributes to the ability of the membrane to partition cellular regions of differing function. It should be noted that the steroid hormones are structurally very similar to the membrane component cholesterol, and one of their important effects is to alter the permeability of the cell membrane.

Third, cell lipids, called glycolipids, are found in combination with sugar molecules, e.g., cerebrosides and gangliosides. These are also utilized in the construction of the cell membrane; it is believed that the lipid components form a major part of the membrane itself, with the carbohydrate component contributing to the surface hydrophilic coat of the membrane (see below under "Cell Membrane").

A substantial amount of lipid is extracted by the standard preparative techniques for histological sections. Lipids can be demonstrated either by the use of a special fixative such as osmium tetroxide, followed by a fat stain such as Sudan black, or by freezing the tissues for sectioning, thus avoiding the solvents used in the paraffin-embedding procedure (Fig. 1-1C).

Carbohydrates

Many of the cell macromolecular compounds which are composed primarily of polymers of sugars, or which are protein-carbohydrate complexes, are exported from the cell. Some become important constituents of the supportive and connective tissues of the organism. Others are components of body lubricants such as the mucus covering the surfaces of cells lining the gastrointestinal tract. Still others are stored within the cell, where they form the most readily available energy reserve in the body. Carbohydrate compounds have been classified in many different ways. It is convenient to divide them into four general categories: (1) polysaccharides, (2) polysaccharide-protein complexes, (3) glycoproteins, and (4) glycolipids (discussed above).

Polysaccharides are polymers of sugars. The simplest polysaccharides are constructed from one repeating hexose unit. Their individuality is imparted by the types of chemical linkages within the polymer and the pattern of branching. The animal polysaccharide glycogen is a complexly branched polymer of glucose, as is plant starch. Both are stored within cells and are then readily available for use when needed (Fig. 1-1D). Polysaccharides excreted by cells generally contain two or more monosaccharide components. Among these are hyaluronic acid (which is a copolymer of glucuronic acid and N-acetyl glucosamine) and chondroitin sulfate (which is a copolymer of glucuronic acid and N-acetyl hexosamine sulfate). These molecules form critically important extracellular lattices in connective and supportive tissues, where they impart appropriate degrees of viscosity and rigidity. When polysaccharide components are attached to a polypeptide component through "weak" chemical bonding, they are frequently termed *mucopolysaccharides*. Chondroitin sulfate-protein complexes occur widely in connective tissue (chapter 5) and account for about 40% of the dry weight of cartilage (chapter 6). Hyaluronic acid-protein complexes are found in the vitreous and aqueous humors and cornea of the eye and in the fluids of joint cavities. The blood anticoagulant heparin is also a mucopolysaccharide.

Compounds containing substantial amounts of protein strongly (covalently) bound to smaller amounts of carbohydrate are usefully termed *glycoproteins* or mucoproteins. These compounds are frequently found on the surfaces of cells. Glycoproteins are especially important in immunological reactions in the body, comprising both the immunoglobulin produced by antibody-forming cells and the antigens responsible for the specificity of the ABO blood group system.

Structural and Functional Organization of Cells

Cells vary greatly in size, shape, and structure, as shown in Figures 1-1, 1-3, 1-9, and 1-44. These variations are adaptations

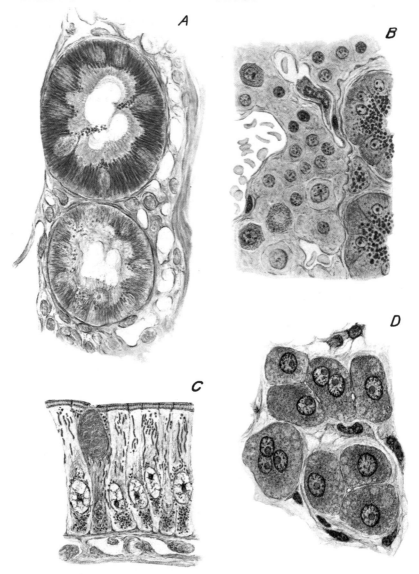

Fig. 1-9. Staining of tissues by various techniques. *A*, kidney of mouse. Contrast the prominence of parallel lined mitochondria in the proximal convoluted tubule *above* with the distal convoluted tubule *below*. Regaud, Altmann acid fuchsin. *B*, island of Langerhans from human pancreas, bordered at *right* by acinar cells, which show chromophilic substance and apical secretion granules. In the island tissue are many B cells (orange), three red granular A cells, and two blue D cells. A polymorphonuclear leukocyte was caught in the upper sinusoid. Helly, modified Masson. *C*, intestinal epithelium of cat, showing one goblet cell among absorbing cells. Note polarized mitochondria and the striated cell border. Champy, modified Masson. *D*, liver cells from rhesus monkey filled with evenly distributed glycogen granules. One cell has two nuclei, another three, which is not uncommon. Biopsy, alcohol, Best's carmine. Camera lucida drawings. (Preparations by Dr. A. E. Severinghaus.)

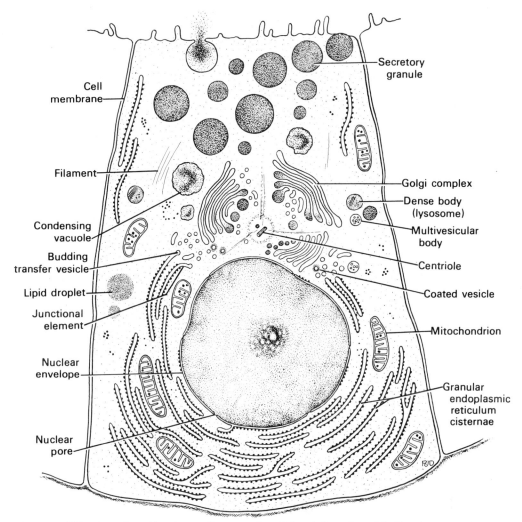

Fig. 1-10. Diagram of a cell as it would appear in a thin section viewed in the electron microscope. All of the organelles depicted here are described in the text. The cell components and their organization indicate that this is a secretory cell. The secretory product is synthesized near the base of the cell in the region of the granular endoplasmic reticulum and is transported to the Golgi region, where it is packaged for release from the upper (apical) surface of the cell.

for the different functions which the cells perform in different tissues and organs, and they are considered in more detail in succeeding chapters. Regardless of specialization, most cells retain a number of features in common (Fig. 1-10). These general characteristics form the subject for the present discussion.

The Nucleus

The nucleus varies in shape and size in different types of cells. In rounded or cuboidal cells, it usually assumes a spherical form (Fig. 1-9D). In tall columnar or spindle-shaped cells, the nucleus is usually elongated, with its long axis corresponding to that of the cell (Fig. 1-9C). In cells whose cytoplasm becomes filled with inclusions, as in mucus-secreting and fat cells, the nucleus is generally flattened against the cell membrane (Fig. 1-1C). It usually reverts to a rounded form after the cytoplasmic inclusions have been extruded.

In some cells, the nucleus becomes lobated, as in neutrophilic leukocytes and megakaryocytes. Cells with a lobed nucleus are often, although not always, in a highly differentiated stage and lack the ability to divide by mitosis (e.g., polymorphonuclear leukocytes). One must not conclude conversely from this that all highly differentiated cells lacking mitotic ability have lobed nuclei.

Although a cell usually has only one nucleus, some types, such as parietal cells of the stomach, liver cells, and surface epithelial cells of the bladder, often have two or more. Osteoclasts of bone usually have a large number of nuclei, five or more.

Structure of the Nucleus. The interphase (nondividing) nucleus is bounded by a *nuclear envelope* and contains one or more *nucleoi*. Particles or clumps of *chromatin* are suspended in the nuclear ground substance.

With the advent of the electron microscope, it was found that the nuclear "membrane" seen by light microscopists was, in fact, a unit of two closely apposed membranes; this unit is called the *nuclear envelope*. At intervals the two membranes curve together and join to form an opening, a *nuclear pore* (Figs. 1-10, 1-11, and 1-17). When the nuclear envelope is sectioned in a perpendicular plane, the pores appear to be spanned by a septum thinner than a regular membrane (Fig. 1-29), but when the pores are viewed face-on in tangential sections of the envelope their structure is seen to be complex (Fig. 1-11). The edge of the pore has an octagonal symmetry and the pore contents display a variable structure. The organization of the pores is of considerable interest because pores are known to play an important role in the exchange of materials between the nucleus and the cytoplasm. The nuclear envelope is related to the cytoplasmic endoplasmic reticulum because (1) ribosomes may be attached to the membrane facing the cytoplasm, (2) continuities between the outer membrane of the envelope and the sacs of endoplasmic reticulum are frequent, and (3) the envelope is reformed from endoplasmic reticulum elements near the end of each cell division.

The *nucleoli* are round, dense, well defined bodies, although they do not have a limiting membrane. In general, there may be from one to four per nucleus, although they vanish temporarily during part of the division cycle. They are composed of RNA and associated proteins. Nucleoli usually stain intensely, but they exhibit a variable basophilia and acidophilia in different cells and at different times, depending on the relative proportions of RNA and basic protein.

The constituents of the nucleolus as seen in the electron microscope are as follows (Fig. 1-12). (1) A *fibrillogranular* ribonucleoprotein component consists of granules enmeshed in a matrix of filaments. These granules contain RNA which is destined for assembly in the cytoplasm into another kind of ribonucleoprotein particle, the ribosome. (2) Other portions of the nucleolus, often the center, consist of dense masses of ribonucleoprotein *filaments* 50 Å thick. (3) Surrounding or extending into the nucleolus are clusters of *deoxy*ribonucleoprotein filaments known as *nucleolus-associated chromatin*. During reformation of the nucleolus after mitosis, the nucleolar components accumulate in association with particular regions of certain chromosomes known as *nucleolus organizers*. It is this organizer region of the chromosome which is seen in association with the mature nucleolus. Finally, it should be pointed out that the ribonucleoprotein components —both the fibrillogranular and filamentous elements—are often aggregated into a meandering thick thread or network called the *nucleolonema*. The associated chromatin may occupy the interstices of the nucleolonema.

Dispersed throughout the nucleus is DNA, the carrier of hereditary characteristics. The DNA double helix (see "Protoplasm") is about 20 Å in diameter; the proteins adhering to this strand increase the diameter to 40 to 50 Å. Basic histone proteins and acid proteins play a role in the expression of activity of DNA, and they lend support to the helix as well. Deoxyribonucleoprotein (DNP) strands are coiled into units 200 to 250 Å in diameter. This is the fundamental structural strand of genetic material, as first proposed by Ris. Masses of these extremely long threads intertwine throughout the nucleus; it has been reported that an individual strand may be as long as 22,000 μm in human lymphocyte nuclei. This thread is too thin to be resolved in the light microscope, thus

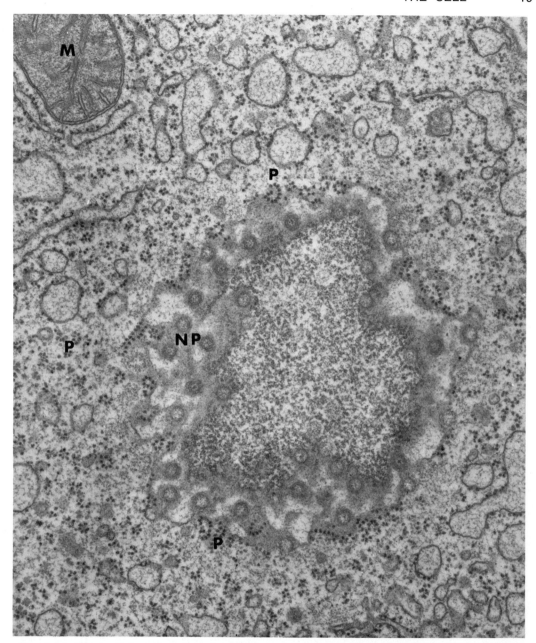

Fig. 1-11. Tangential section through the edge of a nucleus of a developing liver cell. Nuclear pores show internal structure. Polyribosomes are associated with the cytoplasmic surface of the nuclear envelope and also occur free in the cytoplasm. *M*, mitochondrion; *NP*, nuclear pores; *P*, polyribosomes. ×33,800.

explaining why many nuclei appear nearly empty (Fig. 1-1, *A* and *B*).

At certain intervals along the thread, however, the DNP is additionally coiled, forming clumps which can be seen in the light microscope after staining (Fig. 1-13).

These scattered stained clumps and particles are called *chromatin* (from the Greek *chroma,* color), a name derived from the fact that they stain brilliantly with basic coal tar dyes. Chromatin particles occur throughout the nucleus, are often clumped

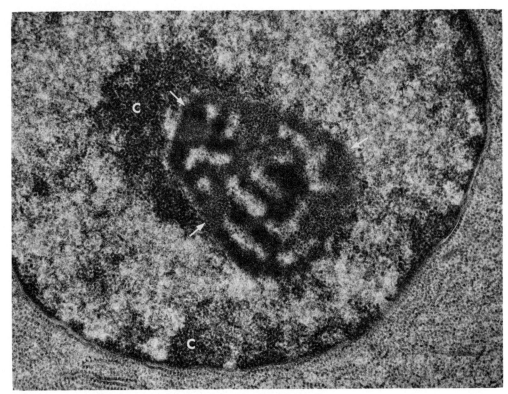

Fig. 1-12. Electron micrograph, showing nuclear chromatin and a nucleolus. The nucleolus, indicated by *arrows,* contains granular and fibrillar elements which may be organized into a dense, meandering strand or network called the nucleolonema. Clumps of chromatin (*c*) abut on the nucleolus and the nuclear envelope. Acinar cell from bat pancreas. ×25,000. (From D. W. Fawcett: The Cell. Its Organelles and Inclusions. W. B. Saunders Company, Philadelphia, 1966.)

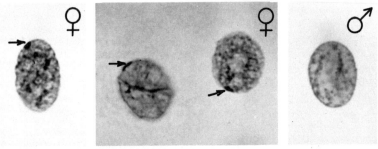

Fig. 1-13. Photomicrograph of four nuclei in a smear of oral mucosa cells from normal adult subjects. The three nuclei on the *left,* obtained from females, each contain a small dense body situated near the nuclear envelope. These Barr bodies are not found in nuclei from males, as shown on the *right.* Thionin staining. ×1800. (From M. L. Barr: *In* Intersexuality, edited by C. Overzier, p. 48, Academic Press, New York, 1963.)

on the nuclear envelope, and are associated with nucleoli, as mentioned above. These particles in the nondividing nucleus are also termed *heterochromatin* (or karyosomes); the DNP not stained, filling the empty-appearing areas, is called *euchromatin.*

The heterochromatin is thought of as *condensed* chromatin, which is inactive metabolically. The euchromatin, on the other hand, is the dispersed or extended form, the state in which chromatin is active. The light microscopist, then, can gain information about the relative activity of the cell by noting the appearance of the chromatin.

This generalization is illustrated by the following examples. In the development of the mammalian erythrocyte, the chromatin is initially dispersed but gradually becomes more condensed; as the cell reaches maturity (and hemoglobin synthesis nears completion), the nucleus is seen to be small, very darkly staining, and homogeneously dense (Fig. 7-11). During maturation of sperm, a similar phenomenon is observed. The nucleus of the mature sperm is filled with "storage" DNP and is, as expected, extremely dense throughout. Once fertilization has occurred, the sperm nucleus inside the egg begins to swell and the chromatin begins to extend for initiation of gene activity.

During division, the chromatin threads become completely coiled or condensed into chromosomes (Fig. 1-14), and division is the only time when the entire length of each chromatin thread is condensed into a unit that is visible by light microscopy. More is said of chromosomes in chapter 2,

in which division is discussed. The configurations, as well as the number, of the mitotic (metaphase) chromosomes are constant, thus allowing their identification. This assumes importance in human disease and is also further considered in chapter 2.

One of the sex chromosomes remains condensed in the interphase cell and is known as the *Barr body*. First described in 1949 by Barr and Bertram, it is the second X chromosome, present normally only in female cells. Female cells contain two X sex chromosomes; male cells contain two sex chromosomes, one X and one Y. Apparently, one X chromosome (but not more than one) must exist in an extended state because it participates in a number of metabolic activities other than that of sex determination. Thus, in the normal situation, when two X chromosomes are present in female cells, one of them remains condensed. It appears as a small stained body (about 1 μm in diameter) beside the nucleolus or adjacent to the nuclear envelope, depending upon the species (Fig. 1-13). The sex chromatin can be seen in sections or smears (from oral mucosa, blood,

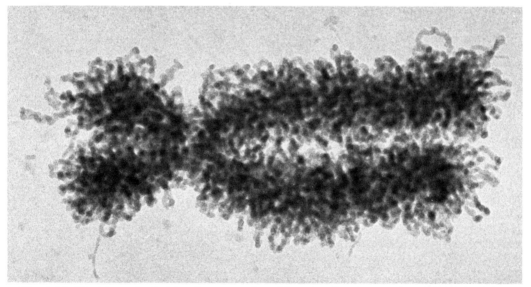

Fig. 1-14. Electron micrograph of an unsectioned human chromosome (no. 12) obtained from a dividing cell. The chromosome is divided in half along its length (into two chromatids) except at the centromere. The chromosome is made up of a unit which varies from 100 to 500 Å in diameter. This chromosome weighs 13.2×10^{-13} g and contains about 4 cm of DNA double helix per chromatid. Some of the looping and coiling which allows the packing of all of this DNA into a chromosome 3 μm in length is visible. ×40,200. (From E. J. DuPraw: DNA and Chromosomes. Holt, Rinehart and Winston, New York, 1970.)

etc.). Identification of Barr bodies aids in the diagnosis of sex in intersexual states and also in studies of congenital diseases related to sex chromatin.

Considering the widely dispersed coiled threads of chromatin, it is not surprising that electron microscopic observations of nuclei in thin sections reveal only a wealth of granules and very short filaments (Fig. 1-12). If chromosomes of the dividing cell are processed for electron microscopy without sectioning, their overall configurations can be appreciated (Fig. 1-14). Visualization of active sites or genes on the chromatin threads is just now beginning to be realized, by careful selection of special systems for study.

For example, during development of an amphibian egg, the chromosomal nucleolus organizer is multiplied and produces about 1000 nucleoli. If these nucleoli are isolated,

dispersed, and then prepared for electron microscopy, thin strands of DNP (100 to 300 Å in diameter) are found; on these fibers are repeating regions (2 to 5 μm long) containing about 100 thin fibrils connected by one end to the fiber and increasing in length from one end of that region to the other (Fig. 1-15). Each region on the DNA axis is one gene, and this gene has sites for the simultaneous production of 100 ribosomal RNA precursor molecules. It has been estimated that, in one of these oocyte nuclei, 3.6 m of DNA double helix contain 2⅓ million of these genes producing ribosomal RNA. This system allows the direct observation of the manufacture of RNA on the DNA molecule.

Functions. The standard histological section offers a few clues regarding nuclear activity. As has been discussed above, the degree of condensation of the chromatin is

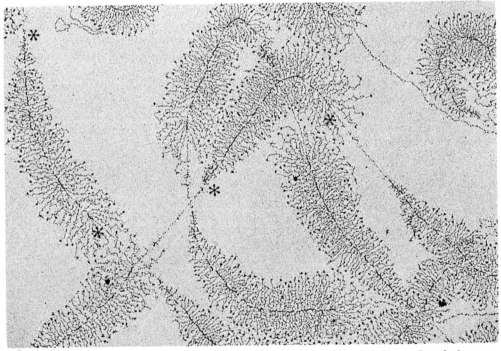

Fig. 1-15. During the development of amphibian oocytes, the DNA increases sharply in amount and is contained within the 1000 or so forming extrachromosomal nucleoli. When this DNA is maximally unwound, it is seen in the electron microscope to be an extremely slender strand with periodic adherent material arranged in a feather-like pattern. Each "feather" (as indicated between *asterisks* in two areas here) is about 2.5 μm long and results from the attachment to the DNA axis of 100 forming ribonucleoprotein molecules in progressive stages of completion. Thus it is shown that about 100 precursor molecules of ribosomal RNA are being formed simultaneously at each gene. × 25,000. (From O. L. Miller, Jr., and B. R. Beatty: Science 164:955, 1969.)

an inverse index of the amount of genetic material that is involved in synthetic activities. Cells with large, pale nuclei containing little condensed chromatin (such as neurons, Fig. 1-1, *A* and *B*) are metabolically very active cells. The size of the nucleolus is also related to cell activity. Nucleoli are small (or absent) in cells which are not actively forming proteins (e.g., mature leukocytes) and generally large in cells which are actively synthesizing proteins (e.g., nerve cells which must replenish their proteins during activity, cells of regenerating tissues, and embryonic cells). These observations are consistent with the more recent knowledge that the nucleolus is the site of formation of ribosomal RNA, and that ribosomes are needed for protein synthesis.

There is now an abundant literature concerning nuclear cytoplasmic relationships. One aspect of this work has involved bisecting unicellular organisms so that only one part retains a nucleus. The part without the nucleus gradually dies, whereas the nucleated portion survives. With the removal of the nucleus, the DNA-RNA-protein production sequence is stopped, and the anucleate part lives only as long as survival time of its protein molecules permits. The overall importance of the nucleus has been nicely stated by Allfrey: "The cell nucleus, central and commanding, is essential for the biosynthetic events that characterize cell type and cell function; it is a vault of genetic information encoding the past history and future prospects of the cell, an organelle submerged and deceptively serene in its sea of turbulent cytoplasm, a firm and purposeful guide, a barometer exquisitely sensitive to the changing demands of the organism and its environment."

The Cytoplasm

Cytoplasm contains a number of formed bodies embedded in a substance which appears translucent and homogeneous in the living cell. This substance has been given a variety of names, such as ground cytoplasm, basic or fundamental cytoplasm, or hyaloplasm. The formed bodies embedded in the cytoplasm are often divided into two groups: *organelles,* composed of living differentiated cytoplasm, and *inclusion bodies,* metabolic or ingested substances which are temporary constituents. The first group includes (1) ribosomes, (2) endoplasmic reticulum with and without ribosomes, (3) Golgi apparatus, (4) lysosomes, (5) peroxisomes, (6) centrosome and centrioles, (7) mitochondria, (8) filaments, and (9) microtubules. The second group includes (1) yolk, (2) fat and carbohydrate (glycogen) deposits, (3) secretion granules, and (4) pigment granules.

Ribosomes. The cytoplasm of many cells contains material which stains with basic dyes, just as does the nuclear chromatin. In certain gland cells, intensely basophilic areas were given the name ergastoplasm (from the Greek *ergaster,* a workman, + *plasma,* plasm) by early workers, because they were thought to be involved in the work of producing secretory granules. This staining is now known to be due to the presence of RNA. With the increased resolution of the electron microscope and the availability of new sectioning techniques, Palade discovered in the early 1950s that these basophilic regions contain a wealth of small, dense granules (averaging 150 Å in diameter). Although these granules frequently are aligned on flattened membranous sacs (endoplasmic reticulum), the granules alone are responsible for the staining. The enzyme ribonuclease abolishes simultaneously the cytoplasmic basophilia and the granules (but not the membranes). The particles are now known to be composed of 60% RNA and 40% protein. Their composition is reflected in their present name, *ribosomes.*

Ribosomes have been found in all animal cells with the exception of adult mammalian erythrocytes (which lose their organelles when they reach maturity). Highly basophilic cells include those engaged in synthesizing secretory proteins, such as pancreatic and salivary acinar cells, and cells in active growth stages, such as lymphoblasts, myeloblasts, and osteoblasts. As mentioned previously, ribosomes occur free in the cytoplasm or are lined up on flattened sacs of endoplasmic reticulum membrane (Figs. 1-16 and 1-17). Those ribosomes associated with endoplasmic reticulum are involved mostly in the formation of proteins for export from the cell, such as the digestive enzymes secreted by the pancreatic acinar cell. When the ribosome is attached to endoplasmic reticulum, the *exportable* proteins produced are delivered into the reticulum cavities rather than into the cytoplasmic matrix (Fig. 1-16). The free ribosomes, on the other hand, are involved primarily in the formation of proteins, including enzymes, *for intracellular use.* In rapidly growing and dividing cells, which

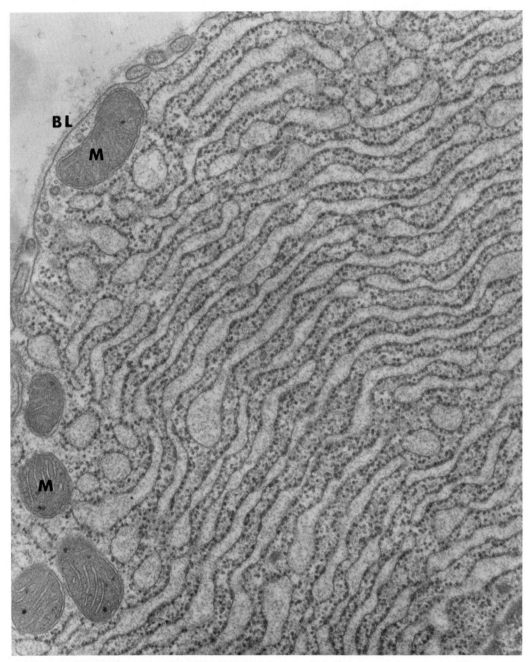

Fig. 1-16. Ribosomes associated with endoplasmic reticulum membranes in a pancreatic secretory cell. The base of the cell with its basal lamina appears at the *upper left. M,* mitochondria; *BL,* basal lamina. ×42,000.

are increasing in cytoplasmic volume, free ribosomes are the most prominent of the cytoplasmic organelles (Fig. 1-17).

The collaborative efforts of cytologists and biochemists employing both in vivo and in vitro systems have led to a new understanding of ribosomes, protein manufacture, and the involvement of various RNAs in the activity. This is an area of investigation which has been aided greatly by the techniques of differential centrifugation (in combination with radioactive tracers) and radioautography at the light and electron microscope levels. When homogenized cells are subjected to differential centrifugation, the nuclei sediment out first, the mitochondria next, and other submicroscopic components last. The submicroscopic material is named the *microsome fraction*. Studies of this fraction under the electron microscope show that it is composed chiefly of fragments of endoplasmic reticulum and adhering ribosomes. The addition of a detergent, deoxycholate, solubi-lizes the membranes, resulting, after additional centrifugation, in a relatively pure preparation of ribosomes. Ribosomal fractions have the capacity to incorporate amino acids into protein molecules.

Polysomal clusters of ribosomes are held together by a single slender strand of RNA called *messenger RNA* (mRNA). In general, the number of ribosomes in a polysome and the length of polypeptide formed are proportional to the length of the mRNA strand. In the immature red blood cell which is synthesizing hemoglobin, polysomes contain an average of five ribosomes, and the polypeptide chains formed contain about 150 amino acids. In developing muscle cells which are producing myosin, an average of 56 ribosomes constitute a polysome involved with assembly of more than 1800 amino acids into the polypeptide chain. The longer mRNA strand has spaces for more ribosomes and requires each ribosome to travel farther, thus providing for the assembly of a greater number of amino

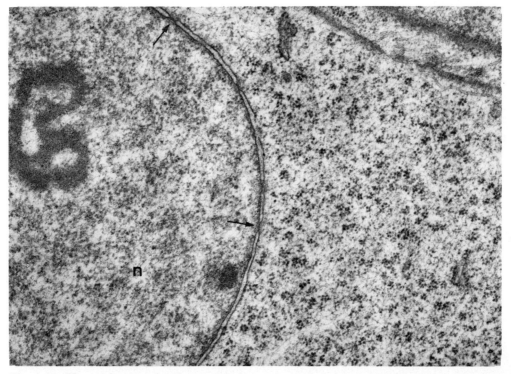

Fig. 1-17. The predominantly ribosomal (polysome) content of the cytoplasm of young developing cells is shown in this electron micrograph of a nerve cell from embryonic rabbit neural tube. The envelope around the nucleus (*n*) has a number of pores (*arrows*). ×32,000. (Courtesy of Dr. Virginia Tennyson.)

acids (as explained in Fig. 1-18). This assembly process, not discovered until the 1960s, is rapid: data from bacteria indicate that only 10 sec are required for the assembly of a protein containing 500 to 1000 amino acids.

Granular Endoplasmic Reticulum. The *endoplasmic reticulum* was first seen in 1945 by Porter, Claude, and Fullam, who were able to examine very thinly spread, cultured fibroblasts in the electron microscope. Because the preparation had not been sectioned, the arrangement of the newly found organelle in a network was quickly recognized. The presence of this lacelike network (or reticulum) in the inner or endoplasmic region of the cytoplasm (although it is not always so distributed) led to the name endoplasmic reticulum. Subsequent study of thin sections added more information. Endoplasmic reticulum exists in the form of tubules and broad, flattened sacs (cisternae) of membrane in reticular sheets interconnected by branchings and anastomoses (Fig. 1-19). Ribosomes may cover much of the endoplasmic reticulum surface; this association of ribosomal granules and endoplasmic reticulum is termed *granular* or *rough endoplasmic reticulum.*

Ribosomes attach both to endoplasmic reticulum membrane and to the outer membrane of the nuclear envelope, with which the endoplasmic reticulum is continuous, and to no other membranes of the cell. When the reticulum membrane is sectioned perpendicular to its surface, the ribosomes dot the surface at more or less regular intervals (Fig. 1-16); when the membrane is sectioned such that patches of its cytoplasmic surface are visible, many of the ribosomes are seen to occur in circle, loop, spiral or rosette arrays which are the membrane-

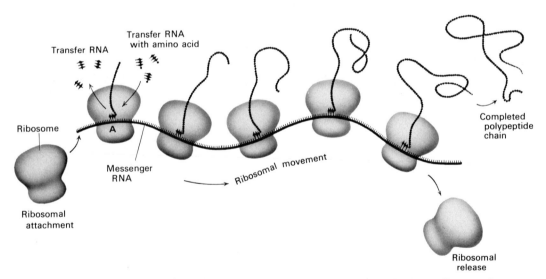

Fig. 1-18. This diagram depicts the role of ribosomes in protein synthesis. A ribosome becomes attached to one end of a strand of messenger RNA (mRNA). The ribosome is known to consist of two subunits of unequal size; it has been speculated that the mRNA strand fits into a groove formed at the junction of these two subunits. A molecule of transfer RNA (tRNA) becomes activated by linking with a specific amino acid; there are some 20 different tRNA molecules, one for each amino acid. The nature of the mRNA sites present in the receiving area of the ribosome (*A*) determines which tRNA, and thus which amino acid, is used. Thus, as the ribosome progresses along the mRNA strand, the code is translated by the tRNAs, which deposit in correct order the amino acids required for the production of a specific protein. The longer the mRNA strand, the farther the ribosome must travel and the greater the number of amino acids assembled. Each ribosome makes a complete chain. That there are five ribosomes in a polysome at a given time, as drawn here, is determined by the mRNA molecule. When the ribosome reaches the end of the strand, it is released and is available for reuse with the same or a different species of mRNA, and the completed polypeptide chain is liberated. (Diagram based upon drawings and descriptions by A. Rich.)

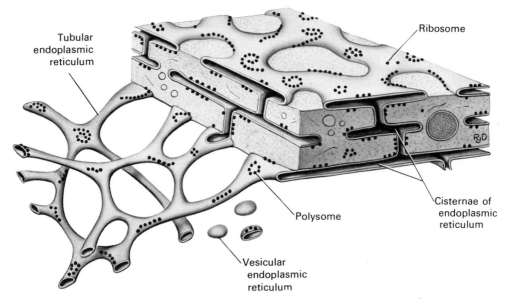

Fig. 1-19. Diagram illustrating the interconnected cisternae and tubules of granular endoplasmic reticulum.

associated polysomes (Figs. 1-19 and 1-20). Occasionally, the proteins synthesized on the ribosomes are visible as dense or filamentous material within the lumina of the reticulum elements (Fig. 1-16).

The amount and configuration of the granular endoplasmic reticulum depend upon the cell type and the physiological state of the cell. Some growing cells, rich in free ribosomes and lacking endoplasmic reticulum, exhibit an intense, diffuse basophilia. Such cells are in the process of elaborating proteins destined to remain within the cell. In many differentiated cells, ribosomes are in large part attached to endoplasmic reticulum, and basophilia may occur only in areas of the cytoplasm rich in that organelle. For example, the pancreatic acinar cell, which synthesizes and secretes exported proteinaceous digestive enzymes (zymogen granules), is highly basophilic in its basal region only. Such an area is filled with numerous granular endoplasmic reticulum cisternae which are closely and regularly packed in parallel rows (Figs. 1-10, 1-16, and 1-22). Relatively few of the ribosomes lie free in the cytoplasmic matrix.

The pancreatic acinar cell is a good system for tracing newly synthesized exportable proteins through the cell, partly because different organelles involved at different times are concentrated in different regions of the cytoplasm. The ribosome-encrusted cisternae of endoplasmic reticulum are located chiefly in the basal portion of the cell, along with the nucleus and mitochondria (an energy source). The apical region of the cell, nearer to the lumen into which the product will be emptied, contains numerous zymogen granules (Fig. 1-9B), interspersed with a few granular reticulum elements. In between these two regions (above the nucleus) there is a well developed network of Golgi apparatus oriented around two centrioles (see diagram, Fig. 1-10). The synthesis, intracellular transport, storage, and discharge of the digestive enzymes have been examined extensively in guinea pigs by administering the radioactive amino acid leucine and examining the pancreatic acini by means of light and electron microscopic radioautography (Figs. 1-21 to 1-24). The path of the exportable protein through the cell was detected by looking for radioactive sites at various time intervals. Sites of radioactivity indicated the presence of the leucine which had been recently used in the synthesis of new exportable protein; unused radioactive leucine had been washed away during preparation. Studies conducted with intact animals and with incubated tissue slices show that the pro-

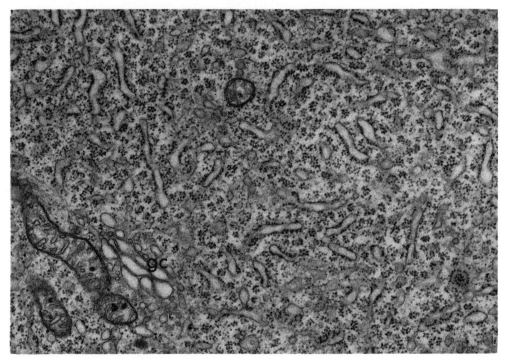

Fig. 1-20. This electron micrograph shows a region containing free ribosomes and granular endoplasmic reticulum in the cytoplasm of a mature neuron. Compare this with the immature nerve cell shown in Fig. 1-17. Where the cisternae are cut *en face* (as at *lower right*), the coiled, looped, or curved arrangement of attached ribosomes in the polysome is clearly seen. Part of a Golgi complex (*gc*) and mitochondria appear at *lower left*. × 29,000.

teins are synthesized on the ribosomes attached to endoplasmic reticulum and are transported within the reticulum to the Golgi zone, where they become concentrated and packaged into zymogen granules for temporary storage. In this manner the digestive enzymes remain isolated from the remainder of the cytoplasm.

The fact that continuities between the granular reticulum and the Golgi apparatus are seldom seen raises a question: how is the newly synthesized protein transported from reticulum cisternae to Golgi elements? In areas of granular endoplasmic reticulum bordering on the Golgi zone, some of the cisternae are partly devoid of ribosomes, i.e., a cisterna may be part rough and part smooth; these cisternae are called *transitional elements*. Interspersed among them are swarms of small vesicles (about 500 Å in diameter) which occasionally appear to be continuous with, or budding from, the cisternae (Fig. 1-25). It now appears that these vesicles, termed *transfer vesicles,* ferry the synthesized product to the Golgi

elements. The newly synthesized proteins are later visualized in *condensing vacuoles* (Fig. 1-24). These vacuoles, found in the Golgi zone, are the sites of progressive accumulation and concentration of protein; they will become the spherical, more dense zymogen granules.

Agranular Endoplasmic Reticulum. Endoplasmic reticulum devoid of ribosomes (*agranular endoplasmic reticulum*; smooth or smooth-surfaced reticulum) is found in a variety of cell types, generally in those lacking a well developed granular reticulum. Unlike the granular reticulum, the smooth reticulum is primarily in the form of tubules which are often interconnected (or merely entangled), tortuous, and very closely packed (Fig. 1-26). Although agranular reticulum elements may be continuous with or derived from rough reticulum, the constituent membrane may differ in that it appears thinner and is more difficult to preserve. The occurrence of agranular reticulum in cells was not recognized before the use of the electron microscope because it

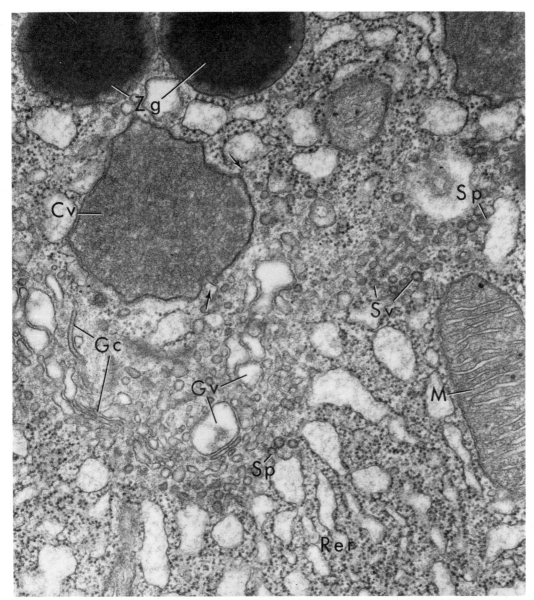

Fig. 1-21. Electron micrograph of a portion of a pancreatic exocrine cell from a slice of a guinea pig pancreas incubated for 3 hr in vitro. The ultrastructure of the incubated cell is approximately the same as that of pancreatic cells fixed at biopsy. Note that the rough-surfaced endoplasmic reticulum (*Rer*) is composed partly of rough-surfaced and partly of smooth-surfaced cisternae. The latter have projections (*Sp*) into the Golgi complex, toward clusters of smooth-surfaced vesicles (*Sv*). Some of the latter are in contact (*at arrows*) with the limiting membrane of a condensing vacuole (*Cv*). *Gc*, Golgi cisternae; *Gv*, Golgi vacuoles; *M*, mitochondrion; *Zg*, zymogen granules. This is a control specimen for comparison with pancreatic slices that were pulse-labeled with radioactive [³H]leucine and then postincubated for varying periods in order to study the secretory cycle by electron microscopic radioautographs. See next three figures. ×43,400. (Courtesy of Drs. J. D. Jamieson and G. E. Palade: J. Cell Biol., vol. 34, 1967).

lacks distinctive staining properties.

The agranular endoplasmic reticulum is known to perform a variety of functions depending upon the cell type in which it resides. In liver cells, this organelle is considered to function in lipid and cholesterol metabolism. (The liver cell is exceptional in that it contains numerous arrays of gran-

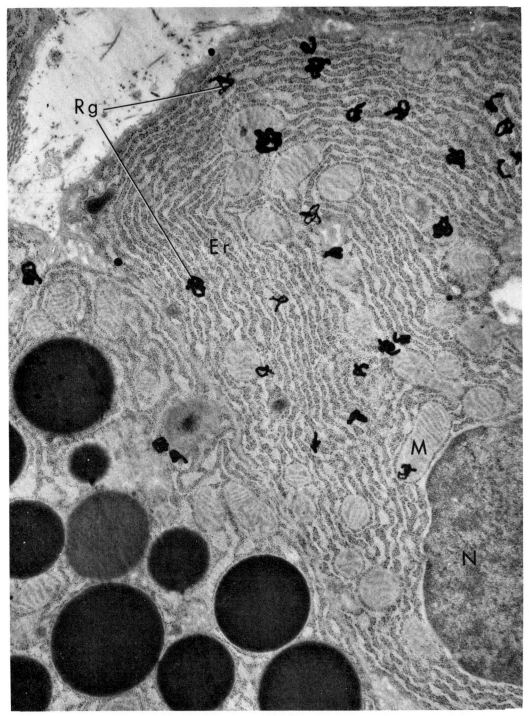

Fig. 1-22. Electron microscopic radioautograph of a pancreatic exocrine cell from a slice of pancreatic tissue that was pulse-labeled in vitro for 3 min with L-[³H]leucine. Note that the radioautographic grains (Rg) are present chiefly over the rough surfaced endoplasmic reticulum (Er). M, mitochondrion; N, nucleus. ×17,500. (Courtesty of Drs. J. D. Jamieson and G. E. Palade, J. Cell Biol., vol. 34, 1967).

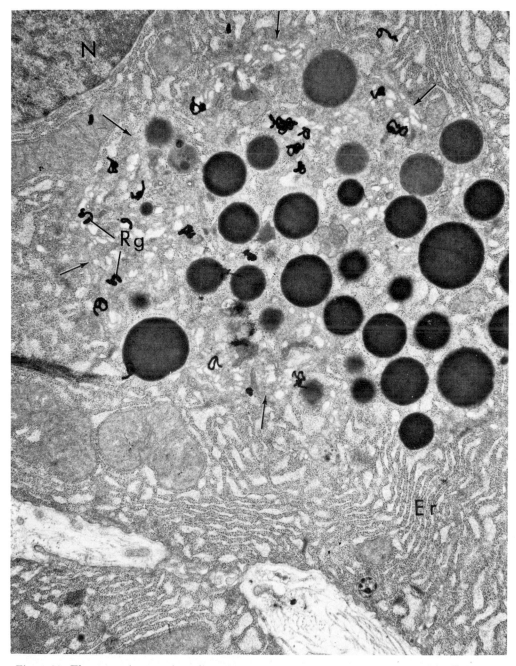

Fig. 1-23. Electron microscopic radioautograph of a pancreatic exocrine cell after 3 min of pulse labeling, similar to that used for the cell shown in Figure 1-22, plus 7 min of postincubation. Note that most of the radioautographic grains (*Rg*), indicating the position of the labeled leucine, are present at the periphery of the Golgi complex (marked by *arrows*). *Er,* endoplasmic reticulum. ×16,700. (Courtesy of Drs. J. D. Jamieson and G. E. Palade, J. Cell Biol., vol. 34, 1967).

ular as well as agranular reticulum, reflecting the manifold activities of these cells.) Agranular reticulum also aids in detoxification processes, e.g., by hydroxylation.

When lipid-soluble drugs such as barbiturates or cancer-producing agents are given to animals, greatly enlarged arrays of smooth reticulum appear in the hepatic

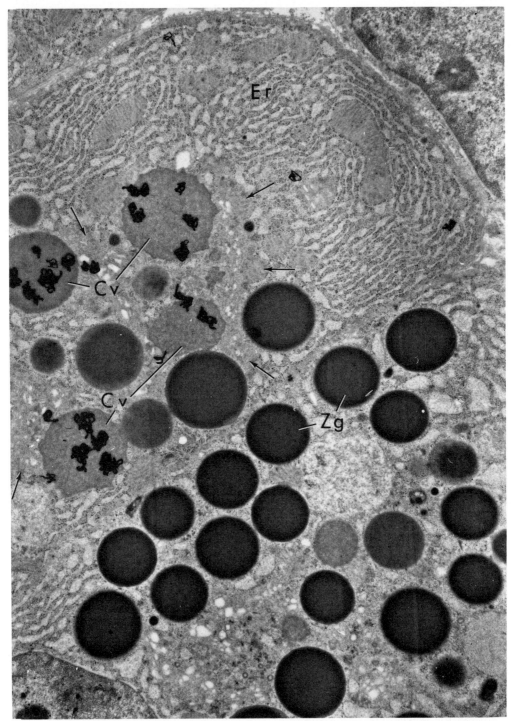

Fig. 1-24. Electron microscopic radioautograph of a pancreatic exocrine cell after 3 min of pulse labeling, as shown in Figure 1-22, plus 37 min of postpulse incubation. The periphery of the Golgi complex is indicated by *arrows*. Note that most of the radioautographic grains are present over condensing vacuoles (*Cv*). This series of radioautographs shows that the secretory material, synthesized from leucine and other amino acids at the sites of ribosomes of the rough-surfaced endoplasmic reticulum, *Er,* is transported via cisternae to the Golgi region, where it is concentrated within condensing vacuoles which become zymogen granules (*Zg*). ×12,500. (Courtesy of Drs. J. D. Jamieson and G. E. Palade, J. Cell Biol., vol. 34, 1967).

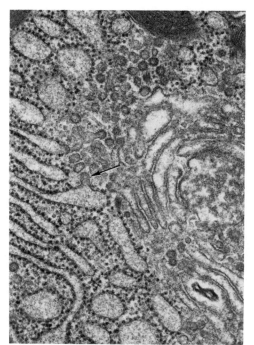

Fig. 1-25. Golgi region of a pancreatic cell showing transfer vesicles between the endoplasmic reticulum and the Golgi membranes. At the *arrow* a transfer vesicle is pinching off from a cisterna of endoplasmic reticulum. × 34,000.

cells. There is a concomitant increase in drug-metabolizing enzymes in smooth membrane fractions isolated from these cells. Investigators speculate that the toxic agent is taken up in the lipid portion of the induced membrane and is thereby brought into contact with the detoxifying enzymes associated with the same membrane. Glycogen particles often are enmeshed within arrays of liver smooth reticulum, suggesting a functional relationship.

In the interstitial cells of the testis, and in the cells of the ovarian corpus luteum and adrenal cortex, the extensive agranular reticulum is considered to participate in cholesterol metabolism and in the production of steroid hormones. The smooth reticulum contained within cells lining the intestine is involved in the metabolism and transport of lipids from components absorbed from the intestinal lumen. The prominent agranular endoplasmic reticulum in the gastric oxyntic cells is thought to participate in the secretion of chloride ions. Finally, the elaborate tubular network

of smooth reticulum (sarcoplasmic reticulum) encasing each striated muscle myofibril functions in the excitation-contraction coupling mechanism (see chapter 8 and Fig. 8-22).

The Golgi Apparatus. The *Golgi apparatus,* discovered by Golgi in 1898, is one of the organelles involved in secretory activity. It is arranged in a reticular network which is either distributed throughout the cytoplasm or confined to a zone near the nucleus, depending upon the cell type. In elongated cells which border on an enclosed space, the Golgi complex lies between the nucleus and the free suface border of the cell. In the light microscope, the Golgi apparatus is visualized after treatment with silver or osmium tetroxide, which is reduced to a black deposit (Fig. 1-27). In cells forming a carbohydrate product, the Golgi region is stained magenta by the periodic acid-Schiff (PAS) technique. Vigorous controversy about the reality of this cell organelle persisted until the era of the electron microscope, when the Golgi apparatus was recognized as a ubiquitous cell structure of consistent form. In the electron microscope, the Golgi apparatus is seen as closely packed stacks of agranular membrane cisternae with associated vacuoles and vesicles (Figs. 1-28 and 1-29). Each stack may be curved; those cisternae on the convex or "outer" face often are more flattened than those on the concave or "inner" face (Fig. 1-28).

Light microscope studies early in this century had indicated that the Golgi apparatus was somehow involved in the elaboration of secretory substances. In 1938 Kirkman and Severinghaus stated, "A great deal of work strongly suggests that the Golgi apparatus neither synthesizes secretory substances nor is transformed directly into them; but it acts as a condensation membrane for the concentration, into droplets or granules, of products elaborated elsewhere and diffused into the cytoplasm."

The role of the Golgi apparatus in concentrating and packaging protein-rich materials has been firmly established with new techniques. The product formed on the ribosomes associated with endoplasmic reticulum becomes contained within the reticulum cisternae and then is transported to

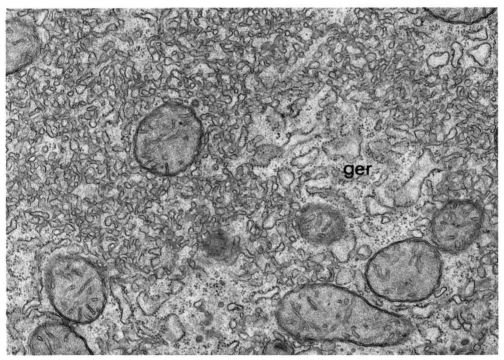

Fig. 1-26. Interspersed among the mitochondria and elements of granular endoplasmic reticulum (*ger*) of this liver cell are slender anastomosing tubules of agranular endoplasmic reticulum. The agranular reticulum is increased in response to the administration of phenobarbital (which is detoxified in these regions). ×26,000. (Courtesy of Dr. Don W. Fawcett.)

Golgi elements via small vesicles which pinch off the reticulum and merge with Golgi membrane. The product, now visible because of increased density, as a rule next appears in the inner Golgi cisternae and leaves the Golgi stack via vesicles or vacuoles which arise as terminal expansions of these cisternae. These vesicles may coalesce, their contents progressively increasing in density, until there is a population of large, dense secretion droplets which move out of the Golgi zone. Because the product is thought to be delivered to the outer cisternae of the Golgi complex in some cells, this aspect is sometimes referred to as the "forming" face; the inner surface is designated the "maturing" face, for it is the region of the maturing secretion droplet. Thus, the protein-rich product is collected and concentrated in the Golgi region and is packaged in Golgi membrane, at all times remaining segregated from the remainder of the cell. In the pancreatic acinar cell, the newly synthesized product is first seen in the condensing vacuoles in the Golgi

region rather than in the cisternae of the Golgi stack.

Almost all proteins exported by the cell contain some sugar moieties, in contrast with those proteins which remain inside. Recent work indicates that it is in the region of the Golgi apparatus that most sugars are added to the protein. The intestinal goblet cell manufactures mucus, a substance composed mainly of protein with a small amount of carbohydrate (glycoprotein). Utilizing electron microscopic radioautography, Leblond and collaborators found that radioactive glucose or galactose administered to rats was added to protein in the Golgi region before the formation of mucus globules. Incorporated radioactivity was first seen over Golgi stacks, at later intervals over mucus globules, and, still later, near the apical cell surface. This work also demonstrated the turnover in Golgi membrane: in spite of successive budding to form globules at the maturing surface, the stack of Golgi cisternae is maintained. Other investigations have indicated that

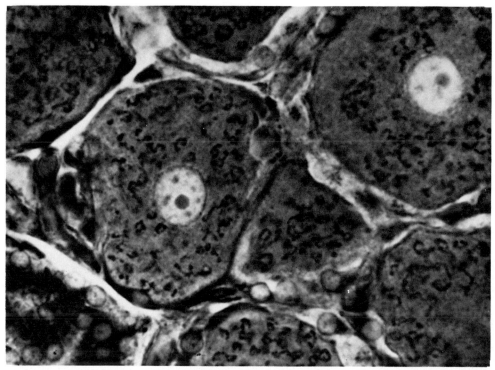

Fig. 1-27. Scattered throughout the cytoplasm of these large neurons are dense ribbon-like deposits revealing the distribution of the Golgi apparatus. Light micrograph of a 5-μm section; Nassonow-Kolatschew technique. ×914. (From W. Hild: Nervensystem. *In* Handb. mikr. Anat. Menschen., edited by V. Möllendorff, part 4, p. 116, Springer-Verlag, Vienna, 1959.)

the Golgi region is also the site of assembly of polysaccharides associated with the plasma membrane or secreted to form extracellular matrix materials. Sulfate is also added to many of these substances in the Golgi region.

It appears now that the Golgi complex is polarized; i.e., different cisternae perform different functions, sometimes at different maturational stages. Working with maturing polymorphonuclear leukocytes from rabbit bone marrow, Bainton and Farquhar have shown that two kinds of granules are formed in a manner similar to secretory granule production, i.e., by the accumulation, condensation, and packaging of product in the Golgi apparatus. But one type of granule (azurophil) arises from the inner surface of the Golgi stack (Fig. 1-28) and the second variety of granule (specific) originates from the outer surface (Fig. 1-29). The granules are formed at different developmental stages and differ in enzymatic content. The polarity of the Golgi appara-

tus is also suggested by osmium impregnation and histochemical investigations. Only the outer cisternae become blackened after prolonged exposure to osmium tetroxide. Histochemists have found that some hydrolytic enzymes are associated with middle cisternae, whereas others are confined only to inner cisternae. Histochemical demonstration of hydrolytic enzymes introduces still another function of the Golgi apparatus, the production of lysosomes.

Lysosomes. By centrifuging the mitochondrial fraction in graded concentrations of sucrose, a class of particles different in enzymatic content from mitochondria was discovered by de Duve in 1955. Enzymatic activity was not fully evident until the membrane bounding the particle became more permeable or was broken—a characteristic of importance for the cell, as discussed below. The dozen or more enzymes associated with these particles are hydrolases, which break down proteins, carbohydrates, and nucleic acids at acid pH (e.g.,

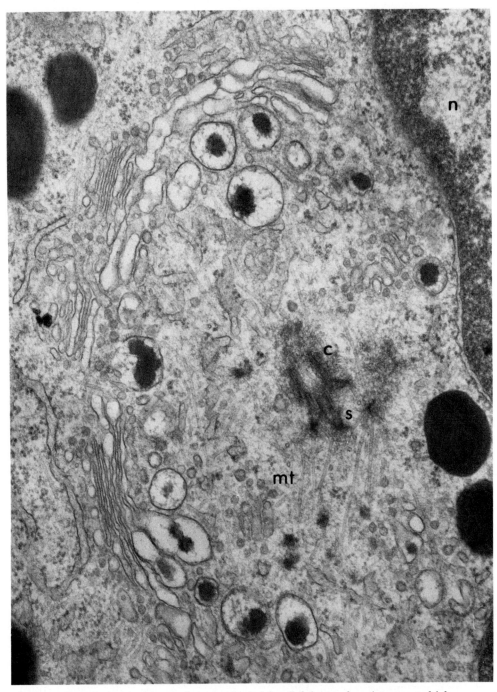

Fig. 1-28. This electron micrograph is dominated by Golgi complex cisternae, which are curved around the centrioles (one of which is indicated at *c*) and toward the nucleus (*n*). Microtubules (*mt*) radiate from densities associated with the centrioles (pericentriolar satellites, *s*) and may be seen as circles (when sectioned transversely) or as double lines (when longitudinally sectioned). The largest dense inclusions here are azurophil granules, typical components of this cell, a polymorphonuclear leukocyte. They arise from the inner (or concave) surface of the Golgi complex by budding off the cisternae. They first appear as dense-centered vacuoles and gradually change into large, dense granules. ×50,000. (From D. F. Bainton and M. G. Farquhar: J. Cell Biol. 28:277, 1966.)

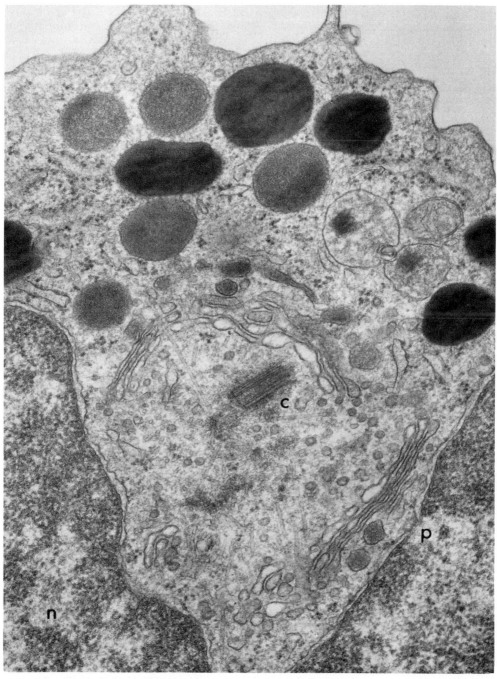

Fig. 1-29. This electron micrograph shows other polymorphonuclear leukocyte granules, the specific granules, in various stages of formation from the outer or convex face of the Golgi complex at a later stage of development than that represented in Fig. 1-28. Beneath the Golgi complex, in the cell center, is a longitudinally sectioned centriole (*c*). Extending from this region are straight profiles of microtubules. In the envelope surrounding the nucleus (*n*) are several pores, one of which is designated *p*. ×50,000. (From D. F. Bainton and M. G. Farquhar: J. Cell Biol. 28:277, 1966.)

cathepsins, glycosidases, sulfatases, phosphatases, ribonuclease, deoxyribonuclease). The lytic activity of these bodies prompted the name *lysosome*.

The search for lysosomes in intact cells led to the realization that they are present in nearly all animal cell types (Fig. 1-30). Lysosomes are heterogeneous in size and content but are always bounded by a single membrane (Fig. 1-31). A lysosome may be identified in tissue sections on the basis of its acid phosphatase content. Acid phosphatase activity is revealed by the presence of a lead product resulting from enzymatic breakdown of an exogenous substrate in the presence of lead ions, the entire reaction

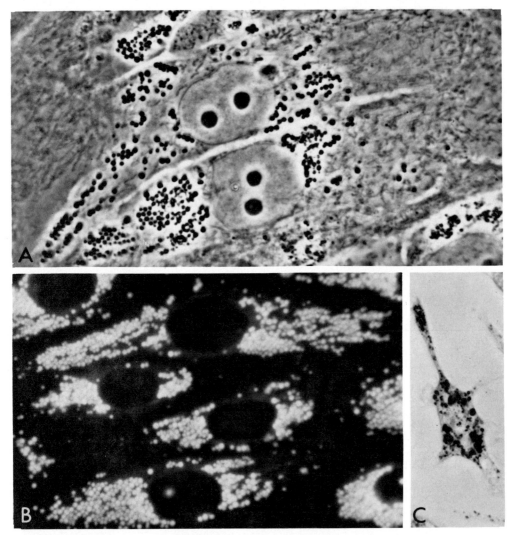

Fig. 1-30. Lysosomes. *A*, as they appear in the phase contrast microscope in living monkey kidney cells. The lysosomes are the small black granules near the nuclei and may be compared to the light gray filamentous mitochondria in the more peripheral cytoplasm. ×1200. *B*, as they appear in the fluorescence microscope. The brightly fluorescing granules are lysosomes which have taken up the fluorescent compound methylcholanthrene administered to similar cells in culture. Nuclei and mitochondria do not fluoresce. ×550. *C*, after the Gomori method, the lysosomes appear as blackened granules in the light microscope. They are "stained" black by the deposition of a reaction product, lead sulfide, which results from the presence of an enzyme (acid phosphatase) characteristic of lysosomes. Mouse macrophage. ×1130. (From A. Allison: Sci. Amer. 217:62, 1967.)

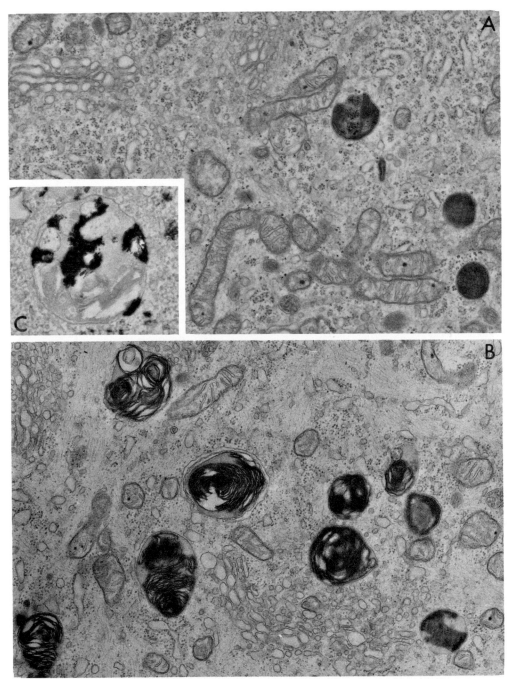

Fig. 1-31. Electron micrographs of lysosomes. *A*, scattered among the granular endoplasmic reticulum, mitochondria, and Golgi complex are dense bodies. In normal tissue, dense bodies appear homogeneous or contain particles and stacked membrane-like structures. If the cultured nervous tissue illustrated here is given a tranquilizer, chloropromazine, the dense bodies increase in number and size and take on a more heterogeneous appearance (*B*), as is typical for lysosomes after a variety of treatments. *C*, a chlorpromazine-induced dense body after the Gomori method as adapted for electron microscopy. The presence of dense patches of reaction product allows this body to be identified as a lysosome. *A* and *B*, ×24,000; *C*, ×34,500. (*B* and *C* from C. F. Brosnan et al.: J. Neuropathol. Exp. Neurol. 29:337, 1970.)

occurring at pH 5.0 (Figs. 1.30C and 1.31C). Lysosomes are also identified by their ability to take up vital dyes (such as acridine orange) or drugs which can be traced intracellularly by fluorescence microscopy (Fig. 1-30B).

The lysosomes perform a variety of important roles for the cell. Intracellular digestion, summarized in Figure 1-32, is one of the most important. Lysis takes place within the confines of membrane-enclosed digestion vacuoles, with no visible damage

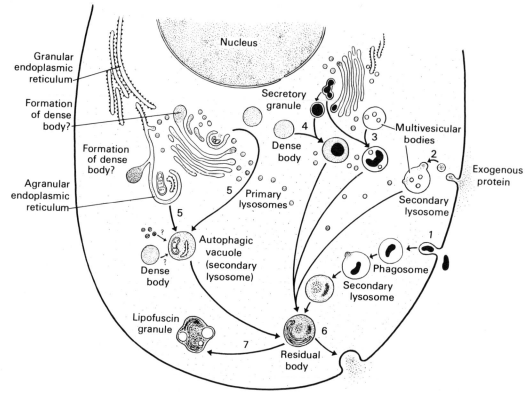

Fig. 1-32. Summary of pathways in the lysosomal or digestive system. A foreign body such as a bacterium is taken into the cell by invagination of the surface membrane, which then pinches off (endocytosis) (1). A *phagosome* thus formed acquires lytic enzymes by fusion with *primary lysosomes,* i.e., lysosomes which have not yet engaged in enzymatic activity. The resulting body is a *secondary lysosome,* i.e., a lysosome in which lytic activity is in progress or has occurred. Exogenous protein macromolecules may be taken up by the cell by means of small pinocytosis vesicles, which form from surface membrane, break away, and flow into the cytoplasm to merge with multivesicular bodies (2). Again, necessary enzymes for processing this material are brought to the multivesicular bodies by primary lysosomes. The digestion of endogenous protein (such as excess secretion granules) may occur in multivesicular bodies or dense bodies (3, 4). Bodies that contain identifiable organelles (such as mitochondria or granular endoplasmic reticulum) are known as *autophagic vacuoles* or cytolysosomes; these bodies are thought to arise by engulfment of organelles by a cisterna of membrane (5). More work is needed to know whether the enzymes are furnished by the cisternae or by fusion with primary lysosomes. The structure resulting from the formation of all of these *digestion vacuoles* is the *residual body,* which looks like a dense body filled with dense particles and whorls of membrane-like structures termed "myelin figures." In some cases, residual body contents may be released from the cell by fusion of the limiting membrane with the cell surface membrane (6). Or the residual body may be retained, participating over and over in digestive activity, growing larger and more heterogeneous in content, and becoming in time a *lipofuscin granule* (7). It is believed that the lysosomal enzymes are produced on ribosomes, after which they are channeled into the granular endoplasmic reticulum and packaged in the Golgi region into primary lysosomes (the small vesicle or the larger dense body type). (Diagram based upon papers by Novikoff and co-workers and Farquhar and collaborators.)

to the cytoplasm outside because the lysosomal membrane prevents enzyme release. An example of intracellular digestion is provided by the polymorphonuclear leukocyte. Its numerous specific granules are in fact lysosomes. When this white cell engulfs bacteria, the granules cluster around the newly formed vacuole, fuse with its limiting membrane, and discharge their content of destructive enzymes into the vacuole. During starvation the lysosomal system may aid cell survival by the sequestration and digestion of organelles (*autophagy*), thus providing reserve nutrients for continued cell life. Autophagy is also involved with normal turnover of organelles and removal of damaged organelles. Substances in excess are digested by the lysosomal system as well; for example, droplets of hormone which are not secreted are broken down by lysosomes of the same cell.

Injurious substances which may or may not be digestible are sequestered within the lysosomal system. Cells exposed to silica or asbestos particles, for instances, are seen in the electron microscope to have lysosomes filled with the dense spheres or rods characteristic of these substances.

The list of compounds known to increase or decrease the permeability of the lysosomal membrane is extensive; as examples, it is known that cortisone decreases the permeability, whereas vitamin A has the opposite effect. When a cell is deprived of oxygen or is damaged in some other way, the lysosomal membrane becomes more permeable or ruptures, thus allowing enzyme release with ensuing digestion of the cell (*autolysis*). Important questions under investigation are whether mitosis might be triggered by lysosomal digestion of a substance which normally represses division and whether certain types of cancer could result from chromosomal breakage by the lysosomal enzyme, deoxyribonuclease.

Related to the lysosomal population are *multivesicular bodies,* membrane-bounded bodies containing smaller membrane-bounded vesicles. Transitional forms between these organelles and dense bodies are often seen. Histochemical procedures have demonstrated that multivesicular bodies contain some acid hydrolases, notably acid phosphatase. Multivesicular bodies may receive exogenous or endogenous protein for breakdown (Fig. 1-32). Small primary lysosomes which bring enzymes to the multivesicular body may be covered with evenly spaced bristle-like structures, and are thus a form of *coated vesicle.* It should be noted, however, that not all coated vesicles represent primary lysosomes. Some coated vesicles are involved in the transport of material from the Golgi apparatus to the cell surface and some are involved with uptake of substances at the cell surface. Recent studies suggest that coated vesicles have a special protein composition (presumably related to the bristle coat) and that they have an important general function in the cell of shuttling membrane from one area to another. This more general function may be only incidentally related to the transport of vesicle contents.

Lipofuscin pigment is now thought to be contained within residual bodies, the end points in the lysosomal digestive system. Not all of the cellular material taken up by lysosomes is digestible, and it is some of this residue that is transformed into pigment. In the electron microscope, the lipofuscin pigment granules are very heterogeneous in appearance (Fig. 1-33), often containing lipid droplets or vacuoles and matrix substance (which contains the lytic activity) as well as the dense pigment. In the light microscope, they are seen as light brown granules in unstained preparations, as darkened bodies after staining with fat-soluble dyes, and as fluorescent particles in ultraviolet light. The pigment granules increase with age, especially in brain and heart tissues; their accumulation may lead to increasing dysfunction of these cells.

Peroxisomes. In the early 1950s, electron microscopy demonstrated a distinct category of small dense bodies in liver and kidney cells; these bodies were referred to by the descriptive term *microbodies*. They resembled lysosomes in being limited by a single membrane, but they frequently contained a dense crystalline or platelike core (Fig. 1-34). Subsequent biochemical studies showed that these organelles contained variable amounts of a few oxidative enzymes but appeared always to contain peroxidase. The universal presence of peroxidase was regarded of sufficient significance to warrant introduction of a new name; these bodies are currently known as *peroxisomes.*

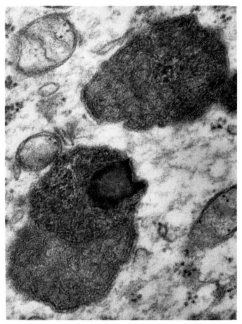

Fig. 1-33. Lipofuscin pigment bodies. In untreated but aging animals, dense bodies may become markedly enlarged, very irregular in contour, and highly heterogeneous in appearance, at which point they are known as lipofuscin bodies or granules. They often contain a wealth of thin, curving, dense bands, as in this figure, and a large, light vacuole. Mature rabbit nerve cell. ×58,000. (Courtesy of Dr. Virginia Tennyson.)

Peroxisomes can be identified positively by utilizing the diaminobenzidine reaction to localize peroxidase activity, but their morphology is also quite characteristic. Recent studies have demonstrated that peroxisomes occur in two size populations and that they are nearly ubiquitous in distribution. They may be present in increased numbers under circumstances that have been correlated with altered lipid metabolism, but their exact function in the cell is not clear. They are thought to arise from smooth endoplasmic reticulum rather than the Golgi apparatus, as do lysosomes, but the relationships of the different categories of peroxisomes to each other and to other cytoplasmic organelles remain equivocal. There is even question now whether all "peroxisomes" do in fact contain peroxidase activity.

Centrosome, Centrioles. The *centrosome* is a specialized zone of cytoplasm that contains the *centrioles*. It usually lies close to or indents the nucleus (Figs. 1-28 and 1-29), although its position varies somewhat in different cell types (Fig. 1-35). In glandular epithelial cells it is situated between the nucleus and the luminal surface. The centrosome is probably present in almost all mammalian cells but is often difficult to demonstrate. It has been observed in living cells, and it can be stained by iron hematoxylin in fixed preparations. Although it is most distinct during cell division, it can be demonstrated during the intermitotic stage. Its most constant feature is the presence of two sharply staining granules or *centrioles,* together called the *diplosome.* This organelle is self-replicating, as is discussed in chapter 2. The centrosome region is more gelatinous and appears more homogeneous than other parts of the cell.

Scrutiny of centrioles in the electron microscope has led to the realization that the two centrioles of a diplosome are oriented perpendicular to each other. Each centriole is a cylindrical organelle, 0.3 to 0.5 μm in length and about 0.15 μm in diameter, apparently closed at one end. The wall of the cylinder is composed of nine evenly spaced, longitudinally oriented, parallel units embedded in a dense material. Each unit consists of three tubular structures joined together. When the centriole is sectioned perpendicular to its long axis, the tubular units are seen as circles (Fig. 1-36). When sectioned parallel to its long axis, the tubules may be visualized as linear elements (Fig. 1-29). Microtubules radiate from the area around the centriole or from closely associated dense clumps of material, which are called *pericentriolar satellites* (Figs. 1-29 and 1-36).

As is indicated later, the centrosome has been clearly associated with the process of mitotic cell division, particularly in the organization of the spindle elements (microtubules). In the nondividing cell, it serves as a center about which other cytoplasmic organelles such as the Golgi apparatus are polarized and, as such, it is termed *cell center, centrosphere,* or *cytocentrum* (Figs. 1-10, 1-28, and 1-29). In addition, a centriole may migrate near the cell surface, where it becomes a *basal body* (kinetosome), which gives rise to a motile cilium or flagellum.

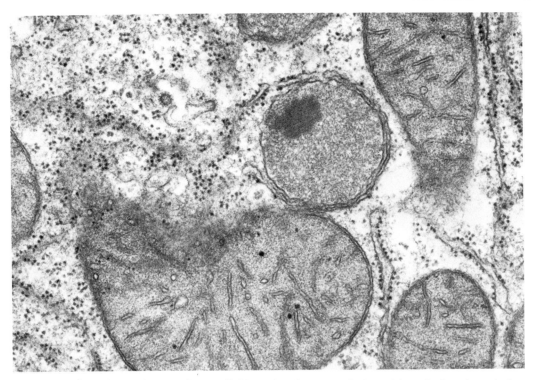

Fig. 1-34. Peroxisome in a rat liver cell. Note the close association with endoplasmic reticulum membranes and the dense crystalline core. ×38,800.

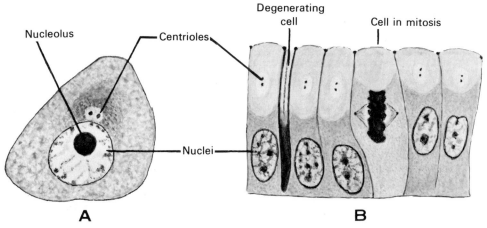

Fig. 1-35. *A,* centrosome in an interstitial cell of human testis. *B,* centrioles in columnar epithelial cells of human stomach. (*A,* redrawn after Petersen; *B,* redrawn after Zimmerman).

The mechanisms by which the centrioles exert their important organizational capabilities are not understood.

Mitochondria. In the 1890s, Altmann and, subsequently, Benda devised improved histological techniques which preserved and stained a population of small cytoplasmic bodies which came to be known as mitochondria (from the Greek *mitos,* a thread, + *chondros,* a grain). These bodies are visible as granules, rods, or filaments in both living (by phase microscopy) and fixed (after special staining) cytoplasm. Mictochondria may be identified in the liv-

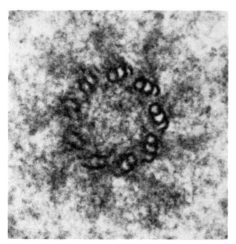

Fig. 1-36. Centriole sectioned perpendicular to its length. The "wall" of the centriole is seen here as a circle of nine units, each composed of three united tubule-like structures. Radiating from these units (resembling a pinwheel) are nine densities called pericentriolar satellites. Electron micrograph of rat ovarian follicle cell. ×140,000. (Courtesy of Dr. Daniel Szollosi.)

ing cell by applying supravital dyes, particularly Janus green B. The ability of these organelles to utilize O_2 and transport electrons maintains the Janus green in its oxidized or colored form, whereas in the surrounding cytoplasm the dye is reduced to a colorless compound. The granules may measure 0.2 to 1 μm or more in diameter, whereas the filamentous mitochondria may be 2 to 4 μm long or, in some cases, up to 10 to 12 μm in length. Mitochondria are present in almost all cell types. Any given cell type as a rule contains a characteristic number of these organelles; a rat liver cell is purported to contain 800 to 1000 mitochondria. The number of mitochondria per cell may be as low as 20 (in sperm) and as high as 500,000 (in giant amebae).

The very plastic and sensitive nature of mitochondria has been realized from observations made on living cells grown in tissue culture. Here the mitochondria are seen to be in constant agitation—expanding and contracting, fusing, dividing, and changing location. They often react more rapidly than any other cell organelle to temperature, metabolic, pH, or osmotic changes. Studies of mitochondrial fractions indicate that mitochondria undergo swelling and

contraction phases related to their physiological activity. Despite these known perturbations, mitochondria appear remarkably consistent in form and in position and orientation in some cell types in situ. In epithelial cells, mitochondria are often polarized such that their long axes are oriented in the direction of the secretory or transport process (Fig. 1-9A).

Electron microscopic studies indicate that each mitochondrion is bounded by two membranes. The inner membrane lies closely apposed to the outer one and, in addition, is thrown into folds (cristae) which protrude inward (Fig. 1-37). Depending upon the cell type, and correlating with physiological activity, the cristae vary in number and form (usually folds or tubules). They may or may not extend all of the way across the mitochondrion interior, and they are oriented either perpendicular (in most cases) or parallel to the long axis. The basic plan of the mitochondrion is nonetheless strikingly similar in all animal forms, ranging from protozoa to mammals. The cristae provide an increase in membrane surface area. An approximate calculation made for the liver cell suggests that the surface area of all of the mitochondrial membrane in that cell is 10 times greater than the surface area of the cell itself. This vast surface area houses the enzymes associated with electron transport and phosphorylation. Studies by Fernandez-Moran and co-workers in the early 1960s demonstrated the presence on crista membranes of any array of particles which were termed "elementary particles" in the belief that each particle represented a fundamental grouping of oxidative enzymes. Later investigations showed that the particles apparently do not contain the oxidative enzymes but do contain mitochondrial ATPase activity (Fig. 1-38).

The interior not occupied by cristae is filled with matrix substance, a finely granular material. Highly dense matrix granules (300 to 500 Å) may be found as well (Fig. 1-37). Their presence and size depend upon the metabolic state and type of cell. These are now known to be, in part, binding sites for ions, particularly cations such as Ca^{2+}. Cytologists puzzled for years over the autonomous behavior of mitochondria and finally were able to demonstrate the presence

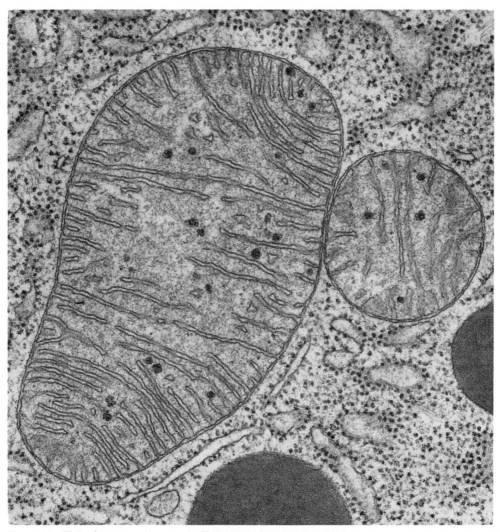

Fig. 1-37. This electron micrograph illustrates the morphological features of mitochondria. The inner membrane, unlike the outer one, is thrown into folds (cristae) which may span the interior. Within the mitochondrial matrix, which fills the area not occupied by cristae, are scattered dense granules. Bat pancreas. ×64,000. (From K. R. Porter and M. A. Bonneville: Fine Structure of Cells and Tissues, 3rd ed., Lea & Febiger, Philadephia, 1968.)

of a circular form of DNA and of RNA in the mitochondrial matrix. These discoveries, of course, provided an explanation for the ability of mitochondria to divide as separate genetic units and to synthesize proteins independently of nuclear control. Mitochondria are not fully autonomous, however, as most of their enzymatic proteins are still synthesized in the cell cytoplasm under nuclear control and transferred to mitochondria secondarily. The self-replicating ability of mitochondria enables the cell to maintain a relatively constant number of these organelles within each daughter cell after division.

Like some of the other cytoplasmic organelles, mitochondria perform diversified functions. Most important, they are the chief source of energy in the cell. During cell respiration, enzymatic breakdown, mostly of carbohydrates but also of fats and amino acids, yields CO_2, water, and energy as end products. The energy freed in this oxidation of foodstuffs is converted

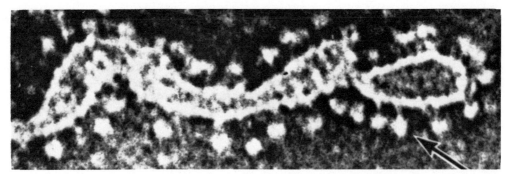

Fig. 1-38. Electron micrograph of a mitochondrial crista, negatively stained. The outer (or matrix) surface of each crista is covered by a regular array of "elementary" particles which are connected by means of slender stalks (*arrow*). Isolated beef heart mitochondria. ×500,000. (From H. Fernández-Morán et al. J. Cell Biol. 22:63, 1964.)

into phosphate bond energy. This energy, bound in adenosine triphosphate (ATP), is required in many different processes, including transport of ions across the cell membrane, protein synthesis, and muscle contraction.

The formation of ATP by the breakdown of glucose involves three different mitochondrial systems. The initial degradation of glucose occurs in the cytoplasm outside the mitochondria. The resulting product, a 3-carbon compound (pyruvate), enters the mitochondrion, where it is processed by a sequence of enzymes known as the *Krebs citric acid cycle*. Liberated hydrogens are fed into a complex chain of flavoproteins and cytochromes called the *electron transport system* or *respiratory chain*. Eventually the hydrogen combines with oxygen, which is thereby reduced to water. At three points along this respiratory chain, sufficient energy becomes available from the transfer of electrons to form ATP by the addition of phosphate to adenosine *di*phosphate (*phosphorylation*). Because oxygen is the oxidizing agent at the terminus of the respiratory chain and the phosphorylation apparatus is intimately *coupled* to this chain, the process is termed *oxidative phosphorylation*.

The respiratory and phosphorylation systems are found in highly ordered recurring assemblies in or bound to the mitochondrial crista membrane. That the membranes hold these essential enzyme systems is reflected in the fact that, in cells requiring more energy, such as insect flight or mammalian cardiac muscle, the cristae are much more densely packed. In such cells, mitochondria also are more numerous and are situated close to the energy-requiring structures.

Contractile protein has been found in mitochondria, suggesting a basis for the contraction observed earlier by light microscopists. Mitochondrial contraction, known to be related to respiratory activity, is thought to aid in mitochondrial movement and in the exchange of substances such as ATP and ions with the cytoplasm. Additional functions of mitochondria now include the accumulation of ions as well as the synthesis of nucleic acids and proteins and the oxidation of fatty acids. These synthetic pathways and the Krebs cycle reactions probably take place in the matrix, in contrast with the respiratory, phosphorylating, active transport, and contractile processes, which occur in relation to the mitochondrial cristae. The outer membrane is the site of monoamine oxidase activity.

Filaments. Slender threads of *filaments* occur in the cytoplasm of virtually all cells. As a rule, they range from less than 30 Å up to 120 Å in diameter and are of indeterminate length. Whether the filaments are randomly scattered throughout the cytoplasm, clustered into wisplike bundles, or aggregated into a meshwork depends upon the cell type. When the filaments occur in bundles, they are visible in the light microscope as *fibrils,* but visualization of individual filaments depends upon the resolution of the electron microscope (Fig. 1-39).

Recently it has become possible to recognize two basic categories of filaments; the

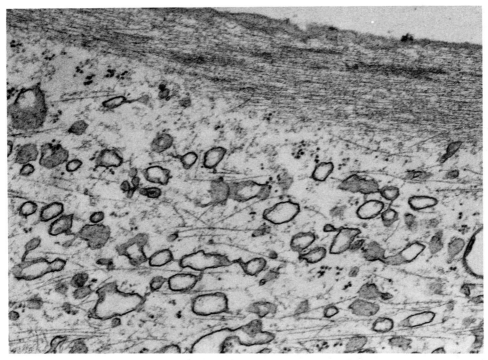

Fig. 1-39. Immediately beneath the cell border (which is shown at *upper right*) is a band of closely packed filaments. Filaments also are scattered throughout other areas of the cytoplasm of this cell grown in culture. ×42,500. (Courtesy of Drs. M. Bunge and D. Bray.)

microfilaments, whose diameters measure less than about 80 Å, and the *intermediate filaments* (or *tonofilaments*), whose diameters range from 80 to 120 Å. Substantial evidence now suggests that at least some, perhaps most, microfilaments are contractile, acting to promote cell shape changes or motility in a wide variety of cells. These are probably relatives of actin filaments, so abundantly deployed in the cytoplasm of all types of muscle. Study of highly motile cells in the living state shows relatively clear pseudopods or a clear, thin, peripheral rim of cytoplasm. This is referred to as *ectoplasm,* known to be more viscous or gelled than the rest of the cytoplasm. It is now known that these areas are full of microfilaments and that the apparent clarity is due to the exclusion of other organelles from these regions. A narrow band of microfilaments just beneath the cell membrane is a prominent feature of the cleavage furrow of dividing cells. Microfilaments are also found appropriately aligned in various embryonic epithelia which are undergoing rapid morphogenetic cell shape changes.

In muscle, the contractile function of actin filaments requires the interaction with another filamentous protein, *myosin.* In the nonmuscle contractile systems, it is still unclear whether myosin-like molecules always accompany the actin-like filaments. Some good evidence suggests that they do, at least in some cells.

Because recent investigations have revealed that these and other actin-like systems are widespread in nature, it is reasonable to presume that microfilament-induced contractility is a common property of most or perhaps all cells. It is a property which is greatly emphasized in muscle cells, traditionally regarded as the only contractile tissues.

Intermediate filaments, on the other hand, are not known to be contractile and usually serve a supportive role in those cells which contain them. Intermediate filaments therefore appear to constitute one important cytoskeletal component, whereas the contractile microfilaments might be considered as intracellular "muscles." Intermediate filaments are exceedingly prominent in the cytoplasm of "wear and tear" epithelia, such as the lining surfaces of the skin and the esophagus. Here they are generally referred to as tonofilaments. In nerve cells, intermediate-sized filaments are a regular component (along with microtubules; see below) of the axons and, to a lesser extent, of dendrites, where they lie parallel to the long axis. In the cell bodies of nerve cells, they are loosely aggregated into gracile bundles. Intermediate filaments are frequently found associated with the firmest sites of adhesion between adjacent cells of epithelial systems, further attesting to their role as a supportive intracellular network important in individual cells and also in transmission of forces among adherent cell populations.

Thus, filaments function in contractile processes, in various types of protoplasmic movement, and in changes in cell shape, as well as in the maintenance of cell form. More work is needed to understand the underlying mechanisms in nonmuscle cells: do the actin-like filaments themselves contract or do they act by sliding past one another or by interreacting with myosin-like molecules or microtubules, as has been suggested?

Microtubules. One of the most active areas of research in recent years has concerned itself with widely occurring, slender, cylindrical structures, the *microtubules.* Their discovery depended not only upon the resolution of the electron microscope but also upon improved preservation with glutaraldehyde fixation. Microtubules vary somewhat in diameter from 180 to 300 Å, but they usually measure about 240 Å, and they have been followed for several microns in thin sections. They are straight or slightly curving, suggesting a rigid structure (Figs. 1-28 and 1-29). When sectioned at right angles to its long axis, the microtubule appears as a circle composed of, on the average, 13 globular subunits, each about 40 to 50 Å in diameter.

Microtubule proteins from diversified sources have been found to be quite similar in their sequences of amino acids, and they closely resemble the muscle protein, actin. These proteins are referred to as *tubulins,* and they are known to circulate between a free monomeric form and an aggregated microtubular configuration. Like actin, tubulin has binding sites for nucleotides. The fact that these proteins also contain specific binding sites for colchicine explains their inability to aggregate and maintain microtubular structure in the presence of this agent. This effect on microtubules accounts for the action of colchicine in blocking mitosis. Microtubules from different locations vary in sensitivity to colchicine, pointing to at least subtle differences in the constituent tubulins.

During cell division, microtubules increase greatly in number, to as many as 3000 per cell, to form the mitotic spindle (which is described in chapter 2). In nondividing cells, microtubules are scattered throughout the cytoplasm. They may converge on centrosomes (Figs. 1-28 and 1-29) and are found in units of three (triplets), forming the framework of the basal body and the centriole (Fig. 1-36). Microtubules form the cores of cilia, flagella, and sperm tails, where they are often organized into nine doublets encircling two centrally situated microtubules (Figs. 4-18 and 4-19). During sperm maturation, hundreds of microtubules are clustered in a very orderly fashion around the nucleus at a time when the nucleus begins to elongate. During the development of chick lens epithelium, when cells may undergo a 4-fold increase in length, microtubules become prominent in the cortical cytoplasm, lying parallel to the axis of elongation. Microtubules are a regular component of the extensions of nerve cells. One of the most striking examples of microtubule arrays was discovered in a spherical protozoan, *Actinosphaerium.* Radiating from the cell body, which is about 100 μm in diameter, are numerous long, needle-like extensions or axopodia, often more than 400 μm long and only 5 to 10 μm in diameter. Each axopodium contains as many as 500 microtubules in a highly ordered arrangement. When these microtubules are disrupted, the axopodia collapse.

Findings like those just mentioned have led to the conclusion that microtubules play a role in maintaining diverse cell shape. Their prominence and orientation during periods of changing cell shape have also suggested that they are active in changing cell form, although no exact mechanism for this postulated role has been established. However, if microtubules are treated with colchicine and thereby prevented from assembly during such a period, normal development may be arrested. As components of the spindle, cilia, and flagella, they not only provide a cytoskeletal framework but also may contribute to the mechanisms by which movement is accomplished. In cilia and flagella, evidence suggests that pairs of microtubules interact directly to cause differential positioning, thereby generating the whiplike motion characteristic of these organelles. Microtubules are also closely associated with actin and, frequently, with microfilaments. It is believed that interactions between microtubules and microfilaments are responsible for at least some kinds of cytoplasmic movement.

Cell Membrane. A membrane, the *plasma membrane* or *plasmalemma,* surrounds the cell, separating the cell contents from the external environment. In this important position it regulates the passage of materials into and out of the cell. This membrane, 70 to 110 Å in thickness, is too thin to be resolved by the light microscope. However, it may be visualized if in an histological section it slants (and is thereby obliquely sectioned) and thus occupies an area wider than its true thickness. In addition, stain taken up by an exterior adherent coating on the membrane may enhance its visibility. Even when a cell membrane is not directly visualized, its presence can be inferred from observations on cells during micromanipulation, when cytoplasm spills out if the membrane is ruptured, and after alterations of the environmental tonicity. When red blood cells are placed in a hypotonic fluid or in water, they swell as a result of the action of osmotically active components of the cytoplasm. They may in fact burst, losing their contents (in this case, hemoglobin).

By treating red blood cells in the manner just described, it is possible to obtain a relatively pure preparation of plasma membrane for biochemical analysis. Such preparations contain about 35% lipid, including phospholipids and cholesterol, 60% protein, and a small amount of carbohydrate. From these data and from estimates of the surface

areas of red cells, it is possible to calculate that there are enough lipid molecules to cover each cell twice. This observation, as well as physical measurements of membrane thickness, birefringence, X-ray diffraction, and surface tension, has lent support to a model of membrane structure proposed by Danielli and Davson in 1935. This model depicts the plasma membrane as a double layer or bimolecular leaflet of lipids sandwiched between two protein coats (Fig. 1-40). The phospholipid molecules of the membrane have both hydrophobic ends, where the fatty acids are located, and hydrophilic ends, where the phosphate groups are attached. It is assumed that the hydrophobic ends appose each other in the middle of the membrane, whereas the hydrophilic ends lie next to the enveloping protein layers. The presence of a continuous hydrophobic region could explain the low permeability of many membranes to water-soluble compounds and their high permeability to lipid-soluble materials.

When the cell membrane is sectioned at right angles to its surface and examined in the electron microscope at lower magnifications, it appears as a dense line. High magnifications and staining make it possible to demonstrate that this line is, in fact, a pair of thinner dense lines separated by a light inner zone, all roughly of similar thickness (Fig. 1-40). This tripartite or *trilaminar* structure seemed to fit the Danielli-Davson model very well; the dense laminae corresponded to the two protein layers and the light intermediate stratum represented the bimolecular leaflet of lipid (Fig. 1-40). The fact that many of the intracellular membranes also exhibited this trilaminar structure (termed "unit membranes" by Robertson) suggested that this was a basic design common to all membranes. Results of freeze fracture studies also support this concept. The fracture planes of rapidly frozen fixed or unfixed cells travel along pathways of lowest resistance. The splitting of membranes internally indicates an area of weak chemical interactions consistent with lipid hydrocarbon chains.

It seems clear, however, that a membrane with continuous lipid leaflets could not pro-

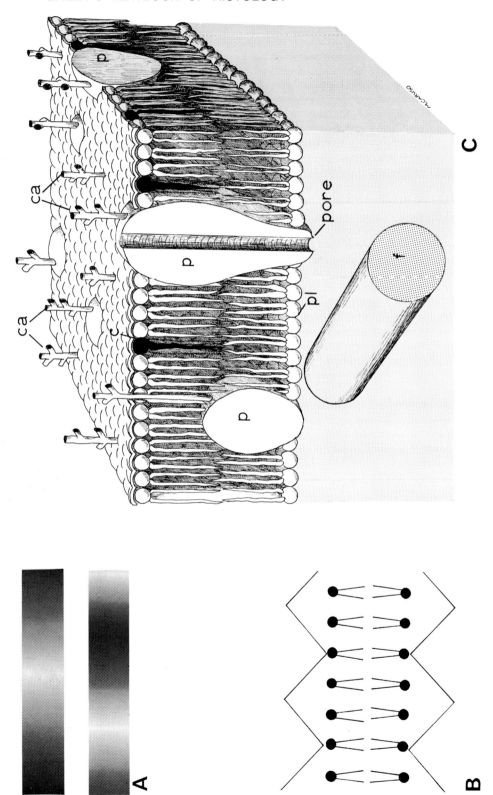

vide for all of the diverse functions that membranes are known to perform. It is now generally believed that, within the basic membrane structure described above, there are scattered sites which provide for special membrane activities as, for example, the attachment of cytoplasmic filaments or the transport of sugars and amino acids across the membrane. At these sites, protein components apparently penetrate the lipid interface of the membrane (Fig. 1-40).

Membranes are known to vary in protein content. In fact, the suggestion has been made that the protein content of membranes provides a rough index or their overall metabolic activity. Membranes, such as those comprising myelin, that have a low protein content (about 20%) have little associated enzymatic activity and function passively in influencing electrical properties of nerve fibers. Mitochondrial membranes, on the other hand, contain dozens of enzymes and are composed of about 65% protein.

Gradually, it is being realized from newer analytical approaches to the study of cell membranes (especially freeze fracturing techniques), that a given cell membrane or territory of membrane is not likely to be a static mosaic in life. Rather, the evidence strongly suggests a "fluid" nature of membranes in which enzymes, attachment points, and reactive or permeability sites can be sequestered or dispersed in patterns or concentrations commensurate with physiological activity. Although the patterns of flux await further elucidation, one should consider the plasmalemma and other cell membranes in an often dynamic rather than static sense, displaying varying rates of renewal and the capability to mo-bilize appropriate molecular components at foci of specified activity.

Freeze fracture techniques have provided a wealth of new information and hold considerable promise for further elucidation of membrane organization. It will be recalled that this method can be applied to unfixed and nondehydrated cells and tissues (as well as to fixed ones), and that it splits individual membranes so that the internal aspects of the cell membrane leaflets can be studied as well as the general contours and interrelationships of various organelles (Figs. 1-7 and 1-41). Freeze-fracture methods reveal characteristic particles on one or the other of the two exposed internal surfaces of a split membrane. It appears that these represent protein and are related to the sites of localized enzymes, foci of attachment, or points of transmembrane transport. The composition and function of these "membrane particles" differ in different kinds of membranes, and these features are being intensively investigated by correlated biochemical and ultrastructural approaches.

On the exterior of the cell, appended to the surface of the cell membrane, is a layer of material containing substantial amounts of carbohydrates which are usually associated with lipids (glycolipids) or proteins (glycoproteins). This coat or *glycocalyx* may be very thick, as over the microvilli of epithelial cells of the intestinal mucosa (Fig. 1-42), or extremely thin, as in the membranes of the myelin sheath, but nevertheless it appears to be universally present on cell surfaces. Ionized groups on the terminal units of the saccharide chains (e.g., sialic acid) give many cell surfaces a negative charge (Fig. 1-40). The presence

---

Fig. 1-40. The appearance of the plasma membrane in electron micrographs is portrayed at *A*. At *B*, the Davson-Danielli bilayer model is shown. The central region of hydrocarbon chains of the phospholipid layers corresponds to the central light space in electron micrographs. *C* depicts additional features of membrane structure. The bimolecular leaflet contains phospholipids (*pl*), cholesterol (*c*), and proteins (*p*). Carbohydrate moieties (*ca*) extend from the external surface, some attached to protein and some to lipid. Some proteins (perhaps most) span the bilayer. Some are thought to form aqueous channels (pores) and some are involved with facilitated transport of certain ions or metabolites. Cytoplasmic filaments (*f*) may be closely associated with the membrane, and some microtubules (not illustrated) terminate near the membrane as well. The membrane bilayer exhibits fluidity, permitting integral proteins to move laterally, thus changing the sites of surface active areas, aqueous channels, and membrane interactions with microfilaments and microtubules.

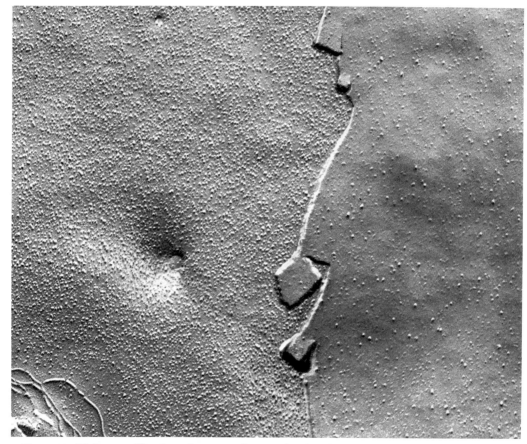

Fig. 1-41. High magnification electron micrograph of a freeze fracture replica showing split membranes of two neighboring cells viewed face-on. On the *right side* of the figure the fracture has split the membrane of one cell, exposing the outer face (E-face), whereas the *left side* shows the inner face (P-face) of the closely neighboring cell. Note the difference in numbers of intramembranous protein particles on the two faces. ×59,250.

of the glycocalyx and the negative charges undoubtedly contribute to the consistent and regular spacing of about 200 Å which occurs between membranes of adjacent cells.

From the above discussion it will be apparent that there may well be as many different kinds of membrane as there are different kinds of cells and cell organelles, and each may be capable of considerable change in life. The importance of membrane within the cell is indicated by the fact that many of the cytoplasmic organelles (endoplasmic reticulum, Golgi apparatus, lysosomal bodies, mitochondria) and the nuclear envelope are constructed of or bounded by membrane. *The intracellular membranes serve vital functions in segre-gating the cytoplasm into compartments for the storage of formed products or the control of interactions of substances in their proper order and in increasing the surface area participating in metabolic processes.*

At the cell surface, the plasma membrane provides for the selection of what enters and what leaves the cell. In addition, in nerve and muscle cells the plasma membrane contains mechanisms to allow for sudden changes in ion permeability in response to changes in its electrical potential or configuration. It also has receptor sites for different kinds of chemicals such as hormones and neurotransmitters (discussed in chapter 10). Its surface characteristics determine how it relates to the surface on which it rests, and how it reacts (by adhesion, repulsion, or fusion) with other cells. The content and the configuration of the surface molecules are important factors in the immunological properties of the cell. The membrane may, in fact, be the most complex macromolecular aggregate in the cell, and the understanding of its structure and function is the key to understanding much of cell biology.

Cytoplasmic Inclusions. The cytoplasm of the cell may contain numerous inclusions of substances which are usually in the nature of raw food materials or the stored products of the cell's metabolic activity. Thus, deposits of proteins, fats, and carbohydrates are characteristic features in certain cells. The storage of *glycogen* by cells of liver and muscle are the outstanding examples of carbohydrate storage (Fig. 1-9*D*). Glycogen is a polymer formed from glucose. It is stained magenta by the PAS reaction or Best's carmine method. In the electron microscope, glycogen (after lead staining) appears as scattered or clustered small dense particles, 150 to 450 Å (Fig. 1-43). Although fat cells are the chief sites of *lipid* storage, many other cell types store some lipid in the form of droplets of varying size. If frozen sections are stained with specific fat-soluble dyes or if the tissue is fixed in osmium tetroxide, the lipid droplets are retained and appear black (Fig. 1-1*C*). In electron micrographs they appear as homogeneous spheres of varying density. Examples of the products of cell activity are *yolk granules* and *secretory granules*.

Another type of cytoplasmic inclusion is the *pigment granule*. Pigment granules possess color without staining. The occurrence of *lipofuscin* is considered above in the section describing lysosomes. Certain cells contain dark brown or black granules which are composed of the pigment *melanin*. In the electron microscope, these granules appear as homogeneous dense bodies. In man they are present in the eye, certain areas of the brain, and the skin (see chapter 14).

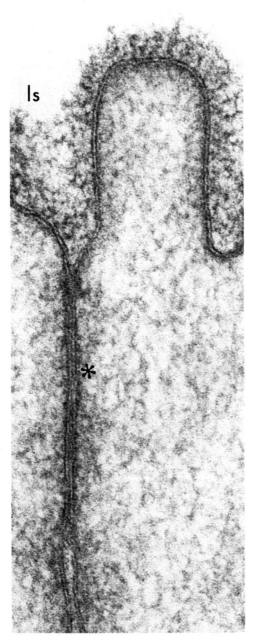

Fig. 1-42. In the digestive tract the luminal surface (*ls*) of the absorbing cells is covered with highly regular finger-like protuberances called microvilli, one of which is pictured here. This electron micrograph clearly illustrates the trilaminar nature of the bounding cell membrane and shows the largely amorphous, "fuzzy" material coating the luminal surface of the cell. Along the lateral cell surfaces the bounding membranes may be more closely apposed than usual (as at *asterisk*). ×180,000. (From K. R.

Porter and M. A. Bonneville: Fine Structure of Cells and Tissues, 3rd ed, Lea & Febiger, Philadelphia, 1968.)

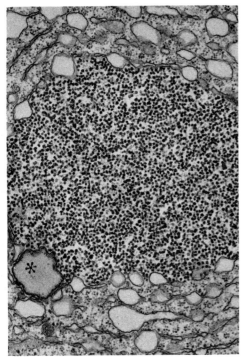

Fig. 1-43. An accumulation of glycogen particles in an X-irradiated neuron. These particles may be compared to the smaller ribosomes scattered among the swollen elements of endoplasmic reticulum. A lipid droplet is marked by an *asterisk*. Electron micrograph of rat nervous tissue in culture. ×25,000. (From E. B. Masurovsky et al.: J. Cell Biol. 32:467, 1967.

General Considerations

Cell Form and Cell Size

The cells of the animal body show a wide variation in size and form, coincident with their adaptation to perform a diversity of specific functions (Fig. 1-44). The tissue cells which have acquired a fixed location in the body become polyhedral, columnar, flat (pavement), fusiform, or spindle-shaped, and they may retain a smooth contour or send out numerous processes. The nerve cell, with its processes sometimes several feet in length, is perhaps the most aberrant type. The laws which control or limit cell size as well as body size are not well understood. Some groups of animals have larger cells than do others, but it does not follow that small animals have small cells and large animals have large cells. The size of the individual is in general determined by the number of its cells, not by their size.

Cell Life and Cell Death

Biologists generally believe that living matter is constructed according to the same basic principles as is the physical world in which it exists. Considering the tenets of physics, particularly thermodynamics, living systems might be expected gradually to decrease in complexity, for energy is always involved in the maintenance of high degrees of organization. Yet the trend in the evolution of living systems is toward greater complexity.

The key to this riddle is, of course, the continual input into living systems of free energy from the sun. This energy was initially used in the synthesis of the simplest of organic substances and is now continuously used to maintain and extend the organization of living things. Many higher organisms do not, of course, use the energy of the sun directly, but feed on lower forms that do.

The process of cell growth can occur with remarkable rapidity, for the chemical reactions within the cell are efficiently catalyzed by the cell *enzymes*. The process of the construction of macromolecules, which is the process of growth, is called *anabolism*. The cell also uses mechanisms of *catabolism* for the breakdown of its components. These catabolic mechanisms can release stored energy for use by the cell, as in the breakdown of fatty acids, and are a necessary part of the ongoing activities of the cell. Both anabolism and catabolism are important for maintaining the proper functional levels of materials within the cell. Several important diseases, called storage diseases, result not from the lack of anabolic activity within the cell but from the failure of the proper enzymatic degradation of cellular constituents. In these conditions, specific cell components accumulate within the cell in abnormal amounts and in time seriously interfere with cell function.

Cell death is an integral part of the growth of tissues and organs. During the development of some tissues, large numbers of cells may die. In these cases there is an

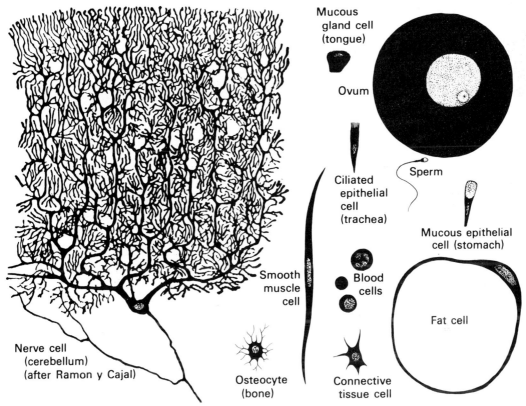

Mucous
gland cell
(tongue)

Ovum

Ciliated
epithelial
cell
(trachea)

Sperm

Mucous epithelial
cell (stomach)

Smooth
muscle
cell

Blood
cells

Fat cell

Nerve cell
(cerebellum)
(after Ramon y Cajal)

Osteocyte
(bone)

Connective
tissue cell

Fig. 1-44. Cells vary widely in size and shape and their nuclei occupy differing positions, as depicted diagrammatically here. All of the cells are drawn to scale (100 μm = nearly 1½ inches), with the measurements based on data from humans.

initial overproduction of certain cell types, and only those required for the functional needs of the tissue survive. Local cell death (*necrosis*) occurs normally in the body, or may be the result of influences which cause disease, such as trauma and inflammation. Morphologically, necrotic tissue can be recognized by the altered structure of the cells and intercellular substance. Coagulation of proteins takes place in the cytoplasm, the latter appearing flocculated or in the nature of a fibrous network. The cells appear fused by the obliteration of cellular boundaries. Or the cell may liquefy, swell, and finally burst (*cytolysis*), the liquefaction being often preceded by the appearance of numerous fat granules. These degradation processes are in many cases caused by intracellular enzymes liberated after the death of the cell (*autolysis*). The nucleus, likewise, shows various forms of structural disintegration. The chromatin may contract into a dense, deeply staining irregular mass (*pyknosis*), it may fragment into a number of small pieces with obliteration of the nuclear boundary (*karyorrhexis*), or it may gradually disappear, as evidenced by the loss of its staining capacity (*karyolysis*).

References

Techniques

ALLFREY, V. The isolation of subcellular components. *In* The Cell; Biochemistry, Physiology, Morphology (Brachet, J., and Mirsky, A. E., editors), vol. I, pp. 193–290. Academic Press, New York, 1959.

BAKER, J. R. Cytological Technique; The Principles Underlying Routine Methods, ed. 5. John Wiley & Sons, Inc., New York, 1966.

BULLIVANT, S. Freeze-etching and freeze-fracturing. *In* Advanced Techniques in Biological Electron Microscopy. (Koehler, J., editor), pp. 66–112. Springer-Verlag, New York, 1973.

COONS, A. H. Histochemistry with labeled antibody. Int. Rev. Cytol. 5:1–23, 1956.

HAMA, K., AND PORTER, K. R. An application of high voltage electron microscopy to the study of biological materials. High voltage electron microscopy. J. Microsc. 8:149–158, 1969.

HAYAT, M. A. (editor). Principles and Techniques of Electron Microscopy. Biological Applications. Vols. 1–6, and Principles and Techniques of Scanning Electron Microscopy, Vols. 1–5. Van Nostrand Reinhold Company, New York, 1970–1976.

PEARSE, A. G. E. Histochemistry, Theoretical and Applied, ed. 3. J. & A. Churchill Ltd., London, 1968.

PEASE, D. C. Histological Techniques for Electron Microscopy, ed. 2. Academic Press, New York, 1964.

POLLISTER, A. W. (editor). Physical Techniques in Biological Research, ed. 2, vol. 3, parts A, B, C. Topics such as phase contrast and interference microscopy, birefringence, microtomy, freeze drying, fluorescence microspectrophotometry and autoradiography are considered. Academic Press, New York, 1966–1969.

ROGERS, A. W. Techniques of Autoradiography. American Elsevier Publishing Company, New York, 1967.

WIED, G. L. (editor). Introduction to Quantitative Cytochemistry. Academic Press, New York, 1966.

General Topics

BRACHET, J., AND MIRSKY, A. E. The Cell; Biochemistry, Physiology, Morphology, 6 vols. Academic Press, New York, 1959–1964.

BRANTON, D., BULLIVANT, S., GILULA, N. B., KARNOVSKY, M. J., MOOR, H., MUHLETHALER, K., NORTHCOTE, D. H., PACKER, L., SATIR, B., SATIR, P., SPETH, V., STAEHELIN, L. A., STEERE, R. L., AND WEINSTEIN, R. S. Freeze-etching nomenclature. Science 190:54–56, 1975.

CASPERSSON, T. O. Cell Growth and Cell Function. W. W. Norton and Company, New York, 1950.

COWDRY, E. V. (editor). General Cytology. The University of Chicago Press, Chicago, 1924.

DARNELL, JR., J. E. Ribonucleic acids from animal cells. Bacteriol. Rev. 32:262–290.

DEROBERTIS, E. D. P., SAEZ, F. A., AND DEROBERTIS, E. M. F., JR. Cell Biology, ed. 6. W. B. Saunders Company, Philadelphia, 1975.

FAWCETT, D. W. An Atlas of Fine Structure: The Cell, Its Organelles and Inclusions. W. B. Saunders Company, Philadelphia, 1966.

FINEAN, J. B. Engström-Finean Biological Ultrastructure, ed. 2. Academic Press, New York, 1967.

GIESE, A. C. Cell Physiology, ed. 3. W. B. Saunders Company, Philadelphia, 1968.

INGRAM, V. M. The Biosynthesis of Macromolecules. W. A. Benjamin, Inc., New York, 1965.

LOEWY, A. G., AND SIEKEVITZ, P. Cell Structure and Function, ed. 2 Holt, Rinehart and Winston, Inc., New York, 1969.

PORTER, K. R., AND BONNEVILLE, M. A. Fine Structure of Cells and Tissues, ed. 4. Lea & Febiger, Philadelphia, 1973.

RHODIN, J. A. G. Histology. A Text and Atlas. Oxford, University Press, New York, 1974.

SMELLIE, R. M. S. The biosynthesis and function of nucleic acids. In The Biological Basis of Medicine (Bittar, E. E., editor), vol. I, pp. 243–281. Academic Press, New York, 1968.

Special Topics

NOTE: In order to reduce the number of references, many of the important earlier papers have not been listed because they are cited in the subsequent reports and reviews given below.

Nucleus

ABELSON, H. T., AND SMITH, G. H. Nuclear Pores: The pore-annulus relationship in thin section. J. Ultrastruct. Res. 30:558–588, 1970.

WISCHNITZER, S. The submicroscopic morphology of the interphase nucleus. Int. Rev. Cytol. 34:1, 1973.

Envelope

GALL, J. G. Octagonal nuclear pores. J. Cell Biol. 32:391–399, 1967.

HEILBRUNN, L. V., AND WEBER, F. (editors). The nuclear membrane and nucleocytoplasmic interchanges (Protoplasmatologia), vol. 5, no. 2. Springer-Verlag, Vienna, 1964. This volume contains a preface by Mirsky, and reviews on the electron microscopy of the nuclear envelope (by Gall), permeability of the envelope (by Loewenstein and by Feldherr and Harding) and nuclear transplantation studies (by Goldstein).

WIENER, J., SPIRO, D., AND LOEWENSTEIN, W. R. Ultrastructure and permeability of nuclear membranes. J. Cell Biol. 27:107–117, 1965.

Nucleolus

BERNHARD, W., AND GRANBOULAN, N. Electron microscopy of the nucleolus in vertebrate cells. In The Nucleus (Dalton, A. J., and Haguenau, F., editors), pp. 81–149. Academic Press, New York, 1968.

BUSCH, H., AND SMETANA, K. The Nucleolus. Academic Press, New York, 1970.

HAY, E. D. Structure and function of the nucleolus in developing cells. In The Nucleus (Dalton, A. J., and Haguenau, F., editors), pp. 1–79. Academic Press, New York, 1968.

PERRY, R. P. The nucleolus and the synthesis of ribosomes. Progr. Nucl. Acid Res. 6:219–257, 1967.

VINCENT, W. S., AND MILLER, JR., O. L. (editors). International Symposium on the Nucleolus, Its Structure and Function. National Cancer Institute Monograph No. 23, United States Government Printing Office, Washington, D. C., 1966.

Genetic Material

BARR, M. L. The significance of the sex chromatin. Int. Rev. Cytol. 19:35–95, 1966.

HARRIS, H. Nucleus and Cytoplasm. Clarendon Press, Oxford, 1968.

HAY, E. D., AND REVEL, J. P. The fine structure of the DNP component of the nucleus. An electron microscopic study utilizing autoradiography to localize DNA synthesis. J. Cell Biol. 16:29–51, 1963.

MILLER, JR., O. L., AND BEATTY, B. R. Visualization of nucleolar genes. Science 164:955–957, 1969.

MIRSKY, A. E., AND OSAWA, S. The interphase nucleus. *In* The Cell; Biochemistry, Physiology, Morphology (Brachet, J., and Mirsky, A. E., editors), vol. 2, pp. 677–770. Academic Press, New York, 1961.

RIS, H. Ultrastructure and molecular organization of genetic systems. Can. J. Genet. Cytol., 3:95–120, 1961.

SWIFT, H. Molecular morphology of the chromosome. In Vitro 1:26–49, 1965.

WATSON, J. Molecular Biology of the Gene. W. A. Benjamin, Inc., New York, 1965.

WATSON, J. D. The Double Helix; A Personal Account of the Discovery of the Structure of DNA. Atheneum Press, New York, 1968.

See also references at end of Chapter 2.

Function

ALLFREY, V. Some chemical aspects of nuclear fine structure—a preface. *In* The Nucleus (Dalton, A. J., and Haguenau, F., editors), pp. ix–xiii. Academic Press, New York, 1968.

BRACHET, J. Nucleocytoplasmic interactions in unicellular organisms. *In* The Cell; Biochemistry, Physiology, Morphology (Brachet, J., and Mirsky, A. E., editors), vol. 2, pp. 771–841. Academic Press, New York, 1961.

BRIGGS, R., AND KING, T. J. Nucleocytoplasmic interactions in eggs and embryos. *In* The Cell; Biochemistry, Physiology, Morphology (Brachet, J., and Mirsky, A. E., editors), vol. 1, pp. 537–617. Academic Press, New York, 1959.

GURDON, J. B. Transplanted nuclei and cell differentiation. Sci. Amer., 219:24–35, 1968.

GURDON, J. B. Nuclear transplantation and the control of gene activity in animal development. Proc. R. Soc. 176:303–314, 1970.

GURDON, J. B., LASKEY, R. A., AND REEVES, O. R. The developmental capacity of nuclei transplanted from keratinized skin cells of adult frogs. J. Embryol. Exp. Morphol. 34:93–112, 1975.

LOCKE, M. (editor). Cytodifferentiation and Macromolecular Synthesis (Society for the Study of Development and Growth, Symposium No. 21). Academic Press, New York, 1963. Included are chapters by Jacob and Monod (genetic repression, allosteric inhibtion and cellular differentiation) and by Gall (chromosomes and cytodifferentiation).

Cytoplasm

Ribosomes, Endoplasmic Reticulum

CARO, L. G., AND PALADE, G. E. 1964. Protein synthesis, storage, and discharge in the pancreatic exocrine cell. An autoradiographic study. J. Cell Biol. 20:473–495, 1964.

EMANS, J. B., AND JONES, A. L. Hypertrophy of liver cell smooth surfaced reticulum following progesterone administration. J. Histochem. Cytochem. 16:561–570, 1968.

FAWCETT, D. W. Structural and functional variations in the membranes of the cytoplasm. *In* Intracellular Membranous Structure (Seno, S., and Cowdry, E.

V., editors), pp. 15–36. Chugoku Press, Okayama, 1965.

HAGUENAU, F. The ergastoplasm: its history, ultrastructure and biochemistry. Int. Rev. Cytol. 7:425–483, 1958.

JAMIESON, J. D., AND PALADE, G. E. Intracellular transport of secretory proteins in the pancreatic exocrine cell. I. Role of the peripheral elements of the Golgi complex. J. Cell Biol. 34:577–596, 1967.

JAMIESON, J. D., AND PALADE, G. E. Intracellular transport of secretory proteins in the pancreatic exocrine cell. II. Transport to condensing vacuoles and zymogen granules. J. Cell Biol. 34:597–615, 1967.

JONES, A. L., AND FAWCETT, D. W. Hypertrophy of the agranular endoplasmic reticulum in hamster liver induced by phenobarbital. J. Histochem. Cytochem. 14:215–232, 1966.

PALADE, G. E. The endoplasmic reticulum. J. Biophys. Biochem. Cytol. 2 (suppl.):85–98, 1956.

PALADE, G. E. A small particulate component of the cytoplasm. *In* Frontiers in Cytology (Palay, S. L., editor), pp. 283–304. Yale University Press, New Haven, 1958.

PALADE, G. Intracellular aspects of the process of protein synthesis. Science 189:347–358, 1975.

PALADE, G. E., AND PORTER, K. R. Studies on the endoplasmic reticulum. I. Its identification in cells *in situ*. J. Exp. Med. 100:641–656, 1954.

PORTER, K. R. The ground substance; observations from electron microscopy. *In* The Cell; Biochemistry, Physiology, Morphology (Brachet, J., and Mirsky, A. E., editors), vol. 2, pp. 621–675. Academic Press, New York, 1961.

PORTER, K. R., CLAUDE, A., AND FULLAM, E. F. A study of tissue culture cells by electron microscopy. J. Exp. Med. 81:232–246, 1945.

RICH, A. Polyribosomes. Sci. Amer. 209:44–53, 1963.

RICH, A. On the assembly of amino acids into proteins. *In* Structural Chemistry and Molecular Biology (Rich, A., and Davidson, N., editors), pp. 223–237. W. H. Freeman and Company, San Francisco, 1968.

SPIRIN, A. S., AND GAVRILOVA, L. P. The Ribosome. Springer-Verlag, New York, 1969.

Golgi Apparatus

BAINTON, D. F., AND FARQUHAR, M. G. Origin of granules in polymorphonuclear leukocytes. Two types derived from opposite faces of the Golgi complex in developing granulocytes. J. Cell Biol. 28:277–301, 1966.

BAINTON, D. F., AND FARQUHAR, M. G. Differences in enzyme content of azurophil and specific granules of polymorphonuclear leukocytes. II. Cytochemistry and electron microscopy of bone marrow cells. J. Cell Biol. 39:299–317, 1968.

BEAMS, H. W., AND KESSEL, R. G. The Golgi apparatus: structure and function. Int. Rev. Cytol. 23:209–276, 1968.

DALTON, A. J. Golgi apparatus and secretion granules. *In* The Cell; Biochemistry, Physiology, Morphology (Brachet, J., and Mirsky, A. E., editors), vol. 2, pp. 603–619. Academic Press, New York, 1961.

KIRKMAN, H., AND SEVERINGHAUS, A. E. A review of the Golgi apparatus. Anat. Rec. 70:413–431 and 557–573, 1938, 71:79–103, 1938.

NEUTRA, M., AND LEBLOND, C. P. The Golgi apparatus. Sci. Amer. 220:100–107, 1969.

RAMBOURG, A. Morphological and histochemical aspects of glycoproteins at the surface of animal cells. Int. Rev. Cytol. 31:57, 1971.

RAMBOURG, A., HERNANDEZ, W., AND LEBLOND, C. P. Detection of complex carbohydrates in the Golgi apparatus of rat cells. J. Cell Biol. 40:395–414, 1969.

REVEL, J. P., AND ITO, S. The surface components of cells. In The Specificity of Cell Surfaces (Davis, B. D., and Warren, L., editors), pp. 211–234. Prentice-Hall, Inc., New York, 1967.

WHALEY, W. G. The Golgi apparatus. In The Biological Basis of Medicine (Bittar, E. E., editor), vol. 1, pp. 179–208. Academic Press, New York, 1968.

Lysosomes, Peroxisomes

ALLISON, A. Lysosomes and disease. Sci. Amer. 217:62–72, 1967.

ALLISON, A. C. Lysosomes. In The Biological Basis of Medicine (Bittar, E. E., editor), vol. 1, pp. 209–242. Academic Press, New York, 1968.

DE DUVE, C. The lysosome. Sci. Amer. 208:64–72, 1963.

DE DUVE, C., AND BAUDHUIN, P. Peroxisomes (microbodies and related particles). Physiol. Rev. 46:323–357, 1966.

DE DUVE, C., AND WATTIAUX, R. Functions of lysosomes. Ann. Rev. Physiol. 28:435–492, 1966.

DINGLE, J. T., AND FELL, H. B. (editors). Lysosomes in Biology and Pathology. John Wiley & Sons, Inc., New York, 1969.

FRIEND, D. S., AND FARQUHAR, M. G. Functions of coated vesicles during protein absorption in the rat vas deferens. J. Cell Biol. 35:357–376, 1967.

HIRSCH, J. G., AND COHN, Z. A. Digestive and autolytic functions of lysosomes in phagocytic cells. Fed. Proc. 23:1023–1025, 1964.

HRUBAN, Z., AND RECHIGL, JR., M. Microbodies and Related Particles; Morphology, Biochemistry and Physiology. Int. Rev. Cytol. Suppl. 1, 1969.

NOVIKOFF, A. B., AND SHIN, W.-Y. The endoplasmic reticulum in the Golgi zone and its relations to microbodies, Golgi apparatus and autophagic vacuoles in rat liver cells. J. Microsc. 3:187–206, 1964.

NOVIKOFF, A. B., ESSNER, E., AND QUINTANA, N. Golgi apparatus and lysosomes. Fed. Proc. 23:1010–1022, 1964.

NOVIKOFF, A., NOVIKOFF, P., DAVIS, C., AND QUINTANA, N. Studies on microperoxisomes. V. Are microperoxisomes ubiquitous in mammalian cells? J. Histochem. Cytochem. 21:737–755, 1973.

PEARSE, B. M. F. Clathrin: a unique protein associated with intracellular transfer of membrane by coated vesicles. Proc. Natl. Acad. Sci. U.S.A. 73:1255–1259, 1976.

SMITH, R. E., AND FARQUHAR, M. G. Lysosome function in the regulation of the secretory process in cells of the anterior pituitary gland. J. Cell Biol. 31:319–347, 1966.

Centrosome, Centrioles

DE HARVEN, E. The centriole and the mitotic spindle. In The Nucleus (Dalton, A. J., and Haguenau, F., editors), pp. 197–227. Academic Press, New York, 1968.

GALL, J. G. Centriole replication. A study of spermatogenesis in the snail *Viviparus*. J. Biophys. Biochem. Cytol. 10:163–193, 1961.

RENAUD, F. L., AND SWIFT, H. The development of basal bodies and flagella in *Allomyces arbusculus*. J. Cell Biol. 23:339–354, 1964.

SZOLLOSI, D. The structure and function of centrioles and their satellites in the jellyfish *Phialidium gregarium*. J. Cell Biol. 21:465–479, 1964.

WOLFE, J. Basal body fine structure and chemistry. Adv. Cell Mol. Biol. 2:151, 1972.

See also references at end of Chapter 2.

Mitochondria

ANDRE, J., AND MARINOZZI, V. Présence, dans les mitochondries, de particules ressemblant aux ribosomes. J. Microsc. 4:615–626, 1965.

ATTARDI, G., AND ATTARDI, B. Mitochondrial origin of membrane-associated heterogeneous RNA in HeLA cells. Proc. Nat. Acad. Sci. U.S.A., 61:261–268, 1968.

BENSLEY, R. R., AND HOERR, N. L. Studies on cell structure by the freezing-drying method. VI. The preparation and properties of mitochondria. Anat. Rec. 60:449–455, 1934.

BORST, P., AND KROON, A. M. Mitochondria DNA: physicochemical properties, replication, and genetic function. Int. Rev. Cytol. 26:107–190, 1969.

HACKENBROCK, C. R. States of activity and structure in mitochondrial membranes. Ann. N. Y. Acad. Sci. 195:492–505, 1972.

HACKENBROCK, C. R., HOCHLI, M., AND CHAU, R. M. Calorimetric and freeze-fracture analysis of lipid phase transitions and lateral translational motion of intramembrane particles in mitochondrial membranes. Bioch. Biophys. Acta 455:466–484, 1976.

HOCHLI, M., AND HACKENBROCK, C. R. Fluidity in mitochondrial membranes: thermotropic lateral translation motion of intramembrane particles. Proc. Natl. Acad. Sci. 73:1636–1640, 1976.

HOGEBOOM, G. H., SCHNEIDER, W. C., AND PALADE, G. E. Cytochemical studies of mammalian tissues. I. Isolation of intact mitochondria from rat liver; some biochemical properties of mitochondria and submicroscopic particulate material. J. Biol. Chem. 172:619–635, 1948.

LEHNINGER, A. L. The Mitochondrion; Molecular Basis of Structure and Function. W. A. Benjamin, Inc., New York, 1964.

MUNN, E. A. The Structure of Mitochondria. Academic Press, New York, 1974.

PALADE, G. An electron microscope study of the mitochondrial structure. J. Histochem. Cytochem. 1:188–211, 1953.

PARSONS, D. F. Recent advances in correlating structure and function in mitochondria. Int. Rev. Exp. Pathol. 4:1–54, 1965.

PEACHEY, L. D. Electron microscope observations on the accumulation of divalent cations in intramitochondrial granules. J. Cell Biol. 20:95–111, 1964.

ROODYN, D. B. The mitochondrion. In The Biological Basis of Medicine (Bittar, E. E., editor), vol. 1, pp. 123–177. Academic Press, New York, 1968.

SWIFT, H. Nucleic acids of mitochondria and chloroplasts. Amer. Natur. 99:201–227, 1965.

TANDLER, B., ERLANDSON, R. A., SMITH, A. L., AND WYNDER, E. L. Riboflavin and mouse hepatic cell structure and function. II. Division of mitochondria during recovery from simple deficiency. J. Cell Biol. 41:477–493, 1969.

TYLER, D. D. The mitochondrion. *In* Cell Biology in Medicine (E. Bittar, editor), pp. 107–149, John Wiley and Sons, New York, 1973.

Filaments

ALLISON, A. C., AND DAVIES, P. Interactions of membranes, microfilaments, and microtubules in endocytosis and exocytosis. *In* Advances in Cytopharmacology, vol. 2, Cytopharmacology of Secretion (Ceccarelli, B., Clementi, F., and Meldolesi, J., editors), Raven Press, New York, pp. 237–248, 1974.

BRODY, I. The ultrastructure of the tonofibrils in the keratinization process of normal human epidermis. J. Ultrastruct. Res. 4:264–297, 1960.

BUCKLEY, I. K., AND RAJU, T. R. Form and distribution of actin and myosin in non-muscle cells; a study using cultured chick embryo fibroblasts. J. Microsc. 107:129–151, 1976.

CLONEY, R. A. Cytoplasmic filaments and morphogenesis: effects of cytochalasin B on contractile epidermal cells. Zeitschr. Zellforsch. 132:167–192, 1972.

GOLDMAN, R. D., LAZARIDES, E., POLLACK, R., AND WEBER, K. The distribution of actin in non-muscle cells. Exp. Cell Res. 90:333–344, 1975.

ISENBERG, G., RATHKE, P. C., HULSMANN, N., FRANKE, W. W., AND WOHLFARTH-BOTTERMANN, K. E. Cytoplasmic actomyosin fibrils in tissue culture cells. Direct proof of contractility by visualization of ATP-induced contraction in fibrils isolated by laser microbeam dissection. Cell Tissue Res. 166:427–444, 1976.

ISHIKAWA, H. Arrowhead complexes in a variety of cell types. Excerpta Medica Congr. Ser. no. 333, pp. 37–50, 1973.

POLLARD, T. D. Functional implications of biochemical and structural properties of cytoplasmic contractile proteins. *In* Molecules and Cell Movement (Inoué, S., and Stephens, R. E., editors), Raven Press, New York, pp. 259–286, 1975.

SANGER, J. W. Intracellular localization of actin with fluorescently labeled heavy meromyosin. Cell Tissue Res. 161:431–444, 1975.

SCHROEDER, T. E. Cell constriction: contractile role of microfilaments in division and development. Am. Zoologist 13:949–960, 1973.

SPOONER, B. S. Microfilaments, cell shape changes, and morphogenesis of salivary epithelium. Am. Zoologist 13:1007–1022, 1973.

TILNEY, L. G. Role of actin in nonmuscle cell motility. *In* Molecules and Cell Movement (Inoué, S., and Stephens, R. E., editors), Raven Press, New York, pp. 339–388, 1975.

WESSELLS, N. K., SPOONER, B. S., ASH, J. F., BRADLEY, M. O., LUDUENA, M. A., TAYLOR, E. L., WRENN, J. T., AND YAMADA, K. M. Microfilaments in cellular and developmental processes. Science 171:135–143, 1971.

Microtubules

ADELMAN, M. R., BORISY, G. G., SHELANSKI, N. H., WEISENBERG, R. C., AND TAYLOR, E. W. Cytoplasmic filaments and tubules. Fed. Proc. 27:1186–1193, 1968.

ALLEN, R. D. Evidence for firm linkages between microtubules and membrane-bounded vesicles. J. Cell Biol. 64:493–496, 1975.

BEHNKE, O. Studies on isolated microtubules. Evidence for a clear space component. Cytobiology 11:366–381, 1975.

BEHNKE, O., AND FORER, A. Evidence for four classes of microtubules in individual cells. J. Cell Sci. 2:169–192, 1967.

BORISY, G. G., AND OLMSTED, J. B. Nucleated assembly of microtubules in porcine brain extracts. Science 177:1196–1197, 1972.

BENTLER, W. L. GRANETT, S., AND ROSENBAUM, J. L. Ultrastructural localization of the high molecular weight proteins associated with in vitro-assembled brain microtubules. J. Cell Biol. 65:237–241, 1975.

FAWCETT, D. Cilia and flagella. *In* The Cell; Biochemistry, Physiology, Morphology (Brachet, J., and Mirsky, A. E., editors), vol. 2, pp. 217–297. Academic Press, New York, 1961.

INOUE, S., FUSELER, J., SALMON, E. D., AND ELLIS, G. W. Functional organization of mitotic microtubules. Physical chemistry of the *in vivo* equilibrium system. Biophys. J. 15:725, 1975.

PORTER, K. R. Cytoplasmic microtubules and their functions. *In* Principles of Biomolecular Organization (Wolstenholme, G. E. W., and O'Connor, M., editors), Ciba Foundation Symposium, pp. 308–345. Little, Brown and Company, Boston, 1966.

SHELANSKI, M. L. Methods for the neurochemical study of microtubules. Res. Methods Neurochem. 2:281–300, 1974.

SLAUTTERBACK, D. B. Cytoplasmic microtubules. I. Hydra. J. Cell Biol. 18:367–388, 1963.

SOIFER, D. (editor). The biology of cytoplasmic microtubules. Ann. N. Y. Acad. Sci., Vol. 253, 1975.

STEPHENS, R., AND EDDS, K. Microtubules: Structure, chemistry and function. Physiol. Rev. 56:709, 1976.

TILNEY, L. G. IV. The effect of colchicine on the formation and maintenance of the axopodia and the redevelopment of pattern in *Actinosphaerium nucleophilum* (Barrett). J. Cell Sci. 3:549–562, 1968.

Cell Membrane

BENNETT, H. S. Morphological aspects of extracellular polysaccharides. J. Histochem. Cytochem. 11:14–23, 1963.

BRETSCHER, M. S., AND RAFF, M. C. Mammalian plasma membranes. Nature 258:43–49, 1975.

DALTON, A. J., AND HAGUENAU, F. (editors). The Membranes. Academic Press, New York, 1968.

DANIELLI, J. F., AND DAVSON, H. A contribution to the theory of permeability of thin films. J. Cell. Comp. Physiol. 5:495–508, 1934–1935.

EDELMAN, G. M. Surface modulation in cell recognition and cell growth. Science 192:218–226, 1976.

GILULA, N. B. Gap junctions and cell communication. *In* International Cell Biology (Brinkley, B. R., and Porter, K. R., editors) pp. 61–69. Rockefeller University Press, New York, 1977.

KORN, E. D. Structure and function of the plasma membrane; a biochemical perspective. *In* Biological Interfaces: Flows and Exchanges. Proceedings of a symposium sponsored by the New York Heart Association, pp. 257–274. Little, Brown and Company, Boston, 1968.

LOEWENSTEIN, W. R. On the genesis of cellular communication. Dev. Biol. 15:503–520, 1967.

LOEWENSTEIN, W. R. Permeability of the junctional membrane channel. *In* International Cell Biology (Brinkley, B. R., and Porter, K. R., editors) pp. 70–82. Rockefeller University Press, New York, 1977.

PINTO DE SILVA, P., AND BRANTON, D. Membrane splitting in freeze-etching. Covalently bound ferritin as a membrane marker. J. Cell Biol. 45:598–605, 1970.

REVEL, J.-P., AND ITO, S. The surface components of cells. *In* The Specificity of Cell Surfaces (Davis, B. D., and Warren, L., editors), pp. 211–234. Prentice-Hall, Inc., New York, 1967.

ROBERTSON, J. D. Unit membranes: a review with recent new studies of experimental alterations and a new subunit structure in synaptic membrane. *In* Cellular Membranes in Development (Locke, M., editor), pp. 1–81. Academic Press, New York, 1964.

ROTHMAN, J. E., AND LENARD, J. Membrane asymmetry. Science 195:743–753, 1977.

SINGER, S. J., AND NICOLSON, G. L. The fluid mosaic model of the structure of cell membranes. Science 175:720–731, 1972.

SJOSTRAND, F. S. A comparison of plasma membrane, cytomembranes, and mitochondrial membrane elements with respect to ultrastructural features. J. Ultrastruct. Res. 9:561–580, 1963.

STEIN, W. D. The Movement of Molecules across Cell Membranes. Academic Press, New York, 1967.

STOECKENIUS, W., AND ENGELMAN, D. M. Current models for the structure of biological membrane. J. Cell Biol. 42:613–646, 1969.

Inclusions

BJÖRKERUD, S. The isolation of lipofuscin granules from bovine cardiac muscle, with observations on the properties of the isolated granules on the light and electron microscopic levels. J. Ultrastruct. Res. Suppl. 5:1–49, 1963.

DELLA PORTA, G., AND MÜHLBOCK, O. (editors). Structure and Control of the Melanocyte. Springer-Verlag, New York, 1966.

DROCHMANS, P. Melanin granules: their fine structure, formation, and degradation in normal and pathological tissues. Int. Rev. Exp. Pathol. 2:357–422, 1963.

REVEL, J.-P. Electron microscopy of glycogen. J. Histochem. Cytochem. 12:104–114, 1964.

CHAPTER 2

Studies of Living Cells, Cell Culture, Cell Differentiation, Cell Division

Fixed and stained preparations have the advantage of being more or less permanent and available for repeated microscopic examination. Unfortunately, fixatives, dehydrating agents, and stains may significantly alter living tissues, and there is always a question of how much artifact the preparative procedures have introduced. It is therefore advantageous to study living cells and tissues whenever possible. In addition, there is the distinct advantage that living cells are observed in action, and functional changes can be observed directly. Studies of living cells also offer the opportunity to control directly the immediate environment of the cell during experimentation.

The living cell is delicate, however, and its study requires great care. The first extensive studies on living tissues were carried out on free-living unicellular organisms and on the eggs and early embryos of lower forms of both plants and animals. Whereas much was learned about the physical properties of the living cell, the methods used could not be applied directly to cells from higher animals, particularly man.

The first human cells studied in detail in the living conditions were blood cells. They were easy to obtain and could be viewed under the highest powers of the microscope while still surrounded by their natural environment, the plasma. Because of the fluid nature of the blood, a thin film could be made between a cover glass and slide. If the coverslip edges were sealed to

prevent evaporation and the stage of the microscope was heated to body temperature, the conditions inside the body were approximated. With this preparation, the various types of white blood cells were recognized and their ameboid and phagocytic activity was observed. This method is still one of the best for the study of blood cells, as well as for an introduction to active living human cells.

This simple procedure cannot be used for the more adherent and interdependent living cells from organized tissues. Attempts have been made to study solid tissues by teasing the tissue apart with fine instruments until it is spread thinly enough to be viewed with the light microscope. Subcutaneous connective tissue can be studied quite effectively in this way, as can muscle and nerve fibers. These preparations are short lived, however, and other methods have been evolved for maintaining living cells for extended periods for repeated direct microscopic examinations.

Cell, Tissue, and Organ Culture

New biological methods often arise out of the need to solve a particular question, and the most dramatic early tissue culture experimentation was devised to solve a problem of nerve fiber growth. Early in this century, histologists were debating whether nerve fibers grew out from the nerve cell body or formed from the fusion of longitudinally arrayed elements within the peripheral nerve. The resolving power of the microscopes available at that time did not allow a clear resolution of this controversy. Harrison attacked the problem directly by placing a part of the developing nervous system of a frog into a clot of sterile lymph and watching nerve fiber formation under the microscope. His experiments provided a clear demonstration that nerve fiber elongation occurs by direct extension and growth of the nerve cell (Fig. 2-1). Soon thereafter many of the tissues of the body found themselves in oddly shaped glass containers surrounded by complex feeding solutions and clots of every sort. Tissue culture was to become, along with the electron microscope, one of the most powerful tools of the cytologist.

Tissue culture (or cultivation in vitro, which literally means "in glass"), is now generally divided into three categories. (1) *Cell culture* refers to growth of continuously dividing cells, which are transferred from vessel to vessel as their numbers continuously increase. (2) *Tissue culture* entails explantation of an immature tissue fragment into culture. The cultured fragment, called the *explant*, generally undergoes some growth and reorganization. Cells growing out from the explant are termed the *outgrowth* (often of the connective tissue variety), whereas other explant cells remain compact and are hard to visualize. To circumvent this difficulty, the tissue may be dissociated (as discussed below) before culture. (3) *Organ culture* generally involves explantation and maintenance of mature tissues or organ fragments. This technique is particularly useful for study of the direct effects of drugs or hormones on various tissues of the body.

Successful in vitro studies require that the tissue be obtained in a sterile state (or that it be treated with antibiotics to render it sterile), for the conditions favoring cell growth are similar to those for bacterial multiplication. At all times the tissues must be handled in a fluid environment with salt concentrations and a pH resembling that of the body fluids. Such salt solutions are called balanced salt solutions (BSS). The tissue may be dissociated into individual cells, often by mild treatment with a digestive enzyme, such as trypsin, which loosens the adhesions between cells, or it may be put out as small fragments. After being washed in BSS, the cells are provided with a nutrient *medium* and maintained either in suspension culture, where the cells are kept floating in the medium by constant

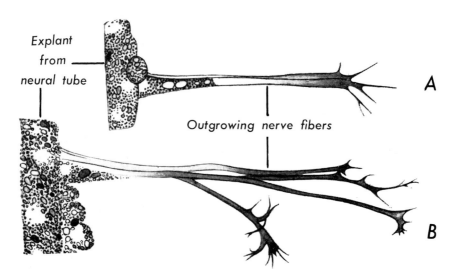

Fig. 2-1. Outgrowth of nerve fibers from pieces of embryonic frog neural tube (which contains the nerve cell bodies) grown in tissue culture. *A*, after 25 hr; *B*, after 34 hr. The expanded tips of the elongating nerve fibers, called growth cones, are regions of vigorous motility. (Redrawn from v. Möllendorff, editor, Handb. mikr. Anat. Menschen., Springer-Verlag, Vienna, after Harrison.)

agitation, or on a surface to which the cells attach. The surface provided for cell growth may be either glass or plastic, sometimes covered with a thin layer of collagen. Sometimes it is advantageous to attach the tissue to this surface (and provide a matrix for growth) by clotting blood plasma around it.

The medium may be completely *defined*, i.e., a mixture of known composition containing vitamins, amino acids, and salts, or *natural*, i.e., a mixture containing one of the complex products of the body, such as blood serum. Certain continuously propagated cell lines can be maintained and continue to grow on completely defined media. The content of one of the simplest of these is given in Table 2-1. For the propagation of certain cells, this medium is often supplemented with 10% serum.

To obtain the fullest possible expression of the organization and functions of certain tissues in culture, it is sometimes necessary to add additional organic ingredients to the medium. The most generally employed substance is embryo extract. In its preparation, embryos are crushed or chopped in an equal quantity of BSS. The solid embryo debris is separated by centrifugation, and a supernatant fluid containing a multitude of undefined cellular constituents is obtained.

Certain specific proteins, called growth factors, have also been discovered; these enhance the growth of specific tissues in culture. A most dramatic example is the stimulation of the growth of certain types of nerve fibers by a factor present in the salivary gland of the mouse. This protein is termed *nerve growth factor* and this puzzling circumstance—a protein present in a digestive gland exerting a very specific effect on nervous tissue—raises many intriguing questions concerning factors which may control appropriate rates of growth in the various tissues of the body. Other instances of specific growth factors are known, but it is not yet clear how frequently they are used in the body as control mechanisms governing normal growth.

Morphology of the Living Cell

The greatest detail in living animal cells can generally be observed in thinly spread

TABLE 2-1

Eagle's minimum essential medium (from H. Eagle: Science, vol. 130:432, 1959)

Components	mg/l
Amino acids	
L-Arginine HCl	126.4
L-Cystine	24.0
L-Glutamine	292.0
L-Histidine HCl · H_2O	41.9
L-Isoleucine	52.5
L-Leucine	52.4
L-Lysine HCl	73.1
L-Methionine	14.9
L-Phenylalanine	33.0
L-Threonine	47.6
L-Tryptophan	10.2
L-Tyrosine	36.2
L-Valine	46.8
Vitamins	
D-Ca-pantothenate	1.0
Choline chloride	1.0
Folic acid	1.0
i-Inositol	2.0
Nicotinamide	1.0
Pyridoxal HCl	1.0
Riboflavin	0.1
Thiamine HCl	1.0
Inorganic salts and other components	
$CaCl_2 · 2H_2O$	265.0
KCl	400.0
$MgSO_4 · 7H_2O$	200.0
NaCl	6800.0
$NaHCO_3$	2200.0
$NaH_2PO_4 · H_2O$	140.0
Dextrose	1000.0
Phenol red	10.0

culture preparations. It is necessary to use a phase contrast or differential interference (Nomarski) optical system to enhance contrast because living cells, being composed chiefly of water, are quite transparent. Even under the best light microscopic conditions, however, only a fraction of the great internal complexity of the cell known from electron microscopic work can be seen (compare Figs. 1-10 and 2-2). The nucleus and its contained nucleoli are clearly visible. It is clear that the cell contents are contained within a very flexible and often very active covering. The cytoplasm is seen to contain varying numbers of dense granules and somewhat less dense, threadlike elements. The dense, particulate granules are elements of the lysosomal system or lipid

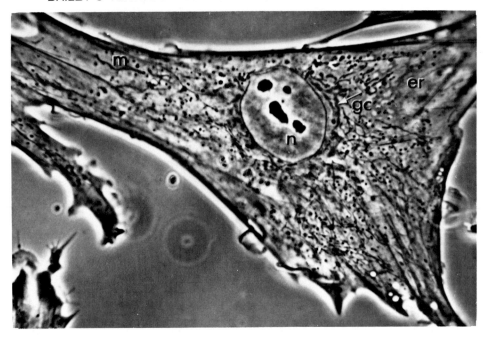

Fig. 2-2. Phase contrast photomicrograph of a living rat embryo cell grown in culture. Many cytoplasmic organelles are visible. The Golgi complex (*gc*) may be seen near the nucleus (*n*). Endoplasmic reticulum (*er*) is visible as a shadowy, branching structure. The long sinuous threads are mitochondria (*m*). ×1450. (From I. K. Buckley and K. R. Porter: Protoplasma 64:349, 1967.)

droplets; the less dense linear organelles are mitochondria. Occasionally the Golgi apparatus and endoplasmic reticulum can be visualized (Fig. 2-2).

When the cell contains substantial arrays of molecules in a patterned orientation, these alter the path of transmitted light, and the manner in which the light is altered gives some clue regarding the basic molecular organization. Thus, with polarizing microscopy, areas containing linear arrays of filamentous material, such as the actin and myosin of muscle cells, can be detected. Similarly, a mass of microtubules such as is found in the mitotic spindle can be dramatically brought into view (see Fig. 2-17).

Experimental Manipulation of Living Cells

Simple observations of living cells have been usefully supplemented with a host of techniques which can be applied more or less directly to living cells.

Vital and Supravital Staining

In *vital staining*, dyes are injected into the living animal so that the activity of certain cells can be demonstrated by their selective absorption of the coloring matter. An outstanding example has been the demonstration of the distribution of highly phagocytic cells throughout the body. When trypan blue is injected into an experimental animal, accumulations of the dye are found in vacuoles in the macrophages of the loose connective tissue, and in the phagocytic cells of lymphatic organs, bone marrow, and liver. This method shows the similarity in function of widely dispersed and morphologically different cells on the basis of their ability to phagocytize foreign particles.

Supravital staining consists of adding dyes to the medium of cells already removed from the organism. When trypan blue is placed on a tissue culture, the macrophages take it up in abundance. Small phagocytic cells have been marked in this way, and their subsequent development into epithelioid and giant cells has been followed. The use of supravital dyes such as neutral red to mark the lysosomal systems of cells is discussed in chapter 1, as is the staining of mitochondria by Janus green.

The selective staining of organelles with a colored dye combined with the high intensities of light available from laser sources provides the opportunity for a new form of *cellular microsurgery.* Laser light, like other visible light, is not much absorbed by living tissue, unless the cells contain pigment granules. If the mitochondria are colored green, however, and laser light of a wavelength absorbed by the green dye is directed at the cell, the light absorption leads to local heating, as well as other effects, and thus to more or less selective destruction of the mitochondria of the cell. If the cone of laser light is restricted to a part of the cell, only some of the mitochondria are damaged. Similarly, chromosomes which have been supravitally stained with acridine orange can be irradiated during mitosis with a laser microbeam. Using this technique, lesions less than 1 μm can be placed on desired sites of individual chromosomes (Fig. 2-3).

Micromanipulation and Microdissection

Several new techniques have been made possible by the development of an instrument, called a micromanipulator, which moves fine glass needles or pipettes with such precision that single cells can be manipulated or dissected. Experiments with the microneedles have made our concept of the physical nature of cells much clearer. Microdissection provided some of the first direct evidence of the presence of a cell

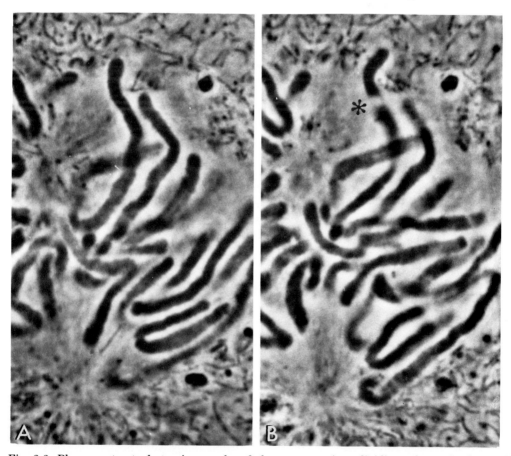

Fig. 2-3. Phase contrast photomicrographs of chromosomes in a dividing salamander lung cell before (*A*) and after (*B*) irradiation with laser microbeam. The cells had been previously treated with a nucleic acid stain, acridine orange, to enhance absorption of the microbeam by the chromosomal material. After irradiation, a discrete lesion is seen (at *asterisk*) in one of the chromosomes. ×2500. (From M. W. Berns et al.: Exp. Cell Res. 56:292, 1969.)

membrane enclosing the cell contents. More recently, micromanipulators have been employed to move or fragment fixed cells while they were being examined under the scanning electron microscope. Thus the value of the technique is being extended to electron microscope levels of resolution.

With these techniques cytoplasm has been shown to be a viscous fluid, its viscosity varying in different cells. The granules, vacuoles, and mitochondria can be moved about within the cell, showing that there is little fixed structure except in highly specialized cells. The nucleus is a bag of fluid which can be indented by the pressure of the needle and which may be pushed about from one part of the cell to another or even, in some special cases, transplanted from one cell to another.

Microelectrodes, which are extremely fine pipettes (tips less than 1 μm in diameter) filled with concentrated salt solutions, may also be mounted in micromanipulators. If these are inserted into cells with great care, the cell membrane will seal around them and allow measurements of the differences in electrical potential between the inside of the cell and the external environment (Fig. 2-4). This technique has been especially useful to the physiologist in the study of nerve and muscle, which employ changes in membrane potentials as a method of signaling (see chapter 10). A related method has been used to detect ionic fluxes across specialized junctions linking adjacent epithelial cells (see chapter 4).

If a microelectrode is filled with a dye carrying a charge and if current of the appropriate polarity is passed into the cell via the electrode, then dye will pass into the cell with the current flow. There are charged dyes which can be made to fluoresce in the light microscope. When injected into cells, these diffuse widely through the cytoplasm. This technique, which may be termed microdye injection, is useful in delineating the contour of individual cells in complexly organized tissues such as the nervous system (Fig. 2-5). Radioactive materials can be similarly employed, but the cell configuration must then be reconstructed from radioautographs of serial sections through the cell.

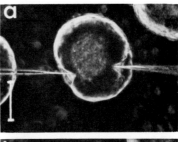
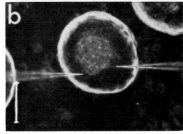

Fig. 2-4. Photomicrographs of frog oocytes being impaled with two extremely fine microelectrodes. The microelectrodes can first be seen to indent the plasma membrane (*a*) and then to penetrate the cell cytoplasm (*b*). This manipulation allows the measurement of intracellular electrical activity. The *bar* indicates 100 μm. (From Y. Kanno and W. R. Loewenstein: Exp. Cell Res. 31:149, 1963.)

Cinematography

Another technique which has been used with tissue culture cells is cinematography, motion pictures taken through the objectives of a microscope. It is useful not only to obtain permanent records of cell activity but also as an experimental aid in the analysis of movement too slow or too fast to be appreciated by the unaided eye. When the exposures are taken at intervals of several seconds and projected on the screen at the usual speed, the photographed processes are speeded up more than 100 times. In such a film, the movements of the macrophages, which are scarcely appreciated by direct observation, become visible. In the division of the cell by mitosis, the shifting of the nucleus during the prophase, the rounded blebs or pseudopodia which are sent out and withdrawn from every part of the surface of the cell, and the violent agitation just before the chromosomes separate are all aspects which cannot be appreciated by any other means. Within the resting cell, the shifting of the granules and

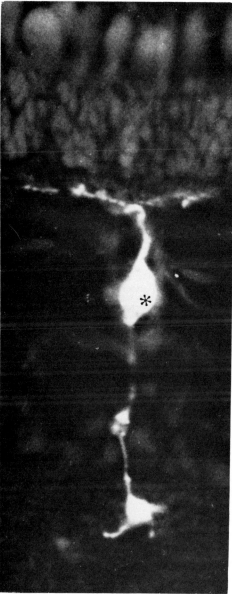

Fig. 2-5. The cell body (*asterisk*) and cytoplasmic extensions of a neuron in the goldfish retina are here demonstrated after the injection of a fluorescent dye (Procion yellow) directly into the cell soma. After injection the tissue is fixed, embedded, and sectioned for viewing in the fluorescence microscope. This technique is useful both in identifying cells penetrated by microelectrodes (which inject the dye as well as record electrical activity) and in delineating the extensions of cells in complex tissues. At the *top* of the figure are rod and cone cells, which fluoresce faintly without dye injection (autofluorescence). Scale: 50 μm = 2 inches. (From A. Kaneko: J. Physiol. 207:623, 1970.)

mitochondria is beautifully demonstrated by these speeded films.

In order to reverse the process and slow activities too quick for the eye, the exposures are taken three or four times as rapidly as they are to be shown on the screen. The movement of cilia has been studied by this method. The contraction of cardiac muscle differentiated in tissue cultures, slowed to one-fourth the actual speed, offers an opportunity to study the mechanism of muscle contraction.

Activities of Living Cells

Application of the techniques discussed above, as well as observations on single cell organisms, has led to the recognition of a variety of types of cellular movements. In the mature mammal, the flagellum of the sperm tail and the cilia of epithelia move, muscle cells contract, and chromosomes move within dividing cells. In addition, certain cells such as leukocytes have the capability of locomotion by other means. All cell types exhibit various intracellular movements.

Intracellular Movements

When one looks inside the living cell, both nuclear motion and movement within the cytoplasm are observed. The simplest form of movement, that is exhibited to some extent by all cells which have been studied adequately, is a shifting about of the elements within the cytoplasm. This is often very slight and so slow that it is frequently overlooked unless cinematography is employed. There are local currents within the cytoplasm which cause the granules and mitochondria to move slowly for varying distances. In addition, one observes rapid linear movements of cytoplasmic particles; this distinctive activity is termed *saltatory movement*. Saltatory activity must not be confused with the more random motions of Brownian movement, which is dampened in healthy cells but which becomes marked in cells after death. Cytoplasmic movement may sometimes involve the transport of materials from the cell body into cell processes and is especially important in cells with long processes such as neurons.

In certain cells, a surprising rotation of the entire nucleus within the relatively immobile cytoplasm has been observed. These periodic rolling motions can be seen when several nucleoli are present to mark the disposition of the nucleus, thus allowing accurate detection of its movements.

Cellular Locomotion

Cellular locomotion means the movement of the whole cell from one place to another. Studies utilizing the tissue culture and cinematography techniques discussed above have revealed at least two quite different mechanisms by which cells move. Amebae locomote by pseudopodial propagated movement. They dispatch long processes in the appropriate direction and then appear to flow into these processes. Among animal cells, leukocytes and histiocytes (i.e., macrophages) appear to move in a similar fashion, i.e., by *ameboid movement*.

Other types of animal cells (such as the mesodermally derived fibroblast and the endodermally or ectodermally derived epithelial cells) exhibit quite different movement patterns. These cells flatten and adhere to surfaces on which they are placed and then glide along this surface without true pseudopodium formation (or gross changes in their overall shape). The membrane along the flattened edges of these cells ruffles, and this ruffling is most active at the edge of the cell marking the direction of movement. The adhesiveness and other properties of the cell surface and of the substrate are important in determining the extent and speed of this locomotion, for movement can be influenced by the shape and properties of the terrain. Changes in the adhesive properties of the cell membrane are especially important during developmental stages of the organism because these properties will influence the migration of cells.

The agencies responsible for the actual movements at the cell border are not clearly understood. These movements may be based on mechanisms similar to those operative in muscle cells, for the active membranes are sometimes underlain by fine filamentous material. It is now known that actin- and myosin-like proteins occur widely in many cell types, suggesting that many cells contain a system that is in some ways similar to the muscle contraction system. The direction of movement of a cell can be influenced by a concentration gradient of some substance in the surrounding solution. The cell is then said to be influenced by *chemotaxis*. Some white blood cells are chemotactically responsive to certain bacteria and move toward any such organism in their vicinity.

An interesting and important aspect of the control of cell movement is the phenomenon of *contact inhibition*. When a moving fibroblast contacts an adjacent fibroblast, its ruffling membrane becomes paralyzed and movement in this region of the cell stops. The cell then reverses its direction of movement, extending an exploring ruffling membrane from its opposite side. When the population of fibroblasts is sufficiently dense, movement of any cell in any direction brings immediate contact. Ruffling then ceases and both movement and proliferation of the cells are suspended. This is called contact inhibition. The cytological significance of contact inhibition is under active investigation, for it has been observed that some cancer (sarcoma) cells, which, like fibroblasts, are derived from mesodermal tissue, are not contact-inhibited when they approach normal inhibited fibroblasts in culture. It is thus possible that the invasiveness of some types of cancer is related to a failure in this type of inhibition.

In some cases where two cells come together and exhibit contact inhibition, the involved membranes are known to form low resistance junctions in regions where cell membranes come into especially close apposition (see Chapter 4). This type of cell-to-cell junction is known to allow small molecules or ions to pass from one cell to another without diffusing into the extracellular spaces. These junctions therefore provide special regions for cell-to-cell communication. This type of junction is known to form, sometimes transiently, during various phases of development and has been postulated to play an important integrating role, determining developmental patterns.

Phagocytosis and Pinocytosis

The term phagocytosis is generally used

to describe the ingestion of solid material by the cell, whereas pinocytosis refers to the ingestion of fluids. Both mechanisms involve a reaction (or adsorption) of the material with the surface coat of the cell membrane, with subsequent invagination of the surface membrane and the sequestration of the ingested material within a vacuole in the cell cytoplasm.

The process of *phagocytosis* (from the Greek *phagein*, to eat) is used by certain single cell organisms for feeding but in higher organisms it is more commonly used as a defense mechanism for the ingestion of particles foreign to the organism. Actively ameboid cells usually have an enhanced capability for phagocytosis. In the case of the more rapidly moving cells, such as neutrophilic leukocytes, engulfment is facilitated by the passage of the cell over the particle, such as a bacterium, to be ingested. The bacteria remain motionless until the leukocyte passes partway over them. Suddenly they begin to move in unison within the interior of the cell and soon appear in small vacuoles which are carried about with the granules in the currents of the cytoplasm. Cells with less rapid locomotion, such as the histiocytes, come in contact with the material to be engulfed by sending out pseudopodia, which adhere to the debris and surround it, either by drawing it toward the cell or by expanding the pseudopodium.

The ingestion of droplets of fluid by cells in tissue culture was described by Lewis in 1931 as *pinocytosis* (from the Greek *pinein*, to drink). A similar process is known to occur in vivo, and the term pinocytosis is now generally used to describe the ingestion of fluids and their contained solutes, whether observed with the light (Fig. 2-6) or the electron microscope. Recent electron microscopic observations indicate that the ingestion of tiny vacuoles below the resolution of the light microscope is a common phenomenon in many cell types. The presence of protein outside the cell generally acts as a stimulus to pinocytosis. Proteins thus ingested are broken down by the lysosomal system of the cell (as discussed in chapter 1). Certain cell types apparently use the process of pinocytosis for the transcellular transport of large molecules (see "Capillaries," chapter 12).

Observation of Living Cells in Situ

The descriptions up to this point have dealt with cells surviving after their removal from the body, but cells have been observed by various methods within the living organism. The earliest attempts were made on the vascular system, on the blood cells circulating in the tadpole's tail fin, in the tongue, foot web, and mesentery of the adult frog, and in the mesentery and omentum of mammals. The transparency of the tail fin of the tadpole is particularly advantageous for the observation of many kinds of cells. Tadpole tail fin has been used to study the outgrowth of nerve fibers and the formation of special sensory nerve endings. The growth of blood vessels and lymphatics and the activity of the endothelium, connective tissue cells, and phagocytes have also been extensively studied.

Mammalian material has been made available for similar observation by the perfection of a technique for inserting a transparent window in the rabbit's ear. Through it, the growth of new blood vessels and lymphatics, the activity of capillaries, the opening and closing of vascular anastomoses, the behavior of the phagocytic cells of connective tissue, and the growth and resorption of other tissues have been studied in detail.

Cytological Analysis in Cell Culture

Cell culture techniques permit certain types of cytological analysis that cannot be undertaken in whole tissues. Several of these are discussed below.

Determination of Karyotype

The chromosomal content of cells is best visualized when the chromosomes are fixed and stained while tightly coiled during mitosis. This is accomplished by placing cells with the capability of multiplication in a medium fostering cell division. An agent (colchicine) which prevents completion of the mitotic process is added, and the cells arrested during mitosis accumulate in the culture. These cells are made to swell by the addition of hypotonic medium and are then flattened with pressure. After staining, the chromosomes may be counted and clas-

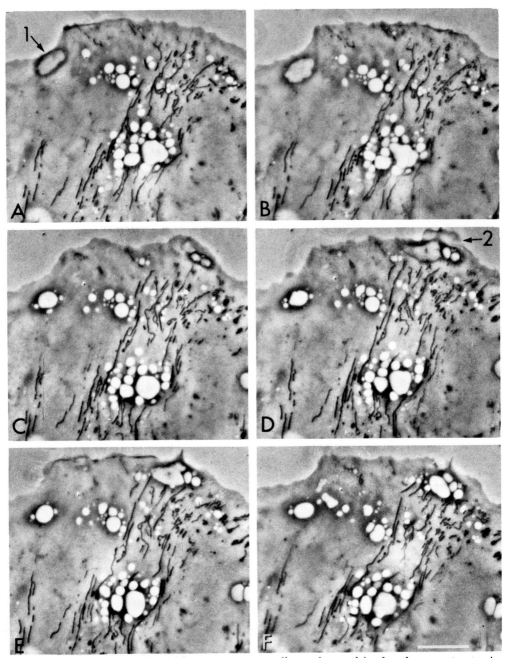

Fig. 2-6. Pinocytosis in cultured human sarcoma cells as observed in the phase contrast microscope. The figures shown here are but a few of those obtained every 2 sec for a time lapse film and were obtained over a 12-min period. Pinocytosis occurs in regions of the cell body which are undulating vigorously. Recent intake of fluid appears as an irregular lake just inside the cell (as at *1A* and *2D*). Secondarily the collected fluid assumes the appearance of more refractile spheroidal droplets which start to migrate interiorly. The *bar* indicates 5 μm. (From A. Gropp: *In* Cinemicrography in Cell Biology, edited by G. G. Rose, p. 279. Academic Press, New York, 1963.)

sified by size and shape. This analysis allows the determination of the *karyotype* of an organism. A normal karyotype for human cells is 46 chromosomes: 22 pairs not

associated with sex determination (autosomes) and 2 chromosomes that determine sex (Fig. 2-7).

A variety of human congenital abnor-

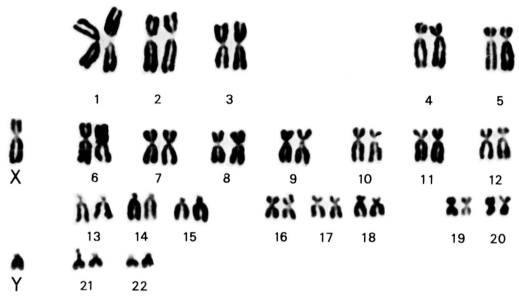

Fig 2-7. A normal karyotype prepared from a human leukocyte dividing in culture. The chromosomes were fixed in acetic alcohol and stained with acetic orcein. When this preparation is viewed in the light microscope the metaphase chromosomes appear in a cluster on the slide. A photograph of these chromosomes is obtained and is then cut up so that the chromosomes may be grouped as shown here. ×1500. (Courtesy of Dr. Orlando Miller.)

malities relate to abnormal karyotypes. For example, the basis for certain types of abnormal sexual development has been traced to abnormalities in sex chromosome number. Thus, if the normal XX sex chromosome pattern of female human cells is altered so that only one X chromosome is present (a condition called Turner's syndrome), or if the normal XY composition of the male is supplemented with a second X to give a XXY complement (a condition called Klinefelter's syndrome), then sexual and other traits of the individual are abnormal. Mongolism is also a condition of abnormal chromosome content; in these cases there is an extra autosome, giving a total chromosome number of 47 instead of the normal 46.

Repeated analysis of cultured cell lines has led to the observation that cells carried for long periods in culture often develop abnormal karyotypes. When cells from normal tissues are set out in culture, they have the number of chromosomes characteristic of the species. For human cells this is 46, the *diploid* number of chromosomes. Cells are termed *euploid* if they contain this number of chromosomes or an exact multiple of it; cells with multiples of the diploid

number also are referred to as *polyploid.* After long periods in culture, many cell types undergo a transformation and the number of chromosomes per cell changes. The cell line is then said to be *aneuploid* (or *heteroploid*) if the cells contain an odd number of chromosomes. The extensively studied HeLa cell lines, derived from a human cervical cancer in 1952 and whose progeny is still carried in many laboratories, may have from 50 to 350 chromosomes per cell.

Various interpretations have been offered for changes in chromosome number in cultured cells. Some investigators believe that it indicates damage to the replicating mechanism resulting from less than optimal culture conditions. Others have suggested that the change from euploid to aneuploid is the mechanism of adaptation of cells to permanent growth in culture, and that if aneuploidy does not occur, cells will not adapt to permanent culture as cell lines. Hayflick has suggested that if cells remain euploid they have a limited life span in culture and undergo only a limited (preset) number of divisions before losing their capacity to survive in culture. This limited life span of euploid cultured cells has been related to an aging process, and the transformation to the aneuploid state has been related to the origin of malignancy, i.e., cancer. When reintroduced into animal hosts, many transformed cells grow as tumors. It should be noted, however, that not all malignant cells are aneuploid.

Cloning

As the above discussion indicates, cells established in culture may be a diverse group, and it is often desirable to select a single cell and to establish it and its progeny as the only cells present in a cell culture line. This process is called *cloning* (from the Greek for twig). It involves isolation of a single cell, either by dissociating and greatly diluting cell populations before culture or by isolating a single cell in a micropipette. These cells are placed in the most propitious culture environment, and as they multiply, their progeny provide, at least for a time, maximally homogeneous cell populations.

Cellular Aggregation

Tissue culture techniques have provided an opportunity to study the reaggregation of cells which have been separated and suspended in a fluid medium. As used by Moscona, this technique allows the dissociation of embryonic organs into individual cells by loosening intercellular adhesions, by treatment with a proteolytic enzyme such as trypsin and/or a reduction in Ca^{2+} concentration of the medium. After dissociation, cells tend to reaggregate, often in structures resembling the tissue of origin. Cells of different organs, and from different species, for example, from kidneys and cartilage from mouse and chick, can be mixed together after dissociation. Under these conditions, kidney cells from both species aggregate in one mass and, similarly, all cartilage cells in another. Cells of a certain organ thus have the ability to recognize cells of similar type and maintain preferential association with them. These observations apply primarily to embryonic organs, for as organs mature the constituent cells lose their capability for cellular reaggregation.

A tissue containing cells from two different sources, for example a mixture of chick and mouse cartilage cells, is called *chimeric*. It is also possible to produce chimeric animals, i.e., animals containing cells from more than one source. Mintz has been able to dissociate the cells of two different mouse embryos at the blastula stage and allow them to reaggregate as one blastula. This is then reintroduced into a pseudo-pregnant mother, and subsequently develops and is delivered normally. If dissociated blastula cells from a strain of black and a strain of white mice are mixed together to form a single blastula, certain of the newborn mice develop alternating black and white areas of hair pigmentation. It is believed that each stripe is derived from a single clone of pigment cells, some clones arising from the cells of the black strain and others from the white.

Heterokaryons

In addition to the possibility of deriving tissues composed of cells from a variety of sources, tissue culture provides the opportunity of producing cells with mixtures of genetic material. Human cells can be cultured together with cells of, for example, chick tissues. If certain types of inactivated virus particles are added to these cultures, the two types of cells fuse together to become one cell with two or more nuclei. It is thus possible to observe the reactions of an inactive nucleus when it is introduced into an active cell (Fig. 2-8). As heterokaryons divide, the nuclei sometimes enter mitosis together and are reconstituted as a single larger nucleus. Cells thus formed contain, within a single nucleus, chromosomes derived from different species. With subsequent divisions certain of these chromosomes may be lost. In man-mouse hybrids, for example, the human chromosomes are gradually reduced in number until in some cases only one remains. This circumstance has been used to determine the localization of certain genes to a specific human chromosome.

Other Uses of Cell and Tissue Culture

Tissue culture has been essential in research on viruses. Functioning cells are necessary for virus growth, and tissue cultures

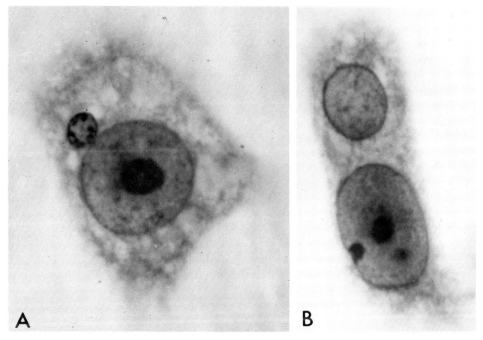

Fig. 2-8. Reactivation of a mature hen red blood cell (RBC) nucleus after introduction into an active HeLa cell. The heterokaryon in *A* contains the large, cultured HeLa cell nucleus (about 10 μm in diameter) and a typical small, dotted RBC nucleus. *B* shows the subsequent enlargements and disappearance of heterochromatin in the hen RBC nucleus. By applying radioautographic techniques to this type of preparation, it is possible to demonstrate that DNA and RNA synthesis (which normally does not occur in the mature RBC nucleus) is resumed in RBC nuclei residing in the cytoplasm of a continuously synthesizing HeLa cell. (From H. Harris: J. Cell Sci. 2:23, 1967.)

offer an opportunity to study virus growth outside the animal host and to prepare large quantities of virus for vaccines. They are also necessary to assay the types and amounts of virus present in any biological preparation.

Observations on Organized Tissue in Culture

With the increasing refinement of tissue culture techniques, it has become possible to establish many of the tissues of the body in culture, often with a high degree of organization and function. Three examples are given here to illustrate the degree of organization that can be achieved by cells maintained in vitro.

Skeletal muscle may be established in culture by taking cells from embryonic muscle before the muscle fibers are fully differentiated. A single cell is selected and, if culture conditions are very carefully controlled, it divides repeatedly, producing a prodigious progeny of like cells. After a substantial amount of cell division has occurred, some of these cells fuse together to form long multinucleated muscle fibers. Normally mitosis does not occur in the cells after they have fused. The muscle fibers thus formed develop cross striations, indicating that the muscle proteins actin and myosin are being formed and aligned within the fiber. The fibers are then capable of contraction. A single muscle cell has thus become a group of functioning muscle fibers (Fig. 2-9).

Nervous tissue in culture may similarly attain an impressive degree of histological organization. Young cells may be taken from the developing nervous system of embryos and placed in chambers, where they can be kept for days, weeks, or even months. Development of the tissue continues in vitro much as it would in vivo (Fig. 2-10). The nerve cells send out processes and these form contacts (synapses) with other neurons. The supporting cells of the

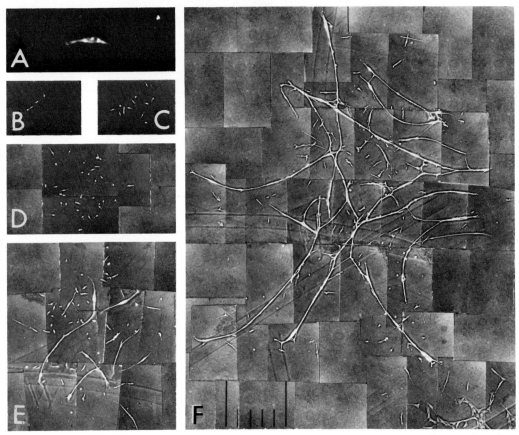

Fig. 2-9. This series of low power photomicrographs records the development of a muscle colony from a single bipolar cell. The colony produced by the single cell in *A* is shown after 1 day (*B*), 2 days (*C*), 3 days (*D*), 5 days (*E*), and 8 days (*F*) of development. After substantial cell division, the cells begin to fuse to form the straplike multinucleate muscle fibers seen in *E* and *F*. The entire muscle mass is a clone because it has arisen from a single cell. In *F*, each division of the scale represents 0.1 mm. (From I. R. Konigsberg: Science 140:1273, 1963.)

neuron form a special ensheathment called myelin, just as they do in vivo. In addition, the nervous tissue in vitro demonstrates many of the electrical properties characteristic of its function in the body.

Gland cells, such as those of the pancreas, can also express their activity in culture. Under proper conditions, this tissue forms zymogen, a complex of digestive enzymes which is one of the characteristic products of the exocrine pancreas in the intact animal.

The list of tissues capable of impressive in vitro performance continues to grow; skin keratinizes, hair and feathers grow, glands secrete, bone is deposited, heart cells beat, blood cells differentiate, collagen forms, and cilia move. The usefulness of

tissue culture techniques in the study of the cell is expanding.

Cell Differentiation

The central problem in the study of development is the question of how a single cell, the fertilized egg, gives rise to the many cell types of the mature organism. The fertilized egg divides rapidly, forming first a ball of cells called a morula; later this mass of cells develops a cavity and is termed a blastula. In mammals this becomes embedded in the uterine wall and is subsequently nourished by the maternal tissues. With time, three classes of cells can be distinguished in the embryonic germ disc of the blastula: the ectoderm or outside layer, the

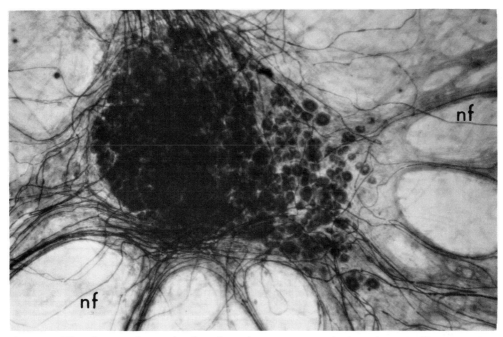

Fig. 2-10. The degree of organization that tissues may attain in culture is illustrated in this photomicrograph of a group of nerve cells which have matured in vitro. Clustered in the *center* are the nerve cell bodies (best seen at the *right*, where they are less concentrated). Radiating from these nerve cells are nerve fibers, often gathered into fascicles. Some individual nerve fibers are visible because their fatty sheaths (the myelin sheaths) are stained with Sudan black; they are best seen when situated singly, as at *nf*. This fat stain colors the neuron cytoplasm more intensely than the nucleus. Whole mount (unsectioned); dorsal root ganglion taken from a rat fetus and grown in culture for more than 6 months. ×100.

endoderm or inside lining, and the mesoderm, the cells between these surface layers. The organization and development of these three fundamental layers of embryonic tissue are discussed in the next chapter. From these layers and from their interaction, ultimately about 100 kinds of cells develop to form the adult mammal. The process of functional and structural specialization of these cells is called *differentiation*. Put another way, differentiation is the process whereby the various cells of a multicellular system acquire, individually or in groups, the structural machinery which allows them to emphasize certain particular functional capabilities. For example, although virtually all cells display some propensity for cytoplasmic contraction, only those cells which we term muscle cells have developed the mechanisms which permit the generation of strong and/or lasting contractile force. Such cells display very elaborate cytoplasmic structure for this

special function. Other functional capabilities are appropriately reduced, but not necessarily eliminated. Muscle cells also display some ability to conduct impulses (an emphasized property of neurons) and to synthesize some collagen (a principal activity of fibroblasts).

The problem of the mechanism and control of differentiation is as broad as the entire subject of embryology and is beyond the scope of the present discussion. It does seem useful, however, in discussing the principles of cytology, to consider how differentiation might be accomplished by an individual cell. In order to differentiate during embryonic development, cells must make a series of small shifts in their potential, as, for example, when a cell of the blastocyst becomes a cell belonging to the endoderm. These then proliferate to make more cells of their own kind. Then another shift is made, and members of this cell group may become either part of the gut wall or part of the lung. If the former occurs, then a third shift ensues, and the cell becomes either absorptive or secretory. Once the fate of the cell is set, the cell is said to be determined. It subsequently becomes structurally differentiated to perform and emphasize specialized functions. What a cell is and what it is capable of doing is largely a matter of the structural proteins and enzyme systems which it acquires.

There can be little doubt that this orderly development rests ultimately on the activities of the genetic material in the cell nucleus, the genes. It is also generally agreed that the basic codes in the genetic material do not change with development, but that different regions of the genome are "turned on" (and others "turned off") as cells develop. The genes are said to be differentially expressed as the cells are progressively determined.

It is also clear that alterations in the use of genetic material during development are not entirely preprogrammed within the cell but are influenced by interactions with other cells. As soon as an organism becomes multicellular the cells begin to react with one another in ways which trigger (or "induce") the onset of appropriate regional differentiation. As will be seen, the trigger may operate by activation of genetic mechanisms or by alteration of the rate or amount of synthetic activity already underway in responding cells. Cells of different stages of maturity may respond differently to normal or abnormal triggering interactions (inductions). The often disastrous effects of the German measles virus and the drug Thalidomide on the embryo, as compared with their mild effect on the older individual, are good examples of abnormal induction processes to which cells of a specific stage are highly sensitive.

The Operon

How do the sequential changes that occur in the cell during development take place? In 1961 the French molecular biologists Jacob and Monod suggested a mechanism by which the expression of genetic material in bacteria might be controlled. Their concept is based on the assumption, now generally accepted, that the genetic information of the organism, encoded in the nucleotide sequence of DNA, is transcribed into messenger RNA (mRNA), as has been discussed above. In union with ribosomes, the nucleotide sequences of mRNA are translated into the amino acid sequence of a specific polypeptide. Jacob and Monod suggest that the synthesis of mRNA on the gene is regulated by specific repressors which are products of other genes, called *regulator genes*. The *repressors* are thought to act by becoming engaged with the operator site of a group of genes. The *operator* plus the "structural" genes it controls is termed the *operon*. When the operator site is open, all of the genes of the operon synthesize mRNA, and when it is closed by the repressor, none do. The affinity of the repressor for the operator site is influenced by the concentration of small molecular weight metabolites within the cell. This scheme is summarized in Fig. 2-11.

This concept explained how an enzyme could be *induced* in a cell at the level of the gene. Suppose a certain type of sugar molecule becomes available in the cell environment and penetrates the cell nucleus. Within the nucleus it can react specifically with a repressor to open an operator site which initiates the synthesis of an enzyme used to break down this type of sugar. The cell is thus provided with a mechanism to use this sugar for its metabolic needs. The student should be able to extrapolate from this example a hypothesis suggesting how one cell could influence the genetic activities of another during development.

Unfortunately, the evidence for the operon mechanism of gene activity has come mostly from bacterial systems, and it is not yet clear to what extent this mechanism is involved in the complex differentiation of higher organisms. Harris has emphasized that a high degree of control of synthetic mechanisms occurs in the cell cytoplasm. Certain cells of lower forms can live, grow, and in fact differentiate after their nucleus has been removed. This is considered possible because the mRNA codes were made before the nucleus was removed and are stable for periods of several days or even weeks after the removal of the nucleus. Cytoplasmic control mechanisms determine when and to what extent the mRNA is to engage in protein synthesis. Thus it is

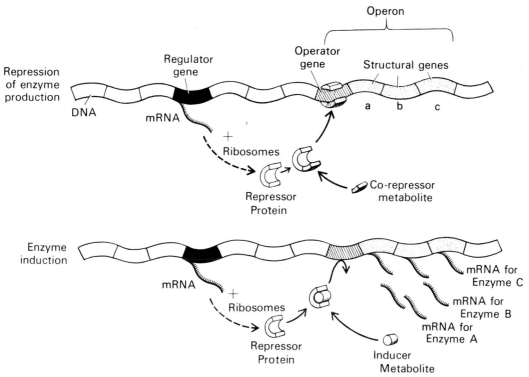

Fig. 2-11. Gene control: the operon concept. According to this concept a regulator gene occupying one site on the DNA strand controls the production of a repressor protein which, in combination with a corepressor substance, inhibits the activity of an operator gene on another site of the DNA strand. In the presence of an inducer compound, the repressor protein is unable to block the operator site. This operator gene controls the activity of adjacent structural genes on which there is assembly of messenger RNA (*mRNA*) molecules involved in enzyme manufacture.

clear that there are many levels of control of genetic expression, both in the nucleus and in the cytoplasm.

Recent work has led to the recognition that differentiation can be a remarkably reversible process in some cell types. One of the most dramatic examples has been provided by the work of Gurdon utilizing techniques introduced in the pioneering studies of Briggs and King. It is possible to destroy the nucleus of an unfertilized frog egg with ultraviolet light and then, using an extremely fine pipette, to introduce a diploid nucleus into the egg to see whether it will be capable of directing the development of the egg (and subsequently the embryo) as the original nucleus would have done. Gurdon has demonstrated that nuclei from fully differentiated intestinal cells in tadpoles can be obtained in a viable state and injected into anucleate frog eggs. In a small number of cases, these eggs developed into normal frogs (Fig. 2-12).

Experiments relevant to this point have also been undertaken by Harris. He has demonstrated, for example, that the nucleus of the highly differentiated chicken red blood cell is dramatically altered upon introduction into a cell already containing an active nucleus (Fig. 2-8). Normally the red cell nucleus does not synthesize measurable amounts of RNA, but in the heterokaryon it resumes RNA synthesis. Both of these experiments indicate that genes are not lost, nor are they permanently inactivated, in the process of differentiation.

This should not be taken to imply that all differentiation is, in the normal animal, reversible. In fact, the various populations of cells in a mature organism can be demonstrated to display varying levels of differentiation as judged by their structure and their varying capability to reverse a course of differentiation or to respond to injury with appropriate repair. The neurons of the mammalian central nervous system do not

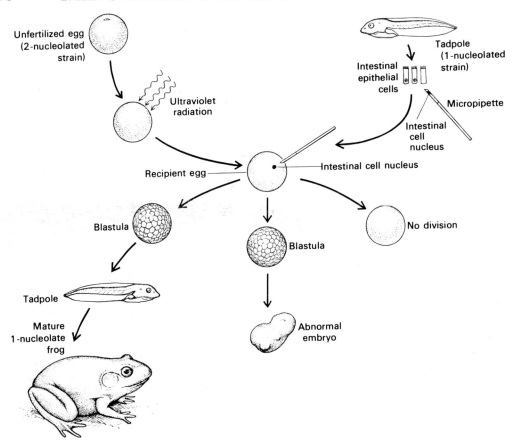

Fig. 2-12. The ability of a nucleus from a differentiated cell to perform all of the basic functions of the unspecialized embryonic nucleus may be demonstrated in the following way. After destruction of the frog egg nucleus by ultraviolet light, a nucleus isolated from an intestinal epithelial cell of a tadpole is substituted by microinjection. In a few cases, development of a normal frog occurs. Because the injected nucleus is the only functional nuclear material it must, in this case, be able to perform all of the functions of the egg nucleus. The use of two different frog strains (one with only one nucleolus in each nucleus and the other with two) allows confirmation of the presence of the intestinal cell nucleus. (After J. B. Gurdon: Sci. Amer. 219:24, 1968.)

reproduce themselves; many have very limited capacities of repair. When nerve cells are lost there is no mechanism for replacement, a point that should not be overlooked in an age which has witnessed an increasing reliance upon adjustment of the activities of the nervous system with drugs of every nature and degree of purity.

Cell-to-Cell Interactions

It is known that there are critical periods during the development of certain cells when exposure to other cells, or to products of other cells such as hormones, is critical for differentiation. Embryonic *induction* involves the interaction between cells or tissues in which one tissue induces a developmental change in another. A classic example is the formation of the lens of the eye. As the brain develops, that part destined to form the sensory portion of the eye bulges laterally and approaches the overlying ectoderm. As this portion of the nervous system comes in contact with the ectoderm, the ectoderm thickens, and its cells elongate and form a lens placode, the precursor of the lens itself. If the nervous tissue is prevented from contacting the ectoderm, no lens is formed. The nervous tissue has induced the formation of the lens. Furthermore, if the nervous tissue destined to form the eye is transplanted under the ectoderm on the back of the animal instead of the head, it will often induce lens formation in this region of the overlying ectoderm.

The development of the pancreas provides one of the best studied examples of tissue interaction. Pancreatic cells first develop in an endoderm derivative, the lining of the primitive gut. Wessels and Rutter have discovered that, at a precise time and at a precise site in the gut wall, some of the lining cells begin to make small amounts of digestive enzymes that mark them unmistakably as pancreatic cells. At this point they bear little histological similarity to mature pancreatic cells. But in terms of gene control a critical change has taken place, for some new region of the DNA code is now being used to transcribe mRNA, and the production of the digestive enzymes is thus possible. Then a puzzling dependence develops. The endoderm from which the pancreas cells are forming requires the close proximity of mesodermal tissue to become fully differentiated into pancreatic tissue. Without mesoderm little further development takes place, but if mesoderm is present the presumptive pancreatic cells greatly multiply their numbers, form definitive gland tissues, and increase their production of enzymes 50-fold—the tissue is now clearly pancreas. After this critical period the pancreatic cells are no longer dependent upon the mesoderm for normal development.

It is clear from this type of experiment that tissue type may be determined before cell division ceases. Cell multiplication of the determined tissue type goes on until a certain volume of tissue is reached. In some tissues the process of cell division is then permanently halted, as with nerve cells or heart muscle cells. In other tissues, cell division may continue at a slower rate to replace tissue elements lost with time, as in the lining of the gut. In other adult tissues, the ongoing needs of rapid cell turnover are met by the division of multipotential "stem cells," cells which themselves do not differentiate but produce progeny that do. An example is the bone marrow myeloblast, which gives rise to many different types of blood cells.

Cell Division

"... Life is an unbroken series of cell-divisions that extend backward from our own day throughout the entire past history of life.... It is a continuum, a never-ending stream of protoplasm in the form of cells, maintained by assimilation, growth and division. The individual is but a passing eddy in the flow which vanishes and leaves no trace, while the general stream of life goes forward."

E. B. Wilson, 1925

Cells arise by the division of preexisting cells. All of the cells of the adult human body, an estimated 10^{14} of them, are derived from just one cell, the fertilized egg. The structure and specificity of cells depend upon the population of proteins therein, and these proteins are assembled under the direction of mRNA. The mRNA carries the code of the genetic material, the DNA, which is contained within the nucleus. Thus it should be apparent that newly formed cells must be endowed with exact replicas of the parent DNA complement. To accomplish this, the parent cell must exactly duplicate its DNA and then precisely divide it and distribute it to two daughter cells. The process by which the DNA molecules are duplicated is called *replication* and the mechanism by which the replicated DNA is divided to supply each daughter cell with its complete and exact complement of hereditary material is termed *mitosis*. The division of nuclear material is referred to as *karyokinesis*; the division of the cytoplasm is called *cytokinesis*.

DNA Replication

To achieve replication, the DNA double helix unwinds, and each strand becomes a template for the assembly of a new one, which then becomes incorporated into a new double helix. The end result, therefore, is two double helices, each composed of one parent and one new strand. This mechanism of replication, termed "semiconservative," is the usual one for mammalian somatic (body) cells. In this manner, the linear arrays of genes are copied exactly if conditions are normal. Utilization of radioactive thymidine, incorporated only into duplicating DNA molecules, has been helpful in studying the mechanism of DNA replication, as well as in discovering the time at which it occurs.

Replication is accomplished before the cell visibly enters mitosis. During the non-dividing (*interphase* or "resting") period, three different phases have been defined: G_1, the gap between the previous mitosis and the start of DNA synthesis (S), and G_2, the gap between the end of S and the beginning of mitosis (M) (Table 2-2). In general, the replication of DNA may occur without cytokinesis, but cell division does not take place without the prefactory replication of DNA. It is known that mitosis is triggered by DNA synthesis, but the stimulus for DNA replication remains a mystery.

Mitosis

The nuclear DNA is contained within chromosomes which are not readily visible by light microscopy in the interphase nucleus. The chromosomal material is actually arranged in dispersed networks of delicate submicroscopic strands collectively referred to as *chromatin*. After staining of the interphase nucleus, only scattered condensed areas of chromatin, the *heterochromatin*, are visible. As the cells prepare for division, the entire chromosome becomes visible, as the term mitosis (from the Greek *mitos*, thread) implies. Each chromosome becomes progressively thicker and shorter by a process of coiling. This extreme

shortening of the chromosomes allows their disentanglement and precise alignment before their division and distribution into daughter cells.

Although mitosis is a continuous process, it is often divided into four stages: *prophase, metaphase, anaphase,* and *telophase*. During a typical mitotic period, prophase may be the longest stage, perhaps 1.5 hr, whereas metaphase, anaphase, and telophase take approximately 20, 4, and 60 min, respectively. In cultured HeLa cells, mitosis is accomplished in about 80 min, the successive stages requiring about 18, 35, 13, and 14 min, respectively.

Prophase. The onset of prophase is recognizable by an increase in the number and density of stainable chromatin particles, which are gradually replaced by slender threads (Figs. 2-13 and 2-14). With continued coiling they become shorter and thickened in girth; the gyres of the threads (chromosomes) increase in diameter and decrease in number. These chromosomes may be studied in appropriately stained, preserved tissue or examined in the living state by means of phase optics or, better still, the Nomarski (differential interference contrast) system (Fig. 2-15).

Each chromosome now contains twice the normal amount of DNA as a result of the replication before the onset of prophase. This doubling becomes visible for the first time when the chromosome ap-

TABLE 2-2

Periods of the cell cycle, i.e., from one cell division to the next

Period	Definition	% of time from one mitosis to the next (generation time*)
Interphase; period of increasing mass with protein and RNA synthesis		
G_1	Gap$_1$: period between previous mitosis and S	30–40% for regularly dividing cells, but time may vary considerably, even lasting the lifetime of the organism
S	Synthesis: period of DNA and histone synthesis	30–50%; this interval usually constant depending upon cell type or state; may be 7 hr in some species
G_2	Gap$_2$: period between S and beginning of mitosis	10–20%; interval fairly constant, lasting up to 2 hr
Division		
M	*M*itosis: period when chromosomes shorten (and thus become visible), are aligned in the middle of the cell, and are divided equally	5–10%; usually lasts 1–2 hr but depends upon the cell type

* The generation time usually ranges from 10 to 30 hr; for certain human cultured cells it is 22 hr, with the S period lasting about 6 hr.

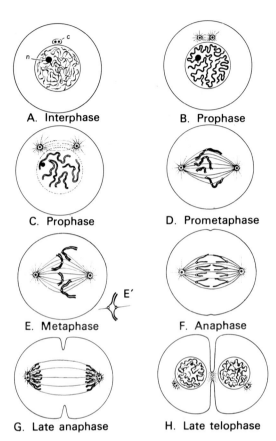

A. Interphase

B. Prophase

C. Prophase

D. Prometaphase

E. Metaphase

E′

F. Anaphase

G. Late anaphase

H. Late telophase

Fig. 2-13. Diagram illustrating the successive cellular events in mitosis, which is described in the text. E′ in an enlargement of the two chromatids of one chromosome, showing completion of separation by detachment at the centromere region. c, centrosome; n, nucleolus.

pears to be divided lengthwise into two parallel, closely apposing units called *chromatids*. As long as they remain attached (in one region only, the *centromere*), they are called chromatids (or "sister chromatids"; Fig. 2-7); once they become separated (at a later interval) they are called "daughter chromosomes." The chromatids coil on themselves rather than around each other.

The organization of the DNA double helix and associated proteins within the chromatid is one of the important questions in cell biology. The basic morphological unit is a 200- to 250-Å diameter strand of DNA-protein, but it remains controversial whether this contains one or two strands of DNA double helix and associated protein. Furthermore, the number (probably

multiple) of these 250 Å units and the manner in which they are constructed into a larger chromatid remain to be clarified. Electron microscope examination of thin sections has not seemed suited for elucidating the structure of these coiled, twisted, folded, and tightly packed filaments and reveals a bewildering array of granules or short segments of filaments which vary only in packing density throughout mitosis. Recently, however, use has been made of the 1 million-volt electron microscope, which allows stereological examination of sections up to 2 μm thick. This method produces three-dimensional images of much longer chromatid filament segments and hence holds promise for reconstruction of an accurate model of chromatid architecture.

During prophase, the nuclear envelope vanishes (thus allowing mixing of nuclear and cytoplasmic contents), the nucleolus disappears, and centrioles start their migration to opposite poles of the cell. Before this, the two *centrioles* (a *diplosome*) have been clustered together, lying at right angles to one another. Between the centrioles a *mitotic spindle* of microtubules begins to enlarge into an array roughly the shape of a football. The centrioles thus act as organizing centers for the spindle and become its two poles. The spindle microtubules converge on, but are not continuous with, the centrioles. A small disclike structure, the *kinetochore*, becomes visible (in electron micrographs) at the centromere region of each chromatid. It is in this region that some of the spindle tubules become attached to chromosomes (Fig. 2-16). The kinetochore is considered to participate in microtubule assembly as well. The spindle structure, which according to recent evidence contains actin- and myosin-like molecules as well as tubulin and microtubules, provides the mechanism for subsequent chromosomal movement.

Metaphase. During *prometaphase* (Fig. 2-13D) the spindle is fully developed and the chromosomes, all in a condensed state and thus visible in their entirety, move into it and become situated midway in the spindle. During metaphase the chromatids continue to condense and shift slightly until they are oriented in a precise manner. Actually, it is the centromere portion of the chromatids

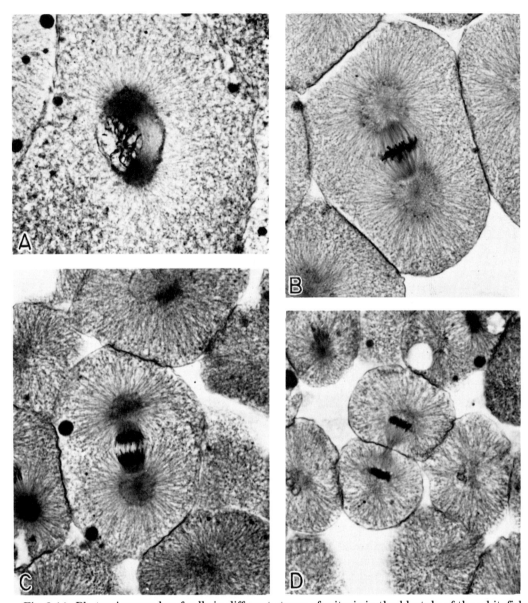

Fig. 2-14. Photomicrographs of cells in different stages of mitosis in the blastula of the whitefish. *A*, late prophase, with chromosomes in coiled threads, nuclear membrane still present, and the cell center divided into two new centers which have moved toward opposite poles of the nucleus; *B*, metaphase, in lateral view; *C*, early anaphase; *D*, telophase. Photographs at ×600, from slides purchased from the General Biological Supply House, Chicago.

which becomes aligned in the *equatorial* or *metaphase plate* of the spindle (Fig. 2-13*E*). The kinetochores of each chromatid pair are oriented perpendicular to the spindle axis and face opposing poles, with the attached microtubules extending toward each pole (Fig. 2-16).

In living cells the spindle microtubules are not visible in the phase microscope, although the spindle area is represented by a clear zone around which are clustered organelles, but they can be detected in the Nomarski system (Fig. 2-15) and appear as birefringent structures in the polarizing microscope (Fig. 2-17). The spindle may be demonstrated in fixed and stained prepa-

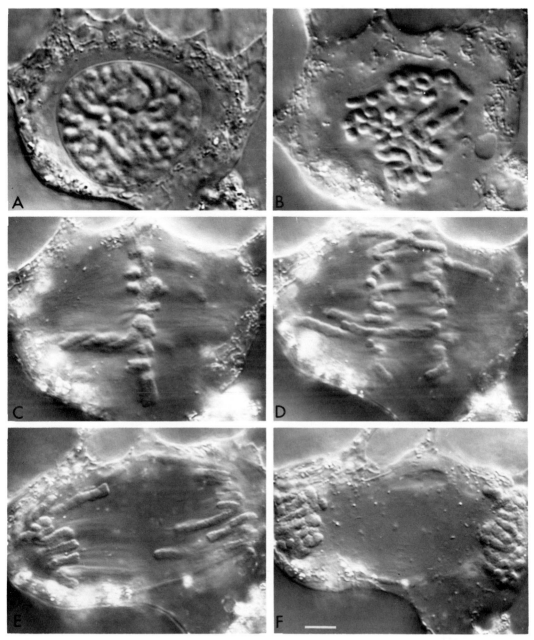

Fig. 2-15. Photomicrographs of successive changes in a lily endosperm cell during mitosis, as seen in the Nomarski optical system. This system has the advantage of revealing spindle fibers in living cells. Time after *A*: *B*, 14 min; *C*, 1 hr 4 min; *D*, 1 hr 14 min; *E*, 1 hr 33 min; and *F*, 1 hr 47 min. Compare with Figure 2-13. The *bar* indicates 10 μm. (From A. Bajer: Chromosoma 25:249, 1968.)

rations (Fig. 2-14) and is beautifully resolved in the electron microscope (Fig. 2-18) as a large array of microtubules which may number in the hundreds or thousands, depending upon the species. A number of microtubules are attached to one kineto-chore and may extend in bundles, which accounts for their visibility in the Nomarski system. There are two types of spindle microtubules: *continuous*, which extend from pole to pole, and *chromosomal*, which extend from the kinetochore to a pole. The

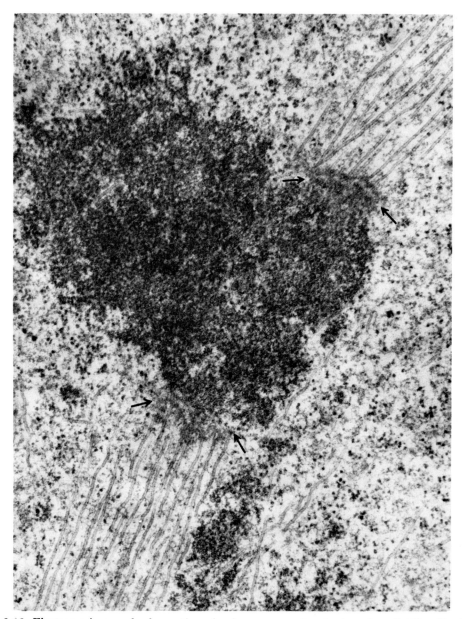

Fig. 2-16. Electron micrograph of a portion of a chromosome at metaphase in a dividing fibroblast in tissue culture. The sister chromatids are still joined in the centromere region shown here. On each chromatid, facing the pole to which it will be drawn, is the kinetochore (*arrows*). The chromosomal spindle microtubules are attached to the chromatid in the kinetochore region. ×45,000. (From B. R. Brinkley: *In* Advances in Cell Biology, edited by D. Prescott, vol. 1, p. 119. Appleton-Century-Crofts, New York, 1969.)

spindle apparatus is highly labile, but it may be isolated from the cell for special study.

When colchicine or related compounds are administered to dividing cells, mitosis is arrested at the beginning of metaphase. Apparently colchicine blocks the migration of the centrioles, presumably because some continuous microtubules cannot be assembled to aid in their poleward movement.

tids neverthele
thus become sh
mal, allowing tl
identification ii
this point, eac
characteristic i
length and the
or *primary con*
mosomes of va
a given species
otype, explaine

Anaphase.
ment in the me
tids are ready
separation of th
of attachment
pair, the two d
their journey t
pears to be pul
the remainder
behind. They a
gions where th
densed and ma
another. At the
dle elongates, a
(in a plane mi
to the spindle
of cytoplasmic

The mechani
daughter chror
poles is not co
been proposed
movement is c
chromosomal n
region. Tubulir
then be availa
subsequent len
tubules, there
overall extensi
studies have s
actin and myos
spindle. These
suggestions tha
mosomal migra
myosin interac
the microtubul
tractile protein
mosomal move
investigation.

Centrioles us
phase or telopl
ter cell with i
Centrioles are
not by division
a template fo

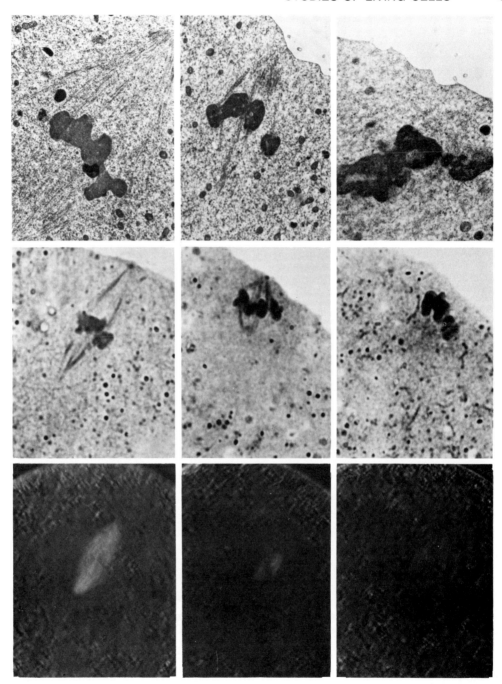

Fig. 2-17. Effect of administering an agent (vinblastine) known, like colchicine, to arrest a dividing cell in metaphase. Division is interrupted because the spindle microtubules disappear, as demonstrated in electron micrographs (*top row, left to right*), light micrographs (obtained by sectioning at 1 μm the tissue prepared for electron microscopy, staining with toluidine blue, and viewing in the phase microscope; *middle row*), and photographs of living cells taken in the polarizing microscope (*bottom row*). This set of pictures also serves to demonstrate that spindle birefringence depends upon the presence of an array of spindle microtubules. Living marine worm oocyte. (From S. E. Malawista et al.: Science 160:770, 1968.)

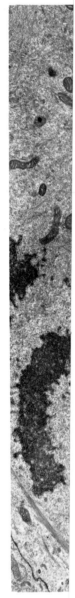

what the metabolic variations may be. The DNA molecule is extremely stable, and this stability is the basis for the continuity of life.

Meiosis

As we have just learned, mitosis is the process by which new daughter cells acquire a complete genetic complement identical to that of the parent cell. In man, the set of 46 chromosomes (the *diploid* number) is thus passed on from generation to generation of daughter cells. If this were the case during the formation of the egg and sperm cells, however, the fusion of nuclei at fertilization would lead to a set of 92 chromosomes. Therefore, a somewhat different division process, *meiosis* (or *reduction division*) is at work in the development of each germ cell to provide for the presence of only 23 chromosomes (the *haploid* number). The diploid number of chromosomes is then restored at the time of fertilization. Meiosis is discussed further in chapter 19.

References

General Topics

DeHaan, R. L., and Ursprung, H. (editors). Organogenesis. Holt, Rinehart and Winston, New York, 1965.

Ebert, J. D., and Sussex, I. M. Interacting Systems in Development. Ed. 2, Holt, Rinehart and Winston, New York, 1970.

Grobstein, C. Cytodifferentiation and its controls. Science 143:643–650, 1964.

Gurdon, J. B. Transplanted nuclei and cell differentiation. Sci. Amer. 219:24–35, 1968.

Harris, H. Nucleus and Cytoplasm. Clarendon Press, Oxford, 1968.

Haynes, R. H., and Hanawalt, P. C. (editors). The Molecular Basis of Life. Readings from Scientific American. W. H. Freeman and Company, San Francisco, 1968.

Jacob, F., and Monod, J. Genetic regulatory mechanisms in the synthesis of protein. J. Mol. Biol. 3:318–356, 1961.

Kennedy, D. (editor). The Living Cell. Readings from Scientific American. W. H. Freeman and Company, San Francisco, 1965.

King, T. J., and Briggs, R. Serial transplantation of embryonic nuclei. *In* Molecular and Cellular Aspects of Development (Bell, E., editor), pp. 171–192. Harper and Row, Publishers, New York, 1965.

Leblond, C. P., and Walker, B. E. Renewal of cell populations. Physiol. Rev. 36:255–276, 1956.

Loomis, W. F., Jr. (editor). Papers on Regulation of Gene Activity during Development. Harper and Row, Publishers, New York, 1970.

Loewenstein, W. R. On the genesis of cellular communication. Dev. Biol. 15:503–520, 1967.

Trinkaus, J. P. Cells into Organs. The Forces that Shape the Embryo. Prentice-Hall, Inc., Englewood Cliffs, New Jersey, 1969.

Wessels, N. K., and Rutter, W. J. Phases in cell differentiation. Sci. Amer. 220:36–44, 1969.

Special Topics

Cell Division

Chromosome Morphology

DuPraw, E. J. Evidence for a "folded-fibre" organization in human chromosomes. Nature (London) 209:577–581, 1966.

Gall, J. Chromosome fibers from an interphase nucleus. Science 139:120–121, 1963.

Moses, M. J., and Coleman, J. R. Structural patterns and the functional organization of chromosomes. *In* The Role of Chromosomes in Development (Locke, M., editor), pp. 11–49. Academic Press, New York, 1964.

Ris, H. Ultrastructure of the animal chromosomes. *In* Regulation of Nucleic Acid and Protein Biosynthesis (Koningsberger, V. V., and Bosch, L., editors), pp. 11–21. American Elsevier Publishing Company, New York, 1967.

Wolfe, S. L. Molecular organization of chromosomes. *In* The Biological Basis of Medicine (Bittar, E. E., editor), vol. 4, pp. 3–42. Academic Press, New York, 1967.

See also references at end of chapter 1

Mitosis

Bajer, A. A. Interaction of microtubules and the mechanisms of chromosome movement (zipper hypothesis). I. General principle. Cytobios 8:139–160, 1973.

Moscona, A. A. (editor). The cell surface in development. John Wiley and Sons, New York, 1974.

Willmer, E. N. (editor). Cells and Tissues in Culture. vols. 1, 2, and 3. Academic Press, New York, 1965.

Tissue Culture

Carrel, A. On the permanent life of tissues outside of the organism. J. Exp. Med. 15:516, 1912.

Fell, H. B. Histogenesis in tissue culture. Cytology and Cell Physiology (Bourne, G. H., editor), Ed. 2, pp. 419–443. Clarendon Press, Oxford, 1951.

Harrison, R. G. Observations on the living developing nerve fiber. Proc. Soc. Exp. Biol. Med. 4:140, 1907.

Experimental Manipulation of Living Cells

Amy, R. L., Storb, R., Fauconnier, B., and Wertz, R. K. Ruby laser micro-irradiation of single tissue culture cells vitally stained with Janus green B. Exp. Cell Res. 45:361–373, 1967.

Fig. 2-18. ... *center* are th... myriads of li... the chromos... pole of the s... Other cytopl... Kangaroo rat...

Because bo... pair do not... the kinetocl... tubules, wit... matids can... chicine is w...

CHAMBERS, R. Micrurgical studies on protoplasm. Biol. Rev. 24:246–265, 1949.

KOPAC, M. J. Micrurgical studies on living cells. *In* The Cell; Biochemistry, Physiology, Morphology (Brachet, J., and Mirsky, A. E., editors), vol. 1, pp. 161–191. Academic Press, New York, 1959.

ROSE, G. G., (editor). Cinemicrography in Cell Biology. Academic Press, New York, 1963.

ZIRKLE, R. E., AND BLOOM, W. Irradiation of parts of individual cells. Science 117:487–493, 1953.

Activities of Living Cells

ALLEN, R. D., AND TAYLOR, D. L. Molecular basis of amoeboid movement. *In* Molecules and Cell Movement (S. Inoué and R. Stephens, editors), pp. 239–258, Raven Press, New York, 1975.

CLARK, E. R. The transparent chamber technique for the microscopic study of living blood vessels. Anat. Rec. 120:241–252, 1954.

FAWCETT, D. W. Transient differentiations associated with surface activity. *In* The Cell. Its Organelles and Inclusions, pp. 389–414. W. B. Saunders Company, Philadelphia, 1966.

FURSHPAN, E., AND POTTER, D. Low resistance junctions between cells in embryos and tissue culture. *In* Current Topics in Developmental Biology (Moscona, A., editor), pp. 95–125. Academic Press, New York, 1968.

GROPP, A. Phagocytosis and pinocytosis. *In* Cinemicrography in Cell Biology (Rose, G. G., editor), pp. 279–312. Academic Press, New York, 1963.

HOLTER, H. Pinocytosis. Int. Rev. Cytol. 8:481–504, 1959.

LEWIS, W. H. Pinocytosis. Bull. Johns Hopkins Hosp. 49:17–27, 1931.

SPEIDEL, C. C. Studies of living nerves. IV. Growth, regeneration, and myelination of peripheral nerves in salamanders. Biol. Bull. 68:140–161, 1935.

Cytological Analysis in Tissue Culture

FITZGERALD, P. H. Chromosomal abnormalities in man. *In* The Biological Basis of Medicine (Bittar, E. E., editor), vol. 4, pp. 133–178. Academic Press, New York, 1969.

HARRIS, H. Hybrid cells. *In* Nucleus and Cytoplasm, Chap. 5, pp. 89–110. Clarendon Press, Oxford, 1968.

HAYFLICK, L. Human cells and aging. Sci. Amer. 218:32–37, 1968.

KONIGSBERG, I. R. Clonal analysis of myogenesis. Science 140:1273–1284, 1963.

MINTZ, B. Genetic mosaicism in adult mice of quadriparental lineage. Science 148:1232–1233, 1965.

MITTWOCH, U. The Sex Chromosomes. Academic Press, New York, 1967.

MOSCONA, A., AND MOSCONA, H. The dissociation and aggregation of cells from organ rudiments of the early chick embryo. J. Anat. 86:287–301, 1952.

PUCK, T. T., MARCUS, P. I., AND CIECIURA, S. J. Clonal growth of mammalian cells in vitro. Growth characteristics of colonies from single HeLa cells with and without a "feeder" layer. J. Exp. Med. 103:273–284, 1956.

Cell Differentiation

FRENSTER, J. H. Mechanisms of repression and derepression within interphase chromatin. In Vitro 1:78–101, 1965.

BRINKLEY, B. R., STUBBLEFIELD, E., AND HSU, T. C. The effects of colcemid inhibition and reversal on the fine structure of the mitotic apparatus of Chinese hamster cells *in vitro*. J. Ultrastruct. Res. 19:1–18, 1967.

CANDE, W. Z., LAZARIDES, E., AND MCINTOSH, J. R. A comparison of the distribution of actin and tubulin in the mammalian mitotic spindle as seen by indirect immunofluorescence. J. Cell Biol. 72:552–567, 1977.

DE HARVEN, E. The centriole and the mitotic spindle. *In* The Nucleus (Dalton, A. J., and Haguenau, F., editors), pp. 197–227. Academic Press, New York, 1968.

DEROBERTIS, E. D. P., SAEZ, F. A., AND DEROBERTIS, E. M. F., JR. Cell Biology, Ed. 6. W. B. Saunders Company, Philadelphia, 1975.

HINKLEY, R., AND TELSER, A. Heavy meromyosin-binding filaments in the mitotic apparatus of mammalian cells. Exp. Cell Res. 86:161–164, 1974.

INOUÉ, S., AND SATO, H. Cell motility by labile association of molecules. The nature of mitotic spindle fibers and their role in chromosome movement. J. Gen. Physiol. 50(Suppl):259–288, 1967.

KORNBERG, A. The synthesis of DNA. Sci. Amer. 219:64–78, 1968.

MAZIA, D. Mitosis and the physiology of cell division. *In* The Cell; Biochemistry, Physiology, Morphology (Brachet, J., and Mirsky, A. E., editors), vol. 3, pp. 77–412. Academic Press, New York, 1961.

MCINTOSH, J. R., HEPLER, P. K., AND VAN WIE, D. G. Model for mitosis. Nature (London) 224:659–663, 1969.

ROBBINS, E., AND GONATAS, N. K. The ultrastructure of a mammalian cell during the mitotic cycle. J. Cell Biol. 21:429–463, 1964.

SCHRADER, F. Mitosis, Ed. 2. Columbia University Press, New York, 1953.

SCHROEDER, T. E. Dynamics of contractile ring. *In* Molecules and Cell Movement, (S. Inoué and R. Stephens, editors), pp. 305–334, Raven Press, New York, 1975.

STUBBLEFIELD, E., AND BRINKLEY, B. R. Architecture and function of the mammalian centriole. *In* Formation and Fate of Cell Organelles (Warren, K. B., editor), pp. 175–218. Academic Press, New York, 1967.

SZOLLOSI, D. Cortical cytoplasmic filaments of cleaving eggs: a structural element corresponding to the contractile ring. J. Cell Biol. 44:192–209, 1970.

CHAPTER 3

General Features of Vertebrate Development

Adult living organisms are vehicles by means of which the germinative cells (ova or sperm) are produced and their genetic complement is transmitted from generation to generation, thereby perpetuating their respective species. Amid all of the living species, those that we characterize as "higher organisms," including man and other vertebrates, display adult body plans that are relatively large and highly complex. They exhibit *sexual* reproduction, a remarkable process which has lent efficiency to the evolution of such complex forms by ensuring variety among the offspring who must contend with new or changing environmental challenges. But sexual reproduction requires that the life of each individual is initiated by the fusion of two tiny cells. From them the new offspring receives the combined set of genetic instructions which dictates all future capabilities. The processes of growth and differentiation convert these cells and their instructions sequentially into the complex reproductive unit which is the adult.

John Tyler Bonner has defined development as the inevitable result of the evolution of *sex* on the one hand and *size* on the other. In other words, successful species, more readily able to invade, feed, locomote, and reproduce in demanding environments, have generally evolved increasingly large, complex, and capable adult forms. Development is the sequence whereby each individual begins life in an appropriately small sexually combined package and gradually converts itself into a much more massive, adaptable adult.

Because the evolution of the vertebrates has been one of continual progression and modification, it is not surprising that, at least as embryos, these animals share many common basic properties. They may all be defined as *triploblastic* (having three fundamental tissue layers), *metameric* (segmented), *eucoelomate* (having true body cavities), and *bilaterally symmetrical*. They all possess, at some stage, a notochord, a dorsal hollow central nervous system, branchial arches and grooves, and pharyngeal pouches.

Early Morphogenesis

Early development (or morphogenesis; the acquisition of form) commences, by definition, with fertilization, although obviously many events involving maturation of sperm and ovum have occurred in anticipation of this event. In human development, fusion of male and female pronuclei within the new, one-celled individual, the *zygote*, is quickly followed by *cleavage*, a series of mitotic divisions (Fig. 3-1). By the time the zygote is transported from the uterine tube into the implantation site on the uterine endometrial wall, it is apparent that the newly derived daughter cells, or *blastomeres*, remain together as an adherent aggregate enclosed by a thin, gradually

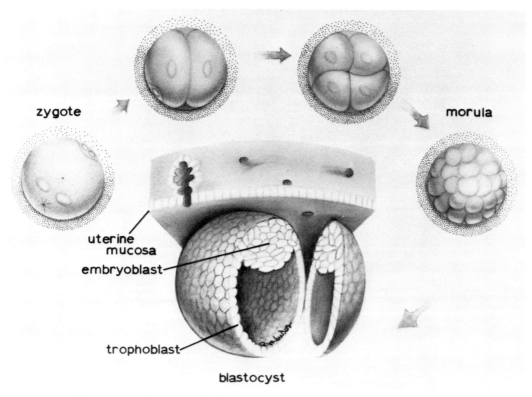

zygote

morula

uterine mucosa

embryoblast

trophoblast

blastocyst

Fig. 3-1. Early stages of human development after fertilization (*left*), through cleavage and morula (*right*). The relationship of the blastocyst and its parts just before the commencement of implantation into the uterine mucosa is shown at *bottom*.

disintegrating extracellular fertilization membrane. The total aggregate, now termed a *morula*, has not increased in mass, but will do so rapidly after attachment to and penetration into the uterine wall. By that time it has formed into a hollow sphere, the *blastocyst*, one side of which is thickened (the *embryoblast* or *inner cell mass*). The rest of the blastocyst is called the *trophoblast*, a surrounding shell of cells, soon fully engulfed into the uterine endometrial wall. Within the embryoblast, certain of the cells can be designated as those which will give rise to the embryo proper, and the rest, together with cells of the trophoblast, are destined to proliferate and provide components of four surrounding extraembryonic membranes; *amnion, chorion, allantois*, and *yolk sac* (Fig. 3-2). The detailed structure and fate of these will be covered in a later chapter.

The region of the embryo proper becomes distinct as a *diploblastic* (bilayered)

plate of cells (the *embryonic disc*) which delaminates away from other embryoblastic cells of amnion and yolk sac destiny. Already a head or anterior end of the plate as well as left and right halves can be defined. The two layers of the embryonic disc are termed the *epiblast* (above) and *hypoblast* (below) (Fig. 3-2). Each layer is epithelial, in the sense of displaying a free surface and possessing definite intercellular junctions which secure adjacent cells within each layer. The epiblast is particularly active mitotically.

Gastrulation

A striking transformation now occurs which is of paramount importance to the modern histologist. It literally sets the stage for all of the organizational features which follow in this book. This is the process of *gastrulation* (Fig. 3-3). Many cells of the epiblast lose attachment with their neigh-

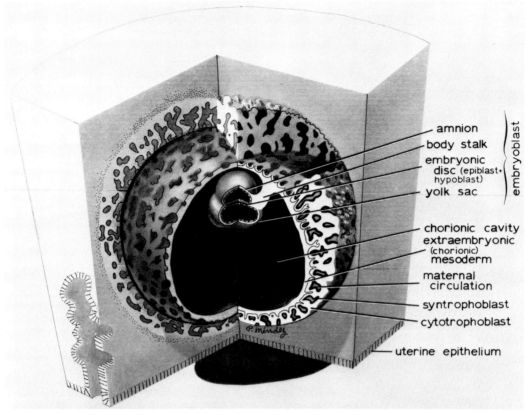

Fig. 3-2. The human blastocyst after implantation into the uterine wall is complete. The inner cell mass has delaminated into amnion, embryonic disc, and yolk sac. Collectively these are suspended from the trophoblast (now chorion) by the body stalk.

bors and migrate inward to become incorporated as a looser population sandwiched between remaining epiblast and hypoblast. Most of this activity occurs along a midline groove in an elongate region of the posterior epiblast, the *primitive streak*, in such a way that the newly freed cells are crowded into the subepiblastic region along the groove. Immediately they commence a lateral migration, forming a spreading sheet or network of cells which progressively separates epiblast from hypoblast. The migrating, spreading network, termed the *mesoblast*, proceeds laterally and anteriorly on either side of the embryonic disc, its two "wings" eventually converging to meet medially at the most anterior portion of the embryonic disc (*dotted arrows*, Fig. 3-3). There the fused mesoblast forms the *cardiogenic plate*. Along the center line, ahead of the primitive groove, a rodlike core of closely adherent mesoblastic cells is laid down as

the embryonic disc elongates and the primitive groove diminishes rapidly in relative dimensions. This core is the future *notochord*.

It is essential to note the vastly different behavior assumed by most of the mesoblastic cells as compared with those left to dwell in the epiblast or hypoblast. Whereas the latter cells remain relatively stationary and locked tightly to each other, mesoblastic cells (other than those of the notochord) display an opposite tendency, migrating rather freely, and, for a time, maintaining a remoteness from their neighbors. The adjective "*mesenchymal*" is often applied to these mesoblastic cells, denoting not only this active, individualistic migratory behavior but also the fact that they are embryonic cells with the potential to proliferate and mature into many diverse types of differentiated cells.

An interesting recently discovered phe-

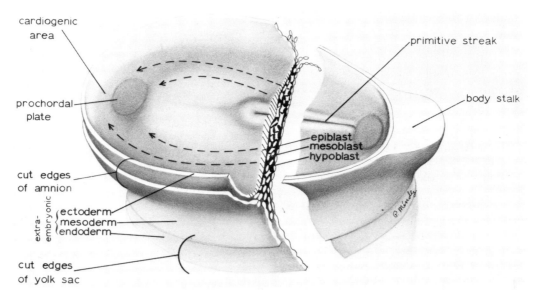

Fig. 3-3. The embryonic disc during the process of gastrulation. The amnion has been cut and lifted off to reveal the epiblastic surface. Cells from the epiblast are entering the mesoblast (primarily in the area of the primitive groove) and migrating anteriorly along the paths indicated by *dotted arrows*. The outline of the notochordal process extending anteriorly from the primitive streak delineates the longitudinal axis of the forming embryo.

nomenon reportedly occurs in chick embryos and perhaps also in mammals. There, cell labeling experiments disclose that some of the newly arrived mesoblast cells near the embryonic midline invade the hypoblast, displacing the original hypoblastic cells laterally. It is now thought that all of the hypoblastic cells which eventually remain in the embryo proper are of this mesoblastic origin. Hence one might say that, at least in the chick, all or nearly all of the cells of the embryo originate from the epiblast.

At the close of gastrulation, when mesoblastic development has achieved a complete or nearly complete intermediate middle layer between epi- and hypoblasts, the embryo is said to be *triploblastic*. Its three fundamental layers are often referred to as the "germ layers." They are: the *ectoderm* (formerly the remaining epiblast); the *endoderm* (formerly the remaining hypoblast); and the *mesoderm* (that mesoblast which has become mesenchymal cells and notochord). The ectoderm and endoderm produce a submicroscopic thin extracellular coating, the *basal lamina*, along their interior surfaces, i.e., surfaces facing the remaining mesoblast. This serves to segregate

them from the mesoblast. Ecto- and endodermal layers can now be defined as *epithelial* (discussed in detail in chapter 4). Similarly, the adherent cells of the notochord enshroud that structure with a basal lamina. The remaining mesoblast (now mesoderm) is trapped in a compartment which is enshrouded by the basal lamina of the ectoderm and endoderm and likewise separated also from the notochord. This compartment can usefully be termed the *mesenchymal* or *mesoblastic compartment*. Unlike the epithelial layers which now surround it and seal it, the mesenchymal compartment contains much extracellular fluid and matrix materials. High volumes of those extracellular fluids and materials are retained in some tissues of mesoblastic origin and lost in others where differentiation involves an intimate secondary clumping of mesenchymal cells.

The cells of each of the three germ layers divide, migrate, group, and differentiate in rather precise patterns, ultimately forming organ systems. In general, the early epithelial cells retain firm, close adhesion with their neighbors and achieve final appropriate shapes by processes of folding, invagination, and evagination of epithelial layers.

Mesenchymal components, by contrast, seem at first to clump or spread, often crowding into nooks formed between ecto- or endodermal epithelial folds. There they form mesodermally derived epithelial linings and/or remain mesenchymal to differentiate further. Thus, most organs are formed by a combination of epithelial linings with mesenchymal compartments packed between. Indeed, as careful analysis has shown, the relationship between mesenchyme and epithelium is virtually always of critical importance, for each plays a controlling or *inductive* influence to signal or direct the appropriate developmental pattern for the other. Likewise, the close proximity of one embryonic epithelium to another may exert reciprocal inductive control in the differentiation of each.

Differentiation and Histogenesis

Tissues from different germ layers, while retaining their individuality, frequently associate in the formation of an organ, inducing each other to express new morphological properties collectively characteristic of that organ. As a result of careful cell marking techniques, we can now trace back (with few exceptions) the original germ layer from which has arisen each and every cell in each organ of the fully developed body (Table 3-1). The process whereby each constituent cell acquires organelles and other properties necessary to emphasize a particular function is termed cellular *differentiation*. The aggregate, integrated differentiation into the specialized cellular patterns of tissues is termed *histogenesis*.

In terms of principal tissue components, the outer epithelia and, as will be seen, the central nervous system develop from ectoderm. The epithelial linings of respiratory passages and gut and the glandular cells of appended organs such as liver and pancreas are of endodermal origin. The smooth muscular coats, connective tissues, and vessels supplying these organs are of mesodermal origin. Mesoderm also differentiates into blood, skeleton, skeletal muscles, and organs of excretion and reproduction. An interesting and important exception is in the case of the gonads, testis or ovary, in which the precursor cells of sperm and ova, the so-called *primordial germ cells*, are now

TABLE 3-1

Major derivatives of the three germ layers and neural crest

Origin	Derivatives
Ectoderm	
	Epithelium of skin, hair, nails, sebaceous, mammary, and sweat glands (including myoepithelial cells of some glands)
	Epithelium of mouth, anus, teeth, taste buds
	Epithelium of nose and nasal glands
	Epithelium of penile urethra
	Epithelium of external auditory canal and membranous labyrinth
	Epithelium of anterior cornea, conjunctiva, lacrimal glands, pars ciliaris, and pars retinae (and related muscle), neural retina, and retinal pigment epithelium
	Brain and spinal cord, epithelial cells of all parts of the pituitary gland
Neural crest ("mesectoderm")	
	Cells of spinal, cranial, and autonomic ganglia; ensheathing cells of peripheral nervous system
	Pigment cells of dermis
	Muscle, connective tissues, and bone of branchial arch origin
	Adrenal medulla
	Cells of meninges
Mesoderm	
	Most connective tissues of body
	Stromal components of all glands
	Lymphatic organs (except Hassall's corpuscles and thymic reticulum)
	All endothelia and mesothelia
	Skeletal, cardiac, and most smooth muscle
	Urogenital epithelia, except urethra and large areas of bladder
	Blood cells and bone marrow
	Adrenal cortex
Endoderm	
	Epithelium of digestive tract except mouth and anus
	Epithelium of glands of digestive tract including liver, gallbladder, pancreas
	Epithelium of thyroid and parathyroid glands and thymic reticulum and Hassall's corpuscles
	Epithelium lining middle ear cavity, inner tympanic membrane, and auditory tube
	Epithelial lining of respiratory tract and its glands (except nostril)
	Epithelium of most of bladder, female urethra, vaginal vestibule, prostatic portion of male urethra, and its glands

believed to be of yolk sac, and possibly endodermal, derivation.

Neurulation

The pattern by which such organ systems

emerge commences with the process of *neurulation*, so named because it involves the establishment of a primitive central nervous system (brain and spinal cord).

As the developing notochord and adjacent mesoblastic cells are mobilized into a central layer beneath the midline ectoderm, an induction occurs which governs a highly coordinated growth and movement of the overlying ectodermal cells, collectively termed the neural plate. In response to the underlying notochord and adjacent mesoderm, there is initiated within these ectodermal cells the activation of specific genes and a resultant synthesis of specific supportive and contractile proteins. These become arranged as intracellular filaments and microtubules (discussed in detail in chapters 1 and 4) which are positioned so as to exert and maintain rather precise changes in the shapes of the induced ectodermal cells. Coupled with regionally specific rates of mitotic activity, directionality in this proliferation, and probably also precise patterns

of cell-to-cell attachment, the shape-changing mechanisms of all of the cells act in harmony to fold the lateral edges of the neural plate upward, between them forming a *neural groove* (Fig. 3-4). This type of response to an inductive stimulus, resulting in individual and collective cell shape changes, can be detected as the basis for shaping of most tissues, organs, and regions. This is particularly true where the newly forming part is largely of epithelial composition. During neurulation, the process begins earliest in the anterior regions, where the mitotic activity is highest; thus the anterior folds are highest and thickest and, with their correspondingly deep groove, they herald the development of the brain. Gradually, the two elevating folds converge toward each other and fuse. First contact occurs in the posterior brain region, and fusion spreads from that point, zipper-like, anteriorly over the brain and posteriorly down the future spinal cord (Fig. 3-5). Fusion of the folds results also in the detach-

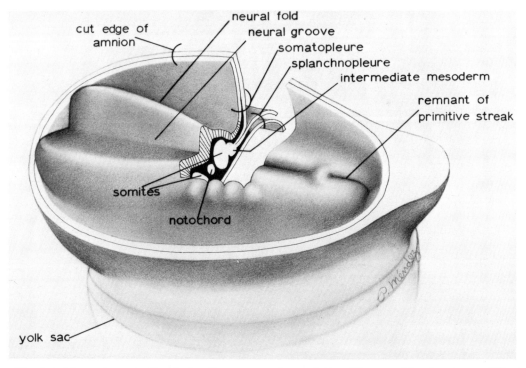

Fig. 3-4. The embryonic disc during the process of neurulation. The mesoblast has begun differentiating into notochord, somites, and intermediate and lateral plate mesoderm. Ectoderm above the somites and notochord has been induced to fold upward. Eventually the lateral margins of the folds will fuse progressively to form the neural tube, the future brain and spinal cord. By this stage of development, the embryonic disc is about twice the length of that depicted in Figure 3-3.

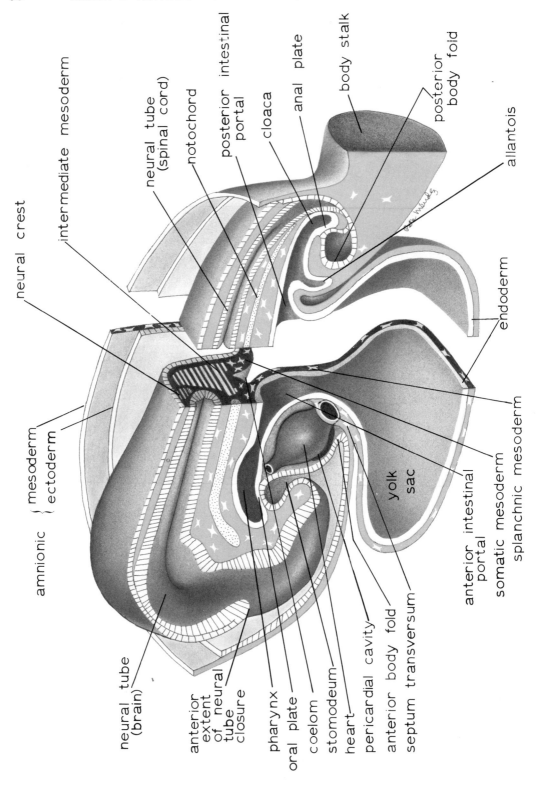

ment from overlying ectoderm of the hollow inner epithelial tube, the *neural tube*, the walls of which will differentiate into the substance of the brain and spinal cord. Note that the spinal cord and posterior brain are immediately underlain by the notochord.

Neural Crest

At the time of neural fold fusion and neural tube detachment, an unusual phenomenon occurs which adds still more cells to the mesenchymal compartment. Certain previously ectodermal epithelial cells residing along the crest of each neural fold suddenly lose their epithelial affinities, disengage, and migrate inward to invade the mesoblast along either side of the developing neural tube (Fig. 3-5). These cells rapidly disperse, making their identification immediately obscure, but special tracer techniques disclose that their numbers are considerable and their derivatives quite important. They are referred to collectively as the *neural crest* and they contribute, among other things, to developing spinal and autonomic ganglia, pigment cells, adrenal medulla, meningeal coverings of the brain and spinal cord, and many skeletal and muscular components of the head.

In a sense, neural crest development is a belated finish to the gastrulation process; the new mesoblastic neural crest cells have arrived in the mesenchymal compartment via a detachment process not dissimilar from that displayed some time earlier by gastrulating mesoblastic cells of epiblastic origin. As they detach from the ectoderm, the neural crest cells penetrate the basal lamina of that layer and become typically mesenchymal in their behavior; they are mitotically active and display a high degree of ameboid migratory capability. Having lost their epithelial attachments, they tend to migrate quite independently, displaying negative affinities toward other mesenchymal cells. Later in their various differentiative patterns, many of them will reverse this property and clump into appropriately shaped groups, such as those giving rise to spinal and autonomic ganglia, or sheets, like the enveloping meninges which eventually surround the neural tube. Many examples of specific neural crest development are portrayed in subsequent chapters of this text.

Somites and the Embryonic Axis

The notocord and neural tube have formed as single midline (or axial) structures which separate right and left halves of the embryo. Each is segregated from the surrounding mesoblastic compartment by the acquisition of basal laminae. Mesenchymal cells immediately lateral to these two components now commence a highly regular pattern of clumping that results in development of sequentially arranged *somites* on either side of the midaxial neural tube and notocord (Fig. 3-4). Some 31 pairs of somites are eventually formed, each representing a first visible representation of the repeating body segment, or *metamere*, which is characteristic of all vertebrate organisms and many invertebrates as well. Somites are compact aggregates of mesenchymal cells whose integrity seems temporarily ensured by a brief encasement in basal lamina material. The encasement is retained only long enough for the somites to achieve their metameric organization; shortly it will disperse as somitic mesodermal cells migrate once again into definite locations and commence differentiation into such serially repeated units of the body as bony vertebrae, axial musculature, ribs, etc. By that time certain neural crest cells have clustered between adjacent somites to give rise to the equally segmentally ordered spinal ganglia.

Somites, spinal ganglia, neural tube, and notochord are regarded as the *embryonic axis*, around which all other elements of

Fig. 3-5. The process of neural tube fusion is nearly complete. The anterior body fold has inverted the cardiogenic region into a position beneath the pharynx. Lateral plate mesoderm has divided to form splanchnic and somatic layers with the interval between identifiable as coelom. Neural crest migration is active. The posterior body fold has rolled anterior to the cloacal membrane so that allantois and body stalk are included in the forming umbilical cord. Communication between the elongating gut and the diminishing yolk sac is still very wide.

the embryo are assembled. From their beginning all components of the axis are mutually interdependent. Each exerts inductive influence upon the others so that spatial and temporal precision is maintained in the shaping of each unit and the axis as a whole. Somites appear first in the thoracocervical levels, where neural tube fusion has just occurred, newer ones arising progressively anteriorly and posteriorly until the entire miniature segmented individual has been laid out. By now (4 weeks), enlargement of the brain and lateral expansion of its walls into ectodermal rudiments of the eyes are apparent. The embryo begins to assume the characteristic shape of a tetrapod vertebrate.

Somatic and Splanchnic Mesoderm

Lateral to the row of somites on each side of the embryonic axis, cells of the mesoblast group into a recognizable, but not distinctly segregated, mesodermal rod. Eventually these two rods elongate to run the full length of the embryonic trunk region. They constitute the *intermediate* mesoderm, an important precursor to the developing excretory system, the gonads, and the inferior vena cava. Lateral to the intermediate mesoderm, the mesoblast extends as a sheet, the *lateral plate mesoderm*, reaching well beyond the boundaries of the embryonic disc, where it continues as the mesoderm of the amnion above, yolk sac below, and the body stalk behind. Within the embryonic disc, this lateral plate mesoderm exists only briefly as a single mesoblastic stratum; small cavitations appearing in its midst eventually fuse, to split the mesoderm into two layers. That layer above, immediately underlying the ectoderm, is termed *somatic mesoderm* (the two together constituting *somatopleure*), and the lower mesodermal layer, lying adjacent to endoderm, is termed *splanchnic mesoderm*. (Combined with the nearby endoderm, it constitutes *splanchnopleure*) (Fig. 3-5). The large mesoderm-coated cavity thus formed between the two layers within the embryo is the first representation of a true *coelom* or body cavity. For a time, the embryonic coelom will remain continuous with the extraembryonic cho-

rionic cavity, or extraembryonic coelom. The mesodermal cells which line the coelom rapidly form attachments and acquire a basal lamina to separate themselves as an epithelial lining layer from the underlying splanchnic or somatic mesenchyme. This special mesodermal epithelial lining of the coelom and its derivative body cavities is referred to as *mesothelium*. Students of histology should note that the term mesothelium refers specifically to the lining epithelium of the true body cavities and *not* to other epithelial linings of mesodermal origin (such as the linings of vessels).

Definition of the above splanchnic and somatic components is important in terms of the patterns of differentiation which occur in each. For example, splanchnic mesoderm will eventually develop into a high proportion of smooth or cardiac nonvoluntary musculature and will be served largely by the autonomic nervous system. Som*a*tic and somite-derived (som*i*tic) mesoderm, on the other hand, will be the source of most skeletal musculature under the voluntary control of somatic neural components.

Body Folds and Formation of the Primitive Gut

As the embryonic disc, with its contained mesodermal and neural tube components, grows in length and width, it becomes elevated into the amnionic cavity. The movement is rather like when a low table, with its enshrouding tablecloth, is lifted above a floor just enough that the cloth drapes down from the table and spreads over the floor. If the table has but a single central pedestal, the tablecloth can next be gathered gradually toward the pedestal. This might conveniently be done by a noose or purse string. The portion of the tablecloth left surrounding the table corresponds to embryonic ectoderm, that spread over the floor is equated with extraembryonic ectoderm lining the inside of the amnionic cavity, and that part of the tablecloth cinched around the pedestal eventually represents ectoderm of the growing *umbilical cord*.

The movement is important to understand, for in the early embryo it gradually delineates embryonic from extraembryonic components, determines the position of the mouth, anus, and heart, and forms the gut and umbilical cord. The ectodermal folds, termed *head, tail,* and *lateral body folds,* are really parts of a single fold, a continuous inpocketing around and beneath the elevated embryo (Fig. 3-5). Eventually this ringlike fold constricts sufficiently in relation to the growing embryo that it constitutes the surface of a narrow neck, the rapidly lengthening umbilical cord. This latter is covered by ectoderm, contains the yolk stalk, allantois, and a mesodermal core, and continues to connect the embryo or fetus with extraembryonic components throughout prenatal life.

One important consequence of the development of the head fold and anterior lateral body folds relates to heart and mouth development. Originally the cardiogenic plate of mesoderm was situated well anterior on the midline of the embryonic disc, so far forward, in fact, that a mesoderm-free *prechordal plate* region separated it from the anterior tip of the notochord and overlying neural plate (Fig. 3-3). During head fold development, the cardiogenic plate, with its overlying ectoderm and underlying endoderm, is inverted and tucked under in such a way that it comes to lie beneath the neural plate and notochord and posterior to the prechordal plate, which has also been inverted. The endoderm is also folded and at the same time evaginated, forming an anterior midline diverticulation above the cardiogenic plate (Fig. 3-5). This diverticulation is the primordium of the *foregut*; its anterior extent is the former prechordal plate (now properly called the *oral plate* or buccopharyngeal membrane). This latter will ultimately perforate to complete the opening of the mouth. Note that the mouth itself is largely lined by ectoderm, a result of its development as an invagination in the oral plate region. This invagination is the *stomodeum* and is the site of origin of several important ectodermal components such as the enamel-forming cells of teeth, some salivary gland epithelia, and the anterior and intermediate portions of the pituitary gland parenchyma.

The endodermally lined foregut remains continuous for a time with a yolk stalk via an *anterior intestinal portal,* and it begins a number of tubular evaginations which will eventually form the secretory or lining epithelia of a number of glands and organs.

Prominent among these are lungs and thyroid glands, and more posteriorly the liver, gallbladder, and pancreas. The pharynx is the most anterior (or superior) part of the foregut, and it develops paired bilateral endodermally lined outpouchings, the *pharyngeal pouches* (Fig. 3-6). Each pouch is met by an inpocketing of ectoderm or *branchial groove,* and occasionally a perforation, a *branchial cleft,* will form at the site of fusion between pharyngeal pouch endoderm and branchial groove ectoderm. Such clefts are usually transitory in mammalian development, but they recall their evolutionary homologues, the gill clefts so prominently retained in present day fishes and other adult lower vertebrates.

On each side of the embryo's developing head, the branchial grooves become apparent in a series of parallel vertical slits. Adjacent grooves bound prominent mesoderm-filled pillars, the *branchial arches,* and these have definite derivates such as the components of the upper and lower jaws, the external ear, parts of the larynx, etc. Their embryonic serial arrangement typifies further the segmented organization now apparent in the head as well as in the trunk of the embryo.

Inside, each pharyngeal pouch displays differentiation of its endodermal lining, which, after extensive invagination, proliferation, and morphogenetic shaping, becomes secretory, supporting, or lining epithelium of such important organs as parathyroid glands, thymus, tonsils, and the middle ear and auditory tube.

While the pharyngeal components take form, the cardiogenic region just beneath undergoes extensive change. Coelom formation extends anteriorly to separate splanchnic from somatic mesoderm; the anterior coelomic pocket thereby formed will ultimately be separated as the *pericardial cavity* (Fig. 3-5). Splanchnic mesoderm of this region forms a single midline tube lined by mesothelium on its outer surface (the visceral pericardial mesothelium) and an *endothelium** on its inside aspect; cardiac muscle will develop in between the two.

---

* The term *endothelium* is specifically used to denote the interior epithelial lining of the heart, blood vessels, and lymphatic channels. All endothelium is of mesodermal origin. The term endothelium should not be confused with either mesothelium or endoderm.

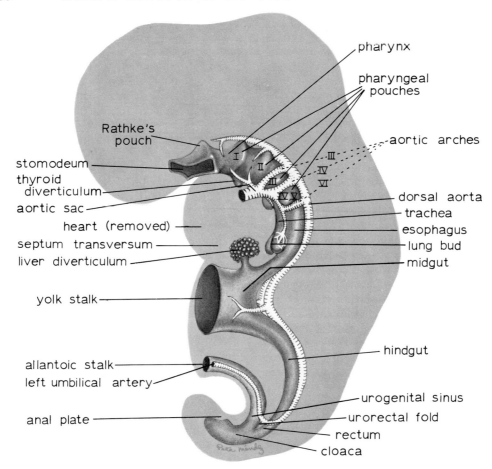

Fig. 3-6. Three-week human embryo showing the extent of development of the endodermal epithelium and major arterial vessels associated with it. Pharyngeal pouches are starting expansion into various epithelial derivatives. Lung primordia are expanding. The cloaca is being divided into urogenital sinus and rectum by development of the urorectal fold. The yolk stalk is still relatively wide.

This tube is attached to and supplied by important venous channels which join it posteriorly. Anteriorly it leads to and feeds paired arterial channels, the *aortic arches*, which course within several of the branchial arches. Quickly this tube initiates a series of contortions and septations which eventually lead to the typical morphology of the four-chambered mammalian heart.

Development of the embryo in the tail fold area has many similarities to that just described in head fold, pharyngeal, and stomodeal regions. A *hindgut* and *posterior intestinal* portal are entrapped within the embryo as the tail fold advances anteriorly, and an *anal plate* is formed by fusion of hindgut endoderm with overlying ectoderm

(Fig. 3-5). This particular ectoderm lies at the bottom of an exterior invagination, the *proctodeum*. The proctodeum is the future anus of the developing embryo, and will become continuous with the hindgut when the anal plate is ruptured during later fetal stages.

The *allantoic stalk*, which took its origin just before tail fold development as a midventral outpouching of hindgut endoderm, is swung ahead of the tail fold, retaining its connection to the hindgut. It opens into an enlarged part of the hindgut, the *cloaca*, in the region of the anal plate (Fig. 3-6). As tail fold development continues, the allantoic stalk is drawn along so that its distal tip finally resides in the umbilical cord.

Later yet, the cloaca will be divided by septation into a *urogenital sinus* (to which the allantoic stalk communicates) and a *rectum* (which drains the hindgut). Before anal plate perforation, the cloacal septation will be completed so that the urogenital sinus (the future urethra and urinary bladder) and rectum will have separate external openings. The urogenital sinus also receives paired *mesonephric* and *ureteric* ducts, which drain the embryonic excretory system developing within the nearby intermediate mesoderm.

As head, tail, and lateral body folds tighten around the belly of the enlarging embryo, the gut is elongated. Suspended within the coelom from the dorsal body wall by a splanchnic mesodermal *mesentery*, the emerging *midgut* elongates even more rapidly than the embryonic tissues around it. For a time during late embryonic and early fetal stages the midgut herniates into a rather wide umbilical cord, where it still communicates with a rapidly narrowing yolk stalk. As the umbilical cord becomes more constricted, the yolk stalk obliterates to a tiny ligamentous remnant, and the midgut is pulled back into the fetus, a process which by necessity involves rotation of the previously herniated midgut limbs. As the midgut continues to elongate and differentiate, it assumes the typical form and position of the small intestine and the proximal part of the large intestine.

Relationship of Histology and Embryology

The foregoing synopsis of early human development is but a glimpse of an obviously complex and highly coordinated series of harmonious events. The histologist must at least be aware of these basic patterns, for they describe the origins of the four basic adult tissue types: *epithelia, contractile tissue* (muscle), *neural tissue,* and *connective* and *supportive tissue* (of which blood is a unique close relative).

The art of histology is greatly enhanced by the ability to appreciate that these four classes of tissues are not completely distinct and exclusive, but rather represent portions of a spectrum of morphological and functional intergradations in cellular differentiation. The *differences* among and within these types are emphasized in the study of adult tissues; their *similarities* and common origins are perceived by a consideration of their embryology.

The adult tissues are not composed of cells only. At very early stages, many cells (especially the nonepithelial cells) become separated from each other by their elaboration of important intercellular substances. These substances also display a spectrum of variation and are just as much a part of the differentiation (and definition) of the emerging tissues as are the cells. Thus, each tissue is an aggregate of cells with its own characteristic amount and variety of intercellular substances (or *matrix*). In some tissues, the intercellular material is scanty (epithelia, muscle) and the cells are closely approximated. In such cases, differentiation relates more to the functional machinery developed within the cells' cytoplasm. In other tissues, the intercellular substances may become the major bulk of the tissue and assume physiological roles of massive proportions (bone, cartilage, connective tissue, blood, lymph). Here differentiation is really defined more by what the cells have constructed outside of themselves. Their cytoplasm may even be relatively nondescript.

Organs of the body are aggregates of the shades and varieties of the basic tissues, blended by appropriate shaping, quantity, and proportion to assume the specialized functions for which organs have evolved. Their construction and synergistic activities can best be appreciated by consideration of embryonic stages when the tissues' relationships are simple and just emerging.

In the chapters ahead, first the basic tissues and then the organs of the body will be examined, not only in terms of final adult microscopic anatomy but also in relation to the embryonic processes and relationships which led to that eventual form. It will be found that adult cells still contain certain organelles which controlled their individual and collective shaping during the embryonic life of their tissue or organ. Likewise it will be seen how both intracellular and extracellular components have gradually been mobilized, first to ensure the inductive tissue interactions controlling development and second, to stabilize and retain the emerging parts of the new individual into its complex, definitive adult form.

References

AREY, L. B. Developmental Anatomy, Ed. 7. W. B. Saunders Company, Philadelphia, 1965.

BONNER, J. T. The Evolution of Development. Cambridge University Press, London, New York, 1958.

GASSER, R. F. Atlas of Human Embryos. Harper and Row, Hagerstown, Maryland, 1975.

HAMILTON, W. J., BOYD, J. D., AND MOSSMAN, H. W. Human Embryology, Ed. 4. Williams & Wilkins, Baltimore, 1972.

HAY, E. D. Organization and fine structure of epithelium and mesenchyme in the developing chick embryo. Chapt. 2. In Epithelial-Mesenchymal Interactions (Fleishmajer, R., and Billingham, R. E., editors), pp. 31–55. Williams & Wilkins, Baltimore, 1968.

JOHNSON, K. E. Gastrulation and cell interactions. Chapt. 6. In Concepts of Developmental Biology. (Lash, J., and Whittaker, J. R., editors), pp. 128–148. Sinauer Assoc., Inc., Stamford, Conn, 1974.

LANGMAN, J. Medical Embryology, Ed. 3. Williams & Wilkins, Baltimore, 1975.

LASH, J. Tissue interactions and related subjects. Chapt. 10. In Concepts of Development. (Lash, J., and Whittaker, J. R., editors), pp. 197–212. Sinauer Assoc., Inc., Stamford, Conn, 1974.

MOORE, K. L. The Developing Human. Ed. 2. W. B. Saunders Company, Philadelphia, 1977.

PATTEN, B. M. Human Embryology, Ed. 3. McGraw-Hill Book Company, New York, 1968.

SPOONER, B. S. Morphogenesis of vertebrate organs. Chapt. 11. In Concepts of Developmental Biology. (Lash, J. and Whittaker, J. R., editors), pp. 213–240. Sinauer Assoc., Inc., Stamford, Conn, 1974.

CHAPTER 4

Epithelium

Chapter 2 has dealt primarily with *cells* as structural and functional units. Basic information on the constituents commonly found in all cells as well as some of the specializations have been discussed. Through the process of cellular differentiation, maturing cells also come to exhibit different and often unique degrees in the development of specific organelles and other cytoplasmic components, and differences in the quantity and quality of extracellular products which they produce. A *tissue* may be defined as a collection of cells and associated intercellular materials specialized for a particular function or functions. It follows, then, that a tissue is the product of the sum total of the properties of its constituent cells. Usually the cells of a given tissue in a given region are relatively uniform in their properties, but from region to region the cellular properties vary, and likewise a given tissue shows gradations in its properties from region to region. Tissues are combined in appropriate patterns and proportions to form *organs*. The organs and organ systems are the subjects of later chapters.

The fundamental properties and patterns of tissues are the subjects of this and the next six chapters. For convenience, tissues are broadly classified into four basic categories: (1) epithelia, (2) connective and supportive tissues, including blood and lymph, (3) contractile tissues (muscle), and (4) nervous tissue. This categorization is tra-

ditional and useful, but there are important overlaps in function. For example, the nervous tissue of the brain and spinal cord can itself be considered an epithelium, a number of epithelial cells are known to display at least subtle degrees of contractility, and in the thymus a major supportive function is carried out by the epithelial component.

In chapter 3 the earliest multicellular stages of an embryo were seen to consist of closely adherent cells. These are shortly segregated into definable layers. Hence, the earliest beginnings of a new individual can be said to be epithelial, because an epithelium may be defined as a layered collection of adherent cells, with very little intercellular material, usually covering internal and external surfaces of the body. It was seen that ectodermal and endodermal epithelial layers cover the external surface of the embryo and its earliest manifestations of a gut. Moreover, and very importantly, these same layers serve as boundaries and seals for the mesenchymal compartment expanding between them. Hence, adhesion in an epithelial system is important not only for the maintenance of topographic integrity but also for the provision of relatively leak-proof seals for the compartments surrounded by those epithelia.

As the organism matures, epithelium covers the outer surfaces of the body as epidermis. Other epithelia line all passages leading to the exterior (the linings of the digestive, respiratory, and urogenital systems, and numerous glands). Epithelia also line most of the closed cavities of the body. Most of these are derived by cavitation of mesenchymal tissues. Their lining epithelial cells are of mesodermal origin. More specifically, the epithelial linings of the pleural, pericardial, and peritoneal cavities are known as *mesothelia,* in view of their mesodermal origin. Likewise the lining of blood and lymphatic vessels is also an epithelium of mesodermal origin. Curiously, this lining has come to be known as *endothelium.*

During development, many embryonic epithelia send invaginating growths into the underlying connective tissues. Many such epithelial invaginations form the parenchymal (functional epithelial) components of glands. These usually contain cavities or passages leading to the surface from which they grew. They are termed exocrine glands (see chapter 15), because the passageway (duct) provides an exit for the products of the epithelial glandular cells. In some of the ingrowths, however, the connection is lost, and deeply lying epithelial cords, follicles, or aggregates of cells are produced and maintained, in spite of the loss of their passages or ducts. Because they must release their secreted products into surrounding connective tissue and thence into the nearby vascular passageways, these are termed *endocrine* glands (see chapter 21).

Epithelia serve widely differing functional demands in different locations. On the surface of the body or along the alimentary canal they are subjected to abrasion, attrition, and drying, and provide protection against these physical demands. In less exposed locations, as in the closed body cavities, the epithelium (mesothelium) is subjected to but little attrition and is covered with a fluid film; in these locations it forms smooth surfaces which glide over each other. In still other locations, epithelia serve not only for protection but also for secretion and absorption. An epithelium may be adapted to great changes in surface area, as in the distensible urinary bladder. Most epithelia are active mitotically throughout the life of the individual, constantly replacing cells which are lost in the normal course of function. In correlation

with the differences in all of these functional demands, there are marked differences in epithelial structure. The epithelia vary in cellular shape, in number of cell layers, in physical and structural characteristics, in their mode of attachment to each other, in their relative mitotic activity, and in their secretory or absorptive potential. In some rather localized circumstances epithelial cells display highly specialized morphology related to sensory reception. It is remarkable that with all of these specialized activities and structural variations, the cells of epithelia maintain themselves as a closely adherent population serving as an appropriately sealed barrier to fluids and other substances which might otherwise leak between the cells and cross the epithelium without being selectively recognized and transported by the cells themselves. More remarkable still is the recently emerging evidence that neighboring cells of many epithelia are in ionic or metabolic communication, i.e., able to signal each other by intercytoplasmic transfer of specific ions or molecules. Hence the cells of epithelia appear to be both physically and functionally adherent and interdependent.

Classification

Because epithelia line surfaces and cavities, they commonly have a free margin which faces the outside environment or the lumen of a particular organ, and a surface which faces underlying or surrounding connective tissue. The free margin is termed the *apical* surface or pole of the epithelium, and the connective tissue-facing pole is termed the *basal* surface. The surfaces of cells which face neighboring epithelial cells within an epithelium are sometimes referred to as the *lateral* cell surfaces. In nearly all epithelia (with some outstanding exceptions), the cells bordering the basal surface secrete a submicroscopically thin extracellular coat, the *basal lamina* (the structure of which is discussed in detail later) along that surface. It serves to separate the epithelium from underlying connective tissue. When the basal lamina is reinforced by layers of connective tissue collagen, the total structure becomes thick enough to be discerned by light microscopy and is referred to as a *basement membrane.*

For convenience, epithelia are classified into different types on the basis of the number of cell layers and the shape of the cells at the apical surface; thus, epithelia of only one layer are termed *simple,* and they are subdivided according to the height of the cells when viewed in cross section, into *simple squamous, simple cuboidal,* and *simple columnar* (Table 4-1 and Fig. 4-1). One often notes cell heights which fall intermediate to those defined strictly by the above terms. The lateral margins of cells also outline specific shapes in many epithelia, although this characteristic is not frequently used in classification. Mesothelial cells, for example (Fig. 4-2), display fairly regular lateral surfaces, whereas the equally simple epithelial cells of kidney tubules have lateral surfaces that are tortuously interdigitated with those of their neighbors (Fig. 18-15).

An epithelium composed of two or more layers is said to be *stratified,* and is subdivided according to thè shape of the cells at the apical surface into *stratified squamous, stratified cuboidal,* and *stratified columnar.* Stratified squamous epithelium is the most commonly found stratified type. In it, only the upper layers are squamous; those along the basal lamina and for a considerable distance above it are columnar and polyhedral (Figs. 4-1 and 14-4). The cells of the basal areas are frequently mitotically active, serving to replenish the layers above. Moreover, the functions served by the cells of various layers may be quite different. This is particularly true in the epidermis of the skin (chapter 14).

The epithelium of some parts of the body consists of a single layer of cells of variable height and arrangement, with all cells resting on the basement membrane, but with only some of the cells reaching the apical surface. The nuclei of these cells are seen at different levels above the basement membrane and, on first inspection, one might conclude that the epithelium is stratified. Only careful study discloses that this epithelium is really composed of only one layer of cells. It has been traditionally classified as *pseudostratified* (Fig. 4-1).

A special modification of stratified epithelium is found in the urinary system, where the number of cell layers and the shapes of the cells vary with distention and contraction of the organ. This type of epithelium is classified as *transitional* (Fig. 4-1).

In addition to the above criteria for classification, epithelia are often described in terms of products they accumulate or release, or in terms of cellular appendages that may characterize the apical surface. Hence, an epithelium which has a high population of specialized cells which syn-

TABLE 4-1

Types of epithelium

No. of cell layers	Shape of surface cell	Examples of location in the body
Simple (one layer of cells)	Squamous	Endothelium of blood vessels, mesothelium of body cavities, thin segment of Henle's loop in kidney
	Cuboidal	Some kidney tubules
	Columnar	Gastrointestinal tract
Pseudostratified (modification of simple; not all cells reach the surface)	Columnar	Trachea, parts of male reproductive system
Stratified (more than one layer of cells)	Squamous	Epidermis, lining of esophagus, vagina
	Cuboidal	Infrequent; found in duct of sweat gland
	Columnar	Infrequent; found in parts of epiglottis and in the male urethra
Transitional (variety of stratified; varies with distention)	Surface cell varies from dome shape in contracted organ to flat in distended state	Lining of renal pelvis, ureter, urinary bladder, and parts of urethra

EPITHELIUM

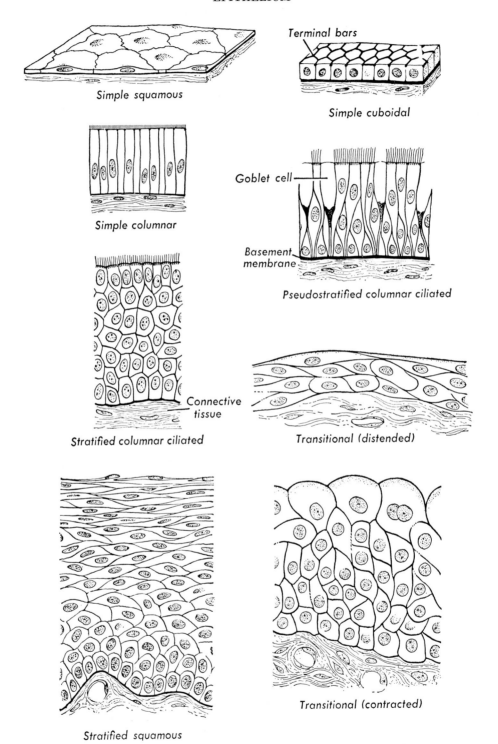

Fig. 4-1. Schematic representation of the various morphological types of epithelium. In each case, the epithelium is shown with some of the underlying connective tissue.

thesize and release mucus into the apical surface (goblet cells) can be termed a *mucous* epithelium. Likewise, because the cells of the apical epidermis accumulate high concentrations of a tough proteinaceous material called *keratin,* this epithelium can be said to be *keratinized.* When the apical surface of an epithelium bears cilia, particularly if they are numerous, the epithelium is said to be *ciliated.* If the same surface possesses large numbers of more minute projections, the *microvilli,* the epithelium is said to have a "striated," "brush," or *microvillous* border.

Combining these various schemes, it is common to describe an epithelium in rather complex fashion. For example, the epidermis of the skin is termed *stratified squamous keratinized epithelium* and the lining of the trachea is a *pseudostratified ciliated columnar epithelium.* The lining epithelium of the intestine is a *simple columnar epithelium* displaying a striated *microvillous* border.

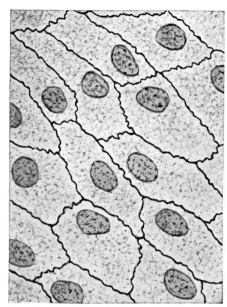

Fig. 4-2. Surface view of mesothelium of mesentery treated with silver nitrate. The cells are sharply outlined by the silver deposit. ×550.

Special Cytological Characteristics

Virtually all substances which enter or leave the body or its components must cross one or several epithelia. Often, materials are sequestered within epithelia to be converted by the cells into specific products. These are subsequently released either apically or basally (see exocytosis, chapter 1). The organelles of epithelial cells are appropriately arranged in a polarized fashion to promote these directional processes; i.e., the cells contain a polarized cytoplasmic content. For example, the Golgi apparatus and accumulated secretion droplets are polarized between the nucleus and the apical border in the parenchymal cells of many epithelial glands. Similarly, rows of mitochondria are arranged between the nucleus and a highly infolded basal surface of the simple epithelial linings in kidney tubules, as part of a polarized mechanism for the pumping of ions across the epithelium. The apical surfaces of many simple epithelia are adorned with cilia and microvilli, whereas such structures are rarely found basally. In stratified epithelia, the progression of young cells from a mitotically active basal

region to replace older cells toward the apex, finally to be cast off at that surface themselves, is also a reflection of epithelial polarization in a somewhat broader sense. Collectively, the polarizations inherent in the many epithelia of an organism underscore the unidirectionality of fluxes necessary to the homeostasis of the many compartments comprising that organism.

The above discussion implies also that the cells of epithelia attain and maintain rather specific shapes. Maintenance of a specific cell shape is requisite not only to the functional polarity of an epithelial cell but also to the mechanical integrity of the epithelium as a whole. Subtle or elaborate cytoskeletal networks of filaments provide an internal scaffolding for this function, and it may be especially well developed in those epithelia that resist wear and tear (for example, the stratified squamous epithelia). This cytoskeleton is composed of 80- to 120-Å cytoplasmic filaments (often termed *intermediate filaments* or *tonofilaments*) which are woven in specific patterns to resist, again on a polarized basis, the forces most frequently applied to the cells. As will be seen, the cytoskeleton is intimately connected to the points of intercellular adhesion within an epithelium.

Other networks of much finer cytoplasmic filaments, the so-called "microfilaments," are also found in epithelial cells. They are well developed components of the more pliable epithelia, epithelia in which absorption or secretion seems emphasized. In fact, much recent evidence strongly suggests that at least some of these microfilamentous populations are actually contractile and exert changes in the shapes of the epithelial cells as a part of normal day-to-day function. Microfilaments are particularly prominent just beneath the microvillous apices of many epithelial cells involved in absorption. It is now believed that they not only control the apical diameter of a given cell but may also be involved with subtle movements of the microvilli themselves. During embryonic stages, the shapes of epithelial invaginations and evaginations are probably promoted by microfilaments within the constituent epithelial cells acting in harmony to provide a very specific result. Again, the shapes achieved and maintained within individual cells through this type of "cytomuscular" activity reflects further the propensity for polarization shown by epithelial cells.

Intercellular Attachment

Most cells invest their plasma membranes to some degree with a glycoprotein or glycosaminoglycan surface coat (sometimes referred to as "glycocalyx"). In epithelia the deposition of this coat may be highly polarized, as seen in the formation of basal lamina. When deposited on the lateral surfaces of epithelial cells, these coatings are much thinner, but they may promote some degree of cell-to-cell adhesion. This type of adhesion seems especially important during initial embryonic stages when the first few cells of an embryo are prevented from dispersing. Rather quickly, however, the early epithelial cells of an embryonic system become attached by firmer sites of intercellular adhesion. These not only serve the function of cell-to-cell mechanical anchorage but also provide the mechanism to seal the epithelial system against the escape of fluids between adjacent cells. Ironically, some of them also provide channels for ionic communication and flux between the cytoplasms of adjacent cells. The details of these attachment mechanisms are submicroscopic and have had to await detailed study by electron microscopy. We know now that a wide spectrum of attachment morphology exists in nature, but for convenience we have classified them into several prominent groups (Fig. 4-3).

One of the most frequent and earliest known types of epithelial attachments is referred to either as a *desmosome* (from the Greek *desmos*, bond, + *soma*, body) or as a *macula adherens* (from the Latin *macula*, spot, + *adhaereo*, to stick). Desmosomes are particularly numerous in stratified epithelium, where they are large and numerous enough to be described from light microscope studies as "intercellular bridges." Their distinctness is often accentuated by preparative techniques which cause the cells to shrink and pull apart except in these regions of adhesion. Electron micrographs show that these are not true bridges, and, in fact, a space of about 200 to 250 Å separates the apposing cell membranes in the desmosomal junction (Fig. 4-4). The cell membrane itself is no thicker in this region than elsewhere, but it may appear so because in each of the adjacent cells there is a dense proteinaceous plaque of cytoplasmic material subjacent to and parallel with the cell membrane (Figs. 4-5 and 4-6). Desmosomes are visible by light microscopy because numerous tonofilaments converge in the region of these plaques and are apparently attached to the plaques and the cell membranes at that point. It was once thought that the tonofilaments terminate at that point or perhaps even proceed into the ad-

Fig. 4-3. Schematic diagram of the range of junctional variation known to exist in cells, based on electron microscopic evidence. The plasma membranes of two apposed cells are depicted, one of which has been split over a short segment at left. There, one leaflet is folded back to display intramembranous components revealed by freeze fracture techniques. The intercalated disc type of junction is characteristic of cardiac muscle, and the chemical synapse is found between neurons; these are discussed in detail in the chapters on muscle and nervous tissue. Septate junctions are found primarily in epithelia of invertebrates. See text for descriptions of each junctional variation.

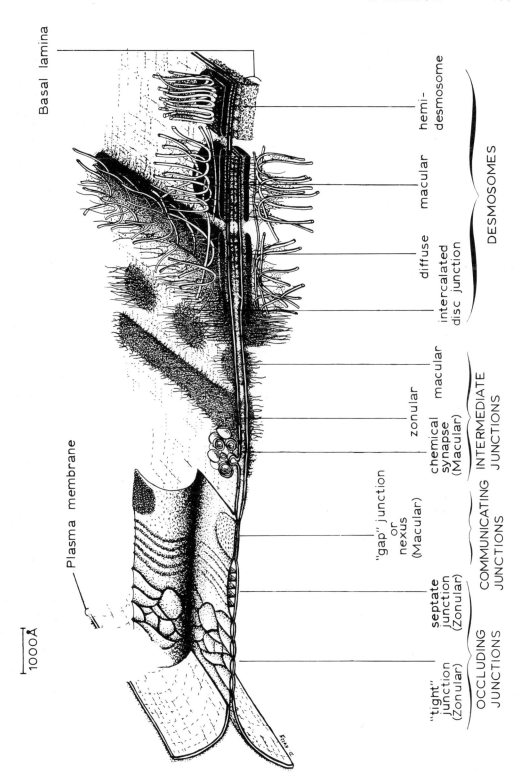

SPECTRUM OF JUNCTIONAL FINE STRUCTURE

1000 Å

Basal lamina

Plasma membrane

hemi-
desmosome

macular

diffuse

intercalated
disc junction

macular

zonular

chemical
synapse
(Macular)

"gap" junction
or
nexus
(Macular)

septate
junction
(Zonular)

"tight"
junction
(Zonular)

DESMOSOMES

INTERMEDIATE
JUNCTIONS

COMMUNICATING
JUNCTIONS

OCCLUDING
JUNCTIONS

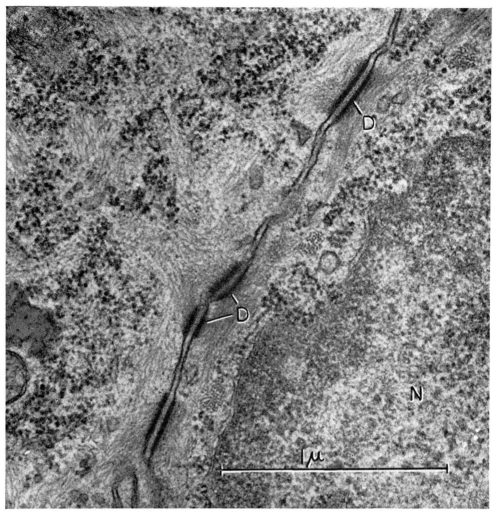

Fig. 4-4. Electron micrograph showing attachments between epithelial cells of stratified epithelium of esophagus of bat. *D*, desmosome or macula adherens; *N*, nucleus. Fine tonofilaments can be seen in the cytoplasm adjacent to the desmosomes and in other regions of the cytoplasm. ×64,000. (Courtesy of Dr. Keith Porter.)

jacent cell, but further studies of high resolution electron micrographs have indicated that many or most of these filaments form shallow or hairpin loops that turn backward into the cytoplasm (Fig. 4-5). In some desmosomes, the filaments course nearly parallel to the plaque, apparently attached to it en route (Fig. 4-6).

The eventual terminus for individual tonofilaments is not known. The extracellular space of desmosomes is filled with an abundance of sialic acid-rich mucoprotein which apparently serves as a strong adhesive, anchoring the membranes of adjacent cells.

It typically displays a dense intermediate line in electron micrographs. This is interpreted by some workers as representing an overlap of the adhesive contribution of the adjacent cells.

It can be seen from the above description that desmosomes represent focalized sites of relatively firm adhesion between adjacent cells, but they are also the focalized sites for anchorage, to cell membranes, of the cytoskeletal filaments within adjacent cells. When viewed over the extent of a given epithelium, it can be seen that the desmosomal-cytoskeletal network within

Looping
tonofilaments

Plasma membrane

dense plaque

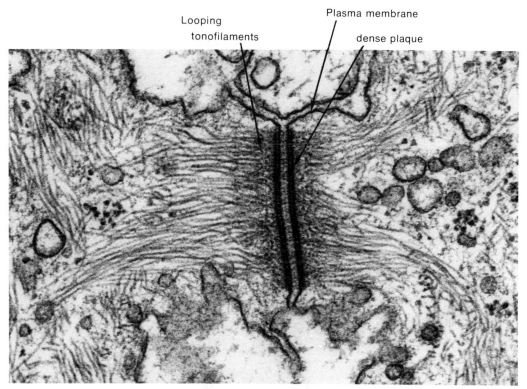

Fig. 4-5. Electron micrograph of a desmosome from stratified squamous epithelium. Note the cell membrane and the presence of an electron-dense plaque in each cell subjacent to the inner layer of the plasmalemma at the level of the desmosome. Tonofilaments of the cytoplasm form loops at or in the dense plaque of the desmosome. In this picture, a thin electron-lucent line can be seen between the dense plaque and the inner border of the cell membrane. Note that a discontinuous midline is present in the material within the intercellular space at the desmosome. From the epidermis of a newt; ×81,000.

an epithelium forms a well engineered, girder-like supportive system for the epithelium.

In the basal cells of an epithelium, this network extends to the basal cell membrane also, although that membrane is not lying adjacent to a neighboring cell, but rather to the basal lamina and underlying connective tissue substrata. Along that surface are found *hemidesmosomes,* which in general morphology closely resemble one-half of the desmosome described above (Fig. 4-7). There are, in fact, notable differences in the morphology of hemidesmosomes as compared to desmosomes, but the main relationships among tonofilaments, plaques, cell membranes, and extracellular adhesive material follow similar principles. Hemidesmosomes are believed to be basal anchorage sites for cytoskeletal filaments and

adhesion points for the basal cell membrane to the basal lamina and connective tissue.

Freeze fracture studies disclose aggregates of intramembranous particles within the leaflets of desmosomal cell membranes (Figs. 4-8 and 4-11). There is some reason to suspect that a mechanism exists for attaching tonofilaments and plaques into the cell membranes, possibly involving these particles, but the exact details of such a mechanism are not fully understood. Hemidesmosomes have also been shown in some species to display intramembranous particles, often of larger individual diameter clustered at the hemidesmosomal site (Fig. 4-8).

Desmosomes are most frequent in those epithelia that resist wear and tear and, as would be expected, in those epithelia that contain the most complex and highly

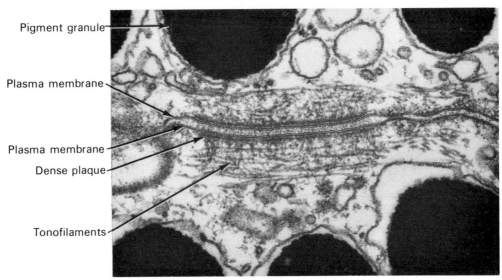

Fig. 4-6. Electron micrograph of a desmosome from epithelium of iris. The outer leaflet of the plasma membrane is specifically more distinct as a result of staining en bloc with uranyl acetate. Note that the tonofilaments approach the desmosome in a horizontal direction, in contrast with the pattern seen in Figure 4-5. See Figure 4-3 for variations of desmosomes. Iris of newt. ×90,000. (Courtesy of Dr. A. Tonosaki).

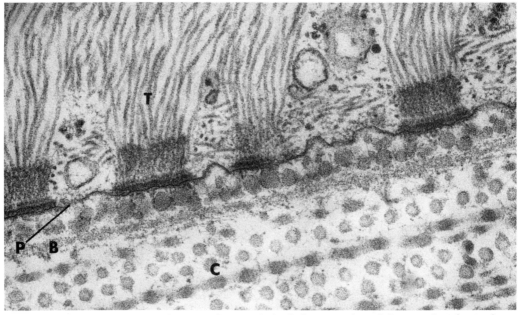

Fig. 4-7. High magnification electron micrograph depicting a portion of the most basal cytoplasm of a basal epidermal cell from a larval salamander. The cytoplasm occupying the upper one-half of the micrograph is separated by a plasmalemma (P) from the underlying dermis (lower half of the micrograph). A basal lamina (B) and layered collagen fibrils (C) support the epidermis. Four hemidesmosomes are recognizable as densities along the plasmalemma. Bundles of tonofilaments (T) converge toward each hemidesmosomal plaque. Presumably, each hemidesmosome is a point of attachment of tonofilaments to the basal plasmalemma and attachment of the plasmalemma to the underlying basal lamina and collagenous substrata. A peculiar, globular lipid-rich layer lies between basal lamina and plasmalemma at this stage of development in this animal. ×74,500.

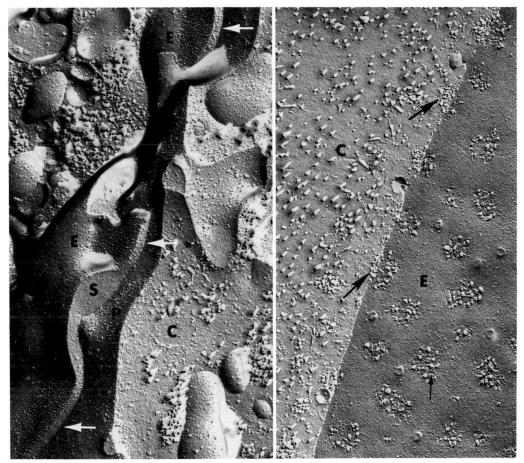

Fig. 4-8. Electron micrographs of freeze fracture replicas of desmosomes (*left figure*) and hemidesmosomes (*right figure*). In the figure at *left*, the fracture plane has passed through the cytoplasms (*C*) of the first of two adjacent epithelial cells. The same fracture next exposes the P-face (*P*) of the plasmalemma of that cell before passing through extracellular space (S) and the E-face (*E*) of the plasmalemma of the adjacent cell. The cytoplasm of that cell is exposed in the *upper left corner*. The fracture plane has passed through three desmosomes (*white arrows*). At these desmosomal sites, it can be seen that closely packed granules occupy the E-faces but are not seen along the P-faces. Hemidesmosomes are similarly revealed in the freeze fracture image to the *right*. The fracture plane has passed through the tonofilament-rich basal cytoplasm (*C*) of an epithelial cell before splitting the basal membrane of that cell to reveal its E-face (*E*). Clusters of densely packed filamentous material can be seen in the cytoplasm adjacent to the cell membrane in the regions of the hemidesmosomes (*large arrows*). Clusters of granules (*small arrow*) are seen on the E-face at points corresponding to hemidesmosomal attachment. Left figure—×55,800; right figure—×45,500. (Micrographs in collaboration with Frances Shienvold).

evolved cytoskeletal filamentous networks.

Nearly all epithelia display a prominent circle of close apposition around the apical neck of each cell which very firmly attaches it to its neighbors. The adjective *zonular* is used to describe this collar-like ring of attachment in contrast to the *macular* or "spot weld" configuration described above for desmosomes. Light microscopists could easily discern this attachment collar in whole mount preparations of mesothelia when the preparations were viewed from the apical aspect and particularly when they were impregnated with silver (Fig. 4-2). In transverse sections the attachment collar appears as a series of distinct spots at the apical margins of each individual cell (Fig. 4-1). The light microscopists termed this attachment collar the *terminal bar, a* designation which is presently in disuse and often replaced by *"junctional complex"* in view of much more detailed knowledge of the components to be found in this region.

In most instances the terminal bar or attachment collar region contains two or sometimes three or four distinct types of attachments (Fig. 4-9). The most universal is the *tight junction* or *zonula occludens.* This tight or occluding junction constitutes the principal seal against passage, between cells, of extracellular materials which might otherwise cross the epithelium. It may be extensively developed along the lateral apical surfaces of cells that are highly impermeable to such passage or it may be sparse and discontinuous in the case of certain epithelia which are relatively and appropriately "leaky." In electron micrographs of transversely sectioned tight junctions (Figs. 4-10 and 4-19), the essential component of the junction is a punctate region where the outer dense leaflet of the cell membrane of one cell comes into direct apposition with that of its neighbor. There

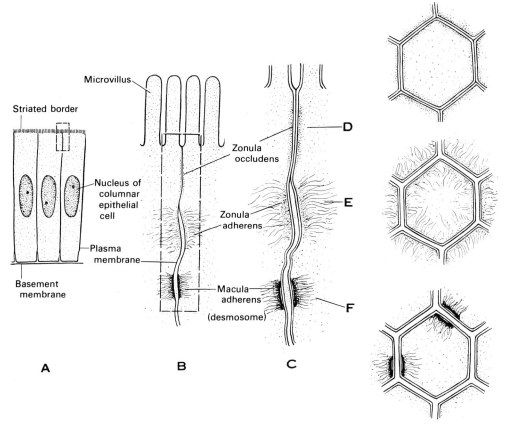

Fig. 4-9. Diagrams of a junctional complex between the adluminal ends of columnar epithelial cells. *A*, the interrelationships of simple columnar epithelial cells of the small intestine as determined by light microscopy. *B*, the structure of the juxtaluminal complex of the region outlined in *A* as determined by electron microscopy. *C*, further details of the junction as determined by high magnification and high resolution electron micrographs. *D, E,* and *F*, the different regions of the junctional complex in transverse sections. Note that the outer leaflets of the plasmalemma of adjacent cells are in contact around the entire circumference of the cell in the region of the zonula occludens, whereas they are separated by a uniform width around the circumference of the cell in the zonula adherens. The maculae adherentes of the junctional complex consist of spots of adhesion. Note that the diagrams of cross sections show the plasmalemma enlarged out of proportion to the cell area; at a similar magnification, the latter would cover more than the width of the page.

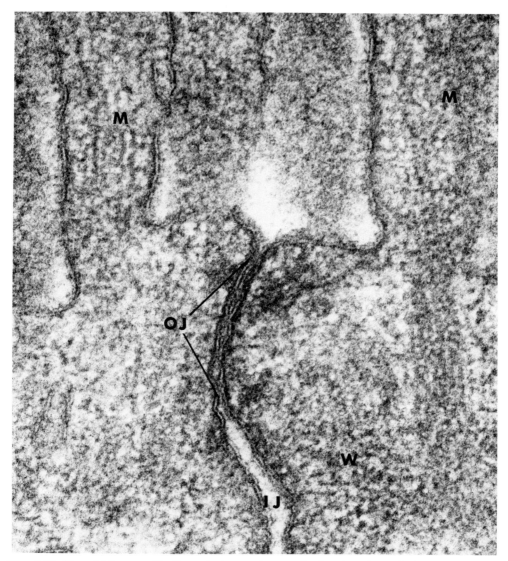

Fig. 4-10. Very high magnification electron micrograph showing the apical junctional region between two intestinal cells of a rat. Microvilli (*M*) of the adjacent cells are visible at the top of the picture. They are covered by plasmalemma which is continuous over the opposed junctional surfaces in the lower center. The section plane has passed through an occluding junction (*OJ*) and an intermediate junction (*IJ*). Microfilaments of the terminal web (*W*) are seemingly attached to the cell membranes at the intermediate junction. The occluding junction displays intermittent points of fusion between the outer leaflets of the plasmalemmas of the two adjacent cells. ×225,000. (Courtesy of Dr. David Chase.)

may be only one or two such points apparent between the cells of leaky epithelia (e.g., kidney proximal tubule), but in relatively impermeable epithelia (e.g., urinary bladder) many such points of apposition are usually found. Freeze fracture study of the membranes in the regions of tight junctions discloses that these points of apposition are really points along ridgelike elevations of the cell surface which fuse with complementary ridges on the surface of the neighboring cell. When viewed face-on in a fracture replica, these ridges form networks of variable extent. In the leaky epithelia there are but a few ridges and they may be discontinuous, whereas in the impermeable epithelia there may be row upon row of such intertwining ridges (Fig. 4-11). Because freeze fracture splits the cell membrane it will be appreciated that the profile of a tight junction consists of ridges on the P-face and corresponding grooves on the E-face. If one were able to look at the true external surface of the cell one would also see ridges. There is current debate as to whether the ridges represent joined members supplied by both cells or a common member shared by the two cells. In either case it is relatively easy to see how this network of adjoined linear elevations along the surfaces of adjacent cells could effectively occlude the potential passageway between them.

Interestingly, the epithelia of invertebrate species display a strikingly different junction in this location. It is termed the *septate junction* because of the presence of multiple parallel ridges of intercellular structure between the adjacent cells. It too is believed to provide a seal against the flux of extracellular materials across the epithelium.

Closely associated with the tight junction region of epithelia is the *intermediate junction* (or *zonula adherens*). This junctional area also encircles the apical-lateral margin of the cells; hence its designation as *zonular* (Figs. 4-10, 4-11, and 4-19). It is also a site of relatively firm adhesion between the adjacent cells, and it displays an extracellular space of about 150 Å. The space contains a mucoprotein adhesive material, although not in the apparent abundance seen in desmosomes. The cytoplasms of the apposed cells at intermediate junctions display a density, but this density is not so distinct

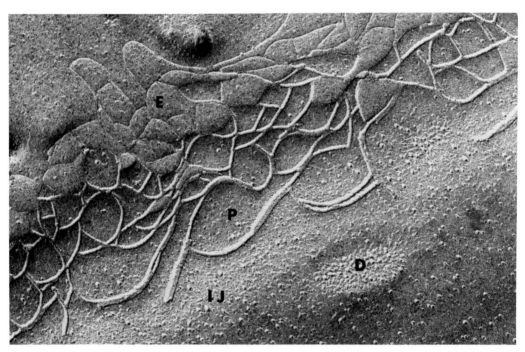

Fig. 4-11. Electron micrograph of a freeze fracture replica taken through the membranes of the apical junctional region of two adjacent cells like those depicted in Figure 4-10. In the *upper left* of the micrograph the fracture plane has split the plasmalemma of one cell, exposing its E-face (*E*). In a line coursing diagonally from the *upper right* to the *lower left* corner of the micrograph, the fracture plane has deviated into the plasmalemma of the adjacent cell, revealing its P-face (*P*) over the *lower right half* of the micrograph. The region of the occluding junction is revealed as a series of entangled grooves on the E-face and corresponding ridges on the P-face of the neighboring cell membranes. The area along the plasmalemma occupied by the intermediate junction (*IJ*) appears somewhat lighter but not otherwise distinctive. An aggregation of granules demarks the location of a desmosome (*D*). Note also widely scattered membrane particles over the exposed P-face. ×84,000.

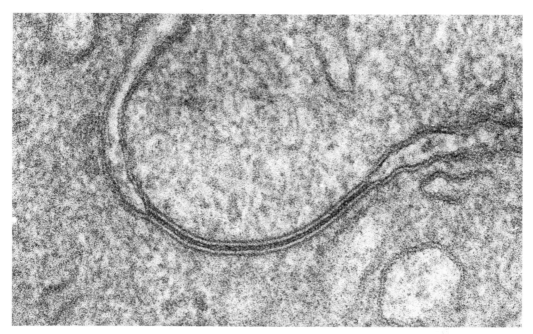

Fig. 4-12. High magnification electron micrograph showing a communicating (gap) junction between two adjacent liver cells of a rat. The cell membranes of neighboring hepatocytes comes into very close proximity in a region shown in the center of the micrograph. Close inspection discloses a 20- to 40-Å gap between the membranes in this region. ×220,000. (Courtesy of Dr. Norton B. Gilula.)

as the plaques of desmosomes. It appears to be the anchorage point for another system of cytoplasmic filaments often concentrated within the apical cytoplasm of these cells, the so-called *terminal web*. Unlike the larger tonofilaments associated with desmosomes, the terminal web filaments are of the *microfilament* variety (less than 80 Å in diameter). The terminal web is particularly well developed in cells that display a microvillous apical border; it is suspected of containing the contractile proteins *actin* and *myosin* and may be involved in minute shape changes at the apex of these cells or within the microvilli themselves. Microfilaments, either continuous or associated with the terminal web, extend as cores into microvilli, where they terminate at the apical tips of those structures. In developing epithelia that are undergoing morphogenetic cell shape changes, similar areas of microfilamentous attachments are found along apical and other surfaces of the cells. Their positioning appears to relate to the specific shapes that will be assumed by the cells as the result of the contractile activity of those microfilaments.

The fourth type of intercellular junction frequently found in epithelia is the "*communicating junction*" (also designated *gap junction, nexus,* or *close junction*). For many years after the introduction of electron microscopy for the study of epithelial junctions, this junction went unrecognized because of its close similarity to regions of tight junctions (Fig. 4-12). When epithelia were treated with small molecular weight, electron-dense tracer particles such as lanthanum (Fig. 4-13) or horseradish peroxidase, it was found that these materials did not penetrate an intercellular space guarded by a tight junction. However, such tracer materials were able to percolate between the two apposed membranes of nearby regions which previously had appeared very similar to the tight junction. It was then recognized that in these latter regions there is a narrow extracellular gap of about 20 Å between the adjacent cells.

Face-on views of such "gap junctions" after treatment with tracer materials revealed the junctional area to be macular in form and also disclosed that the tracer percolates through the gap following a min-

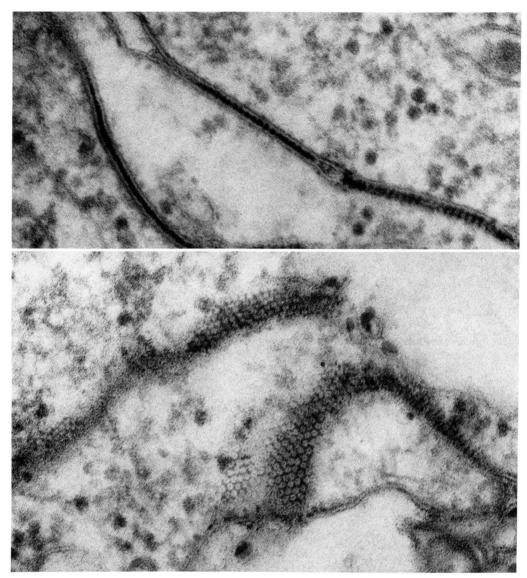

Fig. 4-13. Electron micrographs of communicating (gap) junctions in an invertebrate (*Hydra*). The tissue has been treated with a lanthanum impregnation technique. In the *upper figure,* a colloidal form of the heavy metal lanthanum has been deposited between the adjacent cell membranes of the junctions and appears dense in this cross section micrograph. Lanthanum thereby delineates the intercellular gap, which in this animal is about 40 Å wide. It also reveals in negative image regularly arranged bridging components between the adjacent cell membranes. The bridging components are seen to better effect in the *lower figure,* where the plane of section is parallel to the plane of junction. The bridging components appear as doughnut-shaped profiles arranged in a regular hexagonal array. Lanthanum has percolated into the intercellular space remaining between the bridging components. Both figures ×189,000.

ute hexagonal pattern. Similar images were obtained when areas of gap junction were isolated from epithelial cells and stained with sodium phosphotungstate. Close in-spection of the hexagonal array seen in such face-on views suggests that the junc-tion contains hexagonally arranged sub-units with a center-to-center spacing of about 90 Å. The tracer particles seem to percolate through narrow passages between the subunits.

Freeze fracture study of these junctions confirms such interpretations. When split in the fracture process and replicated, the membranes of gap junctions reveal tightly packed intramembranous particles (Fig. 4-14). In some preparations these are arranged in an hexagonal array along the P-face. The E-face usually displays a complementary array of pits for these particles. There have been a number of interpretations offered as to the molecular arrangement of the proteins presumably comprising the particles and their relationship to the cell membranes. One current model is shown in Figure 4-15. This model depicts the possibility that the particles are manifestations of protein complexes which span the width of each apposed cell membrane and extend extracellularly far enough to join an equivalent member from the adjacent cell. The narrow extracellular space is continuous between the tiny pillars provided by the apposition of these protein complexes. It will be noted that the authors of this model have also portrayed hydrophilic channels coursing through the center of the protein complexes. The presence of such channels is occasionally suggested by the presence of a small dimple or dot in the center of the particles seen in freeze fracture preparations, or a linear density across the membrane in certain special thin sections viewed by transmission electron microscopy. Such images suggest the presence of a communicating pore of approximately 20 Å diameter. However, much more powerful physiological evidence supports the conclusion that some form of an intercytoplasmic channel exists.

It had been known for some years before the discovery of gap junctions that the cytoplasms of cells within a number of epithelia must be ionically coupled. This property can be detected by the insertion of microelectrodes into adjacent epithelial cells or even epithelial cells several cells apart. In either case, an ionic flux can often be detected between the cells under test. This suggests that there are channels interconnecting the cytoplasm of one cell to that

of its neighbor and that these channels are of such minute proportions as to allow only the passage of materials of ionic or small molecular dimensions. Impedance studies indicate the pore diameter to be about 10 Å. Since high calcium concentrations in the cell block ionic flux, this ion may regulate the activity of the pores. The passage of certain low molecular weight (up to approximately 500 to 1100) fluorescent tracers, fluorescein and procion yellow, has subsequently also been demonstrated, and these theoretically require a channel of between 3.5 and 16 Å. Hence, all of the various measurements point toward pore diameters of nearly equivalent ranges.

A number of authors have postulated that such ionic exchanges among cells might serve as mechanisms for coordination of epithelial activities or signals to promote specified changes or new directions during developmental processes. Theoretically, certain ions or other small molecular molecules, such as nucleotides, exchanged between coupled cells should be small enough to be moved very rapidly and yet large enough to carry some reasonably specific code. It has been calculated that a molecular weight of from 300 to 500 falls into the ideal range.

Whereas ionic coupling between epithelial cells has been known from physiological evidence for some time, the exact site of the exchange could not be immediately ascertained. Junctions other than gap junctions have been suspected in the past, but mounting circumstantial evidence has lessened the likelihood that any of them are involved in this activity—at least in vertebrate tissues. Hence, the term "communicating junction" has become a common replacement for gap junction. Investigations utilizing mechanical or chemical dissociation of epithelial cells show that, like tight junctions and desmosomes, communicating junctions are also relatively firm sites of adhesion between adjacent cells. We can infer therefore that in communicating junctions a strong anchorage is maintained between adjacent cells to insure an appropriate level of ionic flux.

Strong morphological and physiological evidence points to the existence of com-

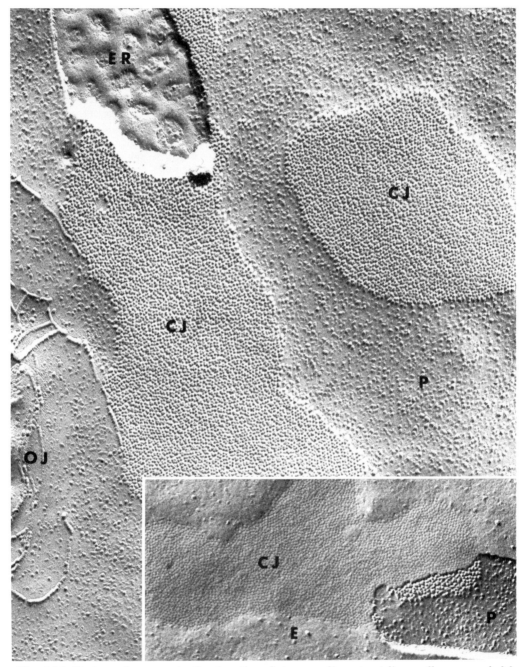

Fig. 4-14. Regions of communicating junctions between adjacent rat liver cells as revealed by freeze fracture and electron microscopy. In the *upper figure* the P-face (*P*) has been exposed to reveal closely packed particles in the region of two communicating junctions (*CJ*). A nearby region of occluding junction (*OJ*) is seen at left. In the *upper part* of the figure, the fracture plane has diverted into the cytoplasm of the liver cell to expose the split membrane surfaces of the endoplasmic reticulum (*ER*). In the *lower figure* the fracture plane has exposed the E-face (*E*) over most of the field of view. An area of communicating junction (*CJ*) is identified by the presence of closely aggregated pits. These pits can be shown to correspond in position to the particles exposed on the P-face (*P*) within the cell membrane of the adjacent liver cell. Both figures ×48,000.

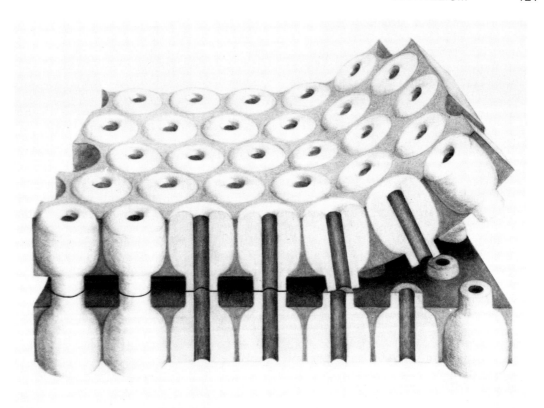

Fig. 4-15. Schematic illustration demonstrating the postulated components within adjacent cell membranes of a communicating junction. Intramembrane particles are seen within each of the two membranes arranged in regular hexagonal pattern. These are the particles revealed by freeze fracture techniques. Each particle represents a molecular aggregate which theoretically contains a pore. The pore provides a communicating channel of approximately 10 to 20 Å between the cytoplasms of the two adjacent cells. This communication is by virtue of the registration across the intercellular gap of extensions of the intramembranous particles from the adjacent membranes. (Courtesy of Dr. Norton B. Gilula.)

municating junctions or nexuses in tissues other than epithelium. They are well developed between adjacent smooth and cardiac muscle cells (chapter 8), where they promote the transfer of contraction-producing excitation from one cell to the next. Nexuses are also common between neuronal cells of lower vertebrate nervous tissue, and occasionally similar junctional morphology has been recorded in the brains of mammals. These junctions are often called "electrotonic synapses," and again presumably serve a function of excitatory transfer (chapter 10).

Our understanding of both the morphology and function of junctions between epithelial and other cells has advanced very rapidly in the past 10 years and promises to continue to do so in the future. It is not presently certain that all of the basic junctional configurations or their subvarieties are known. Certainly, the finest components of junctional architecture require much further elucidation. At this point in our understanding, however, it is possible to realize that a spectrum of junctional morphology exists in nature and that the various basic types we have described, as well as a number of less common subvarieties, fit into that scheme (Fig. 4-3). Potentially all of the junctional configurations can be macular (focalized), diffuse, or zonular. Some of the junctions seem to involve only components of adjacent cellular membranes, whereas others show increasing degrees of involvement of both extracellular and cytoplasmic components. Indeed, the junctions that display the most complex cytoplasmic organization (filaments, plaques, etc.) seem also to display the greatest quantity and complexity of extracellular adhesive materials. Junctions found in other nonepithelial situations can easily be located within the spectrum (for example, intercalated disc junctions of cardiac muscle, chemical synapses of neural tissue), as can the very common septate junction of invertebrate epithelia.

Within epithelia it is typical for many of the junctions to occur together; for example, the type of junctional complex shown diagrammatically in Figure 4-9 is particularly characteristic within the terminal bar region of intestinal, respiratory, and a number of other epithelia. However, tight junctions, intermediate junctions, desmosomes, and gap junctions may also occur independently. In some epithelia the arrangement of the junction permits relatively large intercellular clefts and gaps to be maintained. Good examples are found in the endothelial linings of lymphatic capillaries and vascular sinusoids. These passages become sufficiently large to allow the intercellular passage across the endothelium of large molecules such as plasma proteins or even entire cells (cancer cells, or white blood cells).

Modifications at the Free Surface

Microvilli, or microscopic projections above the free surface, are found in most epithelia. They are usually numerous, often regularly arranged and uniform in length, and particularly well developed in the lining epithelium of the small intestine and other absorptive epithelia. Because the microvilli of the intestine collectively appear vertically striated under the light microscope, the apical surface has been termed a *striated border.* Electron micrographs reveal that the microvilli composing the border are cell membrane-covered cytoplasmic extensions about 2 μm long (Figs. 4-16, 4-19, 16-42, 16-43, 16-45 and 16-46). Each microvillus has a slender core of fine filaments that apparently anchor at the tip of the microvillus and extend into the termi-

nal web. These are believed to provide structural support and, because they are composed of a form of the contractile protein actin, also may interact with myosin molecules of the terminal web area to provide subtle degrees of microcellular movement. Microvilli greatly increase the surface area of the cells in correlation with absorptive functions. Microvilli are also numerous on the free surfaces of the proximal convoluted tubules of the kidney. In this location they are somewhat higher and less uniform than in the small intestine, and they appear as a so-called *brush border* under the light microscope (Figs. 18-13 and 18-14). Epithelia of many other locations, where no border modification is visible by light microscopy, are often seen by electron microscopy to possess short, irregular microvilli.

As indicated above, glycosaminoglycan surface coats (or glycocalyx) are present over the surfaces of epithelial cells, and these extend over the microvilli. In the striated border of the small intestine the surface coat is so well developed that it gives a decidedly fuzzy appearance to the microvilli. These surface coats are glycoprotein in nature and give a positive periodic acid-Schiff reaction. A finely filamentous structure is seen in electron micrographs of such surface coats in the small intestine (Fig. 4-16). Individual filaments are about 25 to 30 Å thick, and they form a radiating and branching network for as much as 0.1 to 0.5 μm above the surface. They are attached to the outer leaflet of the plasmalemma and probably represent an extended integral part of the cell membrane. They are thought to serve a protective role for the free surface of the cell and may also act as a selective barrier allowing colloidal particles and dissolved substances to penetrate between them, while preventing the approach of large particles. Some workers also have postulated that the coat functions as an ion trap, serving to concentrate various small molecular weight charged particles that are to be absorbed by the cells.

Stereocilia are unusually long microvilli found in parts of the male reproductive system (Fig. 4-25) and in sensory regions

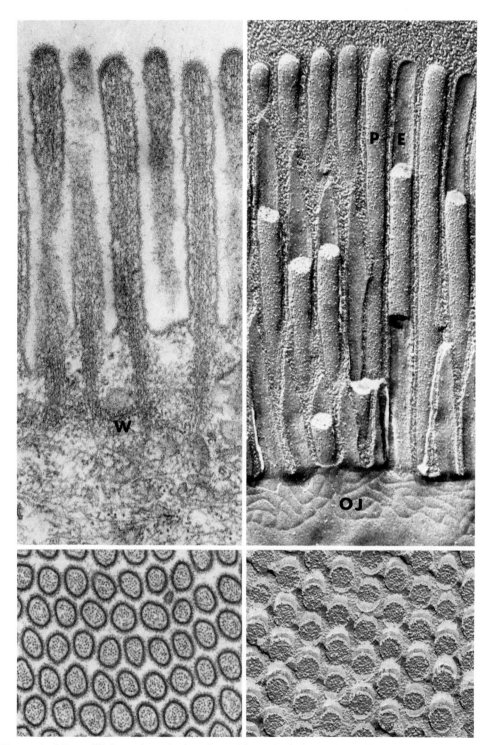

Fig. 4-16. Microvilli from the apical surface of intestinal absorptive cells. In the *left hand* figures, several microvilli are seen by transmission electron microscopy in longitudinal (*upper* figure) and cross section (*lower* figure). Note the continuity of the plasmalemma which covers the surface of each microvillus. The membrane in turn is covered with a fuzzy glycosaminoglycan material. The interior of each microvillus contains microfilaments which are anchored to the plasmalemma at the tip and extend to the apical cytoplasm of the cell, where they engage the microfilamentous terminal web (*W*). In the *right* figures, the same views are shown in freeze fracture preparations. Note that the plasmalemma of each microvillus splits to reveal particle-covered P-faces (*P*) and relatively bare E-faces (*E*). Microfilaments in the core of each microvillus are seen in the cross fracture (*lower* figure). A region of occluding junction (*OJ*) is seen along an E-face in the *upper* figure. All figures approximate ×62,000. (*Upper* figures courtesy of Dr. David Chase, *lower* figures courtesy of Dr. Michael J. Cavey.)

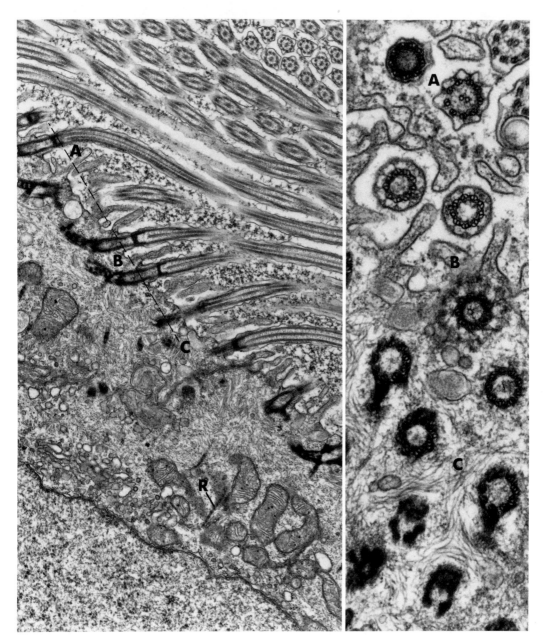

Fig. 4-17. Electron micrograph showing numerous cilia characteristic of the apical surface of the esophagus in a salamander. The shaft of each cilium extends from the surface of the cell, carrying the plasmalemma of the cell with it. At the base of each ciliary shaft a dense basal body can be seen in various planes of section. The basal body contains a centriole capped by a dense plate. Beyond the plate a regular array of microtubules extends into the ciliary shaft. These are seen in various planes of section in the *upper portions* of the figure. Striated rootlets (*R*) radiate from the base of each centriole and extend for some distance into the cytoplasm. Dotted line *ABC* represents the plane of section seen in Figure 4-18. ×19,000. (Micrograph in collaboration with Mary Ann Cahill.)

Fig. 4-18. Higher magnification electron micrograph cut in the plane labeled *ABC* on Figure 4-17. The section plane courses from just outside the cell membrane (*A*) to just inside the apical cytoplasm (*C*). At level *B* the plane passes through the apical plasmalemma. Details of internal ciliary structure are seen at the various levels. At *A*, the dense plate and the typical 9 + 2 arrangement of microtubular doublets, as well as the surrounding plasmalemma, are seen in cross sections of the cilia. At level *B*, the plane passes through the centriolar region of each cilium and discloses a 9 + 0 arrangement of triplets, each displaying an attachment to the cell membrane. Deeper into the centriole (at *C*), the microtubular triplets transition into the basal body and rootlet. ×50,000. (Micrograph in collaboration with Mary Ann Cahill.)

of the inner ear. They do not have the structural characteristics of the true cilia or flagellae. They increase the surface area of the apical cell membrane and may aid in secretion and absorption in the former instance and the reception and transduction of vibratory stimuli in the latter.

Cilia are relatively large, often motile appendages usually formed on the apex of cells. They may be present singly or in massive numbers. Cilia are usually 5 to 10 μm in length and about 0.2 μm in diameter. They are readily seen with the light microscope (Fig. 4-23), but their internal structure cannot be resolved. Electron microscopy discloses that the shaft or free part of each cilium is enclosed by a plasmalemma continuous with that of the cell and

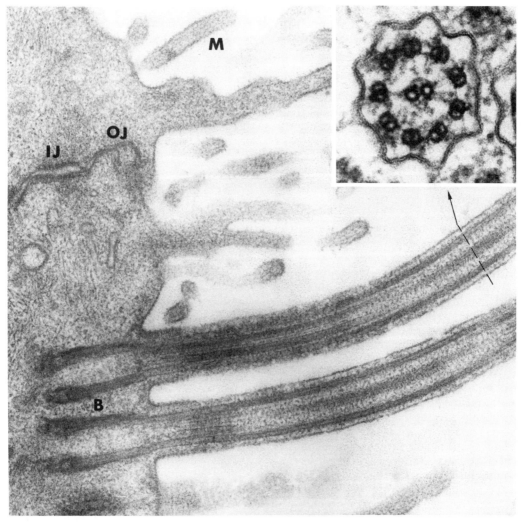

Fig. 4-19. Higher magnification electron micrographs of cilia on the apical surface of the monkey trachea. Centriolar components of two basal bodies (*B*) are seen to be in continuity with the microtubules extending into ciliary shafts. A cross section in the plane indicated at the *arrow* is shown at higher magnification in the *inset*. Here the nine peripheral doublet microtubules and the central pair are well defined, as is the surrounding plasmalemma. Arms can be seen extending from the central member of doublet pairs toward their neighbors. Additional connecting structures extend toward the central pair and the surrounding plasmalemma. Other components of the trachael epithelial apical surface include occasional microvilli (*M*), occluding junctions (*OJ*), and intermediate junctions (*IJ*). ×50,000 (inset ×130,000).

that each contains longitudinal microtubules typically arranged in a constant and orderly manner (Figs. 4-17 through 4-19). Most cilia have two single central microtubules and nine peripheral pairs of fused double microtubules, or doublets. These microtubules extend from near the tip of the cilium to its base. A *basal body* is located in the cytoplasm just inside the free surface of the cell. Each basal body is a modified centriole constituted of a "wall" of nine triplet microtubules. It is quite similar to the centrioles seen in the cell center of many cells and known to play an important role in cell division. In the course of differentiation of a ciliated cell, the centrioles apparently replicate many times to provide a basal body for each cilium. Where the ciliary shaft joins the basal body, the two central fibrils terminate and each of the nine doublets joins a triplet, each doublet continuing as the two central subunits of a triplet. In many instances striated "rootlets" extend from the basal body well into the cytoplasm of the cell. Other fibrous footlike connections may extend onto the nearby cell membrane from the basal body. Both of these modifications are believed to be reinforcing anchorage mechanisms for the cilia. It is interesting that the same fundamental plan of ultrastructural characteristics is found in the cilia of all animals.

Cilia are numerous on the surface cells of the epithelium lining the respiratory tract and on some of the cells of the female reproductive system, for example. In these locations they beat in a coordinated rhythmical wavelike manner, promoting movement of materials over the cell surfaces. The beating of the cilia in the trachea produces an upward movement of mucus with its entrapped dust particles, thus preventing foreign materials from blocking the lower respiratory regions, which must remain unobstructed for proper exchange of O_2 and CO_2. The mechanism which underlies the movement of cilia is currently being elucidated. High resolution electron microscopy and special techniques disclose two arms extending from the central microtubule of each doublet toward the next adjacent doublet (Fig. 4-19). Other less prominent elements extend toward the cen-

tral pair and the surface membrane. The arms are believed to contain an ATPase (*dynein*) whose action promotes bending of the ciliary shaft in a plane oriented to the substructure within the ciliary shaft. Recent evidence suggests that this is accomplished by an ATP-dependent mechanism which causes sliding of the doublets on one side of the cilium with respect to those of the other.

Flagella also have the same axial structure as cilia but are much longer and are usually present as but one or two per cell. The best example of flagella to be seen in the mammalian organism is in the tail of the spermatozoon (chapter 19, Fig. 19-9). Although possessing similar microtubular patterns within their interior, flagellae usually beat in a seemingly more random whip- or wavelike motion.

In certain locations of the body, ciliary projections are highly modified to serve sensory receptor functions. This is strikingly exhibited in the outer segments of the rods and cones of the retina and in some of the hair cells of sensory portions of the inner ear. Such ciliary processes are usually not motile and lack the central pair of microtubules. The nine doublets, however, are retained. In rods and cones, the plasmalemma of the ciliary shaft has been thrown into a highly regular and constantly replaced series of membranous discs. These membranous discs are the site of deposition and action of photosensitive pigments (chapter 22).

Basal Modifications and Developmental Stabilization

With rare exceptions, epithelia secrete a special variety of cell coat (or glycocalyx) along their basal surfaces where they border underlying connective tissues. This material consists of a mucoprotein matrix within which very fine (20 Å) matted filaments of a special type of collagen (Type II, discussed in the next chapter) are embedded. This mat is termed the *basal lamina* (or *basement lamina*). It averages 500 to 1000 Å in thickness and is usually separated from the basal cell membrane by a lucent region of some 500 Å. The basal lamina and its adjacent lucent zone are seldom visible by light microscopy. Current evidence suggests strongly that the basal lamina is a product of the epithelial cells themselves. Frequently it is reinforced with a much thicker layered meshwork of reticular and collagenous fibers embedded in a similar glycosaminoglycan matrix. This layer is termed the *reticular lamina*. Beneath most epithelia it is the combination of the basal lamina and the reticular lamina that constitutes the *basement membrane* which is visible by light microscopy and which has been described beneath epithelia for many years. The basement membrane appears deeply black in silver preparations because of the presence of reticular fibers, and it stains red after periodic acid-Schiff because of its polysaccharides. The basement membrane is easily seen in hematoxylin- and eosin-stained sections of the trachea, where the reticular lamina is exceedingly thick. On the other hand, a similarly disposed layer around the basal surfaces of kidney tubules is almost entirely composed of basal lamina. In that instance it, too, is occasionally thick enough to be discerned by light microscopy. In other locations, such as beneath transitional epithelium, even the basement membrane is so thin as to be unresolvable by light microscopy.

The basal lamina appears as a thin deposit very early in the development of most epithelial rudiments of the embryo. It seems to serve an important function in the segregation of tissues within the embryo. As will be outlined in the next chapter, it becomes the peripheral boundary of a broad and complex connective tissue compartment. However, it should not be considered an impenetrable boundary; it is more analogous to a mesh fence. Many molecules easily diffuse across basal laminae to interact with epithelial cells on the one side and connective tissue components on the other. As noted above, the ultimate seals for preventing fluid loss from these extracellular compartments lie in the tight junctions of the epithelial cells. Figure 4-20 illustrates a vascular channel, the adjacent connective tissue compartment, two basal laminae, and an epithelial region which have been perfused with the tracer

colloidal thorium dioxide, previously introduced into the bloodstream. It can be seen that after an appropriate period of time this molecule has penetrated in clumped aggregates through the endothelium and its basal lamina to occupy the connective tissue compartment. The basal lamina of the epithelium, on the other hand, is more selective and has permitted the diffusion of only the smallest aggregates of thorium dioxide into epithelial extracellular compartments. The larger aggregates are seen clumped along the basal lamina. Hence, in addition to their segregative potential, basal laminae may serve to some extent to regulate the movement of colloidal-sized aggregates or macromolecules among the compartments of an embryo or an adult.

As embryonic epithelial rudiments develop, they assume particular shapes. The initiation of rudiment shaping is probably a function of contractile microfilaments and their associated attachments within the epithelial cells themselves. However, it seems that as the rudiments enlarge, additional reinforcement and stabilization are required to maintain the emergent shapes. The acquisition of basal laminae around these rudiments may be the first step in such an extracellular stabilization construction. Eventually, collagenous and reticular fibers may also be laid down, most frequently through the action of connective tissue cells, eventually reaching reticular lamina proportions. Thus, an extracellular collagenous-glycosaminoglycan encasement for such rudiments serves as a reinforcing framework. It should be realized, then, that the shapes that cells and epithelial rudiments attain and maintain are dependent upon the harmonious interaction of cytoplasmic cytoskeletal (filamentous) networks and their attachments on the one hand and extracellular collagenous stabilizing frameworks on the other.

Epithelia are not the only tissues which deposit basal lamina material. During embryonic development, certain other cells segregate themselves from surrounding connective tissues by the acquisition of similar coats. When the coat completely or nearly completely surrounds such cells, as is the case with smooth, skeletal, and car-

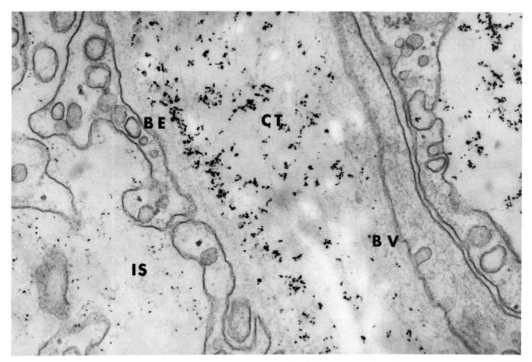

Fig. 4-20. Medium magnification electron micrograph of the connective tissue compartment (*CT*) between a thin-walled blood sinusoid at the *right* of the figure and the basal region of an epithelium at the *left*. There are large intercellular spaces (*IS*) in this epithelium. A heavy metal tracer (colloidal thorium dioxide) has been injected into the blood stream of the animal and allowed to circulate for several minutes. Tracer particles are visible in the sinusoidal lumen at the *right*. They have also leaked through the vessel wall and crossed the vascular basal lamina (*BV*) to occupy the connective tissue. Note that large clusters of the tracer are piled up against the epithelial basal lamina (*BE*) and only fine particles of the tracer have managed to penetrate that basal lamina to gain access to the epithelial intercellular space. The experiment demonstrates that basal lamina material is not impervious to the passage of materials but can serve as a sieve to select the size of molecules that are allowed to pass. ×48,500.

diac muscle as well as fat cells, the encasement is more properly termed an *external lamina*. Reticular lamina is seldom well developed in association with external lamina. Otherwise, the appearance of basal and external laminae is essentially similar. There is some emerging evidence, however, to suggest that there are subtle chemical differences in both the collagen and the glycosaminoglycan found in basal laminae as compared to those in external laminae.

Vascular Supply to Epithelia

Epithelium is avascular. Nutritive materials and oxygen enter it by diffusion through the cells and across basal laminae and basement membranes. Capillaries are present in the epithelium of the stria vascularis of the internal ear, an apparent exception to this rule, and the tissues of the spinal cord and brain might also be considered exceptions on first glance. In these cases, however, blood vessels make only apparent entrance into the epithelia. Close examination by electron microscopy shows that their excursions into the epithelium are looping ones; they carry with them both the basal lamina of the epithelium itself and a basal lamina of the vascular endothelium. Therefore, these vessels do not actually invade the epithelium, but rather remain separated by at least some basal lamina material. This point will be discussed in greater detail in chapters 10 and 11.

Simple Epithelia

Simple Squamous Epithelium

Simple squamous epithelium (*pavement epithelium*) consists of flat scalelike or platelike cells arranged in a layer only one cell thick. On surface view the cells appear as a delicate mosaic, which can be demonstrated especially well by the precipitation of silver at the boundaries of the cells (Fig. 4-2). The edges of the cells are usually slightly interdigitated with those of their neighbors, but may be smooth. The nucleus, situated in the center of the cell, is spherical or ovoid, causing a bulge.

Simple squamous epithelium is widely distributed. It lines the peritoneal, pleural, and pericardial cavities (mesothelium), the heart and all blood and lymph vessels (endothelium), the membranous labyrinth of the internal ear, portions of the uriniferous tubule, and portions of the rete testis.

Endothelium and *mesothelium* are excellent examples of simple squamous epithelium. Pinocytotic vesicles are particularly numerous in the cytoplasm of endothelial cells, and they apparently play a role in the transport of some substances (e.g., large molecules such as proteins) across the cell. The significance of this in relation to other mechanisms for transport is discussed under the circulatory system (chapter 12). According to the best present observations, it appears that regeneration of endothelium, like that of most other types of epithelium, involves multiplication and rearrangement of cells of its own type. Mesothelium differs in that it apparently can be regenerated from cells of the underlying connective tissue. Mesothelial cells can also change into fibroblasts. They seem to be less specialized than other types of epithelial cells and appear to retain some of the multipotency of mesenchyme.

Mesenchymal epithelium is a name sometimes given to the simple squamous cells which line certain other connective tissue-enclosed cavities: the subarachnoid and subdural cavities, the chambers of the eye, and the perilymphatic spaces of the ear. The structure of this epithelium is generally similar to that of mesothelium, although in some sites (e.g., surface of the iris) its cells are more loosely joined to each other.

The cells lining bursae and synovial membranes of joint cavities are associated with collagenous fibers and are more loosely joined to each other than are typical mesothelial cells. They are generally described as fibroblasts, although electron micrographs show that they are somewhat more epithelial than ordinary fibroblasts.

Simple Columnar Epithelium

Simple columnar epithelium (Fig. 4-21) in its various modifications represents the chief secretory and absorptive tissue of the body. It consists of a single layer of tall cells resting on a continuous basal lamina. The height varies considerably and the term *cuboidal* epithelium is applied when height and thickness of the cells are about equal (isodiametric). All transitions from low cuboidal to high columnar types of cells are encountered (Fig. 4-22). The secretory units or *acini* of most glands are lined by cuboidal or columnar epithelial cells whose broad bases rest on the basement membrane and whose apices face the narrow lumen. This is termed *pyramidal* or *glandular* epithelium (Figs. 15-3 and 15-4). In simple columnar epithelial cells, the nucleus is oval and usually placed basally; in cuboidal cells, it is spherical and central. In the basal perinuclear portion of the cytoplasm, there are numerous mitochondria and abundant rough endoplasmic reticulum, particularly in cells that are secretory. The apical portion may contain granules or vesicles of stored products of the cell (zymogen, mucin, etc.). The cytoplasmic constitution varies greatly under different conditions of cellular activity. A striated border may be absent, as in most glandular epithelium, or very prominent, as in the high columnar absorptive epithelium of the small intestine (Figs. 1-9*C* and 4-21).

An important cellular variation found in many columnar epithelia is the goblet cell (Figs. 4-21 and 4-24). This cell is characterized by the accumulation of membrane-bounded mucin droplets and a relative paucity of microvilli. It seems likely that the protein portion of mucin (a glycoprotein)

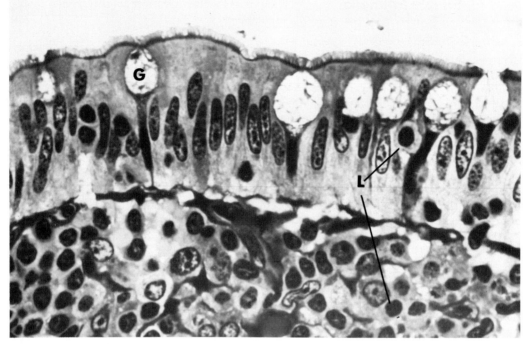

Fig. 4-21. Light micrograph of simple columnar epithelium. All epithelial cells reach both apical and basal surfaces of the epithelium, although some (G) are differentiated as mucus secreting goblet cells. Lymphocytes (L) occasionally invade the epithelium from underlying connective tissue. Monkey intestine. ×1,420.

is synthesized in the rough-surfaced endoplasmic reticulum which is abundant in the basal half of the cell. The carbohydrate moiety of mucin is apparently formed by the Golgi complex, because tritiated glucose injected into laboratory animals appears within minutes, first over the Golgi complex, next within the vesicles of the Golgi complex, later as membrane-bounded mucin droplets in the apical cytoplasm, and finally with the mucus in the intestinal lumen. Protein and carbohydrate moieties of mucin are combined in the Golgi complex; the membranes of the droplets are derived from membranes of Golgi cisternae, which must be replaced continuously. The mucin droplets accumulate in the apical end of the cell and push the nucleus and most of the remaining cytoplasm toward the base. Thus, the cell assumes a goblet shape. The mucin droplets become closely packed but remain membrane-bounded and separate until they escape by exocytosis from the apical end of the cell. Sometimes goblet cells secrete cyclically and at other

times continuously, depending upon the stimuli and demands in a given location. Most mucins are not preserved and stained in the routine preparations for light microscopy. The droplets may wash out of the cell, leaving a clear space, or they may partially dissolve and then fuse into a faintly staining meshwork composed of remnants of mucin and remaining cytoplasm.

Pseudostratified Epithelium

In this type of epithelium (Figs. 4-1 and 4-23 to 4-25), the nuclei lie at different levels, giving it a stratified appearance. All of the cells reach the basement membrane, but not all of them extend to the free surface. Those which do reach the surface are columnar, with one or more thin processes which extend to the basement membrane. These processes are difficult to see in routine histological preparations. Between the slender processes, there are ovoid or spindle-shaped cells. This type of epithelium usually has either cilia or stereocilia. It occurs mainly as the lining of the passages of the respiratory and the male reproductive systems.

Stratified Epithelia

Stratified Squamous Epithelium

Stratified squamous epithelium (Figs. 4-1 and 4-26) is the main protective epithelium of the body and consists of many cell layers. The number of layers varies considerably in different places, but the shape and arrangement of the cells are quite characteristic. The deepest layer, which rests on a basement membrane, is formed by columnar or prismatic cells which in sec-

tions of the tissue appear as a distinct row. Hemidesmosomes are seen along the basal surface of each cell, adjacent to the basal lamina. Nearer to the surface, the cells become irregularly cubical or polyhedral in shape and are usually larger than the cells of the basal layers. Just beneath the free surface, the cells are more flattened and, at the surface, quite squamous. The deeper cells of the basal and polyhedral layers are young, soft cells with relatively large nuclei rich in chromatin. The cytoplasm is finely granular and somewhat basophilic because of its content of RNA. The desmosomal tonofilament bundles are prominent, giving the cell a prickly appearance ("prickle cells," Figs. 14-3 and 14-4).

The extent of change in the superficial

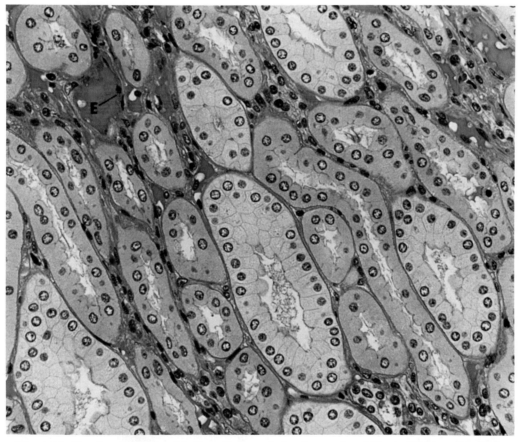

Fig. 4-22. Simple cuboidal epithelium lining tubules in monkey kidney. Some regions appear stratified owing to the plane of section, which courses tangentially through the wall of a tubule. Connective tissue and blood vessels occupy the space between tubules. Close inspection reveals simple squamous endothelium (E) lining blood vessels which are filled with darkly stained blood plasma. ×430.

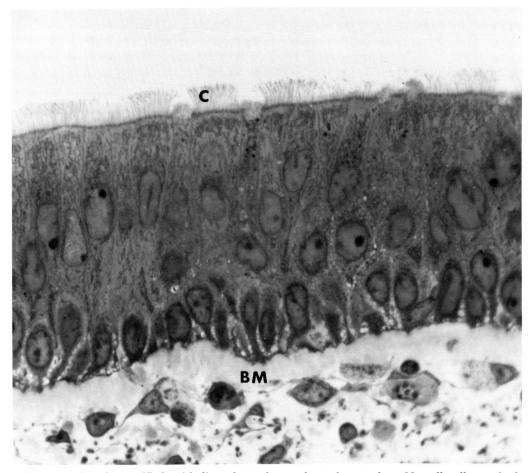

Fig. 4-23. Pseudo-stratified epithelium from the trachea of a monkey. Not all cells reach the apical surface, giving the epithelium a stratified appearance. Note that this epithelium is richly ciliated (*C*) and is characterized by a very thick basement membrane (*BM*). ×1,168.

cells varies with the location and environment of the stratified squamous epithelium. The epidermis, for instance, is subjected to more attrition and drying than is the epithelium of the mouth, pharynx, and esophagus. Its surface cells are nonnucleated, scalelike, and keratinized. On the other hand, the epithelium of moist surfaces such as that of mouth, pharynx, and esophagus is usually not keratinized. The surface cells become very flat, but usually remain nucleated.

The mitotic activity of the cells in the lower layer and the lack of mitosis in the upper layers may reflect the fact that the deeper cells are in closer relation to the underlying capillaries which supply nutri-

tive substances. As new basal cells are formed, their neighbors are pressed upward. Dead scalelike surface cells are constantly cast off, to be replaced by cells from the deeper strata. In man this is a slow and continuous process; in some of the lower vertebrates (e.g., snakes) there is a periodic shedding of the whole superficial layer of the epidermis.

Stratified squamous epithelium covers the entire surface of the body and the orifices of cavities opening upon it. It lines the mucous membranes of the mouth, pharynx, esophagus, portions of the larynx, external auditory canal and conjunctiva, vagina, vestibule, labia majora, and portions of the urethra.

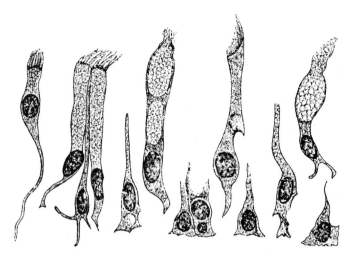

Fig. 4-24. Isolated cells from pseudostratified ciliated epithelium of trachea. Two goblet cells are shown. (Redrawn from Schaffer.)

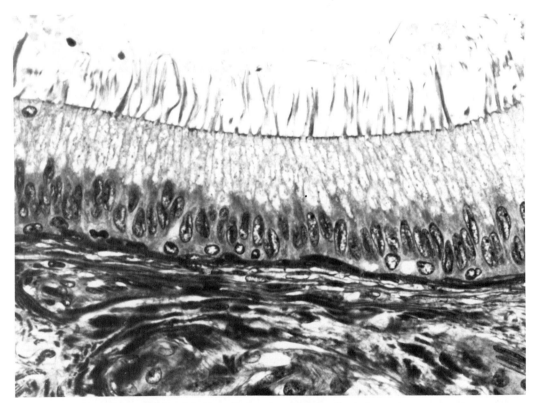

Fig. 4-25. Pseudostratified epithelium lining the epididymis of the male reproductive tract. The cells which do not reach the apical surface are relatively few in number. Their nuclei appear small and located basally. This epithelium bears stereocilia. ×570.

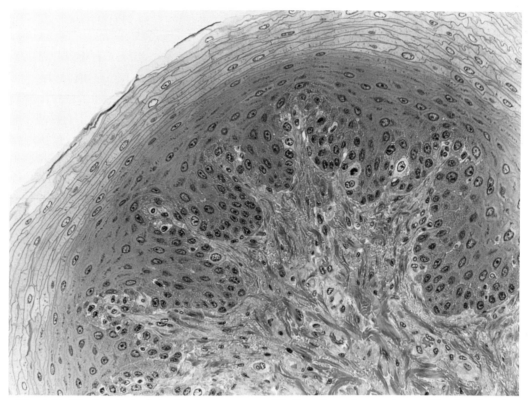

Fig. 4-26. Nonkeratinized stratified squamous epithelium from the esophagus. The basal surface of the epithelium is thrown into folds and contains cells which are distinctly rounded in comparison to the flat-surfaced cells from which the epithelium gains its name. ×465.

Stratified Columnar and Stratified Cuboidal Epithelium

A *stratified columnar epithelium* is comparatively rare. It consists of columnar surface cells which rest on several layers of irregular cubical cells. Stratified columnar epithelium is found chiefly where a stratified squamous adjoins a pseudostratified columnar type, as for instance at the juncture of the oropharynx with the nasopharynx and with the larynx (Fig. 17-5). It is said to occur also in part of the penile portion of the male urethra.

In a few locations, a stratified epithelium has surface cells which are definitely cuboidal, thus forming a *stratified cuboidal epithelium*. Examples are the ducts of salivary and sweat glands (Figs. 4-27 and 14-6) and the lining of the antra of ovarian follicles (Fig. 20-3). The sebaceous glands possess epithelial cells which are polyhedral in shape and several layers in thickness (Fig. 14-13).

The epithelium of seminiferous tubules of the testis is a highly specialized type (Fig. 19-5). Functionally, it is cytogenic; structurally, it probably approximates a stratified cuboidal type more closely than any other, although certain of its cells (cells of Sertoli) are elongated and extend from the basement membrane to the lumen. The shape of the surface cells varies greatly with stages of growth and differentiation.

Transitional Epithelium

All epithelial cells are pliable to some degree, but these properties are especially striking in the transitional epithelium (Figs. 4-1 and 4-28 to 4-30) of the urinary passages and bladder. In the dilated bladder, the epithelium consists of two or three layers of cells. The superficial cells are large, low, cuboidal plates; the lower ones are smaller and irregularly cubical. In the contracted bladder, the epithelium becomes five- or six-layered. The surface cells are large and cuboidal, with a condensed, darkly staining superficial layer of cytoplasm reflective of the abundant microfilaments there. These cells have characteristic convex free surfaces and facet-like indentations in their undersurfaces (Figs. 4-1 and 4-30). The lower cells have rearranged themselves, owing to a reduction of the surface area. They overlap each other and have assumed a flask- or pear-shaped form. The luminal surface of transitional epithelial cells is not smooth in electron micrographs, but rather displays alternating crests and hollows. The apical cytoplasm contains numerous membrane-bounded fusiform vesicles which derive from the surface membrane. When the bladder contracts, the tips of the surface crests rise and join, perhaps under control of the closely related web of subapical microfilaments, pinch off the intervening troughs into the underlying cytoplasm, and reduce the area of the surface membrane. The worn out membranes of the vesicles are supposedly digested by lysosomes, and new membrane material must be added, probably by synthesis in the Golgi complex.

The surface membrane of the bladder has an important function as a barrier to diffusion of water via the cells from underlying tissues into the hypertonic urine in the lumen. The plasmalemma of the luminal surface is unusual in that its outer leaflet is definitely thicker than its inner leaflet, the exact significance of which remains obscure. Diffusion via intercellular routes is prevented by extensive tight junctions between the surface cells. Desmosomes are scarce in the deeper cells; this seems to be correlated with the ability of the cells to adapt during contraction and distention of the organ. Another structural adaptation for contraction and expansion is the presence of numerous interfoldings and interdigitations of the membranes of the deeper cells. The folds tend to disappear when the bladder is distended.

Transitional epithelium is found only in the urinary system—pelvis of kidney, ureter, bladder, and a portion of the urethra.

Other Patterns of Epithelial Organization

In addition to the commonly described epithelial types and configurations noted above, certain other epithelia progress

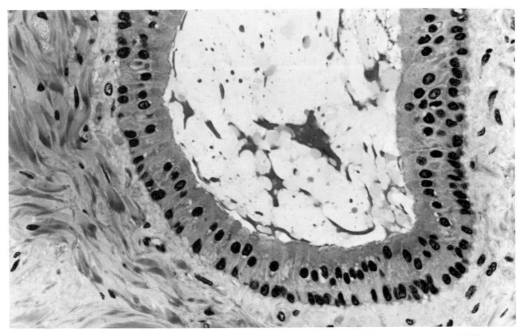

Fig. 4-27. Stratified columnar epithelium. This example of a relatively rare epithelial type is from the duct of a salivary gland. The epithelial cells are cuboidal to columnar in shape and stratified to the extent of two layers. ×475.

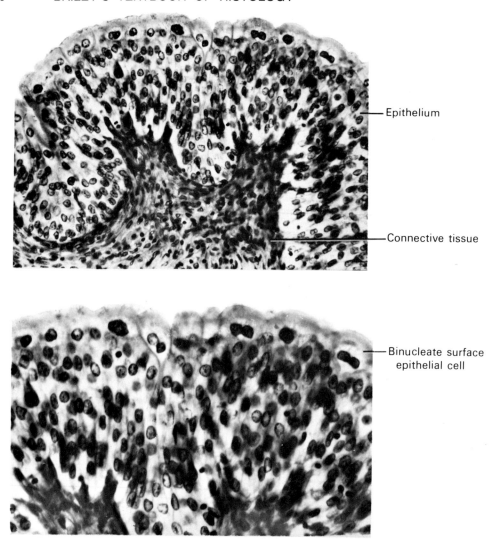

Fig. 4-28. Photomicrographs of transitional epithelium of contracted human bladder. *Upper figure,* ×250; *lower figure,* a portion of the same region, ×390. Note that some of the surface cells have two nuclei and most of the surface cells are umbrella-shaped at their upper border in the contracted bladder. H&E stain.

through patterns of development which alter them considerably. In past years they have been largely ignored because they are hardly discernible as epithelia and because they constitute relatively isolated instances. Recently, however, the importance of their recognition and understanding has become more obvious. A glance at their development aids comprehension.

The derivation of various glands as epithelial invaginations into mesenchymal or connective tissue beds has been discussed above. Retention of the original invagina-

tion stalk, or in some cases the development of a new one, leads to the formation of exocrine glands (Fig. 4-31A). On the other hand, detachment or loss of that stalk gives rise to isolated islands or follicles of epithelial cells which develop into endocrine glands. These must release their secretory products into the surrounding connective tissue and nearby vascular pathways. In this endocrine pattern, the original apical surface of the invaginating cells may either be retained or obscured. The basal surface of the cells in all cases will be retained as that portion of the epithelial mass facing the surrounding connective tissues. When a lumen is retained or emerges secondarily, as is the case in the development of thyroid follicles (Fig. 4-31*B*), a cavity is created which is bounded on all sides by the apical surfaces of lining epithelial cells. In the case of thyroid follicles, the cavity serves as a temporary storage site for secretions first released from the apices of the cells, later to be reabsorbed back through the cells and released basally in the usual endocrine fashion. In this instance it can be seen that both apical and basal surfaces of the epithelium are present in the final adult configuration. In other instances the epithelial

cells may become so closely compacted that a lumen is lost and apical surfaces are pressed against each other and thereby obscured (Fig. 4-31*C*). This is the typical configuration that one sees in the development of cords of parathyroid epithelia and the cords of liver parenchyma, and to a somewhat lesser extent in the pars distalis (anterior lobe) of the pituitary gland. The secretory cells of these organs are all epithelial by derivation and retain some of their epithelial characteristics including an apparent basal surface and typical epithelial cell-to-cell attachment mechanisms.

A further elaboration on this theme is found in the development of thymus (Fig.

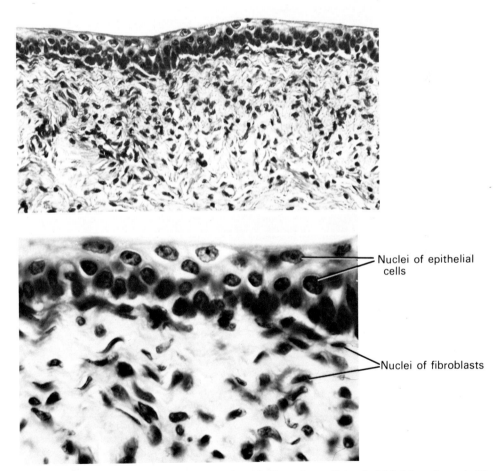

Nuclei of epithelial cells

Nuclei of fibroblasts

Fig. 4-29. Photomicrographs of transitional epithelium from distended bladder of a cat. *Upper figure,* ×250; *lower figure,* a region of the same field, ×90. Note that the cells are arranged in only a few layers and that each stretched surface cell usually covers several of the underlying cells. Transitional epithelium, as indicated by its name, varies in different functional states, and there are numerous gradations between the appearance seen in Figure 4-28 and that seen in Figure 4-29.

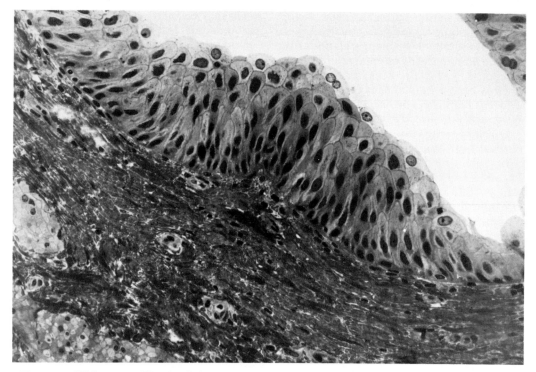

Fig. 4-30. Higher magnification light micrograph of transitional epithelium in a plastic-embedded specimen. This epithelium lines the ureter. Note the rounded free surface of apical cells and the distinct curved boundaries between adjacent epithelial cells. Bundles of smooth muscle are visible at *lower left* amid the connective tissue. ×420.

4-31D). The epithelial precursor of this gland is from endodermal epithelium of one, or perhaps two, pair of pharyngeal pouches. These epithelial masses migrate considerable distances in the embryo, proliferating as they go, to form the eventual epithelial component of the thymus during fetal stages. During this development the epithelial masses lose their apical surfaces and lumina in a manner similar to that decribed above, but in addition the central cells of the epithelial masses become separated from their neighbors so that large intercellular spaces intervene between them. A basal surface around the whole mass is retained and can be identified by the presence of a typical basal lamina.

The internal morphology of such a mass is now sufficiently obscured that its epithelial identity is difficult to appreciate. Electron microscopy, however, discloses that the cells remain attached by desmosomes. By light microscopy the internal parts of such masses bear a distinct resemblance to

reticular connective tissues and cells, and have in the past often been described as such. In the thymus, vascular channels invaginate the mass, particularly in the cortex of that organ, carrying with them a basal lamina of the endothelial cells as well as the basal lamina of the thymic epithelium (or *thymic reticulum*) itself. In subsequent development the intercellular spaces of the reticular epithelium are invaded by lymphocytes, which there proliferate and give the mass the typical histological characteristics of that organ (see chapter 13).

An example similar to the epithelial reticular development outlined in the thymus can be found in the development of tooth buds, wherein the enamel organs proliferating from an epithelial dental lamina also form an enclosed epithelial bag, the central regions of which assume a reticular appearance. Along one basal surface of each of these masses the epithelial cells differentiate as enamel-forming ameloblasts. The other cells of the epithelial mass are retained during development of the crown of the tooth as the so-called *stellate reticulum* (see chapter 16).

Epithelial Repair

Epithelia in certain locations are in a constant state of cellular loss and renewal. The continuous loss of epidermal surface cells with replacement from the deeper layers of stratified epithelium is a case in point. Less obvious, but perhaps just as active, is the loss of columnar cells from the simple epithelium covering the villi, crypts, and other surfaces along the digestive tract. These cells are regularly replaced by mitosis somewhat distant along the epithelium and continual movement of new, maturing cells toward the site of loss. These are normal renewal processes involving little or no

trauma. But many epithelia are also able to respond to injury by a timely increase of mitotic activity and motility in areas adjacent to a wound. The response of epithelium in the healing of wounds in mammals has been more extensively studied in the epidermis than in other types of epithelium.

Both epithelium and the underlying connective tissue are injured in abrasions and most other wounds, and both have a capacity for cell division and for repair, in contrast with more highly differentiated tissue such as nerve cells and skeletal muscle fibers. The response of the epidermis depends somewhat on the size of the injured surface, but there is generally an enlargement and migration of the deeper cells near the wound. These exhibit a sort of ameboid movement, with the formation of tongue-

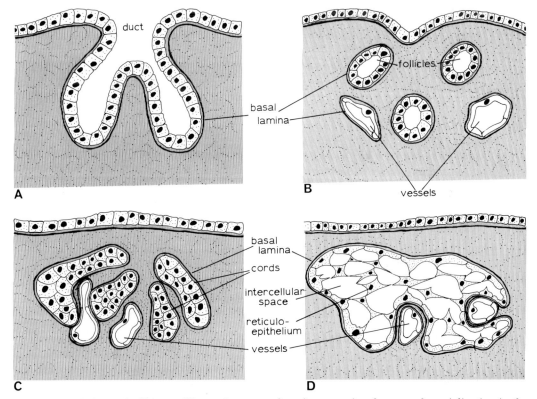

Fig. 4-31. Schematic diagram illustrating examples of progressive degrees of specialization in the development of glandular epithelium: *A*, retention of developmental stalk as the *duct of a gland*; *B*, loss of stalk leading to *follicular pattern*; *C*, loss of stalk and lumen leading to *cord pattern*; and *D*, loss of stalk and lumen but expansion of intercellular spaces resulting in a *reticular epithelial pattern*. Note that in each example a basal lamina is retained, marking the basal surface of the epithelial mass. Blood vessels may indent but not penetrate that basal lamina.

like processes which grow over the denuded area or, if there is a scab, grow under it and help to absorb it. Mitoses are decreased for the first few (4 to 5) days but soon thereafter exceed the normal rate. In wound repair, as in tissue culture, epithelium exhibits the propensity of forming a cellular layer on a surface.

Membranes

Epithelium assumes its full significance only when considered in conjunction with the underlying connective tissue. In that combination, it forms so-called membranes (in the grosser sense) of varying toughness and thickness, as exemplified by the skin and peritoneum. In conjunction with a stratum of connective tissue, it forms the mucosa of the gastrointestinal, respiratory, and genitourinary systems. In general, the connective tissue lying beneath the epithelium is extremely fine but closely woven. This passes gradually into a stratum of coarser, closely woven fibers. The membrane thus formed permits a variable amount of stretching, depending on the location, but prevents an excessive expansion which might separate the epithelial cells. The denseness of the connective tissue varies with the membranes formed; thus, in the mucosa it is not nearly as dense as it is in the skin.

The denser connective tissue of a membrane ultimately grades with no abrupt transition into a looser stratum, which attaches the membrane to the underlying structures and usually permits a movement over them. This underlying zone of looser tissue is well exemplified by the subcutaneous fascia of the skin and the submucosa of the gastrointestinal tract.

Serous Membranes

Serous membranes line the *peritoneal, pleural,* and *pericardial* cavities as the peritoneum, pleura, and pericardium, respectively. A serous membrane consists of mesothelium and an underlying layer of delicate fibroelastic tissue. It should be noted that serous membranes line closed cavities and do not contain glands. They are moistened by a thin fluid similar to lymph.

Mucous Membranes

Mucous membranes (mucosae) line all of those cavities and canals of the body which connect with the exterior; that is, they line the alimentary tract, the respiratory passages, and the genitourinary tract. Although differing in details, the mucous membranes of these various locations all have a similarity in the general plan of their structure. The essential parts are (1) surface epithelium, (2) basement membrane, and (3) a stratum of connective tissue, the *lamina propria.*

Although the name mucous membrane suggests that mucous glands are present, this is not always the case. Both mucous and serous glands are present in the mucous membrane of the alimentary and respiratory tracts, but no glands are present in the mucous membrane of most of the genitourinary tract.

References

BARLAND, P., NOVIKOFF, A. B., AND HAMMERMAN, D. Electron microscopy of the human synovial membrane. J. Cell Biol. 14:29–42, 1962.

BENNETT, H. S. Morphological aspects of extracellular polysaccharides. J. Histochem. Cytochem. 11:2–13, 1963.

BISHOP, G. H. Regeneration after experimental removal of skin in man. Am. J. Anat. 76:153–183, 1945.

BONNEVILLE, M. A., AND WEINSTOCK, M. Brush border development in the intestinal absorptive cells of *Xenopus* during metamorphosis. J. Cell Biol. 49:151–171, 1970.

BRANDT, P. W. A consideration of the extraneous coats of the plasma membrane. Circulation (suppl.) 26:1075–1091, 1962.

CHAMBERS, R., AND DE RÉNYI, G. S. The structure of the cells in tissues as revealed by micro-dissection. Am. J. Anat. 35:385–402, 1925.

CLAUDE, P., AND GOODENOUGH, D. A. Fracture faces of zonulae occludentes from "tight" and "leaky" epithelia. J. Cell Biol. 58:390–400, 1973.

DIBONA, D. R., CIVAN, M. M., AND LEAF, A. The anatomic site of the transepithelial permeability barriers of toad bladder. J. Cell Biol. 40:1–7, 1969.

FARQUHAR, M. G., AND PALADE, G. E. Junctional complexes in various epithelia. J. Cell Biol. 17:375–412, 1963.

FARQUHAR, M. G., AND PALADE, G. E. Cell junctions in amphibian skin. J. Cell Biol. 26:263–291, 1965.

FAWCETT, D. Cilia and flagella. *In* The Cell; Biochemistry, Physiology, Morphology (Brachet, J., and Mirsky, A. E., editors), vol. II, pp. 217–297. Academic Press, New York, 1961.

FAWCETT, D. W. Surface specializations of absorbing cells. J. Histochem. Cytochem. 13:75–91, 1965.

FAWCETT, D. W. An Atlas of Fine Structure. W. B. Saunders Company, Philadelphia, 1966.

GABE, M., AND ARVY, L. Gland cells. *In* The Cell; Biochemistry, Physiology, Morphology (Brachet, J., and Mirsky, A. E., editors), vol. V, pp. 1–88. Academic Press, New York, 1961.

GIBBONS, I. R. Molecular basis of flagellar motility in sea urchin spermatozoa. *In* Molecules and Cell Movement (Inoue, S., and Stephens, R. E., editors), Raven Press, New York, pp. 207–232, 1975.

GOODENOUGH, D. A. The structure and permeability of isolated hepatocyte gap junctions. Cold Spring Harbor Symp. 40:37–44, 1975.

GOODENOUGH, D. A. *In vitro* formation of gap junction vesicles. J. Cell Biol. 68:220–231, 1976.

HICKS, R. M. The fine structure of the transitional epithelium of rat ureter. J. Cell Biol. 26:25–48, 1965.

ITO, S. The surface coat of enteric microvilli. J. Cell Biol. 27:475–491, 1965.

KELLY, D. E. Fine structure of desmosomes, hemidesmosomes, and an adepidermal globular layer in developing newt epidermis. J. Cell Biol. 28:51–72, 1966.

LEBLOND, C. P., AND WALKER, B. E. Renewal of cell populations. Physiol. Rev. 36:255–276, 1956.

MATOLTSY, A. G. Desmosomes, filaments, and keratohyaline granules: their role in the stabilization and keratinization of the epidermis. J. Invest. Dermatol. 65:127–142, 1975.

MOOSEKER, M. S., AND TILNEY, L. G. Organization of an actin filament-membrane complex. Filament polarity and membrane attachment in the microvilli of intestinal epithelial cells. J. Cell Biol. 67:725–743, 1975.

MOOSEKER, M. S. Brush border motility. Microvillar contraction in Triton-treated brush borders isolated from intestinal epithelium. J. Cell Biol. 71:417–432, 1976.

ODLAND, G. F., AND ROSS, R. Human wound repair. I. Epidermal regeneration. J. Cell Biol. 39:135–151, 1968.

OVERTON, J. Cell junctions and their development. Progr. Surf. Membr. Sci. 8:161–208, 1974.

PORTER, K. R., AND BONNEVILLE, M. A. Fine Structure of Cells and Tissues, ed. 3. Lea & Febiger, Philadelphia, 1968.

RAMBOURG, A., HERNANDEZ, W., AND LEBLOND, C. P. Detection of complex carbohydrates in the Golgi apparatus of rat cells. J. Cell Biol. 40:395–414, 1969.

REVEL, J.-P., AND ITO, S. The surface components of cells. *In* The Specificity of Cell Surfaces (Davis, B., and Warren, L., editors), p. 211. Prentice-Hall, Inc. New Jersey, 1967.

ROSS, R., AND ODLAND, G. F. Human wound repair. II. Inflammatory cells, epithelial-mesenchymal interrelations, and fibrogenesis. J. Cell Biol. 39:152–168, 1968.

SATIR, P. Studies on cilia. III. Further studies on the cilium tip and a "sliding filament" model of ciliary motility. J. Cell Biol. 39:77–94, 1968.

SCHAFFER, J. Das Epithelgewebe. Handb. mikr. Anat. Menschen (v. Möllendorff, editor), 2:1–132, Springer-Verlag, Berlin, 1927.

STAEHELIN, L. A. Structure and function of intercellular junctions. Int. Rev. Cytol. 39:191–283, 1974.

WEISS, P. The biological foundations of wound repair. The Harvey Lectures, Ser. 55:13–42, 1961.

CHAPTER 5

The Connective Tissues

The connective and supporting tissues are characterized by cells which function to elaborate and maintain a variety of extracellular materials (matrix) about themselves. These extracellular materials are of such volume that in most cases the cells of connective tissues are rather widely separated, in contrast to epithelia, where cells are closely associated. The character of the extracellular matrix is determined from region to region by the abundance and proportion of fluid, fibers, ground substance molecules, and mineral aggregates. The cells have either synthesized and released these products or promoted their establishment by delicate control of the immediate environment. In connective tissue proper, the extracellular substance is soft; in cartilage, it is firm yet flexible and may be readily cut; in bone, it is rigid because of the deposition of inorganic salts in the matrix.

The cells of one type of connective tissue are often not easily distinguished from those of another on the basis of cytoplasmic structure. Rather, the histologist relies primarily on the appearance and physical properties of the extracellular matrix in assigning a given area of connective or supportive tissue to an appropriate subcategory such as loose connective tissue, dense connective tissue, regular or irregular connective tissue, cartilage, bone, etc. (Scheme 5-1). Even with appropriate criteria, however, such assignments are often difficult. This is so because in the organism the

character of the extracellular matrix may grade imperceptibly from that characteristic of one tissue into that of another. Hence, one is really dealing with a spectrum of connective and supportive tissues rather than a series of easily defined categories.

Embryonal Connective Tissues

The spectral nature of connective tissues is more easily appreciated when one considers their common embryology. All connective and supportive tissues of the body have originated from the mesoblast of the embryo. It will be recalled that, except for the notochord, the original cells of the mesoblast were mesenchymal in their morphology and behavior, dispersing widely and migrating freely as they produced a loose tissue network emphasizing a fluid extracellular matrix interspersed with a network of fine collagenous fibers (Fig. 5-1). The embryonal connective tissue of this stage has classically been referred to as *mucous connective tissue.* Very early in development the mesoblast became a compartment, separated physically from its surrounding epithelial neighbors by the deposition of a basal lamina. This early mesoblastic compartment can be termed the mesenchymal compartment. It is a principal staging area within or around which much further development will occur. The development of many glands and other organs involves extensive invaginations of one or another epithelium into the territory of

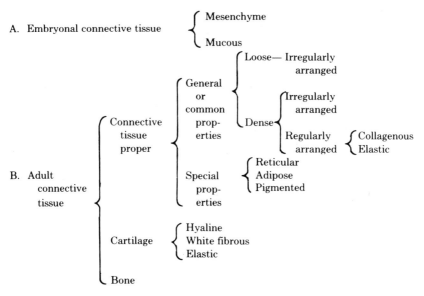

A. Embryonal connective tissue { Mesenchyme
Mucous

B. Adult connective tissue {
Connective tissue proper {
General or common properties {
Loose— Irregularly arranged
Dense {
Irregularly arranged
Regularly arranged { Collagenous
Elastic
}
Special properties { Reticular
Adipose
Pigmented
}
Cartilage { Hyaline
White fibrous
Elastic
Bone

SCHEME 5-1

the mesenchymal compartment. These are sites of intensive epithelial-mesenchymal inductive interaction through which the epithelium is transformed into a functionally differentiated epithelium appropriate to a particular organ (the parenchyma of the organ) and the mesenchymal component differentiates into the appropriate vascular and connective tissue parts (the stroma of the organ). Throughout these processes, separation of the mesenchymal compartment from the epithelial components is maintained by the interposed basal lamina, but it can be seen that the mesenchymal compartment becomes much more restricted and tortuous. A number of cavities also appear within the mesenchymal compartment (coelomic cavities, vascular channels, etc.). In other areas of the body (for example, in areas of muscle differentiation) mesenchymal cells clump together and develop into highly differentiated cells which soon segregate themselves from the mesenchymal compartment by acquiring a basal or external lamina.

The Connective Tissue Compartment

The net result of these types of development is that during later embryonic and early fetal stages, the once simple mesenchymal compartment of the gastrulating embryo is transformed into a tortuous array

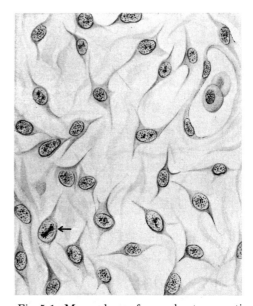

Fig. 5-1. Mesenchyme from subcutaneous tissue from a 10-mm pig embryo. *Arrow* points to a cell in mitosis. The processes of some cells appear to be continuous with those of other cells when viewed under the light microscope, but experimental studies indicate that they are merely in contact. ×650.

of narrow mesenchyme-filled passages interdigitated among the various other epithelial (including endothelial and mesothelial), muscular, and neural components. With very few exceptions, the mesenchymal compartment is separated from those components by a basal or an external lamina which can be visualized as the outer boundary of the compartment. Within this compartment, then, the differentiation of the connective and supportive tissues takes place. The result is the emergence of the connective tissue compartment, an even more complicated compartment whose perimeter remains defined by basal and external laminae. The contents of this compartment are not segregated from each other by basal or external laminae. This is to say that basal and external laminae are not found within connective and supportive tissues. A possible exception to this rule, the case of fat cells, is discussed later.

It is important to recognize the various connective and supportive tissues as intrinsic territories of this single, vast compartment for several reasons. The compartment is one of the body's largest circulating systems. Interstitial body fluids find their way through its most minute passages to bathe all of its cells. Integrity against leakage is maintained by tight junctions between the epithelial cells which guard the perimeter of the compartment. Turnover of the fluid is provided by leakage of blood fluids into the compartment and drainage via venous and lymphatic capillaries. The compartment is the main arena within which the immune mechanisms of the body operate and most storage is achieved. It is literally a channel which must be crossed by most metabolites entering or leaving the cells and tissues of the body. All of these functions, and more, are in addition to the usually emphasized aspects serving skeletal support and structural integrity among tissues and organs.

Adult Connective Tissue

Loose Connective Tissue

Loose, irregularly arranged, or areolar connective tissue is widely distributed in the human body. It forms the superficial and most of the deep fascia; it forms a part of the framework (stroma) of most of the organs; it surrounds blood vessels and nerves and fills in any otherwise unoccupied spaces. It generally contains a varying number of fat cells. When the latter are abundant the tissue is designated as adipose or fat tissue. Subcutaneous tissue (superficial fascia) which is heavily laden with fat cells in many parts of the body is often given a special name, panniculus adiposus.

Loose connective tissue, like all of the other connective tissues, is composed of *cells,* intercellular *fibers,* and *ground substance,* which is the material forming the foundation or background. The composition of ground substance is described later under a separate heading, but it should be noted immediately that the ground substance of loose connective tissue is relatively fluidlike, in contrast with that of cartilage and bone.

The loose connective tissue derives its name from the fact that its intercellular fibers are loosely arranged, in contrast with the closely packed fibers of dense connective tissue. The name *areolar* is descriptive of the general appearance produced by small spaces which contain only an amorphous ground substance.

Loose connective tissue contains most of the types of cells and all of the kinds of fibers found in the other varieties of connective tissue. Hence, a thorough knowledge of its structure serves not only for understanding its own very important functions but also as a basis for understanding the other types of connective tissue.

Connective Tissue Cells. The cells of loose connective tissue have been objects of intensive histological and experimental study. By means of various methods, the following cell types have been distinguished and found to be more or less constant inhabitants of loose connective tissue: *fibroblasts,* or fixed connective tissue cells, *histiocytes* or *macrophages, mast cells, plasma cells, fat cells,* and *wandering cells from the blood.*

Fibroblasts. The *fibroblasts* (Figs. 5-2 and 5-3) are one of the two most numerous cell types of loose connective tissue, the other being histiocytes. Fibroblasts, as their name suggests, are the principal cells responsible for fiber formation. There is evidence that they also form the ground substance.

They are large, somewhat flattened, frequently ovoid cells, with branching processes. Their nuclei are oval and somewhat

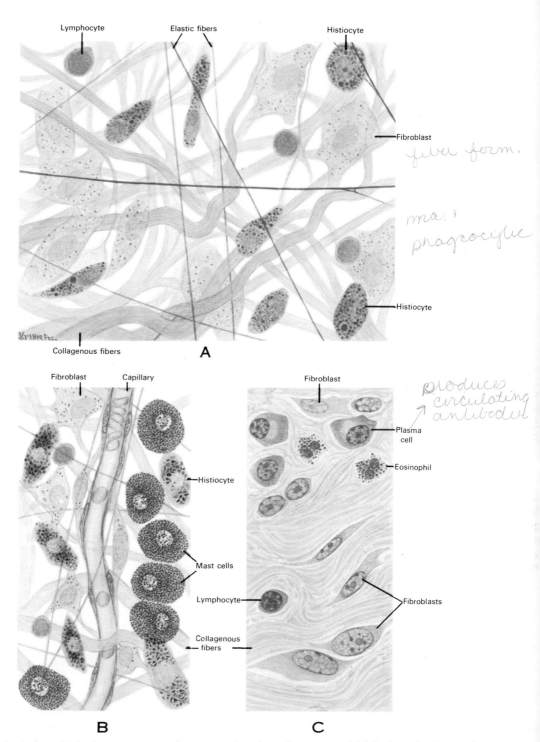

Lymphocyte   Elastic fibers   Histiocyte

fiber form.

Fibroblast

mas! phagocytic

Histiocyte

Collagenous fibers

A

Fibroblast   Capillary

Fibroblast

produces → circulating antibody

Plasma cell

Eosinophil

Histiocyte

Mast cells

Lymphocyte

Fibroblasts

Collagenous fibers

B

C

Fig. 5-2. *A*, spread of subcutaneous areolar connective tissue from a rat which had received several intraperitoneal injections of trypan blue over a period of 2 weeks. The animal was autopsied 1 week after the last injection and the spread was made immediately. After fixation in Bouin's fluid, it was stained with resorcin-fuchsin for elastic fibers and with azocarmine to show cells and collagenous fibers. All of the blue color shown in histiocytes and fibroblasts represents the trypan blue which was taken in by the cells preceding autopsy. No trypan blue is present in the nuclei, although a few vacuoles may appear to be within the nuclei when they are in the overlying cytoplasm. ×650. *B*, subcutaneous spread from the same trypan blue rat, stained with neutral red for mast cells. ×650. *C*, a section through the loose connective tissue of the submucosa of the colon. The field shown is directly beneath the muscularis mucosae. Rhesus monkey. Hematoxylin and eosin-azure. ×1250.

Neutrophil   Plasma cells   Connective tissue

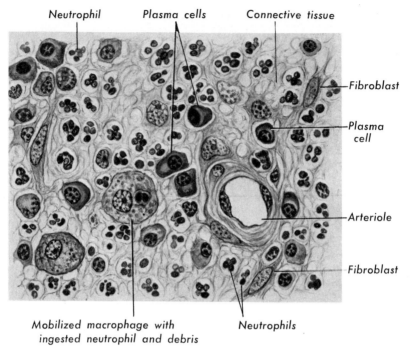

Fibroblast

Plasma cell

Arteriole

Fibroblast

Mobilized macrophage with
ingested neutrophil and debris

Neutrophils

Fig. 5-3. Section of an intratesticular abscess excised 30 days after the initial infection. An intermediate zone of the abscess is figured. Central to the area shown in the figure is a region where neutrophils predominate; peripherally is an extensive fibrosis. Hematoxylin and eosin-azure II. ×753.

flattened, resembling the shape of the cell. They usually stain lightly in fresh connective tissue spreads. In sections prepared by ordinary methods, the fibroblast nuclei are usually shrunken and stain deeply with basic dyes. The chromatin is distributed through the nucleus, with a tendency to become aggregated at intervals along the inner surface of the nuclear envelope. Because the cytoplasm takes little or no stain in its outer (ectoplasmic) region and because the cell membrane is too thin to be resolved under the light microscope, it is difficult to identify the cell boundary.

The appearance of the fibroblast varies in relation to its functional activity. When the cell is actively producing intercellular materials, as in normal development and in tissue regeneration after injury, the cell assumes a more mesenchymal appearance and is enlarged in correlation with an increase in its organelles. The nucleus is larger and the nucleoli are more prominent. The cytoplasm stains more deeply and is basophilic in contrast with the lightly staining, slightly acidophilic cytoplasm of the

relatively inactive cell. Electron micrographs show that there is a marked increase in rough-surfaced endoplasmic reticulum and also in free ribosomes. The Golgi complex is enlarged, and some of its cisternae and vesicles contain electron-dense material. There is also an increase in number of vesicles in other regions of the cytoplasm. The cell membrane is difficult to follow (or resolve) in places where aggregates of filamentous material in the peripheral portion of the cytoplasm face aggregates of extracellular dense material. The significance of these structural changes in relation to fiber formation is discussed further in the section on the origin of fibers. Some investigators prefer to confine the term fibroblast to the active stage of the cell and to use the term fibrocyte for the relatively inactive cell. This seems unnecessary, because they are only different functional states of the same cell.

Histiocytes (Macrophages). The *histiocytes* or *macrophages* (Figs. 5-2 and 5-3) are found in all loose connective tissues. The clasmatocytes and resting-wandering cells of various investigators have been found to be identical with these histiocytes. They are irregularly shaped cells with processes which usually are short and blunt but occasionally are long and slender. The nucleus is more rounded and somewhat smaller and darker-staining than that of the fibroblast. In the resting cell, the cytoplasm, like that of the fibroblast, stains lightly but may contain a few granules and vacuoles. It should be noted that the diagnostic features just listed are minor. The characteristics of the relatively inactive histiocytes do not differ sufficiently from those of the fibroblasts to enable one to distinguish clearly histiocytes from fibroblasts in most light microscope preparations. However, the histiocytes become clearly distinguishable from fibroblasts when they are activated, as in the region of an abscess (Fig. 5-3). The entire cell becomes larger, with a larger nucleus, a more prominent nucleolus, and a cytoplasm more or less filled with granules and vacuoles of ingested material. The histiocytes in an area of inflammation are particularly busy engulfing worn out neutrophilic leukocytes which died in the process of engulfing and destroying bacteria. The neutrophils serve as the "shock troops" and the histiocytes function in "mopping up" operations.

Light microscope studies of macrophages in tissue culture preparations show that foreign material is surrounded by protoplasmic processes and taken into the cell by ameboid-like activity. Electron micrographs show that the ingested materials are membrane-bounded in vesicles named phagosomes. These vesicles combine with primary lysosomes to form secondary lysosomes, as shown schematically in Figure 1-32. Most of the ingested materials are digested by the proteolytic enzymes acquired from the primary lysosomes, but some materials, e.g., carbon particles in the connective tissue macrophages of the lung, are not digestible and may remain in the cytoplasm for a long period.

Objects too large to be engulfed by a single cell are attacked en masse and become surrounded by histiocytes, which eventually fuse to form a *multinucleated foreign body giant cell*. These are not to be confused with blood platelet-producing *megakaryocytes* of bone marrow (Fig. 7-12).

The most commonly used experimental method for identifying histiocytes is to study their physiological reaction in supravital preparations and their intravital response to injected trypan blue, colloidal carbon, etc. Sections of tissue from animals which have had one or more injections of trypan blue show extensive ingestion and segregation of the dye in vacuoles in the cytoplasm of histiocytes and relatively little ingested material in fibroblasts (Fig. 5-2).

Macrophages or histiocytes are widely distributed in the body. They are in loose connective tissue and, therefore, they are present in all fascia. They also occur in the connective tissue which is present in organs, although the proportion of them to fibroblasts may vary considerably in different regions of an organ. The phagocytic cells are also found in specific locations in some organs, e.g., in association with the lining cells of the sinusoids of the liver, lymphatic organs, and bone marrow. These were once thought to be modified endothelial cells, but recent electron microscope studies of tissues after labeling with tritiated thymidine indicate that these cells are probably derived from promonocytes. Together with the histiocytes of loose connective tissue they form the macrophage system, which is discussed in more detail at the end of this chapter.

It has been noted above that macrophages become very *active* in regions of inflammation, as in an abscess (Fig. 5-3). They are also more *numerous* in such areas. The increase may result from (1) multiplication of cells already in the area, (2) migration of histiocytes from neighboring areas, and (3) transformations of monocytes which migrate into the area from the blood vessels.

Plasma Cells. The *plasma cells* (Figs. 5-2, 5-3, and 5-4) are relatively rare in most connective tissues under normal conditions, although they are fairly numerous in the connective tissue of the alimentary mucous membrane and greater omentum. They are also fairly numerous in the reticular connective tissues of blood-forming organs. Their number is greatly increased in areas of chronic inflammation. They are ovoid,

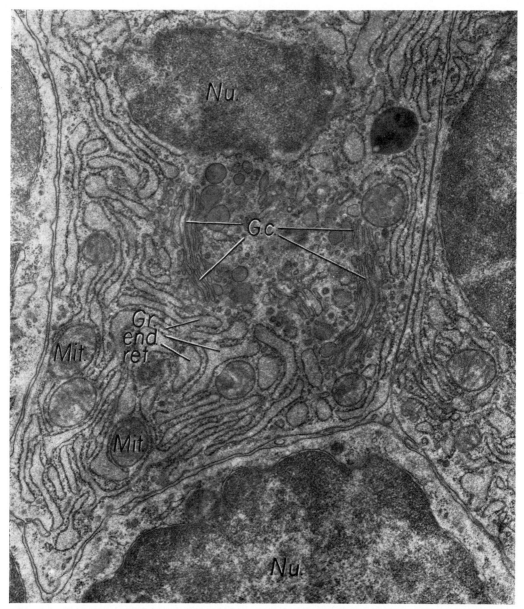

Fig. 5-4. Electron micrograph of a portion of the spleen of a bat, showing parts of two plasma cells (*above*) and a part of a lymphocyte (*below*). *Gc,* Golgi complex; *Gr. end. ret.,* granular endoplasmic reticulum of plasma cell showing relatively wide cisternae and numerous ribosomes associated with the outer surfaces of the membranes of the cisternae; *Mit.* mitochondria; *Nu,* portions of the nuclei. Note that the lymphocyte contrasts with the plasma cell by having very few cisternae of endoplasmic reticulum, although it has numerous ribosomes. ×19,000. (Courtesy of Dr. Keith Porter.)

irregularly shaped cells, smaller than histiocytes but larger than lymphocytes (Fig. 5-2). The nucleus is relatively small and eccentrically placed. The chromatin appears in the form of deep-staining, coarse granules. Because most of the chromatin granules are arranged in a regular manner against the nuclear membrane and only a few are present toward the center, the nucleus has a "cartwheel" appearance.

The cytoplasm of the plasma cell is very basophilic, like that of a lymphocyte, but it has a characteristic unstained or lightly stained area at the side of the nucleus where the cytoplasm is more abundant (Figs. 5-2 and 5-3). The unstained area represents the region of the Golgi complex. In comparison with a lymphocyte, the plasma cell has more cytoplasm in proportion to the size of the nucleus; i.e., the cytoplasmic-nuclear ratio is greater. The cytoplasm of the two types of cells also shows significant differences in electron micrographs. The plasma cell has an extensive endoplasmic reticulum with associated ribosomes, whereas the lymphocyte contains mostly free ribosomes with little reticulum (Figs. 5-4 and 7-3). The Golgi complex is large (Fig. 5-4) and is associated with secretory vesicles that migrate to the surface where they liberate the secretory material by exocytosis in a manner similar to that described for exocrine glands (Fig. 1-10). Some unusually large masses of electron-dense material are seen *occasionally* within the cisternae of the rough-surfaced endoplasmic reticulum; these apparently correspond to the *Russell bodies* first described by light microscopists. They probably represent an aberrant secretory pathway and may forecast degenerative changes in the cell.

The plasma cell precursor (proplasmacyte) has a basophilic cytoplasm which stains well with the red basic dye pyronin, and therefore it is sometimes described as a pyroninophilic cell. The cytoplasm also stains with hematoxylin in hematoxylin and eosin preparations and with Azure II in Azure II-eosin methods. There is considerable evidence that the proplasmacyte is derived from a medium-sized B-type lymphocyte.

It is known from fluorescent antibody techniques and from other lines of evidence that the plasma cell is the major producer of *circulating antibodies.* The mature plasma cell is an end stage, that is, it does not continue to divide. It is derived from pyroninophilic precursors that are actively dividing and reaching stages at which they begin to form antibody. The different roles of the lymphocytes and the macrophages of lymphatic organs in the immune mechanism are discussed in the sections on lymphocytes (chapter 7) and lymphatic organs (chapter 13).

Mast Cells. These cells (Figs. 5-2 and 5-5) occur in varying numbers in most loose connective tissue, being especially numerous along the course of the blood vessels. They are large ovoid cells with relatively small ovoid nuclei and numerous cytoplasmic granules which are usually basophilic. These cells resemble the basophilic leukocytes of the blood in some respects but differ from them in the size and nonsegmented shape of their nuclei. They also differ in the ultrastructural features of their cytoplasmic granules and in function.

Mast cell granules are soluble in water, like those of basophilic leukocytes, and are therefore not very obvious in most routinely prepared hematoxylin and eosin-stained sections. After appropriate fixation the granules stain with most basic dyes and are metachromatic after certain dyes such as toluidine blue; i.e., the granules show a reddish color which is beyond or different from the color of the dye used (Fig. 5-5).

Electron micrographs show that the mast cell has a relatively well developed Golgi complex but relatively few mitochondria and only moderate amounts of free ribosomes and granular endoplasmic reticulum. The secretory granules are membrane bounded and, in the human, the matrices of the granules have varying densities and characteristic patterns resembling scrolls.

The granules contain *heparin,* an anticoagulant, and *histamine,* which produces vasodilation and increases the permeability of capillaries and small venules. The mast cells of a few species, but not of man, also contain serotonin.

The earliest suggestion that mast cells contain heparin came from staining reactions which showed that purified heparin and mast cells are both metachromatic. It was shown later that tissues with numerous mast cells also have more heparin than those with only a few mast cells. Still later, it was found that mast cell tumors of dogs have a very high content of heparin. In more recent studies by radioautography, it has been shown that radioactive sulfur is taken up readily by mast cells.

The evidence that mast cells contain histamine is based on a sequence of studies

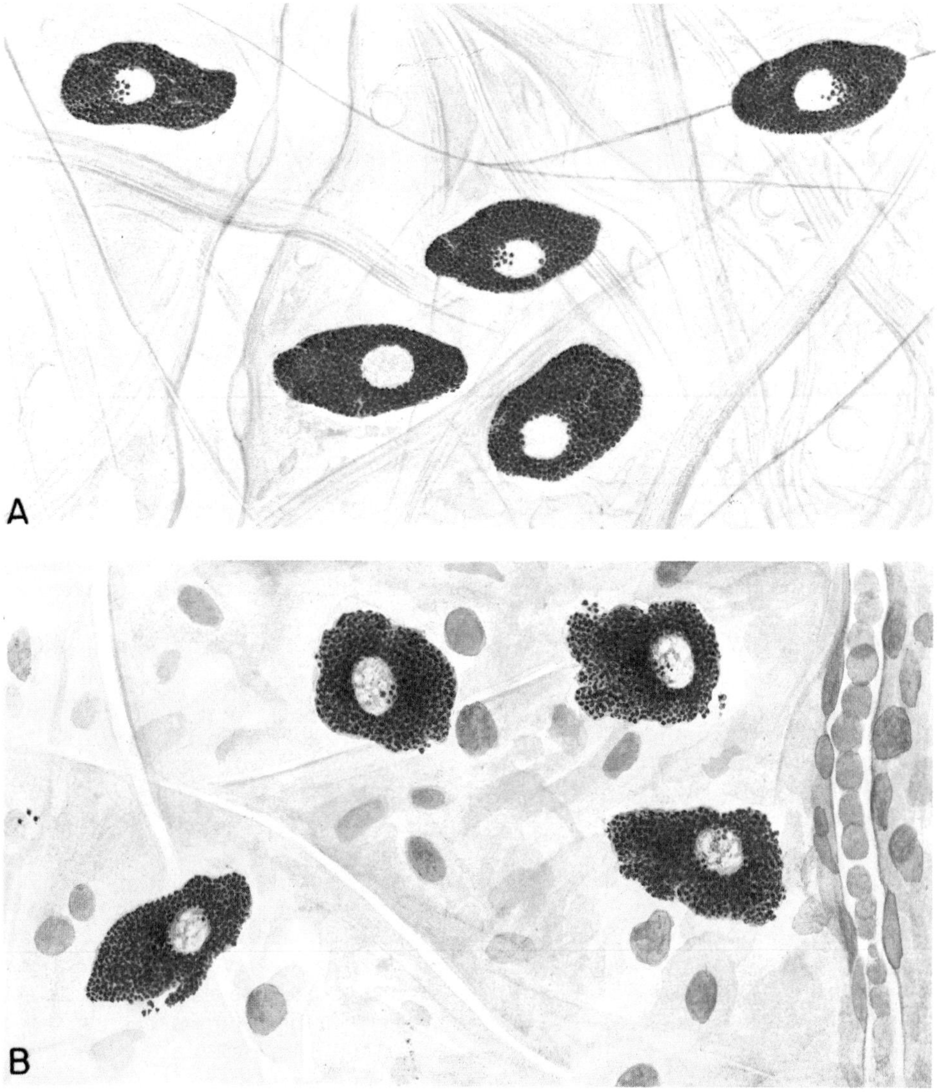

Fig. 5-5. Mast cells in spreads of subcutaneous connective tissue from the inguinal region of a rat. *A*, basophilia of mast cell granules seen after staining with an alcoholic solution of toluidine blue. The pH of the stain was lowered by the addition of HCl and the nuclei of cells remained unstained. Nuclei, connective tissue fibers, and the wall of a capillary are visible in the background by their refraction. ×730. *B*, metachromasia of mast cell granules seen after staining in a dilute aqueous solution of toluidine blue. The mast cell granules give a reddish color with the blue dye. Nuclei of fibroblasts, of histiocytes, and of capillary endothelial cells (*right side of field*) stain blue. Erythrocytes are bluish green. The pH of the stain in this case was relatively high. ×730.

resembling those outlined above for heparin. For example, it was found that tissues containing an abundance of mast cells contain more histamine than those with relatively few mast cells. Later, it was shown by chemical studies that mast cells do produce and secrete histamine.

The importance of heparin as an anticoagulant in clinical work is obvious, but its role in the normal connective tissue remains obscure. The effect of histamine on the endothelium of venules was cited above, and it probably plays a role in the functional relationships of blood vessels and connective tissue under normal circumstances. The role of histamine in relation to antigen-antibody complexes is a subject of active research.

Mast cells, like most other cell types of connective tissue, differentiate from mesenchymal cells during embryonic development. The mast cells are seen in mitosis only occasionally in the adult, and, although it has been suggested that they are long-lived, it seems obvious that some new mast cells in the adult must differentiate from nongranular cells. The cell of origin in this case remains controversial. It was proposed by Maximow and others many years ago that some of the connective tissue cells intimately associated with the blood vessels in the adult have many of the developmental potencies of embryonic mesenchyme. Such "undifferentiated" cells seem the most likely source of mast cells in the adult connective tissues.

Fat Cells. These cells are found singly and in small groups widely distributed in the loose connective tissues. They are similar, except in numbers, to the cells found in masses as *adipose tissue.* The fat content of the cell is dissolved by the reagents generally used in the preparation of sections. Consequently, the cells appear as large empty spaces surrounded by the peripheral portion of the cell and a flattened nucleus (Fig. 5-15).

Fat cells are the only cells generally considered to be connective tissue cells which surround themselves individually with an external lamina.

Wandering Cells from the Blood. Besides the cells enumerated, temporary visitors from the blood and lymph stream are seen in varying numbers. These may include lymphocytes and eosinophilic and neutrophilic leukocytes.

Connective Tissue Fibers. Three types of fibers occur in adult connective tissue. Each of these types is present in loose connective tissue, and thus a study of the fibers in this type of tissue gives an understanding of the fibrillar elements of all adult connective tissue.

White or Collagenous Fibers. The *white* or *collagenous* fibers generally course together in bundles of indefinite length and variable thickness ranging from 10 to 100 μm or more. The individual fibers seen in routine preparations vary in diameter from 1 to 12 μm (Fig. 5-2). When these are studied under the higher magnifications of oil immersion objectives, and particularly after special treatment, it is found that they are composed of smaller fibers, the so-called *fibrils of light microscopy,* only 0.2 to 0.5 μm in diameter. These are held together by an amorphous material which can be dissolved by weak alkalis or by trypsin. They are aligned in a parallel direction, giving the appearance of longitudinal striation. The fibers of the loose connective tissue follow an irregular and undulating course; this allows for movement and flexibility of the other tissues with which they are associated. The collagenous fibers themselves are flexible but so slightly elastic as to be practically nonextensible.

Collagen is a protein which stains with most acid dyes. Hence, the fibers are red in hematoxylin-eosin-stained sections, blue from the aniline blue of Mallory's triple stain, and green or blue in Masson's trichrome, depending on the modification used, i.e., whether the stain contains light green or aniline blue. The fibers are rapidly digested by gastric juice but resist digestion by trypsin in alkaline solution. They swell in dilute acids and are dissolved by strong acids and alkalis. They yield gelatin on boiling; thus, meat with a high content of collagen is made more tender by boiling. Collagen is also a source of glue; animal hides which are composed largely of dense collagenous fibers can be made into leather by tanning.

Electron micrographs show that each of the collagenous fibrils of light microscopy is composed of still smaller *fibrils.* The latter are relatively uniform in diameter in any given connective tissue region but vary in different locations and in different stages of development, ranging from about 200 to 2000 Å. In adult human dermis, they are about 1000 Å in diameter. In regions where collagen is being formed, there are slender collagenous fibrils only about 200 Å in diameter. In these regions, one may also find very thin *microfibrils* (30 to 150 Å) which are collagen-like but lack the characteristic periodicity of collagen.

The electron microscope fibrils of mature collagen have periodic cross bandings at intervals of about 640 Å (Fig. 5-6). Infor-

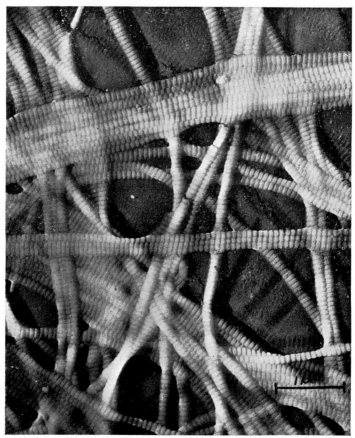

Fig. 5-6. Electron micrograph of collagen fibrils from the adult human dermis. Chromium-shadowed. ×19,300. (Courtesy of Drs. Gross and Schmitt.)

mation on the periodicity and the structure of collagen has evolved from the discovery that collagen can be taken apart in vitro and that its constituent molecules can be reassembled either into their previous native form or into other forms. When young or newly formed collagen is taken from the body and placed in cold neutral salt, it readily dissolves. When the solution is incubated at body temperature, fibers form in vitro which have the same 640 Å periodicity as native collagen. A solution of young collagen can also be made in weak acetic acid. This will yield native 640 Å periodicity collagen by neutralization, or it will give blocks of 2800 Å lengths ("segment long spacing collagen") after treatment with adenosine triphosphoric acid. The same solution will yield 2800 Å segments arranged end to end ("fibrous long spacing") after treatment with glycoproteins. From various

studies of this type, using methods of X-ray diffraction, chemical analysis, and electron microscopy, it has been established that collagen is composed of macromolecules of about 2800 Å in length and 15 Å in width. The substance is named *tropocollagen* (from the Greek *trope,* turning, i.e., turning into collagen). Each macromolecule is composed of three polypeptide chains in the form of a coiled helix (Fig. 5-7). The chains are composed of amino acids and are joined by hydrogen bonding. The macromolecule is structurally polarized and has a characteristic intraband pattern determined by a precise linear sequence of the different amino acid residues in the intramolecular strands. In the development of collagen, the macromolecules become aligned parallel with one another to give the 640-Å periodicity characteristic of collagen. The most commonly accepted expla-

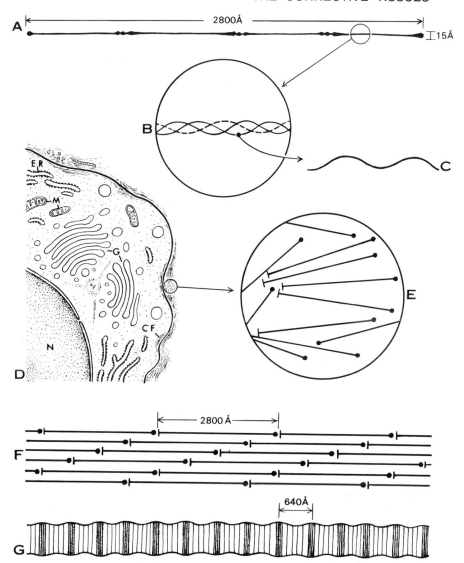

Fig. 5-7. Diagrams of the formation and structure of collagen as determined by electron microscopy, chemical analysis, and X-ray diffraction. *A*, schematization of the tropocollagen macromolecule, showing structural asymmetry along its length. *B*, enlargement of a section of the macromolecule, showing that it is composed of three polypeptide chains, with one (indicated by *broken line*) differing from the other two in amino acid composition. *C*, enlargement of a portion of *B*, showing that each polypeptide chain has a helical configuration. *D*, diagrammatic representation of a portion of a fibroblast, showing a portion of the nucleus (*N*), mitochondria (*M*), rough-surfaced endoplasmic reticulum (*ER*), Golgi complex (*G*), and cytoplasmic microfilaments (*CF*). In the formation of collagen, amino acids taken up by the cell are synthesized into polypeptides at the sites of polyribosomes associated with the endoplasmic reticulum; then the polypeptides are transported via the cisternae of the endoplasmic reticulum to the Golgi complex, where they are assembled into macromolecules which are transported in Golgi-derived vesicles to the cell surface. *E*, enlarged and schematized representation of a small region of material just outside the cell, showing the irregular distribution of tropocollagen macromolecules. *F*, diagrammatic representation of the manner in which the macromolecules are postulated as coming together in an aligned and overlapping pattern to form cross-banded collagenous fibers, as shown in *G*. (*A, B, C, F,* and *G* are redrawn and modified from Gross, 1961 and 1964. *D* and *E* are based chiefly on descriptions by Porter, 1964, and by Gross, 1964.)

nation for the 640-Å periodicity is that the 2800 Å long macromolecules are aligned end to end, but not touching and with the molecules of adjacent rows arranged in a staggered fashion, overlapping by about one-quarter of their length, as shown in Figure 5-7.

Chemically, the tropocollagen macromolecule consists of about 30% glycine and 25% proline and hydroxyproline, with the remainder consisting of other amino acids, including hydroxylysine. Glycine recurs at a constant position and frequency along the alpha chain, whereas the other amino acids recur at variable positions. Because hydroxyproline is not found in any significant amount in any other tissue, a determination of its amount in any organ indicates the amount of collagen in that organ. Proline and hydroxyproline prevent easy rotation of the strand where they are located, and thus they add stability to the macromolecule.

Recent biochemical studies indicate that collagen macromolecules are not identical throughout the body. This stems from the fact that collagen is comprised of three helically intertwined polypeptide chains that can differ individually in their amino acid sequences. These so-called alpha units have now been separated into two basic classes, α_1 and α_2, and, in addition, the α_1 class appears to consist of several *Types*. For example, the collagen macromolecules made by fibroblasts in skin and tendon contain two α_1, Type I polypeptides linked to an α_2 polypeptide, whereas those made by chondroblasts have three α_1, Type II polypeptide chains. Thus, the biochemical information is beginning to provide a sound basis for understanding the difference in collagen appearance at the electron microscope level. Presumably, the polypeptide composition is also directly related to the types and quantity of sugars that are attached, and to the polymerization sequence. Therefore, differences in the morphological appearance of collagen in different locations in the body become more understandable.

Reticular Fibers. These fibers are small, branching fibers which frequently form a netlike supporting framework or reticulum. Their caliber is so small that they are masked by surrounding structures in ordinary stained preparations, but they blacken intensely after silver impregnation (Bielchowsky's method), whereas collagenous fibers are colored yellow or brown. Because they impregnate with silver, reticular fibers are frequently designated as *argyrophilic* fibers.

Reticular fibers are often continuous with collagenous fibers, and it is difficult to obtain any quantity of their substance, known as *reticulin,* for chemical analysis. In most respects, they appear to be chemically similar to collagenous fibers, although they are more resistant to peptic digestion. They also have relatively more carbohydrate, which is apparently associated with each fibril in the form of a surface coat. This explains the fact that reticular fibers give a strongly positive reaction with the periodic acid-Schiff (PAS) technique, whereas collagenous fibers give only a slight reaction. The associated carbohydrate is also responsible for the more intense reaction with certain silver techniques. The reticular fibers have the same 640 Å cross banding as skin-type collagenous fibers and are morphologically similar to them except for diameter. Because collagenous fibers pass through a developmental stage in which they are argyrophilic and apparently identical with reticular fibers, the latter are apparently merely immature stages of the former. In other words, the reticular fibers are not actually a separate fiber type.

These argyrophilic fibers are relatively sparse in adult loose connective tissues, except for regions around muscle fibers (Fig. 8-24) and around blood vessels, nerves, and epithelial structures. They are numerous in glandular organs (Fig. 16-86).

In lymphatic organs and in red bone marrow, the fibers are associated with a special type of cell known as the *reticular cell;* the two elements (reticular fibers and reticular cells) form a type of tissue, the *reticular tissue.* In other locations, reticular fibers, have the same relationship to fibroblasts as collagenous fibers have.

Elastic Fibers. The *elastic* fibers (Fig. 5-2) are highly refractile fibers which are as a rule thinner than the white fibers but may reach a diameter of 10 to 12 μm in some elastic ligaments (e.g., ligamentum nuchae of an ox). They branch and anastomose freely, forming networks. The smaller fibers are round in cross section; the larger are flat or polygonal. They are highly elastic. When seen in large masses (elastic ligaments) in the fresh state, they have a distinctly yellow appearance. In arteries, the elastic tissue often occurs in the form of fenestrated membranes or lamellae.

Elastic fibers are best demonstrated in the fresh condition by immersing the tissue in dilute acid solutions. The collagenous fibers swell and become transparent. The elastic fibers are then seen as highly refractive, shining threads. The elastic fibers react poorly to most stains, but they are colored specifically by certain dyes such as orcein and resorcinfuchsin (Fig. 5-2).

Electron micrographs show that elastic fibers are not made up of cross-banded fibrils as is collagen. In fact, most electron micrographs give the impression that elastic tissue is composed only of an amorphous substance of varying electron density. However, high resolution electron micrographs of thin sections stained with uranyl acetate and lead citrate show that the elastic fiber substance has two components: homogeneous material, *elastin,* and slender *elastic fiber microfibrils* of about 120 Å in diameter.

In the development of an elastic fiber, the microfibrils differentiate earlier than does the elastin, and consequently the microfibrils are more obvious in young elastic tissue. On the other hand, elastin is the most obvious component in mature elastic fibers, and the microfibrils are limited chiefly to the periphery of the fiber, with only a few scattered through the elastin. Whether the elastin appears light or dark in electron micrographs depends on the method of fixation, as noted above. Furthermore, the appearance of the microfibrils may vary not only with the stage of development and method of tissue fixation but also with the functional state of the fiber: it has been postulated that the fibrils are randomly oriented in relaxed fibers and more parallel in stretched fibers.

Chemically, the elastic fiber contains proline, glycine, valine, and a number of other amino acids. It differs, however, from collagen in the proportions of the amino acids. It contains very little hydroxyproline, it has a much higher concentration of valine, and it contains desmosine and isodesmosine, two amino acids not found in collagen. These specialized amino acids are now known to be involved in the cross-linking of elastin. Elastin and the elastic tissue microfibrils differ from each other in the proportions of their amino acids. Elastin has a higher content of valine than the microfibrils, whereas the latter have a much greater content of cystine and completely lack hydroxyproline and desmosine. The microfibrils also contain sugar moieties such as hexose and hexosamine, thus suggesting that they contain glycoproteins.

Elastic fibers are usually formed by fibroblasts, but in certain locations, such as the media of the aorta, they are produced by smooth muscle cells.

The surface of an elastic fiber seems to be continually undergoing changes which involve a turnover of material. In the aging of fenestrated membranes (lamellae) of arteries, small regions of degenerating elastic tissue form seeding sites for mineralization in the peripheral portion of the lamella. In elastic fibers of the skin, age changes occur in the associated mucopolysaccharides. There is an increase in chondroitin sulfate B and keratosulfate in proportion to the other mucopolysaccharides, and this gives a loss of resiliency.

Origin of the Connective Tissue Fibers. The development of connective tissue fibers has been studied extensively, both by light microscopy and by electron microscopy. In locations where connective tissue fibers first appear in embryos, one can see with the light microscope that the accompanying cells differ from the more primitive mesenchymal cells from which they are derived. They have prominent nucleoli and basophilic cytoplasm. They resemble the blast cells characteristically found in other differentiating regions. The name fibroblast, given by early histologists, was based on the belief that the cells participate in some manner in the formation of fibers. Further studies by tissue culture methods showed that the earliest fibers are narrow and that they appear just outside the cell surfaces in at least some instances (Figs. 5-8 and 5-9). However, the best resolution

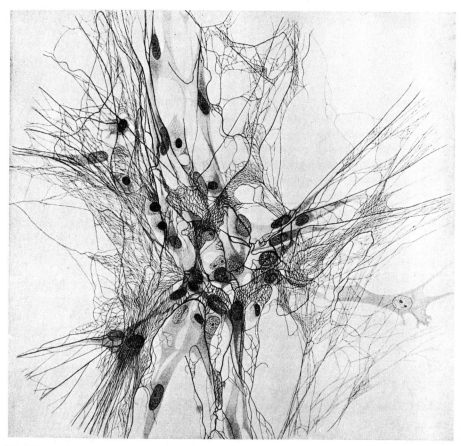

Fig. 5-8. Formation of reticular fibers as seen in a tissue culture preparation. Note that the fibers are closely associated with the cells in some regions and separated from them in others. (After Maximow.)

obtainable by light microscopy left many unanswered questions.

Electron microscopy, in combination with radioautography and biochemical methods, has provided a much better understanding of collagen formation. Among the data obtained from numerous studies of this subject, the results on the formation of collagen by the odontoblasts of the incisor teeth of rats are particularly clear. The odontoblast is a tall columnar cell with the basal end near the blood vessels and with the apical end extending to the newly formed dentin. In other words, the cell is polarized and collagen is secreted in a predictable location. Furthermore, the rat incisor is constantly erupting and collagen formation is a continuing process. In these studies by Weinstock and Leblond (1974), tritium-labeled proline is found over the

ribosomes of the endoplasmic reticulum of the odontoblast within 2 min after intravenous injection. This newly synthesized material is interpreted as *pro-alpha* chains of collagen on the basis of biochemical studies by a number of investigators. The pro-alpha chains, each composed of three polypeptide chains, are irregularly arranged until they reach the Golgi complex, where carbohydrates are added and they gradually become organized into parallel threads of *procollagen*. These are longer than the eventual collagen molecules found outside the cell because they have tailpieces about 130 Å in length that were presumably synthesized at the time the alpha chains were formed. The procollagen threads are transported in vesicles (secretory granules) from the Golgi complex to the cell surface, where the membranes of the vesicles fuse with

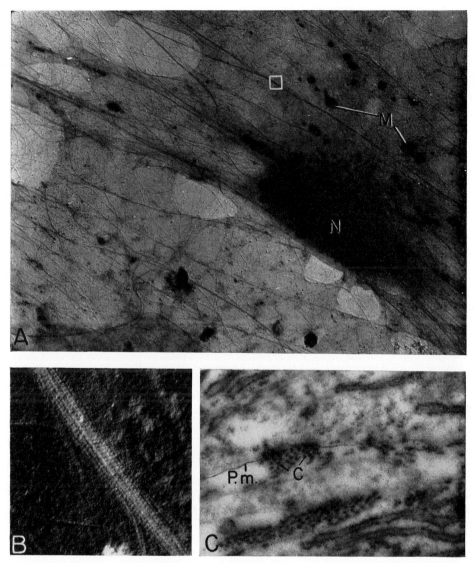

Fig. 5-9. Electron micrographs illustrating the relationship of fibroblasts to collagen fiber formation. *A*, surface view of a fibroblast grown in tissue culture from an explant from the dermis of a 9-
day-old chick embryo. The nucleus (*N*) and mitochondria (*M*) are indicated. Collagen fibers formed
in association with the cell course from *lower right* to *upper left*. ×3,000. *B*, higher magnification of
the fiber shown within the *small square* of *A*. Note that the fiber is composed of many fibrils.
×20,000. *C*, section through cells of the dermis of a 14-day-old chick embryo. A fiber similar to that
illustrated in *B* is shown in a section vertical to the cell surface. No collagen fibrils (*C*) are evident
within the cytoplasm; they appear first on the cell surface (*P.m.*). ×20,000. (Courtesy of Drs. Keith
Porter and G. D. Pappas.)

the cell membranes by exocytosis and the
procollagen threads are released into the
surrounding medium. At or near the cell
membrane, the tailpieces of the procollagen
molecules are sloughed off as the result of
action of a *peptidase enzyme* found near

the cell surface. By the release of the tailpieces, the procollagen molecules become
tropocollagen molecules, which rapidly po-
lymerize to form slender collagenous fibers
described as protofibrils. In the case of the
odontoblast, the entire process from the

time of the initial incorporation of label until the appearance of collagen extracellularly can occur in about 30 min.

The slender "microfibrils" of 30 to 160 Å in diameter observed by some investigators in the electron-dense material at the surface of fibroblasts probably represent early stages of polymerization of tropocollagen into protofibrils. Once they are established, these early protofibrils increase in diameter by the addition of newly polymerized protofibrils at their surface up to a width characteristic for a given tissue, e.g., relatively slender fibers in the lamina propria of the digestive tract and very broad fibers in tendon.

The formation of elastic fibers is outlined in the previous section on their structure. The elastic fibers make their appearance in the embryo later than collagenous fibers, but this is not to be misconstrued to imply that they develop from the latter. Their peripheral microfibrils are morphologically similar to the microfibrils present in regions where collagen is forming, but there is no evidence that they are identical chemically.

In considering the histiogenic functions of fibroblasts, one must not overlook the fact that they secrete the mucopolysaccharides of the intercellular matrix. There is evidence that the protein components are synthesized in the region of the rough-surfaced endoplasmic reticulum and that the carbohydrates are added both in the endoplasmic reticulum and in the Golgi complex, but that sulfation occurs only in the Golgi complex.

Ground Substance. The cells and fibers of connective tissue are embedded in an amorphous background material known as *ground substance*. It is a colloidal substance in the form of a gel of variable viscosity, which binds varying amounts of water. The bound water serves as a medium for diffusion of gases and metabolic substances from the blood vessels to the cells of the tissues, and vice versa. Thus the amorphous matrix and the tissue fluids are intimately associated. Most of the extravascular fluid is bound within the matrix and is not present in any appreciable amount as free water in the connective tissues under normal conditions. Whereas the matrix is normally fluid, it rapidly becomes much

more so in areas of injury and inflammation.

In fresh spreads of connective tissue, the ground substance has the same refractive index as water and isotonic saline solutions, and therefore it is invisible in spreads mounted in these media. The ground substance is quite soluble in the reagents generally used in preparing tissues for sectioning, and it is not seen in the areolar connective tissue of routinely prepared sections. It is preserved best by fresh freezing and freeze-drying techniques, provided that the tissues are fixed subsequently in vapors of ether-formol. In these preparations, the ground substance stains metachromatically, indicating the presence of mucopolysaccharides. In some connective tissues, such as cartilage and bone, it can be preserved by appropriate fixatives in sufficient quantities for histochemical studies. In fact, the mucopolysaccharide content of cartilage and bone is sufficient to affect the tinctorial results in sections routinely prepared and stained with hematoxylin and eosin (chapter 6).

The ground substance contains a number of *mucopolysaccharides* (glycosaminoglycans), which are divided into two main categories, *sulfated* and *nonsulfated,* depending upon whether they are esterified with sulfuric acid. The nonsulfated group includes *hyaluronic acid* and *chondroitin.* The sulfated group includes: *chondroitin 4-sulfate* (chondroitin sulfate A), *chondroitin 6-sulfate* (chondroitin sulfate C), *dermatan sulfate* (chondroitin sulfate B), and *keratan sulfate* (keratosulfate). *Heparin,* produced by mast cells, is also a mucopolysaccharide, and it has a relatively high content of sulfate. Most of the sulfated mucopolysaccharides are very gel-like, and when they are abundant, as in cartilage, they provide support.

Hyaluronic acid is a viscous, fluidlike mucopolysaccharide isolated by Meyer and Palmer in 1934. It is found in synovial fluid, loose connective tissue, etc. (Table 5-1). Because of its capacity to bind water, it probably has a major responsibility for changes in the viscosity and permeability of ground substance. It probably plays a role in preventing the spread of noxious agents in localized infections. An enzyme,

TABLE 5-1*

Main types of connective tissue mucopolysaccharides

Name	Some locations where found	Sulfate/disaccharide unit	Hyaluronidase susceptibility	
			Testicular	Bacterial
Hyaluronic acid	Synovial fluid, umbilical cord, vitreous humor, loose connective tissue, group A streptococci capsules	0	+	+
Chondroitin	Cornea	0		
Chondroitin 4-sulfate (chondroitin sulfate A)	Aorta, bone, cartilage, cornea	1	+	−
Chondroitin 6-sulfate (chondroitin sulfate C)	Cartilage, nucleus pulposus, sclera, tendon, umbilical cord	1	+	−
Dermatan sulfate (chondroitin sulfate B)	Aorta, heart valve, ligamentum nuchae, sclera, skin, tendon	1	−	−
Keratan sulfate (keratosulfate)	Bone, cartilage, cornea, nucleus pulposus	1	−	−
Heparin	Mast cells	2	−	−

* Modified from Spicer et al., 1967.

hyaluronidase, hydrolyzes it, reducing its viscosity with a consequent increase in the permeability of the tissue. For example, subcutaneous injections of India ink to which hyaluronidase has been added spread much more rapidly than injections of ink alone. This enzyme (known as "spreading factor") was first isolated from testicles and snake venom. An enzyme with similar effects on hyaluronic acid is produced by some bacteria. Chondroitin differs from hyaluronic acid by having galactosamine in place of glucosamine.

Chondroitin 4-sulfate differs from chondroitin 6-sulfate only in that the sulfate moiety is attached at carbon 4. Chondroitin 4-sulfate and dermatan sulfate have a number of chemical differences. When they are found in the same location, as in the aorta (Table 5-1), they can be readily distinguished in histochemical preparations by the fact that chondroitin 4-sulfate is susceptible to testicular hyaluronidase, whereas dermatan sulfate is not.

The sulfated mucopolysaccharides are generally much more metachromatic than the nonsulfated ones in toluidine blue-stained preparations. The sulfated group also stains with hematoxylin when it is sufficiently abundant, as in cartilage, to overshadow the associated acidophilic collagenous fibers. Both types of mucopolysac-

charides, sulfated and nonsulfated, give positive PAS reactions.

The PAS Reaction in Connective Tissues. The PAS technique is based on the fact that free aldehydes restore the reddish color to basic fuchsin which has been bleached previously with sulfurous acid. In chapter 1 it is noted that the Schiff reagent (i.e., bleached basic fuchsin) is specific for DNA in the Feulgen reaction because the sections are treated to only a mild hydrolysis which liberates aldehydes from DNA but not from RNA. When a stronger oxidizing agent, such as periodic acid, is used, aldehydes are liberated from polysaccharides in general. Cartilage matrix gives a positive PAS reaction, and the ground substances of other connective tissues also give PAS reactions of varying degrees in different locations. However, *pure* hyaluronic acid is PAS-negative, and the same is apparently true for *pure* chondroitin sulfate. Recent studies confirm that PAS methods do not visualize the acid mucopolysaccharides themselves. The PAS reaction that is given by a number of these carbohydrate-protein complexes is apparently due to the associated carbohydrates, such as hexoses, etc. The PAS-positive reaction given by reticular fibers is apparently due to carbohydrates in the surface coat of the fiber.

Functions of Loose Connective Tis-

sue. Nutrient substances in their passage from the blood vessels to the cells of the body traverse connective tissue, as must also those products of metabolism which reach the blood and lymph capillaries (see Fig. 12-24.) Loose connective tissue loosely binds structures together and holds them in position. It acts as a padding and serves as a pathway for nerves and blood vessels.

The loose connective tissue plays an extremely important role in limiting the spread of localized infections and in the healing process. The localization invokes all elements of the connective tissue. The ground substance, although permeable, tends to inhibit the passage of the noxious agent. In addition to the phagocytic cells (neutrophilic leukocytes and monocytes) which migrate to the area from the blood, the tissue phagocytes (macrophages) multiply and mobilize. The fibroblasts also become active and, after a considerable time, deposit a surrounding barrier of fibers. An area of infection is shown in Figure 5-3. In repair of wounds, the fibroblasts increase in number and form fibers. Sprouts from the blood vessels penetrate into the delicate regenerating tissue, which is known as granulation tissue.

Changes in connective tissues occur in a number of disease states. For example, in a condition known as *scurvy*, collagen is not formed in normal amounts because there is a deficiency of vitamin C which is necessary in order for fibroblasts to hydroxylate normal amounts of proline to hydroxyproline. Many aging changes are closely related to changes in collagen and ground substance. In rheumatoid arthritis, there is an excessive production and abnormal organization of collagen. In fact, the various rheumatic conditions are so intimately related to abnormalities in the formation and repair of connective tissue that they are often spoken of as collagen diseases. Some diseases are clearly related to abnormal function of genes. *Hurler's syndrome*, a condition involving stunted skeletal growth and abnormal fat metabolism, is an hereditary disorder involving an excessive accumulation of dermatan sulfate and heparitin sulfate.

Dense Connective Tissue

Dense connective tissue is chiefly char-acterized by the close packing of its fibers. It occurs in the form of sheets, bands, and cordlike structures. Examples are the dermis, capsules of certain organs, aponeuroses, ligaments, and tendons. Some of the deep fascia is intermediate between dense and loose connective tissue. In most locations, the main component is collagenous fibers, but in a few of the ligaments, elastic fibers predominate.

Dense, irregularly arranged connective tissue is composed chiefly of coarse collagenous fibers, but elastic and reticular fibers are also present. The fibers interlace and form a coarse tough feltwork, and some of them continue into adjacent tissue. Fibroblasts and some macrophages are present but show no special modifications. Examples of dense irregularly arranged connective tissue are dermis (Figs. 5-10 and 14-1), periosteum and perichondrium, and the capsules of some organs. The capsule of the testis (tunica albuginea, Fig. 19-13) is extremely dense.

Dense, regularly arranged connective tissue occurs as cordlike structures and as bands, some of which, as in aponeuroses, may be very broad. The fibers are densely packed and lie parallel to each other, forming structures of great tensile strength. This type of tissue comprises the tendons, ligaments, and aponeuroses.

Tendons are composed almost entirely of white fibrous tissue (Fig. 5-11). The fibers are parallel and are closely packed in bundles which are so dense that they appear almost homogeneous. Fibroblasts are the only cell type present, and they are few in number as compared to loose tissue. In longitudinal sections of tendon, the fibroblasts of tendon cells are elongated and aligned in rows between the bundles of collagenous fibers (Fig. 5-11). In cross sections, the cells appear stellate in shape, with platelike extensions between the collagenous bundles (Fig. 5-12).

Around each bundle of fibers is a small amount of loose tissue, and the whole tendon is surrounded by interlacing fibers.

Aponeuroses have the same composition as tendons but are broad and relatively thin. The fibers may be arranged in several superimposed layers, those of one layer running at an angle to those of adjacent layers. The layers may interweave.

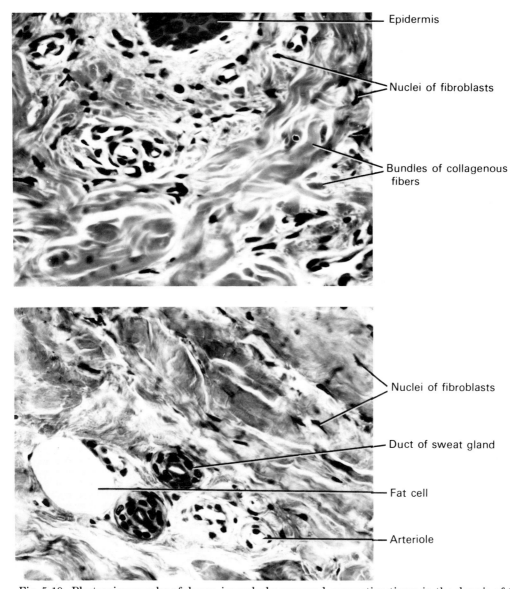

Fig. 5-10. Photomicrographs of dense, irregularly arranged connective tissue in the dermis of the dorsum of the thumb. *Upper figure,* a field just below the epidermis; *lower figure,* a deep region of the dermis just above the subcutaneous tissue. Note variations in the diameter and course of the bundles of fibers in different fields. For example, the bundles of fibers are coarse in the deep portions of the dermis and more slender in the subepidermal region. Even greater variations are found in other parts of the body, and there are many gradations between the loose and dense varieties of irregularly arranged connective tissue. Hematoxylin and eosin-stained section. ×390.

Ligaments in most cases are structurally similar to tendons, being formed predominantly of collagenous fibers, but a few are composed almost entirely of elastic fibers.

The *yellow elastic ligaments* are formed of parallel-coursing yellow elastic fibers which are bound together by a small amount of loose tissue. The elastic fibers may be very large, as in the ligamentum nuchae (Fig. 5-13). The series of ligaments (ligamenta flava) coursing between the arches of the vertebrae are also of the elastic type.

Reticular Connective Tissue

Reticular connective tissue is character-

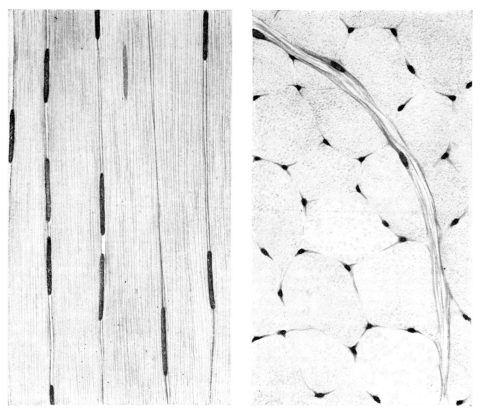

Figs. 5-11 and 5-12. Sections of human achilles tendon. Fig. 5-11 (*left*) is from a longitudinal section and shows rows of dense-staining nuclei of fibroblasts (tendon cells) between bundles of regularly arranged fibrils. Fig. 5-12 (*right*) is from a cross section. Note that the nuclei and the pale-staining cytoplasm of the tendon cells appear stellate in shape. A band of irregularly arranged connective tissue separating tendon bundles is seen in the *right side* of the drawing. Both figures ×575.

ized by a cellular reticulum (reticular cells) and a fibrillar framework and is found primarily in particular locations: namely, in bone marrow, lymph nodes and nodules, and spleen. The fibers are argyrophilic and apparently identical with the reticular fibers formed by fibroblasts in loose connective tissue. However, the reticular fibers of the reticular tissue are formed by reticular cells which differ structurally and functionally from the fibroblasts which form the fibers in the other connective tissues.

The reticular cells are frequently stellate in shape, with processes extending in several directions and often in contact with the processes of neighboring cells (Fig. 5-14). They have a large pale nucleus and fairly abundant lightly staining cytoplasm, but under normal conditions they do not

show cytoplasmic granules and vacuoles that are visible with the light microscope.

Several different functional and developmental potencies have been attributed to reticular cells. It seems likely either that the name includes several distinct types of cells which cannot be distinguished by morphological means alone or that the cells are not all in the same physiological state. Some of them may have retained their embryonic or developmental potencies, whereas others have differentiated into either fibroblastic or phagocytic types of cells. The fibroblastic tendencies are shown by the cells associated with the fibrous elements of the reticular tissue.

The phagocytic activity of reticular cells seemed clearly established on the basis of light microscope studies of lymph nodes of animals injected intravitally with trypan blue. Under the light microscope, the dye appeared to be in flattened reticular cells along the sinusoids and in stellate shaped reticular cells of the cords of lymphatic tissue. However, high resolution electron micrographs show that the sinusoids have an endothelial lining that is relatively non-phagocytic and that the ingested dye is in macrophages closely associated with the endothelial cells and in macrophages dispersed through the cords of lymphatic tissue. The different types of reticular cells and their relationship to the origin of macrophages are discussed in more detail under the heading of Macrophages at the end of this chapter and under Lymphatic Organs, chapter 13.

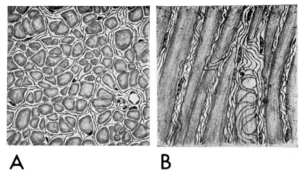

A   B

Fig. 5-13. Ligamentum nuchae of an ox. *A*, tissue cut in cross section; *B*, longitudinal section. Slender and irregularly arranged collagenous fibers are present between the unusually large elastic fibers. ×480.

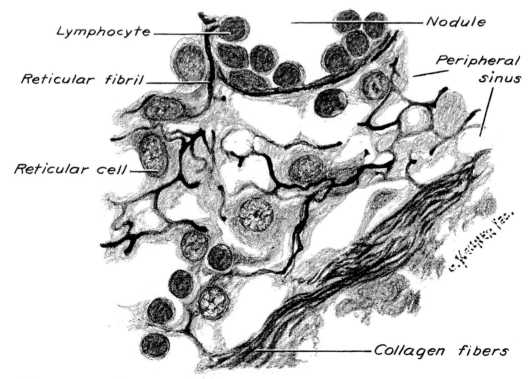

Fig. 5-14. Reticular tissue from lymph node of monkey. Bielschowsky-Foot and eosin-azure. ×1840.

Reticular cells of an undifferentiated type are closely related to mesenchyme and are usually described as having the ability to differentiate into leukocytes and erythrocytes in the hemopoetic tissues. Again, there is a question about this relationship because the morphological characteristics of the stem cell (or cells) in the bone marrow have not been defined.

Adipose Tissue (Fat)

Fat cells are found isolated or in groups in all loose connective tissue, but in certain places they are present in such large numbers and have such an organization as to justify the designation of adipose tissue. The largest deposits of fat are found in the subcutaneous connective tissue (panniculus adiposus), in the kidney region, in the mesenteries and mediastinum, and in the cervical, axillary, and inguinal regions.

Fat is different from the other connective tissues in that the cells, and not the intercellular substance, make up the bulk and determine the nature of the tissue. The cells are large and have an ovoid or spherical shape. The cytoplasm is displaced to the peripheral region of the cell by the presence of a single large fat droplet (Fig. 5-15). The nucleus, flattened and surrounded by a small amount of cytoplasm, is usually found pressed against the periphery. In sections of fixed preparations in which the fat has been dissolved out, the cells appear as empty rings or ovals, or they have a "signet ring" shape if the plane of section passes through the nucleus. When occurring singly or in small groups the cells retain their spherical or ovoid form; in denser masses they become polyhedral as a result of the pressure of adjacent cells. Fat cells are usually arranged in groups or lobules, each lobule being separated from its neighbor by loose connective tissue. Delicate strands of irregularly arranged connective tissue consisting of reticular, collagenous, and elastic fibers surround the fat cells and serve as a bed for the numerous capillaries.

The appearance of the adult fat cell can be best understood by a reference to its histogenesis. In places where fat is to be formed, certain cells of the embryonal connective tissue become grouped in the meshes of a rich capillary network which

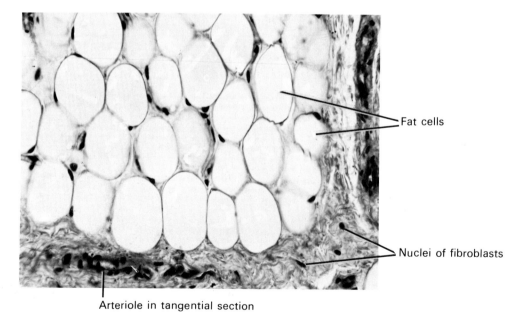

Fat cells

Nuclei of fibroblasts

Arteriole in tangential section

Fig. 5-15. Photomicrograph of fat from human subcutaneous tissue. Because the fat dissolves and escapes from the cell during the dehydration and clearing of the tissue for preparing paraffin sections, the cells appear empty. The cells are large and only a few are sectioned, by chance, in the plane of the nucleus. Hematoxylin and eosin stain. ×250.

marks the end of a small artery. Such groups, each of which is destined to become an adult fat lobule, can be distinguished in man in the 4th month of embryonic life. The cells enlarge, lose their stellate form, become rich in protoplasm, and have the general appearance of secretory cells. Fine fat droplets are formed in the cytoplasm; they increase in number and finally coalesce, forming a larger droplet. By further formation and fusion of fat droplets, the nucleus is pushed to one side and the cytoplasm is gradually reduced to the thin membrane of the adult cell (Fig. 5-15).

Electron micrographs show that the cytoplasm of fat cells contains mitochondria with shelflike cristae, endoplasmic reticulum that is mostly of the smooth-surfaced variety, a few free ribosomes, and a relatively small Golgi complex. Small lipid droplets are occasionally seen at the periphery of the large droplet; these apparently represent small lipid vesicles that have not yet fused with the main droplet. Each fat cell is surrounded by an external lamina, differing in this respect from all other types of connective tissue cells.

The blood supply of fat is rich, and the adult lobule retains its embryonal vascular relations, the vascular supply of each lobule being complete and independent. One artery runs to each lobule, where it breaks up into an intralobular capillary network which in turn gives rise to the intralobular veins, usually two in number.

Chemically, fat consists of the esters of glycerol and certain fatty acids (palmitic, stearic, and oleic). It is not soluble in water or cold alcohol but dissolves readily in ether, chloroform, benzol, and xylol. Because the latter reagents are commonly used in histological technique, the fat is usually dissolved, leaving an empty space or vacuole. When properly fixed, fat and fatlike substances stain black with osmic acid (osmium tetroxide). Other specific stains for fat are certain coal tar dyes, as Sudan III and Scharlach R.

The experimetns of Schoenheimer have shown that the so-called fat deposits of the body are not inactive storehouses. He labeled or "tagged" molecules of carbohydrates and fats with atoms of heavy water, or deuterium, and followed their metabolism in the animal body. He found that mice synthesize fats from carbohydrate on a normal diet without overfeeding or fattening. The fats are rapidly replaced; the turnover in mice requred only about 6 days.

Besides its nutritive value, fat has important mechanical functions. It forms plastic, shock-absorbing pads in the subcutaneous tissue of parts exposed to pressure, such as the gluteal region and the soles of the feet. It packs the orbital cavity and the angles of joints, acting as a guard against exaggerated movements. Such fatty pads are especially prominent in the hip, knee, shoulder, and elbow joints, where they may be retained even in states of extreme emaciation.

As a nonconductor, fat is also an important agent in the conservation of the body heat.

Brown fat, in addition to white fat, is present in numerous species of animals, being particularly prominent in hibernating animals such as the hedgehog and bat. The brown fat of insectivores, bats, and true rodents retains its characteristic appearance throughout life, whereas that of other mammals begins to show variable degrees of regression soon after birth.

Brown fat is well developed in particular regions of the body, e.g., the interscapular region, inguinal area, etc., and it is not distributed widely in the body, as is white fat.

The histological appearance of brown fat is quite different from that of white fat. The nuclei of brown fat cells are round rather than flattened and are often located in the central portions of the cells. The cytoplasm contains numerous lipid droplets which are generally seen as vacuoles after routine histological techniques; thus brown fat is described as *multilocular* in contrast to *unilocular* white fat.

Electron micrographs show that the mitochondria are larger and more numerous in brown fat than in the white variety and that the mitochondrial cristae are more closely packed and extend completely across the organelle. Histochemical studies show that these mitochondria are rich in succinic dehydrogenease and cytochrome oxidase. Rough-surfaced membranes of endoplasmic reticulum are scarce in brown fat cells and smooth-surfaced membranes are less numerous than in white fat. The Golgi complex is also quite small.

Both types of fat are richly vascularized and innervated, but in each case the supply to brown fat exceeds that for the white variety. The postganglionic sympathetic endings have synaptic vesicles of the type that is characteristic for norepinephrine-containing nerves. Recent correlated physiological and electron microscopic studies show that brown fat cells are electrically coupled and are attached to each other by gap junctions. White fat cells do not seem to be functionally interconnected in the same way.

Whereas white fat cells function as storehouses for triglycerides which can be mobilized for fuel by other parts of the body, the masses of brown fat are specialized for transducing the energy stored in fatty acids into heat which warms the blood passing through their capillaries and venules and subsequently increases body temperature. This process is particularly important in newborn and young animals exposed to cold. In this process, which is still a subject of active investigation, there is evidence that the transduction of energy into heat results from a failure of the usual oxidative phosphorylation because of a lack of elementary particles on the mitochondrial cristae in brown fat cells.

Brown fat does not respond to nutritional changes as readily as ordinary fat. On the other hand, hypophysectomy brings about a more rapid lipid depletion in brown than in white fat.

Pigmented Connective Tissue

Pigmented connective tissue cells (melanocytes) occur in the choroid and iris of the eye (Fig. 5-16). The cytoplasm is filled to a varying degree with brown or black pigment, which is usually melanin. Experiments with tissue cultures indicate that pigmented connective tissue cells are a specialized type. The cells form true pigment in the cultures only if they are explanted from a tissue which would have grown pigment in the body. There is considerable evidence that melanocytes are of neural crest origin.

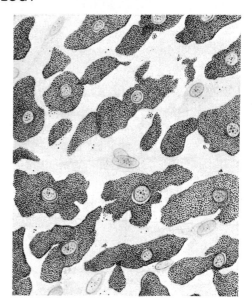

Fig. 5-16. Pigmented connective tissue cells from choroid coat of human eye. Nuclei have been stained with hematoxylin; pigment granules are seen by their natural coloration. A few nuclei of nonpigmented cells are shown among the pigmented cells. ×450.

Blood and Nerve Supply of Connective Tissue

Blood vessels and lymphatics are very numerous in loose connective tissue. The rich capillary plexuses are not, however, in the main destined for the tissue itself but for the more active cells of epithelium and muscle. The connective tissue forms the supporting bed for all blood vessels and incidentally receives its own nutrition from them. In the dense connective tissues and tendons, the blood supply is less abundant. In tendons, the blood vessels follow a straight course between the large collagen bundles and communicate with each other by short branches which run across the bundles, forming a scanty capillary network with oblong meshes. The fibrous membranes of the periosteum and dura mater are more vascular, but here too the blood vessels are mainly destined for bone.

Lymphatics are numerous and form extensive networks, especially in the submucous, subserous, and subcutaneous connective tissue. They are also present in fibrous membranes and tendons, where they form both superficial and deep lymphatic plexuses.

Connective tissue is richly supplied with nerves which end in the tissue itself or go to epithelium and muscle. Special nerve endings are found in the tendons, in fibrous membranes, and in the periarticular connective tissue.

The Macrophage System

It was found by Metchnikoff in the latter part of the 19th century that certain connective tissue cells are markedly phagocytic; he named them *macrophages,* in contrast with the relatively small neutrophilic leukocytes which become *microphages* in the connective tissues during localized inflammations. In the early part of this century, it was found that phagocytic cells are also present along the lumina of liver sinusoids (Kupffer cells) and along the lumina of the venous sinusoids of the spleen and the lymphatic sinusoids of lymph nodes. Aschoff proposed the name *reticuloendothelial system* for the macrophages of the body based on the phagocytic *reticular cells* in the framework of lymphatic organs and the so-called *endothelial cells* of the sinusoids of the liver and lymphatic organs. This term was criticized by Maximow and others on the grounds that reticular refers to only one type of connective tissue macrophage, thus omitting the connective tissue histiocyte. Furthermore, the term endothelial might give the incorrect impression that the endothelial cells of ordinary blood vessels are included. Nevertheless, the term *reticuloendothelial system* was generally adopted as synonymous with *macrophage system.*

The simplest method for identifying the cells of this system is to give living animals injections of certain nontoxic dyes such as trypan blue or of some inert particulate matter such as carbon particles of India ink. The macrophages avidly take up the dye (or particles) and are easily identified in light microscope preparations (Fig. 5-2). Although the cells containing the dye are found in widely separated organs, the reaction is quite specific. Epithelium, nerve cells, and muscle cells take up the dye very slightly, if at all. Fibroblasts take up the dye more slowly and in smaller amounts than do the histiocytes (Fig. 5-2). True endothelial cells of blood and lymphatic vessels either fail to react or react so slightly that when a macrophage is near an endothelial cell a quantitative difference is readily seen (Fig. 16-83). The microglia of the nervous system ingest the dye, and therefore they are included in the system. In fact, all highly phagocytic cells except the leukocytes are included.

Electron micrographs show that macrophages have a well developed Golgi complex and a more or less well developed rough endoplasmic reticulum, dependent on the species (prominent in rodents but present in relatively small amounts in humans). There are, as would be expected in phagocytic cells, numerous cytoplasmic vacuoles, lysosomes, and residual bodies.

Electron micrographs have helped to resolve the relationship between endothelial cells and Kupffer cells of the liver. Although these cells are intimately associated with each other along the lumina of the sinusoids, there is no indication of cells with transitional characteristics even after prolonged stimulation of the macrophage system. Furthermore, the Kupffer cells differ from endothelial cells in that they give a strongly positive reaction for endogenous peroxidase. High resolution electron micrographs of lymphatic organs and bone marrow also cast doubt on the presence of any markedly phagocytic endothelial cells in these organs.

The use of tritiated thymidine, incorporated into DNA only during replication, has been useful in tracing the lineage of Kupffer cells and other macrophages. In testing the role of monocytes, promonocytes from bone marrow were used because the mature monocytes do not usually divide and thus do not usually incorporate DNA. Tissues from various regions of the animals which had received transfusions of labeled promonocytes from compatible strains were fixed and processed for studies by the combined use of radioautography and electron microscopy. Studies of the liver showed the label in a number of Kupffer cells but not in any endothelial cells. It is evident that the new Kupffer cells observed in these studies developed from the labeled promonocytes and not from endothelial cells. The combined evidence from different studies indicates that there is no *endothelial* component of the so-called reticuloendothelial system. The promonocytes from bone marrow used in these studies apparently develop from "stem cells" with morphological characteristics that have not been defined.

There is also a question concerning the *reticular* component of the so-called reticuloendothelial system. Are the highly phagocytic cells of lymphatic organs a functional stage of the reticular cells or are they derived from precursor mononuclear cells brought in by the vascular system? It has not been shown that the phagocytic cells of lymphatic organs participate in the formation of reticular fibers or that the fiber-producing cells change to macrophages. Perhaps they are divergent types from the undifferentiated reticular cells. However, there is increasing evidence in favor of the view that the macrophages of the lymphatic organs, Kupffer cells of the liver, and "dust cells" of the lung develop from mononuclear cells of bone marrow origin. Hence, a more appropriate name for the reticuloendothelial system is *mononuclear phagocyte system* or simply *macrophage system*.

During embryonic development the mesenchyme differentiates into numerous types of cells, including the connective tissue fibroblasts and cells described by Maximow as wandering cells. The latter were considered as relatively undifferentiated and as capable of taking one of several lines of differentiation according to the stimulus of body needs. It was thought at that time that many of the wandering cells become histiocytes of the loose connective tissues and that some remain as *undifferentiated mesenchymal cells*. Cells of a relatively undifferentiated type are identifiable along the blood vessels, where they are known as *pericytes*. These can apparently develop into mast cells, as noted in the preceding section. There is evidence that pericytes can also develop into smooth muscle on regenerating blood vessels, and also into fibroblasts. Although the possibility that some macrophages can develop from the undifferentiated perivascular cells cannot be ruled out, it seems unlikely. Furthermore, there is no evidence that any mac-

rophages develop from lymphocytes or that the monocytes develop from lymphocytes.

The *functional significance* of macrophages is well established. Macrophages normally remove the senile erythrocytes from the circulation, chiefly in the spleen and liver, and store iron, which is reutilized in erythropoiesis. In pathological conditions, they are active in the removal of foreign bodies, bacteria, and damaged cells and tissues. They also process antigens and thus have a very important role in the antigen-antibody response.

References

BENSLEY, S. H. On the presence, properties and distribution of the intercellular ground substance of loose connective tissue. Anat. Rec. 60:93–109, 1934.

BORNSTEIN, P., EHRLICH, H. P., AND WYKE, A. W. Procollagen: Conversion of the precursor to collagen by a neutral protease. Science 175:544–546, 1972.

BRISSIE, R. M., SPICER, S. S., AND THOMPSON, N. T. The variable fine structure of elastin visualized with Verhoeff's iron hematoxylin. Anat. Rec. 181:83–94, 1975.

CARPENTER, J.-C., PERRELET, A., AND ORCI, L. Morphological changes of the adipose cell membrane during lipolysis. J. Cell Biol. 72:104–117, 1977.

CASTRO, C. W., PRINCE, R. K., AND DORSTEWITZ, E. L. Characteristics of human fibroblasts cultivated *in vitro* from different anatomical sites. Lab. Invest. 11:703–713, 1962.

DEMPSEY, E. D., AND LANSING, A. I. Elastic tissue. *In* International Review of Cytology (Bourne, G. H., editor), vol. 3, pp. 437–453. Academic Press, New York, 1954.

EHRLICH, H. P., ROSS, R., AND BORNSTEIN, P. Effects of antimicrotubular agents on the secretion of collagen. A biochemical and morphological study. J. Cell Biol. 62:390–405, 1974.

EVANS, H. M., AND SCOTT, K. J. On the differential reaction to vital dyes exhibited by the two great groups of connective-tissue cells. Carnegie Inst. Contrib. Embryol. 10:1–55, 1921.

FAHIMI, H. D. The fine structural localization of endogenous and exogenous peroxidase activity in Kupffer cells of rat liver. J. Cell Biol. 47:247–262, 1970.

FAWCETT, D. W. A comparison of the histological organization and cytochemical reactions of brown and white adipose tissue. J. Morphol. 70:363, 1952.

FAWCETT, D. W., AND JONES, I. C. The effects of hypophysectomy, adrenalectomy and of thiouracil feeding on the cytology of brown adipose tissue. Endocrinology 45:609–621, 1949.

FOOT, N. C. Chemical contrasts between collagenous and reticular connective tissue. Am. J. Pathol. 4:525–544, 1928.

FURTH, R. VAN, COHN, Z. A., HIRSCH, J. G., HUMPHREY, J. H., SPECTOR, W. G., AND LANGEVOORT, H. L. The mononuclear phagocyte system: a new classification of macrophages, monocytes and their precursor cells. Bull. World Health Org. 46:845–852, 1972.

GLEGG, R. E., CLERMONT, Y., AND LEBLOND, C. P. The use of lead tetracetate, benzidine, o-dianisdine and a "film test" to investigate the significance of the "periodic acid sulfurous acid" technique in carbohydrate histochemistry. Stain Technol. 27: 277–305, 1952.

GODLESKI, J. J., AND BRAIN, J. D. The origin of alveolar macrophages in mouse radiation chimeras. J. Exp. Med. 136:630, 1972.

GOTTE, L., GIRO, M. G., VOLPIN, D., AND HORNE, R. The ultrastructural organization of elastin. J. Ultrastruct. Res. 46:23–33, 1974.

GRANT, R. A., HORNE, R. W., AND COX, R. W. New model for the tropocollagen macromolecule and its mode of aggregation. Nature 207:822–826, 1965.

GROSS, J. Collagen, Sci. Amer. 204: 120–130, 1961.

GROSS, J. Organization and disorganization of collagen. In Connective Tissue: Intercellular Macromolecules, pp. 63–77. J. & A. Churchill Ltd., London, 1964.

HAUST, M. D., AND MORE, R. H. Electron microscopy of connective tissues and elastogenesis. In The Connective Tissue (Wagner, B. M., and Smith, D. E., editors), pp. 352–376. Williams & Wilkins, Baltimore, 1967.

HODGE, A. J., AND SCHMITT, F. O. The tropocollagen macromolecule and its properties of ordered interaction. In Macromolecular Complexes (Edds, M. V., Jr., editor), pp. 19–51. Ronald Press, New York, 1961.

JACKSON, S. F. Connective tissue cells. In The Cell; Biochemistry, Physiology, Morphology (Brachet, J., and Mirsky, A. E., editors), vol. 6, pp. 382–520. Academic Press, New York, 1964.

KAZAYAMA, M., AND DOUGLAS, W. W. Electron microscope evidence of calcium-activated exocytosis in mast cells treated with 48/80 or the ionophores A-23187 and X-537 A. J. Cell Biol. 62:519–526, 1974.

LEBLOND, C. P., GLEGG, R. E., AND EIDINGER, D. Presence of carbohydrates with free 1–2 glycol groups in .sites stained by the periodic acid-Schiff technique. J. Histochem. Cytochem. 5:445–458, 1957.

LEDUC, E. H., SCOTT, G. B., AND AVRAMEAS, S. Ultrastructural localization of intracellular immune globulins in plasma cells and lymphoblasts by enzyme-labeled antibodies. J. Histochem. Cytochem. 17:211–224, 1969.

MAXIMOW, A. A. Bindegewebe und blutbildende Gewebe. Handb. mikr. Anat. Menschen (v. Möllendorff, editor), vol. 2 (Part 1) 232–583, 1930.

MAXIMOW, A. A. The macrophages or histiocytes. Special Cytology (Cowdry, E. V., editor), vol. 2, pp. 709–770, 1932.

MEYER, K. 1946 The biological significance of hyaluronic acid and hyaluronidase. Physiol. Rev. 27:335–359, 1946.

MEYER, K. 1955 The chemistry of the mesodermal ground substances. Harvey Lect. 51:88–112, 1955.

MONIS, B. Variation of aminopeptidase activity in granulation tissue and in serum of rats during wound healing. Am. J. Pathol. 42:301–313, 1963.

MURATA, F., AND SPICER, S. S. Ultrastructural comparison of basophilic leukocytes and mast cells in the guinea pig. Am. J. Anat. 139:335–351, 1974.

NAPOLITANO, L. The differentiation of white adipose cells. An electron microscope study. J. Cell Biol. 18:663–679, 1963.

NOPAJAROOSI, C., AND SIMON, G. T. Phagocytosis of colloidal carbon in a lymph node. Am. J. Pathol. 65:25–42, 1971.

PADAWER, J. Uptake of colloidal thorium dioxide by mast cells. J. Cell Biol. 40:747–760, 1969.

PAPADIMITRIOU, J. M., AND ARCHER, M. The morphology of foreign body multinucleate giant cells. J. Ultrastruct. Res. 49:372–386, 1974.

PORTER, K. R. Cell fine structure and biosynthesis of intercellular macromolecues. In Connective Tissue: Intercellular Macromolecules, pp. 167–196. J. & A. Churchill Ltd., London, 1964.

PORTER, K. R., AND PAPPAS, G. D. Collagen formation by fibroblasts of the chick embryo dermis. J. Biophys. Biochem. Cytol. 5:153–166, 1959.

ROSS, R., AND BORNSTEIN, P. The elastic fiber. I. The separation and partial characterization of its macromolecular components. J. Cell Biol. 40:366–381, 1969.

ROSS, R., EVERETT, N. B., AND TYLER, R. Wound healing and fiber formation. V. The origin of the wound fibroblast studied in parabiosis. J. Cell Biol. 44:645–654, 1970.

SCHMITT, F. O., GROSS, J., AND HIGHBERGER, H. J. Tropocollagen and the properties of fibrous collagen. Exp. Cell Res., 3 (suppl.):326–334, 1955.

SCHOENHEIMER, R. The investigation of intermediary metabolism with the aid of heavy hydrogen. Harvey Lect. 32:122–144, 1937.

SCHUBERT, M. Biochemical and biophysical aspects of collagen. In Connective Tissue: Intercellular Macromolecules, pp. 119–138. J. & A. Churchill Ltd., London, 1964.

SMITH, R. E., AND HORWITZ, B. A. Brown fat and thermogenesis. Physiol. Rev. 49:330, 1969.

SPICER, S. S., HORN, R. G., AND LEPPI, T. J. Histochemistry of connective tissue mucopolysaccharides. In The Connective Tissue (Wagner, B. M., and Smith, D. E., editors), pp. 251–303. Williams & Wilkins, Baltimore, 1967.

STEARNS, M. L. Studies on the development of connective tissue in transparent chambers in the rabbit's ear. Am. J. Anat 67:55–97, 1940.

UDENFRIEND, S. Formation of hydroxyproline in collagen. Science 152:1335–1340, 1966.

WEINSTOCK, M., AND LEBLOND, C. P. Synthesis, migration, and release of precursor collagen by odontoblasts as visualized by radioautography after [³H] proline administration. J. Cell Biol. 60:92–127, 1974.

WEST, G. B. Function of mast cells. J. Pharm. Pharmacol. 14:618–619, 1962.

WISLOCKI, G. B., BUNTING, H., AND DEMPSEY, E. W. Metachromasia in mammalian tissues and its relationship to mucopolysaccharides. Am. J. Anat. 81:1–38, 1947.

WISSE, E. Kupffer cell reactions in rat liver under various conditions as observed in the electron microscope. J. Ultrastruct. Res. 46:499–520, 1974.

YU, S. Y., AND BLUMENTHAL, H. I. The calcification of elastic tissue. In The Connective Tissue (Wagner, B. M., and Smith, D. E., editors), pp. 17–49. Williams & Wilkins, Baltimore, 1967.

CHAPTER 6

The Connective Tissues: Cartilage and Bone

Cartilage

Cartilage, like other regions of the connective tissue compartment, consists of cells, fibers, and ground substance. The last named, however, has physical properties which give to the tissue an elastic firmness, rendering it capable of withstanding a considerable degree of pressure and shear. In some of the lower vertebrates (e.g., elasmobranchs) the whole adult skeleton consists of cartilage, and in the mammals the greater part of the skeleton is first laid down in cartilage. In the adult body, cartilage covers the articular surfaces of bones, and it forms the sole skeletal support of the larynx, trachea, bronchi, and certain other structures.

According to the nature and visibility of the fibrillar elements, cartilage is subdivided into three varieties: (1) *hyaline*, (2) *elastic*, and (3) *fibrous*. Of these, hyaline cartilage is the most widely distributed type.

Hyaline Cartilage

Hyaline cartilage (Figs. 6-1 and 6-2) appears as a bluish white, translucent mass in the fresh condition. It forms the costal cartilages and the cartilages of the nose, larynx, trachea, and bronchi. It is also a major component of the epiphyseal cartilages of growing long bones. In the fetus, nearly all of the skeleton is first laid down as hyaline cartilage and is replaced later by osseous tissue in the formation of the bones.

With the exception of the free surfaces of articular cartilages, hyaline cartilage is always invested by a layer of dense fibrous connective tissue, the *perichondrium* (Fig. 6-1). Hyaline cartilage is composed of cells and an *extracellular matrix* of ground substance and connective tissue fibers.

Cartilage is usually devoid of blood vessels except in areas where vessels may be passing through it to other tissues and in particular zones which are forming ossification centers in intracartilaginous bone development. Exchange of substances between cartilage cells and blood vessels of the perichondrium is mediated by the tissue fluid of the cartilage, i.e., by the bound water which is the dispersion medium of the glycosaminoglycans of the intercellular matrix.

The Cells. The cartilage cells, *chondrocytes*, occupy chambers known as *lacunae* (Figs. 6-1 to 6-3). The cells appear irregularly shaped and shrunken away from the walls of their lacunae in most light microscope preparations because their cytoplasm contains glycogen and lipids which are dissolved by routine techniques. However, the cells fill the lacunae in fresh preparations, as verified by electron microscopic studies of well-fixed material (Fig. 6-4). Although the cell surface is irregular and has short processes extending into depressions in the matrix, there is no obvious space between

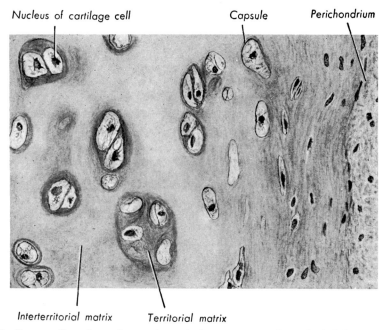

Fig. 6-1. Hyaline cartilage from the trachea of a boy 17 years of age. Delafield's hematoxylin and eosin. ×435.

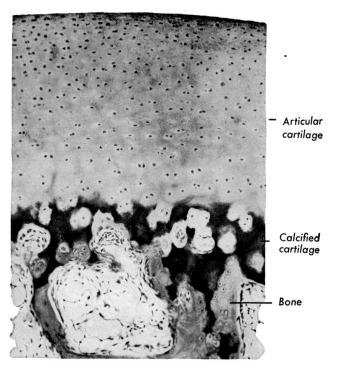

Fig. 6-2. Articular cartilage from a metatarsal bone of a rhesus monkey 2 months old. Photomicrograph. ×165.

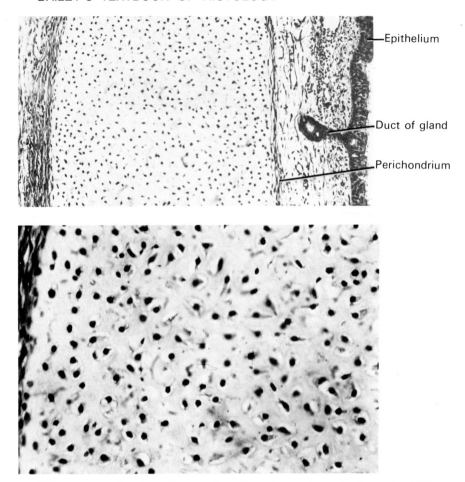

Fig. 6-3. Light micrographs of hyaline cartilage from the trachea of a 5-month-old human fetus. *Upper figure* is at low magnification to cover a relatively large field. Note that the cartilage cells are distributed singly throughout the fetal cartilage, instead of being in groups as they are in later periods (Fig. 6-1). *Lower figure*, a higher magnification of a portion of the field above. Note that the cartilage matrix appears homogeneous and stains uniformly. The irregular shape of the cells is accentuated by the usual shrinkage that occurs during fixation and dehydration for preparing sections. Upper, ×146; lower, ×390.

the cell and its surrounding matrix. Chondrocyte cytoplasm contains, in addition to glycogen and lipid, the usual characteristics of a secretory cell, as described below under Development and Growth.

Chondrocytes and their lacunae vary in shape in relation to their position within the cartilage. For example, the subperichondrial cartilage grades almost imperceptibly into the perichondrium (Fig. 6-1) and hence the cells, like nearby fibroblasts, are flat. Deeper within the cartilage, the cells and their lacunae are usually rounded (Figs. 6-1 and 6-2).

Chondrocytes are often arranged in groups which represent the offspring of a parent cartilage cell (Fig. 6-1). Such groups, termed *isogenous groups*, are found particularly in costal and tracheal cartilages. A special arrangement with the isogenous groups aligned in longitudinal rows is seen in intracartilaginous bone formation (Fig. 6-25).

In embryonal cartilage (Fig. 6-3), the cells are randomly distributed and variable in shape. Some have processes and resemble the mesenchymal cells from which they are derived. Intercellular matrix is relatively scant.

The Intercellular Substance. The in-

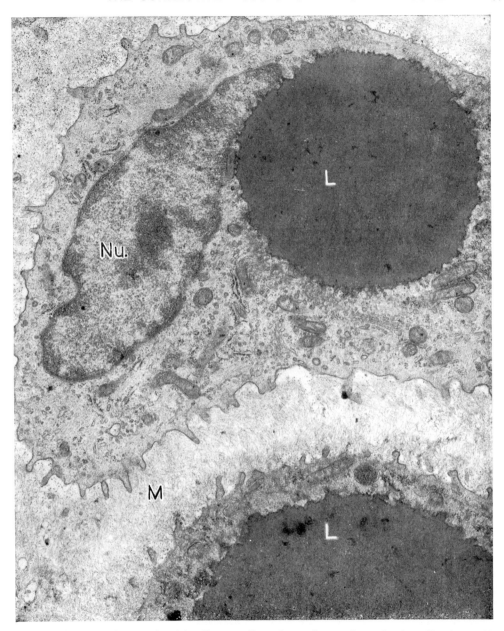

Fig. 6-4. Electron micrograph of hyaline cartilage from the trachea of a bat. Portions of two chondrocytes are seen, one with the nucleus (*Nu*). Large lipid droplets (*L*) are often found in the cytoplasm of mature cartilage cells. Note that the cartilage cells have numerous processes extending into the matrix and that the cells fill the lacunae. A fine feltwork of collagen is seen in the matrix (*M*). ×17,000. (Courtesy of Dr. Keith Porter and the New York Heart Association; Porter, K., Biophys. J. 4, 1964.)

tercellular substance, or matrix, appears homogeneous in the fresh condition and in most routine histological preparations. However, some areas are more basophilic than others and also more metachromatic after toluidine blue staining. For example, each lacuna is surrounded by a thin layer of substance which is strongly metachromatic and presumably composed chiefly of chondroitin sulfate. Such thin metachromatic *lacunar linings* are sometimes described as *capsules*, although this term is ambiguous because the broad zones of basophilic substance around groups of isogenous cells are more frequently described as capsules.

The apparently homogeneous intercellular substance contains fine collagenous fibers which are masked by a ground substance of similar refractive index. Although these fibrils can be detected by light microscopy after treatment of the cartilage with trypsin or dilute acids, our knowledge of their structure is based on biochemistry and electron microscopy. They are mostly slender fibrils of only about 100 to 250 Å in width and they usually lack the 640-Å cross banding characteristic of other collagen. The fibrils are arranged in a feltwork in most of the matrix, but they become parallel with the surface in the subperichondrial region and gradually blend with the perichondrial fibers, which are wider and cross-banded (Fig. 6-5). As noted in chapter 5, the collagen of cartilage differs in chemical nature from that of skin in that it has two α_1-Type II polypeptide chains.

Because the articular cartilages have 640 Å-banded collagen, they are classified by some authors as fibrocartilage. However, they have a hyaline appearance and the overall characteristics of the hyaline type when observed under the light microscope.

The intercellular substance contains *chondromucoids*, which are composed of glycosaminoglycan complexes containing *chondroitin 4-sulfate* and *chondroitin 6-sulfate*. The former is more abundant than the latter in the newborn, but the reverse relationship is attained by adulthood. Some *keratan-sulfate* is present also. It is insignificant in amount at birth but increases with age and may reach relatively high levels in senile, degenerate cartilage.

The basophilia of the cartilage matrix in routine hematoxylin and eosin preparations is due to the basophilia of the sulfate dominating the eosinophilia of the collagen. The matrix just outisde the lacunar lining is generally quite basophilic and is known as *pericellular matrix*. The region around a cell group is also often more basophilic than the general matrix, and is then named the *capsular* or *territorial* matrix (Fig. 6-1).

Intervening regions with less sulfate and more collagen are less basophilic and are known as *interterritorial matrices*.

The ground substance also gives a positive reaction with the periodic acid-Schiff (PAS) technique. Because *pure* chondroitin sulfate is apparently not PAS-positive, it is assumed that the reaction by the cartilage ground substance is due to an undetermined carbohydrate component. The ground substance also contains electron-dense granules of about 100 to 400 Å in diameter known as *matrix granules*. They apparently represent macromolecular complexes of the glycosaminoglycans. *Membrane-bounded vesicles* (*matrix vesicles*) of high electron density are present in the matrix of epiphyseal cartilages in regions where calcification is occurring. These vesicles apparently arise from chondroblasts or chondrocytes by exocytosis, and they range from about 300 Å to 1 μm in diameter. They contain acid phosphatases and are often seen in close association with hydroxyapatites. They apparently indicate sites where initial calcification is occurring (see below).

Development and Growth. As mentioned before, cartilage is a part of the connective tissue spectrum. Like all other connective tissues, it originates within the mesenchymal compartment of the embryo. The blastema of a future cartilagenous mass is first recognized as an area of mesenchymal cell concentration resulting from cell proliferation and enlargement. The cells in the interior of the precartilage blastema show a marked cytoplasmic basophilia resulting from an increase in rough-surfaced endoplasmic reticulum, and they are known as *chondroblasts*. They form the collagenous fibrils and the ground substance of the matrix. As the cells of the central region continue to form more matrix, they become separated from each other and become the chondrocytes, whereas those of the periphery continue as chondroblasts. Electron microscopic studies in combination with isotope techniques have provided information on the manner in which chondroblasts form the matrix chondromucoproteins. The amino acids, such as glycine and proline, are synthesized into peptide chains in the presence of the

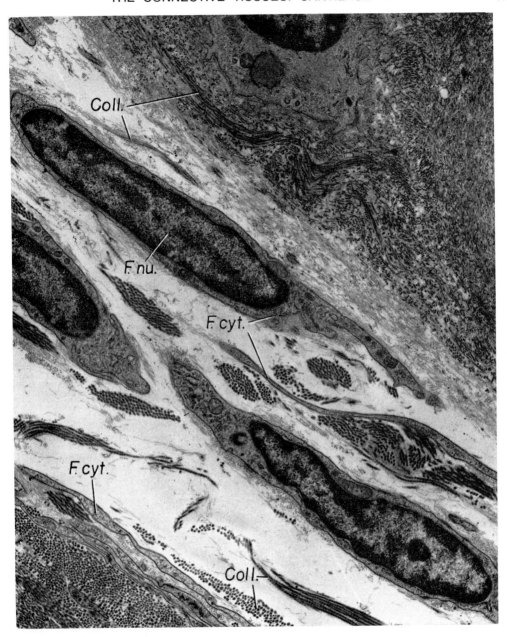

Fig. 6-5. Electron micrograph of junction of hyaline cartilage and perichondrium from the trachea of a bat. A portion of a cartilage cell is seen in the *upper part* of the photograph, and portions of several fibroblasts with their nuclei (*F. nu.*) and cytoplasm (*F. cyt.*) are seen in the *lower part* of the figure. Collagen fibers (*Coll.*) are seen in cross and longitudinal sections. Note that the fibrils adjacent to the surfaces of the fibroblasts are generally smaller than the bundles of fibrils found at some distance from the cells. ×12,250. (Courtesy of Dr. Keith Porter.)

ribosomes of the rough-surfaced endoplasmic reticulum and are then transported to the Golgi complex. Studies of the pathways taken by tritiated glucose and radioactive sulfate indicate that the carbohydrates enter the cell and pass directly to the Golgi complex for synthesis into polysaccharides. The synthesized proteins and polysaccharides are then combined in the Golgi region to form the chondromucoproteins which are secreted by the cells.

Growth of cartilage takes place in two ways: (1) formation of new cartilage by chondroblasts at the surface, known as *appositional growth,* and (2) expansion of the internal mass of cartilage by division of chondrocytes, known as *interstitial growth.*

In appositional growth, chondroblasts of the perichondrium multiply, and some form cartilage matrix as described above whereas others remain as a part of the chondroblast population. In interstitial growth, cartilage cells divide into two, and the daughter cells may divide again, each isogenous group representing the progeny of a single parent cell. The cells become separated from each other, each surrounded by its own capsule and matrix. The old capsules and the territorial matrices merge into the newly formed territorial matrix. Interstitial growth occurs mainly in young cartilage and gradually ceases, further growth being chiefly appositional (subperichondrial).

Nutrition of Cartilage. Cartilage is devoid of vascular and lymphatic channels; hence, nutrition is entirely by diffusion and imbibition. That the matrix is permeable even to coarse particles has been demonstrated. Injection of indigo carmine into the circulation leads to a deposition of the colored particles within the matrix and in the lacunae.

Age Changes. The poor nutrition is probably responsible for certain degenerative changes found in old cartilage, especially in cartilages of considerable thickness. The deeper portions of the cartilage show areas, extending through many cell territories, where the homogeneous matrix is replaced by closely packed coarse fibers. Cavity formation resulting from the softening and liquefaction of these areas may ultimately result.

With old age, cartilage loses its translucency and bluish white color and appears yellowish and cloudy. This change is due to a decrease of acid mucopolysaccharides and an increase in noncollagenous proteins.

Calcification is likewise of common occurrence in old cartilage and is usually associated with degenerative changes of the cartilage cells. Calcification of cartilage is a normal process during bone formation and is described below.

Regeneration and transplantation. Regeneration of cartilage is a slow process and occurs primarily by activity of the perichondrium. When cartilage is broken or injured, the wound is invaded by the perichondrial connective tissue, which gradually develops into cartilage. This type of regeneration depends on the presence of a perichondrium. Regeneration in part, at least, by interstitial growth has been observed but is doubtless comparatively rare. In many instances of cartilage fracture, the pieces become united by dense fibrous tissue which may partly be replaced by a bony clasp.

A high percentage of cartilage *autografts* survive provided that they contain living cells and receive sufficient nutrition. *Homografts* also survive in a fairly high percentage provided that they contain living cells and receive good nutrition. Grafts of cartilage apparently do not stimulate host antibody production to the extent that other tissue grafts do.

Elastic Cartilage

Elastic cartilage appears more yellow and opaque than hyaline cartilage in the fresh condition because of the large number of elastic fibers in its matrix (Fig. 6-6). These branch and course in all directions to form a dense network of anastomosing and interlacing fibers. In the peripheral layers, the fibers are thin and the network is widemeshed; in the deeper portions, they are thicker and more closely packed. The ground substance also contains collagenous fibrils, particularly in the subperichondrial region.

Elastic cartilage develops from a hyalinelike blastema. Elastic fibrils are assembled just peripheral to the cells and traverse the matrix as an elastic network. Growth of the cartilage takes place interstitially and subperichondrially. Calcification of elastic cartilage occurs very rarely, if at all.

Elastic cartilage occurs in the external ear, the Eustachian tube, the epiglottis, and some of the laryngeal cartilages.

Fibrous Cartilage

Fibrous cartilage (Fig. 6-7) is a combination of dense collagenous fibers with carti-

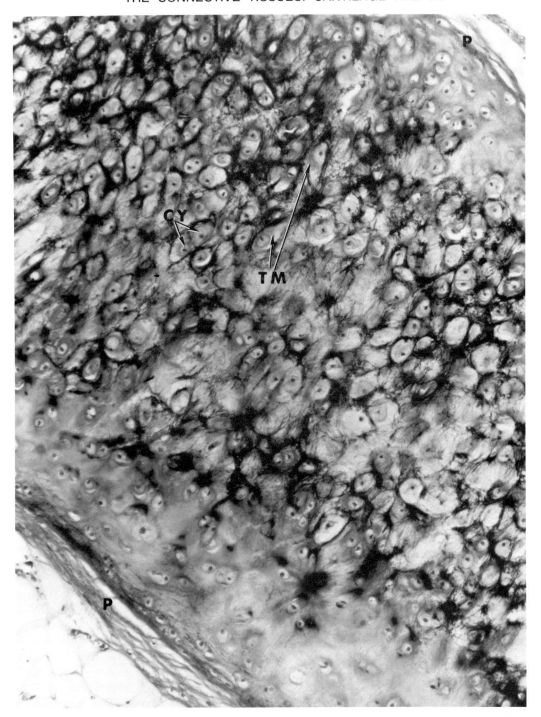

Fig. 6-6. Light micrograph of elastic cartilage from human epiglottis. The mature chondrocytes have condensed nuclei and a vesicular cytoplasm (*CY*). They are surrounded by a territorial matrix (*TM*) that is free from prominent elastic fibers. *P*, perichondrium. Verhoeff's elastic stain. ×195.

lage cells and a scant cartilage matrix. It is generally not circumscribed by a perichondrium. The relative proportions of cells,

fibers, and matrix vary greatly. The cells are frequently in rows, with intervening bundles of collagenous fibers that have the

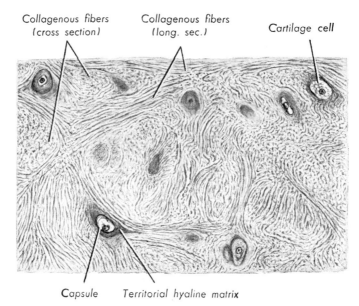

Fig. 6-7. Fibrocartilage from the intervertebral disc of a boy 13 years old. The section was cut transversely to the broad (vertebral) surface of the disc. The part drawn is about 5 mm from the anterior rim of the disc. Near the rim, the tissue is much like tendon. ×435.

characteristic 640-Å cross banding.

Fibrous cartilage is found in considerable amounts in the intervertebral discs, pubic symphysis, ligamentum teres of the femur, glenoid and cotyloid ligaments, and inter-articular cartilages. Because the articular cartilages have numerous fibrils with the 640-Å cross banding, they are classified by some authors as fibrocartilage, even though they have a hyaline-like matrix and other hyaline cartilage characteristics.

The *intervertebral discs* consist largely of fibrocartilage which is continuous above and below with the articular cartilage of the adjacent vertebrae and peripherally with the spinal ligaments. In the center of each disc is a gelatinous ellipsoid mass of variable extent known as the *nucleus pulposus,* a remnant of the embryonic notochord. Its center may contain fluid and cellular debris. Rupture of the disc and herniation of the nucleus pulposus into the spinal canal may be the cause of severe pain and other neurological symptoms.

Bone (Osseous Tissue)

Osseous tissue is a rigid form of connective tissue and is normally organized into definite structures, the bones. These form the skeleton, serve for the attachment and protection of the soft parts, and, by their attachment to the muscles, act as levers which bring about body motion. Bone is also a storage place for calcium ions which can be withdrawn when needed to maintain a normal level of calcium in the blood.

Gross Organization of Bone Tissue

Grossly, two types of bone may be distinguished: the *spongy* or *cancellous,* and the *dense* or *compact.* When a long bone is cut longitudinally (Fig. 6-8), it will be seen that the head, or *epiphysis,* has a spongy appearance and consists of slender irregular bone trabeculae, or bars, which anastomose to form a latticework, the interstices of which contain the marrow. The thin outer shell, however, appears dense. As the shaft, or *diaphysis,* is approached, the irregular marrow spaces of the epiphysis become continuous with the central medullary cavity of the shaft, whose wall is formed by a thick plate of compact bone.

The spongy and compact varieties of bone have the same types of cells and intercellular substance, but they differ from each other in the arrangement of their components and in the ratio of marrow space

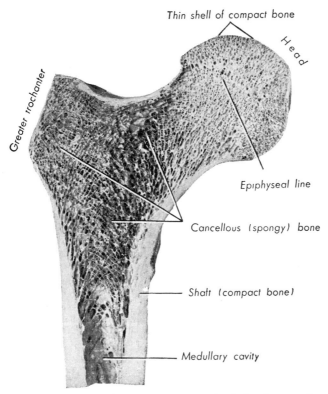

Thin shell of compact bone

Head

Greater trochanter

Epiphyseal line

Cancellous (spongy) bone

Shaft (compact bone)

Medullary cavity

Fig. 6-8. A longitudinal section through the upper end of the femur of an adult male. The epiphyseal line of the great trochanter is not evident. Photograph.

to bone substance. In spongy bone, the marrow spaces are relatively large and irregularly arranged, and the bone substance is in the form of slender anastomosing trabeculae and pointed spicules. In compact bone, the spaces or channels are narrow and the bone substance is densely packed.

With very few exceptions, the compact and spongy forms are both present in every bone, but the amount and distribution of each type vary considerably. The diaphyses of the long bones consist mainly of compact tissue; only the innermost layer immediately surrounding the medullary cavity is spongy. The tabular bones of the head are composed of two plates of compact bone enclosing a marrow space bridged by irregular bars of spongy bone (diploë). The epiphyses of the long bones and most of the short bones consist of spongy bone covered by a thin outer shell of compact bone.

Each bone, except at its articular end, is surrounded by a vascular fibroelastic coat, the *periosteum*. The so-called *endosteum*, or inner periosteum of the marrow cavity and marrow spaces, is not a well-demarcated layer. It consists of a variable concentration of medullary reticular connective tissue which contains osteogenic cells that are in immediate contact with the bone tissue.

Organic and Inorganic Components of Bone

Bone is composed of cells and an intercellular matrix of organic and inorganic substances. The organic fraction consists of collagen and an amorphous component of glycosaminoglycans (protein-polysaccharides) containing chondroitin sulfate. The matrix is acidophilic in stained sections, in contrast to the basophilic reaction of cartilage matrix. This is due to the high content of collagen and low content of chondroitin sulfate in bone. The collagen of bone is generally Type I.

The inorganic component of bone is responsible for its rigidity and may constitute up to two-thirds of the fat-free dry weight. It is composed chiefly of calcium phosphate and calcium carbonate, with small amounts of magnesium, hydroxide, fluoride, and sulfate. The composition varies with age and with a number of dietary factors. X-ray diffraction studies show that the minerals are present as crystals having an *apatite* pattern or structure. More specifically, they are *hydroxyapatites*.

Microscopic Structure

The microscopic structure of bone can be studied either using slices of dried bone ground sufficiently thin to transmit light (ground bone) or using sections made after decalcification by treatment with dilute acids. Although the slices of dried bone contain only the inorganic material, they show considerable detail (Fig. 6-10). The inorganic substance is also retained after the organic constituents are destroyed by burning with free access of air (calcination), but the inorganic material is then very brittle and useless for the preparation of sections.

A characteristic feature of adult bone tissue is its lamellar structure, with the cells and fibers organized in layers or *lamellae*. The osseous tissue of long bones, especially in the compact regions, is also characterized by longitudinal passages or *central canals* (*Haversian canals*) which anastomose

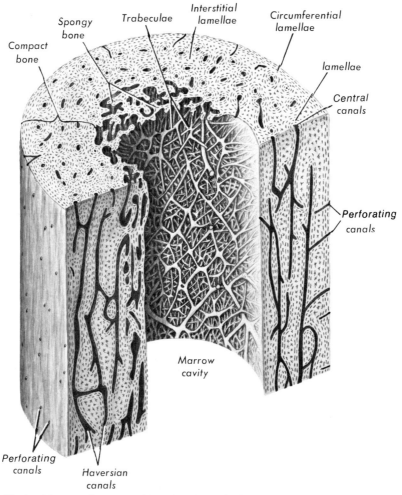

Fig. 6-9. Shaft of human humerus. Drawing is made from undecalcified bone after removal of marrow and other organic components by maceration techniques. (From a chart by H. Poll.)

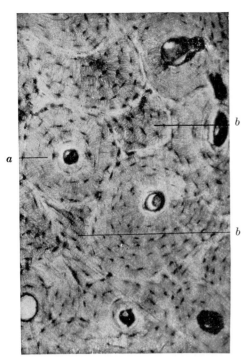

Fig. 6-10. Light micrograph of a transverse section from the shaft of an undecalcified, dried long bone. A slab of the dried bone was ground very thin and then mounted in thick balsam. In the spaces within the bone (lacunae, canaliculi, and some of the central canals), air was imprisoned, so that they appear dark. *a*, osteon; *b*, interstitial lamellae.

with each other by oblique and transverse communications (Fig. 6-9). From the periosteal and endosteal surfaces, somewhat narrower *perforating canals* (nutrient canals, Volkmann's canals) pierce the bone obliquely or at right angles to its long axis and communicate with the central canals, thus establishing a continuous and elaborate system which houses the blood vessels and nerves of the bone.

In a cross section of the bone, the central canals are seen to be surrounded by a varying number (8 to 15) of concentric lamellae and accompanying bone cells. The concentric lamellae of intercellular substance, the cells, and the central canal constitute an *osteon* or *Haversian system* (Figs. 6-10 and 6-11). The whole bone does not, however, consist of such concentric systems. In the periphery, the lamellae run parallel with the surface and form a relatively thin outer

layer of the bone. These are the outer *circumferential* lamellae (Fig. 6-9). A few similarly arranged inner circumferential lamellae separate the osteons from the marrow cavity. Finally, the intervals between the osteons are occupied by more irregular layers of bone, which constitute the *interstitial* lamellae (Fig. 6-10). Adjacent lamellar systems are as a rule delimited from each other by a darkly staining thin layer of modified matrix (cement line, cement "membrane").

Compact bone thus consists of branching and anastomosing concentric tubular lamellae, with intervals filled in by interstitial lamellae, which are covered externally and internally by the more parallel circumferential lamellae. The perforating canals which pierce the bone from its outer and inner surface and become continuous with the central canals are not lined by concentric lamellae.

The bone cells (*osteocytes*) fill the flattened, almond-shaped spaces or lacunae situated between or within the lamellae (Figs. 6-12 and 6-13). Tiny canaliculi course across the lamellae and interconnect neighboring lacunae. The cytoplasmic processes of the osteocytes are found within these canaliculi, but neither the cell processes nor their canaliculi can be traced very far in routine hematoxylin and eosin-stained sections. However, the canaliculi are readily seen after special stains (Fig. 6-12), and the cell processes can be seen in well-fixed and well-stained sections of fetal bone (Fig. 6-13). The full extent of the cell processes has been determined by electron microscopy, which has revealed that the processes of neighboring cells are in contact within the canaliculi by communicating (gap) junctions (see chapter 4).

Electron micrographs show that the osteocytes and their processes do not rest directly on the mineralized matrix but are separated from the walls of their lacunae and canaliculi by an amorphous coat. Histochemical studies show that this material is PAS-positive. It probably serves as an extra medium by which substances can be exchanged between the cells and the blood vessels present in the Haversian canals.

The osteocytes were bone-forming cells (*osteoblasts*) which became imprisoned in the bone as it was deposited. Osteoblasts

Haversian system   Partly destroyed
Haversian system

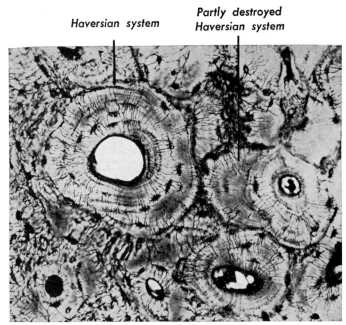

Fig. 6-11. Light micrograph of a transverse section through the shaft of the femur of a young adult rhesus monkey. Decalcified 6-μm section. The walls of the lacunae, canaliculi, and central canals are stained with Schmorl's thionin phosphomolybdic acid method. ×270.

Canaliculi   Haversian canal   Lacuna   Interstitial lamellae

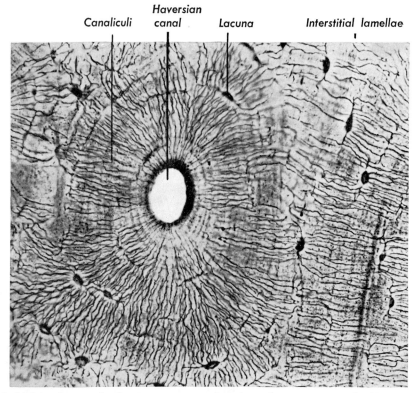

Fig. 6-12. Light micrograph of a transverse section through an osteon and adjacent interstitial lamellae. Decalcified bone from the shaft of the femur of a young adult rhesus monkey, 6-μm section. Schmorl's thionin phosphomolybdic acid method. ×420.

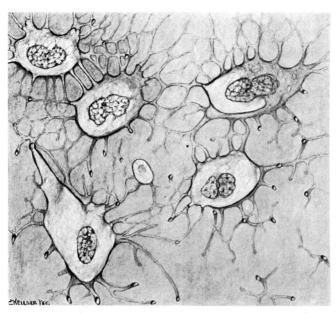

Fig. 6-13. Osteocytes and canaliculi as seen in a tangential section of the peripheral portion of the shaft of the ulna of a 10- to 12-week human fetus. One can follow the extensive network of the canaliculi in the 10-μm section as a result of the staining of the walls of lacunae and canaliculi. Azure II-eosin stain. × 1700.

and osteoprogenitor cells also persist as an incomplete lining of the central and perforating canals and are present in the endosteum and inner layer of the periosteum. With a stimulus such as is supplied by a fracture or physiological stress, they again may become active bone-forming cells.

When the collagenous fibrils are studied in preparations in which precautions have been taken to prevent collagenous swelling, the fibrils are found in delicate fascicles coursing parallel with one another within a single lamella. They follow a helical course in each lamella, with differences in slope and direction in alternate lamellae. This is apparently the reason why transverse sections of osteons show the concentric lamellae alternately striated and punctuated (Fig. 6-12). In the former, the fibrils are coursing circularly at the level of the section and are cut lengthwise. In the punctuated lamellae, the fibrils are parallel to the long axis of the Haversian system at the level of the section and are cut across.

Besides the lamellar fibers, there are found within the outer layers of the bone the coarser, *perforating fibers* of Sharpey (Fig. 6-14). These are continuations of the periosteal fibers and pierce the bone

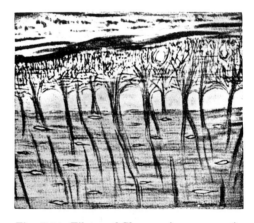

Fig. 6-14. Fibers of Sharpey in cross section of decalcified phalanx from child of 6 years. The fibers of Sharpey are direct continuations of periosteal fibers. (After Petersen.)

obliquely or at right angles to its long axis. They consist of collagenous or fibroelastic bundles with uncalcified or only partly calcified matrix. Purely elastic perforating fibers are likewise found. They extend into the outer circumferential and interstitial lamellae but do not penetrate the osteons. They are especially numerous in places where ligaments and tendons are inserted, and they serve for firmer anchorage of these structures.

Spongy bone shows the same lamellar structure but differs from compact bone in the more irregular arrangement of the lamellae in trabeculae and spicules, and in the presence of relatively few osteons.

Nonlamellar (Woven) Bone

Although the bone of all vertebrates consists of collagen, ground substance, calcium salts, and a permeating system of spaces occupied by cells and their processes, different samples of bone differ in the manner in which their constituents are combined. Thus, the skeletons of fish, amphibians, and birds differ from each other and from those of mammals, and the bone of man shows marked structural changes during ontogenesis. The human embryonic skeleton consists of coarsely bundled *woven bone*; i.e., the collagenous fibers are in coarse bundles and are irregularly woven or plaited, and the lacunae are irregularly dispersed. Stratified or *lamellar bone,* i.e., with fibrils oriented similarly in any given stratum and in different directions in alter- nating lamellae, gradually replaces woven bone, beginning before birth and continuing until only traces of woven bone persist in the adult (for example, in tooth sockets, bony sutures, osseous labyrinth, and regions of tendon-bone attachment). The first bone formed during repair of fractures is of the woven type.

Development and Growth of Bone

According to the embryological origin, there are two types of bone development, *intramembranous* and *intracartilaginous* or *endochondral.* In intramembranous bone formation, the bone develops under or within a layer of connective tissue. It does not involve the removal and replacement of cartilage. In endochondral bone formation, cartilage is first removed, later to be replaced by bone. The development of the flat bones of the skull involves only the intramembranous type of bone formation (Figs. 6-15 to 6-19). The development of the bones of the base of the skull, of the face, and of the axial skeleton involves both types of bone formation: the bone around a cartilage precursor (subperiosteal bone)

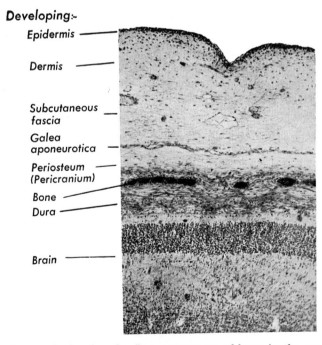

Developing:-
Epidermis
Dermis
Subcutaneous fascia
Galea aponeurotica
Periosteum (Pericranium)
Bone
Dura
Brain

Fig. 6-15. Light micrograph showing the first appearance of bone in the parietal region of the developing skull. Human embryo of about 2½ months. ×60.

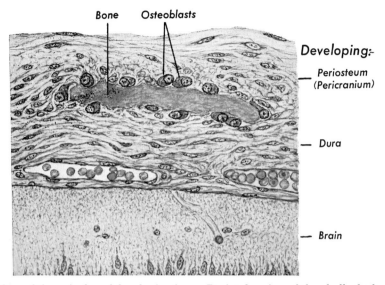

Fig. 6-16. One of the spicules of developing bone. Parietal region of the skull of a human embryo of about 2½ months. Camera lucida drawing. ×420.

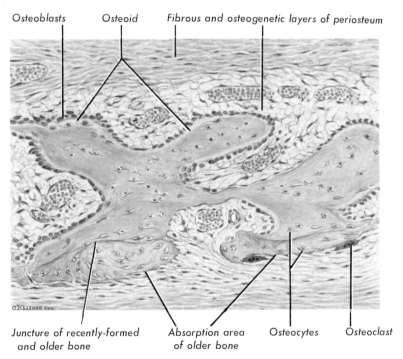

Fig. 6-17. Section through parietal bone of human fetus of 3 months. ×115.

is formed by the intramembranous type, and the bone which directly replaces the cartilage is formed by the endochondral method. It should be kept in mind, however, that *the fundamental process of bone deposition is the same in both types.* In intracartilaginous bone formation, there is simply the additional feature of the removal of portions of the cartilage preparatory to the deposition of the bone.

Cell Types in Osteogenesis

One can identify different types of cells in sites of bone formation as follows: (1)

Osteoid   Osteoblasts   Marrow   Fibrous and osteogenetic
                                      cavity   layers of periosteum

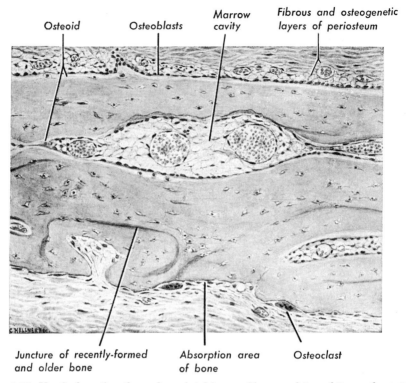

Juncture of recently-formed   Absorption area   Osteoclast
and older bone   of bone

Fig. 6-18. Vertical section through parietal bone of human fetus of 6 months. ×115.

osteogenic or *osteoprogenitor cells,* (2) *osteoblasts,* (3) *osteocytes,* and (4) *osteoclasts.* Because the cells of a given type have similar characteristics regardless of whether they are found in intramembranous or intracartilagenous bone-forming regions, the cytological features of the cell types are described before the topographical aspects of bone formation.

Osteogenic or Osteoprogenitor Cells. In regions of the embryonic mesenchymal compartment where bone formation is beginning and in areas near the surfaces of growing bones, one finds irregularly shaped and somewhat elongated cells which have pale-staining cytoplasm and pale-staining nuclei. They differ structurally only slightly from the mesenchymal cells from which they have arisen. They are identified chiefly by their location and by their association with osteoblasts. They multiply by mitosis, and some of them change into osteoblasts, which change later into osteocytes. It seems established that osteocytes can also change back to osteogenic cells in response to altered conditions in the environment, and

that the various types of bone cells represent different functional states of the same cell. A temporary change of this type is known as *modulation* in contrast with differentiation, which involves a more fixed change.

The osteogenic cells are active during the growing period of bone, and some persist throughout life in the inner portion of the periosteum and in the endosteum of the marrow cavities.

Osteoblasts. These cells are generally larger than the osteoprogenitor cells, and they have a more rounded nucleus, a more prominent nucleolus, and cytoplasm which is much more basophilic (Fig. 6-16). The nucleus is often toward one side of the cell, and close to it, one can frequently see a clear zone which is the negative image of the enlarged Golgi complex (Fig. 6-26). Electron micrographs disclose numerous mitochondria, a well developed rough-surfaced endoplasmic reticulum, (Figs. 6-19 and 6-20), an active Golgi complex with numerous vesicles, and microtubules. The cells have microvillous processes during

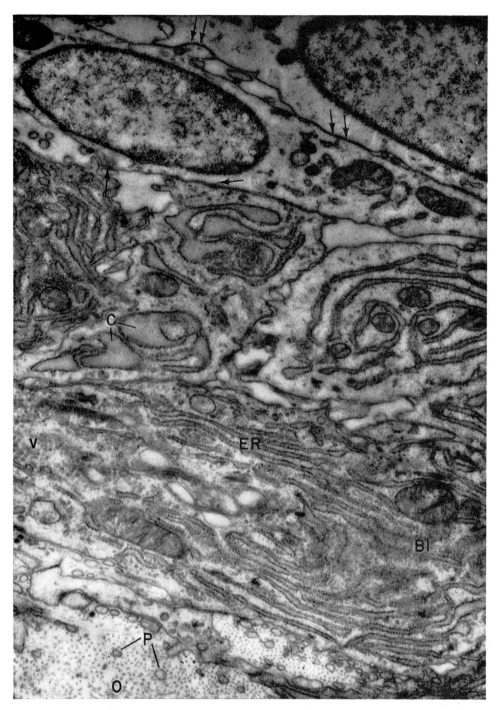

Fig. 6-19. Electron micrograph of developing bone showing layers of osteoblastic cells in relation to osteoid (*O*). Note the increasing complexity of the cytoplasm of the osteoblastic cells as the osteoid is approached. Processes (*P*) of the osteoblasts are seen penetrating the osteoid. Numerous small vesicles (*V*) are dispersed in the cytoplasm (*Bl*) of an osteoblast. The granular endoplasmic reticulum (*ER*) is well developed, and a few cisternae of the reticulum are dilated (*C*). *Arrows* point to two types of junctions between contiguous cells, probably desmosomes and communicating junctions. ×11,000. (Courtesy of Dr. David Spiro, J. Biophys. Biochem. Cytol., 1961.)

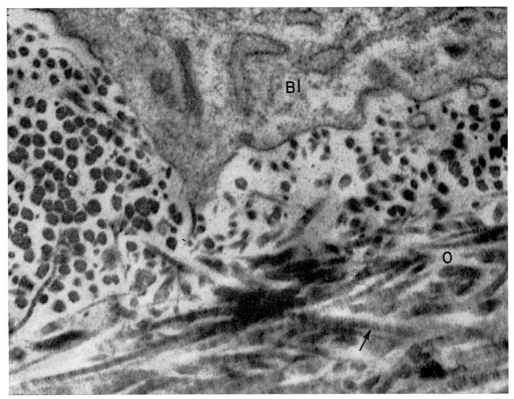

Fig. 6-20. Electron micrograph of developing bone, showing junction of osteoblast (*BL*) with osteoid (*O*). Note that the collagen fibrils adjacent to the cell surface have smaller diameters than those deeper in the osteoid. Fibrils cut lengthwise show a 640-Å repeating periodicity with interperiod bands (*arrow*). ×52,000. (Courtesy of Dr. David Spiro; Dudley and Spiro: J. Biophys. Biochem. Cytol. 1961.)

early development, and some of these elongate and remain as protoplasmic processes within the canaliculi as the matrix increases in amount. The processes of both osteoblasts and osteocytes contain 50- to 60-Å diameter microfilaments which course parallel with the long axes of the processes.

The basophilia of the osteoblasts is due to the abundance of rough-surfaced endoplasmic reticulum, characteristic of cells engaged in protein synthesis. It has been shown by studies in which labeled precursors are used that the osteoblasts secrete the organic components of the matrix, i.e., the collagen fibers and the glycosaminoglycans. From histochemical studies it is known that the cytoplasm of osteoblasts also contains considerable alkaline phosphatase. Although the exact role of this enzyme in calcification is not understood, there is evidence that it is important in

controlling the deposition of calcium. It is known, for example, that calcification continues in growing long bones of animals after the cells have been killed, provided that alkaline phosphatase is added to the solutions in which the bone is kept.

The formation of bone in unusual regions of the adult body (metaplastic bone formation), as in the walls of sclerotic arteries, calcified foci in the lungs, and connective tissue adjoining transplants of transitional epithelium in experimental animals, is difficult to harmonize with the view that bone formation is accomplished specifically by differentiated osteogenic (osteoprogenitor) cells. The most commonly accepted explanation for metaplastic bone formation is that either fibroblasts or persisting primitive mesenchymal cells can differentiate into osteoprogenitor cells under altered environmental conditions.

Osteocytes. These cells are described above under "Microscopic Structure." It has been pointed out that they arise from osteoblasts by modulation. They apparently have a role in maintaining the constituents of the extracellular matrix at normal levels.

Osteoclasts. On the surfaces of bones where resorption is occurring, one frequently finds large, multinucleated giant cells known as osteoclasts (Figs. 6-17, 6-18, and 6-21). They are often found in depressions in the bone (Howship's lacunae).

The number of nuclei in osteoclasts var-

ies greatly. The cytoplasm has a foamlike or vacuolated appearance and gives a variable staining reaction. It is less basophilic than the osteoblast cytoplasm and, in some cells, particularly in the older ones, it becomes slightly acidophilic (Fig. 6-25). Electron micrographs show a paucity of granular endoplasmic reticulum, but reveal clusters of free ribosomes. The mitochondria are relatively short and they are most numerous in the cytoplasm facing the bone. There are multiple paired centrioles corresponding to the number of nuclei and also numerous Golgi complexes. Vacuoles of

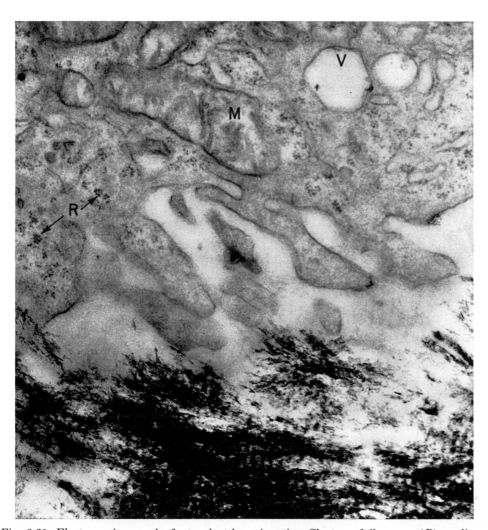

Fig. 6-21. Electron micrograph of osteoclast-bone junction. Clusters of ribosomes (*R*) are dispersed in the osteoclast cytoplasm between mitochondria (*M*) and vacuoles (*V*). Fragments of bone and individual apatite crystals are seen between the processes of the osteoclast. ×40,000. (Courtesy of Dr. David Spiro; Dudley and Spiro: J. Biophys. Biochem. Cytol. 1961.)

various sizes are abundant, as are lysosomes, which often have granules. The surface of the osteoclast facing toward the bone being resorbed has numerous cytoplasmic processes and microvilli, described as a *ruffled border.*

The fact that osteoclasts are often present in depressions where bone is being resorbed supports the view that they have an important role in the process. An increase in the number of osteoclasts when resorption is stimulated by intravascular injections of parathyroid hormone (PTH) also supports this view. Although the mechanisms involved in PTH-stimulated calcium resorption are not fully understood, it is clear from both in vivo and in vitro studies that there is an increased osteoclastic activity. The in vivo changes after PTH apparently accompany increased urinary excretion of electrolytes (including phosphates), which in turn results in resorption of calcium from its storage place in bone in order to maintain a relatively constant level of calcium in the circulating blood. The latter is related to the maintenance of a constant electrolyte balance of calcium in the cytoplasm of the cells of the body and is known as *calcium homeostasis.* In PTH-stimulated resorption, the osteoclasts increase their activity and then increase in size and numbers. This is soon accompanied by increased activity of osteocytes and freeing of the latter from their lacunae.

Osteocytes and osteoclasts appear to be different stages of the same cell type. The latter arise by fusion of osteogenic cells, including those developing from osteocytes when the latter are freed from their lacunae during resorption. The resorption occurs first in the relatively immature trabecular bone. When calcium from bone is no longer needed to maintain calcium homeostasis, osteogenic cells differentiate into osteoblasts, which form new bone to replace that which was resorbed.

Although the origin of osteoclasts has been controversial, the evidence from studies of animals given injections of tritiated thymidine indicate that these cells arise from osteoprogenitor cells. Studies with labeled thymidine also show that there is a turnover of nuclei in osteoclasts. Some of the older nuclei become pyknotic and are extruded from the cell, whereas new nuclei are added by fusion of new osteoprogenitor cells with the osteoclasts.

In regions of cartilage resorption, as in stages of endochondral bone development, there are multinucleated cells with the same characteristics as osteoclasts. Because they are associated with cartilage, they are known as *chondroclasts.* They form by fusion of chondrocytes after the latter are released from their lacunae.

Intramembranous Bone Formation

Because the development of the flat bones of the skull involves only intramembranous bone formation, it is an excellent place to study the structural features of the deposition of osseous tissue uncomplicated by changes in cartilage. In the locations where bone is to be laid down, the mesenchyme becomes richly vascularized, and active proliferation of the mesenchymal cells takes place. Within this primitive connective tissue bed, some of the cells show structural changes which enable one to identify them as osteoprogenitor cells and osteoblasts.

Between the enlarged cells or osteoblasts, an acidophilic hyaline ground substance appears. It masks the fibrils which were already present in the embryonal connective tissue, as well as those that are subsequently formed by the osteoblasts. The intercellular substance, or matrix, which thus is composed of a clear ground substance and collagenous fibers, is usually not calcified at first and is soft and easily cut. It is given the name of *osteoid* (resembling bone) and is the organic part of bone matrix without appreciable inorganic constituent. As the deposition of the matrix progresses, the osteoblasts, with their processes, are imprisoned by matrix being deposited around them; lacunae and canaliculi are thus formed. Because processes of adjoining cells make contact with each other, the canaliculi of adjoining lacunae connect with each other. New osteoblasts, arising by modulation of osteoprogenitor cells, maintain a layer of bone-forming cells at the surface of the newly formed bone. The osteoprogenitor cells multiply by mitosis, and they probably continue to increase for a certain embryonic period by differentiation of undifferentiated neighboring connective tissue cells.

Calcification. In calcification, the minerals are deposited in the form of minute crystals (hydroxyapatites) intimately associated with the collagenous fibers. The crystals are too small to be visible under the light microscope, but electron micrographs show that they appear first on the surfaces of the fibrils and later within them.

Calcification of bone is dependent upon (1) the availability of adequate amounts of minerals, particularly phosphorous and calcium, at the region to be calcified and (2) requisite chemical and physical conditions within the calcification site. The minerals are present in the blood and are carried to the calcification site, where calcium and phosphate ions are present in metastable solution under normal conditions. In some disease states, such as *rickets*, the body lacks an adequate amount of vitamin D, which is essential for absorption and maintenance of the minerals at an appropriate level in the blood. In this condition, collagen and glycosaminoglycans continue to form and the increase of uncalcified osteoid at the growing ends of long bones gives abnormal shapes. The lack of sufficient minerals leads to decreased rigidity.

The local factors responsible for calcification are controlled by the cells in the ossification center. Although many of the details remain obscure, there is evidence on some of the requisites. It is noted in chapter 5 that collagen can be dissolved and reconstituted in vitro, either in its native form or in other types. When different types of reconstituted collagen are exposed in vitro to metastable solutions of calcium phosphate, calcification occurs only in the 640 Å periodicity type. In other words, a "precise stereochemical configuration" is necessary for the initiation of calcification. This raises the question why calcification does not occur in all 640 Å periodicity collagen in the body. Further studies have shown that reconstituted collagen from tendon, which does not calcify in the body, does calcify in metastable solutions of calcium phosphate in vitro, provided that components of the associated ground substance are removed. Apparently, certain glycosaminoglycans associated with collagen have a role in inhibiting and regulating calcification.

The effect of parathyroid hormone (PTH) in stimulating the resorption of calcium from its storage place in bone matrix was discussed above under "Osteoclasts." Another hormone, *calcitonin*, formed by the *parafollicular cells* of the thyroid gland, has an effect opposite to that of PTH; i.e., it inhibits calcium resorption from bone. Moreover, it inhibits the activity of osteoclasts when there is a drop in plasma calcium regardless of whether this is stimulated by PTH or by other factors. For example, patients with various types of metabolic bone disease in which there is a drop in serum calcium have a marked reduction in the number of osteoclasts followed by an increase in number of osteoblasts and osteocytes.

Scurvy is a disease state related to local changes in the calcification site. In this condition, the diet is deficient in vitamin C, which is essential for osteoblasts to form collagen capable of normal cross linkage. The collagen which is formed can become mineralized, but its abnormality affects skeletal growth and maintenance and retards healing of fractures.

Further Growth and Resorption of Intramembranous Bone. Osteogenic cells around the foci of newly formed intramembranous bone continue to multiply and change into osteoblasts and osteocytes. By this process, irregular plates and trabeculae are formed. These enclose spaces (primary marrow spaces) which contain blood vessels, reticular cells, and primitive marrow cells (Fig. 6-18).

During early development of intramembranous bone, osseous tissue is deposited in both the inner and outer surfaces of the flat bones of the skull and also on their peripheral margins. Deposition in the latter area increases the surface area of the bone and also accompanies an enlargement of the cranial cavity to accommodate the growth of the brain. A further increase in the cranial cavity is achieved by resorption along the inner surface, a process which begins relatively early. Continued growth involves new bone deposition, primarily on the outer and marginal surfaces, and resorption, chiefly along the inner surface. However, new bone formation is not entirely absent from the inner surfaces; *the processes of formation and resorption accompany each other in the constant remodeling of bone.*

Intracartilaginous (Endochondral) Bone Formation

In this form of ossification, an embryonal type of hyaline cartilage precedes the formation of bone, and the shape of the bone corresponds more or less closely to that of the prior cartilage. However, it must be realized that the initial cartilaginous model of the bone-to-be is minute in comparison to the eventual mass of the bone. During development, the cartilage is replaced by bone, except at the joint surfaces. This replacement is not completely accomplished, however, until the bone has achieved its full size and growth has ceased.

During the replacement of the cartilage by bone, not only does the supporting function have to be maintained but there is a continual increase in length and diameter as well.

Stages in Intracartilagenous Bone Formation. The first indication of beginning ossification in the cartilaginous model of a long bone is seen near the center of the future shaft, the diaphyseal or *primary ossification center* (Fig. 6-22). The cartilage cells proliferate and hypertrophy, and their lacunae correspondingly increase in number and size. The matrix between the lu-

cunae becomes reduced in amount and forms but thin partitions. These, except for the cartilage capsules, then become calcified by the deposition of lime salts. Such calcified cartilage is not to be confused with mineralized bone. This calcified portion stains more intensely with basic dyes than does the unchanged cartilage at either end of the ossification center.

At about the time that these intracartilaginous changes are clearly evident, the perichondrium assumes an osteogenetic function. Some of the cells of the inner part of the perichondrium change into *osteogenic cells* and, in turn, into *osteoblasts*, which deposit a perforated *bony ring* or *collar* around the cartilage of the ossification center. This bone collar is thin-walled and short at first but becomes progressively thicker-walled and longer as the ossification progresses. It is closely adherent to the cartilage and forms a splint that assists in maintaining the strength of the shaft, which has been weakened by the dissolution of part of the cartilage. It is formed by an intramembranous type of bone development. The perichondrium which surrounded the cartilage has, in this region of ossification, become a periosteum.

Vascular connective tissue from the periosteum, known as *periosteal buds*, grows through apertures in the bone collar and enters the periphery of the changed cartilage matrix (Fig. 6-23). It contains blood vessels and osteogenic cells from the periosteum. These penetrate the thin-walled partitions between the hypertrophied car-

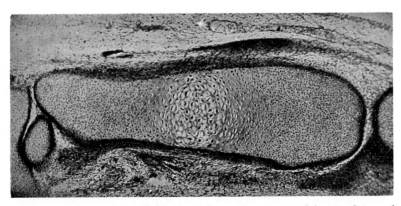

Fig. 6-22. Light micrograph of cartilaginous anlage of metacarpal bone of 4-cm human fetus, showing changes in the central portion preparatory to ossification. The bone collar is beginning to form. ×90.

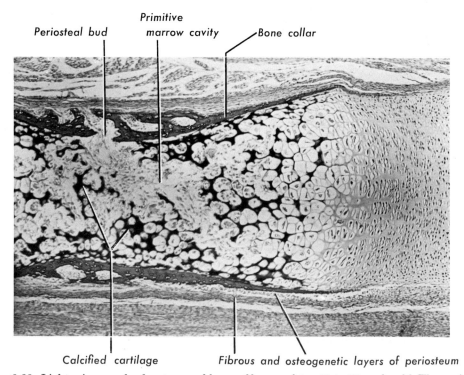

Periosteal bud   Primitive marrow cavity   Bone collar

Calcified cartilage   Fibrous and osteogenetic layers of periosteum

Fig. 6-23. Light micrograph of metacarpal bone of human fetus 10 to 12 weeks old. The periosteal bud is only one of several, as shown by an examination of serial sections. The primary marrow cavity is quite extensive. The zones of cell and lacunar enlargement and of cell multiplication are evident. Only a small amount of reserve cartilage has been included in the figure.

tilage lucunae and thus form cavities, the *primary marrow spaces.* The osteogenic cells multiply by mitosis, and some of them transform into osteoblasts around the periphery of the calcified cartilage remnants.

The hypertrophied cartilage cells of endochondral bone-forming centers become increasingly abnormal and most, perhaps all, of them eventually degenerate. Some authors believe that some of the cells may survive and become osteogenic, because in vitro, isotope labeling at different developmental stages indicates that some of the cartilage cells survive and become chondroclasts and osteoblasts. Furthermore, cartilage cells derived from neonatal mesenchymal cells grown in vitro in association with bone matrix transform into bone cells after subsequent transplantation into isogenic host animals. This type of dedifferentiation and transition into a new type of tissue cell is known as *metaplasia.*

The primitive marrow cavity of developing endochondral bone regularly contains remnants of calcified cartilage matrix on which osteogenic cells align themselves and differentiate into osteoblasts. Thus, the calcified cartilage becomes enclosed first by osteoid and then by mineralized bone. The initial trabeculae of cartilage and bone thus formed is subsequently resorbed as the marrow cavity enlarges during bone growth. Hence, the trabeculae of cartilage and bone serve only as a temporary framework (Figs. 6-24 to 6-26).

The extension of the zone of ossification toward the ends of the cartilage model is accomplished by an orderly sequence of changes in the cartilage similar to those which took place in the formation of the primary ossification center. However, the changes show a more distinct zonal arrangement (Fig. 6-25), and the whole process of bony replacement proceeds as a wave of osteogenic activity toward the extremities of the eventual bone.

Several zones can be distinguished in the cartilage. Beginning at the ends of the cartilage and passing toward the ossification center, these zones, which overlap each other somewhat, are as follows:

Zone of Reserve Cartilage. This zone is relatively long before the formation of the secondary (epiphyseal) centers of ossification which develop in some parts of the skeleton at about the time of birth. After the secondary centers form, the zone of reserve (or resting) cartilage becomes relatively short (Fig. 6-25). The cells are randomly arranged and the growth of the zone is relatively slow.

Zone of Cell Proliferation or Multiplication. In this zone the cells are more or less aligned in rows which course parallel with the long axis of the growing bone. The lacunae containing the daughter cells are broad but flattened, as are the cells, their long axes being perpendicular to the longitudinal axis of the cartilage. By these divisions of cartilage cells and their distribution in rows, the length of the cartilage is increased more than is its diameter as new matrix is formed.

Zone of Cell Maturation and Hypertrophy. In this zone there is no further multiplication of the cells, but they mature and enlarge. This still further increases the length of the cartilage of this region. The cytoplasm of the cells contains considerable amounts of glycogen and alkaline phosphatase at this stage. Poor preservation of glycogen in routine preparations for light microscopy is partly responsible for the vacuolated and lightly stained appearance of the cytoplasm seen in the hypertrophied cartilage cells. The cartilage between adjacent cells within a row, previously small in amount, becomes even thinner.

Zone of Cartilage Calcification. This is a zone of variable length, but is always narrow. The matrix between adjacent lacunae within a row has practically disappeared and the matrix between the rows begins to calcify. The mechanism of calcification in the cartilage matrix has been the subject of much investigation and debate. Recent evidence strongly suggests that prior to their degeneration, hypertrophied chondrocytes release membrane-enclosed vesicles (*matrix vesicles*) containing calcium ions into the surrounding cartilage matrix. These tiny vesicles and their contained calcium serve as nucleation sites for the calcification process. The mechanism by which the large amounts of additional calcium necessary to complete the calcification are made available selectively to the nucleation sites remains unclear.

Zone of Cartilage Removal and Bone Deposition (Zone of Provisional Ossification). In the outer part of this zone, the thin partitions between the lacunae within a row undergo dissolution. This is accompanied by death of the cartilage cells and is apparently aided by an erosive action by blood vessels that grow in from the marrow cavity. Longitudinal canals, filled with vessels and marrow, are thus formed in tunnels surrounded by calcified cartilage matrix. Farther toward the marrow cavity, the calcified cartilage matrix between the newly formed tunnels becomes reduced in amount by resorption, but remnants of calcified cartilage matrix persist; upon these, osteoblasts deposit lamellae of bone (Figs. 6-24 to 6-26). All of the cartilage remnants and their bony coverings are subsequently resorbed as the marrow cavity enlarges during the calcified growth period.

The region where the diaphysis joins the epiphysis, i.e., where the calcified cartilage is being first reinforced and then replaced by bone, is known as the *metaphysis*. This includes the region described above as the zone of cartilage removal and bone deposition.

The overall region of newly formed bone is known as the *spongiosa* on the basis of its spongy appearance. This is subdivided into *primary spongiosa* (equivalent to the zone of provisional ossification) and *secondary spongiosa*. The former is a relatively short region beginning just below the level where the hypertrophic cartilage cells disappear; it is characterized by marrow spaces of fairly uniform width. The secondary spongiosa is a relatively long region with wide and irregularly contoured marrow spaces extending toward the junction of the epiphysis and diaphysis.

While these changes within the cartilage are taking place, the bone collar is increasing in length and in diameter by the deposition of new bone by the osteoblasts of the periosteum. The marrow cavity also increases in size, not only by its longitudinal

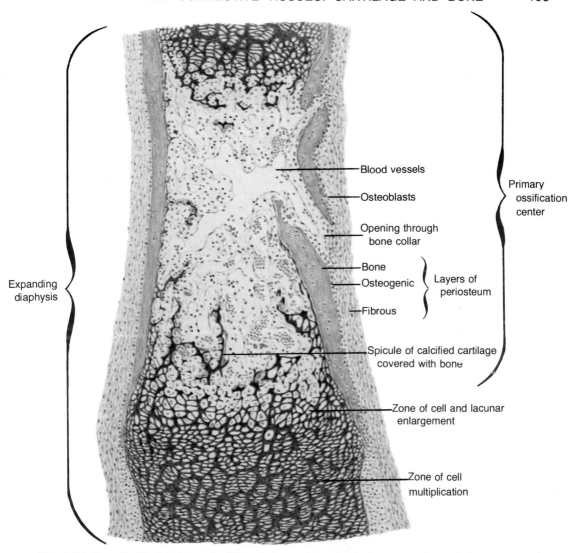

Expanding diaphysis

Blood vessels

Osteoblasts

Primary ossification center

Opening through bone collar

Bone

Osteogenic

Fibrous

Layers of periosteum

Spicule of calcified cartilage covered with bone

Zone of cell and lacunar enlargement

Zone of cell multiplication

Fig. 6-24. Longitudinal section of middle phalanx of finger of a human embryo of about 4 months. Hematoxylin and eosin-azure II. ×80.

extension as a result of cartilage removal, but also in diameter, owing to resorption of the inner part of the bone collar or splint. These processes continue as development proceeds. The zone of reserve cartilage is maintained by continued cell division, as outlined above.

At about the time of birth, additional ossification centers (epiphyseal or *secondary ossification centers*) appear in each end of the long bones. The cartilage in these centers passes through the same changes as seen in the diaphysis. The proliferation of the cartilage cells leads to nearly equal

growth in all directions, however. The cartilage cells, each of which is enclosed in a lacuna, are arranged in irregularly shaped nests and not in rows, and the partitions between the nests run in various directions. As in the diaphysis, the center is invaded by osteogenetic buds, and cartilage removal and bone deposition take place. Bone trabeculae, however, remain in the epiphyseal cavity, giving it grossly a spongy appearance, and the cartilage forming the articular surface persists, anchored to and supported by the underlying bone (Fig. 6-27).

The diaphysis continues its growth in

length long after the epiphyseal centers appear. The cartilage plate which separates it from the epiphysis is called the *epiphyseal plate* (Fig. 6-25).

Eventually, the epiphyseal plate is replaced by bone development on both of its faces (epiphyseal and diaphyseal). At this time, growth of a bone ceases and the diaphysis is bound to the epiphysis by a bony union. The zone of this union is visible in the adult. It is called the *epiphyseal line.*

Osteons. During the growth of the skeleton, some of the spongy bone becomes transformed into compact bone. In this process, lamellae of bone are deposited progressively inward on the surface of the cavities in the spongy bone until they are reduced to narrow canals. Each canal is traversed by blood vessels which originally were in the large cavity. The system of concentric lamellae with its canal and blood vessels forms an osteon (Haversian system).

The osteons of the shafts of long bones are formed by a more complicated process than that described above for transformation in areas of cancellous bone. The first step in the formation of osteons in compact bone is the erosion of tunnels in it by vascular sprouts and osteoclasts from the medullary and periosteal surfaces. The tunnels thus formed (Howship's lacunae) have irregular, roughened surfaces but are of a fairly uniform diameter. When the absorption phase leading to the formation of the tunnel has been completed, osteoblasts arise from the osteogenic cells in the vascular sprouts. They come to lie next to the walls of the tunnel and deposit progressively inward concentric lamellae characteristic of an osteon. A narrow canal containing blood vessels is left: the central canal. Parts of the original circumferential lamellae (ground lamellae) remain between the osteons. However, new generations of osteons keep forming throughout life, although at a reduced rate in later years. In this process, parts of osteons formed earlier, as well as additional parts of the original circumferential lamellae, are destroyed. Stages in the destruction of bone and its replacement by newer osteons are illustrated in Figure 6-28. The osteons have an important function in providing channels for blood vessels through compact bone. They also provide better structural support and presumably make the bone less brittle.

Because bone serves as a storehouse for calcium and phosphate, the rate of bone resorption increases whenever either of these essential elements tends to fall below a normal blood level. This leads to changes in osteons and in the trabeculae at the ends of the long bones. The minerals are not withdrawn independently; both minerals and matrix are withdrawn simultaneously. Destruction of bone can be produced by the experimental administration of parathyroid extract or by a tumor of the parathyroid gland. The latter usually causes pronounced resorption of bone and its replacement by connective tissue (von Recklinghausen's disease).

It has been pointed out that perforating fibers of Sharpey do not enter the osteons. An understanding of the developmental process will make the reason for this clear. Perforating fibers of Sharpey do not grow into bone. Rather they are radially or oliquely directed fibers which have been imprisoned by the advancing deposition of subperiosteal bone in much the same way that a branch of a tree becomes more and more enclosed in the expanding trunk. When a vascular sprout forms a tunnel preceding the deposition of an osteon, the perforating fibers of Sharpey as well as the bone substance are resorbed, and because of their method of formation the perforating fibers are not replaced.

Development of Short Bones

The development of the short bones is similar to that of the epiphyses of long bones. Ossification begins in the center of the cartilage and extends in all directions in the wake of the growing cartilage. Near the end of growth, the endochondral bone is invested with a thin compact layer of subperiosteal bone, except at the articular surfaces which remain cartilaginous.

Remodeling of Bone

Although bone is dense, hard, and rigid, it is able to change somewhat in shape and amount in response to environmental conditions. These changes are not brought

EPIPHYSIS

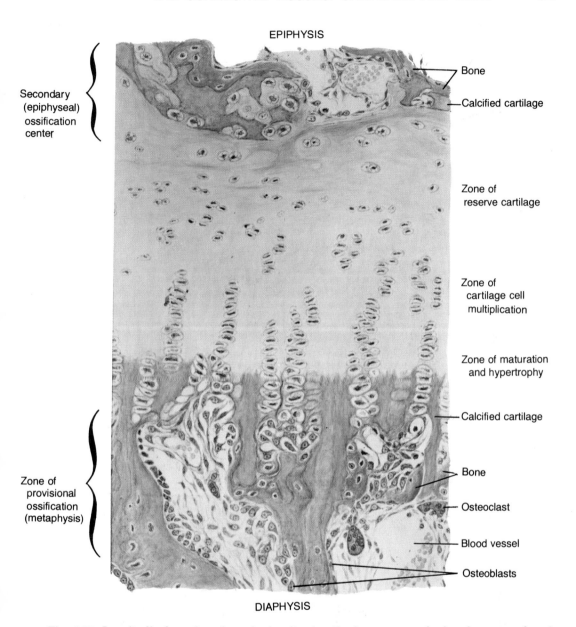

Secondary
(epiphyseal)
ossification
center

Bone

Calcified cartilage

Zone of
reserve cartilage

Zone of
cartilage cell
multiplication

Zone of maturation
and hypertrophy

Calcified cartilage

Zone of
provisional
ossification
(metaphysis)

Bone

Osteoclast

Blood vessel

Osteoblasts

DIAPHYSIS

Fig. 6-25. Longitudinal section through the distal end of a metatarsal of a rhesus monkey 2 months of age. The epiphyseal (secondary) ossification center is well formed. Bone formation is taking place both at the epiphyseal and the diaphyseal surfaces of the epiphyseal plate and is particularly pronounced on the diaphyseal side. Delafield's hematoxylin and eosin. ×280.

about by a remodeling, such as might be done with a plastic wax, but involve the formation of new bone and the removal of bone already formed or the combination of both processes. This capacity to change in shape is well illustrated by the moving of improperly aligned teeth by the orthodon-tist and by the spontaneous movement of neighboring teeth after a tooth is extracted. The bony socket is resorbed ahead of the tooth undergoing movement, and the shape and size of the socket maintained by the formation of new bone in back of the tooth. In other situations, as, for instance, in increased muscular development, bone may be remodeled to meet the additional stresses imposed upon it. In old age, resorption of the surfaces of some bones occurs. The changes in bone are slower and less pronounced in the adult than during the period of growth, but they probably occur to some degree throughout life.

Healing of Fractures

A fracture, like any traumatic injury, causes hemorrhage and tissue destruction. The first reparative changes thus are characteristic of those occurring in any injury of soft tissue. Proliferating fibroblasts and capillary sprouts grow into the blood clot and injured area, thus forming granulation tissue. The area also is invaded by polymorphonuclear leukocytes and later by macrophages which phagocytize the tissue debris. The granulation tissue gradually becomes denser, and in parts of it, cartilage is formed. This newly formed connective tissue and cartilage is designated as a *callus*. It serves temporarily in stabilizing and binding together the fractured bone.

As this process is taking place, the dormant osteogenic cells of the periosteum enlarge and become active osteoblasts. On the outside of the fractured bone, at first at some distance from the fracture, osseous tissue is deposited. This formation of new bone continues toward the fractured ends of the bone and finally forms a sheathlike layer of bone over the fibrocartilaginous callus. As the bone increases in amount, osteogenic buds invade the fibrous and cartilaginous callus and replace it with a bony one. In the replacement of the fibrocartilaginous callus, the cartilage undergoes calcification and absorption, as described in "Intracartilaginous Bone Formation." Typical intramembranous bone formation also takes place. The newly formed bone is at first a spongy and not a compact type. It becomes transformed into a compact type, and the callus becomes reduced in diameter. At the time when this subperiosteal bone formation is taking place, bone also forms in the marrow cavity. The medullary bone growing centripetally from each side of the fracture unites, thus aiding the bony union. The process of repair is, in general, an orderly process, but it varies greatly with the displacement of the fractured ends of the bone and the degree of trauma inflicted. Uneven or protruding surfaces are gradually removed, and the healed bone, especially in young individuals, assumes its original contour.

The Periosteum and Endosteum

The *periosteum* is a fibrous connective tissue investment of the bones, except at their articular surfaces. Its adherence to the bone varies in different places and at different ages. In the young bone, it is easily stripped off. In the adult bone, it is more firmly adherent and especially so at the insertion of tendons and ligaments, where more periosteal fibers penetrate into the bone as the perforating fibers of Sharpey.

The periosteum consists of two layers, the outer of which is composed of coarse, fibrous connective tissue containing few cells but numerous blood vessels and nerves. The inner layer is less vascular but more cellular and contains many elastic fibers. During growth, an osteogenic layer of primitive connective tissue forms the inner layer of the periosteum. In the adult, this is represented only by a row of scattered, flattened cells closely applied to the bone.

The periosteum serves as a supporting bed for the blood vessels and nerves going to the bone and for the anchorage of tendons and ligaments. Its importance for bone regeneration has been a much disputed topic. If the osteogenic layer is considered a part of the periosteum, the latter undoubtedly furnishes osteoblasts for growth and repair. However, the fibrous periosteum of the adult is itself a differentiated end product of the osteogenic layer, and it probably plays no direct part in bone repair but acts as an important limiting layer controlling and restricting the extent of bone formation.

Because both the periosteum and its contained bone are regions of the connective tissue compartment, they are not separated from each other or from other connective tissues by basal laminar material or basement membranes.

The *endosteum* lines the surface of cavities within a bone (marrow cavity and central canals) and also the surfaces of tra-

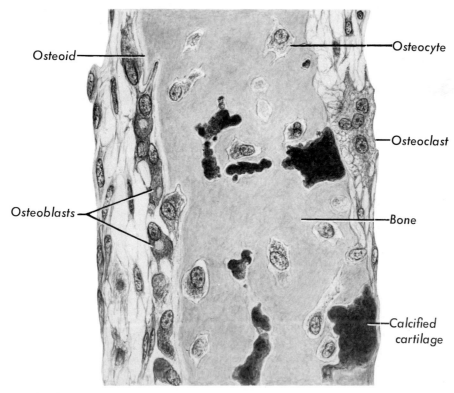

Fig. 6-26. Section of a trabecula in developing endochondral bone. Tibia of human fetus about 3½ months old. Azure II-eosin stain. ×950.

beculae in the marrow cavity. In growing bone, it consists of a delicate stratum of myelogenous reticular connective tissue, beneath which is a layer of osteoblasts. In the adult, the osteogenic cells become flattened and are indistinguishable as a separate layer. They are capable of transforming into osteogenic cells when there is a stimulus to bone formation, as after a fracture.

Marrow

Marrow is a soft connective tissue which occupies the medullary cavity of the long bones, the larger central canals, and all of the spaces between the trabeculae of spongy bone. It consists of a delicate reticular connective tissue, in the meshes of which lie various kinds of cells.

Two varieties of marrow are recognized: *red* and *yellow*.

Red Marrow. Red marrow (Figs. 6-29, 6-30, and 7-11) is the only type found in fetal and young bones, but in the adult it is restricted to the vertebrae, sternum, ribs, cranial bones, and epiphyses of long bones. It is the chief blood-forming organ of the adult body. During the fetal and growth period, it forms part of the osteogenic tissue, which furnishes the osteoblasts for bone development. The architecture of red marrow is discussed below under "Blood Vessels and Nerves," and the cells of marrow are described under "Blood Development," chapter 7.

Yellow Marrow. Yellow marrow consists in the main of fat cells (Fig. 6-27) which have gradually replaced the other marrow elements. Under certain conditions, the yellow marrow of old or emaciated persons loses most of its fat and assumes a reddish color and gelatinous consistency. It is then known as *gelatinous marrow*. With an adequate stimulus, yellow marrow may resume the character of red marrow and play an active part in the process of blood development.

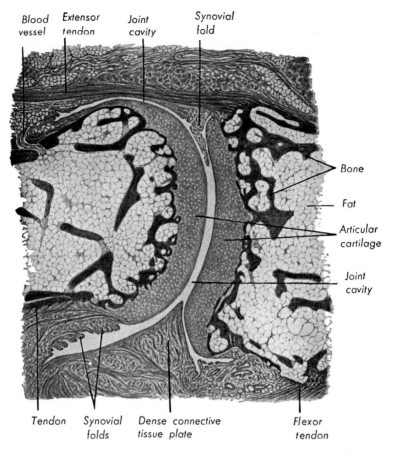

Fig. 6-27. Median sagittal section through the joint between the middle and terminal phalanges of middle toe. Human, 10 years of age. The terminal phalanx is at the *right*. ×14.

Blood Vessels and Nerves

Bone is richly supplied with blood vessels which pass into it from the periosteum. Near the center of the shaft of a long bone, a canal passes obliquely through the compact bone. This is known as the *medullary* or *nutrient* canal, and its external opening is known as the *nutrient foramen*. A medullary artery courses through this canal to the marrow cavity. In its passage through the compact bone, it communicates by branches with the blood vessels of the osteons. On reaching the marrow cavity, the artery divides into ascending and descending branches which supply all portions of the marrow. The terminal branches of the arterioles connect with *sinusoids,* which differ from capillaries by their larger diameter and by their close association with phagocytic cells. There are fenestrations in

the walls of the sinusoids (Figs. 6-29 and 6-30), and the basal lamina is thin and incomplete. Consequently, the sinusoids are more permeable than are ordinary capillaries.

The sinusoids are drained by narrow and thin-walled veins which have no valves. The larger medullary veins pass through the medullary canal accompanying the medullary artery and, like the latter, communicate by branches with the veins of the osteons.

Besides the medullary canals, the bone is everywhere pierced by the perforating canals, which serve for transmission of the numerous smaller vessels. In compact bone, these vessels give rise to a network of branches which run in the osteons. In spongy bone, the network lies in the marrow spaces. Branches from these vessels pass to the marrow cavity and there break

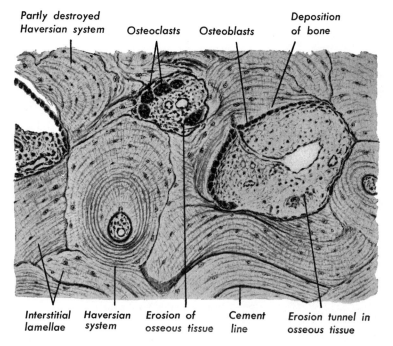

Partly destroyed
Haversian system   Osteoclasts   Osteoblasts   Deposition of bone

Interstitial lamellae   Haversian system   Erosion of osseous tissue   Cement line   Erosion tunnel in osseous tissue

Fig. 6-28. Figure showing the absorption of bone and the formation of an osteon in compact osseous tissue. Proximal phalanx of the thumb of a child 6 years old. ×150. (After Petersen.)

up into a sinusoidal network which anastomoses freely with that formed by the branches of the medullary artery.

Lymphatics. Lymphatics with distinct walls are present in the outer layer of the periosteum. Cleftlike lymph capillaries lined with endothelium accompany the blood vessels in the perforating canals and osteons. The amorphous material which surrounds the osteocytes and cytoplasmic processes in the lacunae and canaliculi serves for the exchange of substances between the cells and blood vessels and as a pathway for lymph.

Nerves. Both myelinated and nonmyelinated nerves accompany the vessels from the periosteum through the perforating canals into the osteons and marrow cavities. Periosteum is highly sensitive to painful stimuli, whereas osseous tissue is relatively insensitive.

Joints (Articulations)

Two main types of connections between bones are distinguished: (1) union without an articular cleft (*synarthrosis*), the joint being immovable or only slightly movable;

(2) connection of bones with an articular cleft (*diarthrosis,* movable joint, Fig. 6-27).

Synarthrosis. In *synarthrosis,* union may be by ligaments or dense fibrous tissue (*syndesmosis*) or by means of cartilage (*synchrondrosis*).

Syndesmosis. In *syndesmosis,* the connecting ligaments may be fibrous or elastic. Of the latter type are the ligamenta subflava which unite the vertebral arches. In the immovable articulations of the cranial bones (*sutures*), short fibers (which are, in the main, continuations of the fibers of Sharpey) unite the serrated edges of adjacent bones.

Synchondrosis. In *synchondrosis,* the cartilage is usually of the fibrous form, except nearest the bone, where it is hyaline (see under "Cartilage"). The intervertebral discs consist of a fibrocartilaginous ring surrounding a central gelatinoid mass, the nucleus pulposus.

Diarthrosis. In *diarthrosis,* the bones are separated by an articular cleft (synovial cavity) and are more or less freely movable. The following structures must be considered: (1) the articular cartilage, (2) the interarticular cartilages, or *menisci,* and gle-

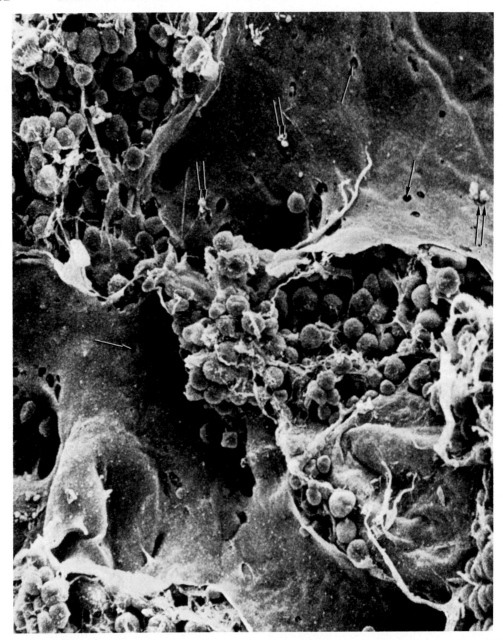

Fig. 6-29. Scanning electron micrograph of rabbit bone marrow showing sinusoids and interstitial tissue. The walls of the sinusoids have fenestrations (*single arrows*). Some of the fenestrations have processes of underlying phagocytic cells extending through them (*double arrows*). Courtesy of Dr. Masayuki Miyoshi. ×1000.

noid ligaments, and (3) the joint capsule.

Articular Cartilage. The *articular cartilage* (Figs. 6-2 and 6-27) covers the ends of the bones and is usually of the hyaline variety, being the remains of the original cartilage in which the bones were formed. No perichondrium is present. The most su-

perficial cartilage cells are flattened and arranged in rows parallel with the surface. In the deeper portion, the cells are rounded and arranged in typical groups. The deepest layer, firmly apposed to the bone, is calcified.

In the acromioclavicular, sternoclavicu-

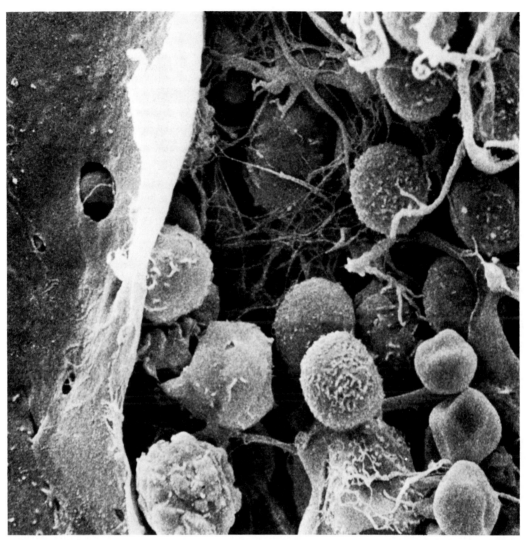

Fig. 6-30. Scanning electron micrograph of rabbit bone marrow showing part of a sinusoid (*left*) and some of the reticular tissue framework filled with hemopoietic, migratory, and phagocytic elements. Courtesy of Dr. Masayuki Miyoshi. ×4200.

lar, and costovertebral articulations, the cartilage is of the fibrous form. The same is true of the cartilage covering the head of the ulna, whereas the surface of the radius which enters into the wrist joints is covered not by cartilage but by dense fibrous tissue.

Articular cartilage, like cartilage elsewhere, is devoid of blood vessels. Metabolic exchange is made by diffusion through the ground substance of the cartilage to and from (1) synovial fluid, (2) capillaries in the periosteum around the periphery, and (3) vessels in the underlying bone. Exchange is chiefly with the synovial fluid.

Interarticular Cartilages. The *interarticular cartilages* and labra glenoidea serve to deepen the sockets for the articular ends; they usually consist of fibrous cartilage.

Joint Capsule. The *joint capsule* consists of two strata: an outer dense *fibrous layer,* which blends with the ligaments and periosteum of the articulating bones, and an inner layer, the *synovial membrane,* which lines the joint cavity, with the exception of the surfaces of the articular cartilages. Prominent infoldings of the synovial membranes are known as *synovial folds* (Fig. 6-27) and more slender projections are known as *synovial villi.*

The synovial membrane consists of an inner layer composed chiefly of cells and an outer layer of variable types of irregularly arranged connective tissue. On the basis of structural variations, the synovial membranes have been classified as fibrous, areolar, and adipose types. In the fibrous type (e.g., over tendons), a thin cellular layer rests on connective tissue fibers that are intimately blended with the fibrous capsule. The adipose type is found over intraarticular fat pads. The areolar type allows mobility of the synovial membrane over the fibrous capsule. Its outer layer contains irregularly arranged collagenous and elastic fibers plus the usual connective tissue cells, including mast cells and macrophages. Its inner cellular layer is thicker than that of the other types and consists of two to four layers of irregularly arranged cells that are usually described as fibroblasts. Electron micrographs show that the cells have numerous cytoplasmic processes, particularly at the adluminal cell surfaces. No basal lamina is seen between the surface cells and the underlying tissue.

The *synovial fluid, synovia,* is apparently secreted by the synovial cells. It is a viscid, mucoalbuminous fluid, rich in hyaluronic acid. It acts as a lubricating fluid, facilitating the smooth gliding of the articular surfaces.

The larger blood vessels of the joint capsule lie in the outer layer of the stratum synoviale, from which smaller vessels and capillaries pass to the inner layer and to some of the villi. The inner layer is richly and the outer layer more poorly supplied with lymph capillaries. Nonmyelinated nerve fibers are found in the connective tissue, some of them ending in end bulbs and Pacinian corpuscles.

References

ANDERSON, H. C. Vesicles associated with calcification in the matrix of epiphyseal cartilage. J. Cell Biol. 41:59–72, 1969.

BARLAND, P., NOVIKOFF, A. B., AND HERMERMANN, D. Electron microscopy of the human synovial membrane. J. Cell Biol. 14:207–22, 1962.

BRIGHTON, C. T., SUGIOKA, Y., AND HUNT, R. M. Cytoplasmic structures of epiphyseal plate chondrocyte. J. Bone and Joint Surg. 55A:771–784, 1973.

CAMERON, D. A., PASCHALL, H. A., AND ROBINSON, R. A. Changes in the fine structure of bone cells after the administration of parathyroid extract. J. Cell Biol. 33:1–14, 1967.

CLARK, S. M., AND IBALL, J. The x-ray crystal analysis of bone. Progr. Biophys. 7:226–252, 1957.

CLARKE, I. C. Articular cartilage: a review and scanning electron microscope study. II. The territorial fibrillar architecture. J. Anat. 118:261–280, 1974.

CRELIN, E. S., AND KOCH, W. E. An autoradiographic study of chondrocyte transformation into chondroclasts and osteocytes during bone formation *in vitro.* Anat. Rec. 158:473–483, 1967.

DAVIES, D. V. The structure and functions of the synovial membrane. Br. Med. J. 1:92–95, 1950.

DUDLEY, H. R., AND SPIRO, D. The fine structure of bone cells. J. Biophys. Biochem. Cytol. 11:627–649, 1961.

GLIMCHER, M. J. The role of the macromolecular aggregation state and reactivity of collagen in calcification. *In* Macromolecular Complexes (Edds, M. V., Jr., editor), pp. 53–84. Ronald Press, New York, 1961.

GODMAN, G. C., AND LANE, N. On the site of sulfation in the chondrocyte. J. Cell Biol. 21:353–366, 1964.

GODMAN, G. C., AND PORTER, K. R. Chondrogenesis, studied with the electron microscope. J. Biophys. Biochem. Cytol. 8:719–760, 1960.

GOMORI, G. Calcification and phosphatase. Am. J. Pathol. 19:197–210, 1943.

HAM, A. W., AND HARRIS, W. R. Repair and transplantation of bone. *In* The Biochemistry and Physiology of Bone (Bourne, G. H., editor), vol. III, pp. 338–397. Academic Press, New York, 1972.

HELLER, M., McLEAN, F. C., AND BLOOM, W. Cellular transformations in mammalian bones induced by parathyroid extract. Am. J. Anat. 87:315–348, 1950.

HOLMGREN, H. Normal morphology of the joint fluid. Acta Orthop. Scand. 20:97–104, 1950.

HOLTROP, M. E. The ultrastructure of the epiphyseal plate. II. The hypertrophic chondrocyte. Calcified Tissue Res. 9:140–151, 1972.

INGALLS, T. H. Epiphyseal growth: normal sequence of events at epiphyseal plate. Endocrinology 29:710–720, 1941.

KIRBY-SMITH, H. T. Bone growth studies—a miniature bone fracture observed microscopically in a transparent chamber introduced into the rabbit's ear. Am. J. Anat., 53:377–402, 1933.

LACROIX, P. Bone and cartilage. *In* The Cell; Biochemistry, Physiology, Morphology (Brachet, J., and Mirsky, A. E., editors), vol. 5, pp. 219–266. Academic Press, New York, 1961.

LEBLOND, C. P., AND WEINSTOCK, M. Radioautographic studies of bone formation. *In* The Biochemistry and Physiology of Bone (Bourne, G. H., editor), vol. III, pp. 181–198. Academic Press, New York, 1972.

MATUKAS, V. J., PANNER, B. G., AND ORBISON, J. L. Studies of ultrastructural identification and distribution of protein-polysaccharide in cartilage matrix. J. Cell Biol. 32:365–375, 1967.

McLEAN, F. C., AND BLOOM, W. Calcification and ossification. Calcification in normal growing bone. Anat. Rec. 78:333–359, 1940.

McLEAN, F. C., AND URIST, M. R. Bone: Fundamentals of the Physiology of Skeletal Tissue, ed. 3. University of Chicago Press, Chicago, 1968.

MEYER, K. The mucopolysaccharides of bone. *In* Ciba Foundation symposium on Bone Structure and Metabolism (Wolstenholme, G. E. W., and O'Connor,

M., editors). Little, Brown & Company, Boston, 1956.

Moss, M. L. (editor). Comparative biology of calcified tissue. Ann. N. Y. Acad. Sci. 109, 1963.

Nogami, H., and Urist, M. R. Substrata prepared from bone matrix for chondrogenesis in tissue culture. J. Cell Biol. 62:510–519, 1974.

Park, E. A. Observations on the pathology of rickets with particular reference to the changes at the cartilage-shaft junctions of the growing bones. Harvey Lect. 34:157–213, 1939.

Peacock, A. Observations on the postnatal structure of the intervertebral disc in man. J. Anat. 86:162–179, 1952.

Pelec, S. R., and Glucksmann, A. Sulphate metabolism in the cartilage of the trachea, pinna and xiphoid process of the adult mouse as indicated by autoradiographs. Exp. Cell Res. 8:336–344, 1955.

Petersen, H. Die Organe des Skelet-systems. Handb. mikr. Anat., Menschen (v. Möllendorff, editor), 2, (part 2):521–676, Springer-Verlag, Berlin, 1930.

Porter, K. R. Cell fine structure and biosynthesis of intercellular macromolecules. In The New York Heart Association Symposium on Connective Tissue. Biophys. J. 4, 1964.

Pritchard, J. J. General anatomy and histology of bone. In The Biochemistry and Physiology of Bone (Bourne, G. H., editor), pp. 1–25. Academic Press, New York, 1956.

Ramagen, W. The bone cell system; form and function. (a review). Beit. Pathol. 150;1–10, 1973

Rasmussen, H., and Bordier, P. The Physiological and Cellular Basis of Metabolic Bone Disease. Williams & Wilkins, Baltimore, 1974.

Revel, J. P., and Hay, E. D. An autoradiographic and electron microscopic study of collagen synthesis in differentiating cartilage. Z. Zellforsch. 61:110–144, 1963.

Robinson, R. A., and Watson, M. L. Crystal-collagen relationships in bone as observed in the electron microscope. Ann. N. Y. Acad. Sci. 60:596–628, 1955.

Salomon, C. D. A fine structural study on the extracellular activity of alkaline phosphatase and its role in calcification. Calcified Tissue Res. 15:201–212, 1974.

Sognnaes, R. F. (editor). Calcification in Biological Systems. A. A. A. S. Publ. No. 64, Washington, D. C., 1960.

Trueta, J. The dynamics of bone circulation. In Bone Biodynamics (Frost, H. M., editor), pp. 245–258. Little, Brown & Company, Boston, 1963.

Weniger, J. M., and Holtrop, M. E. An ultrastructural study of bone cells: the occurrence of microtubules, microfilaments and tight junctions. Calcified Tissue Res. 14:15–29, 1974.

Yeager, J. A., and Kraucunas, E. Fine structure of the resorptive cells in the teeth of frogs. Anat. Rec. 164:1–13, 1969.

Young, R. W. Cell proliferation and specialization during endochondral osteogenesis in young rats. J. Cell Biol. 14:357–370, 1962.

CHAPTER 7

Blood and Lymph

During embryonic development, certain areas of the mesenchymal tissues cavitate and become lined by endothelial cells (see chapter 3). These cavitations coalesce, eventually forming a complex tubular network of vascular passageways—the circulatory system. The endothelial lining of this network is a continuous one, serving not only the venous and arterial vessels but also the lymphatic channels and the chambers of the heart. Within the network the blood and lymph circulate, but it should be realized that the fluids of both blood and lymph also circulate through the connective tissues as interstitial fluid. Basically, fluid components of the blood leak out of certain vascular passages (the capillaries and venules) to supply the interstitial fluid. It is recirculated to the blood via uptake into venules and lymphatic channels. The detailed structure of vascular and lymphatic channels is discussed in chapter 12.

Blood may be considered as a specialized connective tissue consisting of free cells (corpuscles) and a fluid intercellular substance (plasma). Both genetically and structurally, blood is related to the connective tissues. The blood cells develop in the reticular connective tissues of blood-forming organs and enter the bloodstream in a fully formed condition. Although functioning erythrocytes are limited to the bloodstream, the white or colorless corpuscles function in the loose connective tissues and

use the bloodstream merely as a vehicle of transportation.

Because the structural components of mammalian blood are not all true cells, they are sometimes designated as the *formed elements*. They include the red corpuscles (*erythrocytes*), the white blood cells (*leukocytes*), and the *blood platelets* (*thrombocytes*). The total quantity of blood (formed elements and plasma) forms about 8% of the body weight. There are some 5 or 6 liters of blood in a man weighing 150 pounds.

Blood may be studied under the microscope in the living animal in such places as the mesentery and the web of the frog's foot. When small vessels are selected, the blood flow is sufficiently slow to enable one to distinguish the individual corpuscles floating in clear plasma. More detailed observations on living blood cells can be made by placing a fresh drop of blood on a slide beneath a coverslip for studies with the oil immersion objective. By adding relatively nontoxic dyes such as neutral red to a drop of blood, i.e., by the use of supravital staining, one can readily study the reactions of the living cells.

In most of the methods commonly used in clinical work, the blood cells are observed in the nonliving state because they are exposed to special techniques for providing particular kinds of information. Thus, to determine what percentage of total blood consists of formed elements, one centrifuges the blood in a graduated tube—the percentage of formed elements is known as the *hematocrit.*

To determine the number of erythrocytes per cubic millimeter of blood, one uses a special pipette to dilute a known quantity of blood by a known amount of isotonic fluid, and a drop of the mixture is placed in the chamber of a *hemocytometer* slide. The bottom of the counting chamber is ruled in fine squares and is at a known depth beneath the cover slip. Because the cubic dimension of the space over each square is known, one can readily calculate the total number of erythrocytes per cubic millimeter from a count of the erythrocytes lying over a given number of ruled squares. This is known as the *total erythrocyte count,* and is of particular importance in studies of different types of anemia. The *total leukocyte count* is done by a similar method, although less dilution is needed for making the observations in the counting chamber because the leukocytes are not as concentrated in whole blood as are erythrocytes.

To determine the relative proportions of leukocytes, dried blood smears are stained with particular types of compound dyes (e.g., Wright's stain) to give good differentiation of neutrophilic, eosinophilic, and basophilic components of the cells. Details on this technique are given in the discussion of the morphology of the formed elements. The determination of different leukocyte percentages by this method is known as the *differential count.*

Blood Plasma

The plasma is a histologically homogeneous, slightly alkaline fluid. Chemically, it contains globulins, albumins, and inorganic salts, chiefly the chloride, bicarbonate, and phosphate of sodium. Calcium is present in a remarkably constant quantity (1 mg/10 cc of blood). The plasma constitutes 55% of the total quantity of blood and the formed elements constitute 45%; i.e., 45 is the hematocrit value for normal blood. The proportions are altered in a number of pathological conditions: e.g., in microcytic anemia there is a reduction in size and number of erythrocytes, which lowers the hematocrit value.

When blood is exposed to the air or when blood vessels are injured, one of the globulins of the plasma (*fibrinogen*) precipitates out as a network of delicate filaments, the *fibrin,* leaving a clear yellowish fluid, the *serum.* The blood cells become entangled in the fibrin network and a clot is formed. The clot acts as a plug, preventing further hemorrhage. A clot may, however, become of great danger to the individual if it is torn off by the bloodstream and circulates in the blood vessels (embolus), in which case it may block the blood supply of vital organs.

The plasma is the fundamental substance mediating all nutrition. In it are dissolved the nutritive substances derived from the alimentary canal, the waste substances from the tissues, and the secretions of the various endocrine glands. Even the oxygen which is bound by the red blood cells is first dissolved in the plasma before reaching the cells.

The plasma differs from the tissue fluids by the greater constancy of its constituents. The plasma proteins of the blood are seemingly not destined for nutritive purposes but remain as permanent constituents of the plasma. By experimental methods, it is possible to lower the protein content, but in a few days the normal amount is reestablished.

Red Blood Corpuscles (Erythrocytes)

The red blood corpuscles, or erythrocytes, are highly differentiated and specialized for the function of transporting oxygen. In the lower vertebrates, the erythrocyte is a nucleated cell, but in man and all other mammals it is unique in that it normally loses its nucleus, Golgi apparatus, centrioles, endoplasmic reticulum, and most of its mitochondria during the process of maturation before entering the bloodstream as a functional element. When fresh preparations of blood are examined under the microscope, it is seen that the individual red corpuscles have a greenish yellow color (Fig. 7-1C); en masse they give the red color characteristic of blood. In dried smears they are acidophilic and stain orange or pink in Wright's stain.

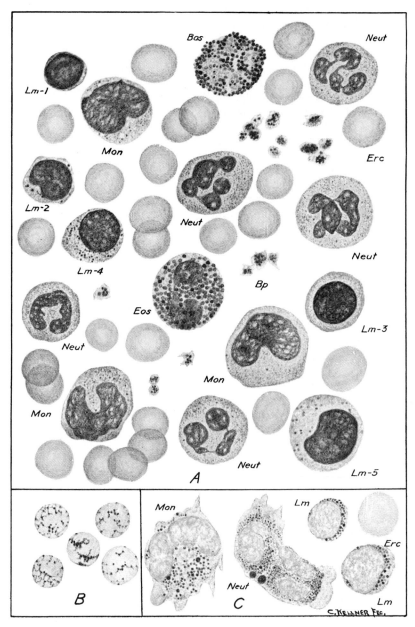

Fig. 7-1. *A*, cells from normal human blood. Wright's stain. *Bas,* basophilic leukocyte; *Bp,* aggregations of blood platelets; *Eos,* eosinophilic leukocyte; *Erc,* erythrocytes; *Lm-1 to 5,* lymphocytes: *1 to 3* are small and medium sizes and *4 and 5* are the less numerous larger forms; *Mon,* monocytes; *Neut,* neutrophilic leukocytes. *B*, reticulocytes from normal human blood stained with dilute cresyl blue. *C*, blood cells as seen after about 20 min of staining with neutral red and Janus green B in a supravital preparation. *Erc,* erythrocyte; *Lm,* small lymphocytes with bluish green mitochondria and a few neutral red granules; *Mon,* monocyte with mitochondria and numerous neutral red granules and vacuoles of varying size; *Neut,* neutrophilic leukocytes with staining of the neutrophilic granules and the formation of a few large vacuoles, which frequently appear after 15 to 20 min of staining. All figures ×1550.

The stains which are commonly used for blood cells consist of mixtures of acidic and basic dyes. The development of this procedure stems from the works of Ehrlich published over the period from 1879 to 1898. He added a solution of orange G (an acidic dye) to a solution of methyl green (a basic dye) until a precipitate was formed, and then he redissolved the precipitate in an excess of the acidic dye for use in staining. Orange G is a sodium salt and methyl green is a chloride. Ehrlich concluded that the mixing of solutions of orange G and methyl green gave sodium chloride plus a new compound, a "neutral" dye consisting of methyl green/orange G, with a dye in both halves of the molecule. He noted that the cytoplasmic granules of some leukocytes took the acidic component of the dye, whereas those of other leukocytes took the basic component, and those of a third group took both components of the neutral dye. Hence, he described the leukocytes as acidophilic, basophilic, and neutrophilic.

Ehrlich's results stimulated other investigators to try other acidic and basic dyes, and a major advance was made by Romanovsky (1891) when he used a mixture of methylene blue and eosin to demonstrate the nucleus of the malarial parasite, which had not been seen before. It soon became evident that this gave superior results for blood cells, and most of the stains currently used for blood smears are modifications of the Romanovsky stain. The best known modifications are those of Giemsa and Wright, the latter being widely employed in clinical work.

The basic dyes used in the preparation of Wright's stain are methylene blue and polychromed (oxidized) methylene blue consisting of methylene azure and methylene violet. When solutions of the basic dyes are added to a solution of the acidic dye eosin, a precipitate is formed. The precipitate is dissolved in acetone-free methyl alcohol and, in usage, the alcoholic solution is placed on the slide and water is added during the staining. The alcoholic solution fixes, or preserves, the cells, and the dilution by water permits dissociation of the dye for differential staining. The dye will eventually precipitate in water, but staining should be completed before this occurs.

In Wright's stained blood smears, the erythrocytes are usually colored buff or orange-pink with eosin, the nuclei of leukocytes are stained metachromatically with methylene azure, and the cytoplasm of lymphocytes and monocytes is stained blue with methylene blue. The cytoplasmic granules of basophils have an affinity for methylene blue and are metachromatic also, whereas the granules of eosinophils have an affinity for the acidic dye. The explanation for the staining of the neutrophilic granules is not understood as clearly. The cells originally received their name because it was thought that their granules stained with the neutral dye. In the case of Wright's stain, the neutral dye is an eosinate of methylene azure. It is likely that most of this is rapidly dissociated when the dye is diluted with water. The granules of the neutrophils in man usually show a lavender color after Wright's stain, probably from methylene azure and methylene violet.

The red corpuscles are biconcave discs. When observed on its flat surface, the corpuscle has a circular outline and the central depression appears as a lighter or darker area, depending on the focus.

Erythrocytes average about 7.7 μm in diameter and 1.9 μm in greatest thickness in dried smears. They are larger in the living state (about 8.6 μm) and smaller in sections (about 7 μm). Although slight variations in size are not uncommon, forms showing marked variations (1 to 2 μm above or below the normal diameter) are relatively rare in normal blood. Large erythrocytes are commonly found in some types of anemia (e.g., pernicious anemia) and are known as macrocytes or megalocytes. Small forms are characteristically present in some other types of anemia (e.g., iron deficiency anemia) and are known as microcytes.

The corpuscles readily change their shape, as may be seen when they squeeze through the narrowest capillaries or pass around the bend of a branching vessel. Another interesting physical characteristic is the tendency of the corpuscles to adhere to each other along their concave surfaces, thus forming rows or rouleaux like piled up coins (Fig. 7-2). Although the cause of this phenomenon is not entirely clear, it is usually explained as the result of surface tension. Rouleaux formation is a transient phenomenon which is not to be confused with "sludging" of erythrocytes. Sludging refers to a clumping of red corpuscles after severe trauma. As a result of burns of the skin and other types of trauma, there is a leakage of fluid from the blood vessels into the surrounding tissue. The trauma may also produce a generalized reaction, in that sludges may circulate and block small vessels in other parts of the body.

Chemically, the erythrocyte cytoplasm consists of a protein and lipoid colloidal

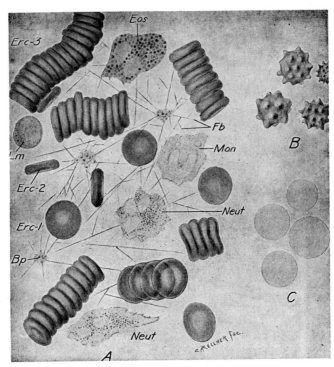

Fig. 7-2. *A*, drawings of human blood cells from a thick film, fresh preparation. (Compare with living cells in thin film preparation, Fig. 7-5.) *Bp*, blood platelets; *Eos*, eosinophil leukocyte; *Erc-1, 2,* and *3*, erythrocytes in surface view (*1*), in profile (*2*), and in rouleaux (*3*); *Fb*, strands of fibrin; *Lm*, small lymphocyte; *Mon*, monocyte; *Neut*, neutrophil leukocyte. *B*, crenation of erythrocytes after the addition of a few drops of 1.5% NaCl to a fresh preparation. *C*, erythrocytes assuming spheroidal shapes and undergoing hemolysis after the addition of a drop of distilled water to a fresh preparation. All figures ×1540.

complex, of which the most important element is *hemoglobin.* Hemoglobin has the remarkable property of binding oxygen in a very loose combination (*oxyhemoglobin*). The hemoglobin becomes saturated with oxygen in the capillaries of the lung, and the circulating blood distributes this oxygen to the cells of the body in exchange for carbonic acid which constantly accumulates as a waste product of metabolism in the tissues. Oxygen is not yielded directly by the corpuscle to the cells, but is first dissolved in the plasma at a level held constant by the erythrocytes.

The contents of the corpuscle are normally in osmotic equilibrium with the plasma; hence the plasma is said to be *isosmotic* or *isotonic.* Isotonic solutions may be prepared for study of the corpuscles outside the body; a 0.85% solution of sodium chloride is approximately isotonic for mammalian blood. When *hypertonic* solutions

are added to blood, the erythrocytes become shrunken and *crenated* (Fig. 7-2*B*). The membranes of the corpuscles are permeable to water and impermeable to sodium and potassium ions, and therefore water passes from the corpuscles to restore partially osmotic equilibrium between the corpuscles and the surrounding medium whenever the latter is hypertonic. A few crenated corpuscles are usually found in fresh preparations of blood studied without the addition of hypertonic solutions; this results from evaporation, which produces a slightly hypertonic solution and an altered pH. It should be added that crenation has also been produced experimentally in isotonic media and may not be entirely dependent on osmotic phenomena.

When blood is placed in distilled water or any *hypotonic* solution, water enters the corpuscles and they assume a spheroidal shape. The corpuscles lose their color by the escape of hemoglobin into the diluted plasma, and the colorless part which remains is known as the *stroma, "blood shadow,"* or *"ghost"* (Fig. 7-2C). Eventually, the shadows may also undergo solution. The process of extraction of hemoglobin is called *hemolysis,* and the substances which effect it are known as hemolysins or hemolytic agents. Hypotonic solutions are not the only substances which produce hemolysis. Of particular interest is the fact that the plasma of one species may hemolyze the erythrocytes of another and that, in man, the serum of certain individuals may produce hemolysis in others. Hemolysis is of interest in clinical work, because one of the types of anemia, *hemolytic anemia,* occurs when the erythrocytes within the body are hemolyzed at a rate which exceeds that of their formation.

Certain substances also bring about an *agglutination* or clumping of corpuscles. Agglutination may occur within the blood stream during certain pathological and experimental conditions and may thus produce a multiple thrombosis of the smaller vessels. Agglutinins present in the serum of some individuals may bring about an agglutination of erythrocytes in others; on this basis, individuals have been divided into several "blood groups." In giving blood transfusions, it is important to select donors from a blood group which is compatible with that of the recipient in order to avoid accidents which would result if the recipient's serum agglutinated the transfused donor cells.

The cytoplasm of the mature erythrocyte appears homogeneous in the fresh condition and is seen as an amorphous, moderately dense material in electron micrographs (Fig. 12-4). The plasmalemma is basically similar in structure and composition to that of other cells. In fact, membranes from red corpuscles served as a source of material for some of the earliest studies of cell membranes. Today the red cell membrane continues to provide important insight into the structure of membranes despite the realization that the organization of the erythrocyte membrane differs from that of conventional nucleated cells (see chapter 1).

A few of the erythrocytes of peripheral blood have a reticulated appearance when supravitally stained with cresyl blue (Fig. 7-1B). They are known as *reticulocytes* or *reticulated erythrocytes.* They are the youngest erythrocytes in the circulating blood, and their reticulated appearance is apparently produced by a clumping of ribosomes by the supravital dye. Electron micrographs of reticulocytes show scattered groups of ribosomes (polysomes) and occasional mitochondria. These cells apparently correspond to the slightly polychromatophilic erythrocytes seen in Wright's stained smears.

The erythrocytes are much more numerous than any of the other formed elements. The average is about 5,000,000/mm^3 of blood in normal adult males (4,500,000 in females), with normal variations ranging from 4,000,000 to 6,000,000. Normal variations occur within the same individual in association with physiological changes, e.g., the increase after exercise. Many of these variations apparently represent a redistribution to the peripheral vessels rather than an actual change in total numbers. Life in high altitudes is accompanied by an increase to about 8,000,000. Whereas the initial change in this case may be a redistribution through an outpouring of red cells from the spleen (chapter 13), there is also a real increase in total numbers in response to the lower oxygen tension. More pronounced variations occur under pathological conditions.

The surface area of a red corpuscle has been given as 128 μm^2. From this, one may calculate that the total surface area of 5,000,000 corpuscles in 1 mm^3 of blood is 640 mm^2 and that in 6 liters of blood the total area available for respiratory function is 3840 m^2. This enormous area suggests the importance and the rapidity of the exchange phenomena between the corpuscles on the one hand and the plasma and air on the other.

Under pathological conditions, not only the number but the size, shape, and hemoglobin content of the corpuscles may vary strikingly. The normal number may be present, but the amount of hemoglobin is reduced, as in some of the *secondary* (chlorotic) anemias. In the *macrocytic anemias,* e.g., pernicious anemia, which results from a deficiency of an erythrocyte maturation factor, vitamin B_{12}, the red cells are reduced in number but are abnormally large, and some cells have an increased content of hemoglobin. In *microcytic anemia,* e.g., iron deficiency anemia, there is a decrease both in the number and in the size of the cells. Under most of these conditions, the cells may show a multiplicity of distortions in shape (poikilocytosis).

White Blood Corpuscles (Leukocytes)

The white blood cells contain no hemoglobin and differ from the red corpuscles in many other important respects. They possess a nucleus and hence are true cells, and they have the power of active ameboid movement, which aids in their passage through the walls of blood vessels and enables them to travel within the connective tissues. They are much less numerous than the red cells, the proportion being about one white cell to 600 red cells, or about 8000/mm³ of blood, with a normal variation from 6,000 to 10,000. Under pathological conditions, the number may be greatly increased (leukocytosis); more rarely there is a reduction in number (leukopenia). At birth the leukocytes are more numerous (15,000 to 18,000/mm³).

The leukocytes, unlike the erythrocytes, perform their functions in the connective tissues. They arise, function, and die outside the bloodstream, which is to them merely a means of transportation from their place of origin to their destination in the connective tissues.

The white blood cells are more or less rounded in shape in fresh preparations and in sections of routinely fixed material. The diameters of the leukocytes in sections of fixed tissue are less than those seen in fresh preparations as a result of shrinkage produced by the technique. On the other hand, the diameters of cells in Wright's stained dried smears are even greater than those seen in fresh preparations because the flattening of the cells more than compensates for the shrinkage caused by the fixation and dehydration. Thus, it is obvious that one is justified in comparing the diameter of one cell type with that of another only when both types are studied by the same method. The diameters given in the following descriptions refer to cells seen in dried smears unless stated otherwise.

The white blood cells may be subdivided into nongranular forms (*agranulocytes*) and granular leukocytes (*granulocytes*). The cytoplasm of the granulocytes is characterized by numerous granules which may be seen in living cells and in fixed and stained preparations. The cytoplasm of some of the agranulocytes contains a few granules which are azurophilic in Wright's stained dry smears, but these are not specific for a particular type of cell, as are the neutrophilic, eosinophilic, and basophilic granules of the cells that are classified as granular leukocytes. Electron microscopic cytochemistry shows that the azurophilic granules are primary lysosomes.

Types of Nongranular Leukocytes (Agranulocytes)

The nongranular leukocytes include the *lymphocytes,* which are mostly small cells about the size of erythrocytes, and a group of larger cells, *monocytes,* which have more cytoplasm and a more indented nucleus. The nongranular leukocytes are comparatively undifferentiated and can reproduce by mitosis. Such division does not usually occur in the bloodstream but rather in the connective tissues and blood-forming organs.

Lymphocytes. The lymphocytes of the normal circulation vary from 6 to 10 μm or more, with the majority being about 7 to 8 μm. They normally constitute about 20 to 25% of the white blood cells (Table 7-1). There is a considerable range for normal individuals, and it is not uncommon to find lymphocyte counts as high as 35 or even

TABLE 7-1
Leukocytes

Type	Size (μm)	% of leuko-cytes
Lymphocytes	6–10	20–45
Monocytes	12–20	3–8
Granulocytes		
Neutrophils	9–12	50–75
Eosinophils	10–14	2–4
Basophils	8–10	0.5–1

45%. They have a relatively large, spherical nucleus which may have a slight indentation on one side. The densely packed chromatin stains intensely. The *nuclei* have a purplish blue color in many Wright's stained preparations (Fig. 7-1). It is important to realize that the nuclear color varies with different batches of Wright's stain and with variations in technical procedures. It is regularly more on the reddish side in immature lymphocytes of blood formation (Fig. 7-14*B*).

The *cytoplasm* of lymphocytes is very basophilic and is a greenish blue in Wright's stain. It varies in amount according to variations in cell size (Fig. 7-1*A*). It is usually homogeneous but may be slightly more basophilic at the border of the cell and paler adjacent to the nucleus. Electron micrographs show an abundance of free ribosomes (Fig. 7-3), relatively few mitochondria, and a rather small Golgi complex. The ribosomes occur throughout the cytoplasm unassociated with the endoplasmic reticulum; in fact, the endoplasmic reticulum is very sparse in the lymphocyte of the circulating blood (Fig. 7-3).

Purplish azurophilic granules are occasionally seen in lymphocytes in Wright's stained dry smears, but they are not specific because they are also found in monocytes and in granular leukocytes. The number of lymphocytes containing these granules varies at different times and in different individuals. A few of the lymphocytes found in blood smears may be as large as 10 to 12

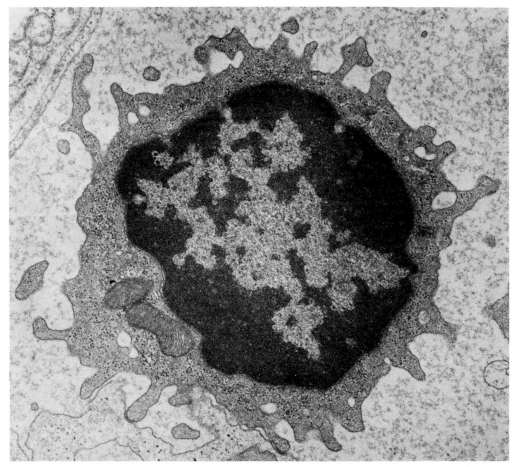

Fig. 7-3. Electron micrograph of a section of a human lymphocyte. Note the numerous free ribosomes, the lack of endoplasmic reticulum, and the condensed nuclear chromatin. Courtesy of Dr. June Marshall. ×25,500.

μm. Most of these resemble the small lymphocytes except for size. However, a few of the large cells have a large nucleus and a cytoplasm which stains readily with the red basic dye pyronin in a manner similar to that described for plasma cells (chapter 5). Some of these cells may be partially differentiated precursors of plasma cells and some may belong to special categories of recirculating cells described below. They are not to be confused with the large lymphoblasts found in blood and blood-forming organs during certain pathological states, e.g., lymphatic leukemia (Fig. 7-14*B*). The latter differ from the normal cells in appearance and function.

When lymphocytes are studied in supravital preparations kept at body temperatures, they are generally stationary for a short time, but after 15 or 20 min they occasionally move in a manner which differs from that of the other leukocytes. They elongate by sending out a blunt pseudopod and advance by a sort of wormlike motion with the nucleus usually in front (Fig. 7-5). In supravital preparations stained with dilute solutions of neutral red and Janus green B, the mitochondria (stained bluish green by the Janus green B) are in the form of granules and rods (Fig. 7-1*C*). Most of the lymphocytes also show a few neutral red granules (probably the azurophilic granules of Wright's stained preparations).

In the description of connective tissue cells (chapter 5), it is noted that plasma cells, the principal producers of circulating antibodies, are derived from lymphocytes. The substances which stimulate the formation of antibodies (*immunoglobulins*) by plasma cells are high molecular weight proteins and carbohydrates known as *antigens*. Although the body accepts new proteins formed during embryonic and fetal life as a part of itself, it develops the ability soon after birth to distinguish new proteins as nonself, or antigens. Some lymphocytes acquire the ability to react against extracellular antigens (exotoxins) produced by bacterial infection. They migrate into lymphatic organs and into the loose connective tissues of particular regions, where they differentiate into plasma cells which in turn secrete antibodies that enter the bloodstream to counteract the toxins; this is known as a *humoral antibody response.* Other lymphocytes reject foreign grafts and react against numerous viral and fungal infections; this is done by a localized cytotoxic response by lymphocytes that have emigrated from the blood vessels, which is known as *cell-mediated immunity.* The lymphocytes which perform these different functions appear to be a homogenous population in light micrographs, but they can be divided into at least two categories by the study of transfused cells identifiable either from isotope labeling or from chromosomal characteristics.

The lymphocytes which function in graft rejection and other types of cell-mediated immunity probably arise embryonically from the yolk sac and seed the thymus by way of the liver and the bone marrow. In the thymus, these lymphocytes multiply and differentiate into *T* (thymus-dependent) *lymphocytes.* In mice, the T lymphocytes have a surface marker known as theta antigen, identifiable by special techniques, but as yet such a marker has not been identified in humans. There is some evidence that in the adult there is a continual reseeding of the thymus with stem cells of bone marrow origin.

The lymphocytes which function as precursors for plasma cells are termed *B lymphocytes* because it was found that, in birds, they develop from a derivative of the cloaca known as the bursa of Fabricius. The bursa apparently provides a special environment for the development for this class of lymphocytes, which is endowed with the ability to differentiate into plasma cells. Mammals lack a bursa of Fabricius, and the exact site of formation of B lymphocytes is controversial. As with T lymphocytes, there is some evidence that, in the adult, a stem cell of bone marrow origin may settle in gut-associated lymphatic tissues, or in particular regions of the lymphatic organs (chapter 13), or in bone marrow itself, and continue to proliferate B lymphocytes. The important point is that the B lymphocyte is not proliferated in the thymus. The T and B lymphocytes cannot be distinguished reliably by their morphological characteristics. Early studies reporting characteristic surface features visible in scanning electron micrographs have not been confirmed.

The recognition of an antigen by a lymphocyte is dependent on the arrangement of the amino acids in its surface membrane. Very slight differences in amino acid sequences are sufficient for recognition or nonrecognition of any given antigen. There are so many different combinations in the gene sequence that at least a few lymphocytes are coded with receptors for every conceivable antigen to which an individual could be exposed in a lifetime. When an individual is exposed to a new antigen, the lymphocytes with the specific receptor respond by multiplication and differentiation. At the first response, there are relatively few cells coded for the particular antigen. Only a few cells at a time leave the vessels to differentiate into antibody-forming plasma cells, and the response is relatively slow; this is known as the *primary response*. Some of the newly formed B cells remain in the circulation as *memory cells*. When the individual is reexposed to the same antigen, there are more cells available and a more rapid response occurs; this is known as the *secondary response*. Repeated injections of small amounts of a toxin are sometimes given to induce an *acquired immunity*. Injections of toxoids, i.e., toxins treated in a manner which destroys their toxic properties while retaining antigenicity, are used to provide *active immunity*.

A reaction against an antigen that stimulates the formation of antibodies by plasma cells involves the collaboration of several types of cells. Bacteria that gain entrance to the body are phagocytosed by neutrophilic leukocytes that die in the process. The dead neutrophils are phagocytosed in turn by macrophages which ingest foreign materials indiscriminately. When a T lymphocyte makes contact with a macrophage it aids in transferring the antigen from the macrophage to a B cell specifically coded for the particular antigen. The T cells of this type are known as "helper" cells; T cells also survive for a long period as memory cells. The B cells generally depend on the collaboration of T cells for differentiation into plasma cells. In further reference to collaboration, it may be noted that eosinophilic leukocytes eventually destroy antigen-antibody complexes.

The exact manner in which T cells function in foreign graft rejection is not fully understood. The cells surround the graft and destroy it but they do not differentiate into plasma cells. They do not react against grafts made from one location to another in the same individual, *autografts,* or against transplants between monozygotic identical twins, *isografts.* They react against grafts between individuals of the same species, *homografts (allografts),* and they give a strong reaction against grafts between animals of different species (*heterografts*).

The T cells form numerous pharmacological agents known as *lymphokines,* that affect cell-mediated immunity. The lymphokines include a macrophage migration-inhibiting factor (MIF), a macrophage aggregating factor (MAF), chemotactic factors (CF), and numerous others.

Antibodies are plasma proteins which belong to a family known as immunoglobulins (Ig). Each molecule is composed of four polypeptide chains which are arranged in pairs with one member of each pair longer than the other, hence they are known as heavy and light chains. The two pairs are joined by several disulfide bridges. The amino acid sequence is constant in the major portion of each chain but variable in the terminal fragment (Fab), which functions in antigen binding. On the basis of differences in the variable portion of the heavy chain, the immunoglobulins are divided into five classes, namely, mu, gamma, alpha, delta, and epsilon (*IgM, IgG, IgA, IgD,* and *IgE*). Experimental studies on mice and other mammals have shown that some of the lymphocytes begin to synthesize IgM during the latter part of fetal life. IgG appears at about the time of birth and can apparently form in the same cells that were previously synthesizing IgM. The IgG-producing cell can apparently also switch to IgA production. The function of IgD is not well documented, but recent studies indicate that it appears in B cells almost as early as IgM does and that the two may be located in the same cell. IgD is scarce in blood serum but present in most B cells that are stimulated by antigens. It has been proposed that proteolysis of IgD is a step in the triggering process for antibody formation. IgE is a reaginic antibody and also functions in allergic reactions. The functional interrelationships of the cells involved in antibody formation is a subject of active research which will undoubtedly lead to a better understanding of Ig formation by the cells.

A high percentage of the lymphocytes present in the bloodstream are recirculating cells. Regardless of whether they initially develop in marrow and circulate by blood vessels to the lymphatic organs or whether they arise by proliferation in the lymphatic organs, they enter (or reenter) the bloodstream via the entrance of the thoracic duct into the subclavian vein and recirculate. They pass through the heart and arteries to the lymphatic organs, where they squeeze between the endothelial cells of postcapillary venules to enter the reticular tissue of the lymphatic organs, commonly referred to as parenchyma.* Although some of the cells proliferate in the lymphatic organs and some differentiate into plasma cells, the majority return to the systemic circulation by way of the efferent lymphatic channels and the thoracic duct.

Because the total number of lymphocytes entering and leaving the bloodstream every 24 hr is several times the number present in the circulation, lymphocytes must enter and leave at an equivalent rate to maintain their approximately constant percentage in normal blood. Studies of transfused labeled cells in mice indicate that approximately 85% of the recirculating cells belong to the T type and that only about 15% are of the B type. A high percentage of the recirculating lymphocytes are long-lived and survive for many months in rodents and for many years in humans. It is thought that the long-lived lymphocytes (both B and T) are the memory cells.

*The term *parenchyma* as applied to animal tissues carries two definitions. The traditional histological definition denotes parenchyma as the functional, cellular component of an organ. Embryologically, the "parenchyma" of an organ is that functional part derived from epithelium. In this context, *parenchyma* is in contrast to *stroma,* which is the mesenchymally derived component of an organ. Both definitions apply well to such organs as glands. The embryological definition, however, is not applicable to such organs as lymph nodes, spleen, and bone marrow, which are totally of mesenchymal origin. In this text, the term parenchyma is avoided in discussing such organs.

Because lymphocytes have a major role in cell-mediated immunity, it is not surprising that they are abundant in connective tissues beneath the epithelial lining of the digestive and respiratory systems. For example, they are aggregated in the Waldeyer's ring of faucial, lingual, and pharyngeal tonsils, in the Peyer's patches of the ileum, and in solitary nodules of other segments of the digestive and respiratory systems. They apparently add to the total body pool of lymphocytes by multiplication in these locations, and they are also strategically situated for their functions.

Monocytes, or Large Mononuclear Leukocytes. Monocytes are large cells which constitute from 3 to 8% of the leukocytes. In dry smears, they usually vary from 12 to 15 μm in diameter, but when extremely flattened and stretched they may reach 20 μm. In supravital preparations, their diameter varies with the activity of the cell. The active monocytes send out numerous pseudopodia and naturally appear larger than the more rounded, inactive forms. The active cells are especially large when flattened in thin film preparations.

The monocyte nucleus is ovoid, kidney- or horseshoe-shaped, very rarely spherical, and usually eccentrically placed (Fig. 7-1). Its chromatin network is finer and stains less densely than that of the lymphocytes. Nucleoli are not obvious within the monocytes in blood smears but are shown in electron micrographs. The cytoplasm is abundant and has a somewhat reticulated or vacuolated appearance; it is slightly less basophilic than the lymphocyte cytoplasm and is more of a grayish blue after Wright's stain. A Golgi apparatus in the cytoplasm near the indentation of the nucleus can be seen by light microscopy after special techniques. There are also some fine azurophilic cytoplasmic granules that are near the limits of resolution of the light microscope.

Electron micrographs (Fig. 7-4) show more rough-surfaced endoplasmic reticulum in monocytes than in lymphocytes but fewer free ribosomes. There are also numerous microfilaments that are associated with cell motility. By a combination of electron microscopy and cytochemistry, it is found that there are membrane-bounded granules that give a positive peroxidase re-

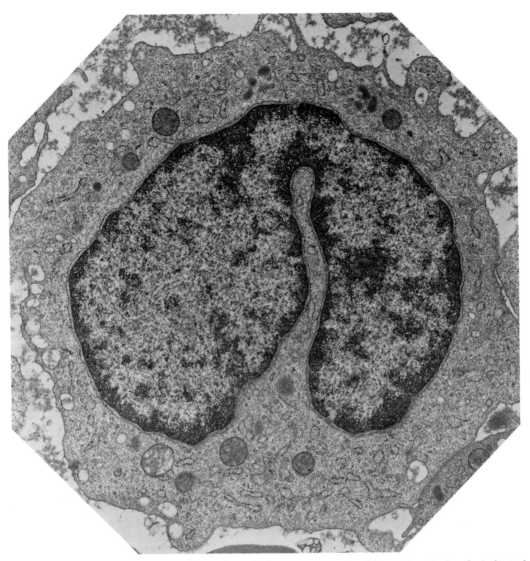

Fig. 7-4. Electron micrograph of a section of a human monocyte. The nucleus is deeply indented and the cytoplasm contains endoplasmic reticulum, vacuoles, and a few small membrane-bounded granules (azurophilic granules). Courtesy of Dr. June Marshall. ×18,000.

action; they are the azurophilic granules of light microscopy and they function as primary lysosomes after the monocytes migrate into the connective tissue. The monocytes do not form any new azurophilic granules after migrating into the connective tissue. However, some additional granules that are peroxidase-negative have been demonstrated by cytochemistry and electron microscopy.

In supravital preparations treated with neutral red and Janus green B, the azurophilic granules are colored by neutral red, and vacuoles of neutral red form by phagocytosis. The vacuoles are often arranged as a rosette around the region containing the cell center, and they increase in size as the supravital staining is continued. Mitochondria are stained bluish green and are usually more numerous around the rim of the rosette than in other parts of the cytoplasm (Fig. 7-1C). Large monocytes are more active than small ones, but none of them travel about rapidly like the neutrophils and eosinophils. The monocytes also exhibit a different type of activity. They continually extend and withdraw pseudopodia and assume an appearance somewhat like an octopus (Fig. 7-5D). The pseudopodia are of different shapes, ranging from threadlike processes to broad membranes, and are very transparent.

In tissue cultures, the monocytes, or promonocytes, can enlarge and take on all of the characteristics of typical *macrophages*. In the body, they migrate readily through the capillary walls into the connective tissues, where they display their phagocytic characteristics. They provide the mobilized macrophages found in areas of focal infection (e.g., abscess, Fig. 5-3). The monocytes also function as the chief cells in combating the bacillus of tuberculosis.

Types of Granular Leukocytes (Granulocytes)

The granular leukocytes are characterized by the presence of specific types of granules in their cytoplasm, and according to the nature of this granulation, they have been subdivided into three groups: the *neutrophilic, eosinophilic,* and *basophilic* leukocytes. They are further characterized by the presence of a many-lobed (polymorphous) nucleus; hence they are called *polymorphonuclear* leukocytes. The lobes of chromatin are connected by very delicate chromatic strands. Occasionally, some of these strands are broken in dry smear preparations, so a few cells may appear to be polynuclear. The granulocytes also differ from the nongranular leukocytes in that they are more highly differentiated and cannot reproduce by mitosis.

Neutrophils. The neutrophilic polymorphonuclear leukocytes (Figs. 7-1 and 7-2) vary in size from 9 to 12 μm in blood smears and are the most numerous of white blood cells. Although they usually constitute about 60 to 70% of the total white blood cells, they have been found to range from 50 to 75% in normal individuals. Under pathological conditions, the range is much

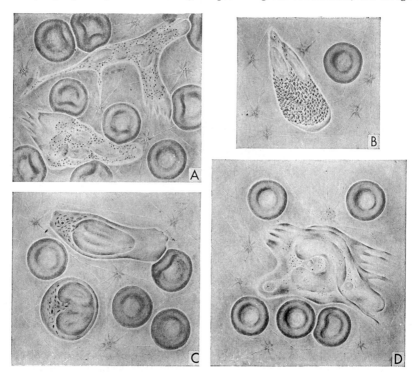

Fig. 7-5. Drawings of living human blood cells from a thin film preparation. *A*, polymorphonuclear neutrophils pushing their way between the red blood cells and the delicate fibrin network extending out from the small platelet masses; *B*, polymorphonuclear eosinophil; *C*, lymphocytes, the round resting stage and the elongated motile stage; *D*, monocyte with pseudopodia in the form of delicate undulating membranes. (Courtesy of Dr. C. M. Goss).

greater. The polymorphic nucleus shows a variety of forms, usually consisting of three to five sausage-shaped masses of chromatin connected by fine threads and arranged in the form of an S or a horseshoe. In blood smears from human females, one can see a small appendage attached to the remainder of the nucleus by a narrow filament, giving a drumstick appearance in almost 3% of the neutrophils (Fig. 7-6). The drumstick is the heterochromatin of one of the two X chromosomes of the female (page 21). It is presumably present in all of the cells in females, but it is closely packed with one of the lobes of the nucleus in most cells and is obscured. Some of the neutrophils of males have hook-shaped and nodule-like appendages, but they generally do not have the drumstick forms.

The cytoplasm is filled with fine granules which are neutrophilic. In some animals, e.g., rabbit and guinea pig, the granules take the acid stain and may be called *pseudoeosinophils*. Because these cells vary in their staining reactions in different species,

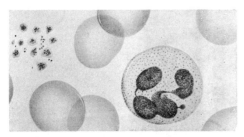

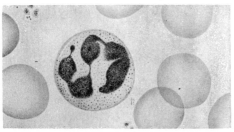

Fig. 7-6. Portions of two oil immersion fields of a Wright's stained blood smear from a human female. Fields have been selected to show the drumstick appearance of the sex chromatin which is seen in a number of the neutrophilic leukocytes in the female. It is seen as a hanging drop of chromatin attached by a thin strand to one of the lobes of the nucleus. A relatively large cluster of blood platelets is seen in the *upper left corner* of the figure. ×1335. (From a preparation made by Miss Karen Fu.)

they are sometimes called *heterophils* rather than neutrophils.

In addition to the neutrophilic granules, there are other granules that have a reddish purple or azure color in Wright's stained smears. The existence of two types of granules has been confirmed by electron microscopy and by biochemical assays of particles separated by differential centrifugation. In many animals there are relatively large electron-dense granules (Figs. 7-7 and 7-8) that correspond to the azurophilic granules of light microscopy and that develop only during the promyelocyte stage of cell differentiation; they are classified as *azurophilic* or *primary granules*. They contain myeloperoxidase and hydrolyases that are characteristic of lysosomes. Another group of granules that are smaller and less electron-dense have a pink color in Wright's stained smears and develop only in the myelocyte stage of leukocyte development; they are known as *neutrophilic* (secondary or specific) granules. They compose about 80% of the granules of the mature neutrophil and contain alkaline phosphatase and some antibacterial constituents but little or no hydrolase. Both types of granules are membrane bounded and both have intracellular functions described below. The mature human neutrophil contains both types of granules, but they cannot be readily distinguished by morphological criteria alone. However, the azurophilic granules contain myeloperoxidase and acid phosphatase and the specific granules contain alkaline phosphatase. These enzymes can be localized by histochemical methods and their presence provides positive identification of the granules.

In differential counts, the neutrophils are sometimes subdivided on the basis of nuclear differentiation. A commonly used classification proposed by Schilling divides the neutrophils into segmented nuclears, about 57% of the total leukocytes, and nonsegmented nuclears, about 4%. The latter group is subdivided into cells with the nuclei either shaped like bands or irregular, shaped like stab wounds, about 3%; juveniles or metamyelocytes with indented or kidney-shaped nuclei, 0 to 1%; and myelocytes, 0%. An increase in relative numbers of nonsegmented nuclears is known as a "shift to the left," whereas an increase in

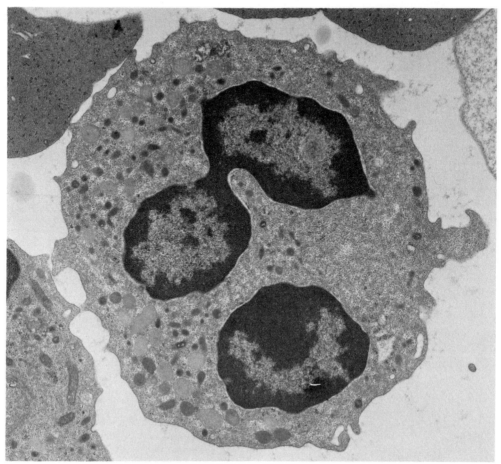

Fig. 7-7. Electron micrograph of a section of a human neutrophil. Three nuclear lobes are obvious. The cytoplasm contains granules of different sizes and densities, mitochondria, free ribosomes, and some strands of endoplasmic reticulum. Some of the granules are probably azurophilic granules, but their positive identification would require histochemical procedures (see text). Courtesy of Dr. June Marshall. ×15,400.

segmented types is known as a "shift to the right." The latter is considered a good sign because it usually indicates that there is no longer any unusual demand on the bone marrow for younger cells.

In supravital preparations, the neutrophilic leukocyte is more active than any other blood cell. It advances by an ameboid movement, usually with the nucleus in the rear. At times, it is difficult to see the strands connecting the nuclear lobes, and the cells may appear to be polynuclear instead of polymorphonuclear. In supravital preparations, the cytoplasmic granules become colored by the neutral red within a few minutes (Fig. 7-1C). After 15 or 20 min, some of the neutrophils form phagocytic

vacuoles of neutral red that occasionally become as large as one of the nuclear lobes. A few small mitochondria stain with Janus green B.

After migration from the bloodstream, the neutrophils phagocytose bacteria and other small particles. They have been called the *microphages,* in contrast with the macrophages, which are larger cells that characteristically engulf larger particles. They are chemotactically attracted by devitalized tissue, bacteria, and other foreign bodies, and they migrate to the site of an infection. They engulf bacteria by endocytosis and form phagosomes. Then the membranes of the azurophilic and neutrophilic granules fuse with the membranes of the

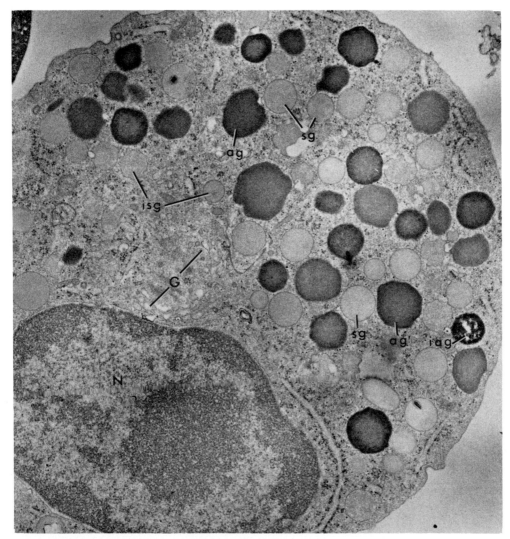

Fig. 7-8. Electron micrograph of a section of a neutrophilic myelocyte from rabbit bone marrow. The tissue was reacted for the enzyme peroxidase during the technical procedure. Note that the reaction product is present in the azurophilic granules (*ag*) but not in the specific granules (*sg*). The reaction product is distributed uniformly throughout most of the mature azurophilic granules, but it is present in flocculent form in an immature azurophilic granule (*iag*) seen at the *right*. Several small and immature specific granules (*isg*) are seen in the vicinity of the Golgi complex (*G*). The nucleus (*N*) is not lobed at this stage. ×18,000. (Courtesy of Drs. D. F. Bainton and M. G. Farquhar: J. Cell Biol. 39, 1968).

phagosomes, thus forming secondary lysosomes. The neutrophilic granules contribute their alkaline phosphatase and antibacterial phagocytin about 3 to 4 min before the azurophilic granules empty. This sequential discharge correlates with the development of a lower pH in the phagosomes by the time the azurophilic granules contribute their peroxidase and lysosomal enzymes which function at a lower pH. These enzymes completely destroy the bacteria, and eventually the neutrophils die in the process and become the pus corpuscles of an abscess. Although the neutrophils serve as the shock troops or as the first line of defense against invading organisms, they are not equally effective against all types of bacteria. For example, they cannot successfully combat tubercle bacilli; in this case, the macrophages are the efficient agents.

Eosinophils. The eosinophilic leukocytes (Fig. 7-1) normally constitute from 2 to 4% of the white blood cells. They are somewhat larger than the neutrophils (about 10 to 14 μm), and are characterized by an abundance of coarse, refractile granules of a uniform size which stain intensely with eosin or other acid dyes.

Electron micrographs show that the granules are membrane-bounded and that they have a matrix of fine particles surrounding an irregularly shaped dense bar or crystalloid (Fig. 7-9). The granules are larger than either the specific or azurophilic granules of the neutrophils. The specific granules of the eosinophils resemble the azurophilic granules of the neutrophils in the sense that they give a positive peroxidase reaction and function as lysosomes.

In supravital preparations, the eosinophils occasionally travel as rapidly as the

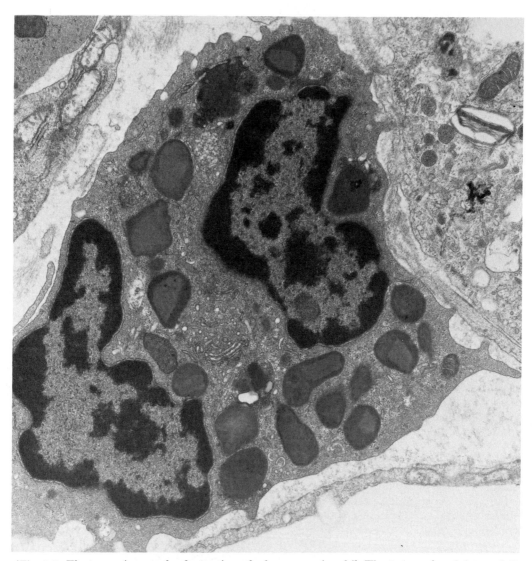

Fig. 7-9. Electron micrograph of a section of a human eosinophil. The two nuclear lobes and the large specific granules containing irregular crystalloid inclusions are characteristic. In this preparation the crystalloids are less dense than the granule matrix. A Golgi region appears between the nuclear lobes. Courtesy of Dr. June Marshall. ×16,400.

neutrophils but not for as long a period. Their granules stain intensely and uniformly with neutral red, and a few mitochondria can be demonstrated with Janus green B.

The eosinophils are more common in the connective tissue of certain areas (e.g., intestinal mucosa) than in the bloodstream. They increase greatly in allergic conditions such as hay fever and asthma, in skin diseases, and in parasitic infestations. Their functional role in these conditions is not entirely clear, but it has been shown that they are particularly phagocytic for antigen-antibody complexes. They contain some histamine, but are not comparable in this respect to connective tissue mast cells and blood basophils. There is a marked reduction in the number of eosinophils in peripheral blood after the administration of adrenal corticosteroids or pituitary hormones which stimulate the adrenal (ACTH). This procedure, often called the Thorn test because of its development by Thorn and his collaborators, provides valuable clinical information on the sites of hormone deficiency.

Basophils. The basophilic leukocytes (Fig. 7-1) are present in blood in an almost negligible quantity, forming 0.5 to 1% or even less of the total number of leukocytes. In size they vary from 8 to 10 μm. The nucleus of a basophil is relatively large and irregularly polymorphous. The lobed nature is not as clearly defined as in other granulocytes, and the chromatin network, which is less compact, takes a lighter stain. The cytoplasm contains a variable number of coarse granules which are basophilic and metachromatic. These granules also vary in size; a few may be as large as or larger than the eosinophilic granules, but the majority are intermediate between the neutrophilic and eosinophilic types. Electron micrographs show that the granules are membrane-bounded structures containing fine particles (Fig. 7-10). Some granules which are more electron dense than others are presumably immature. Because the granules are soluble in water, they are usually not found in sections prepared by the ordinary routine.

In supravital preparations, the basophils are relatively inactive. The basophilic granules are not as refractile as eosinophilic granules, are more variable in size and do not stain as uniformly. Most of the granules give a deeper red reaction with neutral red than do the eosinophilic granules.

Although the blood basophils resemble the connective tissue mast cells in many respects, they have some differential characteristics. For example, they have a more polymorphous nucleus and their cytoplasmic granules have a different ultrastructure. Their main function is to form heparin and histamine, which are stored in their granules before release by exocytosis. They increase in relatively few pathological conditions, e.g., in smallpox, chicken pox, and chronic sinus inflammations. They increase, along with all other leukocytes, in leukemia. Although they normally constitute only about 0.5% of the leukocytes, their total number in an average individual having 6 liters of blood is approximately 200 million. In some of the lower vertebrates (hellbender, mudpuppy, and certain turtles), they are more numerous than the other types of leukocytes.

Blood Platelets

Blood platelets (thromboplastids or thrombocytes, Fig. 7-1) are biconvex disc-shaped bodies 2 to 4 μm in diameter. They arise as fragments of cytoplasm of megakaryocytes of bone marrow, and they are colorless in the fresh state. Because they are small and readily clump when blood is drawn, it is difficult to obtain a precise count, but their number in normal blood is given as 150,000 to 300,000/mm^3. They are found only in mammals. The thrombocytes of lower vertebrates are nucleated cells that are wholly unlike those of man and other mammals.

In Wright's stained blood smears, the platelets are frequently aggregated, but it can be seen that each platelet is composed of a central area (granulomere, chromomere) that stains purple and a peripheral zone which is light blue (the so-called hyalomere). The platelets have numerous granules, a few mitochondria, considerable glycogen, vacuoles, microtubules, and microfilaments. Although the granules are widely dispersed in the cytoplasm, the majority are in the granulomere region. Most of the granules (alpha granules) range from

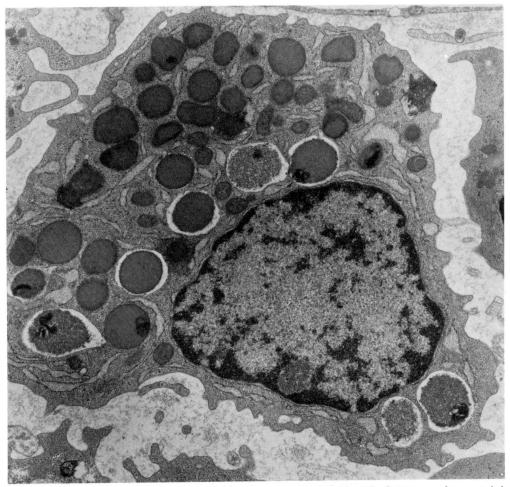

Fig. 7-10. Electron micrograph of a section of a human basophil. Note the large granules containing relatively homogeneous material. Some granules show a separation between the contents and the membrane and a partial dispersion of the contents. Basophilic granules are frequently lost entirely during processing. Note the relatively prominent cisternae of endoplasmic reticulum. Courtesy of Dr. June Marshall. ×14,000.

0.15 to 0.2 μm in diameter. There are numerous microtubules and microfilaments. A particularly prominent bundle of microtubules courses circumferentially just beneath the membrane that encloses the platelet. It is thought that the tubules aid in maintaining the shape of the platelet and that the filaments have a role in contraction. The plasma membrane of each platelet is covered externally by a mucopolysaccharide-rich fuzzy coat. It is thought that this plays a role in the adherence of the platelets to each other.

The platelets presumably liberate an enzyme, *thromboplastin,* which affects the coagulation of the blood. Thromboplastin transforms *prothrombin* into *thrombin,* and the latter, in turn, transforms fibrinogen into fibrin. Thromboplastin is present in the plasma, as well as in the platelets. Blood free from platelets coagulates, although much more slowly, and lymph, which has no platelets, likewise coagulates.

Pathologically, the platelets may by agglutination give rise to colorless intravascular clots or thrombi. Deficiencies of circulating platelets are encountered clinically in various forms of the condition known as thrombocytopenia.

Chylomicrons and Hemoconia

Blood plasma contains very minute globules of fat (chylomicrons, about 1 μm in size) which are best studied by dark field illumination. They are particularly numerous in the plasma after digestion of a meal containing quantities of fat. In addition to the fat globules, blood plasma contains a variable number of small particles which may be observed in dry smears as well as in fresh preparations. These particles are known as hemoconia (blood dust). They are probably produced by disintegration of red corpuscles and leukocytes.

Lymph

Lymph, like blood, consists of a fluid plasma in which are suspended various corpuscular elements. Red blood corpuscles and platelets are entirely missing and granulocytes are few in number, the chief cellular elements being lymphocytes.

The plasma of lymph is similar to that of blood but of less fixed constitution. It carries carbonic acid but very little oxygen.

During digestion, the lymphatics of the intestine become filled with a large amount of fat globules. The lymph assumes a white color and is known as *chyle*. Many of the fat globules are removed and stored temporarily by the lymphatic organs before the lymph reaches the blood stream.

Lymph coagulates, although much more slowly than blood, the fibrin forming a colorless clot in which the cells are entangled.

Disposal of Corpuscles

In contrast with many other cells of the body, the red and white corpuscles of the blood survive for only a relatively short period of time. The life span of the human erythrocyte as determined by tracer doses of radioactive isotopes is about 127 days. From these data, it is obvious that billions of corpuscles are destroyed daily. The destruction is balanced so well by new blood formation that the characteristic number of corpuscles is constantly maintained under normal conditions.

Destruction of erythrocytes frequently begins within the bloodstream itself by a disintegration of corpuscles into small hemoglobin-retaining fragments and is completed by the macrophages of the blood-destroying organs, chiefly by the spleen (see chapter 13). These cells remove the frag-

mented forms and also engulf many senile erythrocytes in toto. The macrophages break up the hemoglobin into an iron-free portion (*globin*) and an iron-retaining part (*hematin*). Hematin is further separated into *bilirubin* and *iron*. The bilirubin is transported to the liver to be excreted in the bile, and the iron (in protein complexes as ferritin and hemosiderin) is conserved by the macrophages to be used again in new erythrocytes developing in the bone marrow.

The life span of the different types of leukocytes is quite variable. The time spent in circulation is also quite variable. The neutrophils spend 8 hr or less in the circulation before migrating into the connective tissue, where they survive for a few days and function as microphages. The lymphocytes generally remain in the bloodstream for only a short period, about 8 hr, at any one time, but some of them (long-lived lymphocytes) recirculate and survive for many years. Monocytes circulate in the blood for only 1 or 2 days and then migrate into the connective tissues, where some of them become macrophages which may survive for many months.

Senile and dead cells are removed by phagocytosis in the spleen and liver. The migration of neutrophils, especially pronounced during infection, and their disintegration in the connective tissues have already been pointed out (page 220). They also escape by penetration through the lining epithelia of mucous membranes, as illustrated by their presence in saliva. Eosinophils show a particular tendency for migration into the connective tissues of the respiratory and gastrointestinal tracts, where they eventually disintegrate. Some of the lymphocytes may undergo dissolution in the circulatory system, some may be destroyed while the blood courses through organs where cells of the macrophage system are particularly numerous, and large numbers migrate into the connective tissues where they apparently disintegrate. Many are lost by migration into the lumen of the intestinal tract.

Development of Blood Corpuscles (Hemopoiesis)

Although the earliest erythrocytes of the embryo develop from extraembryonic mesoderm of the yolk sac and subsequently in the liver and spleen (page 235), erythrocyte development in the adult is normally limited to bone marrow. The development of granular leukocytes is likewise generally limited to marrow under normal conditions. Hence, the erythrocytes and granular leukocytes are described as the *myeloid elements* of the blood. Considerable numbers of lymphocytes and perhaps some monocytes differentiate in the lymphatic organs; therefore, they are classified as *lymphoid elements*. These terms continue to have wide usage even though it is well established that large numbers of lymphocytes and monocytes also develop in marrow.

There is general agreement on most of the cytological characteristics and intercellular relationships of the cells illustrated in Figure 7-11, but numerous controversies have existed in regard to the precursors. According to the *monophyletic* (unitarian) theory, all blood cells are derived from a common stem cell (hemocytoblast). According to the *dualistic* theory, there is one stem cell for the granular leukocytes and erythrocytes and another stem cell for the lymphoid elements. These different theories were based on light microscope studies which indicated that in either case the primitive cell has a basophilic cytoplasm and a rounded nucleus with a prominent nucleolus.

Marked advances in our knowledge of the early stages of blood development have been achieved by the use of new experimental methods. A major advance began with the discovery that rodents in which all blood cells were destroyed by total body X-irradiation would survive provided that they immediately received intravenous injections of bone marrow cells from a closely related animal. Similar results were obtained when one member of a surgically joined (parabiosed) pair received total body irradiation. These findings showed that a cell with the potency to form all types of blood cells circulates in the blood and is not confined to blood-forming organs as previously presumed.

The animals which were X-irradiated and transfused with marrow cells as outlined above frequently developed nodules on the surface of the spleen. The use of suspensions of marrow cells with "marker" chromosomes produced by irradiation showed that each spleen colony represents a clone; i.e., each colony of all types of marrow cells is derived from a single cell, known as a *stem cell*. Suspensions of marrow cells grown *in vitro* in an appropriate medium on agar plates produce colonies similar to those on the spleen; these are known as colony-forming units (CFU). A number of investigators noted a relationship between the number of colonies formed and the volume and concentration of marrow cells. This was verified by counting the number of cells plated as determined by hemocytometer counts of the marrow cells. The proportion of stem cells to the total number of nucleated marrow cells was found to be very low, normally about 1:1000.

The research outlined above provided information on the behavior of stem cells but gave no information on their morphology. A clue to the latter was obtained by differential sedimentation studies which showed that cells from the part of the sedimenting column that contains stem cells have a weight and size comparable with that of lymphocytes. In further studies, samples of cells from the part of the sedimentation column that has stem cell potency were examined by light and by electron microscopy. It was found that the sedimentation column cells have a nucleus which is more irregularly shaped than that of most lymphocytes. The mitochondria are smaller and more numerous than in lymphocytes, and free ribosomes but no rough-surfaced endoplasmic reticulum are present. The characteristics fit those which would be expected of a stem cell which maintains its own population for a lifetime and provides differentiating cells as they are required to replace the mature cells of blood and marrow.

The origin of the stem cell remains controversial. The view that the pluripotential cell arises from reticular cells of bone marrow is questionable. The earliest erythroblasts in the embryo develop from mesenchymal cells of the yolk sac in areas described as "blood islands." There is evidence that undifferentiated cells from the yolk sac reach the liver and other blood-

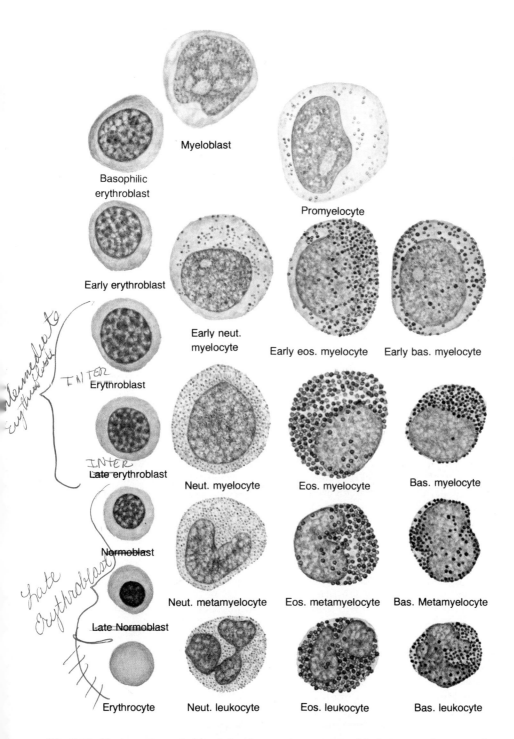

Fig. 7-11. Various stages in blood development as seen in *dried smears* of marrow from a human rib. Wright's stain. ×1560.

forming organs, where they survive as stem cells which proliferate and differentiate into all types of blood cells.

The monocytes have been described as arising from undifferentiated reticular cells, but there is increasing evidence that they develop from promonocytes that also arise from stem cells.

Blood Development in Bone Marrow

Red bone marrow is composed of a framework or stroma of reticular cells and fibers plus free cells located within the meshwork. The stroma also contains a variable number of fat cells. The majority of the free cells are the immature developmental stages of the granular leukocytes and erythrocytes that normally develop only in marrow in the adult. Red marrow also contains megakaryocytes, mature erythrocytes, granular leukocytes, lymphocytes, and plasma cells. The structure and blood supply of marrow with its characteristic network of sinusoids have been described in chapter 6 (page 200).

The Granulocyte Series. The stages of granulocyte development, in order of differentiation, are: *stem cells, myeloblasts, promyelocytes, myelocytes, metamyelocytes,* and *granular leukocytes.*

Myeloblasts. The myeloblasts develop from the pluripotential CFU stem cell, probably by way of a derivative for the granulocyte line (CFU-G). The myeloblasts normally constitute about 2% of the nucleated cells of marrow. Because the stem cell is not specifically characterized by microscopy, it is probably included in this number. However, the stem cells demonstrated by sedimentation studies are present in marrow in the proportion of less than 1 cell/1,000, or less than 0.1%.

The myeloblasts are variable in size, ranging from 8 to 13 μm in diameter. They are characterized by a deeply basophilic cytoplasm and a relatively undifferentiated nucleus. The nucleus is round or ovoid and contains two or more coarse nucleoli. In dried smears treated with Wright's stain, the nucleoli are very pale, and the arrangement of the granular chromatin frequently gives a characteristic sievelike appearance (Fig. 7-11). The nucleus of this same cell type has a very different appearance in sections stained with hematoxylin-eosin-azure (see myeloblasts, Fig. 7-12). Here the nucleoli are stained intensely, and the chromatin shows as a delicate reticulum enclosing pale-staining areas.

The cytoplasm is very basophilic both in sections and in dried smears and is a definite blue of the lymphocyte type after Wright's stain. Electron micrographs show that the myeloblast cytoplasm contains an abundance of free ribosomes but relatively little rough endoplasmic reticulum. They also show numerous mitochondria which are spherical and relatively small.

The myeloblasts of the normal adult marrow arise chiefly by mitotic divisions of their own type and to a lesser extent by differentiation from stem cells. In some pathological conditions they become more numerous in the marrow and also appear in the circulating blood, as in myelogenous leukemia. Here the increase is by accelerated mitotic activity of the myeloblasts and increased rate of proliferation of stem cells.

Promyelocytes. The promyelocytes are more differentiated than the myeloblasts and are somewhat more numerous, about 5% of the nucleated marrow cells. They are usually larger, ranging up to 20 μm or more in marrow smears. The nucleus is rounded or ovoid and occasionally indented. The chromatin is granular and frequently gives a sievelike appearance somewhat like that of the myeloblast. The nucleoli are still prominent. The cytoplasm is even more basophilic than that of the myeloblast and it contains *azurophilic granules,* a distinct difference from the nongranular cytoplasm of the myeloblast. Electron micrographs show an abundance of rough-surfaced endoplasmic reticulum, plus free ribosomes, numerous mitochondria, and a well developed Golgi complex.

Myelocytes. The myelocytes constitute about 12% (range 5 to 20%) of the nucleated marrow cells. There are a number of mitotic divisions and several stages of differentiation within the myelocyte category. The earliest differential feature of the myelocytes is the initial appearance of *specific granules* which differ from the azurophilic granules that form only during the promyelocyte stage. With the appearance of specific granules at the myelocyte stage, the developing granulocytes are distinguishable

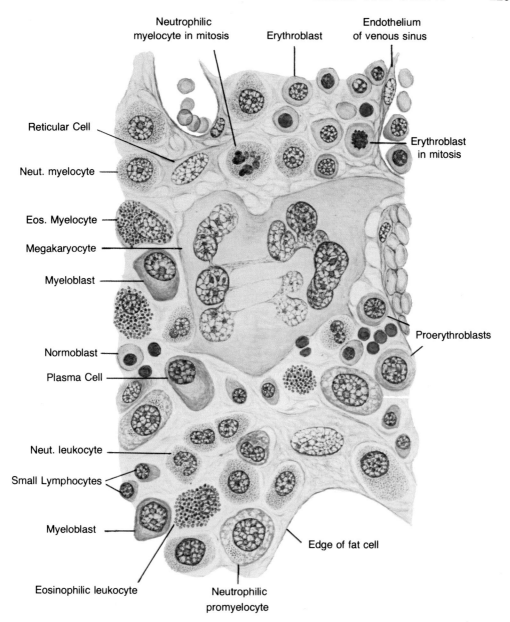

Neutrophilic myelocyte in mitosis

Erythroblast

Endothelium of venous sinus

Erythroblast in mitosis

Reticular Cell

Neut. myelocyte

Eos. Myelocyte

Megakaryocyte

Myeloblast

Proerythroblasts

Normoblast

Plasma Cell

Neut. leukocyte

Small Lymphocytes

Myeloblast

Edge of fat cell

Eosinophilic leukocyte

Neutrophilic promyelocyte

Fig. 7-12. Various stages in blood development as seen in a *section* of marrow from a human rib. Hematoxylin-eosin-azure. ×1365.

as neutrophils, eosinophils, and basophils. Although the types of granules differ structurally and cytochemically, as outlined in the preceding section on types of granulocytes, the course of differentiation is similar in the three types; the neutrophil will be described in more detail as an example.

Electron micrographs show an interesting difference in the manner in which the Golgi complex handles the packaging of the

granules. The azurophilic granules form in the promyelocyte stage, arising by a coalescence of dense-cored vacuoles derived from the inner (adcentriolar) cisternae of the Golgi complex. The specific granules form only in the myelocyte stage and arise by fusion of dense-cored vacuoles derived from the outer cisternae of the Golgi complex (Figs. 1-28 and 1-29, chapter 1). Because the azurophilic granules form only in the promyelocyte stage, their number is reduced by each myelocyte division, and they are greatly outnumbered by the specific granules in the mature cell.

In addition to an increase in numbers of specific cytoplasmic granules during myelocyte maturation, the cytoplasm shows a decrease in basophilia in correlation with a decrease in free ribosomes and rough-surfaced endoplasmic reticulum.

Maturation of myelocytes also involves changes in the nuclei. In the early myelocyte, the nucleus differs only slightly from that of the promyelocyte, but with successive divisions and maturation the nuclei become ovoid and irregular in shape, nucleoli disappear, and the chromatin becomes more dense and compact. The cells eventually reach a stage where they no longer divide, and then they are known as metamyelocytes.

Metamyelocytes. These cells constitute about 22% of the nucleated cells of marrow; the metamyelocyte is the most abundant cell of normal marrow. The nucleus continues its maturation, and in the *neutrophilic metamyelocyte* it becomes increasingly irregular and often assumes a shape known as a *band form.* In further maturation, the cytoplasm shows an increase in glycogen and a decrease in free ribosomes, rough-surfaced endoplasmic reticulum, and mitochondria. The nucleus eventually becomes constricted into two to five lobes, frequently three. The *eosinophilic metamyelocytes* frequently form a nucleus of two lobes, although three or more are not particularly unusual. The chromatin of the nucleus is less dense and less compact than in the neutrophil (Fig. 7-11).

The *basophilic metamyelocyte* differs from the other types of metamyelocytes in the shape of its nucleus and the form of its specific granules. The nucleus does not differentiate into distinct lobes, as it generally does in neutrophils and eosinophils. Therefore, it is difficult to distinguish basophilic metamyelocytes from mature basophilic leukocytes in Wright's stained smears. Furthermore, the basophilic granules, like those of mast cells, are water-soluble and are generally not distinguishable in sections of material fixed in aqueous solutions.

General Considerations of Granulocytopoiesis. When the percentages of the different myelocyte stages are added to the number of mature granulocytes present in marrow (20% or more), it is found that the granular leukocyte line comprises approximately 60% of the cells in normal marrow. Lymphocytes, monocytes, reticular cells, plasma cells, and megakaryocytes may constitute another 10 to 20%, leaving only about 20 to 30% of the marrow cells in the erythrocyte line. Although the literature on differential counts for normal marrow gives an even greater range than that listed above, there is general agreement that the progenitors of the leukocytes outnumber those of the erythrocytes. The numerical preponderance of leukocytogenic over erythrocytogenic cells in marrow, in contrast with the opposite relationship in blood, can be explained partly by the fact that the leukocytes survive for a shorter time in the circulation than do the erythrocytes and also require a longer period for development and maturation in marrow.

Studies of bone marrow cells by the ultraviolet absorption method have shown that ribonucleic acid (RNA) is more abundant in the myeloblast than in any of the other developmental stages of the granulocyte line. The high concentration of RNA is responsible for the marked basophilia of the cytoplasm at the myeloblast stage. The high concentration of cytoplasmic RNA and the prominence of nucleoli are correlated with the rapid formation of cytoplasmic proteins during the early stages. It has been estimated that the total volume of all of the promyelocytes is about 8 times the total volume of the myeloblasts. This follows from the fact that the promyelocytes are more numerous and often larger than the myeloblasts. In the lineage from promyelocyte to myelocyte to metamyelocyte, the cells increase in number with a decrease in size, so that the total volume of all the metamyelocytes is only slightly greater than the total volume of the promyelocytes. Development during these later stages is dominated by differentiation rather than by cell growth. The rapid decrease in cytoplasmic basophilia during these later stages appears to be correlated with the decrease in RNA.

The life span of the granular leukocytes is approximately as follows: about 14 days for differentiation and maturation in bone marrow, about 6 to 10 hr in circulation, and about 1 to 2 days in the connective tissue. A loss of leukocytes from the circulation stimulates an increase in the rate of release of cells from the marrow and a severe loss of cells stimulates an increased rate of differentiation from the stem cell. It is postulated that *leukopoietin,* a stimulating factor carried in the blood, increases the rate of leukocyte production, but the nature of the factor and its mode of action remain obscure.

The Erythrocyte Series. The stages of erythrocyte development are: *stem cells, proerythroblasts, basophilic erythroblasts, polychromatophilic erythroblasts, normoblasts* (orthochromatophilic erythroblasts), and *erythrocytes.*

Proerythroblasts. These are derived by differentiation from the pluripotential (CFU) stem cell by way of a derivative for the erythrocyte line (CFU-E). They are the earliest cells identifiable by light microscopy as a part of the erythrocyte series and they are relatively large, about 12 to 17 μm in diameter. Their nuclei are rounded and have a coarser chromatin structure than that of myeloblasts. Nucleoli are present but less prominent than in the myeloblast. In fresh preparations, or by special techniques, a small amount of hemoglobin can be detected in the cytoplasm of some of the cells, but it is obscured in stained preparations by the basophilia of the cytoplasm because of numerous free ribosomes and polyribosomes.

Basophilic Erythroblasts. After a few divisions, the proerythroblasts differentiate into the basophilic erythroblasts, in which the chromatin is somewhat more coarse and nucleoli are no longer discernible. The cytoplasm continues to be very basophilic because of free ribosomes and polyribosomes. Electron micrographs show little or no rough-surfaced endoplasmic reticulum.

Polychromatophilic Erythroblasts. The basophilic erythroblasts undergo mitotic divisions and give rise to cells in which the hemoglobin is of sufficient quantity to be observed distinctly in stained preparations. There are many generations of erythroblasts and, with each mitotic division, there is a decrease in basophilia of cytoplasm and an increase in quantity of hemoglobin, which is acidophilic.

The cytoplasm of the different generations of cells takes varying amounts of the acid and basic components of Wright's stain; therefore, these cells show a "mixed color varying from purplish blue to lilac or gray" and are called polychromatophilic. A few of these stages are illustrated in Fig. 7-11.

The nucleus of the polychromatophilic erythroblast has a denser chromatin network than that of the basophilic erythroblast, and the coarse chromatin bodies give a checkerboard appearance which is characteristic of developing erythrocytes, as contrasted with the more irregular arrangement of chromatin in the developing granulocytes. The polychromatophilic erythroblasts vary greatly in size but are on the average somewhat smaller than the basophilic erythroblasts. The size variation is related to the number of mitotic divisions any specific cell has undergone by the time of observation; there are several generations within the polychromatophilic stage.

Normoblasts (Orthochromatophilic Erythroblasts). These cells have approximately the same amount of hemoglobin as the erythrocytes. The cells of this stage have usually stopped dividing and are in various stages of maturation. They are only slightly larger than the mature erythrocytes (Fig. 7-11). The chromatin is denser and more compact than in the polychromatophilic cells. Eventually the nuclei become pyknotic, assume bizarre shapes, and are extruded from the cells usually along with a thin coat of cytoplasm and plasma membrane visible in electron micrographs. Small fragments of the nucleus occasionally remain and give rise to deeply staining bodies (Howell-Jolly bodies). The Cabot ring bodies sometimes found in erythrocytes of anemia were once described as remnants of nuclei, but it has been shown that they are induced by hemolytic agents in the solutions used in laboratory techniques.

Erythrocytes. The youngest erythrocytes (*reticulocytes*) contain a delicate reticulum which can be demonstrated by supravital staining with dyes such as cresyl blue (Fig. 7-1*B*). Erythrocytes normally lose their reticular structure soon after leaving the marrow; the normal reticulocyte count of peripheral blood is less than 1% of the erythrocytes. Increased numbers may be called into circulation by repeated hemorrhages. Reticulocyte counts are used as an index of the effectiveness of therapy in pernicious anemia, an increase of reticulocytes after treatment being evidence of an increased production of young erythrocytes.

Normal marrow, in which erythrocytes develop through the stages as described above, is known as *normoblastic marrow.* This contrasts with *megaloblastic marrow,* which occurs in pernicious anemia and other macrocytic anemias.

It has been noted earlier that there is a lack of agreement on terminology for the developmental stages of blood cells. Use of the term normoblast is an example. If one uses normoblast only for cells which have acquired a sufficient amount of hemoglobin to give a cytoplasmic stain almost equal to that of a normal erythrocyte (i.e., for the immediate precursor of a normal erythrocyte), the terms apply as outlined in the preceding description. On the other hand, if one prefers to use the term normoblast for all stages of normal erythrocyte development in contrast with megaloblastic development in anemia, the names for the stages of development become: basophilic normoblasts, polychromatophilic normoblasts, orthochromatophilic normoblasts, reticulated erythrocytes, and mature erythrocytes.

General Considerations of Erythropoiesis. It has been found that ribonucleic acid is more abundant in the basophilic erythroblast than in the later stages of the erythrocyte line. The concentration of RNA is responsible for the marked basophilia of the cytoplasm in the early stages and is apparently correlated with the active synthesis of cytoplasmic proteins during the stages which show the greatest increase in total cell volume.

The normal development of erythrocytes is dependent upon many different factors. Obviously, all of the parent substances which enter into the formation of hemoglobin must be present. The absence of one of these, iron, is responsible for a microcytic type of anemia. Certain additional substances are necessary for the normal maturation of the erythrocytogenic cells. The absence of one of these, vitamin B_{12}, produces pernicious anemia. Vitamin B_{12} has been identified as the antipernicious ane-

mia factor, or liver factor. Actually, the real defect in pernicious anemia is the lack of some substance which is normally present in gastric juice, the *intrinsic factor.* The intrinsic factor facilitates the intestinal absorption of an extrinsic factor present in food (vitamin B_{12} itself). After absorption, B_{12} is stored chiefly in the liver until it is utilized later in bone marrow.

The most potent stimulus for erythropoiesis is hypoxia, or cellular oxygen deficiency. Extracts from plasma of animals made anemic by experimental methods contain a factor which stimulates erythropoiesis when injected into normal animals. The plasma or humoral factor is known as *erythropoietin.*

Erythropoietin is a glycoprotein that is formed by the interaction of *erythrogenin* (a renal factor) and *globin* (hemoglobin protein). Erythrogenin usually forms in the kidney and is therefore known as a renal erythropoietic factor (REF), but it can also form in other locations as demonstrated by studies on animals after bilateral nephrectomy. Hypoxia stimulates the formation of REF and, therefore, increases circulating erythropoietin. Studies of fetal mouse liver cells in vitro indicate that erythropoietin increases the number of hemoglobin-forming cells (erythroblasts) by stimulating the stem cells (CFU-E) to multiply and differentiate into hemoglobin-synthesizing cells (proerythroblasts and erythroblasts).

Iron is present in hemoglobin as *ferritin* and *hemosiderin.* Only a fraction of the iron used in erythrocyte development is obtained from absorption by the intestine; most of it is recycled in the body. Ferritin from degenerating senile erythrocytes is taken up by the macrophage system of the spleen and bone marrow where it is stored. It is released into the circulation as needed and is taken up by the erythroblasts of marrow by a process resembling pinocytosis. The utilization of ferritin in the synthesis of hemoglobin by erythroblasts is dependent on the presence of vitamin B_{12}, but the details of the process are not defined as clearly as are those related to erythropoietin.

Megakaryocytes and Platelet Formation. The megakaryocytes are giant cells (30 to 100 μm) derived from the stem cell, and they apparently give rise to blood platelets. In the normal adult, they are usually said to occur only in marrow. During embryonic development, however, they are also present in other hemopoietic organs (liver, spleen). During the differentiation of a megakaryocyte from a stem cell, the nucleus divides mitotically without accompanying division of cytoplasm. The nuclei usually separate to a late anaphase or early telophase stage and then reunite. In this way a polyploid nucleus is formed with $32N$–$64N$ chromosomes instead of the $2N$ number characteristic of most other cells. The polyploid nucleus is lobulated in a variable and complicated manner, often having only thin strands connecting different lobular units (Fig. 7-12). The megakaryocytes should not be confused with osteoclasts of marrow and foreign body giant cells, which are multinucleated and form by fusion of cells.

The cytoplasm of the megakaryocyte contains the usual organelles and numerous fine granules which apparently form in the Golgi complex. The cell has an irregular shape, with many pseudopodia. From studies with the light microscope, it appeared that platelets form by fragmentation of pseudopodia. Electron microscope studies have clarified the manner in which this occurs (Fig. 7-13). The peripheral regions of the cytoplasm become gradually subdivided by membranes into compartments, each subdivision having granules. When the partitioning membranes become complete, the compartments readily separate from the parent cell to become free platelets, without any rupture of the cell plasmalemma.

Megakaryocytes are limited in their life span, and stages of degeneration are not uncommon. The nucleus becomes smaller and stains more intensely, and the protoplasm degenerates. Some of the fragmented nuclei may find their way into the blood vessels, to be carried through the right side of the heart into the lung capillaries where they degenerate. In pathological conditions, entire megakaryocytes may be carried into the lungs and form an embolism of the vessels.

Development of Lymphoid Elements

Lymphocytes. Studies with labeled cells have shown that an older view, that lymphocytes develop only in lymphatic organs, is incorrect. The lymphocytes develop in bone marrow *and* in lymphatic organs. They differentiate from stem cells and retain the ability to multiply after circulating and migrating to other locations. A relatively undifferentiated lymphocyte, known as a *lymphoblast,* is a relatively large cell with a large nucleus, prominent nucleoli, and very basophilic cytoplasm (Fig. 7-14).

The stages of differentiation resemble those of other leukocytes to the extent that the chromatin becomes more dense and compact, the nucleoli become less obvious, and a few azurophilic granules appear in the cytoplasm of some of the cells. Stages of differentiation are less obvious than in the other leukocyte types, because the nuclei do not become lobed or irregular in shape and there are no specific types of granules.

The lymphocytes which multiply and differentiate in the lymphatic organs may arise from undifferentiated reticular cells, but this seems unlikely. In accordance with recent findings on the origin of stem cells, it is more likely that lymphocytes of lymphatic organs differentiate from stem cells which enter the circulation from bone marrow. The marrow stem cells are probably derived during embryonic development from undifferentiated mesenchymal cells from the yolk sac via the hemopoietic tissue of the liver.

Monocytes. Studies by radioautography and by the chromosome marker technique indicate that the monocytes develop from precursors in the bone marrow. The fact that monocytes constitute only 1 to 2% of all of the nucleated cells in marrow adds to the difficulty in studying the differentiation of this cell type. The promonocyte is described as being 7 to 15 μm in diameter. It has a rounded or oval nucleus with dispersed chromatin and two or more nucleoli. Electron micrographs show that the cytoplasm contains an abundance of free ribosomes and polyribosomes. Some small granules, identifiable as the azurophilic granules of light microscopy, are present near the Golgi complex. The mature monocyte of marrow is about 9 to 11 μm in diameter, and its nucleus is smaller than that of the promonocyte. Electron micro-

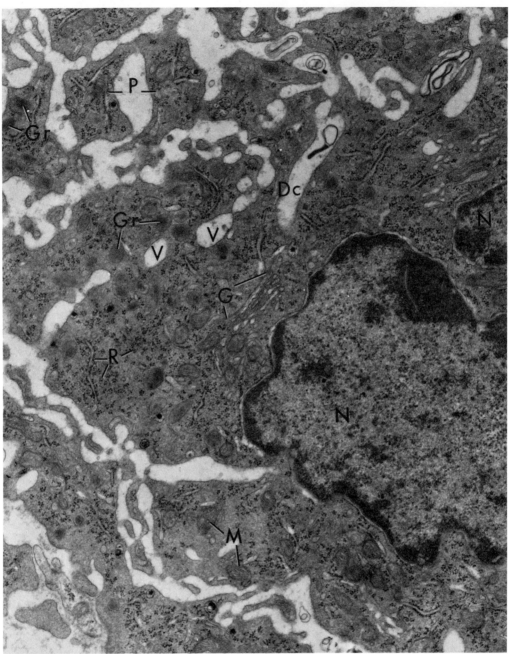

Fig. 7-13. Electron micrograph of a portion of a megakaryocyte. The cell characteristically contains a large multilobed nucleus, but only portions of two nuclear lobes (N) are present within the field of the micrograph. A portion of one of the Golgi regions (G) is seen adjacent to one of the nuclear lobes. Most of the ribosomes (R) are distributed in clusters through the cytoplasm, and only a few are present along the cisternae of the endoplasmic reticulum. Electron-dense granules (Gr) are seen in the cytoplasm of the cell and within the platelets. They are somewhat smaller than the mitochondria (M), and they resemble lysosomes in that they contain acid phosphatase. In the process of platelet formation, portions of the megakaryocyte cytoplasm become partitioned off by membranes. First, membrane-lined vesicles (V) develop; later, platelet demarcation channels (Dc) arise by extension and fusion of the vesicles. Finally, the channels become continuous with one another, and membrane-bounded regions of the cytoplasm become detached as platelets. Precursor stage platelets (P), with only a few remaining attachments, are seen in the upper left portion of the micrograph. From the bone marrow of a mouse. ×20,850. (Courtesy of Drs. K. R. Porter and M. A. Bonneville.)

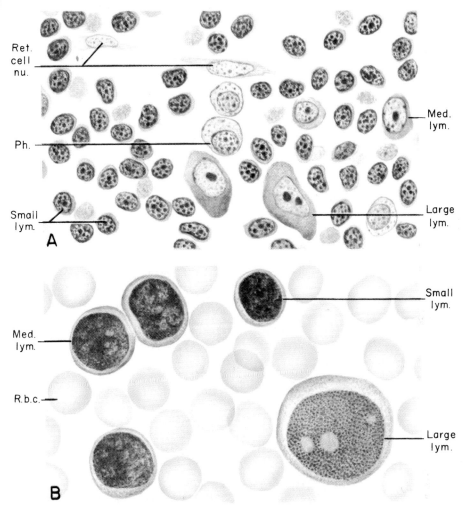

Fig. 7-14. *A*, stages of lymphocyte differentiation seen in a section of the cortex of a monkey lymph node stained with hematoxylin-eosin-azure. Reticular cell nuclei (*Ret. cell nu.*) take a pale stain. Large lymphocytes (*Large lym.*) have prominent nucleoli in an otherwise pale nucleus, with very basophilic cytoplasm. Medium-sized lymphocytes (*Med. lym.*) are intermediate in staining characteristics between the large and the small lymphocytes (*small lym.*). A few phagocytes (*Ph*) are present. *B*, immature lymphocytes in a Wright's stained blood smear from a patient with lymphatic leukemia. The lymphoblast or large lymphocyte (*Large lym.*) has prominent nucleoli which are pale in this stain. Medium-sized lymphocytes, with nucleoli, are more numerous than the small lymphocytes. The size difference between the cells in *A* and *B* is due, in part, to differences in technique: *A* is from a section, *B* from a smear, which flattens the cells. Both figures ×1640.

graphs show fewer ribosomes and more azurophilic granules.

The monocytes usually leave the marrow about 3 days after beginning their differentiation and continue their maturation by forming additional azurophilic granules while they are in the blood. The azurophilic granules of promonocytes and monocytes give a positive peroxidase reaction, a characteristic difference from the azurophilic granules of lymphocytes, which give a negative peroxidase reaction.

Embryonic Development of Blood Cells

Blood cell development in the human embryo begins with the formation of *blood islands* in the extraembryonic mesoderm of the yolk sac during the 3rd week of development. The islands are composed of closely packed mesenchymal cells that differentiate along different lines. The peripheral cells become flattened and adherent, to form endothelium, while the central cells proliferate and differentiate into primitive cells which belong almost entirely to the erythroid line. In the earliest recognizable stage of differentiation observable by light microscopy, the cells have vesicular, pale-staining nuclei with prominent nucleoli and basophilic cytoplasm. They are often described as *hemocytoblasts.* The cells identified as "primitive blood cells" and hemocytoblasts by light microscopy (Figs. 7-15 and 7-16) probably include the erythroid stem cells and proerythroblasts.

The erythroid cells of yolk sac origin differ from bone marrow-derived erythroid cells in that they retain their nuclei throughout their life span. The yolk sac erythroid cells also have a type of hemoglobin that differs from that of the erythroid cells of all other blood-forming organs (liver, spleen, and marrow).

The *liver* becomes the second hemopoietic organ at about 6 weeks and is the most active site of hemopoiesis until the middle of fetal life. Then its activity begins to decrease and normally disappears at about the time of birth. The hemopoietic stem cells of the liver differentiate into both nucleated and nonnucleated erythrocytes plus granular leukocytes and megakaryocytes. At 7 weeks almost all of the circulating red cells are nucleated, but by 11 weeks most are nonnucleated. Studies on fetal mice indicate that the erythroid cell precursors of the liver are derived from mesenchymal cells in the region where the transverse septum and hepatic parenchyma are in contact. The stem cells for the leukocyte line probably arise from mesenchymal cells associated with liver parenchyma, and the mononuclear precursors of macrophages probably arise from a similar source.

The *spleen* is an active blood-forming organ from the latter part of the 2nd month until the 8th month. Erythropoiesis in the spleen ceases soon after birth, but lymphocytes continue to develop in the spleen throughout life.

Red bone marrow is the most important and permanent hemopoietic organ. It be-

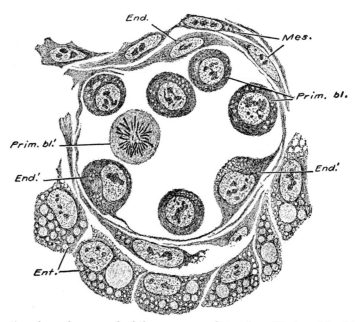

Fig. 7-15. Section through a vessel of the area vasculosa of an 8½-day-old rabbit embryo. *End.,* primitive endothelium; *End.',* primitive endothelial cells rounding off and beginning to differentiate into primitive blood cells; *Ent.,* endoderm; *Mes.,* mesenchyme; *Prim. bl.,* primitive blood cells; *Prim. bl.',* primitive blood cell in mitosis and with cytoplasm showing differentiation toward the primitive erythroblast. (Redrawn from Maximow, Arch. Mikrosc. Anat. 73, 1909.)

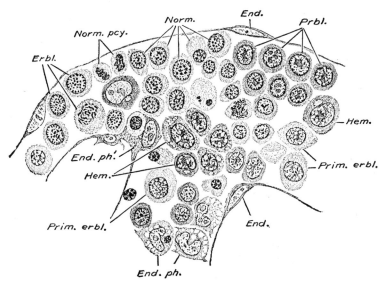

Fig. 7-16. Portion of a vessel from the yolk sac of a 13½-day-old rabbit embryo. *End.*, endothelial cells; *End. ph.*, phagocytic cells which have developed from the primitive endothelium; *End. ph'.*, a phagocytic cell which is still attached to the endothelium; *Erbl.*, erythroblasts; *Hem.*, hemocytoblasts; *Norm.*, normoblasts; *Norm. pcy.*, normoblasts with pyknotic nuclei; *Prbl.*, proerythroblasts; *Prim. erbl.*, primitive erythroblasts. Magnification is slightly less than that of Figure 7-15. (Redrawn from Maximow, Arch. Mikrosc. Anat. 73, 1909.)

comes functional in the 3rd fetal month. The sequence of differentiating cells in fetal marrow is similar to that described under "Blood Development" (page 225). With the advent of marrow as a hemopoietic organ, the number of circulating normoblasts decreases and nonnucleated erythrocytes become predominant.

White (yellow) marrow is composed chiefly of fat cells, but it can readily change to red marrow when there is an increased demand for blood cells (chapter 6).

References

ACKERMAN, G. Cytochemical properties of the blood basophilic granulocyte. Ann. N. Y. Acad. Sci. 103:376–393, 1963.

ACKERMAN, G. A. The lymphocyte: its morphology and embryological origin. *In* The Lymphocyte in Immunology and Haemopoiesis (Bristol Symposium, Yoffey, J. M., editor), pp. 11–30. Edward Arnold, Ltd., London, 1967.

BAGGIOLINI, M., HIRSCH, J. G., AND DE DUVE, C. Resolution of granules from rabbit heterophil leucocytes into distinct populations by zonal sedimentation. J. Cell Biol. 40:529–541, 1969.

BAINTON, D. F. Sequential degranulation of the two types of polymorphonuclear leukocyte granules during phagocytosis of microorganisms, J. Cell Biol. 58:249–264, 1973.

BAINTON, D. F., ULLYOT, J. L., AND FARQUHAR, M. G. The development of neutrophilic polymorpho-

nuclear leukocytes in human bone marrow. J. Exp. Med. 139:907–934, 1971.

BAINTON, D. F., AND FARQUHAR, M. G. Differences in enzyme content of azurophil and specific granules of polymorphonuclear leukocytes. II. Cytochemistry and electron microscopy of bone marrow cells. J. Cell Biol. 39:299–317, 1968.

BAINTON, D. F., AND FARQUHAR, M. G. Segregation and packaging of granule enzymes in eosinophilic leukocytes. J. Cell Biol. 45:54–73, 1970.

BARR, R. D., WHANG-PENG, J., AND PERRY, S. Hemopoietic stem cells in human peripheral blood. Science 190:284–285, 1975.

BENNET, M., AND CUDKOWIZ, G. Functional and morphological characterization of stem cells: the unipotential role of "lymphocytes" of mouse marrow. *In* The Lymphocyte in Immunology and Haemopoiesis (Bristol Symposium, Yoffey, J. M., editor), pp. 183–194. Edward Arnold, Ltd., London, 1967.

BENTFIELD, M. E., NICHOLS, B. A., AND BAINTON, D. F. Ultrastructural localization of peroxidases in leukocytes of rat bone marrow and blood. Anat. Rec. 187:219–240, 1977.

BERMAN, I. The ultrastructure of erythroblastic islands and reticular cells in mouse bone marrow. J. Ultrastruct. Res. 11:291–313, 1967.

BESSIS, M. C. Cytological aspects of hemoglobin production. Harvey Lect. 55:125–156, 1963.

BLOOM, W., AND BARTELMEZ, G. W. Hematopoiesis in young human embryos. Am. J. Anat. 67:21–54, 1940.

BRAHIM, F., AND OSMOND, D. G. Migration of bone marrow lymphocytes demonstrated by selective bone marrow labelling with thymidine-H[3]. Anat. Rec. 168:139–159, 1970.

BRAUNSTEINER, H., AND ZUCKER-FRANKLIN, D. The

Physiology and Pathology of Leukocytes. Grune & Stratton, Inc., New York, 1962.

BRETZ, U., AND BAGGIOLINI, M. Biochemical and morphological characterization of azurophil and specific granules of human neutrophilic polymorphonuclear leukocytes. J. Cell Biol. 63:251–269, 1964.

COOPER, M. D., AND LAWTON, A. R., III. The development of the immune system. Sci. Am. 231:58–77, 1971.

DAVIDSON, W. M., AND SMITH, D. R. A morphological sex difference in the polymorphonuclear leucocytes. Br. Med. J. 2:6–7, 1954.

DEBRUYN, P. P. H. Locomotion of blood cells in tissue culture. Anat. Rec. 89:43–63, 1944.

DOWNEY, H. The myeloblast. In Handbook of Hematology (Downey, H., editor), vol. 3, pp. 1963–2041, 1938.

EDELMAN, G. M. Antibody structure and cellular specificity in the immune response. Harvey Lect. 68:149–184, 1974.

EVERETT, N. B., AND TYLER (CAFFREY), R. W. Lymphopoiesis in the thymus and other tissues: functional implications. Int. Rev. Cytol. 21:205–237, 1967.

EVERETT, N. B., CAFFREY, R. W., AND RIEKE, W. D. Recirculation of lymphocytes. Ann. N. Y. Acad. Sci. 113:887–897, 1964.

FISHER, J. W., AND GORDON, A. S. Conference: erythropoietin. Ann. N. Y. Acad. Sci. 149, 1968.

FORD, C. E., MICKLIN, H. S., EVANS, E. P., GRAY, J. G., AND OGDEN, D. A. The inflow of bone marrow cells to the thymus: studies with part-body irradiated mice injected with chromosome marked bone marrow and subjected to antigen stimulation. Ann. N. Y. Acad. Sci. 129:283–296, 1966.

GLASS, J., LAVIDER, L. M., AND ROBINSON, S. H. Studies of murine erythroid cell development. J. Cell Biol. 65:298–308, 1975.

GORDON, A. S. (moderator). Symposium: studies of leucocyte physiology. Ann. N. Y. Acad. Sci. 136:779–882, 1967.

GOWANS, J. L. The recirculation of lymphocytes from blood to lymph in the rat. J. Physiol. 143:84–85, 1958.

GOWANS, J. L. Lymphocytes. Harvey Lect. 64, 1969.

GOWANS, J. L. Differentiation of the cells which synthesize the immunoglobulins. Ann. Immunol. (Paris) 125 C:201–211, 1974.

HADEN, R. L. Factors influencing the size and shape of the red blood cell. In Blood, Heart and Circulation (F. R. Moulton, editor). A.A.A.S. Publ. no. 13, pp. 27–233. Science Press, Lancaster, Pa., 1940.

HUDSON, G., OSMOND, D. G., AND ROYLANCE, P. J. Cell-populations in the bone marrow of the normal guinea-pig. Acta Anat. 53:234–239, 1963.

KNISELY, M. H. The settling of sludge during life; first observations, evidences, and significances; a contribution to the biophysics of disease. Acta Anat. 44:7–64, 1961.

LERNER, R. A., AND DIXON, F. J. The human lymphocyte as an experimental animal. Sci. Am. 228:82–91, 1973.

LINMAN, J. W., AND BETHELL, F. H. Factors Controlling Erythropoiesis. Charles C Thomas, Springfield, Ill., 1960.

MARCHALONIS, J. J. Lymphocyte surface immunoglobulins. Science 190:20–29, 1975.

MARKS, P., AND RIFKIND, R. A. Protein synthesis: its control in erythropoiesis. Science 175:955–961, 1972.

MAXIMOW, A. The lymphocytes and plasma cells. Special Cytology (Cowdry, E. V., editor), vol. 2, pp. 601–648, 1932.

MENKIN, V. Factors concerned in the mobilization of leukocytes in inflammation. In Symposium on Leukocytic Functions. Ann. N. Y. Acad. Sci. 59:956–985, 1955.

MICKLEM, H. S., ANDERSON, M., AND ROSS, E. Limited potential of circulating hemopoietic stem cells. Nature 256:41–43, 1975.

MOORE, M. A. S., AND MECALF, D. Ontogeny of the hemopoietic system; yolk sac origin of in vivo and in vitro colony-forming cells in the developing mouse embryo. Br. J. Hematol. 18:279, 1970.

NICHOLS, B. A., BAINTON, D. F., AND FARQUHAR, M. G. Differentiation of monocytes. Origin, nature, and fate of their azurophil granules. J. Cell Biol. 50:498–515, 1971.

NICHOLS, B. A., AND BAINTON, D. F. Differentiation of human monocytes in bone marrow and blood: sequential formation of two granule populations. Lab. Invest. 29:27–40, 1973.

NOSSAL, G. J. V. The cellular basis of immunity. Harvey Lect. 63:179–211, 1968.

RIEKE, W. O., EVERETT, N. B., AND CAFFREY, R. W. The sizes and interrelations of lymphocytes in thoracic duct lymph and lymph node of normal and stimulated rats. Acta Haematol. 30:103–110, 1963.

RÖPKE, C., HOUGEN, H. P., AND EVERETT, N. B. Long-lived T and B lymphocytes in the bone marrow and thoracic duct lymph of the mouse. Cell. Immunol. 15:82–93, 1975.

RUBENSTEIN, A. S., AND TROBAUGH, F. E., JR. Ultrastructure of presumptive hematopoietic stem cells. Blood 42:61–80, 1973.

SABIN, F. R. Studies of living human blood cells. Bull. Johns Hopkins Hosp., 34:277–288, 1923.

SCHILLING, V. The Blood Picture (translated by Gradwohl). C. V. Mosby, St. Louis, 1929.

SCHLEICHER, E. M. The origin and nature of the Cabot ring bodies of erythrocytes. J. Lab. Clin. Med. 27:983–1000, 1942.

SHEMIN, D., AND RITTENBERG, D. The life span of the human red blood cell. J. Biol. Chem. 166:627–636, 1946.

SPEIRS, R. S. Cellular aspects of immune reactions. Bioscience 19:411–417, 1969.

SPEIRS, R. S. Lymphoid cell dependence of eosinophil response to antigen. II. Exp. Hematol. 1:150–158, 1973.

THORELL, B. Studies on the formation of cellular substances during blood cell production. Henry Kempton, London. Also Acta Med. Scand. Suppl. 200, 1947.

TYLER, R. W., EVERETT, N. B., AND SCHWARZ, M. R. Effect of antilymphocytic serum on rat lymphocytes. J. Immunol. 102:179–193, 1967.

VIETTA, E. S., AND UHR, J. W. Immunoglobulin-receptors revisited. A model for the differentiation of bone marrow-derived lymphocytes. Science 189:964–969, 1975.

WEISS, L. The hematopoietic microenvironment of the bone marrow: an ultrastructural study of the stroma in rats. Anat. Rec. 186:161–184, 1976.

WINTROBE, M. Clinical Hematology. Lea & Febiger, Philadelphia, 1961.

YAMADA, E. The fine structure of the megakaryocyte in the mouse spleen. Acta Anat. 29:267–290, 1957.

YOFFEY, J. M. (editor). The Lymphocyte in Immunology and Haemopoiesis (Bristol Symposium). Edward Arnold, Ltd., London, 1967.

ZUCKER-FRANKLIN, D. The ultrastructure of megakaryocytes and platelets. In Regulation of Hematopoiesis (Gordon, A. S., editor), vol. 2, pp. 1533–1586. Appleton-Century-Crofts, New York, 1970.

CHAPTER 8

Muscle

Virtually all cells in animal tissues are, at some time in their life cycle, contractile. The degree of contractility may be very subtle or quite obvious, but mobility and cellular shape change is a fundamental property. The tissues which we classify as *muscle* are those which in their differentiation have come to emphasize the property of contractility to a remarkable extent. These tissues are composed of cells whose cytoplasm is literally packed with the machinery necessary to bring about extreme, force-generating, and sometimes quite rapid changes in cell shape. Collectively the cells of muscular tissue are able to provide the motile force for activities as subtle as the constriction of an arteriole, as quick as the beat of a fly's wing, or as massive as the effort of a weight lifter. Indeed, even the morphogenetic cell shape changes and tissue movements associated with molding the proper shape of embryos (chapter 3) involve delicate mechanisms of contractility not unlike the mechanisms found in mature muscle cells.

In nature, there is a wide spectrum of forms and varieties of muscular cells. It ranges from cells which show only small portions of the cytoplasm specialized for contractility to others in which a massive and highly ordered array of organelles performs highly specified degrees and patterns of movement. In mammalian organs, it is possible to recognize three major classes of muscular tissue; *smooth* (or nonstriated),

skeletal, and *cardiac* (the latter two classed together as *striated*). All are derived embryonically from mesenchyme, with a very few interesting exceptions. Most smooth muscle is involuntary in action and takes its origin in splanchnic mesenchyme, but the smooth muscle associated with blood vessels and glands in the periphery of the body is derived from somatic mesenchyme. All skeletal muscle is of somatic mesenchymal origin and most of it is controllable voluntarily. The cardiac muscle of the heart is derived from a rather specialized splanchnic portion of the mesenchymal compartment, and of course it is involuntary.

Smooth Muscle

Smooth muscle is derived from loose mesenchyme, as most massively manifest in the splanchnic mesoderm surrounding the endodermal primitive gut epithelium and its appendages. Smooth muscle of many blood and lymphatic vessels arises from somatic mesenchyme. Exceptions to mesodermal origin are found in the iridic muscle of the eye and in modified muscle cells in the walls of sweat glands which are derived from ectodermal epithelial cells. As differentiation proceeds, some of the cells become recognizable as *myoblasts* by their elongated nuclei and spindle shape. New myoblasts continue to differentiate from mesenchymal cells during the early stages of development. Later, the division of existing myoblasts gradually takes the place of this differentiation in the production of new muscular elements.

As the young muscle cells differentiate, their cytoplasms become crowded with filamentous contractile elements, and the exterior surface of each acquires a surrounding *external lamina*. They are thus individually segregated from the surrounding connective tissue compartment.

Scattered oval nuclei around and among the groups of elongating myoblasts mark the presence of connective tissue fibroblasts. As the muscle cells develop into sheets or bundles, the fibroblasts and/or the muscle cells themselves synthesize and lay down collagenous, elastic, and reticular fibers.

Mature smooth muscle consists of fusiform or spindle-shaped cells with abundant cytoplasm, in whose central thickest portion the nucleus lies. As a rule, the cells are gathered into dense sheets or bands, but they may occur as isolated units scattered among connective tissue fibers in a tissue such as the dartos tunic of the scrotum.

Within the bands, the cells are roughly parallel to each other but irregularly and densely packed, so that the narrow portion of one cell lies against the wide portions of its neighbors. The shape varies according to the organ containing the muscle: for example, very long and slender in the walls of the intestine (Fig. 8-1), short and rela-

tively thick in walls of small arteries, or thrown into irregular folds and twists by elastic fibers in the walls of large arteries. The greatest diameter varies from 3 to 8 μm and the length from 15 to 200 μm, except in the pregnant uterus, where it may exceed ½ mm (500 μm). Outlines of the cells are indistinct in longitudinal views of either fresh material or prepared sections because of the overlapping, but are easily seen in cross sections. Here outlines are round, oval, or flattened and vary in size because the fusiform cells may be cut through thick central portions or at narrow ends (Figs. 8-2 and 8-3). Cells can be separated from one another by teasing after treatment with nitric acid (Fig. 8-1), so that their shape, central nuclei, and faint longitudinal striation can be seen.

The *nucleus* conforms to the outline of the cell, and its shape may therefore be oval, elongated, or flattened (Fig. 8-2). The nuclei of contracted cells usually have a folded or pleated outline, which can be seen in longitudinal sections.

The *cytoplasm* is dominated by longitudinally aligned filaments, which are specialized structures for contraction, but in addition it contains mitochondria, a Golgi complex, centrioles, endoplasmic reticulum, ribosomes, some glycogen, and occasional fat droplets. The filaments are not clearly visible in routine sections, but they can be detected as "fibrils" in fresh preparations after maceration in nitric or trichloracetic

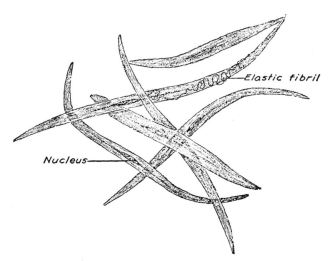

Fig. 8-1. Smooth muscle cells teased from intestine treated with nitric acid. Unstained. ×800.

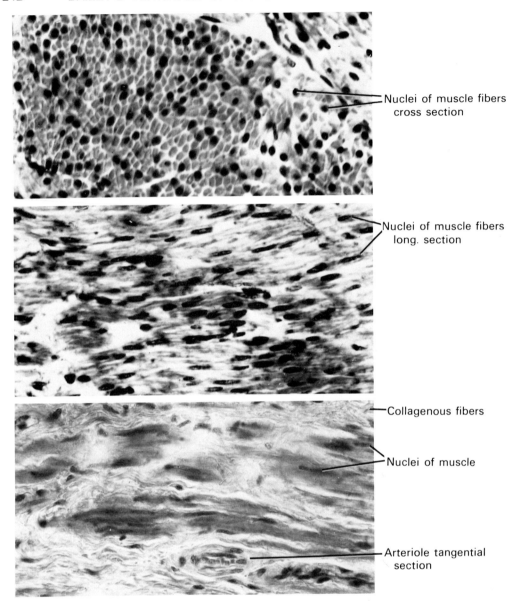

Nuclei of muscle fibers
cross section

Nuclei of muscle fibers
long. section

Collagenous fibers

Nuclei of muscle

Arteriole tangential
section

Fig. 8-2. Photomicrographs of smooth muscle. The *upper figure* shows the muscle fibers cut transversely; the *central* and *lower figures* show the fibers cut longitudinally. In the *central figure,* the fibers are seen in compact arrangement, with a minimum of associated connective tissue, whereas in the *lower figure* the fibers are interspersed with considerable connective tissue. *Upper* and *central* micrographs are from human urinary bladder; *lower* micrograph is from human rectum. All figures ×390.

acid. They represent aggregates of *myofilaments,* which can be seen in electron micrographs (Fig. 8-4). The filaments of smooth muscle cells differ from those in striated muscle in that they are not arranged in registered order (see under "Skeletal Muscle") and are not readily preserved.

Chemical studies show the presence of both contractile proteins, *actin* and *myosin,* in the filamentous fractions of smooth muscle. However, most of the filaments seen in electron micrographs of vertebrate smooth muscle cells correspond to the *thin* (actin) filaments of striated muscle. Coarse fila-

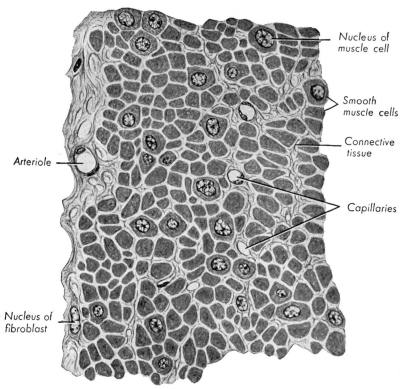

Fig. 8-3. Smooth muscle cut transversely, from the muscularis externa of human stomach. Hematoxylin and eosin. ×1665.

ments, identified as *thick* (myosin) filaments, can be seen in vertebrate smooth muscle, contracted or relaxed, after special fixation procedures (Fig. 8-5). They have not been visible in most of the routine electron micrographs published to date (Fig. 8-4). Therefore, some workers have postulated alternatively that most of the myosin of vertebrate smooth muscles is present in an unaggregated form, and furthermore that aggregation into visibly thick filaments occurs during tension production, a state requiring special fixation procedures for preservation. Thick and thin filaments are seen more readily in invertebrate than in vertebrate smooth muscle cells, and some of the so-called smooth muscle cells of invertebrates are intermediate in type between smooth and skeletal. The actin filaments of smooth muscles (vertebrate and invertebrate) often course obliquely in the cell and generally attach in characteristic dense condensations along the inner surface of the plasmalemma. Because the filaments are responsible for contraction of the mus-

cle cell, the generation of force by such an arrangement must also have an oblique component. Electron-dense regions are seen at intervals along the bundles of thin filaments and at places where the filaments attach to the plasmalemma. These dense areas form attachment sites for both the actin filaments and transversely oriented tonofilaments. They have been likened to the Z discs of striated muscle that appear to hold actin filaments in register (see below).

In routine hematoxylin and eosin-stained sections, the cytoplasm usually appears more or less homogeneous. The color tone of the muscle cytoplasm differs slightly from that of nearby collagen fibers because the ribosomes in the eosinophilic muscle cytoplasm bind hematoxylin, giving the muscle a slight purplish tint, in contrast with a more pure eosin color in collagen. These reactions are variable and the identification of the tissues should be based more on morphological characteristics than on tinctorial reactions. Masson's trichrome

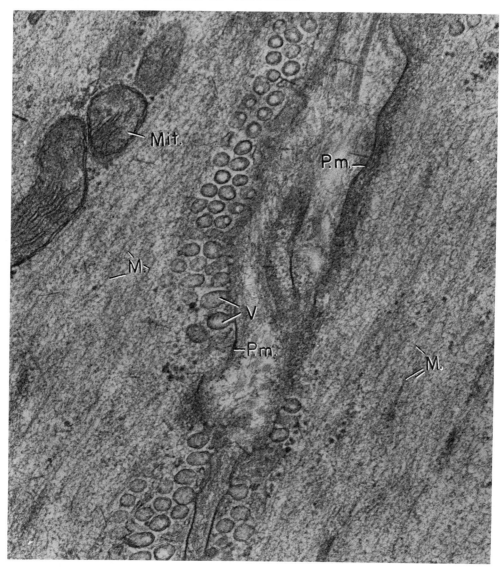

Fig. 8-4. Electron micrograph of portions of two smooth muscle cells from the esophagus of a bat. Note fine myofilaments (*M.*), mitochondria (*Mit.*), pinocytotic vesicles (*V.*), and plasma membranes (*P.m.*). ×57,750. (Courtesy of Dr. Keith Porter.)

stain simplifies the differentiation of smooth muscle from collagen because muscle is usually stained red in this technique, whereas collagen is colored blue or green, depending upon the stain modification used. Identification of smooth muscle in routine preparations stained with hematoxylin and eosin is further complicated when some of the cytoplasmic constituents are not preserved. Consequently the cytoplasm of smooth muscle cells often appears vacuolated and pale and is easily confused with

bundles of nerve fibers.

The *plasma membrane* of the smooth muscle cell in high resolution electron micrographs resembles that of most other animal cells, although the densities along its internal aspect plus the prominent external lamina over its outer surface give it a notably thickened appearance. In certain localized regions where adjacent muscle cells come into macular apposition, the external lamina is lacking and the adjacent membranes form *nexuses,* or *gap junctions* (chapter 4, Figs. 4-12 through 4-15). The nexuses of smooth muscle do not encircle the cells, as do the zonulae of epithelial cells; they probably facilitate transmission of impulses for contraction from one cell to another.

The external lamina of each smooth muscle cell forms a complete covering, except for the regions of nexuses, and appears to aid in holding the cells together. It is composed of an amorphous substance with many fine fibrils which blend peripherally with reticular and collagenous fibrils of the connective tissue. The reticular fibers can be demonstrated for light microscopy either by Bielchowsky's silver method or by the periodic acid-Schiff (PAS) technique. By resorcin-fuchsin, neighboring elastic fibers can be demonstrated. These are occasionally seen in macerated preparations as tiny coils around the cells (Fig. 8-1). Between the larger bundles of smooth muscle cells, coarser collagenous and elastic fibers are found (Figs. 8-2 and 8-3). Because smooth muscle in mammals either ends in soft parts or forms more or less continuous circular or spiral bands, there is no specialized connective tissue attachment such as the tendon of skeletal muscle.

The *contraction* of smooth muscle is apparently dependent upon a sliding interaction of thick and thin myofilaments, but details of the contractile mechanism are not as well understood as they are for skeletal muscle. The thick filaments are considerably longer (~2.2 μm) than those of skeletal muscle and are disposed in a ratio of about 1 thick filament/15 thin filaments. Although the filaments are apparently not arranged in orderly register, as they are in striated muscle, the contraction still appears to be basically dependent upon an interaction of myosin and actin. As will be seen in the discussion of striated muscle contraction, this interaction requires activation on the part of calcium ions released into the cytoplasm. The calcium reservoir is known in striated muscle, but not in smooth muscle. However, some evidence points toward the possibility that calcium ions are sequestered into smooth muscle cells through the action of numerous caveolae and vesicles which line the plasmalemma (Fig. 8-4).

The contraction of smooth muscle is slow and sustained; it contrasts with the range of skeletal muscle activity, which is generally more rapid and fatiguing. Two types of contraction have been observed. Each individual cell may contract in its entirety, or the contraction may pass over the cell in a wave, only part of each cell being in a state of contraction at a given instant. The oblique direction of the filaments and their attachment at the side of the cell, rather than a longitudinal end to end arrangement, seems to correlate with the ability for localized contraction. When the cells have been caught in a completely contracted state by the fixative, they appear shortened and stain more intensely by light microscopy. If a wave has been caught passing over the cell by the fixing reagent, the contracted portion is bulged and shortened and is more heavily stained than the rest of the cell, so that it looks like a swollen dark segment of the cell. These *contraction bands* have a tendency to extend in lines across the whole sheet of muscle so that the contracted swelling involves the center of one cell and the narrower extremities of its neighbors at the same time (Fig. 8-6).

There are *nerve endings* about smooth muscle cells, but motor terminations for every cell have not been demonstrated. It seems, therefore, that a supplemental type of transmission must be utilized to activate the cells distant from nerve endings. This might involve: (1) communicating junctions or nexuses as described above; (2) mechanical pull of a contracting cell on its neighbors by their connective tissue investments; and (3) action of chemical agents.

Smooth muscle is not as richly supplied with blood vessels as is skeletal or cardiac muscle. The arteries and veins are carried in the coarser septa of connective tissue. The capillaries lie in connective tissue between thin layers or small groups of cells rather than about individual cells. Connective tissue cells are rare or absent among the reticular fibrils between the muscle cells, unless associated with the blood vessels or larger connective tissue laminae.

Smooth muscle is found in the wall of the alimentary canal from the middle of the esophagus to the anus; gallbladder and hepatic ducts; dorsal wall of trachea and

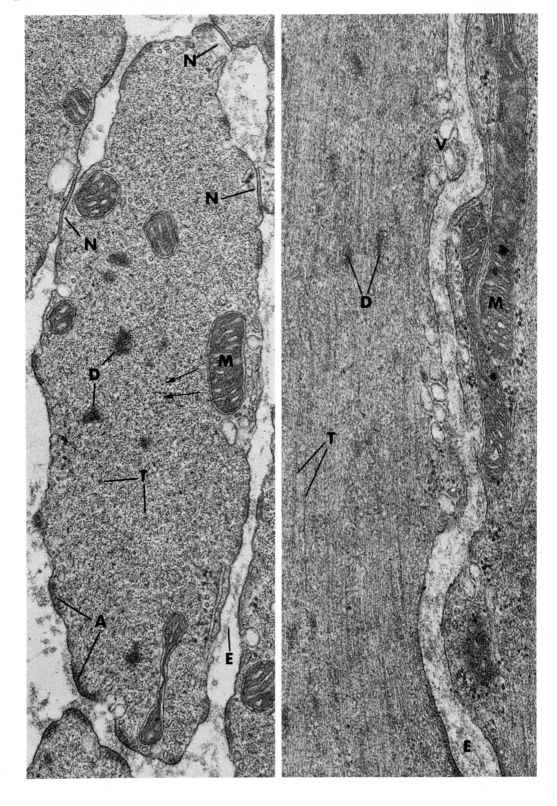

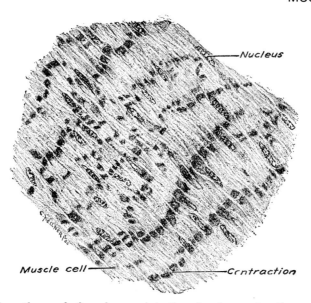

Fig. 8-6. Smooth muscle from human intestine showing contraction nodes. ×500.

whole bronchial tree; ureter, bladder, urethra, corpora cavernosa, testes and ducts, prostate and Cowper's glands; broad ligament, oviduct, uterus, and vagina; blood vessels; and larger lymphatics and spleen. It also is found in the skin in connection with hairs (arrectores pilorum) and occasionally in other places (e.g., corrugator cutis ani), and in the iris and ciliary body of the eye.

Proliferation of smooth muscle cells by mitotic division has been found in the uteri of virgin rabbits treated with female sex hormone, and formation of new muscle cells from undifferentiated cells during pregnancy has been described. The regenerative powers of the muscle coats of the alimentary tract are limited, however, and healing of wounds takes place principally by scar formation. The muscle cells of the walls of new blood vessels associated with healing processes have been described as coming from primitive types of perivascular connective tissue cells.

Skeletal Muscle

The smallest independent cellular units of mature skeletal muscle are called *fibers*. Although they are frequently referred to as cells, the more specific term fiber is preferable. They are grossly more complicated than the cells of smooth muscle; they have many nuclei and are larger than most cells. The fibers are grouped together into bundles called *fasciculi*. In some muscles (gluteus maximus, deltoideus), the bundles become larger than in others, giving the muscle a coarse-grained appearance when seen with the naked eye. The larger muscles are composed of many fasciculi.

The skeletal muscles of the trunk are derived from myotomal mesoderm of the embryonic segments or somites. Their

Fig. 8-5. Electron micrographs of smooth muscle from rat small intestine. The cells in the *left figure* are cut transversely. Thick (140-Å) filaments (*T*), perhaps consisting of myosin, are seen distributed among numerous thin (50-Å) actin filaments. Near the center of the *left micrograph*, a cluster of a third class of filaments, the noncontractile 100-Å intermediate filaments, can be identified (*arrows*). Note the nexuses (*N*) between adjacent smooth muscle cells and attachment placques (*A*) which may anchor filaments to the cell membrane. In the *right figure* the smooth muscle cells are cut longitudinally. Thick filaments (*T*) are seen paralleling the numerous thin filaments. Cytoplasmic dense bodies (*D*), which may function as anchoring devices among the thin filaments, are observed in both figures. Note also pinocytotic vesicles (*V*), external lamina (*E*), and mitochondria (*M*). ×67,200. (Courtesy of Dr. Richard M. Bois.)

eventual innervation and action reflects this segmental (*metameric*) origin. The limb muscles are formed from the mesenchyme of the limb buds. Muscles of the tongue are formed from head mesenchyme, and many muscles of the face, jaws, neck, and shoulders derive from mesenchyme of the branchial arches (the *branchiomeric musculature*). Head and branchial mesenchyme may be of neural crest origin.

As in the case of smooth muscle, the first evidence of differentiation is the elongation of the nuclei and cell bodies to form myoblasts (Fig. 8-7). Then an unusual step occurs. Fusion of myoblasts gives rise to multinucleated *myotubes*. Growth occurs by continued fusion of myoblasts and myotubes. There is no evidence of nuclear division either by amitosis or mitosis in the new multinucleated muscle cells (fibers). The specialized *myofilaments* make their appearance in the cytoplasm during or shortly after the fusion of myoblasts. Actin and myosin filaments appear separately and are arranged randomly at first. They generally arise in scattered regions of the cytoplasm and gradually become aligned into *myofibrils* as they accumulate, first as irregular bundles of filaments, and later with filaments aligned in lateral register at Z discs of the fibrils (see below). It has been shown that the cytogenesis of skeletal muscle in vitro is similar to that in vivo and that the organelles essential for contraction (myofilaments, T tubules, etc.) can differentiate in the absence of any nerve supply to the muscle.

The number of muscle fibers apparently does not increase significantly during the last month of fetal life or after birth. Increase in the overall size of a muscle is then brought about by the increase in diameter

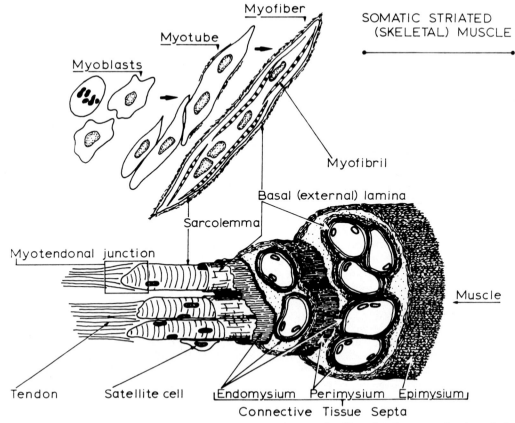

Fig. 8-7. Schematic representation of the stages in muscle fiber development (*top*) and the eventual organization of adjacent muscle fibers and their connective tissue ensheathments and attachments. (Drawing courtesy of Dr. Michael J. Cavey.)

of the fibers through the formation of more myofilaments. As myotubes differentiate into uniform muscle fibers, they invest themselves, individually or in groups, with external lamina, thus segregating themselves from surrounding connective tissue.

Not all of the primitive muscle fibers survive. Many of them fail to establish themselves as necessary units of the muscle and degenerate.

Fibers

The *fibers* are cylindrical structures which vary greatly in length. A common average length for a fiber in man is 3 cm, but lengths of 4 cm or more are not uncommon, and the shortest fibers in small muscles (e.g., stapedius) are less than 1 mm in length. Lengths of individual fibers can be studied best in teased preparations of excised muscles, particularly in those removed after rigor mortis has set in. The separation is made easier by treatment with nitric acid, which destroys the connective tissues that bind the fibers together. Three types of fibers can be dissected out with care and patience: (1) those extending from one end of the fasciculus to the other; (2) those beginning at one or the other end of the fasciculus and terminating within the substance of the bundle; and (3) those having both ends within the muscular substance (Fig. 8-8). Actually, each muscle is composed of many fasciculi, and the connections from the different fasciculi to the main tendon are via interfascicular, dense, regularly arranged connective tissue (i.e., by subdivisions of the main tendon).

The diameters of fibers vary from 10 to 100 μm, so that, in many cases, the fibers are visible to the naked eye. Although fibers of different thickness are intermingled in the same muscle, there is a more or less typical size for each muscle, and some correlation has been found between the heaviness of the work a muscle performs and the thickness of its fibers. Fibers in the delicate ocular muscles are much smaller than those of a bulky muscle like the gastrocnemius (Fig. 8-9). The fibers of a well nourished individual are thicker than those of one who is emaciated. Moreover, the increase in size of a muscle which takes place during the growth of an individual or which is brought about by exercise, is due to an increase in the size of its fibers rather than an increase in their number.

Skeletal muscle fibers also vary in diameter in different classes of vertebrates. For example, the fibers of amphibians and fishes are generally thicker, whereas those of birds are thinner, than those of mammals.

When a fresh muscle fiber is teased and broken, a thin, transparent covering membrane known as the *sarcolemma* (from the Greek *sarx,* flesh, + *lemma,* husk) is visible under the light microscope. Electron micrographs reveal that it is composed of a plasmalemma plus an external lamina and occasional reticular fibers. Nevertheless, it has become common to use the term *sarcolemma* for the plasmalemma of muscle cells. Inside the sarcolemma are the nuclei and the massive cross-striated contractile organelles, the *myofibrillae.* Surrounding the fibrillae and accumulated near the nuclei is the more fluid portion of the fiber, which is called the *sarcoplasm.* It corresponds to the background cytoplasm of other cells.

Because of its unique mode of development, each skeletal muscle fiber comes to

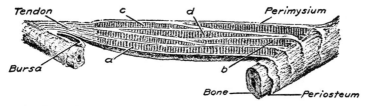

Fig. 8-8. Diagram of muscle attachment to skeleton and relation of fibers to each other within a fasciculus. *a,* fiber extends the length of fasciculus; *b,* fiber begins at periosteum but ends in muscle; *c,* fiber begins at tendon but ends in muscle; *d,* both ends of fiber within the muscle (Redrawn from Braus.)

possess many *nuclei,* several hundred appearing within a fiber of average size. The characteristic position for these nuclei in mammals is directly under the sarcolemma (Figs. 8-10, 8-11, and 8-13), but occasionally a fiber may be found with some nuclei in the interior. The nuclei are flattened, oval, frequently elongated, and of approximately the same size as the nuclei of neighboring connective tissue cells. They are scattered along the fiber in irregular spirals or longitudinal rows. In fresh muscle, they are difficult to see by light microscopy, faintly outlined against the background of striated substance. In fixed preparations, they show a loose network of chromatin threads and granules. The interior position is more frequently encountered in less differentiated

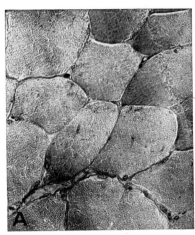 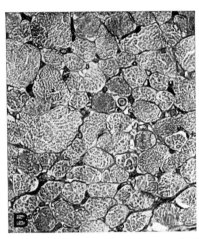

Fig. 8-9. Relative diameters of human muscle fibers. *A*, gastrocnemius; *B*, ocular muscle. The muscles were taken from the same subject, a middle-aged adult, and were photographed at the same magnification. ×335.

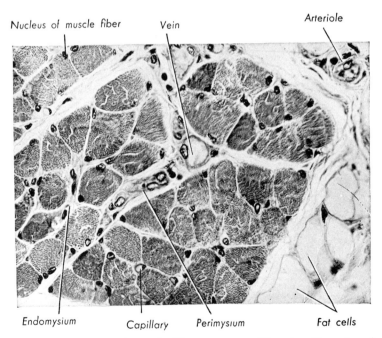

Nucleus of muscle fiber   Vein   Arteriole

Endomysium   Capillary   Perimysium   Fat cells

Fig. 8-10. Cross section of skeletal muscle. Human tongue. Hematoxylin and eosin. Photomicrograph, ×510.

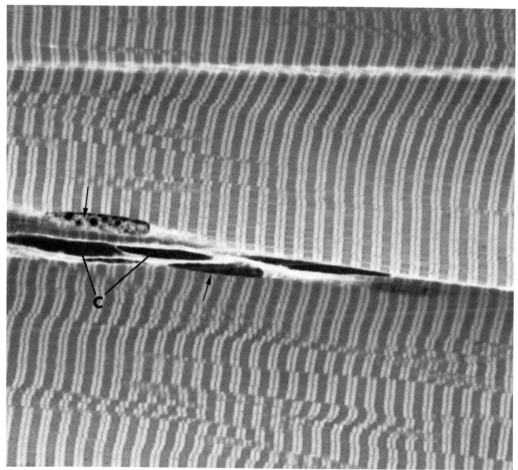

Fig. 8-11. High magnification light micrograph of plastic-embedded longitudinally sectioned skeletal muscle. Portions of three fibers are visible. Flattened myonuclei (*arrows*) lie beneath the cell membranes of two of the fibers. Equally flattened connective tissues cells (*C*) lie nearby. Although it is difficult to discern individual myofibrils, the registered banding patterns which form the cross striations of each fiber are obvious. A bands are dark and wide and I bands are light and of about equal width. Each I band is bisected by a narrow dark line, the Z disc. Close inspection reveals a slightly lighter midportion of each A band, the H band. In a few regions a faint dark line, the M band, can be discerned midway within H bands. ×2,000.

muscles, particularly in the so-called dark fibers or those rich in sarcoplasm. Interior nuclei are of common occurrence in the lower vertebrates, and in skeletal muscles of insects it is usual for the nuclei to form an axial column in the center of the fiber.

Myofibrils

Skeletal muscle examined with comparatively low magnification has a striking and characteristic appearance resulting from the regular alternation of light and dark stripes or striations across each fiber (Figs.

8-11 and 8-12). These striations are visible whether the muscle is living, freshly removed from the body, or fixed and stained, and in either ordinary transmitted light or polarized light. The bands are produced by the side-by-side alignment of alternating light and dark segments of longitudinally oriented myofibrils. *Myofibrils* range from 1 to 2 μm in diameter for the most part but may be as small as 0.2 μm.

In a cross section of a fiber, the myofibrils are usually visible as punctate densities with individual size and shape. They are separated from each other by narrow re-

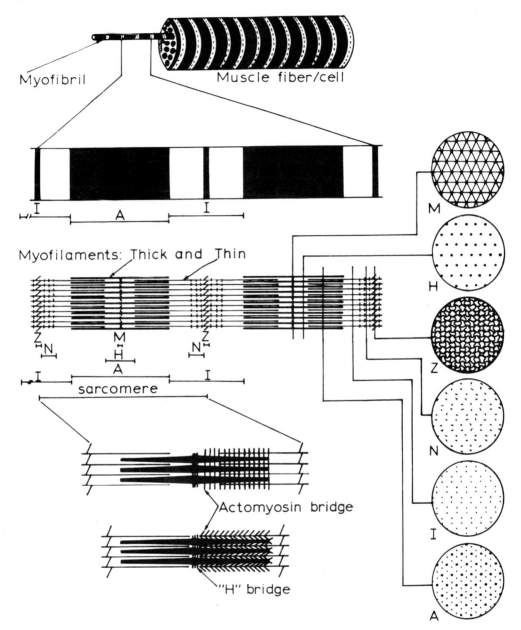

Fig. 8-12. Schematic representation of the organization of two sarcomeres along a myofibril removed from a muscle fiber. Details of the sarcomeres and their bands as revealed by electron microscopic techniques are shown in the *lower portion* of the diagram. The *circled images* to the *right* represent thin cross sections through various regions of a sarcomere. At *bottom left,* component filamentous parts of a single sarcomere are shown in relaxed and contracted states. (Diagram courtesy of Dr. Michael J. Cavey.)

gions of clear *sarcoplasm* (Fig. 8-10). When the sarcoplasm is distributed irregularly, the fibrils seem segregated into groups known as Cohnheim's fields.

The *cross striations* are a property of the myofibrillae, and they usually stand out clearly in longitudinal sections of fixed muscle. They color readily with a variety of dyes. The more refractive segments are deeply colored, whereas the less refractive ones are pale. The broad darkly staining band is doubly refractive or *anisotropic* when studied under polarized light, and therefore it is known as the *A band*. The light-staining band is relatively monorefringent or *isotropic* when studied under the polarizing microscope, and therefore it is known as the *I band*. Each of these bands is bisected by a narrow zone. It is dense in the I bands and designated Z line or disc (from the German *Zwishenscheibe*, between disc). The line bisecting the A band is pale and is designated H (both from the German *Hell*, light, and from the name of the discoverer, Hensen) (compare Figs. 8-11 and 8-12).

The portion of fibril between two successive Z discs is the fundamental unit of contraction along each myofibril. Each such unit is called a *sarcomere*. Its length in relaxed mammalian muscle is 2 to 3 μm. It may be stretched to a greater length, and in greatly contracted fibers it may be reduced to about 1 μm. Insect muscles with sarcomeres 14 μm long have been described.

With the electron microscope all of the cross bands or discs observed with the light microscope are revealed, plus some additional bands (Fig. 8-12). Moreover, the sarcomeres of each myofibril can be seen to be an orderly assembly of much finer filaments. Two filament types predominate; these are known collectively as *myofilaments* because their interaction results in the generation of contractile force. One of the myofilament types has a diameter of about 100 Å, whereas the other type is only 50 Å in diameter. The *thick (myosin) filaments* have a length of approximately 1.5 μm and extend from one end of the A band to the other. The *thin (actin) filaments* extend from either side of the Z line, across the adjacent I band, and into the A band as far as the H zone (Figs. 8-12 to 8-15). Thus, the cross bands seen with the light microscope are related to the distribution and overlap of interdigitating myofilaments as revealed by the electron microscope.

The distribution of the myofilaments can be seen to advantage in electron micrographs when the myofibrils are sectioned transversely (Figs. 8-16 and 8-17). Sections across the I band show only thin filaments, those through the extremities of the A band have both thick and thin filaments, and those through the H zone have only thick filaments. The two types of filaments have a precise relationship to each other in the A band regions where they interdigitate. As seen in cross sections, they have a remarkably constant hexagonal arrangement, with one thick filament in the center of a hexagon of six thin filaments (see also Fig. 8-18). The thick filaments are arranged as triangles with one thin filament at the center of each triangle. Close inspection reveals thin cross bridges extending from each myosin filament to link it with its neighboring actin filaments.

Actin filaments terminate at the Z disc, a filamentous network which serves as an orderly attachment of the actin filaments of one sarcomere to those of the next. Z disc filaments appear reinforced with a dense sarcoplasmic matrix material in many striated muscles. Although the pattern of filamentous arrangement within the Z disc can be deduced from high resolution electron micrographs (Fig. 8-19), the precise molecular mechanism for actin-to-actin linkage there is not well understood. Various models have been proposed; some anticipate direct actin-to-actin interaction, whereas others rely upon the presence of intermediary linking molecules such as tropomyosin. According to the most obvious model, there are separate filamentous attachments across the Z disc linking the tips of the actin filaments. An alternative structure could be that adjacent actin filaments or tropomyosin associated with them join in the form of hairpin loops in the Z disc region, and that the loops from adjoining sarcomeres are interlinked.

Myosin filaments seem held in register by virtue of some form of attachment in the center of the H band, the so-called M line or disc (Figs. 8-12 and 8-14). Here each myosin filament is connected with its neighboring myosin filaments by slender, transversely oriented filaments about 40 Å in diameter, and these latter filaments may be interconnected and supported by other slender filaments that course parallel to the myosin filaments. Like smooth muscle cells, striated muscle is known to contain 100-Å supportive filaments, or tonofilaments. However, the exact architecture of this noncontractile cytoskeleton and its relation to the contractile system have not been well resolved. Microtubules may also play an important supportive role, particularly in myoblasts and myotubes. None of these filaments and microtubules are to be confused with cross bridges between myosin and actin filaments, which have an important role in the mechanisms of contraction.

Further details on actin and myosin fila-

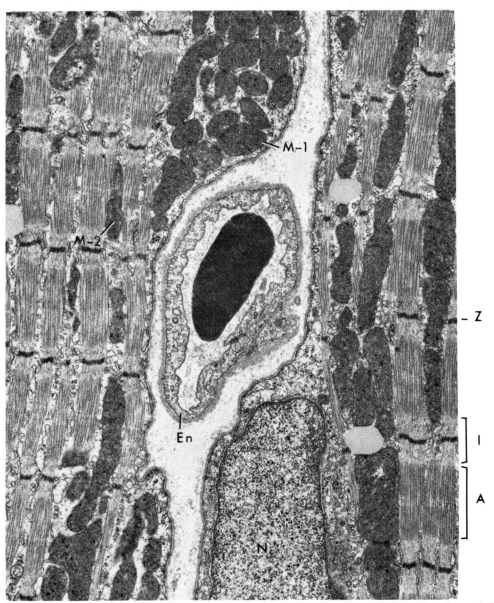

Fig. 8-13. Electron micrograph showing portions of two skeletal muscle fibers. The plane of the section cuts only one of the muscle fiber nuclei (*N*). Numerous mitochondria (*M-1*) are seen in the sarcoplasm of the subsarcolemmal region of each fiber and additional mitochondria (*M-2*) are present in the sarcoplasm between myofibrils. The anisotropic or A bands (*A*) of each myofibril are dark and the isotropic or I bands (*I*) are relatively light. Each of the latter is bisected by a dense Z disc (*Z*). Caveolae and vesicles can be seen in the cytoplasm of the endothelium (*En*) of a capillary located in the connective tissue between the muscle fibers. Extrinsic eye muscle of slow loris. ×14,000. (Micrograph, in collaboration with Mary Ann Cahill.)

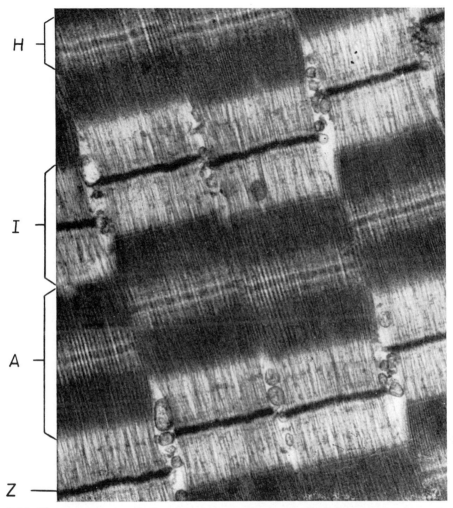

Fig. 8-14. Electron micrograph showing portions of four myofibrils from skeletal muscle, taken from rabbit psoas muscle. The anisotropic bands (*A*) are dense for most of their extent; they are bisected by lighter bands (*H*), within which there is a thin dense M band (unlabeled). The isotropic bands (*I*) are light regions, each bisected by a relatively dense, narrow line (*Z*). ×26,000. (Courtesy of Dr. H. E. Huxley.)

ments have been obtained by electron microscope studies of negatively stained, isolated filaments and from X-ray diffraction studies (Fig. 8-20). Each actin filament is composed of two strands of *F actin* (fibrous actin) coiled in a helix. Each F actin filament is a polymer of about 200 small globular units, *G actin* monomers. *Tropomyosin* and *troponin,* newly described regulatory proteins, are associated with the actin filaments. Tropomyosin is believed to be helically wound along the grooves of the F actin double helix and troponin is thought to occupy specific active sites as globular

molecules inserted at each half-turn of the same helix.

Myosin filaments are composed of long molecular subunits consisting of *light meromyosin* and *heavy meromyosin.* The former are packed together longitudinally, to form the rigid backbone of the myosin filament. Each is extended by the addition of a more flexible heavy meromyosin subunit. Heavy meromyosin subunits consist of a rodlike portion with a globular head. The rod portion lies parallel to the backbone myosin filament in relaxed muscle, and the globular head extends laterally as

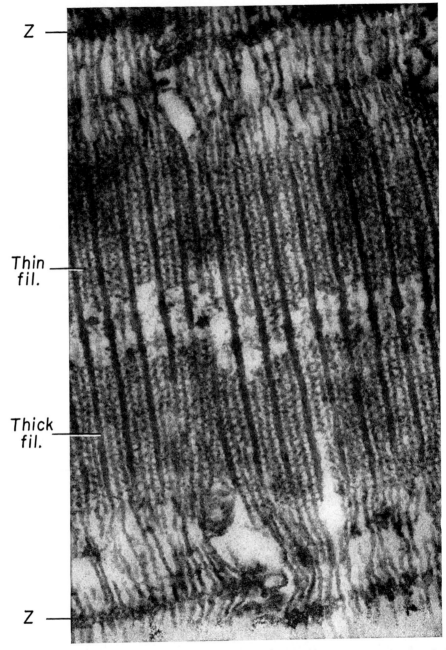

Fig. 8-15. High magnification electron micrograph of longitudinal section of relaxed skeletal muscle, taken from rabbit psoas muscle. The thick myosin filaments (*Thick fil.*) extend throughout the length of the A band and the thin actin filaments (*Thin fil.*) are found in the I band and in a part of A; they do not continue through the H band, although there is some indication of a connecting protein of undetermined nature linking thickened portions of the thick filaments in the center of the H band (M line). The actin filaments are twice as numerous as the myosin ones, but they are seen in this manner only when the section passes through the fibers in a plane, as indicated in Fig. 8-18. Heavy meromyosin cross linkages from myosin to actin are visible. ×148,000. (Courtesy of Dr. H. E. Huxley.)

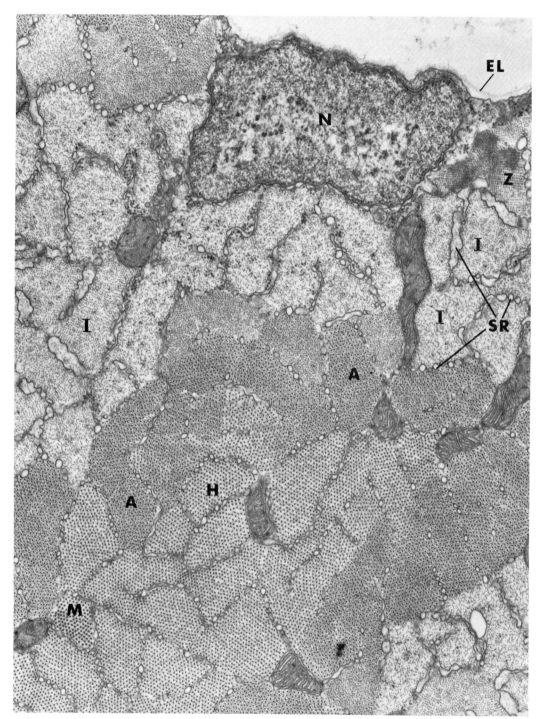

Fig. 8-16. Electron micrograph of a cross section of a small portion of a "fast" skeletal muscle fiber. The nucleus (*N*) lies just inside the sarcolemma and the external lamina (*EL*). *Z, I, A, H,* and *M* refer to planes of section through corresponding bands of sarcomeres (compare to diagram in Fig. 8-12). The sarcoplasmic reticulum (*SR*) is abundant and forms an ensheathment around individual myofibrils. Note that the tubular sarcoplasmic reticulum expands into terminal cisternae in regions where it approaches the Z disc. This sample is from amphibian skeletal muscle. ×32,500. (Micrograph in collaboration with Mary Ann Cahill.)

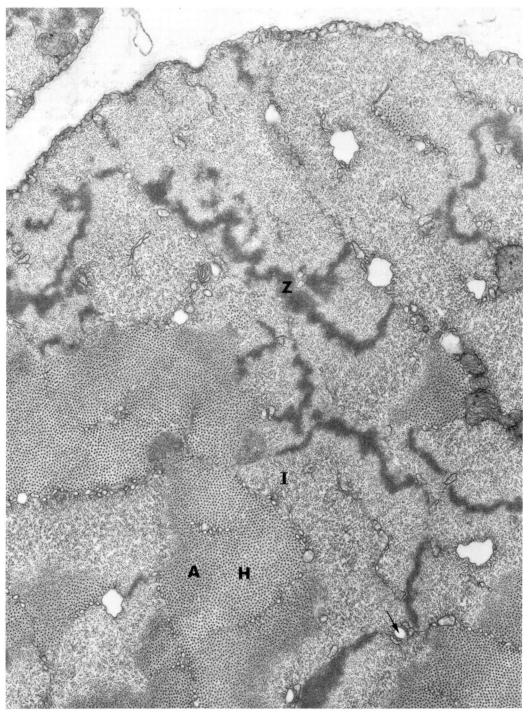

Fig. 8-17. Electron micrograph of a cross section through a small portion of amphibian tonic ("slow") skeletal muscle. Note that the cross sectional appearance of A, H, and I bands is essentially identical to that of fast muscle, as shown in Fig. 8-16. However, the Z disc (*Z*) is much more dense in its matrix component and irregular in profile. The sarcoplasmic reticulum is also more sparse, and individual myofibrils are less distinct in cross sectional view. A T tubule (*arrow*) is seen wedged between two small sarcoplasmic reticulum terminal cisterns. Other T tubules are visibly and probably artifactually dilated in this specimen. ×32,500. (Micrograph in collaboration with Mary Ann Cahill.)

MUSCLE

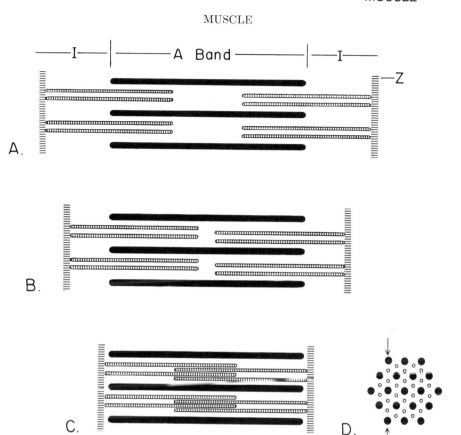

Fig. 8-18. Diagram showing changes in fine structure of skeletal muscle during contraction. *A*, resting muscle; *B*, partially contracted; *C*, contracted; and *D*, arrangement of myofilaments as seen in a cross section through the anisotropic band. Note that longitudinal sections (*A, B, C*) show the thick (myosin) filaments separated by two thin (actin) filaments when the plane of the section corresponds with that shown by the *arrows*; in sections perpendicular to the one indicated, two actin filaments usually are superimposed and appear as one thin filament for each thick one. Note that the isotropic (*I*) band shortens and disappears during contraction, whereas the anisotropic (*A*) band maintains its length over a wide range of muscle lengths. In extreme contractions, beyond that illustrated, the ends of the myosin filaments of one sarcomere meet with those of adjacent sarcomeres and crumple along the *Z* line, giving rise to new band patterns. Not illustrated is the fact that sarcomeric girth is increased concurrently with contracture. (Diagrams based on illustrations and descriptions by H. E. Huxley.)

a cross bridge from the thick myosin filament to the actin (Figs. 8-20 and 8-15). The myosin molecules are polarized in the sense that the heavy meromyosin subunits are always aligned with their globular heads directed away from the midpoint of the backbone filament. Thus they face in opposite directions on opposite sides of the M lines in relaxed muscle. It is of interest that the cross bridges are absent from the M line itself, where the myosin filaments are held in register by their own connecting

latticework. Adenosine triphosphatase and actin-binding sites are apparently located in or on the globular region of the heavy meromyosin.

In a given muscle there is established during development an appropriate proportion of fibers which contract rapidly (*phasic* fibers) and ones which contract in a slower and more prolonged fashion (*tonic* fibers). Although these have been occasionally rigidly classified as "fast" and "slow," respectively, it now appears that there is a fairly

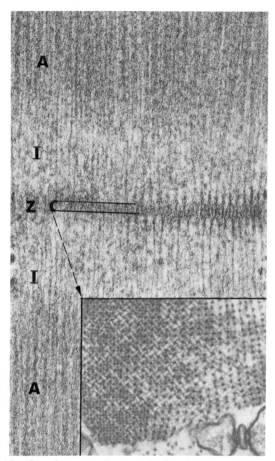

Fig. 8-19. High magnification electron micrograph showing a portion of a Z disc (*Z*) as seen in a longitudinal section of skeletal muscle. The Z disc is flanked by its adjacent I band (*I*) and nearby A bands (*A*) of two adjacent sarcomeres. The *inset* depicts details of the Z disc when seen in a cross section, the plane and thickness of which is indicated by *brackets* and *arrow*. A nearby T tubule and two terminal cisterns are seen in the *lower right* of the *inset*. Amphibian skeletal muscle. ×90,000. (Micrograph in collaboration with Mary Ann Cahill.)

continuous range in speed of contraction, and the extremes of the range display obvious corresponding fine structural differences in their myofibrillar makeup (compare Figs. 8-16 and 8-17). In fact, over the breadth of muscle that we commonly describe as skeletal there are far more variations than are usually implied in histology textbooks.

The Sarcoplasm

This is the cytoplasm of muscle fibers which fills all of the interstices between the myofibrils, around the nuclei, and beneath the sarcolemma. It contains a Golgi complex, variable amounts of mitochondria, en-

doplasmic (sarcoplasmic) reticulum, and a few ribosomes. It also contains glycogen and occasional lipid droplets.

Fibers which are rich in sarcoplasm tend to be slower (tonic) and have a dark appearance in the fresh state, whereas faster (phasic) fibers have less sarcoplasm and are lighter in color. In some species, e.g., turkey, the dark fibers are characteristically predominant in particular muscles and the light fibers predominate in other muscles. The two types of fibers as well as intermediate varieties are appropriately intermingled in human and most other mammalian muscles.

The *sarcoplasmic reticulum* is seen in electron micrographs as a network of cis-

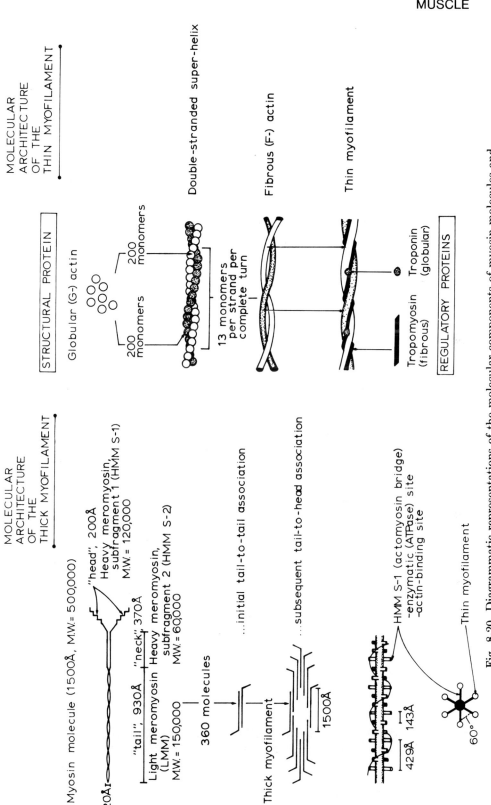

Fig. 8-20. Diagrammatic representations of the molecular components of myosin molecules and filaments (*left*) and actin molecules and filaments (*right*). The probable location of tropomyosin and troponin in relation to actin helices is also shown. See text for further explanation. (Diagrams courtesy of Dr. Michael J. Cavey.)

terns or membranous tubules which course between and around the myofibrils (Figs. 8-16 and 8-21 to 8-23). It is described as an agranular reticulum because the relatively few ribosomes present are scattered through the cytoplasm and are not aligned on the membranes. The cisterns course chiefly in a longitudinal direction, i.e., parallel with the direction of the myofibrils. In frog skeletal muscle, in which the sarcoplasmic reticulum has been studied extensively, it is found that lateral anastomoses between longitudinal cisterns form a perforated collar around the myofibrils at the level of the H band and broad *terminal cisterns* on each side of another membranous component, the *transverse tubule,* at the level of the Z line (Figs. 8-22 and 8-23). Each transverse tubule and its closely apposed two terminal cisterns constitute a *triad.* Studies of mammalian skeletal muscle show a similar triadic organization but often with transverse tubules and accompanying terminal cisterns at the level of each A-I junction, rather than at the Z disc. This provides two sets of tubules and terminal cisterns per sarcomere.

The transverse tubules are now known to be invaginations of the cell plasmalemma. Their lumen is open to the connective tissue around the muscle fiber and is actually extracellular space. They do not appear to open into the sarcoplasmic reticulum, but in the triads their lining membranes form junctions, or *couplings,* with the membranes of the terminal cisterns. The precise structure and relationship of the membranes in the junctional components that maintain a triad have not been resolved. However, it now seems clear that an action potential traveling along the transverse tubule membrane is able to signal the terminal cisterns across the junc-

tions. Transverse tubules, therefore, serve for rapid transmission of impulses from the exterior to the deepest regions of the cell, thus giving coordinated activity of all myofibrils.

In the study of longitudinal sections, it appears that Z discs, sarcomeres, and triads are aligned in perfect lateral register—from myofibril to myofibril—across the breadth of a muscle fiber. However, recent evidence gained from high voltage stereo electron microscopy of thick sections and serial reconstructions discloses that there is actually a slight displacement of register from one myofibril to the next such that the alignment of Z discs and triads courses spirally along the fiber, rather like the alignment of steps down a spiral staircase. The slight variation is thought to function in integrating and smoothing the contractions of sarcomeres throughout a given muscle cell.

The *mitochondria* or *sarcosomes* are found beneath the sarcolemma, around the nuclei, and in the sarcoplasm between the myofibrils (Figs. 8-13 and 8-21). In the last location, they are generally aligned with their long axis parallel to the direction of the myofibril, although they may be found encircling the myofibril transversely, particularly in the region overlying the Z disc.

Changes during Contraction

Morphological changes associated with contraction have been studied both in living and in fixed muscle. In both cases, the fiber as a whole becomes shorter and broader when it contracts. Each sarcomere also becomes shorter and broader (Fig. 8-18). The isotropic or I band becomes shorter as the sarcomere becomes shorter, and it disappears when the fibers are stimulated to

Fig. 8-21. Electron micrograph depicting portions of two fibers of amphibian skeletal muscle. The picture shows the interfibrillar components of the muscle fiber in addition to the fine structure of the myofibrils. Note the external lamina (*El*), the mitochondria (*M*), the longitudinally oriented elements of the sarcoplasmic reticulum (*Lsr*), and the dilated terminal cisterns (*Tcr*) of the reticulum. The transverse tubules (*Tt*), invaginations of the sarcolemma, are also seen. The *inset, upper left,* shows, at higher magnification and in a plane perpendicular to the rest of the plate, the relationship of a transverse tubule to the terminal cisterns of the reticulum. The transverse tubule with a dilated cistern on each side constitutes a triad. A nerve ending (*Ne*) on a muscle fiber is seen in the *lower half* of the picture. Note the presynaptic vesicles (*psv*) in the nerve terminal and the junctional folds (*Jf*) of the sarcolemma. ×27,300; *inset,* ×61,870. (Micrograph in collaboration with Mary Ann Cahill.)

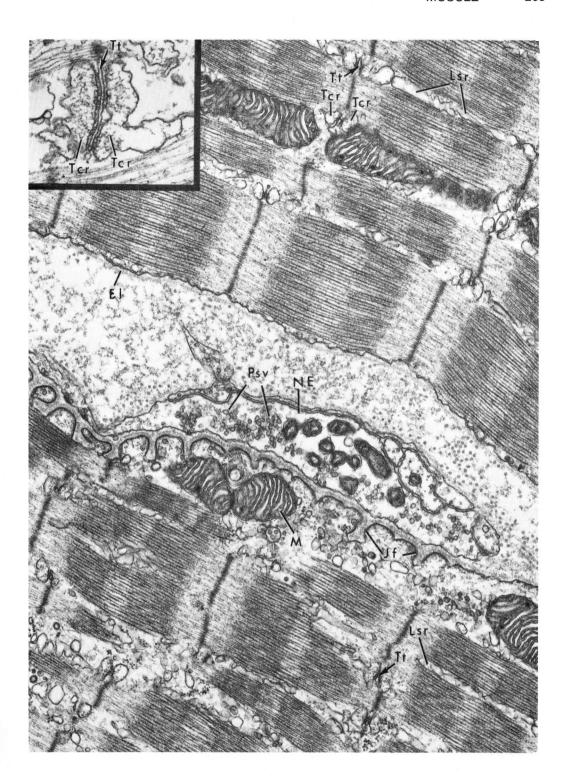

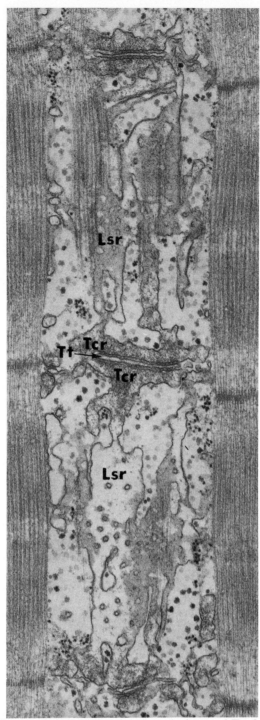

Fig. 8-22. Electron micrograph of the sarcoplasmic reticulum and T tubular system of amphibian skeletal muscle. The section plane in this micrograph has passed just to one side of a myofibril, thus intersecting the nearby sarcoplasmic reticulum. Adjacent myofibrils are shown in longitudinal section on *left* and *right* edges of the micrograph. Longitudinal elements of the sarcoplasmic reticulum (*Lsr*) are seen to be perforated by tiny round cytoplasmic passageways. The adjacent sarcoplasm contains densely stained glycogen granules. Each longitudinal element can be traced into a terminal cistern (*Tcr*) which is filled by a dense flocculent material. At the level of the Z disc, two terminal cisterns flank a transverse tubule (*Tt*) which has been cut lengthwise. Hence, the triad formed by these elements is seen face on in this section. Similar images are seen at the levels of the next Z discs (top and bottom). Compare this electron micrograph with Figure 8-23. ×34,000. (Micrograph in collaboration with Mary Ann Cahill.)

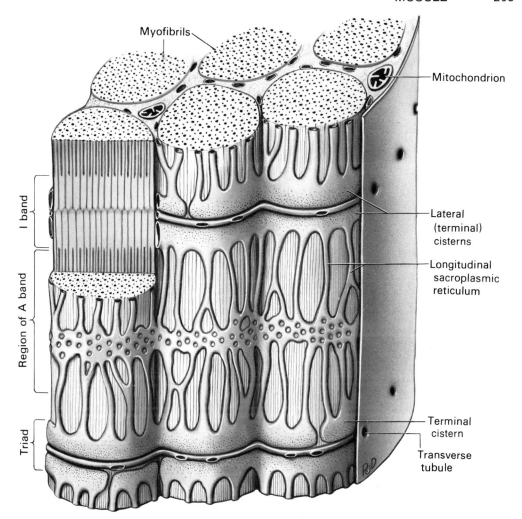

Fig. 8-23. Diagrammatic three-dimensional drawing to show the interrelationships of myofibrils, transverse tubules (T tubules), and elements of the sarcoplasmic reticulum in skeletal muscle. The diagram is based on studies of frog skeletal muscle in which the T tubules are located at the level of the Z line. In man, the T tubules are located at the level of the AI junctions, with two T tubules per sarcomere. The T tubules of cardiac muscle are located at the level of the Z line, as diagrammed here for skeletal muscle. The T tubules of cardiac muscle, however, are of much larger diameter than those of skeletal muscle and the cisterns of the sarcoplasmic reticulum are in a plexiform pattern that is continuous from one sarcomere to another. (Redrawn and modified after Peachey.)

contract to about 50% of their resting length. The H zone of the A band gradually disappears concurrently. The total length of the A band, on the other hand, remains constant during normal cycles of contraction and relaxtion. The A band seems to shorten only when contraction is so extreme that it produces a concentration of dense material along the Z disc, forming a darkly staining *contraction band*. It is postulated that this is due to overlap of the ends of the thick (myosin) filaments against the Z disc.

Electron micrographs of *contracted* muscle show an interdigitation of the thick and thin filaments throughout the length of the sarcomere, in contrast with the arrangement seen in resting muscle. Based on these findings, Hanson and Huxley first proposed a *sliding filament* mechanism of contraction (Fig. 8-18). In resting muscle, the thick and thin (myosin and actin) filaments are presumably not firmly attached to each other because a relaxed muscle can be stretched mechanically beyond its normal rest length. During muscle contraction, the cross bridges of the myosin filaments connect progressively with increasing numbers of active sites on neighboring actin filaments, and the actin filaments are drawn farther into the A band. The heavy meromyosin heads of the cross bridges each appear to attach to and interact with one active site after another along the actin filament helix as the latter is pulled into the A band.

When a nerve to a muscle is stimulated, a depolarization wave (action potential) spreads rapidly over the muscle cell membrane and over the membranes lining the T tubules to the deepest regions of the cell. Presumably a change in the membrane potential of the T tubules induces, in some manner, a reaction in the adjacent terminal cisterns. The result is that calcium is released from its storage place in that part of the sarcoplasmic reticulum into the sarcoplasm immediately bathing the myofibrils. Such freed calcium is necessary for the actin-myosin interaction to occur. According to one of several current theories, calcium operates by invoking a steric conformational change on the protein *troponin*, which otherwise acts as a safety catch, preventing activation of myosin adenosine triphosphatase by actin (when calcium is absent). The activation occurs as soon as calcium can be bound by troponin. Adenosine triphosphatase, as noted earlier, is present in the cross bridges, or globular heads, of heavy meromyosin molecules. The latter then readily swing to join with active actin sites by reason of the flexible or hingelike neck attaching the heavy meromyosin to the light meromyosin filament. In the process of contraction, adenosine triphosphate (ATP) is changed to adenosine diphosphate (ADP), with the release of energy. Apparently a phosphate group is split from ATP each time a cross bridge goes through a cycle of attachment and release at each successive actin binding site. When removal of phosphate groups from ATP stops, there is no further action of myosin-actin cross bridges, and the muscle returns to its resting state. At the same time, calcium is withdrawn from the sarcoplasm back to the sarcoplasmic reticulum. ADP is rephosphorylated into ATP before the muscle is ready for contraction again. Sarcosomes (mitochondria) carrying the enzymes of the citric acid cycle have an important role in the formation and maintenance of ATP.

Connective Tissue

Surrounding each muscle fiber is an external lamina and then a sheath of very delicate, irregularly woven reticular fibrils plus their surrounding ground substance fluids and other molecules (Fig. 8-7 and *center*, Fig. 8-21). It is called the *endomysium*. At many points, the delicate fibrils combine into stronger strands, which merge with collagenous connective tissue fibers. The collagenous fibers, mingled with elastic fibers, form a more or less complete connective tissue sheath about groups of a dozen or more muscle fibers to make up a *fasciculus*. The fasciculi are in turn bound into larger and larger orders of bundles, and the entire muscle has as its outer investment the deep fascia seen in gross anatomy. The outermost sheath of connective tissue is called the *epimysium*, and the tissue surrounding the fasciculi and dividing the muscle by septa is called the *perimysium*.

Muscle-Tendon Attachment

At the ends of a muscle, its fibers are attached securely either to tendon, to periosteum, or to some fibrous connective tissue structure. In light microscopic sections stained with ordinary dyes, the fibrils of the muscle fiber often appear to be continuous with those of the tendon. The striations of the muscle fiber decrease in distinctness, so that the exact point at which they disappear and the tendon fibers begin is uncertain. Sections stained for reticular fibers by the Bielschowsky silver method show that the reticular fibers associated with the sarcolemma become aggregated into strands as they converge around the end of the muscle fiber, and that the strands become continuous with fiber bundles of the tendon (Fig. 8-24). Connective tissue fibers do not penetrate the sarcolemma but merely extend into indentations. Electron micrographs have confirmed these conclusions and have shown in detail how the connective tissue fibers are inserted into invaginations of the sarcolemma (Fig. 8-25). There they are apparently attached firmly to the external lamina, which in turn is adherent to the sarcolemma. Within the muscle fiber, the actin (thin) filaments distal to the last sarcomere are drawn out and anchored by an as yet obscure mechanism to the cell membrane. Hence tension generated by the series of sarcomeres aligned in a fibril is transmitted successively to the cell membrane, to the external lamina, and then to collagen fibers of the tendon.

Blood Vessels

The larger branches of the arteries penetrate the muscle by following the septae of the perimysium. The arterioles which penetrate the fasciculi give off capillaries at abrupt angles. The capillary supply is very rich (Fig. 8-26), several capillaries having contact with each muscular fiber. The veins follow the arteries; even their smallest branches have valves.

Lymphatic capillaries are not found between the individual muscle fibers. They are present, however, in the connective tissue septa and along the blood vessels.

Nerves

Every skeletal muscle fiber receives at least one motor nerve ending from the central nervous system. The minute anatomy of the *motor end plates* is described in chapter 10. The sensory or afferent fibers are principally associated with specialized end organs known as *neuromuscular spindles*, also described in chapter 10.

Regeneration

In adult mammals, regeneration of skeletal muscle seems quite limited. However, regeneration of vertebrate skeletal muscle can occur after certain chemical, mechanical, or disease-mediated injuries. In most cases, shortly after injury, mononucleated myoblasts appear between the external lamina and the underlying degenerating muscle fiber. Subsequent stages of regen-

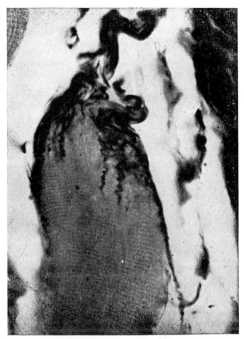

Fig. 8-24. Photomicrograph showing attachment of muscle to tendon. The muscle fiber is enclosed by a network of argyrophilic (reticular) fibers which project into invaginations of the sarcolemma at the end of the muscle fiber, thus giving a firm attachment of muscle and tendon. The argyrophilic fibers become continuous with bundles of collagenous fibers which are seen coursing toward a tendon at the *upper right* part of the micrograph. Monkey. Bielschowsky silver and Masson's stain. ×600. (After Goss.)

eration closely parallel embryonic myogenesis in that myoblasts proliferate and then undergo fusion to form multinucleated myotubes. Myotube differentiation is characterized principally by synthesis of contractile proteins leading to the maturation of a myofiber. Although motor end plates typically develop in association with the regenerating muscle fibers, complete return of functional activity is usually limited by the amount of scar tissue, which also develops within the regenerating muscle. The major source of regenerating myoblasts, at least in young mammals, appears to be *satellite cells* (Fig. 8-27), a small population of morphologically undifferentiated cells located between the external lamina and sarcolemma of uninjured muscle fibers. Satellite cells are probably derived from embryonic myoblasts. During postnatal muscle growth

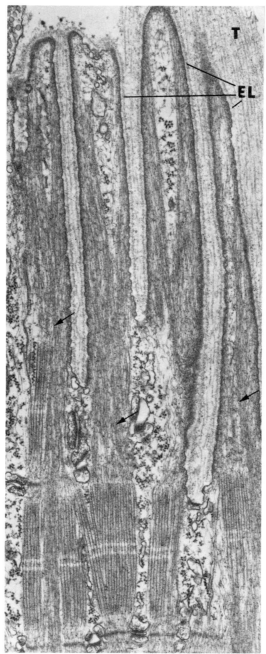

Fig. 8-25. Electron micrograph showing a longitudinal section through a myotendonal junction. The sarcolemma and its surrounding external lamina (*EL*) are folded into long finger-like extensions which interdigitate with collagen of a tendon (*T*). Actin filaments (*arrows*) of the last sarcomeres are drawn out into long filamentous extensions which attach to the sarcolemma along the faces of the interdigitations. ×24,600. (Micrograph in collaboration with Mary Ann Cahill.)

they fuse with their adjacent growing my-ofiber, resulting in an increase in the number of myonuclei. However, not all satellite cells fuse during muscle growth, and those that remain in adult skeletal muscle may have an important role in the repair and regeneration that does occur in mature skeletal muscle.

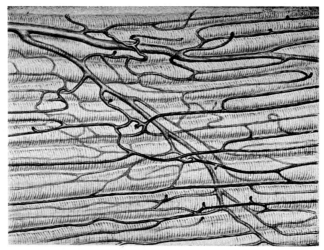

Fig. 8-26. Arterioles and capillaries in skeletal muscle. The vessels were filled with gelatin colored with carmine. ×140.

Cardiac Muscle

The heart muscle, or *myocardium,* is derived from splanchnic mesoderm and, as noted in chapter 3, is recognizable at a very early age in mammals. The mesenchymal primordium of the heart is at first sequestered well anterior to the neural plate in the early embryo, but with development of the head fold, it is swung into a position just beneath the developing foregut. Here it is formed into a three-layered tube which will ultimately be contorted and partitioned into the definitive four-chambered heart. The three layers are: an internal endothelial lining, which together with underlying connective tissue constitutes the *endocardium*; an external mesothelium, which together with its adjacent connective tissue comprises the *visceral pericardium*; and between those two layers, a mesenchymal bed, the so-called "*cardiac jelly,*" around which differentiation of cardiac myoblasts takes place. The result of the latter process is the formation of the myocardium, a distinct layer surrounding all of the chambers of the heart but much thicker around the ventricles than around the atria. Cardiac muscle fibers arise by differentiation and growth of single cells, not by a fusion of cells, as is the case for skeletal muscle fibers. Growth of the fibers occurs by formation of new myofilaments, particularly in the peripheral portion of the cytoplasm.

The myocardium of vertebrate hearts is therefore composed of *non-syncytial* muscle fibers (cells) which adjoin in an irregular manner to form a branching network. In mammals, the network of cells is partially subdivided by connective tissue into bundles and laminae that wind about the heart in long spirals, particularly in the ventricular walls. The fibers within a bundle are roughly parallel, but the bundles themselves course in different directions in the deeper and more superficial layers, so that any section through the myocardium presents groups of fibers cut longitudinally, transversely, and with varying degrees of obliquity.

Fibers

The cells or fibers of adult cardiac muscle fit together so tightly that under the light microscope they give the false impression of comprising a syncytium (Figs. 8-28 and 8-30). Electron micrographs show, however, that cardiac muscle is difinitely composed of elongated, branching cells with irregular contours at their junctions. The fibers are usually about 14 μm in diameter in a normal adult heart, but they vary during normal growth and under pathological conditions. In a newborn, the fibers are only 6 to 8 μm, or approximately one-half the diameter of those of an adult. In hearts showing hypertrophy, the fibers may be 20 μm or more in diameter.

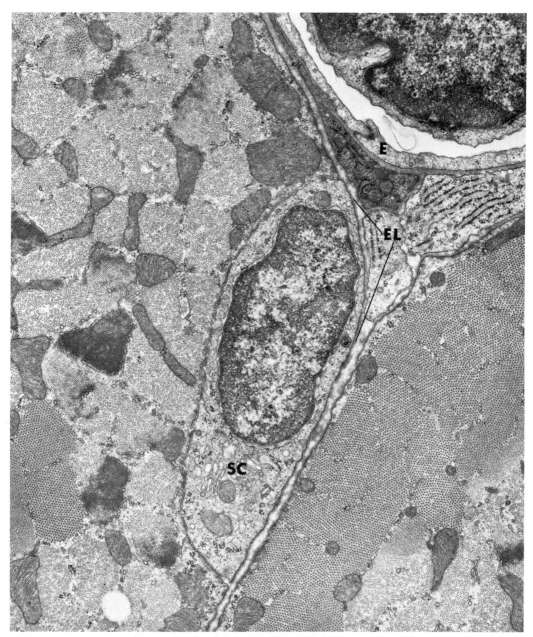

Fig. 8-27. Electron micrograph showing a satellite cell (*SC*) positioned between two skeletal muscle fibers, shown here in cross section. Note that the satellite cell lies entirely within the external lamina (*EL*) of the muscle fiber to the *left*. The endothelium (*E*) of a capillary and several processes of connective tissue cells are seen in the *upper right corner.* ×11,500. (Courtesy of Dr. Mikel H. Snow.)

Each fiber is enclosed by a *sarcolemma* which is similar to that of skeletal muscle. The structure seen with the light microscope includes a cell membrane, an external lamina outside the plasmalemma, and associated reticular fibers.

The nuclei, unlike those of skeletal muscle, are generally located in the central portion of the fiber, and number one per cell, or occasionally two, in contrast with the multinucleated condition in skeletal muscle. They are oval in shape and quite large, sometimes one-half of the diameter of the fibers (Figs. 8-28 and 8-30).

The fibers contain two types of *myofilaments, myosin,* and *actin,* arranged into *sarcomeres* similar to those in skeletal muscle. The filaments course in longitudinally oriented bundles or fascicles, generally known as *myofibrils.* However, the myofibrils course more irregularly than in skeletal muscle, and they frequently branch. Sarcomeres and bundles of myofilaments of one myofibril often become confluent with those of an adjacent myofibril. Consequently, the myofibrils are not as well demarcated as they are in skeletal muscle. In cross sections, the arrangement of the cut ends of the myofibrils often gives the appearance of bands or spokes of a wheel (Fig. 8-29). In longitudinal sections they diverge around the nucleus leaving a paler-staining zone of *sarcoplasm* at each pole of the nucleus (Fig. 8-30). This zone contains the usual organelles plus some bundles of specialized myofilaments. It has a sarcoplasmic reticulum (endoplasmic reticulum), fat droplets, and glycogen. Lipochrome pigment granules may be present

in older hearts. *Mitochondria* are much more abundant than in skeletal muscle and are characterized by their numerous cristae. They are clustered in the area around the nucleus and are also distributed beneath the sarcolemma and between the bundles of myofilaments. In the latter region, there are usually one or two per sarcomere.

The Golgi complex is also located near the nucleus. Curiously, in atrial fibers this region is often rich in dense, membrane-bounded granules, whereas ventricular fibers seldom display this organelle. The functional significance of these "*atrial granules*" is unknown (Fig. 8-31).

The *sarcoplasmic reticulum* consists mainly of smooth-surfaced membranes, but small segments occasionally have polyribosomes attached. The cisterns tend to course longitudinally, but they anastomose so frequently that they give a plexiform pattern. The reticulum is continuous from one sarcomere level to another, and there are no dilated terminal cisterns around the Z disc or at any other level. The membranes of the cisterns come into close association

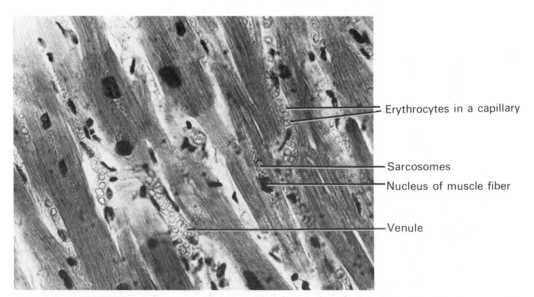

Fig. 8-28. Photomicrograph of a longitudinal section of cardiac muscle fibers from human ventricle. Note that the fibers branch and become apposed to each other in a complicated pattern. The intercalated discs at the sites of intercellular attachment are not obvious in this section, and they are frequently obscured in hematoxylin and eosin-stained preparations of human cardiac muscle. Cardiac muscle has a rich blood supply and the capillaries and venules are seen clearly in this preparation. The 10-μm section is sufficiently thick to show some of the vessels winding around and over the muscle fibers. ×390.

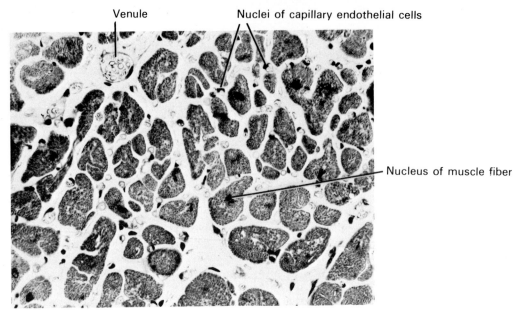

Venule   Nuclei of capillary endothelial cells

Nucleus of muscle fiber

Fig. 8-29. Photomicrograph of a transverse section of cardiac muscle from human ventricle. Note the central position of the nuclei and the irregular contour of branching fibers cut in cross section. The myofibrils are also cut in cross section, giving the cytoplasm of each fiber a stippled or punctate appearance. Hematoxylin and eosin. ×390.

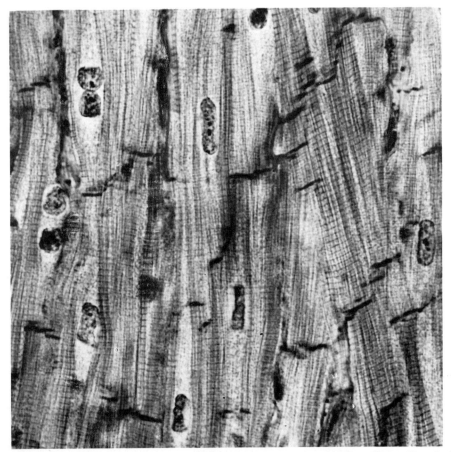

Fig. 8-30. Longitudinal section of muscle from left ventricle of monkey. The wider dark cross lines are intercalated discs. Mitochondria occupy the clearer areas adjacent to the nuclei. Photomicrograph, ×920.

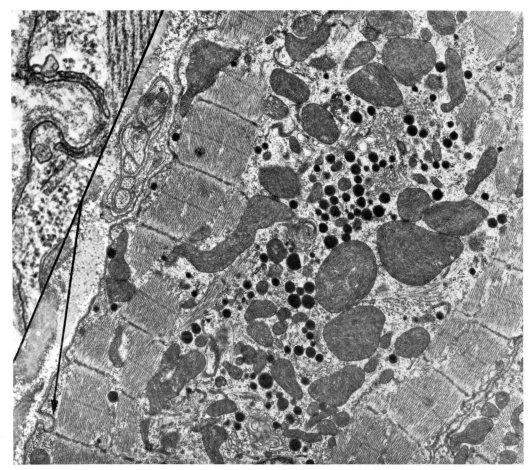

Fig. 8-31. Electron micrograph of cardiac muscle from the wall of the atrium. Large mitochondria plus smaller, dense "atrial granules" are prominent cytoplasmic features. A small nerve bundle courses within surrounding connective tissue at *left*. The *inset* and *arrow* display at higher magnifications the details of a diadic peripheral coupling and the opening of a wide T tubule onto the surface of the myocardial cell. ×11,200. Inset ×50,400. (Courtesy of Dr. David Chase.)

at various points with the membranes of wide and less regularly arranged *transverse tubules* (T tubules) and with the sarcolemma at the cell surface.

In those mammals studied thus far, it appears that cardiac T tubules are formed during neonatal stages as invaginations of the sarcolemma which extend into the deepest regions of the fiber. The tubules course mainly in a transverse direction but are often interconnected by longitudinally oriented branches. T tubules are generally seen at the level of the Z disc in all vertebrates studied; this location is similar to that in frog skeletal muscle and different from that in mammalian skeletal muscle. The transverse tubules of cardiac muscle

have a much wider lumen than those of skeletal muscle, and unlike skeletal muscle T tubules, they contain external lamina-like material. Their openings at the surface of the fiber are quite large and obvious in electron micrographs of glutaraldehyde-fixed material (Fig. 8-31). The tubules do not open into the cisterns of the sarcoplasmic reticulum, but their membranes become closely associated at various points and in various patterns with the cisternal membranes. The membranes are separated by a space of about 150 Å, in which poorly defined densities are observed. Because most transverse tubules are associated with only one cistern at any point, the most frequent association is called a *diad,* in distinction from *triads* of skeletal muscle, in which a transverse tubule is located between two terminal cisterns. The membranes of the transverse tubule transmit the stimulus for contraction from the surface of the fiber to all depths of the fiber, and the *couplings* at the diads presumably effect a response within the lumen of the sarcoplasmic cisterns that results in the release of stored calcium to the sarcoplasm around the bundles of myofilaments. The presence of calcium is necessary for the actin-myosin reaction in contraction, as described for skeletal muscle.

Cisterns of the sarcoplasmic reticulum lying just beneath the sarcolemma often have couplings with the sarcolemma. These are also diads, and they function as *peripheral couplings*. Because the membrane of the transverse tubule is invaginated sarcolemma, the sarcoplasmic cisterns associated with the T tubules, as well as those associated with the surface of the fiber, are actually all *subsarcolemmal cisterns*.

The cytological changes during contraction of cardiac muscle are similar to those in skeletal muscle. The sliding of actin filaments farther into the A band during contraction occurs by the same sequence of events. However, there are a number of differences in the functional reactions of these two types of muscle, such as differences in speed and strength of contraction, in factors affecting contraction, and in autorhythmicity. For example, the heart muscle is more dependent upon calcium in the surrounding medium than is skeletal muscle. This may be correlated with the fact that heart muscle lacks the dilated terminal cisterns of skeletal muscle and has less space for internal storage of calcium. The contraction of cardiac muscle is relatively prolonged, somewhat like that of tonic skeletal fibers. In this respect, it is interesting that the myofilaments of both tonic skeletal and cardiac muscle are arranged in less distinctly defined myofibrils. The ability of cardiac muscle to contract rhythmically at an intrinsic basic rate in the absence of a nerve supply or other external stimulus remains unexplained. Skeletal muscle usually contracts only after an external stimulus that is provided under normal conditions by the motor nerve endings.

Intercalated Discs

Intercalated discs are peculiar to cardiac muscle. They are seen by light microscopy as cross bands 0.5 to 1 μm thick (i.e., less than a cross striation or sarcomere) and are strongly refractive in fresh muscle and deeply stained in fixed material (Fig. 8-30). They often follow an irregular course, giving the appearance of a step formation. Electron micrographs show that the intercalated discs represent specialized cell junctions with a complex pattern and with a variety of structural characteristics (Figs. 8-32 and 8-33). In some regions, particularly where branches of the muscle fibers are firmly anchored end to end, the cytoplasm along the inner surfaces of the membranes of adjacent cells is densely filamentous. Here also the cells are separated by a uniform 150- to 200-Å space. This portion relates to the attachment of actin filaments to the sarcolemma and the transmission of contractile force from cell to cell. The structure of this region resembles that encountered on the cytoplasmic side of myotendonal junctions (page 266). Such intercalated disc junctions are focal, but otherwise not greatly dissimilar from intermediate junctions; hence their occasional classification as *fascia adhaerentes*. Until recently, many authors have referred to these as "intercalated disc desmosomes," although only in lower vertebrates is their structure really very desmosome-like (see also Fig. 4-3). All of the electron-dense regions have sufficient width to be seen collectively as the intercalated discs of light microscopy. Other true desmosomal portions of the intercalated disc regions apparently function chiefly for additional firm cell adhesion and the anchorage of noncontractile cytoskeletal tonofilaments. In still other regions, in or near the intercalated disc, particularly where the cells meet laterally, there are focal nexuses or gap junctions. These junctions are currently believed to provide electrotonic coupling among the cardiac muscle cells and thus contribute to a network of communicative pathways over which the overall rhythmic activity of the heart may be coordinated.

Connective Tissue of Cardiac Muscle

In the mammalian heart, a net of reticu-

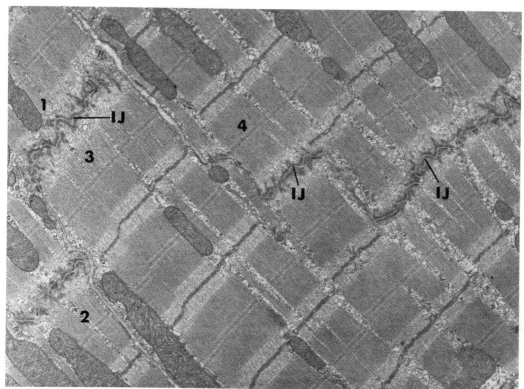

Fig. 8-32. Low magnification electron micrograph showing a longitudinal section in the region of intercalated disc joining four myocardial cells (*1, 2, 3,* and *4*). Note the stepwise arrangement of the junctional faces, in register with Z discs, as well as shallow interdigitations in each junctional area (*IJ*). ×12,600. (Courtesy of Dr. N. Scott McNutt.)

lar fibers and fine collagenous fibers surrounds each muscle fiber and its external lamina (Fig. 8-34). This net corresponds to the endomysium of skeletal muscle, but it is more irregular in its arrangement because the cardiac muscle cells are apposed to each other in a complicated pattern. Between bundles of muscle fibers, there are coarser collagenous and elastic fibers. These regions correspond to the perimysium of skeletal muscle. The connective tissue is particularly dense at the atrioventricular junction. The topographical arrangement of the connective tissues in the heart is described in chapter 12.

Blood Vessels and Nerves of Cardiac Muscle

Branches of the coronary arteries and cardiac veins penetrate the myocardium by coursing among the collagenous and elastic fibers of the larger bundles of connective tissue. An extensive plexus of blood and lymph capillaries is found in the connective tissue network surrounding each muscle fiber. The blood supply of cardiac muscle surpasses that of skeletal muscle.

Branches of sympathetic and parasympathetic nerves follow the connective tissue pathways and terminate in fine endings on the muscle fibers. The frequency of muscle contraction is accelerated by stimulation of the sympathetics and retarded by the parasympathetics.

Conduction System

Cardiac muscle fibers, because of their intimate network of junctional contacts and their inherent capacity to conduct, are capable of transmitting a contractile impulse over the entire heart. However, some of the fibers are modified in structure and conduct at a rate surpassing that of the typical cardiac fibers. These special con-

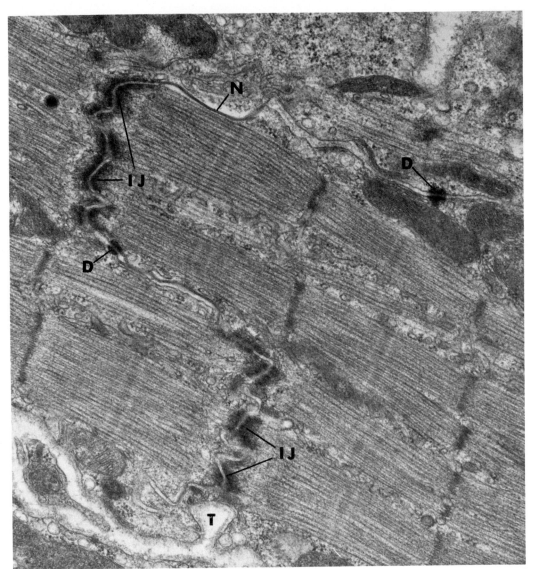

Fig. 8-33. Electron micrograph showing a longitudinal section through a portion of an intercalated disc. Intercalated disc junctions (*IJ*) anchor the actin filaments of abutting myocardial cells at areas of firm intercellular adhesion. True desmosomes (*D*) and nexuses (*N*) are also found, mainly along the lateral surfaces of the intercalated disc interdigitations. The opening of a T tubule (*T*) is visible on the surface of one myocardial cell. ×33,000. (Courtesy of Dr. David Chase.)

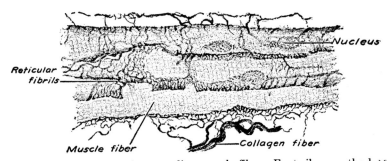

Fig. 8-34. Reticular fibrils about cardiac muscle fibers. Foot silver method. ×900.

duction elements are known as *Purkinje fibers*; a description of their structure and distribution is given in chapter 12.

Regeneration of Cardiac Muscle

There is little or no regenerative capacity of cardiac muscle fibers after injury or destruction. Healing is accomplished by scar formation.

Hypertrophy of the heart after any condition which places an excessive functional demand on the organ is accomplished by an increase in the size of the fibers rather than by an increase in their numbers. Likewise, growth of the heart during childhood is accomplished by an increase in the size of the fibers.

References

ASHTON, F. T., SOMLYO, A. V., AND SOMLYO, A. P. The contractile apparatus of vascular smooth muscle: intermediate high voltage stereo electron microscopy. J. Mol. Biol. 98:17–29, 1975.

BENDALL, J. R. Muscles, Molecules and Movement. (An Essay on the Contraction of Muscles). American Elsevier Publishing Company, Inc., New York, 1969.

BENNETT, H. S. The structure of striated muscle as seen by the electron microscope. *In* The Structure and Function of Muscle (Bourne, G. H., editor), vol. 1, pp. 137–181. Academic Press, New York, 1960.

BOIS, R. M. AND PEASE, D. C. Electron microscopic studies of the state of myosin aggregation in the vertebrate smooth muscle cell. Anat. Rec. 180:465–480, 1974.

BOURNE, G. H. (editor). The Structure and Function of Muscle. Three volumes. Academic Press, New York, 1960.

BOZLER, E., AND COTTRELL, C. L. The birefringence of muscle and its variation during contraction. J. Cell Comp. Physiol. 10:165–182, 1937.

BRANDT, P. W., LOPEZ, E., REUBEN, J. P., AND GRUNDFEST, H. The relationship between myofilament packing density and sarcomere length in frog striated muscle. J. Cell Biol. 33:255–263, 1967.

DEAMER, D. W., AND BASKIN, R. J. Ultrastructure of sarcoplasmic reticulum preparations. J. Cell Biol. 42:296–307, 1969.

DEWEY, M. M., AND BARR, L. Intercellular connection between smooth muscle cells: the nexus. Science 137:670–672, 1962.

EISENBERG, B., AND EISENBERG, R. S. Selective disruption of the sarcotubular system in frog sartorius muscle. A quantitative study with exogenous peroxidase as a marker. J. Cell Biol. 39:451–467, 1968.

FAWCETT, D. W. The sarcoplasmic reticulum of skeletal and cardiac muscle. Circulation 24:336–348, 1960.

FAWCETT, D. W., AND MCNUTT, N. S. The ultrastructure of the cat myocardium. I. Ventricular papillary

muscle. J. Cell Biol. 42:1–45, 1969.

FISHMAN, A. P. (editor) The myocardium; its biochemistry and biophysics. Circulation 24(2) and American Heart Association, New York, 1960.

FORBES, M. S., AND SPERELAKIS, N. Myocardial couplings: their structural variations in the mouse. J. Ultrastruct. Res. 58:50–65, 1977.

FRANZINI-ARMSTRONG, C. The structure of a simple Z-line. J. Cell Biol. 58:630–642, 1973.

GODMAN, G. C. On the regeneration and redifferentiation of mammalian striated muscle. J. Morphol. 100:27–82, 1957.

GOSS, C. M. The attachment of skeletal muscle fibers. Am. J. Anat. 74:259–289, 1944.

HALL, C. E., JAKUS, M. A., AND SCHMITT, F. O. An investigation of cross striations and myosin filaments in muscle. Biol. Bull. 90:32–50, 1946.

HANSON, J., AND HUXLEY, H. E. The structural basis of contraction in skeletal muscle. Sympos. Soc. Exp. Biol. 9:228–264, 1955.

HODGE, A. J. The fine structure of striated muscle. J. Biophys. Biochem. Cytol. 2(Suppl.):131–142, 1956.

HUXLEY, H. E. The fine structure of striated muscle and its functional significance. Harvey Lec. 60:85–117, 1964.

HUXLEY, H. E. The mechanism of muscular contraction. Science 164:1356–1366, 1969.

ISHIKAWA, H. Formation of elaborate networks of T-system tubules in cultured skeletal muscle, with special reference to the T-system formation. J. Cell Biol. 38:51–66, 1968.

ISHIKAWA, H., AND YAMADA, E. Differentiation of the sarcoplasmic reticulum and T-system in developing mouse cardiac muscle. *In* Developmental and Physiological Correlates of Cardiac Muscle (Lieberman, M., and Sano, T., editors), Raven Press, New York, pp. 21–35, 1975.

ISHIKAWA, H., BISCHOFF, R., AND HOLTZER, H. Formation of arrowhead complexes with heavy meromyosin in a variety of cell types. J. Cell Biol. 43:312–328, 1969.

JOHNSON, A. J., AND SOMMER, J. R. A strand of cardiac muscle. Its ultrastructure and the electrophysiological implications of its geometry. J. Cell Biol. 33:103–129, 1967.

KELLY, D. E. Models of muscle Z-band fine structure based on a looping filament configuration. J. Cell Biol. 34:827–839, 1967.

KELLY, D. E. Myofibrillogenesis and Z-band differentiation. Anat. Rec. 163:403–425, 1969.

KELLY, R. E., AND RICE, R. V. Ultrastructural studies on the contractile mechanism of smooth muscle. J. Cell Biol. 42:683–694, 1969.

KNAPPEIS, G. G., AND CARLSEN, F. The ultrastructure of the Z disc in skeletal muscle. J. Cell Biol. 13:323–336, 1962.

KNAPPEIS, G. G., AND CARLSEN, F. The ultrastructure of the M-line in skeletal muscle. J. Cell Biol. 38:202–211, 1968.

LEGATO, M. J., AND LANGER, G. A. The subcellular localization of calcium ion in mammalian myocardium. J. Cell Biol. 41:401–423, 1969.

MCNUTT, N. S., AND WEINSTEIN, R. S. The ultrastructure of the nexus. J. Cell Biol. 47:666–688, 1970.

MOMMAERTS, W. F. H. M., WITH BRADY, A. J., AND ABBOTT, B. C. Major problems in muscle physiology. Ann. Rev. Physiol. 23:529–576, 1961.

MONOMURA, Y. Myofilaments in smooth muscle of guinea pig's taenia coli. J. Cell Biol. 39:741–745, 1968.

PANNER, B. J., AND HONIG, C. R. Filament ultrastructure and organization in vertebrate smooth muscle. Contraction hypothesis based on localization of actin and myosin. J. Cell Biol. 35:303–321, 1967.

PANNER, B. J., AND HONIG, C. R. Locus and state of aggregation of myosin in tissue sections of vertebrate smooth muscle. J. Cell Biol. 44:52–61, 1970.

PEACHEY, L. D. The sarcoplasmic reticulum and transverse tubules of frog's sartorius. J. Cell Biol. 25:209–231, 1965.

PEACHEY, L. D. Structure and function of T-system of vertebrate skeletal muscle. In The Nervous System, vol. 1, The Basic Neurosciences (Tower, D. B., and Brady, R. D., editors), Raven Press, New York, pp. 81–90, 1975.

PEACHEY, L., AND PORTER, K. R. Intracellular impulse conduction in muscle cells. Science 129:721–722, 1959.

PORTER, K. R. The sarcoplasmic reticulum in muscle cells of Amblystoma larvae. J. Biophys. Biochem. Cytol. 2(Suppl.):163–170, 1956.

RICE, R. V., MOSES, J. A., McMANUS, G. M., BRADY, A. C., AND BLASIK, L. M. The organization of contractile filaments in a mammalian smooth muscle. J. Cell Biol. 47:183–196, 1970.

ROSENBLUTH, J. Fine structure of epineural muscle cells in Aplysia californica. J. Cell Biol. 17:455–460, 1963.

ROSENBLUTH, J. Obliquely striated muscle. II. Contraction mechanism of Ascaris body muscle. J. Cell Biol. 34:15–33, 1967.

SHIMADA, Y., FISCHMAN, D. A., AND MOSCONA, A. A. The fine structure of embryonic chick skeletal muscle cells differentiated in vitro. J. Cell Biol. 35:445–453, 1967.

SNOW, M. H. Myogenic cell formation in regenerating rat skeletal muscle injured by mincing. I. A fine structural study. Anat. Rec. 188:181–200, 1977a.

SNOW, M. H. Myogenic cell formation in regenerating rat skeletal muscle injured by mincing. II. An autoradiographic study. Anat. Rec. 188:201–218, 1977b.

SOMMER, J. R., AND WAUGH, R. A. The ultrastructure of the mammalian cardiac muscle—with special emphasis on the tubular membrane systems. Am. J. Pathol. 82:191–232, 1976.

SPIRO, D. The ultrastructure of heart muscle. Trans. N.Y. Acad. Sci. 24(Ser.2):879–885, 1962.

SZENT-GYORGYI, A. Chemical Physiology of Contraction in Body and Heart Muscle. Academic Press, Inc., New York, 1953.

CHAPTER 9

Organization of Nervous Tissue

Nervous tissue is characterized functionally by its ability to transmit impulses from one part of the body to another, often over long distances. The structural unit immediately responsible for this functional capability is a cell type known as the *neuron*. Neurons, however, cannot function without the support and protection of other neighboring cells of the nervous tissue known as *glia* (or *neuroglia*). Together neurons and glia provide for the capability of the generation and conveyance of a form of electrical activity called a nerve impulse along the length of a neuron. These impulses provide a means of rapid signaling between the various regions of the body. Combining many neurons into the intricate circuitry of the nervous system, the organism is able to receive information about its environment and its internal state, analyze this information, and respond in an appropriate manner.

As noted in chapter 3, neurons and their supporting glial companions take their origin embryonically from two sources, later to be combined into development of the total nervous system. The first and most massive source of nervous tissue appears on the dorsal surface of the embryonic disc shortly after gastrulation. Here an oval plate of surface ectoderm (the *neural plate*) thickens along the embryonic axis and soon folds along its lateral margins to form a deep median longitudinal groove. Eventually, this groove closes over and becomes a long hollow tube (the *neural tube*) extending over the entire length of the developing embryo (Figs. 9-1 and 3-4). This tube is epithelial at its origin, is epithelial during its development, and, although highly modified, will always retain basic epithelial characteristics. Eventually it becomes the substance of the brain and spinal cord, i.e., the *central nervous system* (CNS). Differential proliferation along the internal aspect of this tube leads to a rapid increase in the number of its epithelial cells. More massive proliferation anteriorly heralds the formation of the brain (Fig. 3-5); posteriorly the thickening of the neural tube is less apparent (Fig. 9-3), but a rather precise developmental pattern is established and persists in the spinal cord (Figs. 9-2 and 9-4). Some of the newly proliferating cells (*neuroblasts*) of the epithelial neural tube are destined to become neurons, and others (the *glioblasts*) will differentiate into various glial elements.

As cellular proliferation proceeds, three concentric regions become apparent within the wall of the tube (Fig. 9-2). The most internal (subventricular) region is termed the *ependymal* or *matrix* layer and contains actively dividing cells. After division, the nuclei of daughter cells take up positions in the intermediate (or *mantle*) layer; those which differentiate as neuroblasts send processes toward the exterior. These axons may grow out of the neural tube (e.g., to form ventral root motor fibers), or they

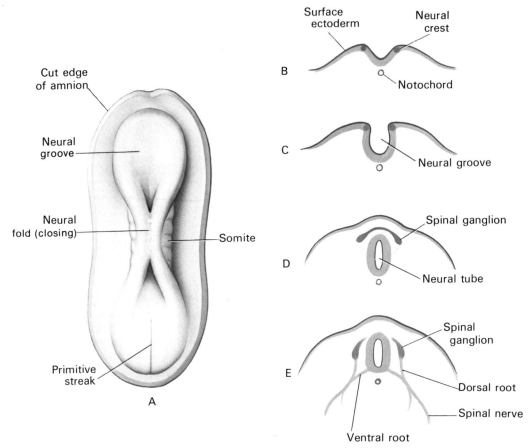

Fig. 9-1. Surface and cross sectional views of the development of the neural tube on the dorsal surface of the embryo. The lips of the neural fold fuse to enclose a hollow tube, the neural tube. This fusion progresses anteriorly and posteriorly until the neural tube is completely shut off from the amnionic fluid. Parts *B, C, D,* and *E* show cross sections through the neural tube at various stages of development. The derivation of the spinal ganglion from the neural crest and the joining together of the dorsal and ventral nerve root to form the spinal nerve are shown.

may course up or down the tube to form the relatively anuclear outermost *marginal* layer. In the fully differentiated CNS, these three layers (marginal, mantle, and ependymal) become, respectively, (1) the white matter, (2) the gray matter, and (3) the ependyma and an immediately subjacent layer in which proliferation of glial cell precursors continues into adulthood. Within these layers, the neurons develop first, the astrocytes later, and the oligodendrocytes last.

The enlarged upper (or anterior) end of the neural tube develops three dilations which form the forebrain, the midbrain, and the hindbrain of the CNS. In these regions, additional cell proliferation and cell

migration lead to the development of surface (cortical) areas containing large numbers of neurons.

Concurrent with the development of the neural tube, a second source of nervous tissue arises in a peculiar fashion. Along the lips of the neural groove some of the ectodermal cells which originally lay just lateral to presumptive neural tube separate from the ectodermal epithelium to invade the underlying mesenchymal compartment. Their release from the ectoderm coincides closely with the time of closure of the neural tube. These cells are termed *neural crest* and can be found migrating lateral to the neural tube along its entire length (Fig. 9-1).

Neural crest cells are at first quite mesenchymal in their behavior and unrecognizable from other mesenchymal cells around them. Eventually, they can be shown to give rise to a number of specific derivatives, not all of which are nervous tissue. A very large number of them will, however, contribute to the peripheral nervous system.

The first indication of this differentiation is the clumping of some neural crest cells in a repeating serial fashion along either side of the neural tube between adjacent somites. These are rudiments of spinal *ganglia*. A ganglion (singular) is a clumped group of neurons lying outside the CNS, i.e., within the peripheral nervous system. Similar clustering will occur later in a more ventral position, giving rise to ganglia of the *sympathetic* portion of the autonomic nervous system. Other parasympathetic ganglia will arise from neural crest clumping in various regions to be discussed later. Within each ganglion, growth will occur by proliferation, and some of the new cells will differentiate into neurons, whereas others will differentiate into supportive compo-

nents not dissimilar from the glia emerging within the neural tube. Hence, populations of neuroblasts and glioblasts can be found in both neural tube and neural crest derivatives. That is to say, *both* neural tube epithelium and neural crest cells give rise to neurons and glia.

Other cells of the mesenchymal compartment, at least some of which are of neural crest origin, surround and ensheath the neural tube. These are the protective and nourishing meningeal layers (*meninges*) of the CNS. As will be seen, these are continuous with similar protective coverings of elements of the peripheral nervous system.

The CNS (at this stage, the neural tube) is brought into contact with other parts of the body through development of the peripheral nervous system. Extensions of neurons (the longest of which are termed *axons* or *fibers*) grow out from certain regions of the brain and spinal cord to make functional contact with the *effectors* of the body—the muscles or glands. These outgrowing fibers constitute one portion of the peripheral nervous system and will carry

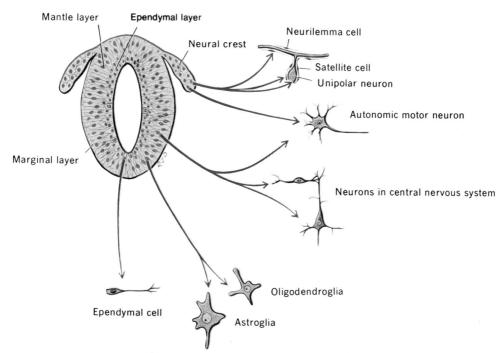

Fig. 9-2. This schematic diagram indicates the cells which derive from the neural tube and the neural crest. Note that mitotic activity in the neural tube is restricted to cells near the ependymal layer. (From Noback, C.: The Human Nervous System, McGraw-Hill, New York, 1967.)

output impulses from the CNS to peripheral structures. They are called *efferent* or *motor* because they control the activities of the outlying tissues. Neuroblasts within spinal ganglia develop fibers which course in two directions—to the periphery and toward the neural tube. The latter penetrate the neural tube and establish connections with neurons of the CNS. These fibers are thus able to provide an input of signals from the periphery to the CNS. They are therefore termed *afferent* or *sensory*. It can be seen that motor and sensory neurons and their fibers become intermixed to form *cranial* and *spinal nerves* of the *peripheral nervous system* (Figs. 9-3 and 9-4). It is clear also that fibers of some CNS neurons extend into the peripheral nervous system and fibers from some ganglionic neurons extend into the CNS. In this way the basic integration of the two components is established.

Although neurons exhibit a great variety of shapes and forms, each is characterized by having one or more cytoplasmic processes. Some of these are specialized to receive signals from other neurons. These processes are called *dendrites*, or the *dendritic zone* of a neuron; this part of the neuron constitutes most of the receptive portion. Neurons also develop a main trunk or principal process which generates the nerve impulse (frequently termed the *action potential*) and conducts this impulse along the length of the neuron to its most distant regions. This main trunk is the *axon* (or *neuronal fiber*). The termination of an axon most frequently forms a special contact, a *synapse*, with the dendritic portion, axon, or the cell body of another neuron, or it may form a similar contact (*myoneural junction*) with a muscle cell. Many neurons receive a great number of signals from a variety of sources on their dendritic, or receptive, surface. Those incoming signals may be either *inhibitory* or *excitatory*. The summation of these influences will determine whether the neuron will fire (i.e., generate its own action potential) and thus influence the dendritic portion of the next nerve cell in the pathway.

Basic Organization

An arrangement whereby a motor and a sensory neuron are linked together synaptically as a receptor-effector mechanism constitutes the simplest type of *reflex arc*. An example of this type of combination is illustrated in Fig. 9-4*A*, which represents a cross section through the spinal cord and a spinal nerve. The cell body of the sensory neuron is located outside the spinal cord, where, together with other similar cell bodies, it forms a spinal ganglion. The sensory neuron is *unipolar*; that is, it has only one process. A short distance from the cell body, this single process, which is structurally an axon, divides into a peripheral process with a receptor ending in the skin and a central process which enters the spinal cord by way of the *dorsal root* of the spinal nerve. The central process may terminate in contact with either the dendrites or the cell body of a *multipolar* motor neuron located in the ventral part of the cord. The axon of this second neuron leaves the cord by way of the *ventral root*, joins the sensory fibers to form the *spinal nerve*, and courses peripherally to terminate on an effector (skeletal muscle, in the example illustrated in Fig. 9-4*A*).

The two-neuron reflex, described above, although theoretically possible, is a much more simple arrangement than that which is usually found in mammals. More commonly, a series of neurons is interposed between the sensory and motor neurons of the basic reflex arc. These are commonly called *interneurons* (or internuncial neurons). Simpler nervous systems, as in some invertebrates, often have relatively few interneurons interposed between receptors and effectors, and the reactions of the organism are quite stereotyped and predictable. In higher animals, the pathways provided by interneurons can be very complex; nerve impulses generated in receptors in the periphery are carried to many levels of the nervous system, including the highest centers (the cerebral cortex) of the brain. In the various parts of the brain, incoming information is sorted, stored, and used in determining the appropriate motor responses. Complex interneuronal pathways lead from the brain back to the cranial or spinal motor neurons and are influential in determining whether these neurons will fire, i.e., generate a nerve impulse (and thus cause a muscle to contract or a gland to

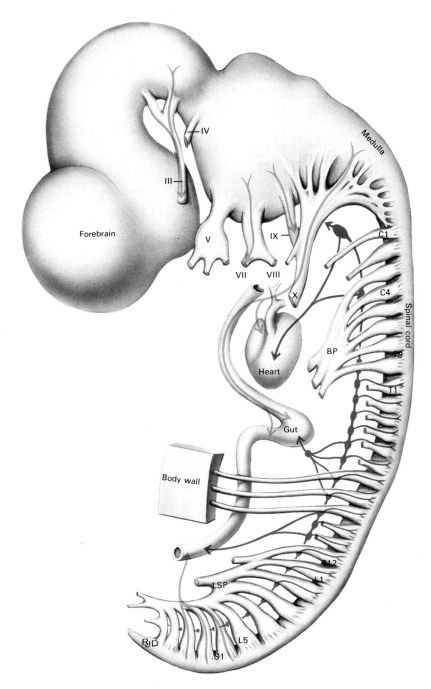

Fig. 9-3. Diagram of derivatives of the neural tube after brain parts have begun to form and after the cranial and spinal nerves have developed. Cranial nerves are given *Roman numerals,* and spinal nerves of the cervical (*C*), thoracic (*T*), lumbar (*L*), and sacral (*S*) regions are indicated by *numbers.* The craniosacral (*blue*) and thoracolumbar (*red*) parts of the autonomic nervous outflow are derived from the "head and tail" and the "middle" part of the neuraxis and provide dual innervation to visceral structures. The dominance of the vagus nerve (*X*) in the innervation of the trunk viscera is apparent. The fact that autonomic outflow is always a two-neuron system is not shown.

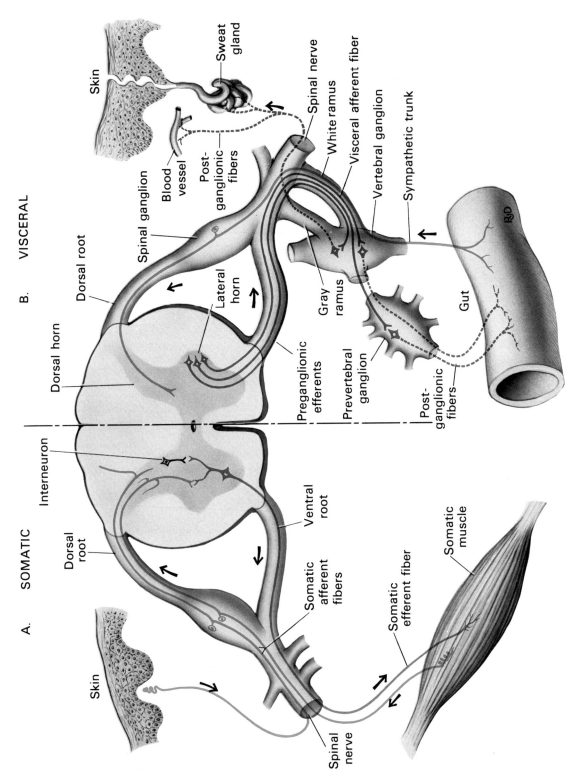

Fig. 9-4. *A*, somatic nerves. *B*, visceral nerves. A cross section of spinal cord is shown connected via dorsal and ventral roots to the spinal nerve and to one of the ganglia of the autonomic system. The patterns of afferent (*blue*) and efferent (*red*) nerve fibers in both the somatic and visceral system may be directly compared. For details see text.

secrete). In the vertebrate nervous system, the cranial or spinal motor neuron is the chief executive; these cells constantly receive "advice" in the form of hundreds or thousands of inhibitory and excitatory synapses applied to their dendritic portion or to their cell bodies. These motor neurons provide the *final common pathway* from the CNS to its effector organs. Once they fire, there is no mechanism of recall; the muscle contracts or the gland secretes.

It is clear that the basic reflex arc is not controlled by local sensory influences alone but by information converging on the motor neurons from many levels of the CNS, including the cerebral cortex, the midbrain, and the hindbrain. How these complex synaptic networks become organized is one of the most challenging questions in neurobiology. There is no doubt that some synaptic contacts are genetically determined, for certain synapses form in nerve tissue completely isolated from the other tissues of the body and from sensory influences. Some investigators believe that, after having been guided to the correct region by mechanical forces and by chemical gradients, the axon makes contact with another neuron because of affinities of surface macromolecules. Certain synapses appear to require some degree of use to be retained, others do not. Are most synapses permanent? Are new synapses formed with learning? Are some synapses superfluous? Are more synapses formed in animals exposed to an "enriched" environment? Is memory stored in our nervous systems? These are some of the questions that present neurobiological experimentation is attempting to answer.

The Spinal Nerve

The arrangement of the nerve cells and fibers within the spinal cord makes it possible to differentiate two distinct areas of tissue: a thick peripheral layer of *white matter* and a central column of *gray matter* (Fig. 9-3). The white matter is composed primarily of longitudinally directed nerve fibers, many of which are covered by white lipid-rich sheaths provided by the membranes of certain glial cells. Such membranous sheaths are termed *myelin*. The gray matter is composed principally of nerve cells and their fibers and glial cells. Many of the fibers of the gray matter are unmyelinated, but a considerable number of myelinated ones are present also. In transverse section, the gray matter is shaped like the letter H. Its dorsal wings constitute the *dorsal horns* and its ventral ones the *ventral horns* (in which lie the cell bodies of the motor neurons). The two lateral gray areas are connected across the midline by a transverse bar, the *gray commissure*, in which lies the small central canal, the remnant of the previously wide neural tube lumen. It is, of course, evident that the dorsal and ventral horns seen in cross section actually are continuous columns of gray matter extending the length of the cord.

The *dorsal roots* are composed of the afferent or sensory fibers; these fibers have their cell bodies grouped into an enlargement of the dorsal root called the *dorsal root ganglion* (Fig. 9-4). The *ventral roots* contain the efferent or motor fibers, and these join the dorsal root to make up the *spinal nerve*. Those afferent fibers which are distributed to sensory endings in the body, exclusive of the viscera, are termed *somatic afferent* fibers; those providing the sensory innervation of the viscera are the *visceral afferent* fibers. Both functional types have their cell bodies in the spinal ganglia (Fig. 9-4).

A great many of the efferent fibers are distributed to the voluntary skeletal muscle of the body and are therefore termed *somatic efferent* fibers. Other efferent fibers terminate on smooth or cardiac muscle and glandular epithelium of visceral structures; these are the *visceral efferent* fibers.

The Autonomic Nervous System

The visceral efferent components of both the cranial and the spinal nerves pursue a different course than do the somatic efferent fibers, for two neurons are always involved in the conduction of a visceral impulse from the CNS to the effector organ. They also differ physiologically in that the essentially visceral reflexes which they mediate are often not subject to direct voluntary control and are also more or less diffuse, rather than localized, in their effects. Because of these and certain other differences, it has been found convenient to consider the visceral efferent neurons of the body as a separate physiological system for which the name first given by Langley, the *autonomic nervous system,* is commonly used. According to the original definition, the autonomic system included only the visceral efferent (motor) innervation and did not include either the visceral afferent (sensory) fibers or those higher centers in the CNS which influence the visceral activities. In recent years, however, the use of the term "autonomic" generally has included all of the neural apparatus concerned with visceral function. In this sense, the term becomes more synonymous with "visceral" or "vegetative."

It must be emphasized that the autonomic nervous system is purely a functional grouping of efferent neurons and is in no sense an anatomical division. Some neuron cell bodies lie within the CNS; others are located in visceral ganglia in distant regions of the body. Autonomic nerve fibers are present in all spinal nerves and in most of the cranial nerves. The reflexes which they govern may be initiated by sensory impulses flowing over somatic afferent or visceral afferent fibers or coming from any receptor organ. The stimuli may be in the external environment or they may arise within the body.

The efferent fibers to visceral structures leave the CNS at three levels, making it possible to recognize three divisions of the autonomic nervous system (Fig. 9-5). In the *cranial division,* autonomic fibers leave by way of cranial nerves III, VII, IX, and X. Other visceral efferent fibers emerge through the thoracic and the upper lumbar spinal nerves; these constitute the *thoracolumbar division.* The *sacral division* includes visceral efferent fibers that leave by way of sacral spinal nerves 2, 3, and 4.

Whatever their level of origin, all visceral efferent pathways involve two successive neurons (Figs. 9-4 and 9-5). The first of these has its cell body within the central nervous system and its axon terminating in a peripheral autonomic ganglion; it is therefore termed a *preganglionic* neuron. In the ganglion, it makes synaptic connec-

tion with a second multipolar neuron, the *postganglionic neuron,* whose axon terminates on an effector organ (muscle or epithelium).

In the cranial and sacral divisions, the preganglionic fibers generally end in *terminal* ganglia which lie near or within the walls of the structures that they innervate. In this and other respects, as well as in their response to certain drugs, the cranial and sacral divisions resemble each other and differ from the thoracolumbar components. They are therefore grouped together as the craniosacral or *parasympathetic* division of the autonomic nervous system.

The thoracolumbar visceral efferent outflow is the *sympathetic* division of the autonomic nervous system. Its preganglionic fibers terminate in either *vertebral* or *prevertebral* ganglia. The vertebral ganglia are a series of ganglia, connected linearly by nerve fibers, that lie along the ventrolateral aspects of the vertebral column and thus form two *sympathetic trunks* extending on either side the length of the vertebral column. The prevertebral, or *collateral,* ganglia are aggregations of postganglionic neurons associated with visceral nerve plexuses in the abdomen (Figs. 9-4 and 9-5).

In general, most visceral organs are innervated by both the parasympathetic and sympathetic divisions, the effects of which are usually, but by no means always, antagonistic. For example, the parasympathetic fibers to the heart transmit impulses which tend to slow the heart rate; impulses from the sympathetic fibers, on the other hand, accelerate it. In the stomach, parasympathetic impulses excite muscular contraction, and sympathetic impulses inhibit it. The stimulation of the parasympathetic contributes to the conservation of bodily energy; the stimulation of the sympathetic assists the body in meeting emergencies.

Sympathetic Division

The sympathetic trunks are composed of a series of vertebral ganglia containing the cell bodies of postganglionic neurons and connected in linear order by ascending or descending nerve fibers (Figs. 9-3 to 9-5). In the cervical region there are three ganglia: the *superior cervical* ganglion, which

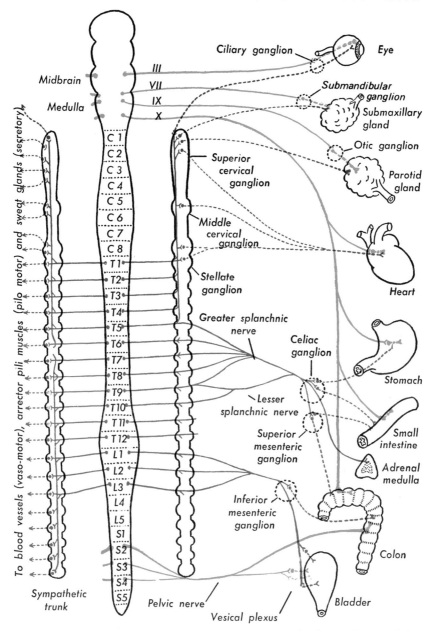

Fig. 9-5. Diagrammatic representation of some of the chief conduction pathways of the autonomic nervous system. For clearness, the nerves to blood vessels, arrector pili muscles, and sweat glands are shown only on the *left side* of the figure and the pathways to other visceral structures are shown only on the *right side*. The sympathetic division is shown in *red*, the parasympathetic division in *blue*. *Solid lines* represent preganglionic fibers; *broken lines* represent postganglionic fibers.

is the largest; the *middle cervical,* sometimes absent; and the *inferior cervical,* which may be fused with the first thoracic to form the *stellate ganglion.* In the thoracic region, the ganglia, 10 or 11 in number,

are segmentally arranged. Three or four ganglia are associated with the lumbar level and four or five with the sacral region.

Each sympathetic trunk is connected with the spinal nerves of its side by a series of communicating rami composed of nerve fibers. These are of two types. One type, the *gray communicating rami,* consists of fibers mostly devoid of myelin; these are found connecting the trunk to every spinal nerve. The other type, the *white communicating rami,* is limited to the thoracic and first three or four lumbar nerves and is not present at cervical or sacral levels (Fig. 9-5).

Preganglionic fibers of the sympathetic division have their cell bodies located in the *intermediolateral cell column (lateral horn)* of the thoracic and upper lumbar levels of the spinal cord (Fig. 9-4). The myelinated fibers emerge through the ventral roots and reach the nearby sympathetic trunk by way of the white communicating rami. Within the sympathetic trunk the preganglionic fiber may take one of three courses:

1. It may terminate in this level of the trunk in synaptic relation to a *postganglionic neuron* whose nonmyelinated axon joins the corresponding spinal nerve by way of the gray communicating ramus. The postganglionic fiber courses peripherally to terminate in the smooth muscle of a blood vessel (vasomotor), in the arrector pili muscle of a hair (pilomotor), or among the epithelial cells of a sweat gland (secretory) (Fig. 9-4).

2. Many of the preganglionic fibers from the white rami pass directly through the sympathetic trunk without interruption and continue to the prevertebral (collateral) ganglia, from which postganglionic fibers course to the visceral organs. Preganglionic fibers such as these emerge as branches from the sympathetic trunks. Those from the 5th to 10th thoracic ganglia form the *splanchnic nerves* and terminate in the *celiac ganglia,* which are prevertebral. The postganglionic fibers contribute to the formation of the celiac plexus and pass directly to their terminations in the viscera.

3. A great many of the preganglionic fibers, upon reaching the sympathetic trunk, course either caudally or cranially in this trunk before they have a synaptic juncture with postganglionic neurons. These fibers form the pathways for the visceral efferent outflow to regions of the trunk which do not possess white rami. For example, preganglionic fibers originating at levels as low as the seventh thoracic terminate in the superior cervical ganglion. From this ganglion, nonmyelinated postganglionic nerve fibers run to various visceral structures. Some accompany the internal carotid artery as the internal carotid plexus and furnish the pathway by which impulses reach the dilator pupillae muscle of the eye. Other fibers form the superior cervical cardiac nerve to the cardiac plexus and conduct impulses which accelerate the rhythm of the heart.

Other pathways of the sympathetic division are shown diagrammatically in Figure 9-5.

Parasympathetic Division

The cranial parasympathetic preganglionic neurons lie in the midbrain and medulla, sending their axons out over the oculomotor, facial, glossopharyngeal, vagus, and accessory cranial nerves (Fig. 9-3). These preganglionic fibers are myelinated and course in their respective nerves to terminal ganglia located near or within visceral structures.

In the case of the oculomotor nerve, the preganglionic fibers enter the orbit with this nerve but diverge to reach the ciliary ganglion, forming its short motor root. The ciliary ganglion, which lies against the lateral surface of the optic nerve, contains the postganglionic neurons whose axons course in the short ciliary nerves to the eyeball. In the eyeball, they are distributed to the ciliary muscle of accommodation and the sphincter muscle of the iris. The antagonistic action of parasympathetic and sympathetic nerves is here evident, for the parasympathetic fibers bring about contraction of the pupil; sympathetic postganglionic fibers from the superior cervical ganglion cause dilation of the pupil.

The vagus nerve contains many preganglionic fibers. The cell bodies lie in the medulla, and many of the fibers pass to the cardiac plexus and terminate in synaptic relation to ganglion cells located on the surface of the atria and roots of the great vessels or in the subepicardium of the atrial walls. The axons of these cardiac ganglion cells are short postganglionic fibers which end in the heart muscle. They are inhibitory in function.

The parasympathetic innervation of the gastrointestinal tract and other abdominal viscera is through efferent fibers of the vagus nerve and also the pelvic nerve, which arises from nerve cells in the lateral horn of the second, third, and fourth sacral segments of the spinal cord. These are preganglionic fibers. Those which innervate the gastrointestinal tract course without interruption to terminate in its wall. Here they are synaptically related to postganglionic neurons, which, with associated plexuses of nerve fibers, form two extensive ganglionated plexuses, the *enteric ganglionated plexuses*. One of these, the *myenteric plexus* or *plexus of Auerbach*, is situated between the longitudinal and circular layers of muscle. The other, the *submucosal plexus* or *plexus of Meissner*, lies in the submucosa. These plexuses are composed of small ganglia connected to each other by strands of nerve fibers. Other strands connect the plexuses with each other.

Preganglionic fibers which pass to pelvic reproductive and urinary organs terminate in synaptic relation to the cell bodies of postganglionic neurons located in or near the walls of these viscera.

The nerve fibers of the enteric plexuses fall into the following classes:

Postganglionic Sympathetic Fibers. These are derived from postganglionic neurons located chiefly in prevertebral ganglia. They end on the smooth muscle of the gut and among epithelial cells. Their impulses usually inhibit gastrointestinal activity.

Preganglionic Parasympathetic Fibers. These are fibers of the vagus or, in the descending colon and rectum, the visceral branches of sacral nerves. They end in synapses with the ganglion cells of the myenteric or submucosal plexuses.

Postganglionic Parasympathetic Fibers. These are axons of the above mentioned ganglion cells. They innervate smooth muscle and epithelium of the gut,

and their impulses usually excite gastrointestinal activity.

Visceral Afferent Fibers. These fibers are sensory and intermingle with the visceral efferent fibers. They play an important part in gastrointestinal reflexes. Some of the sensory fibers from the gut course in the vagus to the sensory ganglia of this nerve and from there to the medulla. Other sensory fibers course in the visceral nerves, then through the vertebral sympathetic ganglia and the white rami communicantes to their cell bodies in the spinal ganglia and then to the spinal cord (Fig. 9-4).

References

ARIËNS KAPPERS, C. U., HUBER, G. C., AND CROSBY, E. C. The Comparative Anatomy of the Nervous System of Vertebrates, Including Man. 3 volumes. Hafner Publishing Company, New York, 1960.
BOURNE, G. H. (editor). The Structure and Function of Nervous Tissue. 3 volumes. Academic Press, New York, 1968–1969.
BULLOCK, T. H., AND HORRIDGE, G. A. Structure and Function in the Nervous Systems of Invertebrates. 2 volumes. W. H. Freeman and Company, San Francisco, 1968.
CANNON, W. B. The Wisdom of the Body. W. W. Norton & Co., New York, 1939.
CANNON, W. B., AND ROSENBLUETH, A. Autonomic Neuro-effector Systems. Macmillan, New York, 1937.
CARPENTER, M. B. Human Neuroanatomy, Ed. 7. Williams & Wilkins, Baltimore, 1977.
CROSBY, E. C., HUMPHREY, T., AND LAUER, E. W. Correlative Anatomy of the Nervous System. Macmillan, New York, 1962.
HERRICK, C. J. An Introduction to Neurology. W. B. Saunders, Philadelphia, 1931.
KUNTZ, A. The Autonomic Nervous System. Lea & Febiger, Philadelphia, 1953.
NOBACK, C. R. The Human Nervous System: Basic Principles of Neurobiology, Ed. 2. McGraw-Hill, New York, 1975.
PATTON, H. D., SUNDSTEN, J. W., CRILL, W. E., AND SWANSON, P. D. Introduction to Basic Neurology. W. B. Saunders, Philadelphia, 1976.
RAMON Y CAJAL, S. Histologie du Système Nerveux de l'Homme et des Vertébrés. 2 volumes. A. Maloine, Paris, 1909–1911.
RHODIN, J. Nervous system—organization. Chapter 12. *In* Histology, A Text and Atlas. Oxford University Press, 1974.
WHITE, C., SMITHWICK, R. H., AND SIMEONE, F. A. The Autonomic Nervous System. Macmillan, New York, 1952.

CHAPTER 10 ▮▮▮▮▮▮▮▮▮▮▮▮▮▮▮▮▮▮▮▮▮▮

Nervous Tissue

In higher animals, the great majority of neurons are within central nervous tissue. The histology of this tissue reflects its origin. Like other epithelia, its cells are closely packed, with little extracellular space or substance, and are connected by frequent cell-to-cell junctions. Unlike most epithelia, however, nervous tissue is comprised of enormous numbers of cells, many of great complexity, and it contains a special type of junction: the *synapse* (from a Greek word meaning clasp.) All neurons participate in synaptic contact, and must be so connected to survive. The human brain contains billions of neurons, and certain of these receive thousands of synapses. The enormous number of neurons in the human body and the complexity and specificity of their circuitry provide for the functional capabilities of the nervous system and give man his rich variety of reaction and behavior.

In the central nervous system (CNS), the neuronal cell bodies are the most conspicuous elements. They tend to occur in groups called *nuclei* (not to be confused with the nucleus of a single cell) if they occur as a cluster, *layers* if they occur in a laminar array, and *columns* if they occur in a linear configuration. Related to the nerve cell bodies are great entanglements of nerve cell processes (axonal and dendritic) called *neuropil,* where many of the synaptic contacts occur. Nerve fibers (generally axons) grouped into bundles that travel to other parts of the nervous system are called *tracts.*

Special techniques are required to work out the circuitry of nervous tissue, but in standard preparations, neurons can generally be identified and their organization into nuclei, layers, and columns can be analyzed. More specialized techniques delineate the whole of the neuronal contour, demonstrate synapses, or detect certain types of neurotransmitters; other procedures demonstrate degenerating cell processes. Only when electron microscopy is used in addition to these basic techniques, however, does the full complexity of the nervous system begin to be apparent.

The CNS epithelium is marked by compactness, in contrast with the peripheral nervous tissues, in which nerve cell bodies and nerve fibers are interspersed with distinctive connective tissue investments. Supportive cells—the *neuroglia*—are the helper cells of all neurons. These cells include the various neuroglia cells of the central nervous system, the Schwann cells of the peripheral nerve fibers, and the satellite cells of the craniospinal and autonomic ganglia. Connective tissue forms part of the membranous meninges surrounding the entire CNS and provides tubular investments around peripheral nerves. It also contributes to the capsules of the ganglia and is associated with the sensory nerve fiber endings in the formation of sense organs.

The Neuron

The neuron may be defined as the nerve cell body with all of its extensions. Neurons

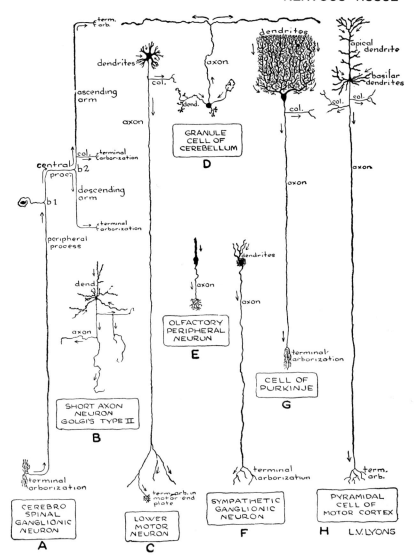

Fig. 10-1. Some of the principal forms of neurons. The sheaths are not shown. The axons, except in *B*, are shown much shorter in proportion to the size of body and dendrites than they actually are. The direction of conduction is shown by the arrows. *Col,* collateral branch; *proc,* process; *term. arb,* terminal arborization.

are generally elongated—some may be over 5 feet long—to provide for their function of communicating between various regions of the body (Fig. 10-1). Despite their elongation, neurons seldom are multinucleated, and it is important to recognize the portion of the nerve cell which surrounds the nucleus, the *perikaryon,* or cell body, for this region is vital for the survival of the entire cell. The processes extending from the perikaryon are specialized for three primary functions (Fig. 10-2): (1), *reception* of various stimuli—this is generally the function of the dendrites, although areas of the cell body or the axon may also receive signals from other cells; (2) *conduction* of the nerve impulse to regions distant from the receptive area—this is generally the function of the axon, but some dendrite regions and cell bodies may also propagate impulses; and (3) *synaptic transmission* of the signal to subsequent neurons in the neural pathways or to muscle or gland. This *effector* function generally occurs in the nerve terminals, where minute amounts of chemical compounds called *neurotransmitters* are

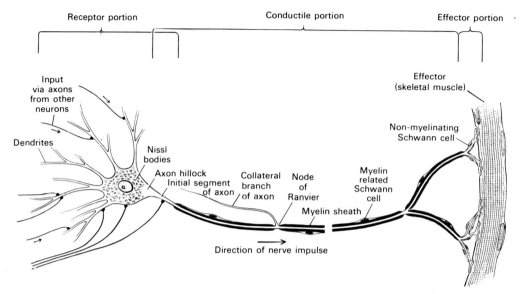

Fig. 10-2. This diagram illustrates the receptor, conductile, and effector portions of a typical large neuron. The effector endings on skeletal muscle identify this as a somatic motor neuron; in many neurons the effector endings are applied to the receptor portions of other neurons. The presence of the myelin sheath on the conductile portion of the neuron (the axon) increases conduction velocity. The axon is shown to be interrupted, for it is much longer than can be illustrated here.

released. Each neuron is thus equipped to receive information, to act on the basis of this information to signal its distant portions, and then to influence other neurons or other tissues.

Classification of Neurons by Shape

The general form of the neuron is best studied after staining thick sections of nervous tissue with heavy metals such as silver or gold (Fig. 10-3). Adaptation to different functional needs in various parts of the body leads to a great spectrum of neuronal shapes and sizes (Fig. 10-1). *Multipolar neurons* (Fig. 10-1, *B, C, D, F, G,* and *H*) frequently have a number of dendritic processes arising directly from the cell body. The axon may also arise from the cell body or from the proximal part of one of the dendrites. The axon sometimes branches soon after its formation to provide recurrent collateral branches which return to the region of the cell body (Fig. 10-2). Except for these collaterals, there is often no further branching until the axon reaches the region of terminal arborization and transmitter release (Figs. 10-1 and 10-2). In *bipolar neurons,* one process emerges from

each pole of an elongated cell body (Fig. 10-1*E*). The receptor and effector portions of these cells are often limited to the extreme ends; the entire intermediate portion, including the cell body, is conductile in function. In *unipolar neurons* (as found in most sensory ganglia), the nerve cell body possesses a single process which divides not far from the cell body into two branches, one proceeding to some peripheral structure and the other entering the CNS (Fig. 10-1*A*). Both arms of the single process have the structural and functional characteristics of an axon; together they form the conductile portion of the cell. The receptor part is located in some peripheral sense organ and the central part arborizes within the CNS to provide effector influence upon the dendrites of various CNS cells. It should also be noted that in various specialized areas of the CNS there appear to be cells which do not possess axons. These are small cells, called *anaxonic neurons,* which have both receptor and effector regions on their dendritic portions. They thus require no conductile portion to convey receptor influences to distant regions. One example, the amacrine cell of the retina, is discussed in chapter 22.

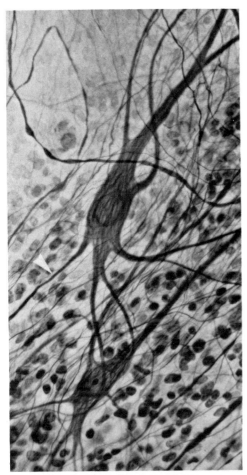

Fig. 10-3. This photomicrograph shows two large neurons that have matured in tissue culture. The culture has been fixed and then stained with silver. In the *lower neuron* the nucleolus is stained deeply, as are many of the nuclei of the surrounding supporting cells. Within the neurons neurofibrils are seen interlacing in the nerve cell body and extending into the numerous dendrites. The axon of the *upper neuron* is indicated by a *white arrowhead.* ×310. (Courtesy of Dr. C. D. Allerand.)

The Nerve Cell Body

As in most other cells, the nerve cell body consists of a mass of cytoplasm, the perikaryon, surrounding a nucleus. There is little distinctive in the content of the nerve cell body, for the usual cell organelles are present; it is the quantity of certain components and their disposition which indicate the special functional capacities of the neuron. The generally accepted *neuron doctrine* states that the vertebrate neuron cell body, with its nucleus, is the genetic center of the neuron, and that the various nerve cell processes depend on this cell body for their survival. If these processes are cut off from the nucleated portion, they degenerate and ultimately disappear.

Nerve cell bodies vary considerably in size. The small granule cells of the cerebellum are about 4 μm in diameter, whereas large motor cells in the ventral horn of the human spinal cord may attain diameters of 135 μm (certain invertebrate neurons may be 4 times this size). The size of the neuron cell body generally reflects the amount of cytoplasm being supported in the cell processes. Thus, some of the largest neuronal cell bodies are those with the longest and thickest axons.

Nucleus of the Nerve Cell

The *nucleus* of the nerve cell is spherical in form, and its size is generally proportional to the size of cell it occupies. It is generally pale, with widely dispersed chromatin, suggesting a high volume of transcriptional activity. Certain large neurons are known to contain a tetraploid amount (i.e., twice the normal amount) of DNA. Usually the nucleus is situated approximately in the center of the cell body in large nerve cells, the most striking exceptions being its eccentric position in the cells of Clarke's column in the spinal cord and in cells of sympathetic ganglia. Eccentric nuclei are also seen in various pathological conditions and when the axon of the cell is injured. Although most neurons have a single nucleus, some binucleate neurons are generally present in sympathetic ganglia and a few are occasionally present in sensory ganglia.

The *nucleolus* is relatively large and appears particularly prominent because the remainder of the nucleus stains lightly. In tissues from females, the sex chromatin (or Barr body) is often clearly visualized within the lightly staining nucleoplasm. In some animals (such as the cat, in which it was first observed), this body is seen as a satellite of the nucleolus about 1 μm in diameter; in human females it is adjacent to the nuclear envelope. The appearance of this body is described in chapter 1 on the cell and in chapter 7 on the blood.

Cytoplasm of the Nerve Cell Body

The cytoplasm surrounding a neuron's nucleus is termed the *perikaryon*. It contains chromophilic or Nissl substance (ribosomes and endoplasmic reticulum), Golgi apparatus, mitochondria, filaments, microtubules, lysosomes, and cytoplasmic inclusions such as fat, glycogen, lipofuscin, and sometimes the pigment melanin.

When neurons are grown in tissue culture and visualized in the living state by phase microscopy, exceptionally clear regions in the cytoplasm may be observed (Fig. 10-4). These are distinct from the granular lysosomes and mitochondria or the clear linear aggregates of filaments and microtubules. These regions absorb the same wavelengths of ultraviolet light as do nucleic acids, and stain strongly with basophilic dyes except after prior treatment with ribonuclease (Fig. 10-5). The German histologist Nissl first noted that these distinctive areas in fixed neurons stain with basic aniline dyes.

He called the stained material chromophilic substance, and noted that it appears as very small granules clumped together in a variety of shapes (Fig. 10-5), usually larger in motor than in sensory neurons. The *Nissl substance,* as these areas are now commonly called, is one of the hallmarks in identifying neurons. Nissl substance is found in the perikarya and in the proximal parts of the dendrites of all large and many small neurons but not in the axon and the axon hillock (Figs. 10-2 and 10-5A).

Electron micrographs show that the Nissl substance is composed of clusters of endoplasmic reticulum plus ribosomes (Fig. 10-6) bound to the outer surfaces of cisternae or free in the cytoplasm between. Free ribosomes frequently are arranged in rosettes or linear arrays of five or more granules (Fig. 10-7). The basophilia depends upon the presence of RNA in the ribosomes, not upon components in the endoplasmic reticulum. Certain cisternae of endoplasmic reticulum come to lie unusually close to the plasma membrane of the perikarya. These *subsurface cisternae* are a distinctive characteristic of neurons visible only in electron

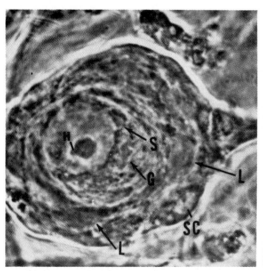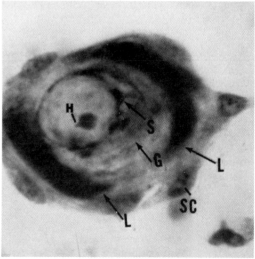

Fig. 10-4. Photomicrographs of the same neuron before (*left*) and after (*right*) fixation and staining of Nissl substance. The picture on the *left* is of a living chick neuron in tissue culture photographed with a phase microscope. The large, relatively homogeneous masses (*L*) apparent in the phase microscope are seen to be heavily stained by the basic dye employed to stain Nissl substance (*right*). *S* marks a patch of Nissl material often found near the nuclear envelope and commonly called the nuclear cap. *H* calls attention to heterochromatin adjacent to the nucleolus. *G* points to some granular material seen in the living state that proved not to be Nissl material after staining. *SC* marks a satellite cell nucleus. *Left,* ×1800; *right,* ×2000. (From: Deitch, A. D., and Murray, M. R.: J. Biophys. Biochem. Cytol. 2:433, 1956.)

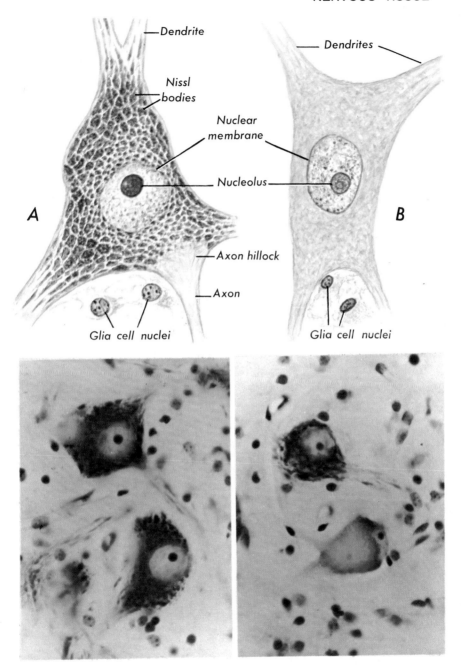

Fig. 10-5. These neurons from the ventral horn of the spinal cord are stained for Nissl substance by the toluidine blue method. *A* is a drawing of a normal neuron illustrating the absence of Nissl substance in the axon hillock region; *B* is a drawing of a neuron similarly stained after treatment with the enzyme ribonuclease to remove RNA. This preparation is counterstained with erythrosin. The pictures *below* are photomicrographs showing three normal neurons and one neuron showing chromatolysis in response to axon section several days earlier (*lower right*). The comma-shaped nucleus is at the cell body periphery, and the center of the perikaryon stains very lightly. *Above,* ×1,000; *below,* ×750.

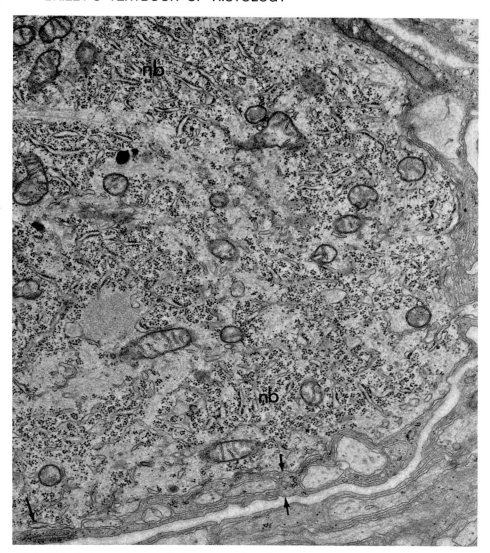

Fig. 10-6. This electron micrograph shows a portion of a neuron perikaryon ensheathed by satellite cell processes. The Nissl substance seen in Figure 10-5 is shown here to be aggregates of ribosomes and endoplasmic reticulum cisterns (as at *nb*). Light, often linear areas (sometimes called roads) separate the Nissl material. Cisterns of endoplasmic reticulum lying very near the surface of the neuron are referred to as subsurface cisterns (*single arrow*). The width of the satellite cell investment is indicated by the *paired arrows*. Rat sensory ganglion neuron. ×21,500.

micrographs (Fig. 10-6).

The fact that neurons exhibit a large nucleolus and abundant granular endoplasmic reticulum indicates that they are actively synthesizing proteins. This may seem surprising, because mature neurons are not increasing in size or number. However, most protein synthesis for the nerve cell and its extensions is accomplished in the region of the cell body (and the proximal dendrites). Material constantly moves from

these areas of production to the farthest reaches of the axon and dendrites.

After repeated electrical stimulation or after amputation of a substantial part of the axon the disposition of the chromophilic substance in the nerve cell body is altered. In this condition, known as *chromatolysis,* the nucleus becomes eccentrically located and the basophilic material in the cytoplasm is concentrated in the cell periphery (Fig. 10-5). Certain types of neu-

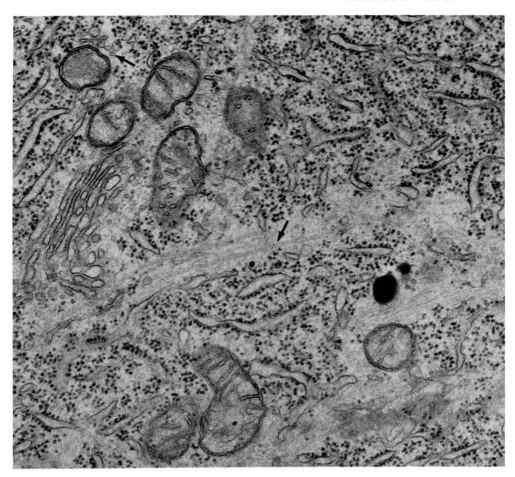

Fig. 10-7. A typical region of neuronal cytoplasm is shown in this electron micrograph. Within Nissl substance, many of the ribosomes are in polysomal aggregates that either lie free in the cytoplasm or are arrayed on cisternal membrane. Also illustrated are a Golgi region (*left*), microtubules in cross and longitudinal section (*arrows*), and two small, dense lysosomes. Rat sensory ganglion neuron. ×43,000.

rons undergo this change as a prelude to degeneration, but others are able gradually to reverse the chromatolytic pattern, regenerate amputated parts, and return to their former organization. Chromatolysis may be observed as early as the 1st day after an axon is cut and is most marked at about 2 weeks. There is little change in the total quantity of RNA in the perikaryon during the early stages of regeneration, although its concentration decreases, because the cell imbibes water and increases in volume by more than 200%. In neurons capable of axonal regeneration, the amount of RNA and protein in the neuron increases after several days, and the amputated part is slowly regenerated. The neuronal cyto-

plasm then returns to normal. The extent and rapidity of the changes depend upon the type of neuron and the nature and location of the injury: an injury near the cell body causes more effect than one at a distance. Injury near the cell body is more likely to lead to cell death.

Clear areas of neuronal cytoplasm between Nissl substance (Fig. 10-6), as well as in both axons and dendrites, contain numerous minute *filaments* and *microtubules*. The microtubules are 200 to 300 Å in diameter and are similar to those found in other cell types. Typically, the filaments are linear elements about 70 Å in diameter, occurring in groups interspersed with microtubules (Fig. 10-7). They are often called *neurofilaments,* but it is not clear whether they are chemically distinct from filaments in other cell types. Filaments and the prominent Nissl substance are the most characteristic features of the nerve cell cytoplasm. The filament content of neurons varies between species and between regions of the nervous system. The success of microscopic silver staining is sometimes related to these variations. Successful silver preparations characteristically show dark, slender elements called *neurofibrils.* The neurofibrils visible in the light microscope are aggregates of filaments on which silver has been deposited. These neurofibrils course parallel with one another in the axon and dendrite but cross and interlace in the cell body (Fig. 10-3). The frequent association between filaments and microtubules and their location among Nissl substance and in axons and dendrites suggest a possible role in intercellular transport (described below under "Axoplasmic Transport").

The *Golgi apparatus* is limited to the perikaryon. Its prominence in neurons remains unexplained because much of the protein manufactured by the neuron is not channeled through the Golgi region, as it is in secretory cells. The protein that does pass to the Golgi region in neurons may be related to the lysosomal system (see chapter 1). *Mitochondria* are plentiful in the perikaryon, as well as in the dendrites and axons. Neither the mitochondria nor the lysosomal elements of nerve cells are morphologically distinctive. *Lipofuscin pigment granules* begin to appear at an early age and increase in number and distribution with advancing age; hence they are known as "wear and tear pigment." This pigment is yellow or brown and stains with lipid dyes. These granules are apparently secondary lysosomes (chapter 1) which represent the end product of incessant lysosomal activity during the long life of the nerve cell. Their accumulation has been postulated to inhibit eventually the normal function of some neurons—a normal part of the aging process.

Some nerve cells contain granules of dark brown pigment, *melanin.* This occurs in certain cells of the olfactory bulb, the locus ceruleus in the floor of the fourth ventricle, the substantia nigra of the midbrain, and certain cells of the reticular formation. Melanin is also present in some spinal and sympathetic ganglion cells.

Dendrites

Like a tree spreading its limbs to allow each leaf exposure to the sun, the highly branched dendrites (from the Greek *dendron,* tree) allow an expansion of the neuron surface for the reception of many axon terminals. Dendrites are generally shorter than axons, but they branch repeatedly and their surface is often studded with fine spiny or knobbed excrescences (*spines* or *gemmules,* Fig. 10-8); this elaboration of surface area allows large neurons to receive as many as 100,000 separate axon terminals on their dendritic surfaces. At the point of axonal contact, the dendritic membrane is often modified (see "Synapses," below). These axonal inputs are not randomly arranged; axons from one source occupy a specific region of the dendritic tree, whereas axons from another source terminate elsewhere. The contents of the dendrites resemble those of the cell body except that Nissl substance is generally restricted to the more proximal regions. Microtubules and mitochondria are conspicuous, and there are a few microfilaments (Fig. 10-9). The dendrites, like the axons, also contain a few channels of smooth membranes.

Axons

Axons (sometimes termed axis cylinders) arise either from the nerve cell body (Fig. 10-3) or from the proximal part of a dendrite. They are slender extensions with a smoother contour and a more uniform diameter than dendrites have. The axon may have side or *collateral* branches along its length, but its most prominent branching generally occurs shortly before its termination. These terminal branches are termed *telodendria,* and the actual point of ending, where the axon is frequently enlarged, is called the *terminal.* The plasma membrane of the axon is often termed the *axolemma*; morphological specializations of this membrane have been observed in the region of the initial segment of the axon, at nodes of Ranvier (see below) and at the terminals.

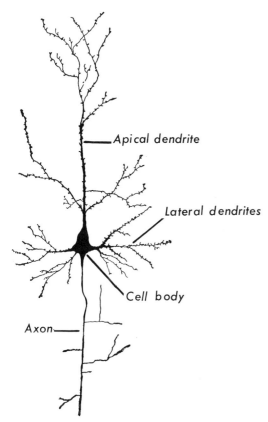

Fig. 10-8. This drawing shows part of a pyramidal cell from human cerebral cortex, including the dendritic portion, the cell body, and the proximal part of the axon. The tiny protuberances on the dendrites are called spines or gemmules. Gold chloride method.

The axonal contents are termed the *axoplasm*; this cytoplasm differs from that of the cell body in that the only formed organelles normally observed are mitochondria, filaments, microtubules, and channels of smooth membrane. Nissl substance and Golgi elements are lacking. At the point of egress of the axon from the nerve cell body (or dendrite), there is generally a region of cytoplasm from which Nissl substance is conspicuously absent (Fig. 10-2). This region marks the emerging process as the axon (rather than a dendrite) and is called the *axon hillock*.

That portion of the axon between the cell body and the point at which the myelin sheath begins is termed the *initial segment* (Figs. 10-2 and 10-10). In many neurons, this region is known to have a much lower

threshold of electrical excitability than does the dendrite or the perikaryon (see below). Morphologically, it is characterized by three special features: (1) a dense layer of finely granular material undercoating the axolemma, (2) scattered clusters of ribosomes but no discrete Nissl substance and (3) microtubules gathered into slender fascicles (Fig. 10-10).

Axoplasmic Transport

Although there is evidence that some axons contain minute amounts of nonmitochondrial RNA and that they undertake a small amount of protein synthesis, the acknowledged protein assembly center of the neuron is the cell body. The transport of manufactured material into the processes of the cell, especially the long axon, presents special problems. From observations on constricted axons, and from radioautographic studies after labeling of the proteins formed in the cell body, it is known that materials constantly travel from the cell body into the axon and are transported peripherally. The microtubules (and perhaps the filaments) are believed to be involved in this process. A small amount of material travels rapidly (at rates of 40 mm/day or more), but the bulk moves slowly, at a rate of about 1 mm/day in mammals. The latter figure is also the approximate rate of axonal regrowth after cutting. Normally, the transported materials are presumed to be destined for replenishment of proteins involved in the ion transport mechanisms of the axolemma, in the release and uptake mechanisms for neurotransmitters, and perhaps in the trophic effect of nerve on innervated tissues (see below). There is also thought to be transport of some material or signal from the periphery back to the cell body, for the nerve cell body responds to changes in the distal region of the axon.

Axon Terminals, Synapses, Receptors, and Neurotransmitters

As the action potential of an axon is carried into the region of its terminal, the mechanism of signaling is generally changed from electrical to chemical. In certain spe-

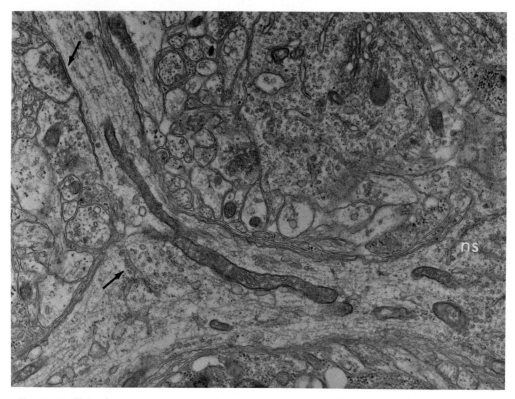

Fig. 10-9. This electron micrograph shows a primary dendrite arising from a cell body (*right*) and branching into two secondary dendrites (*left*). Nissl substance in the periphery of the parent neuron is marked *ns*. The *upper arrow* indicates an axodendritic synapse. The *lower arrow* points to endoplasmic reticulum related to ribosomes within the dendrite. Note that the dendritic shaft is covered in many places by flattened processes of astrocytes. The compactness and complexity of the cellular elements is characteristic of central nervous tissue. Rat spinal cord. ×17,000. (From: Bunge, R. P., et al.: J. Cell Biol. 24:163, 1965.)

cial terminals, however, the electrical signal may be carried directly to an adjacent cell via a communicating junction (gap junction or nexus). In neural tissues, such junctions are also frequently termed *electrical synapses, electrotonic junctions,* or *ephapses.* These junctions are akin to those observed in various epithelial cell layers, in smooth muscle, and in particular portions of the intercalated discs of the heart. Here the membranes of both cells are brought into especially close contact (Fig. 10-11), and special channels are established between the two cells to allow ionic currents involved in the electrical signal to pass directly between cell interiors with little resistance (see chapter 4 for details). This type of cell-to-cell communication has the advantage of great rapidity.

More commonly, the signal entering the axon terminal has no direct electrical effect on the adjacent cell. Instead, it causes the release of a neurotransmitter from the axon terminal. This chemical diffuses across a narrow (200-Å) intercellular space to react with a specialized *receptor* region on the adjacent cell. Interaction of neurotransmitter with receptor leads to electrical activity in the second cell. The site at which this "chemical" form of transmission (as opposed to the "electrical" transmission discussed above) takes place is called a *synapse.*

A synapse is defined as a region of specialized attachment between nerve cells or between nerve cells and effector organs. Light microscopic observations disclose synapses to be areas of axon enlargement containing mitochondria and neurofibrillar material. Electron microscopy reveals that

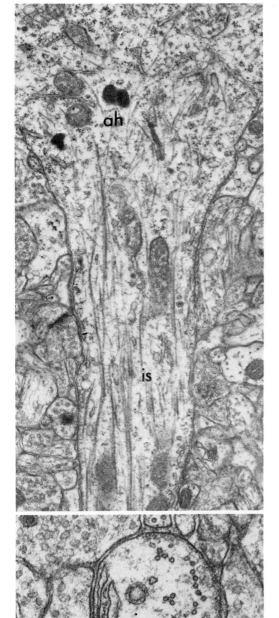

the axon characteristically contains clusters of tiny vesicles in the region of the synapse and that the plasma membrane of both the axon and the contacted cell is often modified in this area. These modifications consist of dense material applied to the inner surface of one or both of the apposed membranes, in addition to the presence of demonstrable extracellular material between the apposed membranes (Figs. 10-12 and 10-13). Unlike epithelial junctions such as desmosomes, the intracellular dense material is not disposed similarly on both membranes. This difference and the presence of vesicles in the axon make the synapse asymmetrical. This asymmetry is thought to correlate with the physiological observation that the synapse transmits the nerve signal in one direction only—from the axon to the cell contacted. The electrotonic junctions discussed above are thought to transmit the impulse with equal efficacy in either direction.

At the *synapse,* the axon is termed the *presynaptic* element, the cell being contacted is called the *postsynaptic* element, and the intervening extracellular space is designated the *synaptic cleft* (Figs. 10-12, 10-13, and 10-15). At synapses, axonal enlargements are called *boutons terminaux* (or end feet) if they are terminating, or *boutons en passage* if they continue on to make additional contacts elsewhere (Fig. 10-12). Thus, a single axon may display synapses with many different neurons. The dense material within the synaptic cleft apparently attaches the pre- and postsynaptic elements. This attachment is strong

Fig. 10-10. Electron micrographs of the initial segment of an axon of the cerebral cortex of a rat. The *upper figure* shows a longitudinal section through the initial segment (*is*) arising from the axon hillock (*ah*). Note the absence of Nissl substance and only occasional free ribosomes, the presence of dense material undercoating the axolemma, and fascicles of microtubules. The *lower figure* shows a cross section of the initial segment beyond the level of the axon hillock. In the field shown, the initial segment is partially surrounded by a large axonal terminal that forms a synaptic complex in the region marked by an *asterisk, lower right.* Two flattened cisterns surrounded by dense material are seen on the *left side* of the segment; similar structures are sometimes found in dendritic spines. *Upper figure,* ×23,000; *lower figure,* ×49,000. (From: Peters, A., et al.: J. Cell Biol. 39:604, 1968.)

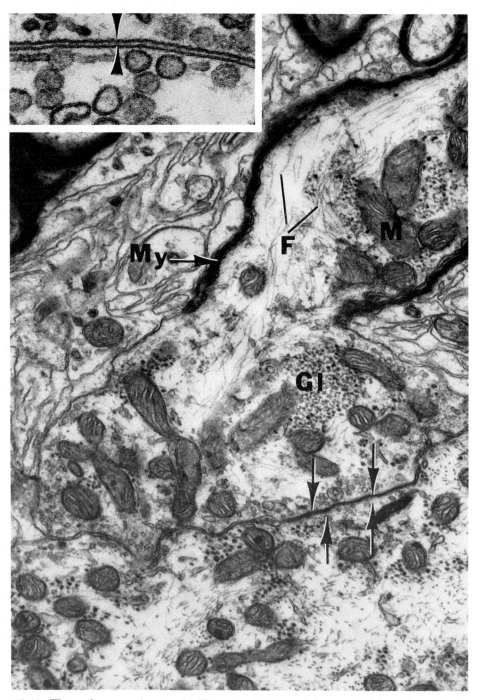

Fig. 10-11. These electron micrographs illustrate the type of close apposition of cell membranes that allows direct electrical coupling between nerve cells. This is a section of an axosomatic electrotonic synapse from the medulla of a gymnotid fish, Sternopygus. Filaments (*F*), mitochondria (*M*), and glycogen (*Gl*) are present in the axon. Termination of the myelin sheath (*My*) may be seen. At the *paired arrows* the axonal membrane and the membrane of a neuron cell body are very closely apposed. The *inset* (*upper left*) shows a similar junction at higher magnification to illustrate the closely apposed membranes (at *arrows*). ×27,500; inset, ×110,000. (Courtesy of Dr. George Pappas.)

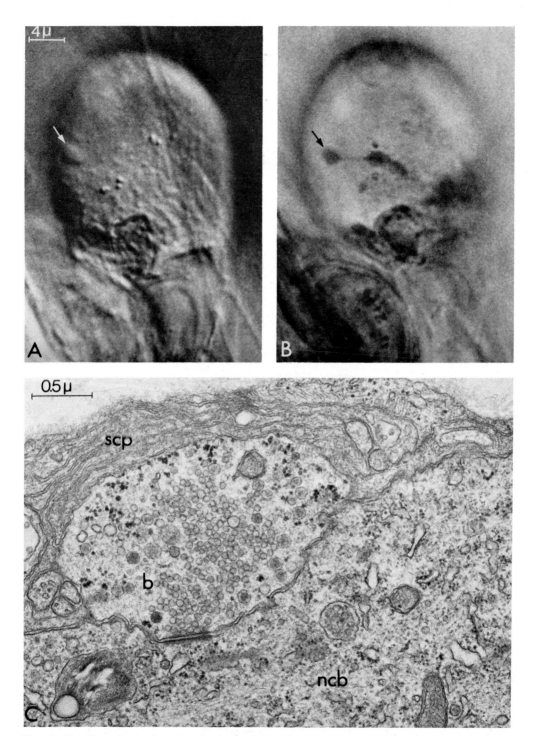

Fig. 10-12. These three photographs show a synaptic bouton in living tissue (*A*), after vital staining
(*B*), and after preparation for electron microscopy (*C*). *A* shows a bouton (*arrow*) on the cell body
of a parasympathetic neuron in the interatrial septum of the frog heart. The septum has been
removed from the heart, pinned out in tissue culture medium, and viewed with a Nomarski
differential interference contrast optical system. *B* shows the same nerve cell 15 min after adding a
dilute solution of methylene blue to the medium. The terminal synaptic bouton (*arrow*) seen in *A*
and two others (apparently boutons en passage) not visible in the unstained preparation have taken
up the dye. *C* is an electron micrograph of this type of bouton. A bouton (*b*) contains a mitochondrion,
glycogen particles, a few granular vesicles, and numerous small agranular vesicles, some of which
are clustered next to a region of specialized membrane. Layers of Schwann cell processes (*scp*)
cover the bouton, except where it is in contact with the postsynaptic nerve cell body (*ncb*). (From:
McMahan, U. J., and Kuffler, S. W.: *In* Excitatory Synaptic Mechanisms, edited by P. Andersen
and J. K. S. Jansen. p. 57, 1970.)

enough to survive tissue homogenization and differential centrifugation, and it is possible to prepare a tissue fraction comprised, in large part, of the axon terminals still attached to cleft substance and postsynaptic membrane. Such preparations are termed *synaptosomes* and are now widely used in biochemical studies.

Synapses may be classified on the basis of (1) position, (2) membrane specialization, or (3) organelle content. On the basis of position, they are termed *axodendritic, axosomatic,* or *axoaxonic,* thus indicating whether an axon abuts upon a dendrite, a nerve cell body, or another axon. Axoaxonic synapses are most often found on the initial segment region or near the axon terminal. Some axodendritic synapses are distinguished by an increased amount of dense material coating the cytoplasmic side of the synaptic membranes and a widening of the synaptic cleft (Fig. 10-14).

Variations in the quantity and quality of *synaptic vesicle* content of the axon terminal also aid in the classification of synapses. Although the vesicle content of the terminal is often not homogeneous, one type generally predominates. At neuromuscular junctions (where nerve contacts skeletal muscle) and in many CNS terminals, the majority of synaptic vesicles are 300 to 600 Å in diameter and are spherical with apparently clear centers (Figs. 10-12 and 10-13). In axon terminals of autonomic nerve fibers supplying smooth muscle (as in the intestine and ductus deferens), the synaptic vesicles may be slightly larger. They are also round but contain a prominent dense particle or short rod (Fig. 10-48). This allows the distinction between terminals with "clear" and those with "dense-cored" (or granular) vesicles. It has been observed that synapses known to release the neurotransmitter acetylcholine (i.e., *cholinergic* synapses) contain clear vesicles, whereas terminals known to release noradrenalin (i.e., *adrenergic* synapses) contain vesicles with dense cores. Aldehyde fixation of nervous tissue produces varying images of endings which contain predominantly clear vesicles. In these preparations, the clear vesicles in certain axonal endings appear smaller and are disc-shaped instead of spherical. Clusters of this type of vesicle have been observed in axonal terminals that are known

to be inhibitory in function (Fig. 10-15), but this has not been a consistent correlation, and hence the demonstration of this type of vesicle is not considered sufficient evidence to identify a synapse as inhibitory. Rather, the varying synaptic vesicle morphology may be due to osmotic effects. The matter awaits clarification.

The demonstration of vesicles in axonal endings and the physiological observation that certain transmitters are released in "packets" (i.e., in pulses of several thousand molecules rather than in a continuous stream) have together led to the suggestion that the vesicles contain or bind the neurotransmitter. It was also suggested that vesicles release the neurotransmitter by dumping it into the synaptic cleft after fusing with the presynaptic membrane, i.e., by pinocytosis in reverse (Fig. 10-13). It seems certain that neurotransmitters are located in synaptic vesicles, but the mechanism of their release is not as clear and may differ in cholinergic and adrenergic synapses.

The synaptic complex is also known to contain mechanisms for the breakdown and/or uptake of released neurotransmitter. Certain cholinergic synaptic areas are known to contain the enzyme acetylcholinesterase in the pre- and postsynaptic elements, in the synaptic cleft, and in the adjacent tissues. This enzyme hydrolyzes acetylcholine with the formation of acetate and choline. Part of the choline is taken up by the presynaptic element and reutilized in subsequent acetylcholine synthesis. In adrenergic endings, the transmitter has not been observed to be similarly broken down; it is simply taken up intact from the surrounding extracellular spaces for reuse.

The number of clearly identified neurotransmitters is few, including *acetylcholine, norepinephrine* (noradrenaline), *γ-aminobutyric acid, serotonin,* and possibly *glycine* and *dopamine.* These are all small molecules which, after release, combine with specific areas on the postsynaptic membrane called *receptor sites.* The receptor sites react with a specific neurotransmitter and not with others, and this reaction engenders a permeability change to certain ions. If this permeability change leads to a decrease in the electrical polarization of the postsynaptic membrane, the effect is *excitatory,* making it more likely

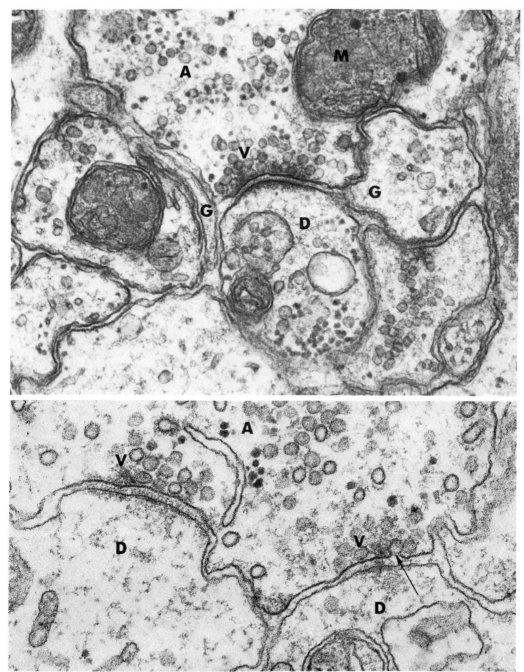

Fig. 10-13. Electron micrographs showing synaptic regions from the brain of a salamander. In the *upper figure,* an axonal terminal (A) is in synaptic juxtaposition with a dendritic terminal (D). The presynaptic cytoplasm of the axon is characterized by clustered presynaptic vesicles (V). A filamentous web can be seen along the postsynaptic (dendritic) side of the contact zone. A dense intercellular material occupies the synaptic cleft between axonal and dendritic surfaces. Glial cell processes (G) appear to encircle and seal the synaptic cleft. Dense glycogen granules are found within both axonal and dendritic cytoplasms, and mitochondria (M) are characteristic of axonal terminals. In the *lower figure,* an axonal terminal (A) abuts upon portions of two dendrites (D). Two synaptic sites are characterized by presynaptic vesicles (V), one of which appears to have been fixed at the moment of its continuity with the presynaptic plasma membrane (*arrow*). Upper figure, ×71,000; lower figure, ×81,000.

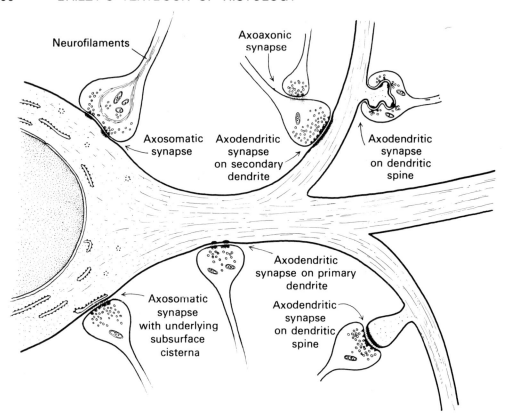

Fig. 10-14. The types of synapses occurring on various parts of the neuron are depicted here. Note that the degree of membrane "thickening" varies in different types of synapses, and that the material applied to the cytoplasmic side of the presynaptic membrane is often seen as a regular pattern rather than as a solid plaque. Variations in synaptic vesicle morphology are not shown.

that the postsynaptic element will generate an action potential. When recording from the postsynaptic cell, the physiologist observes an excitatory postsynaptic potential (often abbreviated EPSP). If the effect is to increase electrical polarization of the membrane, making it less likely that the postsynaptic element will "fire," the effect is said to be *inhibitory* and an inhibitory postsynaptic potential (IPSP) is recorded. The specificity of synaptic action depends upon the receptor site rather than on the neurotransmitter, for a transmitter may have an excitatory influence at one synapse and an inhibitory effect at another.

It seems certain that molecules other than neurotransmitters must also pass between cells at synaptic junctions, for many synapses also have a *trophic action* on the postsynaptic element. The normal state of skeletal muscle, for example, is dependent upon the continuing presence of neuromus-

cular junctions; if the nerve is cut, the neuromuscular contact degenerates and the electrical, chemical, and anatomical properties of the muscle fiber are permanently altered unless nerve regeneration occurs. Certain neurons of the CNS do not survive if a substantial portion of their synaptic input is removed.

The junction between nerve terminal and skeletal muscle has many of the properties of the basic synaptic apparatus described above. The functional relationship between nerve and cardiac or smooth muscle, on the other hand, presents some basic differences; these are discussed below under the heading of "Nerve Terminations."

Neurons, like many other cells, maintain a negative electrical potential across their plasma membrane, the inside of the cell being about 70 mv more negative than the outside. If this potential is made progressively less negative, a point is reached at

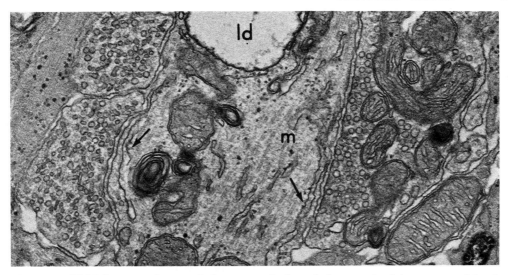

Fig. 10-15. This electron micrograph from rat spinal cord shows a dendrite contacted by three axonal boutons. The dendrite contains microtubules (*m*), mitochondria, a large lipid droplet (*ld*) and cisterns of endoplasmic reticulum underlying its surface membrane (*arrows*). Note that the axonal terminal on the *right* contains predominantly round synaptic vesicles, whereas the two terminals on the *left* contain vesicles that are generally somewhat smaller and somewhat flattened. These differences in synaptic vesicle morphology are revealed only after primary fixation in aldehyde. ×46,000. (From: Bunge, M. B., et al.: Brain Res. 6:728, 1967.)

which major permeability changes in the surface membrane cause the generation of an action potential; once generated, this action potential tends to be propagated rapidly and with little loss of amplitude over the neuron surface. On many neurons, however, there is a limited number of sites at which action potentials are generated. The dendritic tree and the cell body are often not very excitable. The action of synaptic contacts in these areas leads to transient local shifts, some inhibitory and some excitatory, in the properties of the postsynaptic membrane. Generally, only when several excitatory synaptic inputs act together (and are not canceled by inhibitory influences) does a change in membrane potential reach sufficient strength to be carried down over the dendrite and cell body to excite the initial axonal segment. In most neurons, this region is much more sensitive to membrane potential shifts than is the dendrite or the cell body, and it is here—at the initial segment—where the all or none action potential of the axon is initiated.

Neuroglia

Most organs of the body have an internal connective tissue framework which not only serves as a vascular bed but also provides a supporting skeleton for the particular cellular elements of the organ. Peripheral nerve has such a framework, albeit rather specialized (as discussed below), whereas the CNS does not. This is not difficult to appreciate if one recalls that the CNS is an epithelium and that epithelia are segregated from connective tissues. The brain and spinal cord are "floated" in a fluid environment: the cerebrospinal fluid. Connective tissue associated with the CNS is limited to the enveloping membranes (the meninges) and to a small amount which accompanies blood vessels. The neuroglia (from the Greek *neuron*, nerve, + *glia*, glue) or more simply, glia, form the nonneuronal interstitial tissue of the nervous system. The neuroglia are thought to assist the neurons in their activities. For example, certain glial cells invest axons with a myelin sheath, dramatically increasing the speed of impulse conduction. Other functions of glia are less clear. It has been suggested that they provide direct assistance for the metabolic activities of neurons by providing high energy compounds, or by assisting in control of neuronal environment (by reacting to changes in ion concentration in the extracellular spaces or by aiding in the elimination of CO_2). Glial cells do not generate action potentials, and they have never been observed to provide or to receive synapses. Studies of glial function are presently a fertile frontier in neurobiological research.

Before the era of the electron microscope, neuroglia could be studied only by special and often difficult selective staining procedures. Electron microscopy has provided the means for studying all elements of nervous tissue simultaneously and for delineating the relationships of cell membranes. Hence, many of the features described below are seen only in electron micrographs.

In routine preparations of CNS tissue, many of the nuclei seen with the light microscope do not belong either to nerve cells or to vascular tissue (Fig. 10-5). These nuclei belong to the glial cells, and careful study of their morphology often permits identification of particular cell types. However, the identifying characteristics observable by light microscopy are not equal to those seen by electron microscopy. Glial cells within the CNS have traditionally been divided into the following classes: (1) *astrocytes,* (2) *oligodendrocytes,* (3) *microglia,* and (4) *ependyma* (Fig. 10-16). These are the derivatives of the *neural tube glioblast* population. The *neurolemma cells* (or *cells of Schwann*) of peripheral nerves and the *satellite cells* which surround the cell bodies of the spinal and cranial ganglia are the glial elements of the peripheral nervous system, the *neural crest glioblast* derivatives.

Astrocytes

As the name implies, the astrocytes are stellate cells with many cytoplasmic processes (Figs. 10-16 and 10-17). They are often divided into two general types, *protoplasmic* and *fibrous,* which have in common their shape (which provides a large surface area), the presence of characteristic cytoplasmic filaments and glycogen, a generally loosely packed cytoplasm, and a tendency to have one or more processes terminating in the immediate vicinity of a blood vessel (perivascular feet). In both astrocytic types, the nucleus is irregularly ovoid and less compact than in other glial cell types.

Protoplasmic Astrocytes. These are found principally in the gray matter of the brain and spinal cord. In addition to their perivascular cellular extensions, these cells also provide flattened processes which cover much of the nonsynaptic neuronal surface, and they circumscribe synaptic zones, suggesting that they may function to separate the activities of synaptic regions from adjacent tissues (Fig. 10-13). In some areas of the brain, protoplasmic astrocytes are connected to one another by low resistance communicating (gap) junctions. There are also isolated reports of similar junctions between the membranes of neurons and astrocytes. The significance of such junctions is not obvious in terms of the present state of knowledge.

Fibrous Astrocytes. These differ from the protoplasmic type in having fewer processes which are much straighter and longer (Fig. 10-16). They possess many more filaments coursing in bundles through their cytoplasm (Fig. 10-18). When specially stained in light microscopic preparations, these bundles appear as straight, unbranched "astroglial fibers." Fibrous astrocytes are found chiefly in the white matter. They have been observed to be attached to each other by communicating, intermediate, and desmosomal types of junctions. Fibrous astrocyte processes are particularly numerous near the periphery of the brain and spinal cord. Here their end feet form the continuous outer perimeter of the neural tissue. As such, this *astrocytic border* (or *outer glia limitans*) abuts directly upon the basal lamina surrounding the entire CNS, including those regions (*perivascular space*) where that basal lamina courses deeply into the brain or cord to accompany blood vessels. *Hence, the astrocytic border constitutes the basal, cellular surface of the entire CNS epithelium.*

Fibrous astrocytes are the scarring cells of the nervous system, filling in gaps after tissue is lost in various disease processes. Connective tissue may also participate in CNS scarring. The result is generally a hardened mass of tissue within the normally soft brain tissue. This scarring process is termed *sclerosis* ("hardening").

Oligodendrocytes

These cells are also called oligodendroglia (from the Greek *oligos,* few, + *dendron,*

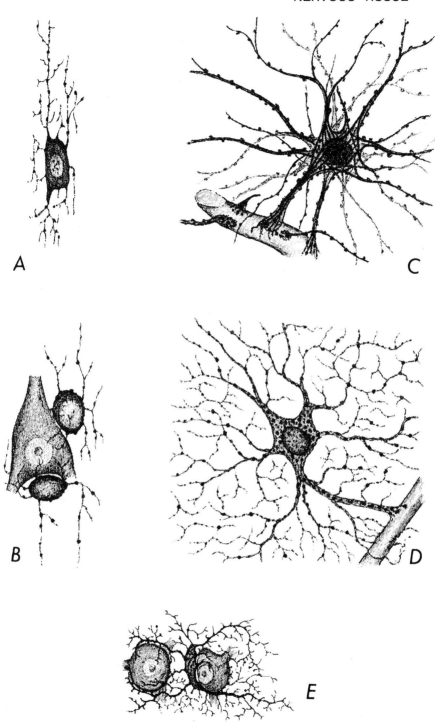

Fig. 10-16. *A*, oligodendrocyte in white matter (interfascicular form) (see also Fig. 10-33); *B*, two oligodendrocytes lying against a nerve cell (perineuronal form); *C*, astrocyte of fibrous type with processes forming foot plates against a neighboring blood vessel. Astrocytic fibrils (bundles of filaments) are visible in the cell body and the processes. *D*, astrocyte of protoplasmic type with foot plate on blood vessel; *E*, microglial cell in vicinity of two nerve cell bodies. Redrawn from a preparation by Penfield; del Rio-Hortega's modified silver method.

tree, + *glia,* glue). They were given their name by del Rio-Hortega because of the fact that their branches are small and few as compared with the astrocytes. They differ from astrocytes in the following ways: (1) their nuclei are generally smaller, rounder, and denser than astrocytic nuclei—this is the chief identifying characteristic in the standard histological preparation; (2) the entire cell body is smaller and the processes are fewer and more delicate; (3) their cytoplasm is denser, containing chiefly ribosomes, mitochondria and microtubles, and the filaments and glycogen prominent in astrocytic cytoplasm are absent (Figs. 10-19 and 10-20).

Oligodendrocytes are of three general types. When found in groups adjacent to blood vessels, they are termed *perivascular;* their function in this position is unknown. When found directly adjacent to neuron cell bodies (as in gray matter), they are termed *perineuronal* (or gray matter

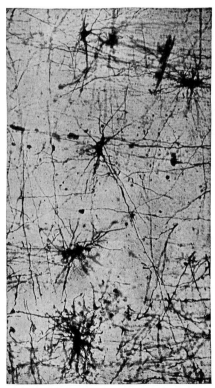

Fig. 10-17. This photomicrograph shows several astrocytes in the white matter of spinal cord. The straight unbranched processes are characteristic of the fibrous astrocytes of this region. Golgi's chrome-silver method.

satellite cells). This close relationship suggests some type of symbiosis between glia and neuron, but efforts to identify positively what might exchange between them have not yet been successful.

When oligodendrocytes are found in white matter, they are termed *interfascicular.* Many, perhaps most, of these are directly related to myelin formation and maintenance in a manner in many ways similar to that of the peripheral Schwann cell (discussed below). The anatomical connection between the myelin supporting oligodendrocyte cell body and the myelin sheath is narrow and joins one oligodendrocyte with several myelin sheaths—a connection thought to be permanent and to provide a route through which may pass the necessary materials for the maintenance of the myelin sheath. Thus, such myelin sheaths appear to be metabolically related to the oligodendrocyte cell body in much the same way that the axon is related to the neuron cell body (Fig. 10-35).

Certain of the smaller cells in nervous tissue (which may be classified as small oligodendrocytes) may be multipotential reserve or "stem" cells capable of reacting to various types of nervous system damage and providing whatever type of glial cell is needed for repair.

Microglia

This glial type has usually been described by light microscopists as a small, densely staining cell with a rounded, deeply staining nucleus. In preparations stained by special silver techniques, the cells identified as microglia have delicate and tortuous cytoplasmic processes with delicate spines (Fig. 10-16*E*). High resolution electron micrographs reveal very few cells that can be identified as microglia in normal nervous tissue, and it seems likely that many of the cells identified as microglia by silver techniques are varieties of oligodendrocytes. The microglia are generally considered to be macrophages and hence derived from promonocytes (see "The Macrophage System," chapter 5). Although there is some controversy concerning this interpretation, it seems clear that (1) there are relatively few macrophages present in normal nervous tissue, (2) mononuclear precursors of macrophages circulat-

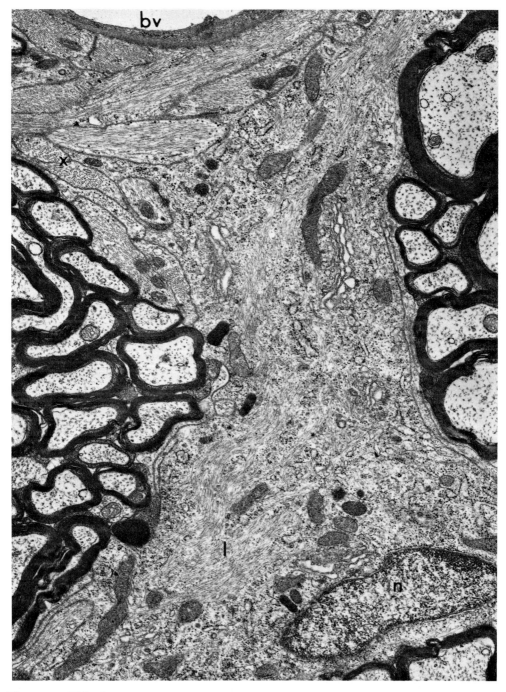

Fig. 10-18. This electron micrograph from rat optic nerve shows a fibrous astrocyte interposed between myelinated axons (cut in cross section). Part of the astrocyte nucleus (*n*) is shown, as well as astroglial filaments cut in longitudinal (*l*) and in cross (*x*) section. A series of filament-filled astrocytic processes are applied to the basal lamina surrounding a blood vessel (*bv*) at the *top* of the picture. Some of these processes contain glycogen particles. ×15,000. (From Vaughn, J. E., and Peters, A.: J. Comp. Neurol., 133:269, 1968.)

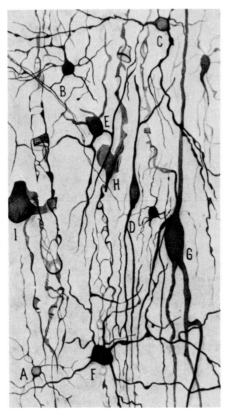

Fig. 10-19. This drawing by del Rio-Hortega shows the various types of oligodendrocytes found in white and gray matter. Note that the cells have few processes but that these may be very complex. The elaborate interfascicular forms of oligodendrocytes shown at *H* and *I* are depicted in more detail in Figure 10-33. (From: del Rio-Hortega, P.: Mem. Real. Soc. Espan. Hist. Nat., 14:5, 1928.)

ing in the bloodstream rapidly enter the nervous tissue after injury, and (3) most of the neuroglial cells can participate to some extent in the activities required for the removal of cell debris. In many cases of minimal injury the astrocyte can dispose of the debris, and invasion by macrophage precursors is not required.

In extensive injury when a great deal of dead tissue must be disposed of, the phagocytic cells become greatly enlarged and stuffed with debris, so that the nucleus appears compressed or indented (Fig. 10-21). These cells are called compound granular corpuscles or gitter cells (lattice-like cells). Most of the cells of this type are derived from cells that migrate from the

bloodstream, and whether some also differentiate from glial cells remains controversial. These cells are capable of taking up impressive amounts of cellular remnants (especially myelin); laden with this material, they take up positions around blood vessels, and the contained material is slowly digested over several weeks or months.

Ependyma

The ependyma (Figs. 10-22 and 10-23) in ordinary preparations appears to consist of closely packed cells with elongated nuclei, lining the cavities of the spinal cord and brain (central canal and ventricles). Their long axes are perpendicular to the cavity, and although they present the appearance of a columnar or cuboidal epithelium, this is a false impression. Ependymal cells are in reality derived as the most apical cells of the neural tube epithelium. In the adult, therefore, they are closely adherent cell bodies lining the apical (ventricular) surface of the CNS epithelium; the basal surface is the outer perimeter of the brain and cord. These cells have inner processes ramifying more or less deeply into the epithelial walls of the CNS and sometimes providing end feet to the outer glia limitans or to perivascular areas. Ependymal processes are not unlike those of fibrous astrocytes in their fine structure. They may have, in certain forms and in certain places at least, cilia which protrude into the neural cavity (Fig. 10-23).

Peripheral Glia

As peripheral axons course among various body tissues, they are found everywhere in association with companion cells which provide various types of axonal ensheathment. When these companion cells are in association with a nerve cell body (as in the peripheral ganglia of the autonomic or sensory system), they are called *satellite cells;* when they provide ensheathment for axons, they are called *neurilemma cells* or *cells of Schwann.* During development, these companion cells arise from neural crest and migrate peripherally along the outgrowing axons. They provide a sheath which everywhere encloses the nerve, except at certain axon tips, as dis-

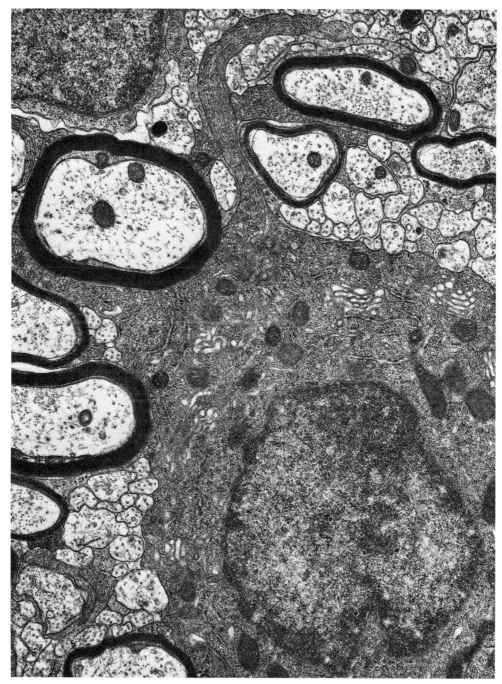

Fig. 10-20. This electron micrograph from neonatal rat spinal cord shows an oligodendrocyte in apposition to both myelinated and unmyelinated axons. Oligodendrocytes present this dense appearance after aldehyde fixation. They characteristically contain many ribosomes and microtubules and lack bundles of filaments. The slender processes of this cell are related to myelin segments (as is shown schematically in Fig. 10-35). ×16,000. (Courtesy of Drs. P. L. Hinds and J. E. Vaughn.)

cussed below (Fig. 10-45). The basic form of ensheathment provided for the axon is shown in Figures 10-24 and 10-25. The

Schwann cell embraces the axon and cradles it in a trough formed from its plasma membrane. The axons remain outside the

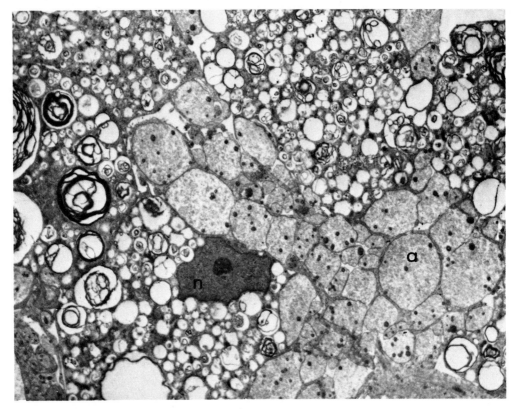

Fig. 10-21. Microglial cells (gitter cells) engorged with remnants of degenerating myelin are shown in this electron micrograph from a demyelinating lesion in cat spinal cord. Cross-sectioned axons which have lost their myelin sheaths occupy the *lower right* and *central* areas of the picture (e.g., *a*). The remainder of this field is filled with the cytoplasm of four microglial phagocytes. These become so engorged with debris that the nucleus may be indented (as in *n*). ×4500. (From: Bunge, R. P., et al.: J. Biophys. Biochem. Cytol. 7:685, 1960.)

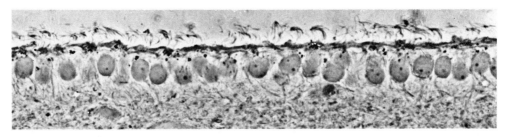

Fig. 10-22. This photomicrograph shows the row of ependymal cells lining the wall of the third ventricle of an adult rabbit brain. Bundles of cilia protrude from the ventricular surfaces of these cells. (From: Tennyson, V. M., and Pappas, G. D.: *In* Pathology of the Nervous System, edited by J. Minckler, p. 518, McGraw-Hill, New York, 1968.)

Schwann cell cytoplasm but are surrounded by its plasma membrane. The region in which the lips of the encircling Schwann cell processes approach each other is termed the *mesaxon* (Figs. 10-25 and 10-26). Each Schwann cell extends over a distance of several hundred micrometers along the axon, and the external surface of each Schwann cell becomes encased in basal lamina to separate it from surrounding connective tissue. This basic pattern of ensheathment, with a single Schwann cell embracing from one to a dozen separate axons, is found throughout the peripheral nervous

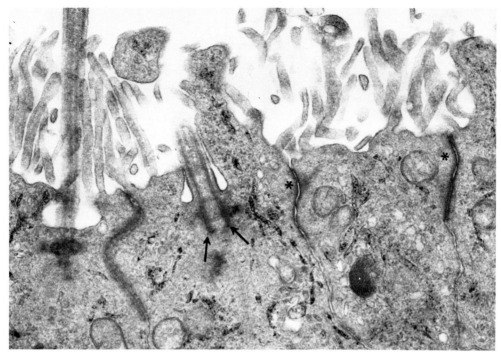

Fig. 10-23. This electron micrograph shows both microvilli and cilia projecting from the surface of ependymal cells lining the spinal cord central canal in a human fetus. The *arrows* indicate a basal body at the base of the cilium. Junctional complexes (*) occur between lateral cell borders near the free cell surface. ×23,500. (From: Tennyson, V.: *In* Developmental Neurobiology, edited by W. A. Himwich, p. 47, C. C. Thomas, Springfield, Illinois, 1970.)

systems of both invertebrates and vertebrates. In many species, this is the highest form of peripheral nerve ensheathment found.

Nerve fibers ensheathed in this manner are termed *unmyelinated;* they comprise the majority of the postganglionic axons from the autonomic ganglia and axons from the smaller neurons of the sensory ganglia. These unmyelinated peripheral nerve fibers are sometimes called C fibers or fibers of Remak. They conduct nerve impulses at the rate of about 1 m/sec. In light microscopic observations of routine histological preparations, these smaller diameter unmyelinated fibers are often not directly visible, but the presence of a nerve fascicle in the tissue can be distinguished by the elongated nuclei of the ensheathing Schwann cells, as well as by the connective tissue layers, discussed below, which are external to the Schwann cell ensheathment (Fig. 10-24). The function of Schwann cell ensheathment of unmyelinated nerve fibers is not known, but it is known that the axolemma,

and not the plasmalemma of the Schwann cell, is the membrane responsible for the propagation of the action potential.

Peripheral Myelination

The majority of the peripheral nerve fibers have a diameter of more than 1 μm; these fibers become ensheathed by myelin, which is actually the spirally disposed plasma membrane of the Schwann cell, compacted to provide a highly resistant but regularly interrupted sleeve of insulation around the axon. During development of the sheath, the apposing lips of a single embracing Schwann cell slide by one another, forming a spiral membrane as the original mesaxon elongates (Fig. 10-25, *B* to *D*).

There is some evidence that this "jelly roll" configuration of myelin is accomplished by the repeated circumnavigation of the axon by the outer mass of Schwann cell cytoplasm—that part containing the nucleus. This leaves behind a great length

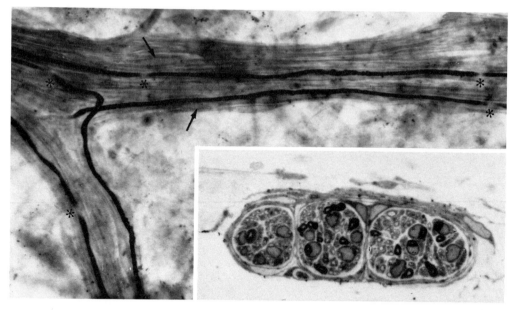

Fig. 10-24. These light micrographs show a small nerve fascicle viewed longitudinally (*above*) and in cross section (*inset*). The tissue has been fixed in OsO₄, which preserves and blackens myelin. In the *upper picture,* individual segments of myelin are delineated by nodes (*). The remainder of the fascicle is composed of unmyelinated nerve fibers and their associated Schwann cells. Cell nuclei (*arrows*) are not stained but are visible as elliptical structures between the nerve fibers. In the cross section, a perineurial sheath is seen around each of three small nerve fascicles. Myelin sheaths, some with related Schwann cell nuclei, and individual unmyelinated fibers with Schwann cell investments are shown. ×500; *inset,* ×1600.

of spiraled and specialized plasma membrane which becomes compacted together into lamellae to form myelin. As compaction occurs, the outer surface of the membrane from one turn of the spiral is applied to the outer surface of the membrane from the next, to form the *intraperiod line* of compact myelin; the apposition of the cytoplasmic surfaces as the cell cytoplasm is eliminated forms the *major dense line* of the myelin sheath (Fig. 10-25). By this mechanism, one Schwann cell forms one segment or *internode* of the myelin of one axon, with the Schwann cell nucleus located external to the compacted lamellae and about midway along the myelin segment. The Schwann cell also invests its external surface with a basal lamina as myelination proceeds toward completion. At each end of the internode, there is a gap of a few micrometers, which is called a *node of Ranvier,* and then another internode of myelin begins (Fig. 10-24). As nerves elongate during growth, the diameter of the axon is further increased and the segments of myelin are increased in length and in diameter,

so that the thickest axons will eventually have the longest (and thickest) segments of myelin and thus the greatest distance between the interrupting nodes of Ranvier.

One might suspect that a very narrow extracellular space might wind itself between the layers of myelin, thus providing a spiral path for the flux of extracellular material from outside in to reach the axon. However, this possibility seems negated by recent freeze-fracture evidence that discloses a narrow occluding junction that seals the gap at its outer margins, i.e., along outer- and innermost mesaxon and along the edges of the nodes of Ranvier (Fig. 10-27).

Figures 10-28 and 10-31 illustrate that myelin is an integral part of the Schwann cell and that Schwann cell cytoplasm is retained both external and internal to the compact myelin layers and in the paranodal areas. The amount of cytoplasm in these regions decreases with development, but substantial amounts remain in the region of the Schwann cell nucleus and near the nodes of Ranvier. The cytoplasm external

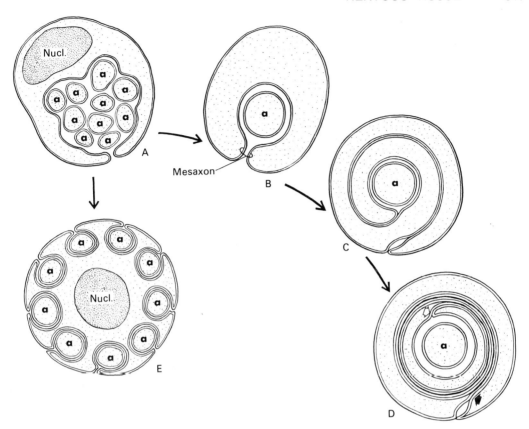

Fig. 10-25. Forms of ensheathment in peripheral nerve. During development, the small embryonic nerve fibers are surrounded in groups by Schwann cells (*A*). Those fibers which will become myelinated enlarge and become ensheathed by individual Schwann cells (*B*). The encircling lips of the Schwann cell slide by one another, and the mesaxon is elongated (*C*). As the mesaxon is compacted (*D*), myelin is formed. Note that the apposition of the cytoplasmic surfaces of the plasma membrane forms the major dense line of the myelin sheath; the apposition of the external surfaces of the plasma membrane forms the intraperiod line (*D*). Axons which will not be myelinated remain small and obtain ensheathment within individual troughs in the Schwann cell (*E*). *a* = axon; *nucl.* = nucleus; inner mesaxon marked by *white arrow;* outer mesaxon marked by *black arrow.*

to the compact myelin is visible in the light microscope and has frequently been termed the neurilemma sheath. Unfortunately, this term has also been used in the past to include various connective tissue elements external to the Schwann cell, including the basal lamina that borders all Schwann cells. It is important to distinguish between the cytoplasm of the myelin-related Schwann cell and the adjacent connective tissue.

At the node of Ranvier, the lamellae ofmyelin also appear more widely separated because Schwann cell cytoplasm has been retained. Each myelin lamella is brought successively into contact with the axon, so that the outermost lamellae of myelin approach the axon nearest the node. At the node itself, loosely interdigitating Schwann cell processes partially fill the nonmyelinated interval (Figs. 10-30 and 10-31). The basal lamina surrounding one internode is directly continuous with that of the next internode, thus bridging the node of Ranvier.

Initially, the myelin segment is quite smooth and regular. If not injured, the myelin-Schwann cell unit, like the neuron, is thought to be maintained for the lifetime of the individual. As it ages, myelin develops distortions and redundancies in its basic tubular form. In addition, there develop oblique, funnel-shaped clefts, called *Schmidt-Lanterman* clefts, which interrupt the smooth contour of the internode. These

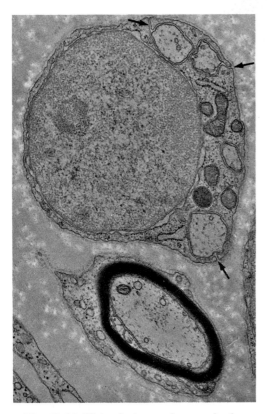

Fig. 10-26. This electron micrograph shows four unmyelinated nerve fibers ensheathed by one Schwann cell. The mesaxons (where the trough of Schwann cell membrane is open to the extracellular space) are marked by *arrows*. A myelinated axon appears below. Rat peripheral nerve. ×23,000.

clefts have been observed in the living myelin sheath, and electron microscopic examination has established that they are focal areas along successive layers of myelin where there is incomplete membrane compaction and Schwann cell cytoplasm is retained (Fig. 10-28).

The finer details of the myelin sheath are not visible in the routine histological preparation. If a fixative that preserves lipid (such as osmium tetroxide) has been used, the compacted regions of myelin are visualized as a sleeve around the axon. In preparations involving the use of lipid solvents, much of the myelin sheath is dissolved, leaving a proteolipid residue called *"neurokeratin."* In silver-stained preparations, the axon appears in cross sections as a central density apparently surrounded by a space because the myelin has been largely

extracted. These points are illustrated in Fig. 10-29.

Myelin-containing tissues can be fractionated and a relatively pure myelin preparation recovered. This is found to contain about 80% lipid, including cholesterol, phospholipids, glycolipids, and plasmalogens, and about 20% protein, including some proteolipids. The high lipid content gives myelin a whitish appearance in the fresh state. This explains the whiteness of peripheral nerves (e.g., the white rami of the autonomic nerves, as compared with the gray rami that contain primarily unmyelinated fibers), as well as the distinction between white and gray matter of the CNS.

The myelinated axon is the superhighway of the nervous system, the periodic interruptions at the nodes of Ranvier providing the "limited access" to current flow which allows myelin ensheathment to speed greatly the process of impulse conduction. In the typical myelinated nerve fiber, the action potential is first generated in the initial segment of the axon (Fig. 10-2). This current flows through the axon to depolarize and "fire" the first node of Ranvier. The action potential thus generated forces a pulse of current into the axon interior. Because of the high resistance and low capacitance of the surrounding myelin, the current remains confined to the axon and flows forward, not radially, until the next node is reached. Thus, the myelinated fiber forces ionic currents to flow great distances before regeneration of the action potential. Both physiological and morphological evidence now suggests that the axonal plasmalemma is far richer in sodium channels in the nodal region. It appears that specific proteins termed *ionophores* are accumulated and maintained in the membrane at each node, each such molecule providing an ion pump or pore for ionic influx or outflux associated with excitation of the axonal membrane of each successive node. This leaping or jumping of the current has led to the term *saltatory conduction*. This process is not only faster than the sequential deplorization of unmyelinated fibers but also more economical of ionic interchange between the inside and outside of the fiber.

Myelinated fibers vary considerably in size, from large (10 to 20 μm in overall

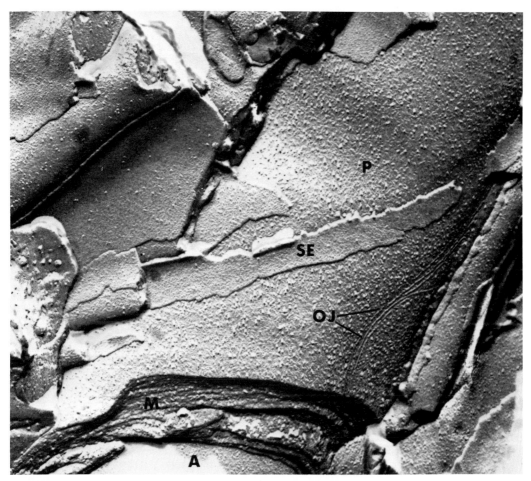

Fig. 10-27. Electron micrograph of a freeze fracture replica from the brain of a salamander. A myelinated axon (*A*) has been exposed at the *lower edge* of the picture after its myelin investments (*M*) and much of its Schwann cell have been cleaved away. The P-face (*P*) of the outermost myelin lamella is exposed to view, as is a small slip of Schwann cell membrane E-face (*SE*). Ridges of an occluding junction (*OJ*) are seen on the myelin P-face near the area of the outer mesaxon. ×60,000.

diameter) to medium (4 to 10 μm) to small (2 to 4 μm) (Fig. 10-29). In recent physiological classification, the large and medium fibers are type A, the small myelinated fibers are type B, and unmyelinated fibers are type C. The largest diameter fibers have the longest myelin segments (between 1 and 2 mm); they thus have the greatest spacing between nodes and hence the fastest nerve conduction rates (up to 140 m/sec).

Central Myelination

The major differences between peripheral myelin and that within the CNS are: (1) there is little cytoplasm associated with the mature central myelin sheath; (2) the cell body which forms central myelin—the oligodendrocyte—is not as directly apposed to central myelin segments as is the Schwann cell in the periphery; and (3) the myelin supporting oligodendrocyte may be related, at least during development, to more than one axon and to more than one segment of forming myelin (Figs. 10-33 to 10-35). In addition, there is no basal lamina associated with myelin sheaths in the CNS. This is expected because the CNS is an epithelium and basal lamina material is deposited only outside epithelia. Whereas the overall pattern of myelin deposition is the same, the relation of the oligodendrocyte to more than one axon indicates that

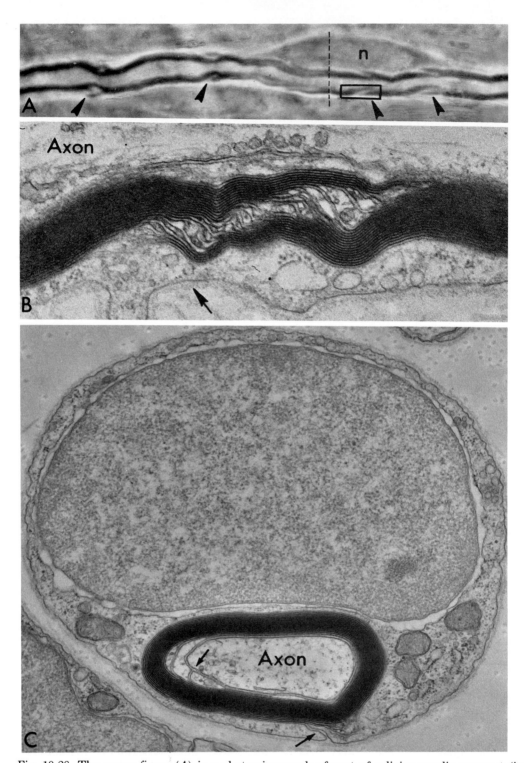

Fig. 10-28. The *upper figure* (*A*) is a photomicrograph of part of a living myelin segment (in tissue culture) displaying a series of Schmidt-Lanterman clefts (*arrowheads*) and the nucleus (*n*) of the Schwann cell related to this internode. In an electron micrograph (*B*) a cleft, as in the box in *A*, is seen to be a region where the myelin lamellae are separated by cytoplasm but retain their continuity. The *arrow* in the *middle picture* indicates the basal lamina external to the Schwann cell. *C* is an electron micrograph of a myelin sheath cut in cross section at the level of the *dotted line* in *A*. The *arrows* indicate the inner and outer mesaxons, the points where the membrane spiral which forms the compact myelin begins and ends. Rat peripheral nerve. *A*, ×3,000; *B*, ×60,000; *C*, ×30,000.

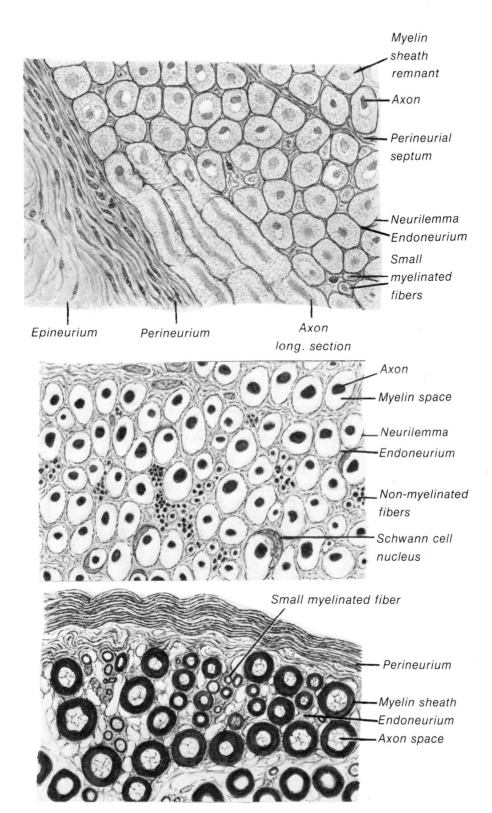

Myelin
sheath
remnant

Axon

Perineurial
septum

Neurilemma
Endoneurium

Small
myelinated
fibers

Epineurium

Perineurium

Axon
long. section

Axon

Myelin space

Neurilemma
Endoneurium

Non-myelinated
fibers

Schwann cell
nucleus

Small myelinated fiber

Perineurium

Myelin sheath
Endoneurium
Axon space

Fig. 10-29. These drawings illustrate cross sections of peripheral nerve after standard histological preparation and H & E staining (*top*), after silver staining to show the axons (*middle*), and after fixation with OsO_4 to preserve the myelin sheaths (*bottom*). The spoke-like remnants of myelin seen in H & E preparations are called neurokeratin.

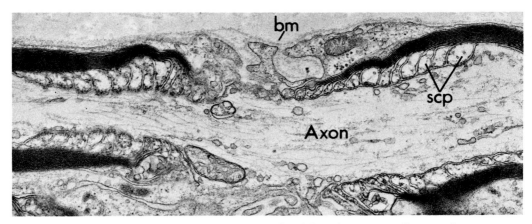

Fig. 10-30. This electron micrograph shows a node of Ranvier on a small axon of a rat sensory ganglion cell. The myelin lamellae terminate in loops in which a small amount of Schwann cell cytoplasm is retained. The innermost lamellae terminate farthest from the node. *bm* = basal lamina; *scp* = Schwann cell processes. ×27,500.

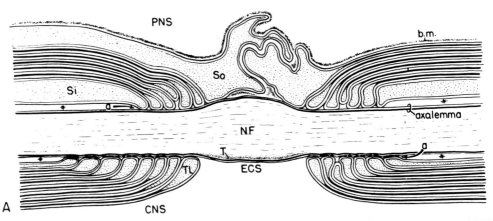

Fig. 10-31. This drawing compares nodal regions from the peripheral nervous system (*PNS*), (*above*) and *CNS* (*below*). In the PNS the Schwann cell provides both an inner collar (*Si*) and an outer collar (*So*) of cytoplasm in relation to the compact myelin. The outer collar (*So*) extends into the nodal region as a series of loosely interdigitating processes. Terminating loops of the compact myelin come into close apposition to the axolemma in regions near the node, apparently providing some barrier (*arrow* at *a*) for movement of materials into or out of the periaxonal space (*). The Schwann cell is covered externally by a basal lamina. In the CNS the myelin ends similarly in terminal loops (*tl*) near the node, and there are periodic thickenings of the axolemma where the glial cell membrane is applied in the paranodal region. These thickenings may serve to confine material in the periaxonal space (*) so that movement in the direction of the *arrow* at *a* would be restrained. At many CNS nodes there is considerable extracellular space (*ECS*). (From: Bunge, R.: Physiol. Rev. 48:197, 1970.)

the myelin membrane spiral cannot be formed by cell circumnavigation around the axon; the actual mechanism of central myelin deposition is unknown.

The very small amount of cytoplasm external to the central myelin sheath has led to the frequent statement that there is no neurilemma cell in the CNS. There is, in fact, some cytoplasm related to central

myelin both internally and externally and at the nodes of Ranvier (Figs. 10-31 and 10-35), but it is too scant to be seen in the light microscope. Myelinated central fibers have no connective tissue coats, as found in peripheral nerves (Fig. 10-35).

The integrity of myelin depends upon both the axon (as discussed below) and the myelin-supporting cell—the Schwann cell

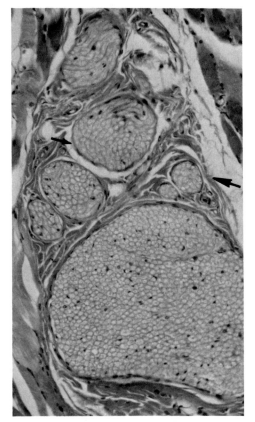

Fig. 10-32. This photomicrograph shows seven peripheral nerve fascicles of varying sizes within the muscles of the tongue. At places, the encasing epineurium (*large arrow*) is separated from the underlying perineurium (*small arrow*). The nuclei of Schwann cells and endoneurial cells are visible as darkly stained elements within the fascicles. The outline of individual myelinated fibers is seen, but much of the myelin has been extracted in the tissue preparation. H & E stain. ×130.

or the oligodendrocyte. If the myelin-supporting cell is damaged, as in certain demyelinating diseases, the myelin will break down even though the axon is preserved. If the axon is preserved, remyelination sometimes occurs in both central and peripheral nervous tissue.

The Peripheral Nerves

The nerve fibers, coursing from their cell bodies to their terminations in some peripheral structure or the CNS, are grouped together in bundles to form the peripheral nerves. The fibers connected with the

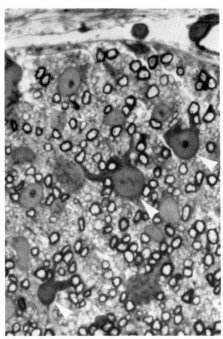

Fig. 10-33. Photomicrograph of 5-day old kitten spinal cord with the surface of the cord above. Myelin sheaths in varying stages of formation have been cut in cross section. Three myelin-related cells (*white arrowheads*) each display two processes which appear to extend to at least two different myelinated axons. A 1-μm section of OsO_4-fixed material embedded in plastic and stained with toluidine blue. ×1200.

spinal cord form the spinal nerves and those connected with the brain comprise the cranial nerves.

When the spinal cord is viewed grossly, it is readily observed that the rootlets of a peripheral nerve are associated with both its dorsal and its ventral regions. The dorsal root is distinguished from the ventral by an enlargement containing nerve cell bodies, the *dorsal root ganglion*. The dorsal root contains the sensory or afferent nerve fibers from both somatic and visceral structures; the ventral root contains the motor or efferent fibers to somatic muscles and fibers to the visceral effectors. These are smooth muscle (as in the wall of the gut), cardiac muscle, and glands (Fig. 9-4). The dorsal and ventral roots join together to form the spinal nerves; the spinal nerve is thus a mixed nerve of both sensory and motor fibers. Some of the sensory fibers are myelinated, whereas others are not; the same applies to motor fibers. For this rea-

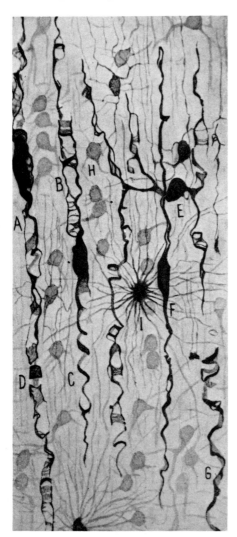

Fig. 10-34. Diagram by del Rio-Hortega of the oligodendrocytes in white matter of cat central nervous tissue. The cells labeled *AD, BC, E, F,* and *G* are related to underlying myelin sheaths, which are not stained in this preparation. Oligodendrocytes that appear not to be related to myelin sheaths are labeled *H,* and an astrocyte appears at *I.* (From: del Rio-Hortega, P.: Mem. Real. Soc. Espan. Hist. Nat., 14:5, 1928.)

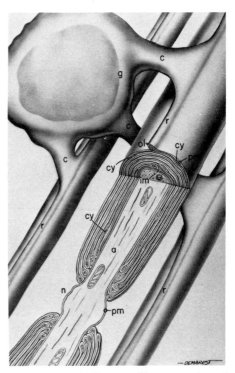

Fig. 10-35. This diagram illustrates the relationship of the oligodendrocyte to the central myelin sheath. The trilaminar plasma membrane (*pm*) is here designated as two lines separated by a space, except in the mitochondrion, where it is represented by a single line. The inner mesaxon (*im*), formed as a glial process completes the initial turn around an axon (*a*) and starts a second, is retained after myelin formation is completed. Some cytoplasm of the glial process is present here. Cytoplasm is trapped occasionally at *cy.* On the fully formed sheath exterior, a bit of glial cytoplasm is also retained. In transverse sections, this cytoplasm is confined to a loop (*ol*), but along the internode length, it forms a ridge (*r*) which is continuous with a glial cell body (*g*) at *c.* When viewed transversely, the sheath components are oriented in a spiral, only the innermost and outermost layers ending in loops; in the longitudinal plane, every myelin unit terminates in a separate loop near a node (*n*). Within these loops glial cytoplasm is also retained. (From: Bunge, M., et al.: J. Biophys. Biochem. Cytol. 10:67, 1961.)

son, it is generally not possible in the standard histological preparation to distinguish afferent from efferent fibers or visceral from somatic fibers.

Of the cranial nerves, some are purely efferent, others are purely afferent, and still others contain both efferent and afferent fibers. The same fundamental relations hold for the cranial nerves as for the spinal nerves. The afferent fibers arise from cell bodies in ganglia outside the CNS and the efferent fibers arise either from neuron bodies lying within the brain or from cells in autonomic ganglia. The optic "nerve" and parts of certain other cranial nerves form exceptions to this statement. The optic nerve actually is a fiber tract connecting the retina—an outlying evaginated part of the neural tube—with the brain.

Epineurium

In all peripheral nerves, the delicate nerve fibers, both myelinated and unmyelinated, are strengthened and protected by substantial connective tissue investments (Fig. 10-32). In histological sections, the connective tissue sleeves in which the nerve fibers course are often the most conspicuous elements. Enclosing the entire nerve is a thick sheath of connective tissue, the *epineurium*. It is composed of irregularly arranged collagenous and elastic fibers, together with fibroblasts and histiocytes. When the nerve fibers are arranged in several distinct fascicles, as is often the case, these bundles are separated by extensions of the epineurium.

Perineurium

Inside the heavy epineurial layer is a more delicate sleeve of connective tissue, the *perineurium*. Recent studies indicate that flattened cells on the inner aspect of this layer form continuous epithelioid

sheets, neighboring cells being joined by well developed occluding junctions. The perineurium may be several such layers thick, each layer surrounded by basal lamina material. As such, the perinuerium provides an effective barrier to the penetration of material into or out of the nerve (Fig. 10-36). Thus, when marker proteins are applied to the nerve externally, they are excluded from the inner regions not by the heavy and coarse connective tissue of the epineurium but by the occluding junctions of the continuous cellular sleeves of the inner part of the perineurium.

Endoneurium

Inside the perineurium are the scattered cells (fibroblasts and histiocytes) and the delicate connective tissue fibers of the *endoneurium*. A basal lamina surrounding the neurilemma (or Schwann cell) separates the latter from the surrounding endoneurium (Figs. 10-27 and 10-28). Hence, it can be seen that the relatively loose, fluid connective tissue of the endoneurium constitutes a connective tissue well isolated from the general connective tissues of the body, except at the distal tips of nerves. This endoneurial space is of potential impor-

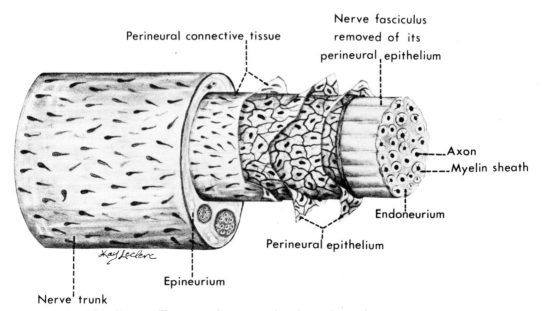

Fig. 10-36. This diagram illustrates the connective tissue sheaths around a peripheral nerve. The perineurial cells are seen disposed as an epithelium, and thus form a barrier against penetration of certain materials into the nerve fascicle. (Courtesy of Drs. T. R. Shantha and G. H. Bourne.)

tance in the metabolism and conductance of its contained axons and may present a pathway for viral or bacterial infection. Further aspects of this compartmentalization are discussed in relation to the meninges.

The Ganglia

Cranial and Spinal Ganglia

The cranial and spinal ganglia consist of aggregates of afferent neuron cell bodies situated on the sensory roots of their respective nerves. Each ganglion is surrounded by a connective tissue capsule which is continuous with the epineurium and perineurium of the peripheral nerve. Connective tissue trabeculae extend from the capsule into the ganglion, and the neurons are separated into irregular groups by strands of connective tissue and by bundles of nerve fibers (Figs. 10-37 and 10-38).

Each ganglion cell is invested with both cellular and fibrous connective tissue elements. The inner aspect of this investment consists of flattened cells closely applied to the plasma membrane of the neuron. These cells are the *satellite cells*; they form a mosaic which completely envelops the neuronal cell body. These cells are akin to the Schwann cells of the nerve fibers; both are peripheral glial cells and both are derived

from neural crest tissue. Satellite cells have been reported to myelinate sensory ganglion neuron cell bodies in the guinea pig, further attesting to their similarity to Schwann cells. As with Schwann cells, the outer aspect of the satellite cell investment is made up of a basal lamina reinforced externally by connective tissue fibers intermingled with flattened fibroblasts (sometimes called *capsule cells*) (Fig. 10-39). The connective tissue elements outside the satellite cell basal lamina are continuous with the endoneurium of the contiguous nerve fibers.

The nerve cells of the cranial and spinal ganglia are unipolar neurons whose cell bodies vary in size from 15 to 100 μm. The smaller neurons, which give rise to unmyelinated fibers, contain closely packed Nissl substance, giving these cells a dark appearance in conventional stains. The large neurons, on the other hand, have Nissl substance separated into groups by microtubules and neurofilaments which course through the cell body and extend into the axonal process. The "dilution" of the Nissl material by these poorly staining elements gives these cells a lighter appearance (Fig. 10-38).

The ganglion cells have one principal myelinated process, which at some distance from the cell body, divides into a peripheral branch which courses in the peripheral

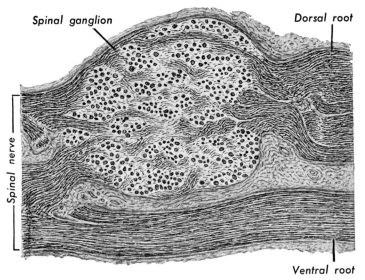

Fig. 10-37. Longitudinal section through a spinal ganglion of an infant, 2 months of age. Cajal silver. ×28.

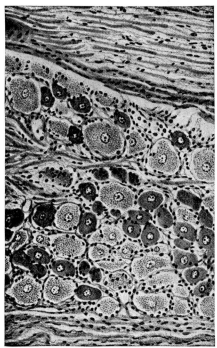

Fig. 10-38. Drawing of a section of a human spinal ganglion. Two principal types of ganglion cells are shown: a large clear type with well marked Nissl bodies and a smaller more darkly staining type. This dichotomy reflects a closer packing of Nissl material in the smaller neuron. The nuclei of the surrounding satellite cells are also evident. (Ph. Stohr, Jr., from v. Mollendorff, Handbuch der mikroskopischen Anatomie des Menschen.)

nerve and a central branch which enters the CNS. The course of the axon in the neighborhood of the cell body varies for different neurons. In some cases, the axon is coiled and looped around the cell body to form an intracapsular "glomerulus"; in other cases, it follows a relatively straight course from its cell body to the point where it divides into a central and a peripheral process. The majority of the large ganglion cells have axons of the "glomerular" type, whereas most of the small, darkly staining cells have the uncoiled type. These cell bodies do not receive synapses; the sensory ganglion is not an integrative center.

The Autonomic (Sympathetic and Parasympathetic) Ganglia

The majority of the autonomic ganglia resemble the cranial and spinal ganglia in having a similar connective tissue capsule and framework. Unlike sensory ganglia, these ganglia contain synapses, for they are the way stations where certain of the first neurons of the two-neuron efferent system form a synapse with the second neuron of the visceral motor pathway (Fig. 10-12).

The neurons are multipolar cells with numerous branched dendrites and a single axon which forms the unmyelinated postganglionic visceral efferent fiber (Fig. 10-40). The cell bodies vary in size from 15 to 60 μm. The nucleus is relatively large and pale, round or oval in shape, and often eccentrically placed. Binucleate cells are not uncommon. The Nissl substance may be distributed uniformly throughout the cytoplasm or may be confined either to the perinuclear zone or to the peripheral cytoplasm. Lipofuscin granules are somewhat more frequent here than in corresponding sensory ganglia. In the larger ganglia, each cell is surrounded by a layer of satellite cells, as in the spinal ganglia (Fig. 10-40). Often, two ganglion cells may share a single satellite cell-connective tissue investment.

Located in a confusing array throughout these ganglia are frequent axosomatic and axodendritic synapses. The preganglionic elements contain numerous round, clear vesicles, as would be expected in a synapse known to be cholinergic (see above). It has recently been demonstrated that there are small, densely staining interneurons in certain sympathetic ganglia which apparently allow some integrative activity within the ganglion itself.

It will be recalled from the discussion in chapter 9 that the synaptic contact between the first and second neuron of the parasympathetic system is frequently not in a discrete ganglion but directly in the wall of the organ innervated (heart, gut, bladder, etc.). Here presynaptic fibers make contact with neurons in isolated groups. The postsynaptic neurons often have no definitive dendrites. The synapse frequently occurs on the cell body of the second neuron; it is the activity of the axons of this postsynaptic neuron, then, that results in neurotransmitter release in relation to the smooth muscle or glands of the visceral structures of the body (Fig. 10-12).

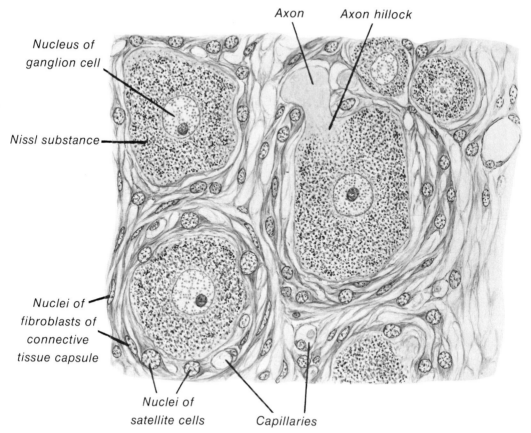

Fig. 10-39. Unipolar nerve cells from a Gasserian (cranial) ganglion stained by the Nissl method. Human, 19 years of age. ×835.

Degeneration and Regeneration of Nerve Fibers

The individuality of the neuron and the interdependence of its parts are strikingly exemplified by its behavior when injured. When a nerve trunk is cut across, certain changes take place in the cut ends for a short distance on either side of the cut. These are degenerative changes of a traumatic nature, involving necrosis of the injured parts. On the proximal side of the injury (toward the cell body), degenerative changes may extend the distance of a few internodes, but very soon regenerative processes are initiated, leading to a new growth from the end of this central stump.

Distal to the site of injury, however, the degenerative changes are progressive and in time lead to the complete breakdown and disappearance of this portion of the nerve fibers, including their terminal arborizations. This process is known as *second-ary* or *Wallerian degeneration*. This means that an axon cut off from its cell of origin degenerates and disappears; this behavior of the axon accords with the fact that the cell body is the trophic center of the neuron.

The first changes seen in the distal portion of the cut nerve occur in the axons themselves. They lose their uniform contour and swell intermittently, and the nerve fiber takes on a beaded appearance. Within 3 to 5 days after section of a peripheral nerve, the axons break up into irregular, twisted segments which finally undergo complete disintegration. In the CNS, this axon breakdown is often very much slower, and special stains (e.g., the Nauta stain) which selectively delineate the degenerating axons and their terminals are useful in tracing fiber pathways in neuroanatomical studies.

Coincident with these changes in the axon are degenerative changes in the mye-

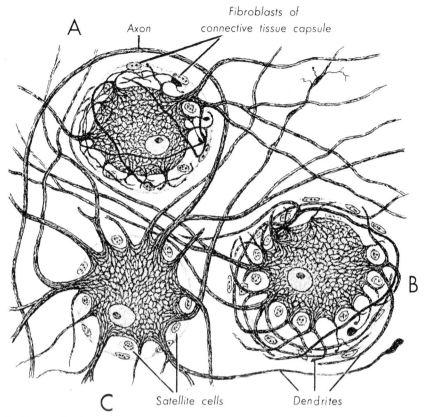

Fig. 10-40. Sympathetic nerve cells, human, 36 years of age. Cajal's silver stain. *A* and *B*, cells whose dendrites form a pericellular plexus. *C*, cell with long dendrites. Redrawn from Cajal.

lin sheath. During the first few days, there is a fragmentation of the myelin, so that it becomes broken into spherical, oval, or elongated segments which surround the fragments of the axon (Fig. 10–41). In the succeeding days, these myelin fragments undergo further breakdown within Schwann cells or invading histiocytes. The myelin fragments appear as smaller and smaller droplets until finally they disappear (Fig. 10–41). The chemical changes taking place as the myelin is digested are the basis of the selectivity of the Marchi stain for degenerating myelin. This stain allows degenerating tracts (which contain myelin) to be identified, and it is a useful adjunct to the axonal stains mentioned above.

In peripheral nerve tissue, the degeneration of the axon and myelin sheath occurs within the confines of the connective tissue framework. The endoneurial elements which originally surrounded the axon-Schwann cell unit forms a tubular envelope within which the reacting Schwann cells are confined (Fig. 10–41). While the breakdown and digestion of axon and myelin are progressing, certain Schwann cells enlarge and undergo mitosis. Confined by the sleeve of connective tissue mentioned above, these cells accumulate in tubular or bandlike arrays ("band fibers" or "protoplasmic bands") along the length of the nerve. This tubular framework is very important in supplying pathways for regenerating axons as they grow out of the proximal and into the distal stump of the damaged nerve.

The extensive degenerative processes in the proximal and peripheral stump are not the only changes which follow nerve section. Degenerative changes also occur in the neuron body itself. An apparent *chromatolysis* may be observed as early as the 1st day after nerve section and is marked at about 2 weeks. The cytological changes that characterize chromatolysis have been discussed above. It should be noted that this response to axon section is another useful anatomical tool in identifying neu-

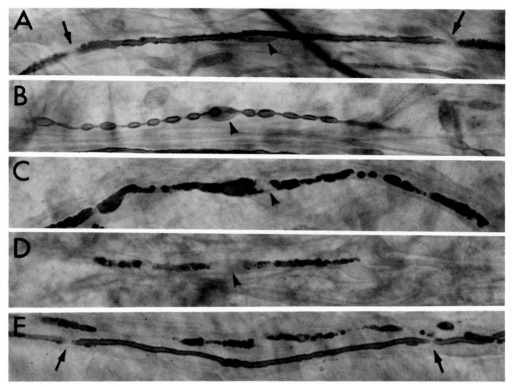

Fig. 10-41. *A*, normal short myelin segment delineated by two nodes of Ranvier (*arrows*) and showing the myelin-related Schwann cell nucleus (*arrowhead*). Myelin segments are shown breaking down several hours after the axon has been cut (*B*), several days later (*C*), and about 1 week later (*D*). In each case the Schwann cell involved in disposal of the myelin remnants is marked by an *arrowhead*. *E* is a small nerve fascicle containing one normal myelinated nerve fiber and remnants of a myelinated axon severed about 1 week earlier. If larger amounts of myelin must be digested, macrophages invade the tissue and assist the Schwann cells. Cultured rat sensory ganglia fixed in OsO_4 and stained with Sudan black. ×520.

rons with damaged axons. Thus, if a neuron is observed in chromatolysis after a particular neurological lesion, it is presumed that this neuron supported an axon which coursed through the lesion area.

Regrowth from severed axons is generally considered to be vigorous in the autonomic nervous system and active in the somatic peripheral nervous system but minimal and generally ineffective in the CNS. If the neuron cell body which supports nerve fibers within the peripheral nervous system survives, regeneration can be expected. The axons of the proximal stump of the severed nerve form bulbous enlargements and axonal sprouts within a few days (Figs. 10-42 and 10-43). Usually it takes about 2 weeks for the axonal sprouts to cross the scar to enter the endoneurial tubes of the distal stump of the severed

nerve. The growing tip of the axonal sprout advances more rapidly after it has entered the endoneurial tube. Axonal growth across the scar is facilitated by bridges which are formed chiefly by proliferation and migration of the Schwann cells and fibroblasts. The axonal sprouts are unable to cross the gap when it is too long or when it becomes filled with dense collagenous fibers. Nerve transplants are made in order to facilitate the growth of axonal sprouts across gaps of any appreciable size (e.g., after gunshot wounds); the transplanted nerve provides the important guiding connective tissue framework and thus may be effective even though it contains no viable cells.

Each sprout from the proximal end of a severed nerve usually splits into a number of branches, sometimes as many as 50. This increases the chance of appropriate connec-

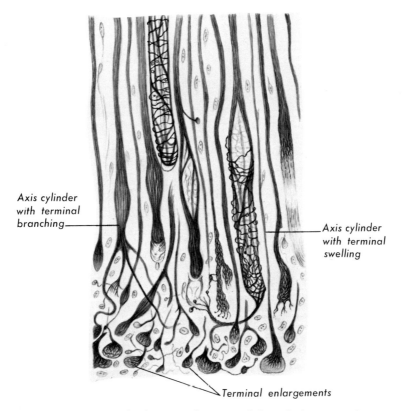

Axis cylinder with terminal branching

Axis cylinder with terminal swelling

Terminal enlargements

Fig. 10-42. Regenerating axons in the central stump of the sciatic nerve of a cat 2½ days after section of the nerve. (Redrawn from Ramon y Cajal.)

tions. A number of branches may enter a single Schwann tube. Some of these branches enlarge; others degenerate. In fibers which will become myelinated, generally only one axon is left per tube.

When only a fraction of the nerve fibers of a peripheral nerve are cut, the remarkable process of *collateral sprouting* appears. If 75 of 100 nerve fibers innervating a region are cut, the 25 remaining fibers sprout numerous collateral branches (at the point of the node of Ranvier in myelinated fibers), and these attempt to take up the positions of the 75 lost fibers. This attempt is often at least partially successful, and the 25 remaining fibers then have expanded regions of nervous influence. In practical terms, this means that the number of muscle fibers supplied by each motor nerve fiber is increased, or that the field of sensation served by a sensory neuron is enlarged. This type of regeneration is common after motor neuron loss in poliomyelitis and helps to ex-

plain the partial recovery of motor function that occurs.

In the CNS of mammals, where Schwann cells are lacking and no band fibers are formed, regeneration does not occur as readily as in the peripheral nervous system. Recent studies have shown, however, that axons bridge the gap between the cut ends of a transected spinal cord in mammals when special efforts are made to prevent connective tissue from growing into the gap. Even under the best conditions, however, effective regeneration accompanied by functional recovery does not occur.

Nerve Terminations

The axons which form the peripheral nerve fibers terminate in peripheral structures to which or from which they convey nerve impulses. The *efferent* fibers terminate in tissues in which they excite activity by releasing a neurotransmitter. In the so-

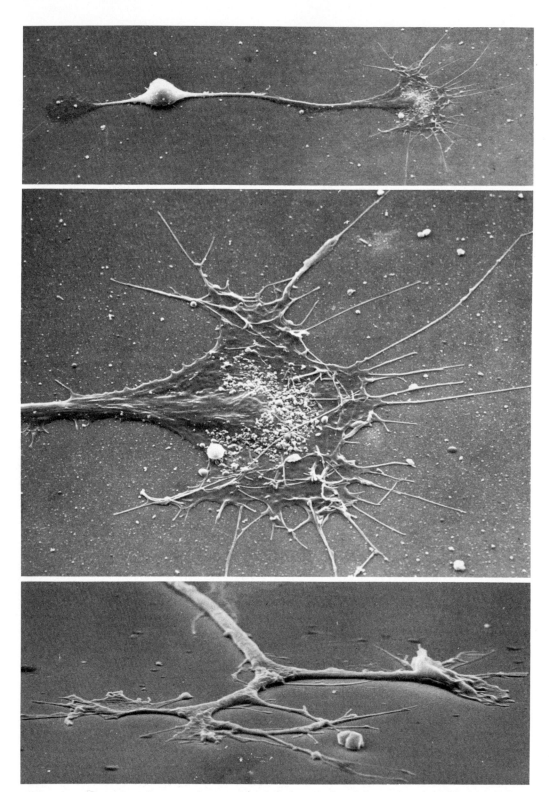

Fig. 10-43. Scanning electron micrographs of neurons isolated from an 8-day-old chick embryo and grown in culture. In the *upper* figure, a parasympathetic neuron from the ciliary ganglion displays its cell body toward *left center* and a growth cone at the tip of its axon toward the *right*. The growth cone is shown at higher magnification in the *center figure*. It displays many active microvillus-like microspikes which move about over the free surface of the growth cone, appearing

matic effectors (skeletal muscle), the transmitter released is acetylcholine. By reacting with special sites on the muscle membrane, acetylcholine causes the generation of an action potential in the muscle fiber, with subsequent muscle contraction. In many of the visceral effectors, two different transmitters are involved: acetylcholine released by the parasympathetic nerve terminals and nonrepinephrine released by sympathetic endings. It should be recalled that in the former case the endings contain small, round, clear vesicles; in the latter case they contain dense-cored vesicles of slightly larger size. The dual autonomic innervation provides for shifts in organ activity; parasympathetic nerves stimulate digestive action in the intestine after eating, whereas sympathetic nerves inhibit intestinal activity during exercise. In the case of afferent fibers, on the other hand, the receptor portions are located throughout the body, where nerve fibers end freely in the tissues or in specially organized structures. In either case, they received stimuli which cause them to convey nerve impulses to the CNS.

Terminations of Somatic Efferent Fibers

The cell bodies of these fibers lie in the ventral gray matter of the spinal cord or in the motor nuclei of cranial nerves in the brain. The axons are myelinated and form part of the ventral roots and efferent fibers of the peripheral nerves, terminating in the skeletal muscles of the body and head. The nerve fibers enter the perimysium, in which they may bifurcate several times, thus permitting one neuron to innervate more than one muscle fiber. A motor neuron and the muscle fibers innervated by it constitute a *motor unit*. The finer muscles that are concerned with precise movement have an abundent nerve supply. For example, muscles which move the eyeball often have a 1:1 ratio of neuron to muscle fiber, whereas the motor units of many regions may include as many as 1600 muscle fibers.

After repeated branchings in the perimysium, the nerve fibers pass to the individual muscle fibers, where they terminate in structures known as *motor end plates* (Fig. 10-44). At the end plate region, the myelin is lost and the endoneurium becomes continuous with a layer of reticular fibers over the sarcolemma. The fiber terminates in a series of bulbous expansions, and in these regions the Schwann cell covering (which has replaced the myelin as an axon sheath) is withdrawn from between the nerve and muscle fiber (Fig. 10-45). At the regions of termination, the nerve indents the plasma membrane of the muscle fiber, forming a "synaptic gutter." Within the nerve terminal are a multitude of small, round, clear vesicles about 450 Å in diameter, and an abundance of mitochondria. Details of this junction, which has many similarities to the synapses of the CNS, are shown in Figures 10-46 and 10-47. It has been suggested that the general configuration (rather than the ultrastructural details) of nerve endings on "fast" muscle fibers differs from that of endings on "slow" fibers and, in fact, that the "tropic" characteristics of the nerve terminal determine whether the muscle fiber contacted is of the slow or fast type.

In the part of the muscle fiber beneath the motor end plate region, there is an increase in number of muscle nuclei. In ordinary sections, the muscle nuclei may appear adjacent to or even between some of the Schwann cell nuclei where nerve fibers course in grooves of the muscle fiber, but electron micrographs have clearly shown that the axon terminals do not penetrate the sarcolemma and therefore do not intermingle with the constituents of the muscle cell (Fig. 10-45).

Termination of Visceral Efferent Fibers

Postganglionic visceral efferent fibers from the autonomic ganglion cells termi-

---

and disappearing as the axonal process is extended. This type of growth cone may move over a substratum at a rate of 50 to 150 μm/hr. The growth cone contains smooth endoplasmic reticulum, but no ribosomes or other granules. Cytoplasmic particles do appear in culture to move up and down the axon to and from the growth cone, presumably reflecting active axonal flow patterns. In the *lower figure*, a growth cone on the axon from a dorsal root ganglion neuron has split during its extension to form two subsidiary growth cones (*right* and *left center*). Upper figure, ×850; center figure, ×2850; lower figure ×4400. (Courtesy of Dr. Norman Wessells).

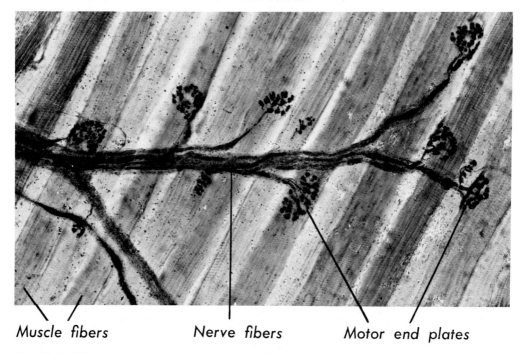

Muscle fibers   Nerve fibers   Motor end plates

Fig. 10-44. Photomicrograph of motor nerve ending in intercostal muscle. Gold chloride method. ×315.

nate in the following effectors: heart muscle (cardiomotor); smooth muscle of viscera (visceromotor), of blood vessels (vasomotor) and of hairs (pilomotor); and glandular epithelia (secretory). These axons are unmyelinated.

In heart muscle and in smooth muscle, the fibers form plexuses around the muscle bundles. From these plexuses, fine nerve fibers course in relation to individual muscle fibers. Electron microscopic examination indicates that no special junctions are formed but that bulbous enlargements of the nerve fiber in the vicinity of, and in some cases directly adjacent to, smooth muscle fibers contain aggregates of synaptic vesicles (Fig. 10-48). Some enlargements contain the small, clear vesicles; others contain the larger, dense-cored variety. The former are considered characteristic of parasympathetic fibers; the latter are components of sympathetic nerve fibers (see above). Apparently, neurotransmitter released from these areas is able to influence responsive cells in the surrounding tissues without establishing discrete neuromuscular junctions.

In glandular epithelium, the visceral efferent fibers form a plexus beneath the basement membrane, through which the fibers pass to terminate in relation to individual gland cells.

Classification of Terminations of Afferent Fibers

Those parts of the body which receive stimuli and contain the terminations of peripheral afferent fibers are known as receptors. The receptors have the function of responding to various physical and chemical stimuli, and furthermore, certain receptors have the function of reacting primarily to one particular kind of stimulus. The mechanism of reception must provide for the initiation of a nerve impulse, and in this sense the action of a receptor is considered analogous to the chemical excitability of the dendritic portion of the typical neuron. In some receptors (as in the taste bud), special cells receive the stimulus and respond with receptor potentials which, in turn, activate the nerve ending. In other receptors (as in the Pacinian corpuscle), the nerve ending itself receives the stimulus and develops a *generator potential* which

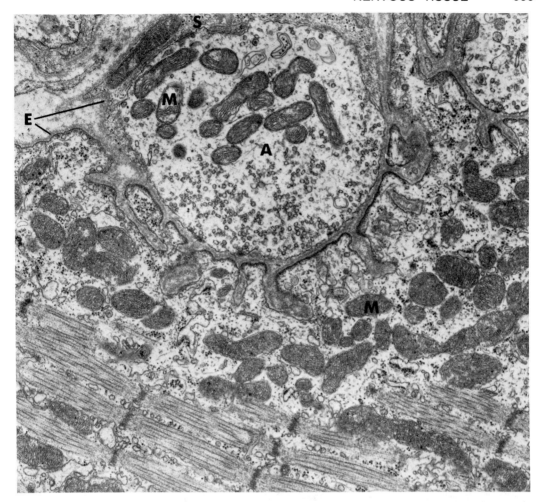

Fig. 10-45. Electron micrograph showing a portion of a motor end plate along a skeletal muscle fiber in the extraoccular muscle of a mammal. An axonal terminal (*A*) is seen in cross section situated in an indentation of the surface of the muscle cell. A small portion of the terminus of its Schwann cell (*S*) is visible at the *upper edge* of the micrograph. The axonal terminal displays numerous vesicles similar to those seen in other cholinergic synaptic endings. Both the axonal terminal and the nearby muscle cell cytoplasm are richly endowed with mitochondria (*M*). Note that the external lamina (*E*) of both the Schwann cell and the muscle cell course into the indentation occupied by the axonal terminal. Several folds are seen along the muscle cell surface within the indentation. These also contain external lamina material. ×22,700.

triggers the action potential of the nerve fiber. The concept that each type of sensation (touch, heat, etc.) has its own specific receptor has been modified, for it has been observed that different receptors may respond to the same stimulus (e.g., both Pacinian corpuscles and free nerve endings respond to tactile stimuli).

The receptors may be classified in several more or less overlapping ways:

1. Some receptors are found widely distributed over the body. These may be collectively termed receptors of general body or *somaesthetic* sensibility (touch, pressure, pain, temperature, position, movement). Other receptors are found aggregated only in certain places in the head, where they constitute the *organs of special senses* (smell, sight, taste, hearing, and head position and movement).

2. Another distinction may be made between *exteroceptors*, the receptors affected

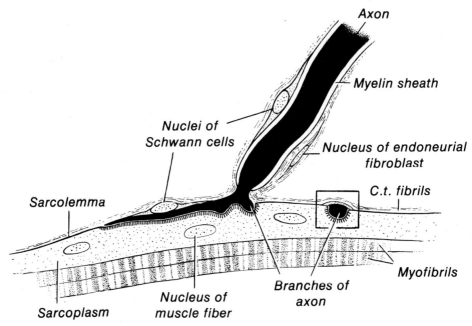

Fig. 10-46. Somatic motor nerve ending on a skeletal muscle fiber. The myelin ends just before the axon reaches the muscle fiber. Schwann cells associated with myelin end at the same point. Other Schwann cells continue onto the branches of the axon. Their cytoplasm is so thin that it can be seen under the light microscope only at the level of the nuclei. The branches of the axon lie in invaginations of sarcolemma known as primary synaptic clefts. The subneural sarcolemma and subjacent sarcoplasm, often described as a "subneural apparatus," may appear as a series of rodlets in special preparations under the light microscope.

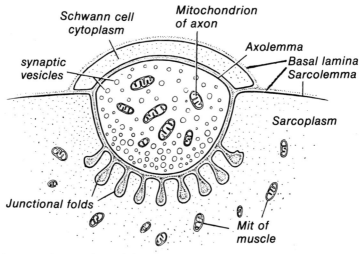

Fig. 10-47. Diagram of a portion of the motor end plate (enclosed in the box in Fig. 10-46) showing a branch of an axon in a synaptic indentation as seen in electron micrographs (Fig. 10-45). Secondary clefts or junctional folds extend inward from the primary cleft or gutter. The axon is covered by a thin layer of Schwann cell cytoplasm on the side away from the muscle, but no Schwann cell cytoplasm extends into the indentation. The space between the axolemma and sarcolemma contains an amorphous material, continuous with the basal lamina material around the muscle cell. (Diagram based on descriptions and illustrations by Robertson, 1960, and Couteaux, 1947 and 1960.)

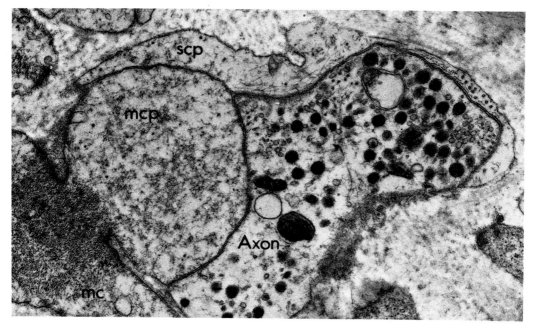

Fig. 10-48. Electron micrograph of a region of contact between a smooth muscle cell and a nerve fiber in the small intestine of a toad. A bulbous process (*mcp*) protrudes from the muscle cell (*mc*) containing conspicuous fine filaments. This process is in direct contact with an axon containing a variety of vesicles, including many granule containing vesicles. The axon is partially covered by a Schwann cell process (*scp*). In this type of "visceral" neuromuscular junction neither membrane specialization nor vesicle accumulation near the presynaptic membrane is apparent. ×22,500. (Courtesy of Dr. J. Rosenbluth.)

by external stimuli (touch, light pressure, cutaneous pain and temperature, smell, sight, and hearing); the *proprioceptors*, which are affected by stimuli arising within the body wall, especially those of movement and posture; and the *enteroceptors*, which are affected by stimuli arising within the viscera. In receptors, the modes of termination of the peripheral processes of the cranial or spinal ganglion cells are so varied and complicated as to make impracticable any structural classification except in the broadest sense. The terminal arborizations of the afferent fibers, however, follow one of two structural arrangements. Either they terminate freely among the body tissues or they are surrounded by special connective tissue capsules. The distinction can thus be made between *free* or *nonencapsulated* sensory endings and *encapsulated* ones.

Nonencapsulated Afferent Endings. These endings are found in practically all epithelia of the body, in connective tissue, in muscle, and in serous membranes. They are the most common type of sensory ending in the body.

In the skin and in those mucous membranes which are covered by stratified squamous epithelium, the nerve fibers of a given branch separate as they approach the epithelium, lose their myelin sheaths, and form a subepithelial plexus. From this plexus, axons or their branches enter the epithelial layer and split into minute arborizations, which terminate between the cells in little knoblike swellings. In the skin, the nerve endings do not penetrate beyond the cells of the stratum granulosum.

Essentially similar free nerve endings are seen in other epithelial surfaces, such as the mucosa of the respiratory tract (Fig. 10-49).

Another form of free nerve ending is the *peritrichial* ending, in which sensory fibers encircle the hair follicle and terminate principally in the connective tissue sheath and vitreous membrane of the follicle. Fine nerve fibers may also extend into the outer epithelial root sheath.

In general, these intraepithelial endings terminate among epithelial cells that do not differ from the adjoining epithelial cells.

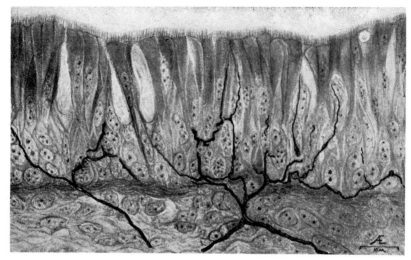

Fig. 10-49. Nerve endings in bronchial epithelium (pseudostratified ciliated columnar epithelium). Reduced silver method of Cajal. (After A. Elftman.)

In deeper epithelial layers of the skin, however, are leaflike expansions of a nerve terminal, each of which forms a *meniscus* in contact with an epithelial cell which stains differently from the other cells. This is a *tactile cell*, and the whole apparatus is known as a *tactile corpuscle of Merkel*.

Sensory fibers also terminate diffusely in connective tissue. They all end variously by a branching of the sensory fibers among the fibers and cells of the connective tissue. Such endings are found extensively in the dermis and subcutaneous tissue and in the connective tissue of mucous and serous membranes, the periosteum, and the blood vessels, to name a few instances.

In addition to arborized terminations in the interstitial connective tissue of muscle, nonencapsulated sensory nerve endings are also found around the individual muscle fibers themselves (Fig. 10-50).

Encapsulated Afferent Endings. These include such structures as the *end bulb*, the *tactile corpuscles of Meissner*, the *Pacinian corpuscles*, the *muscle spindles*, and the *tendon organs* (or *organs of Golgi*).

Of the encapsulated sensory endings, probably the simplest are the so-called end bulbs. These are spherical or oval in shape and consist of a thin, lamellated capsule of flattened connective tissue cells and fibers surrounding a central cavity, the *inner bulb*. Within the inner bulb, the naked axons of one or more myelinated fibers end. In some inner bulbs, the axon may terminate in a number of branches which twist and interlace to form a spherical, skeinlike mass known as a glomerulus. An example of this type is seen in the *end bulbs of Krause* in the conjunctival connective tissue.

End bulbs are found in the lips, in the mucous membranes of the tongue, cheeks, soft palate, epiglottis, nasal cavities, lower end of rectum, peritoneum, serous membranes, tendons, ligaments, connective tissue of nerve trunks, synovial membranes of certain joints, and the external genitals, especially the glans penis and clitoris.

The *tactile corpuscle of Meissner* (Fig. 10-51) offers an example of a more complex encapsulated tactile corpuscle. It occurs especially in the hairless portions of the skin and is most numerous in the finger tips, the palms of the hands, and the soles of the feet. Lying within the connective tissue of the dermal papillae, these corpuscles are oval bodies which are composed of flattened connective tissue cells in the form of horizontal lamellae surrounded by a connective tissue capsule. Two or more myelinated nerve fibers are distributed to each corpuscle. As the fibers reach the corpuscle, the connective tissue sheath of the nerve joins the connective tissue capsule, the myelin sheaths disappear, and the naked axons pass into the corpuscle, where they

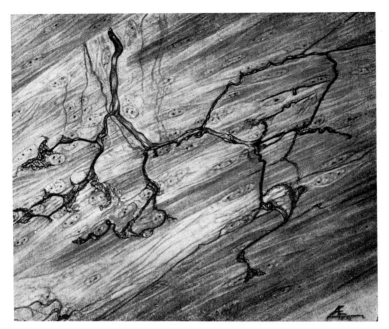

Fig. 10-50. Afferent nerve endings in muscle (smooth) of one of the larger bronchi. Seven-day-old puppy. Reduced silver method of Cajal. (After A. Elftman.)

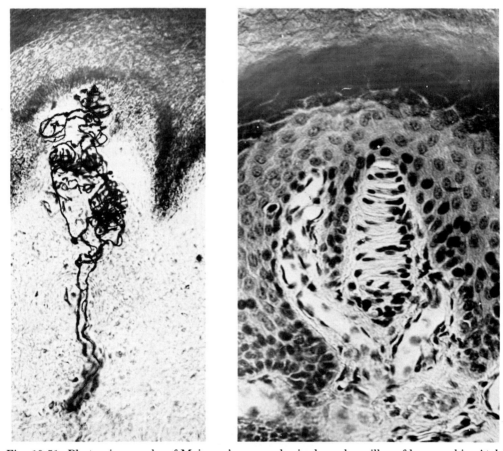

Fig. 10-51. Photomicrographs of Meissner's corpuscles in dermal papillae of human skin. At *left,* stained with silver, showing the axon; at *right,* stained with hematoxylin and eosin, showing the connective tissue elements of the nerve ending. Only a portion of the epidermis is included in the field. (Courtesy of Dr. A. Elwyn.)

branch and pursue a spiral course among the connective tissue elements. In addition to the myelinated fibers, many tactile corpuscles and other encapsulated receptors may also contain the endings of unmyelinated fibers, the significance of which is not known. The corpuscles of Meissner are known to respond to tactile stimuli.

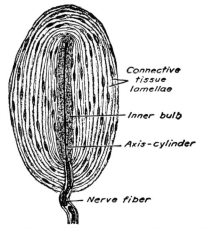

Fig. 10-52. Pacinian corpuscle. Human. (Redrawn from Cajal.)

The *Pacinian corpuscles* are laminated eliptical structures which differ from the simpler end bulbs already described chiefly in the greater development of the connective tissue capsule. They are relatively large structures which are visible to the naked eye (Fig. 10-52). The capsule is formed by a large number of concentric lamellae; each lamella consists of connective tissue fibers lined by a single layer of flat connective tissue cells. The lamellae are separated from one another by a clear fluid or semifluid substance. As in the simpler end bulbs, there is a central cavity within the capsule known as the inner bulb. Each Pacinian corpuscle is supplied by a single myelinated nerve fiber. After losing its myelin sheath, the axon extends through the center of the inner bulb, terminating in a knoblike expansion.

Fine blood vessels enter the base of the corpuscle along with the nerve fiber and break up into capillary networks among the lamellae. They do not enter the inner bulb.

Pacinian corpuscles are found in deeper subcutaneous connective tissue, especially

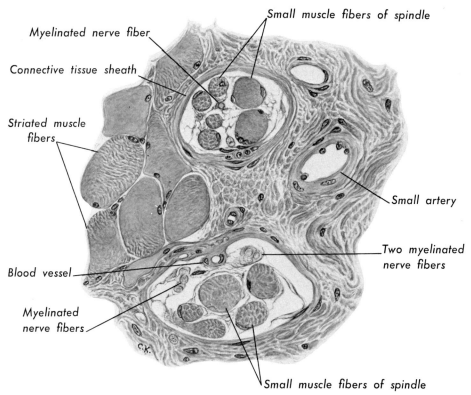

Fig. 10-53. Cross section of two muscle spindles in skeletal muscle of monkey.

of the hand and foot, in parietal perito- neum, pancreas, mesentery, penis, clitoris, urethra, nipple, mammary gland, and in connective tissue in the vicinity of tendons, ligaments, and joints. Their form and to some extent their position indicate that they are stimulated by deep or heavy pressure.

In skeletal muscle, sensory nerves terminate in end bulbs and in complicated end organs called *muscle spindles*. The muscle spindle (Figs. 10-53 and 10-54) is an elongated cylindrical structure within which are one or several small muscle fibers, connective tissue, blood vessels, and myelinated nerve fibers. The whole is enclosed in a connective tissue capsule which is pierced at various points by one or more nerve fibers. The thinner nerve fibers are generally motor fibers and end on the muscle fibers in typical motor end plates. The thicker myelinated fibers are sensory fibers, which lose their myelin as they branch re-

peatedly within the spindle. The axons then terminate around the enclosed muscle fibers in close apposition to the sarcolemma. Frequently, the ending is in the form of a spiral; it may also form a series of rings or an arborization. The whole structure functions as a unit in reflex regulation of muscle tone.

The muscle fibers of the spindle are thinner than usual and richer in sarcoplasm. They also contain more nuclei, particularly in the regions surrounded by nerve fibers. They are referred to as *intrafusal fibers*, as opposed to the *extrafusal fibers* of the muscle proper. The motor neurons of the spinal cord that innervate the intrafusal fibers are termed *gamma motor neurons*; the motor neurons supplying the remainder of the muscle fibers are termed *alpha motor neurons*. Details of the structure of the muscle spindle are given schematically in Figure 10-55. The polar regions of each intrafusal fiber are striated and contractile,

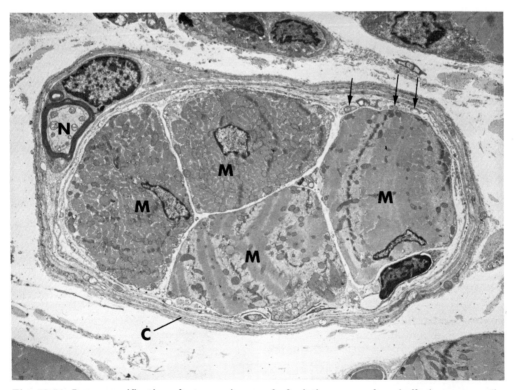

Fig. 10-54. Low magnification electron micrograph depicting a muscle spindle in cross section. Four small intrafusal muscle fibers (*M*) are visible within the connective tissue capsule (*C*). A large myelinated primary afferent axon (*N*) and its Schwann cell are seen penetrating the capsule. Small unmyelinated (probably efferent) axons are visible within the capsule (*arrows*). ×3000. (Courtesy of Dr. Mikel Snow and Amy Erisman.)

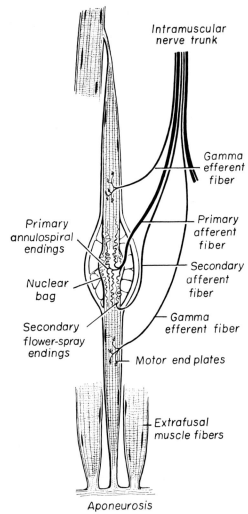

Fig. 10-55. Diagram of muscle spindle. Each spindle contains several slender muscle fibers (intrafusal) enclosed by a connective tissue sheath which becomes continuous at its ends with the connective tissue endomysium of regular muscle fibers (extrafusal). For purposes of clarity, only one intrafusal fiber is shown. (Diagram based on illustration from Barker, D.: Q. J. Microsc. Sci. 89:143, 1948.)

whereas the central region of each fiber is expanded and contains more nuclei; hence it is known as the nuclear bag. In the latter region, the connective tissue sheath is separated from the sarcolemma by a space filled with tissue fluid and traversed by connective tissue fibers and nerve fibers. The intrafusal muscle fibers are supplied by three types of nerve fibers: (1) small *efferent* fibers (gamma efferents) which ter-

minate in motor end plates; (2) primary *afferents*, which are large and wind around the muscle fibers to form annulospiral endings; and (3) secondary *afferents*, which are small and branch to terminate in clusters known as flower spray endings.

Because the intrafusal fibers are parallel with the extrafusal fibers, they are stretched and their afferent nerves are stimulated whenever the extrafusal fibers of the muscle as a whole are stretched. Hence, the spindle afferents function as stretch receptors. Contraction of extrafusal fibers reduces tension on the muscle spindle, whereas localized contraction in the poles of the intrafusal fibers under stimulation of gamma efferents increases tension on the nuclear bag region and stimulates the stretch receptors.

The afferents have their neuron cell bodies in the spinal ganglion. The central processes from the cells with annulospiral receptors form synapses in the spinal cord with alpha motor neurons which send axons to motor end plates on extrafusal muscle fibers. Thus, a two-neuron (monosynaptic) path is established, functioning as a stretch or myotactic reflex. This type of reflex activity maintains muscle tonus and provides a background for voluntary movements after stimulation of the alpha motor neurons from higher centers. Stretch receptor

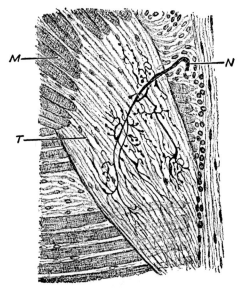

Fig. 10-56. Musculotendinous bundle from a 6-month human fetus. *M*, muscle fibers; *N*, nerve fiber; *T*, tendon fibers. (Redrawn from Tello.)

reflexes associated with the flower spray endings are more complicated and involve polysynaptic pathways.

At the junction of muscle and tendon are found the elaborate sensory structures known as the *tendon organs* or *organs of Golgi* (Fig. 10-56). These are spindle-shaped bodies composed of several tendon bundles covered by a thin capsule. Into this there enter one or several afferent nerve fibers which break up into complicated arborizations upon the tendon bundles.

The proprioceptive stimuli of position and movement resulting from the constant or varying tension of voluntary muscles and their attached tendons are received by muscle spindles and tendon organs. The information gathered in these receptors guides the CNS in governing the attached muscle in the fine degrees of contraction or relaxation necessary for precise motor control.

References

AKERT, K., SANDRI, C., WEIBEL, E. R., PEPER, K., AND MOOR, H. The fine structure of the perineural endothelium. Cell Tissue Res. 165:281–295, 1976.

AKERT, K., AND WASER, P. G. (editors). Mechanisms of synaptic transmission. Progr. Brain Res. 31, 1969.

BARKER, D. (editor). Symposium on Muscle Receptors. Hong Kong University Press, Hong Kong, 1962.

BODIAN, D. The generalized vertebrate neuron. Science 137:323–326, 1962.

BOURNE, G. (editor). Structure and Function of the Nervous System, vols. 1 and 2. Academic Press, New York, 1968, 1969.

BUNGE, R. Glial cells and the central myelin sheath. Physiol. Rev. 48:197–251, 1968.

CAUSEY, G. The Cell of Schwann. E. and S. Livingstone, Ltd., Edinburgh, 1960.

CLEMENTE, C. D. Regeneration in central nervous system. Int. Rev. Neurobiol. 6:257–301, 1964.

COUTEAUX, R. Motor end-plate structure. In The Structure and Function of Muscle (Bourne, G. H., editor), vol. 1, pp. 337–380. Academic Press, New York, 1960.

DAVIS, H. Some principles of sensory receptor action. Physiol. Rev. 41:391–415, 1961.

DEITCH, A. D., AND MURRAY, M. R. The Nissl substance of living and fixed spinal ganglion cells. J. Biophys. Biochem. Cytol. 2:433–444, 1956.

DE ROBERTIS, E. D. P. Histophysiology of Synapses and Neurosecretion. The Macmillan Company, New York, 1964.

DOUGLAS, W. W., AND RITCHIE, J. M. Mammalian nonmyelinated nerve fibers. Physiol. Rev. 42:297–334, 1962.

DROZ, B. Protein metabolism in nerve cells. Int. Rev. Cytol. 25:363–390, 1969.

ECCLES, J. C. The Physiology of Nerve Cells. Johns Hopkins Press, Baltimore, 1957.

ECCLES, J. C. The Physiology of Synapses. Academic Press, New York, 1964.

GASSER, H. S. Properties of dorsal root unmedulated fibers on the two sides of the ganglion. J. Gen. Physiol. 38:709–728, 1955.

GEREN, B. B. Structural studies of the formation of the myelin sheath in peripheral nerve fibers. In Cellular Mechanisms in Differentiation and Growth (Rudnick, D., editor), pp. 213–220. Princeton University Press, Princeton, 1956.

GLEES, P. Neuroglia; Morphology and Function. Charles C Thomas, Springfield, Ill., 1955.

GRAY, E. G., AND GUILLERY, R. W. Synaptic morphology in the normal and degenerating nervous system. Int. Rev. Cytol. 19:111–182, 1966.

GUTH, L. Regeneration in the mammalian peripheral nervous system. Physiol. Rev. 36:441–478, 1956.

HILD, W. Das Neuron. In Handbuch der mikroskopischen Anatomie des Menschen (von Möllendorff, W., and Bargmann, W., editors), Springer-Verlag, Berlin, vol. 4, part 4, pp. 1–184, 1959.

HYDÉN, H. The Cell. In The Cell; Biochemistry, Physiology, Morphology (Brachet, J., and Mirsky, A. E., editors), vol. 4, pp. 215–323. Academic Press, New York, 1960.

HYDÉN, H. (editor) The Neuron. Elsevier Publishing Company, Amsterdam, 1967.

KATZ, B. Nerve, Muscle and Synapse. McGraw-Hill Book Company, New York, 1966.

KUFFLER, S. W., AND NICHOLLS, J. G. The physiology of neuroglial cells. Ergebn. Physiol. 57:1–90, 1966.

LANGMAN, J. Medical Embryology, ed. 3. Williams & Wilkins, Baltimore, 1975.

MORALES, R., AND DUNCAN, D. Specialized contacts of astrocytes with astrocytes and other cell types in the spinal cord of the cat. Anat. Rec. 182:255–266, 1975.

MUGNAINI, E., AND WALBERG, F. Ultrastructure of neuroglia. Ergebn. Anat. Entwicklungsgesch. 37:194–236, 1963.

MURRAY, M. R. Nervous tissue in vitro. In Cells and Tissues in Culture (Willmer, E. N., editor). vol. 2, pp. 373–455. Academic Press, New York, 1965.

NOBACK, C. R. The Human Nervous System. McGraw-Hill Book Company, New York, 1975.

PALAY, S. L., AND PALADE, G. E. The fine structure of neurons. J. Biophys. Biochem. Cytol. 1:69–88, 1955.

PAYTON, B. W., BENNETT, M. V. L., AND PAPPAS, G. D. Permeability and structure of junctional membranes at an electrotonic synapse. Science 166:1641–1643, 1969.

PENFIELD, W. (editor). Cytology and Cellular Pathology of the Nervous System, vols. 1, 2 and 3. Paul B. Hoeber, New York, 1932.

PENFIELD, W. Neuroglia: normal and pathological In Cytology and Cellular Pathology of the Nervous System (Penfield, W., editor), vol. 2, pp. 421–479. Paul B. Hoeber, New York, 1932.

PETERS, A., PALAY, S., AND WEBSTER, H. de F. The Fine Structure of the Nervous System. The Neurons and Supporting Cells. W. B. Saunders, Philadelphia, 1976.

QUARTON, G. C., MELNECHUK, T., AND SCHMITT, F. O. The Neurosciences. Rockefeller University Press, New York, 1967.

RAMON Y CAJAL, S. Degeneration and Regeneration of the Nervous System. Oxford University Press,

London, 1928.

RICHARDSON, K. C. The fine structure of autonomic nerve endings in smooth muscle of the rat vas deferens. J. Anat. 96:427–442, 1962.

ROBERTSON, J. D. The ultrastructure of adult vertebrate peripheral myelinated nerve fibers in relation to myelinogenesis. J. Biophys. Biochem. Cytol. 1:271–278, 1955.

ROBERTSON, J. D. The ultrastructure of Schmidt-Lanterman clefts and related shearing defects of the myelin sheath. J. Biophys. Biochem. Cytol. 4:39–46, 1958.

ROSENBLUTH, J. Intramembranous particle distribution at the node of Ranvier and adjacent axolemma in myelinated axons of the frog brain. J. Neurocytol. 5:731–745, 1976.

SCHNAPP, B., PERACCHIA, C., and MUGNAINI, E. The paranodal axo-glial junction in the central nervous system studied with thin sections and freeze-fracture. Neuroscience 1:181–190, 1976.

SHANTHAVEERAPPA, T. R., AND BOURNE, G. H. Perineural epithelium: a new concept of its role in the integrity of the peripheral nervous system. Science 154:1464–1467, 1966.

SPERRY, R. W. Chemoaffinity in the orderly growth of nerve fiber patterns and connections. Proc. Nat. Acad. Sci. USA 50:703–710, 1963.

UZMAN, B. G., AND NOGUEIRA-GRAF, G. Electron microscope studies of the formation of nodes of Ranvier in mouse sciatic nerves. J. Biophys. Biochem. Cytol. 3:589–598, 1957.

WEISS, P. (editor). Genetic Neurology; Problems of the Development, Growth, and Regeneration of the Nervous System and Its Functions. University of Chicago Press, Chicago, 1950.

WEISS, P., AND HISCOE, H. B. Experiments on the mechanism of nerve growth. J. Exp. Zool. 107:314–395, 1948.

WINDLE, W. F. Regeneration of axons in the vertebrate central nervous system. Physiol. Rev. 36:427–440, 1956.

WOLSTENHOLME, G. E. W., AND O'CONNOR, M. (editors) Growth of the Nervous System. Little, Brown and Company, Boston, 1968.

YOUNG, J. Z. The functional repair of nervous tissue. Physiol. Rev. 23:318–374, 1942.

CHAPTER 11

The Spinal Cord, Cerebellar Cortex, and Cerebral Cortex

The central nervous system is an array of various types of cell assemblies specialized to carry out their specific functions. Groups of nerve cell bodies carrying out similar functions are termed *nuclei.* If linearly arranged (as in the spinal cord), such cell groups may be termed *columns.* Groups of nerve fibers interconnecting these neuronal groups are called *tracts.* Myelinated tracts form the *white matter* of the central nervous system (CNS). When neuronal cell bodies occupy layers at the surface of the brain, these areas are termed cortical regions or *cortex.* The CNS is covered with connective tissue and supported in a special fluid, the cerebrospinal fluid (CSF). The purpose of this chapter is to present the cytology of several typical CNS regions and to describe the connective tissue investments that act both as a subcompartment for the CSF and as a protective covering for the fragile CNS tissues.

Investments of the Brain and Cord and the Fluid Spaces

The brain and spinal cord are enclosed by two connective tissue investments, the *dura mater* and the *pia-arachnoid,* the latter usually being subdivided into two layers, the *pia mater* and *arachnoid* (Figs. 11-1 and 11-2). These "membranes" are collectively known as the *meninges,* the dura mater being the *pachymeninx* and the pia-arachnoid the *leptomeninx,* or *leptomeninges.*

The *dura mater,* which is the outer of the two investments, consists of dense fibrous tissue (Fig. 11-2). The *cerebral dura* serves both as an investing membrane for the brain and as periosteum for the inner surfaces of the cranial bones. It consists of two layers. The inner layer is composed of dense connective tissue lined on its inner surface by a single layer of flat cells. The outer layer, which forms the periosteum and is similar in structure to the inner layer, is much richer in blood vessels and nerves. The *spinal dura* corresponds to the inner layer of the cerebral dura; the vertebrae have their own separate periosteum. It contains more elastic tissue than the inner layer of the cerebral dura but otherwise resembles it in structure. The outer surface of the spinal dura is covered with a single layer of flat cells and is separated from the periosteum by the *epidural space,* which contains anastomosing, thin-walled veins lying in connective tissue rich in fat (Fig. 11-1). The inner surface of the spinal dura is also lined by a single layer of flat cells. Beneath the spinal dura, between it and the arachnoid, is the *subdural space,* a narrow cleft containing fluid. It has no apparent direct communication with the subarachnoid space.

The *pia mater* (Fig. 11-2) closely invests the brain and cord, extends into the convolutions of the brain, and protrudes into the ventricles at the thin-walled portions of the brain, where, in combination with modified ependymal cells, it forms the cho-

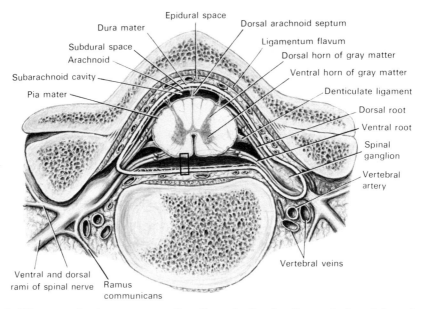

Fig. 11-1. Diagram of a transverse section through the fourth cervical vertebra showing the coverings of the spinal cord and related structures. An area comparable to that within the *box* is shown at higher magnification in Figure 11-2. (From Rauber-Kopsch, Anatomie.)

roid plexuses (described below). The pia consists of fibrous tissue and contains the blood vessels that send branches into the nerve tissue. The basal lamina of the CNS separates pial and perivascular connective tissue from the fibrous astrocyte end feet (outer glia limitans) that comprise the basal surface of brain and spinal cord. Pial connective tissue is continuous with the perivascular connective tissue that accompanies vessels which loop into the walls of the CNS. That connective tissue comprises a narrow space (*perivascular space*) between CNS basal lamina on the one side and vascular endothelial basal lamina on the other. As a vessel extends more deeply into the CNS wall, the perivascular space narrows until it disappears, and the two basal laminae are fused around the deepest smallest vessels.

The *arachnoid* (Fig. 11-2) passes over the convolutions of the brain without dipping into them. It is partly separated from the pia by a substantial space, across which trabeculae pass, connecting pia and arachnoid. This is the *subarachnoid space*, and it is filled with a clear fluid, the CSF. The trabeculae and arachnoid contain delicate strands of connective tissue covered with a layer of flat or low cuboidal cells which

also extends over the outer pial surface. This layer of cells is epithelioid and lines the subarachnoid spaces. The cells ordinarily have large, pale, oval nuclei. Recent evidence discloses that, like the cells of the perineurium, the outer arachnoid cells are attached by occluding junctions. Hence, they seem to serve as the outermost seal for the CSF-filled subarachnoid space. This cellular layer may be continuous with the perineurium at nerve roots. If so, a narrow continuity may exist between endoneurium and subarachnoid space or pial connective tissue.

The spinal dura and the inner layer of the cerebral dura are poor in blood vessels. The outer layer of the cerebral dura, forming as it does the periosteum of the cranial bones, is rich in blood vessels, which pass in to supply the bones. The pia is quite vascular, especially its inner aspect, from which vessels pass into the brain and cord. The arachnoid is nonvascular (Fig. 11-2).

The Cerebrospinal Fluid

The CSF in the subarachnoid space is in continuity with the CSF of the brain cavities (the ventricles) and the central canal of the spinal cord. This continuity is ef-

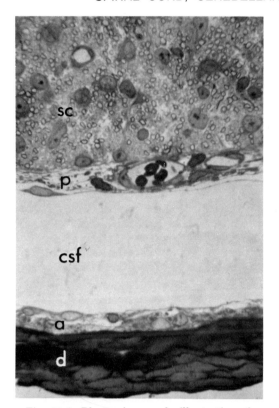

Fig. 11-2. Photomicrograph illustrating the histology of the region outlined by the *box* in Figure 11-1. The white matter of the spinal cord (*sc*) shows a variety of neuroglia cells in the process of forming myelin. Many small myelin sheaths are seen in cross section. Immediately overlying the cord tissue is the pia mater (*p*), containing two blood vessels, one of which contains several red blood cells. The space between the pia mater and the arachnoid (*a*) contains the cerebrospinal fluid (*csf*). The heavy connective tissue layers of the dura mater (*d*) form the outermost investment. The arachnoid is shown in its normal close apposition to the dura; only in abnormal conditions does fluid accumulate in the potential space between these two membranes. Kitten spinal cord.

fected through an aperture in the caudal part of the thin roof of the fourth ventricle (the foramen of Magendie) and an aperture in each of the thin-walled lateral recesses of the fourth ventricle (the foramina of Luschka).

The CSF is a clear, colorless fluid which is slightly viscous and of low specific gravity (1.004 to 1.006). It contains small quantities of inorganic salts, chiefly sodium chloride and potassium chloride, as well as small amounts of dextrose and traces of proteins. It normally contains very few cells. Its quantity in an adult man is about 150 ml. The bulk of the CSF is probably formed by the activity of the epithelial cells lining the choroid plexus, from which it passes into the ventricles and thence by the foramina of Magendie and Luschka into the subarachnoid spaces. Because adjacent ependymal cells lining the walls of the ventricles and spinal cord are joined by junctions that do not appear to be everywhere tight, CSF probably also percolates between those cells and through the intercellular spaces of the brain and cord. Some workers believe that substantial amounts of the CSF or certain of its components are produced by cells of the neural tissue, to pass into the ventricles, spinal canal, or perivascular spaces. If so, CNS tissue may be considered to have not only its interior and exterior surfaces, but also its interstices and individual cell surfaces, bathed in CSF. The drainage of the fluid back into the bloodstream appears to be chiefly by passage through the walls of arachnoid villi (see below) and into the cerebral venous sinuses.

Choroid Plexuses

Certain parts of the wall of the brain are composed solely of modified ependymal cells forming a thin epithelial membrane, a lamina epithelialis, which is covered externally by a highly vascularized pia mater. These two layers together constitute the *telae choroideae*, which form the roof of the fourth ventricle, the roof of the third ventricle, and parts of the walls of the lateral ventricles. Projecting into the ventricles are complex folds and invaginations from the telae choroideae containing tortuous networks of small vessels and capillaries, the *choroid plexuses* (Fig. 11-3). The term "choroid plexus" is often used in referring to the entire mass of infolded membranes, rather than to the network of blood vessels alone.

The modified ependymal epithelium covering the choroid plexuses is a simple cuboidal to low columnar type with a rather granular cytoplasm. In electron micrographs, the free surface of the cells appears to be thrown into fine irregular cytoplasmic projections, resembling a brush border. These cells play an important role in the production of the CSF. The cells of this

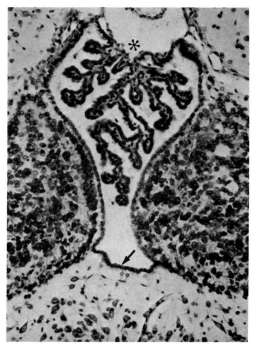

Fig. 11-3. Photomicrograph showing tufts of choroid plexus protruding downward from the roof (*) of the third ventricle into the ventricular cavity. The *arrow* points to the ependymal cells that form the lining of the third ventricle. Rat brain. ×130.

modified ependyma, unlike ependyma elsewhere, are joined together along their lateral borders by occluding junctions. Thus, although the capillaries of this region are known to be quite "leaky" (as compared with capillaries elsewhere in brain parenchyma), extravascular material is prevented from entering the CSF directly because of the seal along the lateral edges of the cells of the choroid plexus epithelium.

The Arachnoid Villi

In certain places, the arachnoid sends prolongations into the dura which protrude into a venous sinus or venous lacuna. The prolongations contain spaces, traversed by trabeculae, which may be regarded as continuations of the subarachnoid space. These arachnoidal outgrowths, which are covered with the usual layer of low cells, are known as *arachnoid villi* (Fig. 11-4). They are most numerous along the longitudinal fissure of the cerebral hemispheres, where they protrude into the superior longitudinal venous sinus. They are also sometimes found along the transverse, cavernous, and superior petrosal sinuses. It is thought that these villi have small one-way valves which permit the intermittent flow of CSF from the subarachnoid space into the venous sinuses (which have a very low fluid pressure).

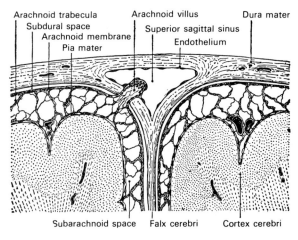

Fig. 11-4. Schematic diagram of coronal section of meninges and cerebral cortex, to show relation of arachnoid villus to dural venous sinus. The potential subdural space is necessarily shown of greater size than is normal; the subarachnoid space is also increased in width to illustrate the character of the subarachnoid mesh. The nuclei of the cells lining the subarachnoid space are faintly shown. (After Weed.)

The Fluid Compartments and the Blood-Brain Barrier

As is pointed out in the above discussion, the CSF occupies both the cavities of the CNS and the spaces around the brain and spinal cord. Because neither the lining of the brain ventricles (the unspecialized ependyma) nor the covering of the brain surface (the pia) provides a tight barrier against the entry into or egress of fluids from the substance of the brain, the narrow extracellular clefts between neurons and glia of the CNS are also in continuity with CSF (Fig. 11-5). Clinical sampling of the CSF with analysis of its composition provides a useful index of cellular changes in CNS diseases.

Perivascular spaces are also thought to be in continuity with this fluid system (Fig. 11-5). Near the surface of the brain, where pial tissue is carried down into brain substance with the penetrating blood vessels, this perivascular space is substantial and provides a common site of cell invasion in brain disease. Deeper within the brain wall, the pericapillary spaces are scarcely larger than the other cleftlike intercellular spaces of nervous tissue. In these deeper areas, the basal lamina of the capillaries is often surrounded by flattened cellular extensions of astrocytes, the outer glia limitans. This application of astrocytic processes to the capillary wall led to the suggestions that (1) these "suckerfeet" are avenues of nutrient passage from blood vessel to neuron, and/or (2) the mosaic of applied cellular processes constitutes the barrier for the passage of materials from blood vessels to brain parenchyma (*the blood-brain barrier*).

The use of the electron microscope has

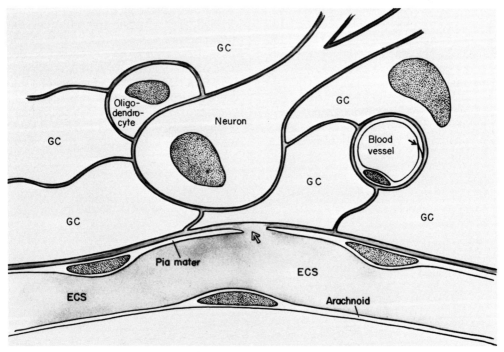

Fig. 11-5. Diagram illustrating the continuity between the cerebrospinal fluid within the subarachnoid space and the fluid filling the extracellular space within the nervous tissue parenchyma. Protein markers placed in the cerebrospinal fluid pass between the cells of the pia mater (*hollow arrow*) and into the narrow extracellular space of the nervous tissue. On the other hand, markers placed within the blood vessels of nervous tissue are confined to the vessel lumina by the presence of occluding junctions between the overlapping processes of endothelial cells (*solid arrow*). Thus the cerebrospinal fluid represents a type of extracellular fluid (*ECS*) for nervous tissue cells. *GC* = neuroglial cell. (From: Bunge, R.: The Neurosciences: Second Study Program, edited by F. O. Schmitt, p. 782, Rockefeller University Press, New York, 1970.)

demonstrated the precise site of the blood-brain barrier for certain types of molecules. When certain marker proteins (which can be rendered visible in the electron microscope) are injected into the vascular system, their entry into brain tissue is prevented by the minute occluding junctions between the lateral edges of the endothelial cells. When these protein markers are placed within brain substance, they pass between all cells (including the perivascular astrocyte processes and even through synaptic clefts) but do not enter blood vessels. Thus, the blood-brain barrier for these proteins is in the wall of the CNS capillaries and is not provided by the perivascular tissues (the astrocytic processes, connective tissue, or basal lamina). Whether the perivascular astrocytic feet function in nutrient transport is not known (see chapter 10).

The Spinal Cord

In transverse section (Fig. 11-6), the spinal cord appears oval in shape and slightly more flattened on its ventral than on its dorsal surface. It is surrounded by the pia mater spinalis, which extends into the deep longitudinal *ventral median fissure*. Dorsally, the cord is partitioned longitudinally by the *dorsal median sulcus*, which is composed principally of neuroglia

and over which the pia mater passes without entering. At the entrance of the dorsal root fibers on either side, there is a *dorsolateral groove* or *sulcus*.

The *gray matter* occupies the central part of the section, where it is arranged somewhat in the form of the letter H. Dorsally, the gray matter extends almost to the surface of the cord as the *dorsal gray columns* (*posterior horns*). The *ventral gray columns* (*anterior horns*) are shorter and broader and do not so nearly approach the surface of the cord. Surrounding the gray matter is the *white matter*, which, in each lateral half of the cord, is divided by the dorsal column into two parts. The part lying between the horn and the dorsal median septum is the *dorsal funiculus* (*dorsal* or *posterior white column*); the other part, comprising the remainder of the white matter, is the *ventrolateral funiculus* (*ventrolateral* or *anterolateral white column*).

The ventrolateral white column is again divided, rather indefinitely, by the ventral horn and nerve roots into a *lateral funiculus* (*lateral white column*) and a *ventral funiculus* (*ventral* or *anterior white column*). In the thoracic segments of the cord there is usually a lateral protrusion of the gray matter slightly dorsal to the dorsal boundary of the ventral horn. This region is called the *lateral horn*; it contains the

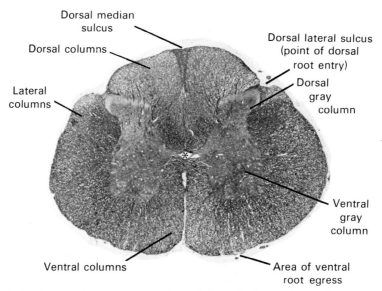

Fig. 11-6. Photomicrograph of a cross section of the spinal cord in the lumbar region of a cat. The H-shaped central region is the gray matter, surrounded by the tracts of nerve fibers which form the white matter. The central canal is marked with an *asterisk*.

nerve cell bodies of the CNS neurons of the thoracodorsal portion of the autonomic nervous system.

Gray Matter

In the cross portion of the H structure is seen the *central canal*, usually partially obliterated in the adult and represented only by a group of ependymal cells. The central canal divides the gray matter connecting the two sides of the cord into a *ventral gray commissure* and a *dorsal gray commissure*.

The components of the lateral portions of the H are, as noted above, the *dorsal horns*, which are primarily concerned with sensory input, and the *ventral horns*, which are concerned with motor activity. Between these two, and lateral to the gray commissures, is the *intermediate* (or *middle*) *gray*, which is associated largely with visceral innervation. The neuron cell bodies in these regions of gray matter are arranged in longitudinal columns, each a linear aggregate of neurons specialized for a particular function.

The dorsal horn contains three major nuclear groups specialized for the reception of the sensory impulses carried into the spinal cord by the axons of dorsal root ganglia. The various modalities of somatic sensation are handled differently in this region, some of the incoming axons synapsing locally and others being carried upward toward the brain before synapsing. Thus the sensory information available to the organism via the *first order* sensory neurons of the dorsal root ganglia is carried to *second order* sensory neurons and is distributed widely throughout the CNS.

Visceral sensibilities, on the other hand, appear to be channeled primarily to the poorly defined nuclear columns of the intermediate gray. As has been noted, in certain regions of the cord this same intermediate zone contains motor neurons of the visceral system (in the lateral horn cell column). Thus, the visceral areas of the gray matter are generally more medially located than are the somatic regions.

The ventral horn contains many motor cells (ventral or anterior horn cells) arranged in columns in relation to the portion of the body musculature that they innervate. Motor neurons providing fibers to trunk musculature are more medially disposed in ventral gray matter, and motor neurons to the muscles of the limbs are located laterally. Certain of these motor neurons are the largest neurons in the spinal cord. Their dendritic portions, which are generally multipolar, extend several millimeters up or down the cord to receive a variety of signals from local (spinal) interneurons as well as axons from distant (e.g., cortical) parts of the CNS. In higher animals, very few first order sensory neurons make direct contact with motor neurons. The large axons of the motor neurons can be seen passing out through the ventrolateral white matter to form, along with the fibers of the visceral motorneurons in the intermediate gray, the ventral spinal root at the surface of the cord.

White Matter

In order to carry nerve signals to and from gray matter at different levels of the spinal cord and to the higher centers in the brain, fibers must course up and down the long axis of the cord. These fibers (axons) leave the gray matter and form the more superficial white matter. The white matter is thus composed of myelinated and a few unmyelinated nerve fibers and neuroglia, along with blood vessels and inward continuations of the pia mater. White matter contains no neuron cell bodies or dendrites. If the section has been cut through a *dorsal* (*posterior*) *nerve root*, a small bundle of *dorsal root fibers* can be seen entering the white matter of the cord along the dorsal and medial side of the posterior horn. Ventral to the anterior gray commissure is a bundle of transversely disposed myelinated fibers, the *ventral white commissure*. In the dorsal part of the dorsal gray commissure there are also fine, similarly disposed myelinated nerve fibers, the *dorsal white commissure*. Both of these commissures are composed of fibers crossing from one side of the spinal cord to the other.

The Cerebellar Cortex

General Structure

The cerebellum, connected with the rest of the brain by its three peduncles, consists of two lateral lobes or hemispheres connected by a median lobe, the vermis. These are divided by transverse fissures into lobules, each lobule consisting of a median portion belonging to the vermis and two winglike extensions belonging to the hemispheres. The surfaces of the lobules are marked by folds (*laminae* or *folia*) running approximately parallel to the fissures and thus transversely to the longitudinal axis of the brain. The surface of the cerebellum is composed of gray matter, the cortex, which envelops the white matter.

In the *cerebellar cortex* there can be distinguished, with ordinary stains (hematoxylin-eosin, Nissl), an outer or *molecular layer* containing few cells and no myelinated fibers, an inner *granular layer*, and, between the two, a single row of large flask-shaped cells, the *cells of Purkinje* (Fig. 11-7). Below the granular layer is an area of white matter containing the fibers that carry signals to or from the neuronal machinery of the cortex.

The major input of nerve fibers to the cerebellum arrives in the granule cell layer. With routine stains, this layer appears to be comprised of closely packed cell nuclei, but there are clear spaces here and there which are called *islands* or *glomeruli*. The cell nuclei belong to small neurons, the *granule cells*, and the glomeruli are regions where the granule cell dendrites receive synapses from axons arriving from outside the cerebellum. The incoming fibers, which are highly branched, are called *mossy fibers* (Fig. 11-8). Each granule cell possesses three to six short dendrites for the reception of the mossy fiber input.

The granule cell sends its fine, unmyelinated axon to ascend into the molecular layer, where it divides into two branches running longitudinally along the folium and terminating in varicosities (Fig. 11-8). These are the *parallel fibers* of the molecular layer. They thus run at right angles to and through the dendritic expansions of the Purkinje cells, and their cross sections, together with the terminal dendritic arborizations of the Purkinje cells, give the molecular layer its punctate appearance. During their course in the molecular layer, the parallel fibers make synaptic contact (known to be excitatory) with dendrites from a number of different Purkinje cells.

The Purkinje dendrite also receives ex-

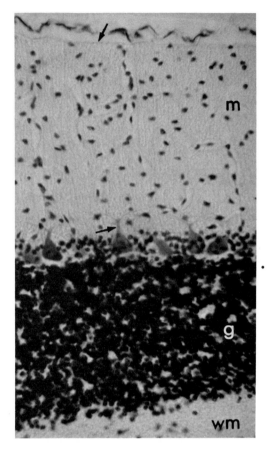

Fig. 11-7. Photomicrograph showing the layers of neurons within the cerebellar cortex of a rat. The *upper arrow* indicates the surface of the cerebellum, which is covered by remnants of the pia. The *lower arrow* indicates the dendrite of a Purkinje cell. The soma of this cell and adjacent Purkinje cells are also visible. The molecular layer (*m*) contains a considerable number of capillaries. *g*, granule cell layer; *wm*, white matter. Compare with Figure 11-8.

citatory input from *climbing fibers*, many of which are recurrent collaterals from neurons of the deep cerebellar nuclei (see below). These climbing fibers, which entwine the dendritic trunk (Fig. 11-8), have a powerful excitatory influence on the Purkinje cell.

Other granule cell axons are known to make contact with smaller neurons, the *basket cells*, which are located in the region of the Purkinje layer. These cells are so named because their axons form basket-like skeins around the bodies and initial axonal segments of the Purkinje cells (Fig. 11-8).

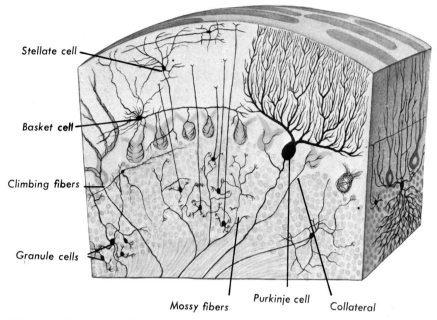

Stellate cell

Basket cell

Climbing fibers

Granule cells

Mossy fibers   Purkinje cell   Collateral

Fig. 11-8. Schematic diagram of structure of cerebellar cortex. (After Bargmann.)

They are thus well disposed to exert an inhibitory influence on Purkinje cell activity. We have thus described two excitatory inputs and one inhibitory input to the Purkinje cell.

The Purkinje cell possesses several main dendrites, which enter the molecular layer and form a remarkably rich arborization extending to the surface. The dendritic arborization is fan-shaped, extending at right angles to the laminae. The axon is given off from the end of the cell opposite to the dendrites and passes into the granular layer. Here axon collaterals may turn back to enter another part of the cerebellar cortex, but the main axon continues on to neurons deep within the cerebellum that form the deep cerebellar nuclei. The influence of the Purkinje axons on the neurons of the deep cerebellar nuclei is thought to be inhibitory. It is the neurons of the deep cerebellar nuclei that have axons leaving the cerebellum to provide the cerebellar output to other regions of the nervous system.

As complex as the above interneuronal connections may appear at first reading, the cerebellar circuitry is actually more complex than this short review indicates. This complexity is achieved not by unique cytology but by repetition of basic neuro-cytological components (elaboration of the cell surface to provide a dendritic zone, development of basic synaptic types, extension of the cell as an axon with specializations at the axon terminal). The same statement can be made regarding the more complicated cerebral cortex discussed below.

Function

The cerebellum contributes to nervous system function by serving to modulate and coordinate skeletal muscle activity. Among other activities, it assists in preventing muscle "overshoot" so that a muscle contraction once started will not become too gross by being carried too far; thus, fine movements are facilitated. The cerebellum is not involved in sensation or in intellectual processes.

Even a beginning understanding of how the cellular assemblies of the cerebellar cortex participate in this type of control must await the student's study of the origins of the fibers that enter the cerebellum and the destinations of fibers that comprise the cerebellar output.

From the viewpoint of the neurocytologist, it is interesting that after aldehyde fixation, the cells known to provide inhibitory influences (e.g., the basket cell contacts with Purkinje cell bodies) have often been found to contain primarily flattened synaptic vesicles in their nerve endings, whereas cells known to provide excitatory influences (e.g., the climbing fiber contacts with Purkinje dendrites or granule cell contacts with Purkinje dendritic spines) have been found to contain primarily spheroid synaptic vesicles (see discussion of this point in chapter 10).

The Cerebral Cortex

General Structure

The cerebral cortex (or pallium) is the external layer of gray matter covering the convolutions and fissures of the cerebral hemispheres. It has an area of about 200,000 mm^2 and varies in thickness from about 1.5 to 4.0 mm. It contains, in addition to nerve fibers, neuroglia, and blood vessels, the bodies of nearly 14 billion neurons. The older, less elaborate olfactory cortex is termed the *allocortex*; the rest is the *neocortex* or *isocortex*.

The chief types of neurons found in the cortex are (1) *pyramidal cells*, (2) *stellate* or *granule cells*, (3) *horizontal cells*, and (4) inverted or *Martinotti cells* (Figs. 11-9, 11-10). The pyramidal cells (Fig. 11-10) are characterized by a pyramid-shaped perikaryon with an apical dendrite directed toward the surface of the brain and an axon leaving the base of the perikaryon to course into the white matter as a projection or association fiber. These axons provide the principal output of the cortex. The granule or stellate cells are characterized by their relatively small size, numerous dendrites coursing in various directions, and a relatively short axon. Many of the axons providing an input to the cortex are thought to end on their dendrites. The horizontal cells, found mostly in the outer layer, are characterized by their horizontally disposed dendrites and axons, which presumably serve to interconnect neighboring cortical regions. The inverted or Martinotti cells, which are located in the deeper cortical layers, have axons directed toward the surface, to be distributed entirely intracortically.

When viewed in a section cut perpendicular to the cortical surface, the most strik-

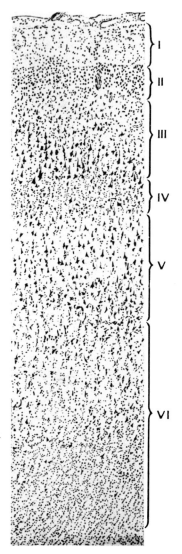

Fig. 11-9. Photograph of cell layers of Nissl-stained preparations of cerebral cortex. (After Bargmann.)

ing aspect of the cerebral cortex is the lamination of its cellular components in layers horizontal to the surface. The neocortex is characterized by a laminated appearance in which six layers can be identified (Fig. 11-9): (1) The outermost *molecular layer*, made up chiefly of cell processes and of horizontal cells; (2) the *external granular layer*, composed chiefly of small, triangular neurons; (3) the *pyramidal layer*, composed chiefly of relatively large pyramidal cells plus many granule cells; (4) the *internal granular layer*, made up chiefly of the stel-

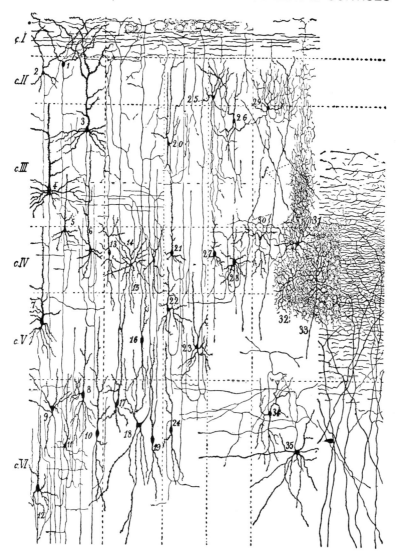

Fig. 11-10. Various forms of nerve cells of the cerebral cortex. From various figures of Cajal, especially of the temporal cortex. *cI*, zonal layer of cortex; *cII*, external granular layer; *cIII*, pyramidal layer; *cIV*, internal granular layer; *cV*, ganglionic layer; *cVI*, multiform layer. *1* to *12*, cells, mostly pyramidal, whose axons enter the white matter (corticofugal cells); *13* to *35*, cells whose axons do not leave the gray matter (or cortex); *13* to *19*, cells with directly ascending axons; *20* to *24*, cells with arciform ascending axons; *25* to *28*, cells with short descending axons, with or without ascending collaterals; *29*, *30*, short axon cells, properly speaking (Golgi's type II); *31* to *33*, cells with bushy axons (bipenicillate and neuroglia form), some forming terminal nests around the small granule cells; *34*, *35*, large stellate cells of layer *VI* with extensively branching axons, especially extending horizontally; *f*, fibers of unknown origin. On the *right* are shown corticopetal fibers and their terminal plexus, especially dense in layer *IV*. (After Bonne.)

late or granule cells; (5) the *ganglionic layer* of large and medium-sized pyramidal cells; and (6) the *multiform layer*, containing neurons of widely varying shape, including Martinotti cells.

The laminar arrangement of cortical neu-

rons so clearly visible in histological sections is deceptive in view of the known functional properties of certain cortical regions. The functional organization of some cortical areas receiving sensory stimuli (e.g., the cortex at the back of the head, which receives signals from the visual system) involves *columns* of neurons oriented vertical to the cortical surface. Stimuli arriving in this cortical region activate a specific column of cells, each column 0.3 to 0.5 mm in diameter. The intrinsic morphological basis for these functional columns has not been clearly defined.

The thickness of the various cell layers differs considerably in different areas of the cerebral cortex. Some areas exhibit such marked modification in the layers of cells that they are known as *heterotypic*, in contrast with *homotypic* areas, which show all of the six layers outlined in Figure 11-9. On the basis of differences in structure and function, the cortex has been mapped into a number of areas. In some regions, the cytoarchitecture of a particular area of cortex corresponds quite precisely to the functional modality known to be processed in that cortical region. This is true, for example, in cortical regions concerned with vision and with hearing. In other cases, cortical regions of different function have virtually identical cytological arrangements.

The input to the cortex comes from a great variety of sources. Many of the sensory modalities have representation in discrete cortical regions which provide surface representations for the different body parts. Other cortical regions are concerned with the initiation and/or control of motor activities; these regions are also *somatotopically* organized, each part of the body being represented in a discrete area of cortex. There are also discrete cortical regions associated with special faculties, e.g., speech. In the human, there are in addition substantial cortical areas, called association areas, which have connections with the motor and sensory regions of the cortex. These association areas provide additional orders of circuitry to assist in the analysis of sensory input and the programming of motor output.

Function

The discussion of nervous tissue begins in chapter 9 with the suggestion that higher animals use multiple sets of interneurons to effect their more discriminating and exact behavior. Between the primary sensory neurons in various sensory ganglia and the motor neurons of the "final common path," there are interposed, in the higher animal, circuit upon circuit of neuronal "wiring." By these circuits, sensations reach cortical levels. This wiring system provides for the convergence and association of many kinds of stimuli from all parts of the body. This cortical mechanism not only associates many stimuli before the performance of a motor activity, but it also dissociates, i.e., discriminates, and thus, by inhibition, it enables motor activity to be limited only to the necessary movements. There is also plasticity in cortical mechanisms, for the neurons are somehow changed by their activities. Whatever their nature, the acquired changes of the cortex, because of its plasticity and consequent capacity for "learning," affect the action of subsequent stimuli reaching the cortex and furnish the basis of memory, of personal experience, and of individually acquired neural mechanisms, as opposed to germinal or inherited neural mechanisms. Cortical mechanisms are also involved in the transmission, by educational processes using complex symbols, of acquired experience to the plastic cortex of other individuals. Animals other than man "learn," i.e., acquire and utilize individual experience, but it is doubtful that any animal other than man significantly *summates* experience, i.e., transmits it to other individuals and generations. The cortex is thus, in a sense, the organ of human culture and conduct. This supermaze of neuronal interconnections provides for the origin and expression of the highest faculties of the mind. If it is possible for the human cerebral cortex to understand the mechanisms of its own function, the concentrated study of many generations will certainly be required to accomplish this task.

References

BRIGHTMAN, M. W., AND REESE, T. S. Junctions between intimately opposed cell membranes in the vertebrate brain. J. Cell Biol. 40:648–677, 1969.

CARPENTER, M. B. Human Neuroanatomy, ed. 7. Williams & Wilkins, Baltimore, 1976.

CHOW, K. L., AND LEIMAN, A. L. The structural and functional organization of the neocortex. Neurosci. Res. Progr. Bull. 8:157–220, 1970.

CROSBY, E. C., HUMPHREY, T., AND LAUER, E. W.

Correlative Anatomy of the Nervous System. The Macmillan Company, New York, 1962.

ECCLES, J. C., ITO, M., AND SZENTAGOTHAI, J. The Cerebellum as a Neuronal Machine. Springer-Verlag, New York, 1967.

ECONOMO, C. The Cytoarchitectonics of the Human Cerebral Cortex. Oxford University Press, London, 1929.

LAJTHA, A., AND FORD, D. H. (editors). Brain Barrier Systems. Progr. Brain Res. 29, 1968.

NOBACK, C. R. The Human Nervous System. McGraw-Hill Book Company, New York, 1975.

PETERS, A., PALAY, S. L., AND WEBSTER, H. The Fine Structure of the Nervous System. The Neurons and Supporting Cells. W. B. Saunders, Philadelphia, 1976.

SHOLL, D. A. The Organization of the Cerebral Cortex. Methuen and Company, London, 1970.

WEED, L. H. Certain anatomical and physiological aspects of the meninges and cerebrospinal fluid. Brain 58:383–397, 1934.

WISLOCKI, G. B. The cytology of the cerebrospinal pathway. Special Cytology (Cowdry, E. V., editor), vol. 3, pp. 1485–1521, 1932.

CHAPTER 12

The Circulatory System

The circulatory apparatus consists of a blood vascular system and a lymph vascular system. The *blood vascular system* consists of (1) the *heart,* which is a pump for propelling the blood, (2) the *arteries,* which are tubes for conveying the blood toward the organs and tissues, (3) the *capillaries,* which are anastomosing channels of small caliber with thin walls providing for much of the interchange of substances between the blood and tissue fluids, and (4) the *veins,* which in their initial segments also provide for blood-tissue fluid interchange but in addition serve for the return of blood to the heart.

The lymph vascular system consists of lymphatic capillaries and various-sized lymphatic vessels which ultimately drain into main trunks, the thoracic duct and the right lymphatic duct, which empty into the large veins in the neck.

The Blood Vascular System

The entire system—heart, arteries, veins, capillaries—has a common and continuous lining which consists of a single layer of endothelial cells. This single layer of cells forms the main component of the wall in the capillaries, but some additional cells and tissues are usually present. Accessory coats of muscle and connective tissue become prominent in the larger vessels and the heart. Because the structure of the capillary is simpler than that of the other parts

of the system, it has become customary to describe the capillaries first.

Capillaries

The capillaries are delicate tubes with an average diameter of about 7 to 9 μm. They branch extensively without much change in caliber, and the branches anastomose to form networks which vary in density and pattern in different tissues and organs. The tissues with the highest metabolic activity have networks of elaborately branched and closely packed capillaries. This is so in the lungs, liver, kidney, and most glands and mucous membranes. The capillaries of the network nearest to the arterioles supplying them are called arterial capillaries, and those nearest to the venules draining them are called venous capillaries.

The capillary network between arterioles and venules often contains a central or *thoroughfare channel,* where the blood flow is continuous, in contrast with the branches of the network, where the flow tends to be intermittent (Fig. 12-1). The proximal portion of the central channel, i.e., the part just beyond the arteriole proper, is known as a *metarteriole* (from the Greek *meta,* beyond). The metarteriole has isolated smooth muscle cells dispersed at intervals along the outer surface of its endothelial cells. These smooth muscle cells are surrounded by a glycoprotein coat which is continuous with the basal lamina of the

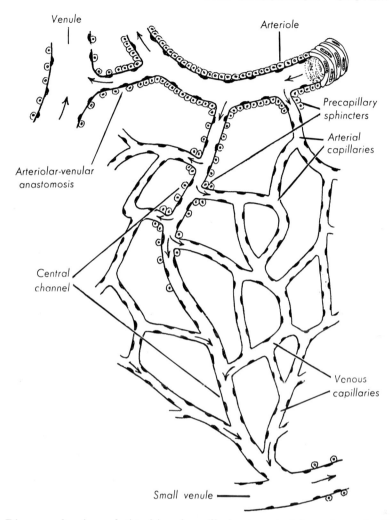

Fig. 12-1. Diagram showing relationship of capillaries to arteriole and venule. The proximal portion of the central channel through a capillary bed is surrounded by scattered smooth muscle fibers and has been named the "metarteriole"; the distal portion of the central channel is structurally a true capillary.

endothelium. They have branching processes and tend to be oriented longitudinally on the vessel (Fig. 12-2), in contrast with the transversely oriented muscle cells of the arterioles proper (Fig. 12-8). The venous end of the thoroughfare channel resembles other capillaries except for its wider lumen.

The thoroughfare channels differ from the branched portions of the capillary networks in their functional behavior, and they can be differentiated more readily in living than in fixed preparations. The thoroughfare channels convey an active flow of blood at all times, although the amount of flow varies with vasoconstriction and vasodilation of the metarteriolar segment. Flow in the branches of the network is intermittent during relatively inactive metabolic periods; in other words, the branches do not all function at once, except when there is an increased demand. The amount of blood entering the branches is controlled by the state of contraction of smooth muscle cells of the *precapillary sphincters,* which are located where arterial capillaries arise from arterioles, whether from metarterioles or from arterioles proper. The number of thoroughfare channels in proportion to the number of branched capillaries differs for different regions of the body; in skin, for example, the direct channels are numerous, whereas in skeletal muscle they are relatively infrequent in comparison with the branches of the meshwork.

The wall of the capillary is composed of a single layer of endothelial cells which rests on a basement membrane (basal lamina and lamina reticularis), plus a thin adventitia which consists of some connective tissue fibers along with a discontinuous layer of connective tissue cells. Two endo-

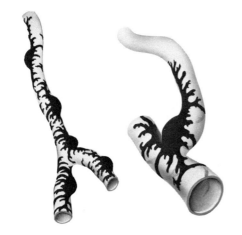

Fig. 12-2. Modified smooth muscle cells on precapillary arterioles (metarterioles) of human heart. The cells and their processes are demonstrated by a chrome silver impregnation method. *Left*, several muscle cells with their processes surrounding a metarteriole; *right*, higher magnification of one muscle cell at junction of metarteriole and capillary. (Redrawn and modified from Zimmermann.

thelial cells, and occasionally only one, generally suffice for the complete circumference of small capillaries, but three to five cells are often required for larger ones. In surface view, the endothelial cells are seen as a delicate mosaic when their cell boundaries are demonstrated by the precipitation of silver at the cell margins (Fig. 12-3). The cells usually have irregular borders and tend to be arranged with their long axes parallel with the long axes of the tubes. In routinely prepared sections for light microscopy, the cytoplasm appears clear or finely granular and the cells bulge into the lumen in the regions where the nuclei are located. This condition is generally accentuated by shrinkage of the vessels and their cells during fixation for light microscopy.

Electron micrographs of specially prepared tissue show that the endothelial cells have a thin glycoprotein layer over their luminal surface (endocapillary layer), some short microvilli, and the usual organelles, including a relatively small Golgi and some scattered mitochondria. They also have a variable number of specific granules of about 0.1 to 0.2 μm in diameter. These granules, like most organelles, are membrane-bounded and contain an electron-dense matrix which frequently contains some small tubular structures. The function of these granules has not been clearly defined. Electron micrographs also show that the capillary endothelial cells often have pinocytotic vesicles ranging in diameter from about 600 to 1000 Å (Fig. 12-4). Some of the vesicles are found entirely within the cell cytoplasm, whereas others are open either at the inner (luminal) surface or at

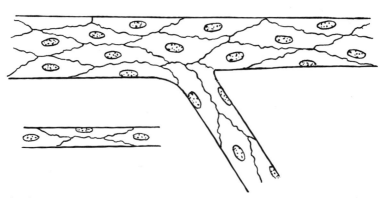

Fig. 12-3. Surface view of large and small capillaries stained with silver nitrate and hematoxylin to show outlines of endothelial cells and their nuclei.

the outer (tissue) side; the open vesicles are also known as *caveolae*. The view that pinocytotic vesicles function in transporting materials, such as macromolecules, is supported by electron micrographs of tissues from animals which had received intravascular injections of colloidal particles which serve as markers. However, other mechanisms have a major role in the transport of substances across endothelium, as discussed below under "Structure and Function." It has also been proposed that caveolae may be involved in the elaboration of an endocapillary glycoprotein substance and may serve as the site for enzymatic activation of angiotensin in the capillaries of the lung (see chapters 17 and 18).

Adjacent endothelial cells may meet in a simple end-to-end pattern, but more often the edge of one cell overlaps that of another along an oblique course or in complicated S-shaped patterns. The walls of adjacent cells are separated from each other by about 200 Å along parts of their course, but at intervals they come into closer association by junctions which differ somewhat from the junctional complexes of simple columnar epithelium (chapter 4). Fairly extensive areas of occluding junctions are present in cerebral capillaries and in the thymic cortex, but these junctions are less well developed in capillaries of other regions. Recent studies using freeze fracture techniques show branching or staggered strands representing the occluding junctions, but no communicating (gap) junctions were detected. The occluding junctions apparently do not form rings of complete occlusion at the adluminal ends of the cells.

Pericapillary cells are closely associated with the capillaries. This category includes *fibroblasts, histiocytes,* and *pericytes.* Fibroblasts and histiocytes are present in the connective tissue associated with the capillaries in most parts of the body, but there are some locations where the capillaries are so closely related to the tissues with which they function that there is little or no intervening space for connective tissue. For instance, in the glomeruli of the kidney, the basal lamina of the endothelium is fused with the basal lamina of the epithelium of the visceral layer of Bowman's capsule. *Pericytes* are irregularly shaped, isolated

cells distributed at intervals along the capillaries in a pattern resembling that of the modified muscle cells on metarterioles. In electron micrographs, the pericytes appear enclosed by the basal lamina of the endothelium because each pericyte is surrounded by an electron-dense coat which is continuous with the basal lamina portion of the endothelial cells (Fig. 12-5).

In the literature on capillaries, the term pericyte is sometimes used synonymously with Rouget cell. This is misleading because the cells described by Rouget (1875) as contractile units along vessels in the nictitating membrane of the frog eye *in vivo* were apparently smooth muscle cells on vessels that are now classified as metarterioles (Figs. 12-1 and 12-2). The cells currently identified as pericytes in electron micrographs are relatively undifferentiated in the sense that they apparently can develop into several different cell types, including smooth muscle. The endothelial cells themselves are contractile and can change their shape and reduce the diameter of the capillary lumen, but their contractility is not equivalent to that of smooth muscle.

Types of Capillaries. The vessels joining arterioles and venules can be divided into different categories on the basis of their ultrastructure and function as follows: (1) *continuous capillaries,* (2) *fenestrated capillaries,* (3) *sinusoidal capillaries,* (4) *sinusoids,* and (5) *venous sinuses.*

In the *continuous capillary,* there is a complete layer of cytoplasm throughout each endothelial cell (Fig. 12-4). This type is found in muscle and in many other locations. The *fenestrated capillary* differs from the continuous type in that its endothelial cells have numerous fenestrae of about 700 to 1000 Å in diameter where the cytoplasm is absent and the cell wall consists solely of a porous diaphragm thinner than the cell membrane (Figs. 12-5 and 12-6). The cytoplasm of the endothelial cells of fenestrated capillaries also differs histochemically from that of the continuous capillaries of muscle in that it generally fails to show any alkaline phosphatase enzyme activity. The fenestrated type is found in locations known for their fluid transport, although fenestrae do not provide the only route for fluid transport. Good examples of

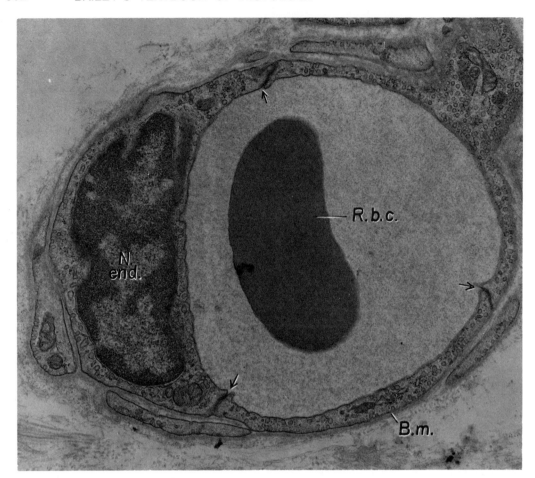

Fig. 12-4. Electron micrograph of blood capillary from lamina propria of bat esophagus. Junctions of endothelial cells are indicated by *arrows*. The nucleus (*N. end.*) of one endothelial cell is seen. Within the cytoplasm of the endothelial cells, there are numerous vesicles. These are particularly clear in the *upper right corner* of the photograph, where the plane of the section is tangential to the surface of the cell. Basal lamina material (*B.m.*) surrounds the endothelium and also encloses some processes of pericytes, shown on the *left*. A red blood cell (*R.b.c.*) is seen in the lumen of the vessel. ×13,000. (Courtesy of Dr. Keith Porter.)

this type of vessel are found in the intestinal villi, ciliary processes of the eye, and choroid plexuses. A special variety of the fenestrated type of endothelium is present in the glomerular capillaries of the kidney (chapter 18).

Sinusoidal capillaries (e.g., endocrine glands, carotid and aortic bodies) differ from both the continuous and fenestrated type in that they are wider and their basal and reticular laminae are less prominent (Figs. 21-5 and 21-11). Their fenestrae also may be somewhat larger than those of the fenestrated capillaries. They differ from sinusoids in that they have no intercellular

gaps and no macrophages closely associated with their endothelial cells (Table 12-1).

The *sinusoids* of the liver and bone marrow differ from sinusoidal capillaries in a number of respects: they are wider, and their basal lamina is scanty and often absent (Fig. 12-7). The sinusoids of the liver also differ in that they have macrophages known as Kupffer cells closely associated with their endothelial cells (chapter 16).

The *venous sinuses* of the spleen are wider than the sinusoids of the liver and differ in other respects, as listed in Table 12-1. They are described in detail in chapter 13.

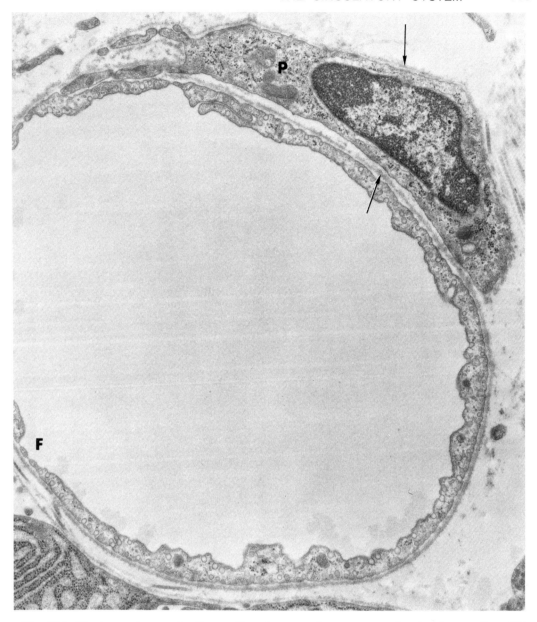

Fig. 12-5. Electron micrograph of a capillary from monkey pancreas showing fenestrations (*F*) and a pericyte (*P*). Note the basal lamina on both sides of the pericyte (*arrows*). ×14,500.

Correlation of Capillary Structure and Function. Exchange of substances between the blood vessels and surrounding tissues occurs chiefly in the capillaries and small venules. The passage of fluid across the capillary wall is partially dependent on the blood pressure within the capillaries and on the colloid osmotic pressure of the blood. The former factor promotes passage from the vessels to the tissues, and the latter factor favors reabsorption. The blood pressure in the arterial capillaries is normally higher than in the venous capillaries, and the blood pressure on the arterial side also exceeds the colloid osmotic pressure of the blood plasma. Based on the pressure relationships, fluids normally pass by diffusion from the vessels to the tissues in the arterial part of the capillary bed and return to the vessels via the venous capillaries,

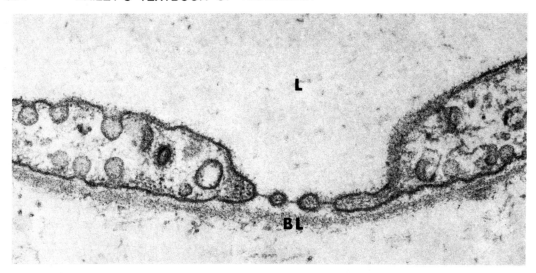

Fig. 12-6. Electron micrograph of a fenestrated capillary wall showing fenestrae with a thin diaphragm and the continuous underlying basal lamina. *L*, lumen of capillary; *BL*, basal lamina. ×67,500.

TABLE 12-1

Diagnostic properties of blood capillaries, sinusoids, and venous sinuses

Parameter	Continuous capillary	Fenestrated capillary	Sinusoidal capillary	Sinusoid	Venous sinus
Cross sectional diameter	Small	Small	Intermediate	Large	Larger
Regularity of cross section	Regular	Regular	Variable	Irregular	Variable
Intercellular gaps	Absent	Absent	Absent	Present and variable	Variable
Fenestrations	Absent	Numerous	Numerous and larger	Variable	Absent
Basal lamina	Prominent and continuous	Prominent and continuous	Continuous	Scanty or absent	Discontinuous
Lamina reticularis	Prominent	Prominent	Variable	Absent	Variable
Avid macrophages associated with endothelium	Absent	Absent	Absent	Common	Questionable

small venules, and lymphatic channels. Pressure within the capillaries can be modified at the local level by vasoconstriction and vasodilation through contraction and relaxation of smooth muscle cells in the walls of arterioles, metarterioles, and precapillary sphincters (Fig. 12-1).

Electron microscope studies of tissues fixed after transfusion of substances of different molecular weight (e.g., horseradish peroxidase, molecular weight 40,000, and ferritin, molecular weight 500,000) have provided a better understanding of the permeability of vessels of different regions.

It is known, for example, that the cerebral capillaries which have occluding junctions and relatively few pinocytotic vesicles are impermeable to macromolecules and also to horseradish peroxidase, which has a low molecular weight and a diameter of only about 50 Å. At the other extreme of permeability, there are the sinusoids of the liver and bone marrow and the venous sinuses of the spleen, which have relatively wide spaces between the cells, large and irregularly distributed fenestrations, and no or only an incomplete basal lamina; these permit the passage of larger molecules and

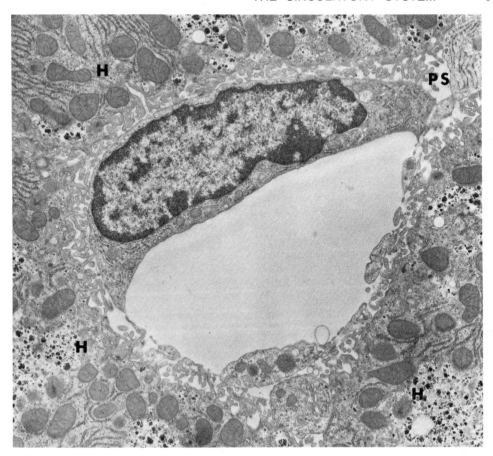

Fig. 12-7. Electron micrograph of a portion of a hepatic sinusoid showing the discontinuous or fenestrated endothelial lining. There is no basal lamina beneath the endothelium in this region. *H*, hepatic cells; *PS*, perisinusoidal space. ×7750.

even whole cells such as erythrocytes.

As already mentioned, the majority of the capillaries of the body lack the well developed occluding junctions; in these, the exchange between the blood vessels and the surrounding tissue can occur via intercellular clefts plus pinocytotic vesicles, fenestrae, or both, according to the type of endothelium. Some authors assign a major role to the pinocytotic vesicles, but more recent studies of the capillaries of cardiac and skeletal muscle have shown that the amount of fluid transported across the endothelium in a given period of time greatly exceeds the amount that can be accounted for by the number of pinocytotic vesicles present. Fluid exchange apparently occurs chiefly by the intercellular clefts. When vascular permeability is increased by injections of substances such as histamine and endo-

toxin, relatively large intercellular gaps appear in the endothelium of the venous capillaries and small venules. This is correlated with an even more sporadic occurrence of occluding junctions than is found in the nonstimulated capillaries. Under conditions of inflammation, substances pass from the blood to the surrounding tissues chiefly on the venous side of the capillary bed.

Lipid-soluble substances such as oxygen and carbon dioxide can readily diffuse through the endothelial cell membrane. Lipid-insoluble substances cannot diffuse through the cell membrane; they are transported across the endothelial cells by routes described by physiologists as a *small pore system* for low molecular weight substances such as water and a *large pore system* for macromolecules. The pinocytotic vesicles may represent the small pore system in part, but, as noted above, the amount of water transported over a given period of time in some tissues greatly exceeds the amount that could be accounted for by the number of pinocytotic vesicles present.

Considerable evidence has accumulated in support of the view that fluid transport across the capillaries of muscle, for example, is via the intercellular clefts of about 150 to 200 Å in width and that these correspond to the small pore system described by physiologists. It has also been reported, however, that in some vessels the pinocytotic vesicles may fuse to form patent transendothelial channels that could correspond to the small pore system where they occur. The cytological equivalent of the large pore system remains controversial, although evidence has been accumulating in support of the view that pinocytotic vesicles and fenestrae 600 to 1000 Å in diameter (when present) are the counterparts of the large pore system of physiologists.

Arteries

As mentioned previously, the walls of capillaries are composed mainly of endothelium, but scattered perivascular cells and a delicate connective tissue framework are also present. In larger vessels, the accessary cells and connective tissue become organized so that three tunics or coats become recognizable. These coats are most distinct in arteries of medium caliber. (1) The innermost coat, the *intima*, consists of an endothelial lining continuous with that found in the walls of the capillaries, an intermediate layer of delicate connective tissue, which is absent in the smaller vessels, and an external band of elastic fibers, the *internal elastic lamina*, which marks the boundary between the intima and media. (2) The middle coat, or *media*, consists mainly of smooth muscle cells with varying numbers of elastic and collagenous fibers. (3) The outer coat, *adventitia* or *externa*, is composed chiefly of connective tissue.

The structure and relative thickness of each of the tunics varies according to the size of the artery. Although the changes along the arterial tree are gradual and never abrupt, one may readily distinguish different types of arteries according to size, structure, and function. Following the blood vessels from the heart to the capillaries, we recognize (1) large, elastic arteries, (2) medium-sized, muscular arteries, and (3) small arteries and arterioles. Working backward from the capillaries which have been described, we will consider the structure of the arterioles first.

Arterioles and Small Arteries. The transition from a capillary to an arteriole is marked by the appearance of isolated smooth muscle fibers which are arranged spirally. These small arterioles of transitional type are called precapillary arterioles or metarterioles (Fig. 12-1). As the vessels become larger, the muscle cells increase in number and form a complete coat of one or two layers of circularly arranged fibers (Figs. 12-8 and 12-9). Outside of the muscle, the connective tissue is condensed to form a fibrous layer which is composed of flattened fibroblasts and longitudinally arranged collagenous fibrils. Thus, in the walls of the *arterioles,* the three coats are already distinguishable: an endothelial intima, a muscular media, and an adventitia of connective tissue. Although a few scattered elastic fibers can be demonstrated in the walls of very small arterioles, an internal elastic membrane sufficiently thick to be visible under the light microscope does not begin until the vessels have reached a diameter of about 40 μm.

The endothelial cells often have footlike processes that extend through the basal lamina and the internal elastic lamina to make contact via gap junctions with the innermost layer of smooth muscle cells of the media; these are known as *myoendothelial junctions.* They are also present, but less numerous, in the medium-sized and large arteries. It has been suggested that they facilitate metabolic or informational exchange between the lumina of the vessels and the muscle cells of the media.

The coats of the vessels increase in thickness and become more organized as the vessels increase in caliber. In vessels of about 130 μm in diameter, the media has three or four layers of muscle cells and a more prominent elastic lamina. When the vessels reach a diameter of about 300 μm, their walls show all of the structural features of medium-sized vessels.

Some authors use the term arteriole for small arteries ranging in caliber from about

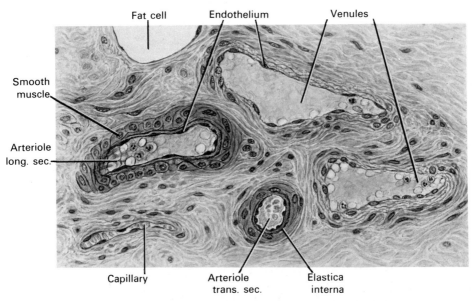

Fig. 12-8. Arterioles and accompanying venules from the submucosa of a human rectum. The arteriole at the *left* is cut longitudinally in the central part of its course, where its walls show the circularly arranged muscle fibers cut across, but farther to the *left*, where it passes out of the plane of the section, the wall of the arteriole is cut tangentially and shows muscle fibers extending over the lumen. The vacuoles in the blood plasma just beneath the endothelium of the vessels are artifacts produced by shrinkage. ×325.

300 μm to the very small precapillary vessels. Under this definition, the term arteriole encompasses most of the small, unnamed arteries and consists of vessels in which the tunica media ranges in thickness from one to several layers of muscle cells. Other authors use the term arteriole for vessels which have only one or two layers of muscle cells (Fig. 12-1) and the term small artery, for vessels which connect the arterioles proper with the medium-sized or muscular arteries. The latter usage seems preferable.

The arterioles are able to regulate the distribution of blood to different capillary beds by vasoconstriction or vasodilation in localized regions. Widespread vasoconstriction or vasodilation of the arterioles alters the peripheral resistance to flow from the larger arteries and hence plays an important part in regulating blood pressure. The arterioles and small arteries are structurally adapted for vasoconstriction and vasodilation, because their walls are composed primarily of circularly arranged muscle fibers which are controlled by the autonomic nervous system. Elasticity is not as important in these vessels as in the larger arteries,

in which the blood pressure is much higher. Arterioles are not directly involved in interchange between blood and tissue fluids, and the walls are relatively impermeable. This is accompanied by well developed occluding junctions between the endothelial cells. Hence, the sparseness of elastic tissue and the presence of well developed occluding junctions in arterioles are examples of correlation between structure and function.

Medium-Sized Arteries. These include all of the named arteries of gross dissections except the very large ones. There is a gradual transition between the branches of the medium-sized arteries and the small arteries described above. Examples of medium-sized arteries are the radial, tibial, popliteal, axillary, splenic, mesenteric, and intercostal arteries. The walls of these blood vessels are relatively thick, mainly as a result of the large amount of muscle in the media (Fig. 12-10). They are therefore called *muscular* arteries, in contrast with the *elastic* arteries like the aorta, in the wall of which elastic tissue predominates. The muscular arteries have also been called *distributing arteries* because they distribute the blood to different organs and, by contraction or

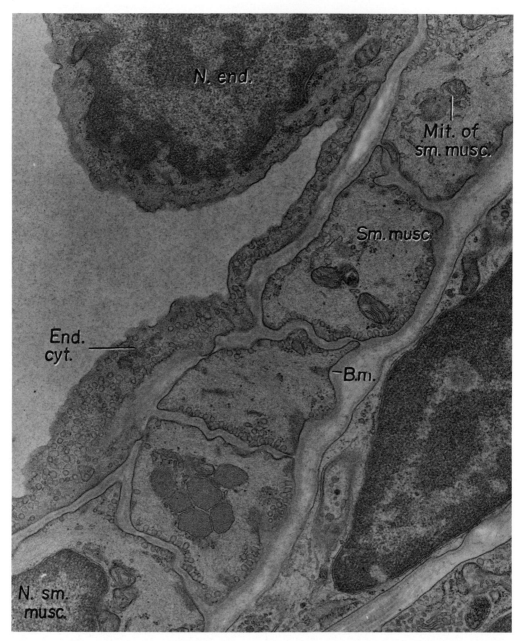

Fig. 12-9. Electron micrograph of a portion of an arteriole from the cervical region of a bat. The nucleus (*N. end.*) of one endothelial cell is seen, and numerous pinocytotic vesicles are present in the cytoplasm of the endothelial cells (*End. cyt.*). Because the circularly arranged smooth muscle cells are cut transversely, one may conclude that the plane of the section is longitudinal to the axis of the vessel. A nucleus (*N. sm. musc.*) is seen in one of the muscle cells, and their mitochondria (*Mit. of sm. musc.*) are shown. Numerous vesicles are seen at the periphery of the muscle cells. Basal lamina material (*B. m.*) is seen beneath the endothelium and around muscle cells. Fibroblasts and fine connective tissue fibrils are seen in the adventitial coat at the *right*. ×22,500. (Courtesy of Dr. Keith Porter.)

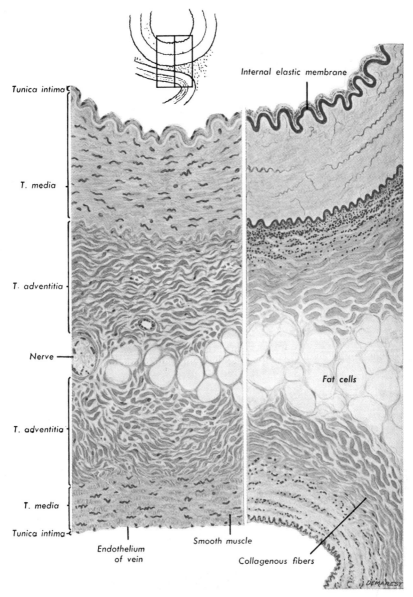

Tunica intima

T. media

T. adventitia

Nerve

T. adventitia

T. media

Tunica intima

Endothelium of vein

Smooth muscle

Internal elastic membrane

Fat cells

Collagenous fibers

Fig. 12-10. Two cross sections of the same medium-sized artery and vein (intercostal artery *above*, vein *below*). The *line drawing* at *upper left* gives orientation of regions drawn. Section on the *left* is stained with hematoxylin-eosin, that on the *right* with resorcin-fuchsin to show elastic tissue. *T.*, tunica. ×215.

relaxation, aid in regulating the supply to different regions in response to different functional demands.

The *intima* of the medium-sized arteries is composed of three layers: *endothelium, intermediate layer,* and *internal elastic lamina.* The endothelial layer is similar to that described above for small arteries. The intermediate layer consists of delicate collagenous fibers and a few elastic fibers embedded in a connective tissue matrix. Isolated and longitudinally oriented smooth muscle fibers are present in the intermediate layer, especially in places where the vessels branch. Some of these were mistakenly identified by light microscopists as fibroblasts, but electron micrographs show practically no fibroblasts within the intima of normal vessels. Prominent bundles of longitudinally oriented smooth muscle fibers are present in the intima of some of the larger muscular arteries (femoral, popliteal, axillary, hepatic, splenic, renal, and coronary).

The *internal elastic lamina* of the medium-sized artery is a fenestrated band of closely interwoven elastic fibers. In the smaller vessels of this type, the internal elastic layer is prominent and often split into a double membrane. It is intimately connected with the media and marks the boundary between the latter and the intima. This membrane often shows longitudinal folds in sections of fixed tissue; this is due chiefly to the postmortem contraction of the smooth muscle of the vessels.

The *media* is the thickest coat, consisting of 25 to 40 layers of circularly disposed muscle fibers. The thickness of the muscle coat is to some extent proportional to the size of the vessel, but there are considerable variations in arteries of the same size. Between the layers of muscle, there are small amounts of connective tissue composed of elastic, collagenous, and reticular fibers. Because there are apparently no fibroblasts within the media, it is assumed that the connective tissue fibers of this layer are formed by the smooth muscle cells. Furthermore, the intercellular mucopolysaccharides are apparently also formed by the smooth muscle cells.

The smooth muscle cells of the medium-sized arteries, like those of other types of arteries, are in communication with each other by means of gap junctions, described in chapter 4. Because most of the neuromotor nerve fibers terminate in the outermost part of the media and in the adjacent adventitia, the effect of the neurotransmitter substances on the innermost layers of the media may be via the gap junctions of the muscle fibers as well as by diffusion via intercellular substance.

The amount and distribution of elastic tissue in the media are closely correlated with the caliber of the vessel. In the smaller vessels, the elastic fibers are scattered between the muscle cells, but in the larger vessels they form circularly oriented elastic nets together with a few radially oriented fibers. In the larger vessels of the group there is a fenestrated membrane or network of elastic tissue, the *external elastic lamina,* at the junction of the tunica media with the adventitia (Fig. 12-10). The largest vessels of the group contain circularly disposed fenestrated membranes of elastic tissue (Fig. 12-11); hence, these vessels are transitional between the muscular and elastic types in structure.

The *adventitia* is a coat of considerable thickness, occasionally as thick as the media. It is composed of connective tissue containing collagenous and elastic fibers, most of which course longitudinally. The elastic fibers are concentrated in the inner layer of the coat, where they form a coarse network. The outer layer of the adventitia blends gradually with the surrounding connective tissue which attaches the artery to other structures.

A few longitudinal smooth muscle fibers are occasionally found in the inner layer of the adventitia, between the elastic fibers. In some arteries (splenic, dorsalis penis), bundles of longitudinally disposed muscle fibers occur in close proximity to the media.

Large Arteries. The large arteries belong to the *elastic* type. They have also been called *conducting arteries,* because they conduct the blood from the heart to the medium-sized distributing arteries. The walls of these vessels are relatively thin in proportion to their diameter; this is accompanied by an increase in elastic tissue and a decrease in smooth muscle. Whereas the various elements are generally arranged either circularly or longitudinally in the medium-sized arteries, they tend to follow a spiral course in the large arteries. The aorta is the chief representative of this group (Fig. 12-12). Other vessels of the type include the innominate, common carotid, subclavian, vertebral, and common iliac arteries. The transition in histological structure from large arteries to those of the medium-sized (muscular) type is gradual rather than abrupt.

The *intima* is thicker in large arteries than in the other types, and is lined by endothelial cells which tend to be short and polygonal in shape. The connective tissue immediately beneath the endothelium is composed of fine collagenous fibers together with some elastic fibers. The deeper

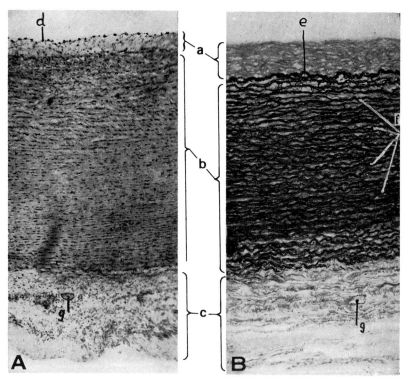

Fig. 12-11. Cross section through internal carotid artery. Retouched photograph. ×85. *A* stained with hematoxylin-eosin; *B* with resorcin-fuchsin; *a*, intima; *b*, media; *c*, adventitia; *d*, endothelium; *e*, internal elastic lamina; *f*, elastic lamina in media; *g*, vasa vasorum.

portion of the intima contains connective tissue fibers and a few longitudinally oriented smooth muscle fibers (Fig. 12-12). The amount of elastic tissue and the character of the internal elastic lamina change with age. Because the inner elastic lamina is usually split into two or more lamellae which merge with other similar layers in both the intima and the media, it is difficult precisely to identify this lamina in the aorta.

The *media* is distinguished by numerous fenestrated elastic sheets which course spirally and anastomose to form complex nets. The elastic layer at the junction of the media with the adventitia does not differ from the elastic tissue found throughout the media; hence it is not as clearly demarcated as the external elastic lamina of medium-sized arteries. The narrow spaces between the lamellae are permeated by a finer elastic network, in the meshes of which the muscle fibers are contained. The muscle tissue is greatly reduced in amount, and its fibers are short, flat cells of irregular out-

line. They unite to form branching bands which, like the elastic lamellae, pursue a spiral course. The muscle fibers are surrounded and supported by a small amount of collagenous and reticular fibers.

The *adventitia* is a thin coat consisting of connective tissue composed mostly of collagenous fibers arranged in longitudinal spirals. It contains relatively few elastic fibers. A few longitudinally arranged smooth muscle fibers are occasionally found in the adventitia of some of the large arteries. A few ganglion cells are also occasionally present.

Because the blood is propelled through the blood vessels by the rhythmic contractions of the heart, the rate of flow is not uniform. When the heart contracts and forces blood into the aorta, the walls of the elastic arteries stretch and a part of the force of the beat is converted into potential energy in the form of increased elastic tension. During diastole of the ventricles, the potential energy of the expanded arterial walls is transformed into kinetic energy,

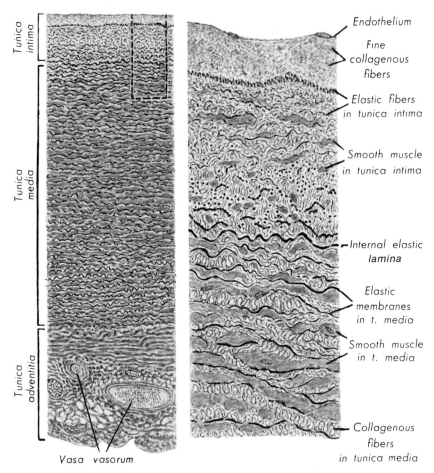

Fig. 12-12. Cross section through ascending aorta, human, age 23 years. Low power view at *left* shows layers of tissue present in total thickness of vessel. Region outlined by *broken line* is enlarged in the figure at the *right* to show structure of tunica intima and a portion of the adjacent media. Weigert's elastic tissue and Van Gieson's stains to differentiate elastic fibers, collagenous fibers, and smooth muscle. Left, ×60; right, ×285.

which keeps the blood moving forward. Thus, the elasticity of the large arteries makes the blood flow less irregularly than it would if the vessels were rigid tubes. The most marked irregularity is found at the beginning of the arterial system; the flow becomes more uniform in the terminal parts of the arterial system.

Special Forms of Arteries. There are certain arteries which exhibit pronounced structural peculiarities. The *cerebral* and *dural* arteries, which are protected from external mechanical forces, are thin-walled for their caliber. They have a well developed internal elastic lamina but almost no elastic fibers in the media. The adventitia is poorly developed and consists mainly of collagenous fiber bundles.

The arteries of the *lung* have thin walls, owing to a reduction of both muscle and elastic tissue. This is probably associated with the lower blood pressure in the pulmonary circulation.

In the *penile* and *pudic* arteries, a hyperplasia of the intima and media manifests itself after puberty, whereas the adventitia remains relatively thin. The intima especially becomes greatly thickened and contains many longitudinal muscle fibers in its outer layer.

The *umbilical* arteries have a media composed of two muscle layers, an inner longitudinal and an outer circular. The internal elastic lamina is indistinct and missing in some places. A true adventitia is lacking in the segment within the umbilical cord and is poorly developed in the intraabdominal segment.

Aging of the Arteries. The arteries undergo age changes which differ in type and degree in different vessels of the same individual. The elastic arteries, especially the aorta, show more changes than do the muscular arteries of the extremities such as the femoral or brachial. Particularly pronounced and early changes occur in the arteries of the brain and heart.

In a 4-month-old human fetus, the aorta has a tunica intima composed only of endothelium and one elastic lamina. By the end of fetal life, the internal elastic lamina has become thicker, and after birth it splits into two or more layers. Additional elastic and collagenous fibers develop between the endothelium and internal elastic lamina, and the elastic layers of the media also increase in number. The layers of the aorta are not completely differentiated until about 25 years of age. It is difficult to separate some of the final stages of differentiation from regressive changes resulting from use. In fact, some authors think that arteriosclerosis may be a physiological rather than a pathological process. In the aging or wearing out process, the tunica intima becomes thicker, the elastic layers of the media change chemically and become less elastic, and fat gradually accumulates between the elastic and collagenous fibers.

The anterior descending branch of the left coronary artery furnishes another interesting example of age changes. In this vessel, the internal elastic lamina is already split at the time of birth, definite hyperplasia of the elastic tissue occurs during the first decade, and calcification of the media begins in the third decade. It is interesting to note that similar changes in another branch of the coronary arteries—the posterior descending branch of the right coronary—do not occur until considerably later. The calcification of the media is one of the main changes in the arteries of muscular type.

The Carotid and Aortic Bodies. These structures were once included with the endocrine system because their cells were erroneously thought to resemble those of the paraganglia and adrenal medulla. They have been described subsequently as chemoreceptors because their secretory activity changes in response to changes in O_2 and CO_2 in the blood.

The *carotid bodies* are small, paired organs located near or in the bifurcation of each common carotid artery. They have an abundant vascular supply and contain numerous sinusoidal capillaries. The *glomus cells* (principal cells of the globular shaped organs) show no particularly distinguishing characteristics in the usual hematoxylin and eosin-stained sections, but they have cytoplasmic granules which stain well with neutral red and with other basic dyes. Two main types of cells can be identified in electron micrographs. The *Type I glomus cell* is the most numerous. It is relatively large and has a rounded nucleus and numerous membrane-bounded dense-cored granules that are relatively small. The *Type II glomus cell* is less numerous and has an oval-shaped nucleus with rather densely staining heterochromatin and few or no cytoplasmic granules.

The Type I cells are generally described as secretory units, with Type II cells serving in a supporting role. However, there have been numerous questions about the manner in which the Type I cells work. For example, because the Type I cells lose their ability to respond to changes in O_2 tension and degenerate after the carotid body branch of the 9th cranial nerve is cut, it is evident that they are supplied with efferent nerve endings rather than solely with afferents as once believed. Furthermore, electron micrographs show that the nerve endings on the Type I cells have the cytological characteristics of efferents. Recent electron microscope studies explain some of these supposed contradictions by showing that the nerve fibers of the Type I cells have synapses of both afferent and efferent types. The nerve endings are cup-shaped and fit closely around the basal end of the cell. Whether the afferent or efferent synaptic endings predominate in function depends on the proportion of O_2 and CO_2 in the blood. When the blood vessels of the medullary region of the brain which function in respiratory control are carrying blood with a normal level of O_2 (normoxia), the glomus cells secrete dopamine at a high level. Under these conditions, the afferent synapses discharge spontaneously, i.e., they arc endogenously active, and their rate of discharge is controlled by an inhibitory feedback mechanism. When the O_2 tension of the blood is low (hypoxia), there is a decrease in the inhibitory feedback mechanism and also a stimulus of the efferent synapses which release a neurotransmitter, perhaps ACH.

The *aortic bodies* have not been studied as extensively as the carotid bodies, but apparently they function in the same manner, i.e., as *sensors* for responding to changes in oxygen tension in the blood. In the rabbit, where the structure and innervation of these bodies has been studied in some detail, the right aortic body is in the angle formed by the subclavian and common carotid, whereas the left aortic body is closely applied to the roof of the arch of the aorta. The aortic bodies are innervated by a branch of the 10th cranial nerve.

The Carotid Sinus. This sinus is an enlargement at the bifurcation of each common carotid. In this region, the media of the wall of the artery is relatively thin and the adventitial layer has a rich supply of specialized sensory nerve endings derived from the carotid sinus branch of the glossopharyngeal nerve. The nerves have reticulated swollen endings in contact with the cells of the adventitial layer and appear as terminal menisci. They are stimulated by distention of the vessel wall (by an increase in blood pressure), and they bring about reflex dilation of splanchnic vessels, slowing of the heart, and a fall in systemic blood pressure.

Veins

The caliber of veins is as a rule larger than that of arteries, but their walls are much thinner because of a great reduction of the muscular and elastic elements. The collagenous connective tissue, on the other hand, is present in much larger amounts and constitutes the bulk of the wall. The relatively sparse circular muscle of the media is more loosely arranged and separated into layers by abundant collagenous fibers. The internal elastic lamina is not a compact fenestrated layer but rather consists of a network of elastic fibers which becomes distinct only in the larger veins. The three coats—intima, media, and adventitia—are present, but their boundaries are often indistinct. The entire wall is flabbier and more loosely organized than in arteries, and it tends to collapse when not filled with blood.

A histological classification of veins is difficult, as their structure varies extensively. The variations are not always related to the size of the vessels, but rather depend on local mechanical conditions. A description of the venous wall can therefore enumerate only the most general features.

Small Veins. The transition from capillary to vein is a very gradual one, the connective tissue elements appearing first and the smooth muscle cells somewhat later. The smallest veins (*venules*) are endothelial tubes surrounded by an outer sheath of collagenous fibrils with a few fibroblasts (Fig. 12-8). These vessels are highly permeable and are important sites of exchange between blood and tissue fluids. Occluding junctions are poorly developed between their endothelial cells. Postcapillary venules have a special morphology and functional significance in many of the lymphatic tissues (see Chapter 13).

Isolated, circularly disposed muscle fibers make their appearance in vessels of 40 to 50 μm, although the presence of muscle fibers is variable and is not always dependent on caliber. In venules of 0.2 to 0.3 mm, the circular muscle fibers form a continuous layer and the adventitia is a relatively thick coat of longitudinally disposed collagenous fibers and a few scattered elastic fibrils.

Medium-Sized Veins. This category includes most of the veins of gross anatomy, with the exception of the main venous trunks (large veins) of the thoracic and abdominal cavities.

The *intima* is a thin layer (Fig. 12-10) consisting of: (1) an endothelial lining and (2) a delicate subendothelial zone of thin bundles of collagenous fibers interspersed with a few elastic fibers which form an internal elastic lamina in the larger vessels of this category.

The *media* is considerably thinner than that of a corresponding medium-sized artery and consists chiefly of circularly arranged smooth muscle fibers interspersed with collagenous fibers and a few elastic fibers. The latter are often arranged longitudinally and are particularly distinct in the outer portion of the media when the tissue is appropriately stained for elastic tissue (Fig. 12-10). The media is thickest in the veins of the lower extremity and thin in the veins of the head and abdomen.

The *adventitia* is well developed and forms the bulk of the wall. It consists of collagenous and elastic tissue and often contains a few bundles of longitudinal muscle fibers.

Large Veins. In the large venous trunks of the thoracic and abdominal cavities the tunica media is relatively thin and poorly defined, whereas the adventitia is relatively thick. The media contains numerous collagenous fibers, a few elastic fibers, and scattered smooth muscle fibers that tend to be circularly arranged. The adventitia contains numerous bundles of longitudinally oriented smooth muscle fibers intermingled with irregularly distributed collagenous and elastic fibers (Fig. 12-13). Unusually stout bundles of longitudinally oriented muscle fibers are found in the portal vein and heptic portion of the inferior vena cava. The category of large veins includes the superior and inferior venae cavae, the innominates, the internal jugulars, and the portal, splenic, azygos, superior mesenteric, renal, adrenal, and external iliac veins.

Special Features of Certain Veins. Very little or no muscle whatever is found in the following veins: the subpapillary veins ("giant capillaries") of the skin and nail bed, the trabecular veins of the spleen, the dural sinuses, most pial and cerebral veins, the veins of the retina and of the bones, and the deeper veins of the maternal placenta.

Especially rich in muscle are the veins

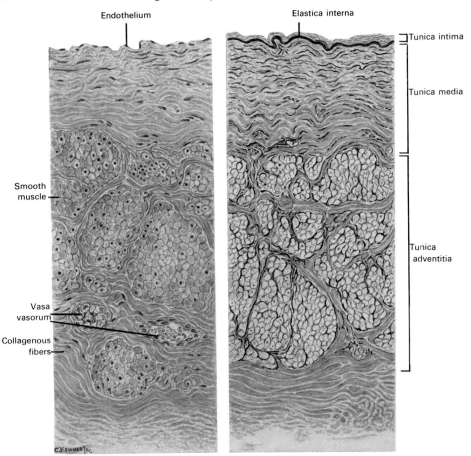

Fig. 12-13. Two cross sections of the same internal jugular vein; *left*, stained with hematoxylin-eosin; *right*, stained with resorcin-fuchsin and picro-fuchsin to differentiate elastic fibers, collagenous fibers, and smooth muscle. ×180.

of the *gravid uterus,* which contain muscle fibers in all three coats. The *umbilical* vein has an inner longitudinal and outer circular muscle layer. The latter is occasionally interspersed with longitudinally oriented muscle fibers.

Longitudinal smooth muscle fibers are found in the intima of the saphenous, popliteal, femoral, basilic, cephalic, median, internal jugular, umbilical, and some mesenteric veins, and in the veins of the gravid uterus.

Near their entrance into the heart, the adventitia of the venae cavae and pulmonary veins is invested with a layer of cardiac muscle, the fibers coursing spirally or circularly around the tube.

Valves. Veins over 2 mm in diameter are provided at intervals with valves (Figs. 12-14 and 12-15). These are semilunar flaps or pockets which project into the lumen, their free margin being directed toward the heart. As the blood flows toward the heart, it flattens the flaps against the wall and thus passes without obstruction toward the heart, but if it starts to flow in the reverse direction, the valves float up, approach each other, and occlude the cavity.

The valves are derived from the intima and consist of connective tissue covered by a layer of endothelium. Beneath the endothelium of the surface of the valve directed against the blood current is a rich network of elastic fibers continuous with the elastic tissue of the intima. The connective tissue of the side facing the wall of the vein is entirely free from or contains but few elastic fibers. Adjacent to the valve, on the side toward the heart, the wall of the vein is usually distended and thin; this region is called the *sinus of the valve.* The smooth muscle of the vein at the base of the valve and along the sinus region runs mostly in a longitudinal or spiral direction. Valves are especially numerous and strong in the larger veins of the lower extremities. They are absent from the veins of the brain and spinal cord and their meninges as well as from the umbilical vein, most of the visceral veins, with the exception of some branches of the portal, and the superior and inferior venae cavae and their branches.

Portal Vessels

In most parts of the body, arteries are connected with veins via capillary plexuses. Modifications of this pattern occur in some locations in adaptation to special functions. When capillaries lead to vessels which in turn supply a second set of capillaries (or sinusoids) before returning the blood to the

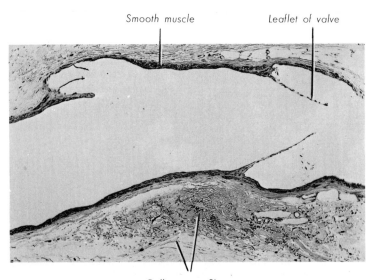

Smooth muscle   Leaflet of valve

Collagenous fibers

Fig. 12-14. Longitudinal section of a vein from human subcutaneous tissue showing valves. The valve at *upper left* is in a small tributary which curves out of the plane of the section. A part of the lower leaflet of the valve at *right* is enlarged in Figure 12-15. Photomicrograph. ×84.

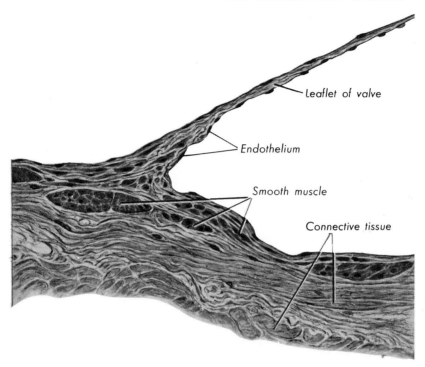

Fig. 12-15. Higher magnification of a part of the valve of the vein shown in Figure 12-14. ×447.

systemic veins, the arrangement of vessels is known as a *portal system.* The liver is an example of a *venous portal system,* with a set of capillaries between veins. In this instance, the portal vein receives blood by its tributaries from the capillaries of most of the abdominal viscera and empties into the hepatic sinusoids that lead to the hepatic veins. The anterior pituitary gland is another example of a venous portal system. Capillaries from the infundibulum drain into veins which supply the sinusoidal capillaries of the anterior lobe.

The kidney glomerulus is an example of an *arterial portal system,* with a capillary plexus between arteries. In this case, afferent glomerular arterioles supply glomerular capillaries which drain into efferent glomerular arterioles and thence to a capillary plexus around the uriniferous tubules.

Arteriovenous Anastomoses

In addition to the capillary and sinusoidal connections of vessels already described, arteries sometimes empty directly into veins—*arteriovenus anastomoses.* Such connections may be found in pathological conditions resulting from injury, in vascular neoplasms, and in developmental anomalies. They also occur normally in certain parts of the body. They are especially numerous in the sole of the foot, in the palm of the hand, in the skin of the terminal phalanges, and in the nail bed. The arteriovenous anastomoses are usually surrounded by a connective tissue sheath, and the arterioles generally follow a convoluted course, forming a structure known as a *glomus* (chapter 14, Fig. 14-17). The smooth muscle fibers are modified in shape and structure and are epithelioid in appearance.

When the arteriovenous anastomoses are open, they shunt a considerable amount of blood directly into the veins and decrease the flow through adjacent arterioles leading to the capillary bed, but in the normal behavior of the peripheral vessels they are contracted a large part of the time.

Blood Vessels, Lymphatics, and Nerves of the Blood Vessels

Vasa Vasorum. Arteries and veins with a diameter over 1 mm are supplied with small nutrient blood vessels, the *vasa vasorum.* These vessels branch and form capillary networks within the adventitia.

Branches also continue into the deepest layers of the media of the veins, whereas they penetrate only to the periphery of the media in arteries. The exchange of metabolites between the cells of the tunica media of arteries and the plasma of blood vessels is by diffusion through the interstitial material of the media. This exchange can be made with the blood within the capillaries of the tunica adventitia and also with the blood within the lumen of the artery itself.

Lymphatics. Lymphatics have been found in the adventitia of many of the larger arteries and veins. Extensive *perivascular lymph spaces* surround the thin-walled blood vessels of the pia-arachnoid of the brain and spinal cord.

Nerves. The walls of blood vessels have a rich nerve supply. The nerve fibers are mainly unmyelinated axons from sympathetic ganglia and are known as vasomotor nerves because they control the caliber of the blood vessel. The fibers form a plexus in the adventitia and terminate chiefly within the peripheral portion of the media, where they have delicate knoblike endings associated with the muscle fibers. Neurotransmitter substances released at the nerve endings may reach the more deeply situated muscle cells by diffusion through the intercellular material. The gap junctions between the muscle fibers may also transmit responses from the outer layers of muscle cells to those situated closer to the lumen.

Besides the vasomoter nerves, the blood vessels receive myelinated sensory nerve fibers which are the peripheral arms of spinal or cranial ganglion cells. The larger fibers run in the connective tissue surrounding the blood vessel. They enter the adventitia, divide repeatedly, lose their myelin sheaths, and terminate in free sensory endings.

The Heart

The heart is a pump for propelling the blood through the blood vessels. It is composed of four chambers in the following sequence in relation to blood flow: (1) the *right atrium* receives venous blood from the superior and inferior venae cavae and from the coronary sinus; (2) the *right ven-* *tricle* receives blood from the right atrium through the right atrioventricular (AV) orifice, which is guarded by the tricuspid valve, and it pumps blood into the pulmonary artery; (3) the *left atrium* receives blood from the pulmonary veins and opens into the left ventricle via the left AV orifice guarded by the bicuspid (mitral) valve (Fig. 12-16); and (4) the *left ventricle* pumps blood into the aorta.

Although the different chambers of the heart vary to some extent in their microscopic structure, the arrangement of tissues in each conforms to a general plan. The wall of each chamber consists of three layers: an inner layer or *endocardium,* a middle layer or *myocardium,* and an outer layer or *epicardium.* The myocardium forms the main mass of the heart.

Endocardium. The endocardium is a glistening layer covering the inner surface of the atria and ventricles. It is thick in the atria, especially in the left atrium, and thin in the ventricles; this explains the whiter color of the inside of the atria as contrasted with the red appearance of the inside of the ventricles, where the color of the cardiac muscle shows readily through the thin endocardium. At the arterial and venous orifices, the endocardium becomes continuous with the intima of the vessels with which it is comparable in structure. It is lined by an endothelium of irregularly shaped, polygonal cells with oval or round nuclei. Beneath the endothelium is a thin layer of fine collagenous fibrils and, outside of this, a stouter layer containing abundant elastic tissue and varying numbers of smooth muscle cells (Fig. 12-17). In most parts of the heart, the deepest layer of the endocardium is composed of loose connective tissue which binds the endocardium proper to the myocardium. This layer, often referred to as subendocardium, coutains collagenous fibers, elastic fibers, and blood vessels. In the ventricles, it also contains some of the specialized muscle fibers of the impulse-conducting system. This layer is absent from the papillary muscles and chordae tendinae.

Myocardium. The myocardium consists of a special form of striated muscle tissue already described as cardiac muscle (chapter 8). Its thickness varies in different parts

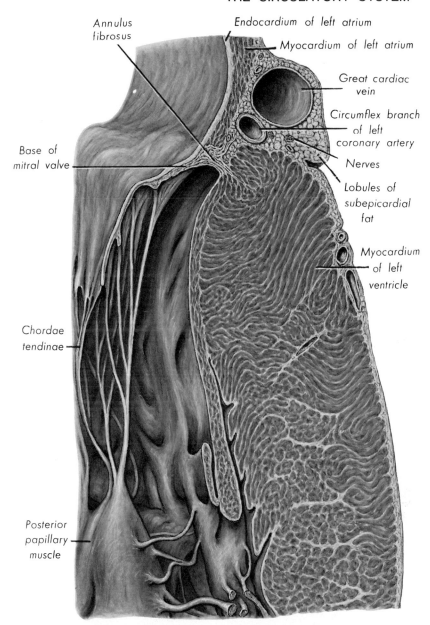

Fig. 12-16. Low power three-dimensional view of the zone of junction of the left atrium with the left ventricle in the human heart. The region illustrated is from the posterior part of the heart and shows the posterior papillary muscle and the posterior cusp of the bicuspid (mitral) valve. ×3.5.

of the heart; it is thinnest in the atria and thickest in the left ventricle. The atrial muscle tends to be arranged in bundles in a sort of latticework with spaces where the connective tissue of the endocardium joins with that of the epicardium. The muscle bundles of the outer part of the atrial wall are oriented chiefly in a transverse or oblique direction and continue over both atria. The bundles in the deeper portions of the atrial wall are more independent for each atrium and are oriented approximately at right angles to the bundles of the outer layer. The innermost bundles stand out as ridges (pectinate muscles) in the auricular portions of the atria.

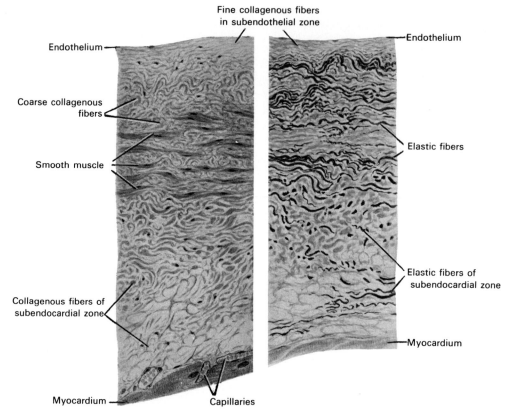

Fig. 12-17. Cross sections through the endocardium of the left atrium of an adult. Section on the *left* is stained with hematoxylin and eosin; the one on the *right* is stained for elastic fibers. ×230.

The disposition of the muscle tissue of the ventricles is much more complicated. It is usually described as composed of several layers, the fibers of which run in different directions. The arrangement of these fiber layers can be readily determined by dissecting hearts in which the connective tissue has been broken down by maceration. The muscle of the ventricles consists mainly of two sets of fibers, a *superficial* set and a *deep* set. These run at approximately right angles to each other. Both sets of fibers take their origin from fibrous connective tissue of the AV rings. The superficial fibers follow a spiral course from the base of the ventricles to the apex of the heart, where they turn inward to terminate in the papillary muscles. The deeper layers follow a circular course on each ventricle, with some of the fibers making an S-shaped pattern as they pass from one ventricle to the other by way of the interventricular septum.

The cardiac muscle of the atria is separated from that of the ventricles by strong fibrous rings, the *annuli fibrosi,* which surround the AV orifices. The fibrous rings are composed mainly of dense bundles of collagenous fibers. They also contain some elastic fibers, fibroblasts, and fat cells which become continuous with the accumulation of adipose tissue in the region of the coronary sulcus (Fig. 12-16).

The fibrous rings show structural variations in different persons and at different ages. They exhibit more marked variations in different species, e.g., they contain hyaline cartilage in sheep and bone in the ox.

The *annuli fibrosi of the atrioventricular orifices* form a part of a dense connective tissue supporting structure known as the *cardiac skeleton.* Other parts of this skeleton are: the *annuli fibrosi at the arterial foramina,* the *trigona fibrosa,* and the *septum membranaceum.*

Epicardium. The epicardium is the visceral layer of the pericardium. It is lined by a single layer of mesothelial cells, which may be flat or cuboidal, depending on the contraction state of the heart. Below the mesothelium is a layer of connective tissue containing a considerable number of elastic fibers in its deeper portion. At the venous and arterial openings, the connective tissue fibers pass over into the adventitia of the blood vessels. The deep layer of the epicardium contains blood vessels, nerves, and varying amounts of fat; it is often described as a subepicardium although it is a part of the epicardium. Fat is especially abundant in the subepicardial tissue of the atria and is particularly prominent near the AV junction (Fig. 12-16).

Valves of the Heart. The atrioventricular valves (tricuspid and mitral) are attached at their bases to the annuli fibrosi (Figs. 12-16 and 12-18). They consist of folds of endocardium covering a central plate of dense bundles of collagenous fibers which are continuous with the fibrous tissue of the annuli fibrosi and chordae tendinae. The endocardium is thicker on the atrial than on the ventricular side and contains more elastic tissue. Scattered bundles of smooth muscle extend into the endocardial layer on the atrial sides of the valve (Fig. 12-18). There are normally no blood capillaries beyond the region penetrated by the smooth muscles.

The semilunar valves of the pulmonary artery and aorta resemble the AV valves in their microscopic structure, but they are much thinner and contain no smooth muscle fibers. They also lack blood and lymphatic capillaries.

Impulse-Conducting System. Besides its ordinary musculature which furnishes the energy for the movement of the blood, the heart possesses a system of special muscle fibers whose function is to regulate the proper succession of contractions of atria and ventricles. It is known as the impulse-conducting system. A part of the system extending from the right atrium into the

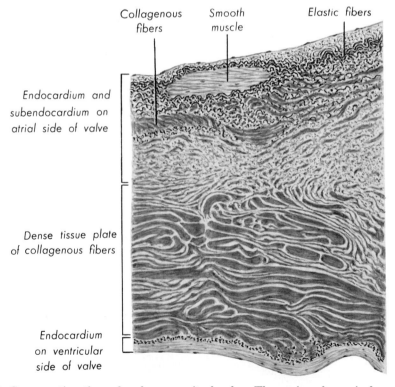

Collagenous fibers   Smooth muscle   Elastic fibers

Endocardium and subendocardium on atrial side of valve

Dense tissue plate of collagenous fibers

Endocardium on ventricular side of valve

Fig. 12-18. Cross section through a human mitral valve. The region shown is from the base of the valve, with the *right* side of the illustration facing the AV junction and annulus fibrosus. (Compare with Fig. 12-16 for orientation.) Weigert's elastic tissue and Van Gieson's stains to differentiate elastic fibers, collagenous fibers, and smooth muscle. ×110.

ventricles may be easily demonstrated by gross dissection and is known as the *atrio-ventricular bundle* or *bundle of His*. This bundle has its origin in the *atrioventricular node* which is found in the subendocardium of the median wall of the right atrium close to the termination of the coronary sinus (Fig. 12-19). From the node, a common bundle or stem, the *crus commune,* is continued into the membranous septum of the ventricles, where it divides into two trunks which go, respectively, to the left and right ventricles. Small accessory bundles have also been described. Each trunk of the main bundle sends branches to the papillary muscles of its respective ventricle and divides to form an extensive network in the subendocardial tissue of each ventricle. Branches from the subendocardial plexus continue into the myocardium, where they continue to subdivide and eventually become continuous with the regular cardiac muscle fibers.

The fibers that form the AV bundle and its branches are modified muscle fibers generally known as Purkinje fibers. Although the differences between these fibers and ordinary cardiac muscle fibers are less pronounced in humans than in ungulates, they are usually sufficient for identification in routinely prepared slides (Fig. 12-20). In comparison with ordinary cardiac fibers, the distinguishing characteristics of Purkinje fibers are: their myofibrils are reduced in number and usually limited to the periphery of the fiber; they contain relatively more sarcoplasm; their nuclei are more rounded and more often in groups of two or more; they usually have a larger diameter, particularly in the peripheral branches of the system; they apparently lack the transverse tubules of cardiac muscle; they give a positive reaction for acetylcholinesterase; and they generally have more glycogen. The myofibrils resemble those of ordinary fibers in that they are cross-striated. Electron micrographs show that the Purkinje fibers, like ordinary cardiac muscle fibers, are separate cells and that the intercalated discs seen under the light microscope are electron-dense areas along the membranes of cell junctions. The Purkinje fibers ultimately lose their specific characteristics and terminate by coming into contact with ordinary cardiac fibers (Fig. 12-21).

The AV node is composed of a group of irregularly arranged, branching fibers (*nodal fibers*) which have a smaller diameter and fewer myofibrils than ordinary cardiac muscle fibers (Fig. 12-22). On the side of the AV node adjacent to the AV fibrous ring, the nodal fibers become continuous with Purkinje fibers of the AV bundle; on the opposite side of the node, they are continuous with cardiac muscle fibers of the atrium. The junctions of the AV nodal fibers and Purkinje fibers occur at different

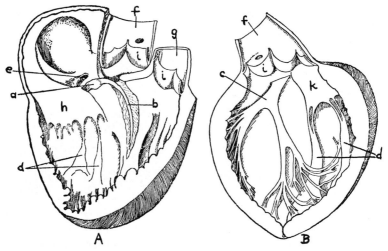

Fig. 12-19. AV bundle of human heart. *A*, view of right heart; *B*, view of left heart. *a*, AV node; *b*, right trunk of bundle; *c*, left trunk of bundle; *d*, papillary muscles; *e*, coronary sinus; *f*, aorta; *g*, pulmonary artery; *h*, flap of tricuspid valve; *i*, semilunar valve; *k*, flap of mitral valve. (After Tandler.)

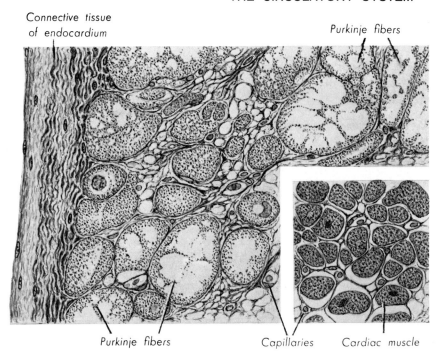

Connective tissue of endocardium

Purkinje fibers

Purkinje fibers   Capillaries   Cardiac muscle

Fig. 12-20. Purkinje fibers from the subendocardial region of a human moderator band cut transversely. The cardiac muscle illustrated in the *inset* is taken from the same section as the Purkinje fibers but is located at a greater distance beneath the endocardium. The magnification of the two figures is the same, ×500. (Redrawn from preparations of Truex and Copenhaver.)

levels ranging from those within the node itself (Fig. 12-22), to others within the AV bundle. In the latter instance, the nodal fibers are aligned longitudinally like the Purkinje fibers, but the two types are usually distinguishable by their morphology.

Another division of the specialized system, the *sinoatrial* (SA) *node* is found in the deep epicardium at the junction of the superior vena cava and right atrium in the region of the terminal sulcus. (Fig. 12-23). This node is composed of slender, fusiform fibers which have the general structure of the fibers of the AV node. A plexus of fibers extends from the SA node into the myocardium of the right atrium.

It is well established that the stimuli for cardiac contraction are normally initiated in the SA node. Because some of the fibers of this node come into close association with the typical cardiac muscle fibers and because the latter, as already described, are arranged as a meshwork of contiguous cells, the impulse initiated in the SA node may spread as a contraction wave over the typical cardiac fibers of both atria and then into the special fibers of the AV node. On the other hand, electrophysiological studies of canine and rabbit hearts indicate that the impulse initiated in the SA node is transmitted by special pathways to the AV node. The preferential atrial conduction pathways described from physiological and pharmacological studies are located chiefly in regions which were at the junctions of the sinus venosus and atrium in the embryonic heart. They are also closely related with pathways of nerve fibers. Many of the muscle fibers of the preferential pathways have cytological characteristics that are intermediate between those of nodal fibers and typical myocardial fibers. Results of microscopic studies to determine whether the fibers of the atrial conduction pathways differ cytologically from the ordinary atrial fibers remain controversial.

After the conduction impulse reaches the AV node, it is conducted at a relatively slow rate through the node to reach the AV bundle of His, where it travels rapidly to the ventricles. If this bundle is injured or destroyed, the normal rhythm in the

Cardiac
muscle

Transition of Purkinje fibers
into cardiac muscle

Purkinje
fibers

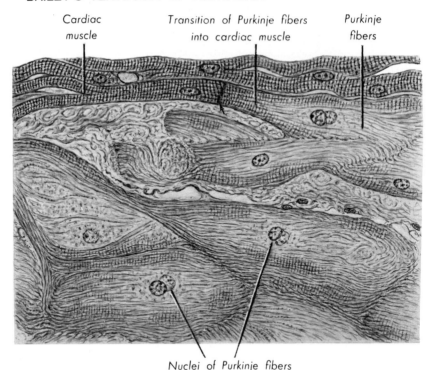

Nuclei of Purkinje fibers

Fig. 12-21. Longitudinal section of a beef moderator band showing transition of Purkinje fibers into cardiac muscle fibers in the myocardial portion of the band. The transition occurs near cell junctions and does not indicate a syncytium of cells. An intercalated disc can be identified in the region indicated by the *arrow*, although the discs are not stained in most parts of this preparation. ×500. (Redrawn from preparation of Truex and Copenhaver.)

succession of atrial and ventricular beats is lost. Branches of the bundle transmit the impulse at a relatively high velocity over both ventricles and terminate with typical cardiac fibers. The branches of the bundle are composed of typical Purkinje fibers with structural characteristics distinctly different from those of typical cardiac fibers.

Blood Vessels. Blood for the nutrition of the heart is supplied through the two coronary arteries. The distribution of the branches of the coronary arteries is quite variable; for example, the SA node of the human heart is supplied entirely by branches from the right coronary artery in about 70% of the cases studied, by the left coronary in a much lower percentage, and by both right and left branches in a few cases. However, regardless of variations in the blood supply for particular regions, the total amount of blood supplied by the left coronary greatly exceeds that supplied by the right coronary, in correlation with the

greater work load and larger muscular mass on the left side.

The venous return is partly by venules that drain into the coronary sinus and partly by *venae cordae minimae* that empty directly into the heart chambers. Numerous vessels of this type, also known as Thebesian veins, open directly into the right atrium. Vessels of similar type also open into the left atrium and into both ventricular cavities. Retrograde flow, that is, flow from the ventricular cavities into the venae cordae, occurs under conditions of altered pressure relationships.

The AV valves apparently have only a few or no vessels in the dense, fibrous central plates. The supply in the subendothelial layers differs for the different leaflets of the valve: it is richer in the aortic cusp of the mitral valve than in others. The supply is also richer in infants than in normal adults.

The bundle of His is, according to some investigators, supplied by special fine

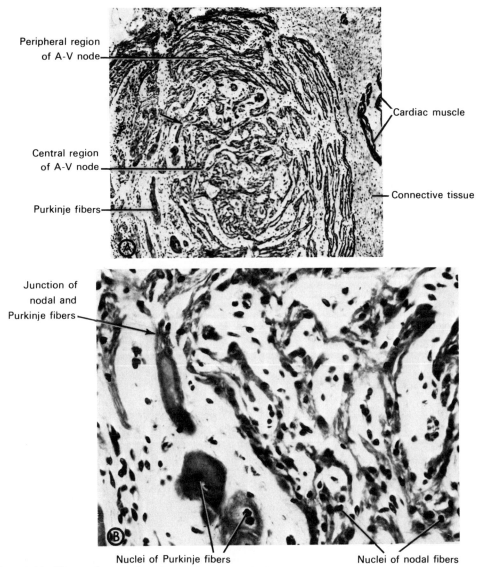

Peripheral region of A-V node

Cardiac muscle

Central region of A-V node

Connective tissue

Purkinje fibers

Junction of nodal and Purkinje fibers

Nuclei of Purkinje fibers   Nuclei of nodal fibers

Fig. 12-22. Photomicrographs of a section through the AV node of a sheep heart. A, low magnification micrograph of an area from the wall of the right atrium medial to the opening of the coronary sinus and just above the origin of the AV bundle. Only a few atrial muscle fibers are seen in this section. The junctions of nodal fibers with atrial fibers occur chiefly in the preceding sections, at a greater distance above the origin of the AV bundle. B, higher magnification micrograph of a portion of the field seen in A. For orientation, note that the *arrows* to the junctions of nodal fibers with Purkinje fibers are directed to the same cells in A and B. The fibers of the AV node are very similar in size and structure to those of the SA node but are arranged in a different pattern. The presence of Purkinje fibers of large diameter in the AV nodal area is characteristic of hearts of ungulates; the special conduction fibers of the human heart do not attain the large diameter typical of ventricular Purkinje fibers until the branches of the AV system are reached. Hematoxylin and eosin. A, ×63; B, ×116. (From preparations of Copenhaver and Truex: Anat. Rec. 114, 1952.)

branches of the coronary arteries. The capillary net is less dense than in the ordinary musculature of the heart.

Lymphatics. The heart is supplied with

lymph channels which form networks in the endocardial, myocardial, and subepicardial layers.

Nerves. The heart receives nerve fibers

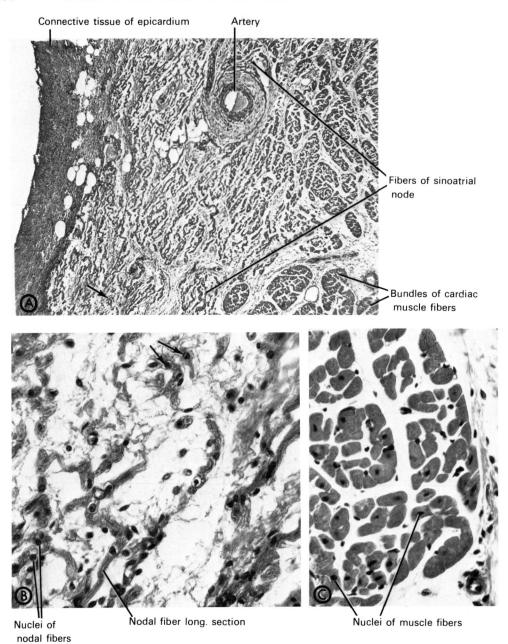

Fig. 12-23. Photomicrographs of a section through the SA node and adjacent cardiac muscle of a sheep heart. *A*, low magnification micrograph of an area from the wall of the right atrium near the junction of the atrium and the superior vena cava. *B*, a portion of *A* at higher magnification. For orientation, note that the *arrows* in *B* point to the same nodal cells that are indicated by the *arrow* in *A*. *C*, section of typical atrial myocardial fibers at the same magnification as that of the nodal fibers in *B*. Note that the diameter of the nodal fibers is less than that of the atrial muscle fibers. The nodal fibers are also interspersed with more loose connective tissue and course in a very irregular pattern. With higher magnification, one would also see that the myofibrils are less numerous and more irregularly arranged within the nodal fibers than they are in the atrial muscle fibers. Hematoxylin and eosin stain. Greater contrast between the fiber types can be obtained by the use of special stains. *A*, ×63; *B* and *C*, ×146. (From preparations of Copenhaver and Truex: Anat. Rec. 114, 1952.)

from the vagus and the sympathetic division of the autonomic system. These fibers form an extensive cardiac plexus at the base of the heart. The vagus and sympathetic fibers have antagonistic functions; the former inhibits and the latter accelerates the action of the heart.

The efferent vagus fibers do not go directly to the cardiac muscle but arborize around parasympathetic ganglion cells scattered in the wall of the heart, chiefly in plexuses in the deep epicardium. These cells are especially numerous in the dorsal wall of the atria, in the coronary sulcus near the larger coronary vessels, and at the base of the aorta and pulmonary artery. The ganglion cells send out delicate, nonmyelinated nerve fibers which branch and end in terminal varicosities on the muscle fibers.

Some of the sensory nerve fibers are derived from the vagus; others have their cell bodies in the spinal ganglia of the first to the fourth thoracic nerves. The fibers of the latter group pass through the white rami, up the sympathetic trunk to the cervical sympathetic ganglia, and thence to the heart by way of the cardiac nerves.

The Lymph Vascular System

Besides the blood vessels, the body contains a collateral system of endothelium-lined channels which collect tissue fluid and return it by a circuitous route to the bloodstream. The fluid in these vessels is called lymph. Unlike the blood, the lymph circulates in one direction only, from the periphery toward the heart. The *lymphatic capillaries* end blindly in the tissues from which the lymph is collected (Fig. 12-24). They, as well as the larger vessels which conduct the lymph to the bloodstream, freely anastomose along their course, gradually fuse to form fewer lymph channels, and are ultimately gathered into two main trunks, the large *thoracic duct* and the smaller *right lymphatic duct*. The thoracic duct empties into the left subclavian vein, and the right lymphatic duct drains into the right subclavian, in each case near the point where the subclavian joins with its

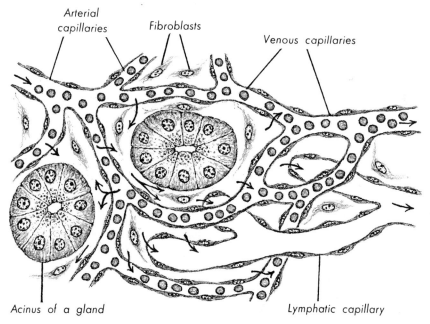

Arterial capillaries   Fibroblasts   Venous capillaries

Acinus of a gland   Lymphatic capillary

Fig. 12-24. Diagram showing the relationship of lymphatic capillaries to blood capillaries and to the tissue fluids around the acini of a gland. Similar relationships exist in most of the organs of the body. *Arrows* indicate the direction of flow of fluid leaving the arterial capillaries, permeating the connective tissue spaces as tissue fluid, and reentering the blood capillaries on the venous side. The lymphatic capillaries supplement the venous capillaries in the drainage of fluid from the tissues to the circulatory system.

respective internal jugular vein. In the pathways of the lymph vessels there are groups of lymph nodes containing lymph sinuses in which the lymph is filtered before reaching the thoracic and lymphatic ducts.

Lymphatic capillaries and vessels occur in most tissues and organs. They have not been demonstrated in the central nervous system, the bone marrow, the intralobular portion of the liver, the coats of the eyeball, the internal ear, and the fetal placenta.

Lymph Capillaries. The lymph capillaries, like those of the blood, are delicate tubes with walls which consist of a single layer of endothelial cells. The tubes are larger, however, and instead of having a uniform diameter, they vary greatly in caliber within short distances. The exceedingly thin cells have a flattened, oval nucleus and an irregular outline which can be demonstrated with silver impregnations. Electron micrographs of lymphatic capillaries show no endothelial pores (fenestrae) but instead display fairly numerous micropinocytotic vesicles. Junctional complexes are rare and gaps readily appear between the cells under altered conditions. The basal lamina is usually absent or, at most, present only in spots. The outer surface of the endothelium is attached to the surrounding connective tissue at intervals by fine filaments that are perpendicular to the course of the capillary; these are known as *anchoring filaments*. They presumably aid in keeping the lumen from closing when the vessel is empty.

The lymph capillaries anastomose to form extensive networks in the spaces between the blood capillaries. In the skin and in the mucous and serous membranes, the lymph capillaries are usually more deeply placed than are the blood capillaries.

Lymph Vessels. The lymph vessels resemble the veins in structure, but their walls are as a rule thinner than those of veins of a corresponding caliber. In the smaller lymph vessels, the endothelium is surrounded by collagenous and elastic fibers and a few smooth muscle cells. In the larger ones, three coats may be distinguished: intima, media, and adventitia. The intima is composed of the endothelial lining, underneath which is a delicate network of elastic fibers disposed longitudinally.

The media consists mainly of circularly disposed smooth muscle fibers and a few longitudinal ones. Between the muscle fibers are relatively few, delicate, elastic fibrils. The adventitia, which is the thickest coat, is composed of longitudinally coursing collagenous fibers, among which are bundles of longitudinal muscle and elastic fibers.

The lymph vessels contain numerous valves which are usually arranged in pairs and whose free margins are always directed centrally, i.e., in the direction of the lymph flow. The valves are infoldings of the intima.

Thoracic Duct. The thoracic duct has a considerable amount of muscle tissue. The *intima* consists of an endothelial lining, a thin intermediate layer of fibroelastic tissue in which are bundles of longitudinal muscle fibers, and an internal elastic lamina composed of a longitudinal network of elastic fibers. The elastic lamina is best developed in the caudal portion of the duct and is much thinner or missing altogether in the cervical portion.

The *media* is the thickest coat and consists of longitudinal and circular muscle bundles, the former predominating. The muscle bundles are separated by abundant connective tissue composed mainly of collagenous fibers. Elastic fibrils are scarce in the inner layer of the media but become more numerous in the outer portion.

The *adventitia* is poorly defined. Near the media is a layer of coarse collagenous fibers, mainly longitudinally disposed and containing considerable elastic tissue and occasional longitudinal muscle fibers. The outer layer is more finely fibrillar and merges with the surrounding connective tissue.

Development of the Circulatory System

Blood Vessels and Heart

The myocardium of the heart develops from bilaterally localized regions of splanchnic mesoderm. The endothelium of the heart and vessels differentiates from mesenchymal cells derived from mesoderm. The heart and the main trunks of its accompanying large vessels (e.g., aorta) develop independently of the peripheral vessels, with which they unite later. While the heart develops within the embryo, the earliest vessels and earliest blood cells develop from extraembryonic mesenchyme. The earliest vessels have the structure of capillaries. They appear first near the periphery of the area vasculosa which surrounds the developing embryo. Here groups of cells known as *"blood islands"* differentiate from the rest of the mesenchymal cells, appearing in the chick by the end of the 1st day of incubation. The superficial cells of these islands flattened to form the endothelium; the central cells develop into the primitive blood cells. The channels, which are at first unconnected, anastomose and give rise to a network of channels which are the earliest capillaries. These develop rapidly in the area vasculosa, and some of them increase in size to become arteries and veins, the smooth muscle and connective tissue of their walls being differentiated from the surrounding mesenchyme. This differentiation progresses toward the embryo where the vascular lumina unite with intraembryonic vessels which also have developed from mesenchyme in situ. After a primary system of closed vessels has been established and after the embryonic circulation has been initiated, new vessels develop as outgrowths from preexisting vessels. New vessels arise by a similar method in the adult, e.g., the outgrowth of new vessels into granulation tissue.

The *heart* in the earliest human embryos (2 to 3 mm) consists of an *endothelial tube* surrounded by a layer of splanchnic mesoderm which forms the *myoepicardial mantle*. The two layers are at first separated by a considerable space filled with a gelatinous fluid (cardiac jelly). As development proceeds, the two layers become firmly united, the endothelium now forming the lining of the myoepicardial mantle. The endothelium and its underlying connective tissue form the endocardium. From the myoepicardial mantle are formed both myocardium and epicardium.

Lymphatics

The earliest lymphatic vessels arise by differentiation of mesenchymal cells into endothelium-lined spaces in situ. These spaces secondarily establish connections with venous plexuses, but the only connections which persist are via the thoracic duct on the left and the smaller right thoracic duct. In their development, the lymphatic plexuses arise first in the thoracic and abdominal regions and subsequently grow into the head and extremities.

References

BENNETT, H. S., LUFT, J. H., AND HAMPTON, J. C. Morphological classification of vertebrate blood capillaries. Am. J. Physiol. 196:381–390, 1959.

BRUNS, R. R., AND PALADE, G. E. Studies of blood capillaries. I. General organization of blood capillaries in muscle. J. Cell Biol. 37:244–276, 1968.

CHAMBERS, R., AND ZWEIFACH, B. W. Topography and function of the mesenteric capillary circulation. Am. J. Anat. 75:173–207, 1944.

CLARK, E. R., AND CLARK, E. L. Observations on changes in blood vascular endothelium in the living animal. Am. J. Anat. 57:385–438, 1935.

CLEMENTI, F., AND PALADE, G. E. Intestinal capillaries. I. Permeability to peroxidase and ferritin. J. Cell Biol. 41:33–58, 1969.

COPENHAVER, W. M., AND TRUEX, R. C. Histology of the atrial portion of the cardiac conduction system in man and other mammals. Anat. Rec. 114:601–626, 1952.

DAVIES, F. The conducting system of the vertebrate heart. Br. Heart J. 4:66–76, 1942.

DAVIES, F., AND FRANCIS, E. T. B. The conduction of the impulse for cardiac contraction. J. Anat. 86:302–309, 1952.

FRENCH, J. E., FLOREY, H. W., AND MORRIS, B. The absorption of particles by the lymphatics of the diaphragm. Q. J. Exp. Physiol. 45:88–103, 1960.

HOFFMAN, B. F. Physiology of atrioventricular transmission. Circulation 24:506–517, 1961.

HOFFMAN, B. F. Atrioventricular conduction in mammalian hearts. *In* Comparative Cardiology (Hecht, H. H., and Detwiler, D. K., Conference Chairmen). Ann. N.Y. Acad. Sci. 127:105–112, 1965.

HOGAN, P. M., AND DAVIS, L. D. Evidence for specialized fibers in the canine right atrium. Circ. Res. 23:387–396, 1968.

HOLLINSHEAD, W. H. A cytological study of the carotid body of the cat. Am. J. Anat. 73:185–215, 1943.

JAMES, T. N. Anatomy of the cardiac conduction system in the rabbit. Circ. Res. 20:638–648, 1967.

JAMES, T. N., SHERF, L., AND URTHALER, F. Fine structure of the bundle-branches. Br. Heart J. 36:1–18, 1974.

KARNOVSKY, M. J. The ultrastructural basis of capillary permeability studied with peroxidase as a tracer. J. Cell Biol. 35:213–236, 1967.

LANDIS, E. M. The passage of fluid through the capillary wall. Harvey Lect. 32:70–91, 1937.

LANDIS, E. M., AND PAPPENHEIMER, J. R. Exchange of substances through the capillary walls. *In* Handbook of Physiology (Hamilton, W. F., and Dow, P., editors), sect. 2, vol. 2, pp. 961–1034. American Physiological Society, Washington, D. C., 1963.

LEAKE, L. V., AND BURKE, J. F. Ultrastructural studies on the lymphatic anchoring filaments. J. Cell Biol. 36:129-149, 1968.

MAJNO, G., PALADE, G. E., AND SCHOEFL, G. I. Studies on inflammation. II. The site of action of histamine and serotonin along the vascular tree: a topographic study. J. Biophys. Biochem. Cytol. 11:607-626, 1961.

MAJNO, G., SHEA, S. M., AND LEVENTHAL, M. Endothelial contraction induced by histamine-type mediators. An electron microscopic study. J. Cell Biol. 42:647-672, 1969.

NONIDEZ, J. F. The aortic (depressor) nerve and its associated epithelioid body, the glomus aorticum. Am. J. Anat. 57: 259-301, 1935.

OSBORNE, M. P., AND BUTLER, P. J. New theory for receptor mechanism of carotid body chemoreceptors. Nature 254:701-703, 1975.

PALADE, G. E. Blood capillaries of the heart and other organs. Circulation 24: 368-384, 1961.

PALADE, G. E., AND BRUNS, R. R. Structural modulations of plasmalemmal vesicles. J. Cell Biol. 37:633-649, 1968.

PAPPAS, G. D., AND TENNYSON, V. M. An electron microscope study of the passage of colloidal particles from the blood vessels of the ciliary processes and choroid plexus of the rabbit. J. Cell Biol. 15:227-239, 1962.

PAPPENHEIMER, J. R. Passage of molecules through capillary walls. Physiol. Rev. 33:387-423, 1953.

PHELPS, P. C., AND LUFT, J. H. Electron microscopical study of relaxation and constriction in frog arterioles. Am. J. Anat. 125:399-428, 1969.

RAVIOLA, E., AND KARNOVSKY, M. J. Evidence for a blood-thymus barrier using electron-opaque tracers. J. Exp. Med. 136:466-498, 1972.

REESE, T. S., AND KARNOVSKY, M. J. Fine structural localization of a blood-brain barrier to exogenous peroxidase. J. Cell Biol. 34:207-217, 1967.

RHODIN, J. A. G. The ultrastructure of mammalian arterioles and precapillary sphincters. J. Ultrastruct. Res. 18:181-223, 1967.

RHODIN, J. A. G. Ultrastructure of mammalian venous capillaries, venules, and small collecting veins. J.

Ultrastruct. Res. 25:452-500, 1968.

ROBB, J. S., HISS, F., AND ROBB, R. C. Localization of cardiac infarcts according to component ventricular muscles. Am. Heart J. 10:287-292, 1935.

SIMIONESCU, M., SIMIONESCU, N., AND PALADE, G. E. Segmental differentiation of cell junctions in the vascular endothelium. The microvasculature. J. Cell Biol. 67:863-885, 1975.

SIMIONESCU, N., SIMIONESCU, M., AND PALADE, G. E. Permeability of muscle capillaries to small heme peptides. Evidence for the existence of patent transendothelial channels. J. Cell Biol. 65:586-607, 1975.

SIMIONESCU, N., SIMIONESCU, M., AND PALADE, G. E. Recent studies on vascular endothelium. Ann. N.Y. Acad. Sci. 275:64-75, 1976.

SOMMER, J. R., AND JOHNSON, E. A. Cardiac muscle. A comparative study of Purkinje fibers and ventricular fibers. J. Cell Biol. 36:497-526, 1968.

TRUEX, R. C. Anatomical considerations of the human atrioventricular junction. In Mechanisms and Therapy of Cardiac Arrythmias (Dreifus, L. S., and Likoff, W., editors), pp. 333-340. Grune & Stratton, New York, 1966.

TRUEX, R. C., AND ANGULO, A. W. Comparative study of the arterial and venous system of the ventricular myocardium with special reference to the coronary sinus. Ant. Rec. 113:467-492, 1952.

TRUEX, R. C., AND COPENHAVER, W. M. Histology of the moderator band in man and other mammals, with special reference to the conduction system. Am. J. Anat. 80:173-201, 1947.

WALLS, E. N. Dissection of the atrioventricular node and bundle in the human heart. J. Anat. 79:45-48, 1945.

WEARN, J. T. Morphological and functional alterations of the coronary circulation. Harvey Lect. 35:243-269, 1940.

WILLIAMS, M. C., AND WISSIG, S. L. The permeability of muscle capillaries to horseradish peroxidase. J. Cell Biol. 66:531-555, 1975.

ZIMMERMAN, J., and AND BAILEY, C. P. The surgical significance of the fibrous skeleton of the heart. J. Thorac. Cardiovasc. Surg. 44:701-712, 1962.

CHAPTER 13

Lymphatic Organs

Protection of the body against deleterious effects of invading foreign substances, cells, or microorganisms is a critical function which necessarily involves the activity of many organs and tissues. Components of the so-called "immune system" are spread over most parts of the body, in some regions being definable as discrete organs (lymphatic organs), in other areas spread throughout the connective tissue as lymphatic tissue. Lymphatic tissue is less highly organized and will be considered first.

Lymphatic Tissue

Lymphatic (lymphoid) tissue is not one of the fundamental tissue types of the body. Rather, it is a special variety of reticular connective tissue that is regularly infiltrated with lymphocytes. With the exception of the thymic reticulum, lymphatic tissue seems solely derived from mesenchyme, and its cells and fibers are not separated from other connective tissue by a basal lamina. Regions where the lymphocytes are not closely packed are identified as *loose lymphatic tissue,* in contrast with *dense lymphatic tissue,* in which the lymphocytes are closely aggregated. There are numerous gradations between these two varieties of lymphatic tissue, and there is also gradation between the loose lymphatic tissue and regions where widely scattered lymphocytes infiltrate into the connective tissue.

Regions where closely packed lymphocytes are in spherical aggregations are known as *lymphatic nodules* (lymphatic follicles). After birth, such nodules often have lighter-staining areas known as *germinal centers* (secondary nodules) that are described in more detail under "Lymph Nodes."

Solitary lymphatic nodules are widely scattered in the digestive, respiratory, and urinary tracts. Particularly prominent aggregations of nodules form the Peyer's patches found in the wall of the small intestine on the side opposite to the mesenteric attachment. The aggregations of lymphatic tissue that are identified as separate lymphatic organs include the lymph nodes, tonsils, thymus, and spleen. They are defined by the presence of a dense connective tissue capsule which isolates the enclosed lymphatic tissue from the surrounding tissues. The tonsils are examples of only partially encapsulated aggregations of nodules.

The chief characteristic common to all lymphatic organs is the presence of large numbers of lymphocytes pervading a framework of reticular cells and fibers. The lymph nodes are the only lymphatic organs located in the course of lymphatic vessels; that is, they are the only ones that have both afferent and efferent lymphatic vessels. They are also the only ones that contain lymphatic sinuses, and they are the only structures which filter the lymph. The spleen, thymus, and tonsils resemble most other organs in their relationship to lymphatic vessels. They have efferent lymph vessels draining from them, but they have neither afferent lymphatic vessels nor lymphatic sinuses.

The Lymph Nodes

The lymph nodes are variable in number but are more or less constantly found in certain definite regions of the body such as the mesentery, axilla and groin. They are frequently in groups or in a series, as in the inguinal and axillary regions. They vary in size, ranging from minute bodies to as much as 2.5 cm in length. They are usually oval or bean-shaped, with an indentation, the *hilus,* on one side, where the blood vessels enter and leave the node. The lymphatic vessels leaving the node, the *vasa efferentia,* are also found at the hilus, but the entering vessels, the *vasa afferentia,* are found at various points along the convex surface of the node.

Lymph nodes are covered by a *capsule* of connective tissue which blends with the surrounding connective tissue and holds the organ in position. The capsule consists of rather closely packed bundles of collagenous fibers and scattered elastic fibers. A few smooth muscle fibers can be found in the capsule around the points of entrance and exit of lymphatic vessels. At the hilus, there is a depression where the capsule is thickened and extends deep into the node. At various points over the surface of the

node, the capsule gives off septa or *trabeculae* that extend into the substance of the organ. The trabeculae of connective tissue and the elements of the lymph tissue are arranged differently in the outer or cortical and the inner or medullary regions. However, there are also numerous similarities between the regions, and the structure of the organ can be understood best by considering the cortex and medulla together.

Cortex and Medulla

In the cortex, the trabeculae are more or less perpendicular to the surface, and they partly subdivide this region into compartments which are continuous centrally with the more irregularly arranged anastomosing subdivisions of the medulla (Figs. 13-1 and 13-2). The cortical compartments also communicate laterally with each other through spaces between the trabeculae. The degree of development of the trabeculae and of separation into compartments varies in nodes taken from different parts of the body and in nodes of different animals. In some of the other mammals (e.g., ox), the trabeculae are more highly developed than in man and mark off more distinct compartments.

The lymphocytes are closely packed in the cortical regions of the nodes and often form spherical aggregations, the *cortical nodules* (*primary nodules* or *follicles*), which are continuous centrally with anas-

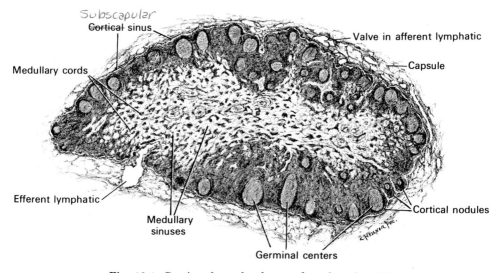

Fig. 13-1. Section through a human lymph node. ×10

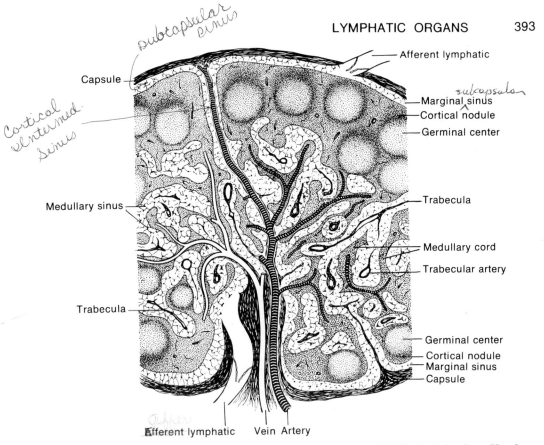

subcapsular sinus (handwritten annotation)

Capsule —

Cortical el internud Sinus (handwritten annotation)

Medullary sinus —

Trabecula —

— Afferent lymphatic

subcapsular (handwritten annotation)
—Marginal sinus
—Cortical nodule
—Germinal center

—Trabecula

—Medullary cord
—Trabecular artery

— Germinal center
— Cortical nodule
— Marginal sinus
— Capsule

after (handwritten annotation)
Efferent lymphatic   Vein Artery

Fig. 13-2. Diagram of a lymph node. (Modified after a drawing by M. Heidenhain, from Heudorfer.)

tomosing cords of lymphatic tissue in the medulla known as *medullary cords.* The dense lymphatic tissue of the cortex is separated from the capsule by a lymphatic channel known as the *marginal sinus (subcapsular sinus).* This sinus is continuous around most of the circumference of the node except where it is interrupted by connective tissue trabeculae. The marginal sinus is continuous with other lymphatic channels, *trabecular sinuses,* which extend centrally between the connective tissue trabeculae and the aggregations of cortical nodules. In the deep cortical region, these latter channels continue as *paracortical (parafollicular) sinuses.* Paracortical sinuses become continuous with the anastomosing *medullary sinuses,* located between the medullary cords of lymphatic tissue and the connective tissue trabeculae (Fig. 13-2). There are generally several afferent lymphatic vessels leading into the marginal sinus along the convex surface of the node opposite the hilus, and usually

only one or two efferent vessels that exit at the hilus.

Although the dense lymphatic tissue of the cortex commonly surrounds the medulla except at the hilus, it varies in thickness in nodes from different locations and also within the same nodes at different times. The nodules are often arranged in a single layer around the periphery, but they may also be found in layers where the cortex is thickened.

The cortical nodules often contain lighter-staining central areas known as *germinal centers* (secondary nodules, *reaction centers*). They were named germinal centers in recognition of the fact that they are more active in lymphocyte proliferation than are other parts of the node. It was also noted many years ago that the germinal centers appear during certain types of inflammation; hence the name reaction center. The framework of the center, like that of other parts of the node, is composed of reticular cells and reticular fibers. The reticular cells of the germinal centers are relatively large and have particularly long protoplasmic processes; hence they are often described as *dendritic cells.* These cells have large, pale-staining nuclei and cytoplasm which is only lightly basophilic. The lymphocytes of the germinal center consist chiefly of the medium-sized and large varieties known as *lymphoblasts;* these range up to 15 μm or more in diameter. The nuclei of these cells contain considerable heterochromatin, which takes a relatively pale stain, thus counteracting the overall effect of the basophilic cytoplasm. The centers also contain a number of macrophages with cytoplasm that is only lightly basophilic. This combination of staining characteristics of the cells accounts for the light appearance of the germinal centers in comparison with the more darkly staining borders of small lymphocytes that surround the centers (Figs. 13-1 and 13-3). The center itself often appears relatively dark on the side facing the medulla and lighter on the side facing the marginal sinus (Fig. 13-4). The darker-staining zone (cap) contains a higher proportion of dividing cells and more closely packed cells.

Germinal centers contain a number of plasma cells in addition to the other cell types described above. It is well established that plasma cells form antibodies and that they differentiate from lymphocytes of the B type (bursa-derived type, chapter 7). It is also known that the lymphocytes of the germinal centers belong to the B type. Although plasma cells are not as numerous in the germinal centers as in the medullary cords (Fig. 13-5), it seems evident that the centers have a major role in the secondary response in antigen-antibody reactions. The centers do not appear until after birth, in response to antigen. They disappear in the absence of antigen and reappear in the same region after subsequent stimulation from antigens. When animals are kept in a germ-free environment from the time of birth, the centers fail to develop. They also remain inactive in animals thymectomized at birth. No

The interrelationships of reticular cells and endothelial cells lining the lymphatic sinuses have been studied extensively. It was once thought that the linings of the sinuses consist chiefly of reticular cells that are more flattened than those which form the framework of the cortical nodules and medullary cords of lymphatic tissue. However, more recent electron microscope studies indicate that the portions of the cortical

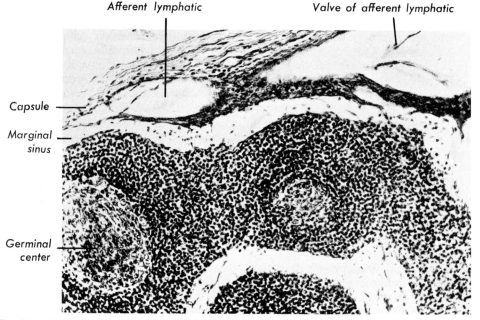

Afferent lymphatic   Valve of afferent lymphatic

Capsule

Marginal sinus

Germinal center

Fig. 13-3. Portion of cortex of human lymph node. Photomicrograph. ×260. (After Petersen.)

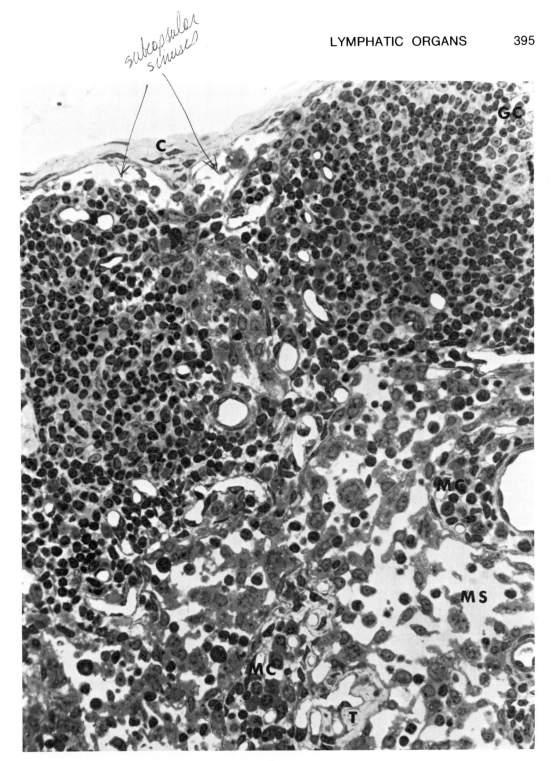

subcapsular sinuses

Fig. 13-4. Light micrograph of a lymph node from monkey showing cortex and medulla. The capsule (*C*) in the *upper left* is underlain by marginal sinus. A germinal center (*GC*) of a cortical nodule is at the *upper right*. Medullary cords (*MC*), medullary sinuses (*MS*), and a trabecula (*T*) appear at the *lower right*. ×400.

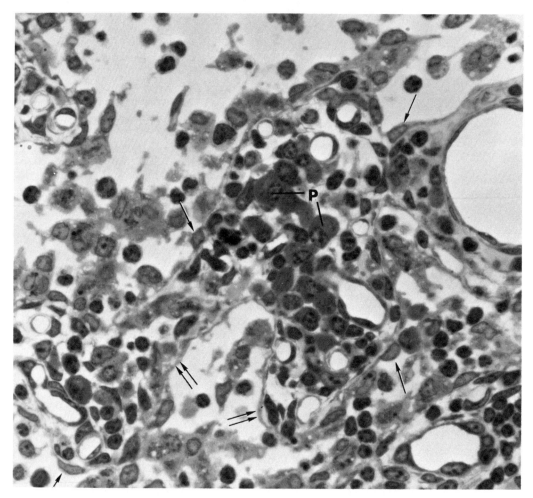

Fig. 13-5. Light micrograph of a section through a medullary cord and medullary sinuses of a lymph node from monkey. Endothelial cells lining the medullary sinuses surrounding the cord. are indicated by the *arrows* (*single arrows* show nuclei and *double arrows* show thin cytoplasmic extensions). *P,* plasma cells. ×640.

and medullary sinuses that abut against the capsule and trabeculae, respectively, are lined by endothelial cells with gaps between them (Fig. 13-6). The walls of the cortical and medullary sinuses which abut, respectively, against cortical nodules and medullary cords (Figs. 13-5 and 13-6) are also lined by endothelial cells with intercellular gaps, but these endothelial cells are more frequently associated with reticular cells and macrophages than are the cells on the capsular and trabecular sides of the sinuses.

The reticular cells which are associated with the endothelial cells of the sinus, as well as those which form a framework across the lymphatic cords and sinuses, are intimately associated with reticular (argyrophilic) fibers, and the protoplasmic processes of these cells form a thin, but complete, covering of the fibers. Recent electron microscope studies using transfused labeled cells indicate that the reticular cells are generally not very phagocytic, contrary to earlier views. Most of the macrophages seen in lymph nodes are apparently derived from mononuclear cells (promonocytes) which are closely associated with the reticular cells of the framework and with the endothelial cells lining the sinuses. Although animals given repeated injections of colloidal dyes (e.g., trypan blue) for a

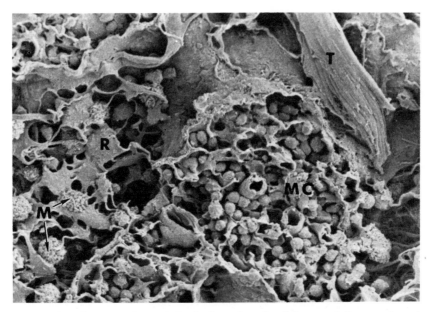

Fig. 13-6. Scanning electron micrograph of a lymph node of dog, medullary region. A trabecular sinus opens into a medullary sinus at the *upper center*. Note the relatively continuous nature of the lining of the sinuses. *MC,* medullary cord; *M,* macrophages; *R,* reticular cell; *T,* trabecula. Courtesy of Masayuki Miyoshi. ×750.

relatively long period often show a few small vacuoles of ingested material in the reticular cells of their lymph nodes, the dye is not segregated and concentrated into large vacuoles, as it is in macrophages. The reticular cells and macrophages of lymph nodes differ from each other in their reaction to colloidal dyes in a manner rather similar to the difference exhibited by fibroblasts and macrophages in connective tissue (chapter 5, Fig. 5-2, *A* and *B*).

The lymphocytes of the lymph node consist of large, medium-sized, and small varieties. The largest cells, known as lymphoblasts, range up to 20 μm in diameter. They have a large, pale-staining nucleus with one or two prominent nucleoli and a very basophilic cytoplasm; this same cell type is present in other lymphatic organs (e.g., germinal centers of the spleen). Large lymphocytes are numerous in the germinal centers, but some may be found throughout the node.

The small lymphocytes are the most numerous variety in the node. Although they seldom divide, they may be readily stimulated to enlarge into the medium-sized and large varieties, which are active mitotically. In studies of transfused labeled lympho-

cytes, it is found that the lymphocytes of the germinal centers and their caps consist entirely of the B type (bursa-derived type, chapter 7). On the other hand, the lymphocytes of the deep (paracortical) region of the cortex belong to the T type (thymus-dependent type, chapter 7). Other portions of the node contain mostly the B type.

Lymphatic Vessels and Sinuses

Several lymphatic vessels pierce the capsule on the convex side of the node and open into the marginal sinus which continues into the parafollicular and medullary sinuses. The lymph circulates slowly through the cortical and medullary sinuses, which afford a greatly enlarged area for circulating lymph in comparison with that provided by the afferent lymph vessels. From the medullary sinuses, lymph vessels course through the connective tissue of the hilus and form the efferent lymphatics, which are wider but less numerous than the afferent lymphatics.

The flattened lining cells of the sinuses become continuous at the periphery of the node with the endothelial cells lining the afferent and efferent lymph vessels. The lining cells lack a basal lamina and often have gaps between the cells. As mentioned earlier, the lining cells are closely associated with reticular cells, but they are apparently endothelial in nature and not flattened reticular cells as described in the earlier literature on this subject.

Blood Vessels

Arteries enter the nodes through the connective tissue at the hilus, and some of the arterial branches course in the trabeculae to the capsule. Other arterial branches leave the trabeculae soon after entering the node and course into the medullary cords. These supply capillaries to the medulla and continue into the cortex, where arterioles penetrate the cortical nodules, giving off capillaries to the lymphatic tissue. The vessels of the germinal centers apparently consist of capillaries only. The venules that drain the cortex have a typical squamous endothelial lining in their course through the outer cortex but the venules from the deep (paracortical) cortex are lined by cu-

boidal endothelial cells (Fig. 13-7). These particular venules facilitate the passage of lymphocytes from the blood vessels into the lymphatic tissue for recirculation via the lymphatic and thoracic duct back to the blood vessels. The lymphocytes of the recirculating type are apparently able to recognize the cuboidal endothelial cells of the postcapillary venules as the site for migration. The migration has been described as occurring either by an intercellular route or by an intracellular (transcellular) course. Current evidence favors the intercellular route (Fig. 13-8).

The blood vessels draining the blood from all portions of the node other than the paracortical region consist of veins and venules lined by the usual squamous type of endothelium. They follow the same general course as the arteries and exit at the hilus.

Nerves

The nerves, which are not abundant, en-

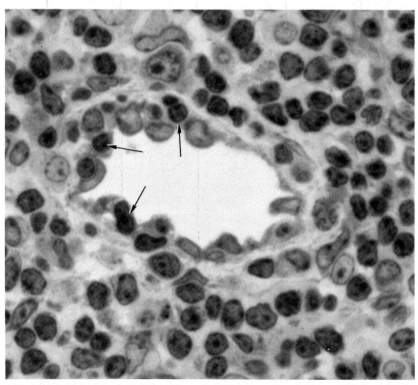

Fig. 13-7. Light micrograph of a postcapillary venule from the deep cortical region of monkey lymph node. Note the nuclei of endothelial cells bulging into the lumen. Dense nuclei of migrating lymphocytes appear at the *arrows*. ×975.

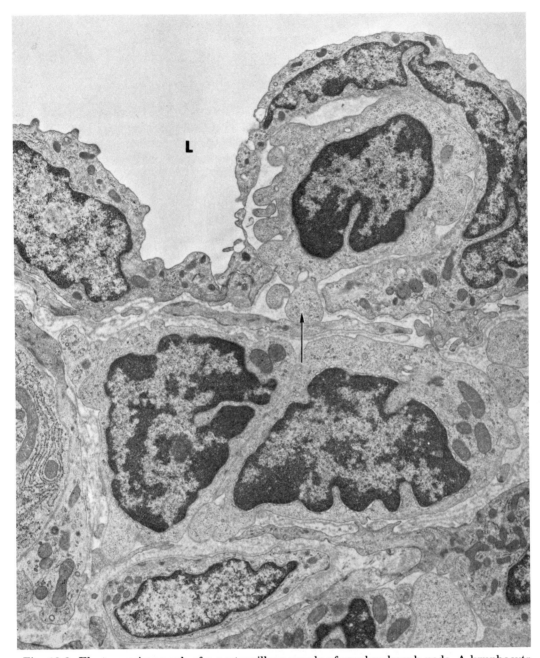

Fig. 13-8. Electron micrograph of a postcapillary venule of monkey lymph node. A lymphocyte is seen nearly surrounded by cytoplasm of an attenuated endothelial cell. A process of the lymphocyte penetrates the basal lamina (*arrow*). From this micrograph it cannot be ascertained whether the lymphocyte has migrated between endothelial cells or through a single cell. Two other lymphocytes lie beneath the endothelium partially surrounded by basal lamina material. *L*, lumen of venule. ×9200.

ter the node at the hilus and accompany the blood vessels. Some of them terminate in the trabeculae and capsule, whereas others form perivascular networks that follow the vessels into the lymphatic tissue.

Functions

The lymph nodes participate in the production of lymphocytes as evidenced by numerous mitoses of lymphoblasts within the node, particularly within the germinal centers. However, the presence of more lymphocytes in the efferent than in the afferent vessels is more closely related to the recirculation of lymphocytes. Studies with transfused labeled cells show that approximately 95% of the lymphocytes leaving the node belong to the recirculating type. These cells leave the postcapillary venules of the subcortical (juxtamedullary) region of the cortex and enter the lymph circulation, to be carried by the thoracic duct to the systemic circulation. The postcapillary venules of the nodes are lined by a cuboidal endothelium which facilitates the migration of the cells into the nodes, as described above under "Blood Vessels."

The lymph nodes also have an important role in phagocytosis of foreign material, which readily passes from the interstitial fluid of connective tissues into lymphatic capillaries via the gaps between their endothelial cells. The bronchial nodes are good examples of this. Inhaled carbon particles which pass through the epithelial lining of the alveoli of the lungs enter the connective tissue, then pass into lymphatic capillaries of the lung, and thence move on into bronchial lymph nodes by the afferent lymph vessels. The foreign material accumulates especially in the medullary regions of the node but may blacken the entire node after extensive and prolonged exposure. Because the lymphatic capillaries are permeable to large molecules and even to entire cells, the lymph node sinuses may contain erythrocytes that escape from blood vessels by internal hemorrhage. Unfortunately the great permeability of the endothelium of lymphatic capillaries also allows cancer cells to enter the lymph nodes; eventually these cells reach the blood circulation via the thoracic duct.

One of the major functions of lymph nodes is the production of antibodies. There are various ways in which antigens may be handled by the body. Some may be excreted, some may be taken up by macrophages and be subjected to degradative enzymes, and some may be processed by adherence to macrophages for reactions with lymphocytes, which lead to the differentiation of lymphocytes into antibody-forming plasma cells, as discussed under "Lympho-

cyte Functions, chapter 7," and under "Functions of the Thymus" in this chapter.

Development

Recent studies of well-fixed lymph nodes from human fetuses ranging from 26 to 245 mm in length have clarified the manner by which lymph nodes arise by partitioning of lymphatic sacs. Primordia of the nodes are first recognizable when some connective tissue, along with some blood vessels and lymphocytes, invaginates the endothelial walls of the sacs in certain locations (Fig. 13-9). Several nodes usually form from a single lymphatic sac; hence, the nodes are usually in groups. The invaginating connective tissue forms the capsule of the node and surrounds it everywhere except where lymphatic vessels and blood vessels enter and exit. Connective tissue trabeculae are present at an early stage and become more pronounced as development progresses. The medullary region differentiates into its characteristic morphology earlier than the cortical region does. The latter does not attain its characteristic pattern until relatively late in fetal life. Germinal centers do not usually appear until after birth, and usually only after stimulation by antigen.

Hemolymph Nodes

In certain animals, structures have been described that are similar to lymph nodes, except that afferent and efferent lymphatic vessels are absent and the sinuses contain blood instead of lymph. True hemal nodes of this type occur in the sheep. In the pig, hemolymph nodes have been described which have sinuses connected with both lymphatic and blood vessels, so that they appear to be intermediate between lymph nodes and the hemal nodes of sheep. In man, the occurrence of organs of this type has been questioned and seems very doubtful. Normal lymph nodes usually contain a few red blood cells, some of which may have been brought in by the afferent lymphatics, whereas others probably enter from the blood vessels within the node by diapedesis. It is true that nodes may be found in man with considerable numbers of red blood cells, but there have been no descriptions of connections between the si-

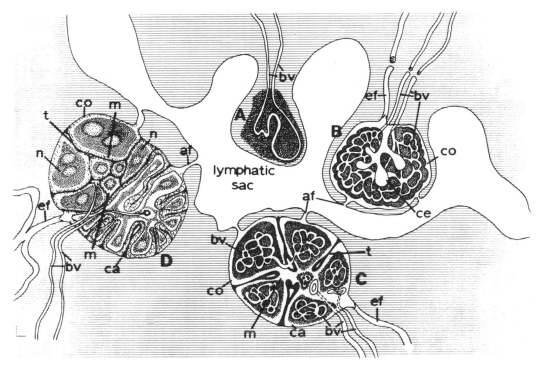

Fig. 13-9. Diagram of several stages of lymph node differentiation. *A,* early stage, showing aggregation of lymphatic tissue around a capillary loop and invagination of the complex into the lymphatic sac lumen. *B,* later stage, showing formation of central and cortical lymphatic sinuses and the efferent drainage channel. *C,* later stage showing formation of trabeculae. *D,* final stage showing formation of definitive morphology. This mode of formation permits several nodes to form simultaneously in association with a single lymphatic sac and accounts for the usual grouping of nodes. *BV,* blood vessels; *CO,* cortical sinus; *CE,* central sinus; *CA,* capsule; *AF,* afferent lymphatics; *EF,* efferent lymphatics; *N,* nodules; *M,* medullary sinuses; *T,* trabeculae.

nuses and the blood vessels. It seems very probable that the presence of an unusual number of erythrocytes may be the result of hemorrhage from vessels either within the node or in the neighborhood of the afferent lymphatics.

The Tonsils

The Palatine Tonsils

The palatine tonsils are paired, oval-shaped bodies located in the oropharynx between the glossopalatine and pharyngo-palatine arches. They consist of dense accumulations of lymphatic tissue in the connective tissue of the mucosa. They are covered on their free surface by a stratified squamous epithelium which is continuous with the epithelium of the rest of the pharynx. This epithelium has the same structure

as elsewhere in the pharynx: flat surface cells, beneath which are irregular cells, whereas the deepest cells are cuboidal or more or less columnar and rest upon a basal lamina. A thin layer of fibrous connective tissue with papillae is usually found between the basal lamina and the underlying lymphatic tissue. At various places on the surface of the tonsil, deep indentations or pockets occur. These depressions, 10 to 20 in number, are known as the *crypts* of the tonsil (Fig. 13-10) and are lined by a continuation of the surface epithelium that becomes thinner as the deeper part of the crypt is reached. Passing off from the bottoms and sides of the main or primary crypts are frequently several secondary crypts, also lined with the same type of epithelium.

Surrounding each crypt is a zone of varying thickness, consisting of a rather diffuse

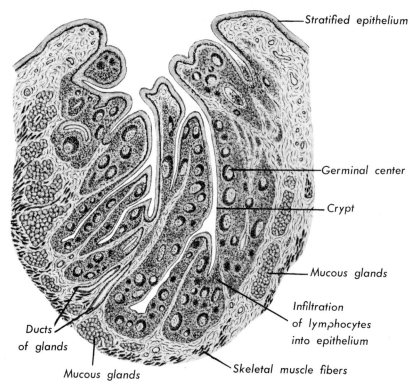

Fig. 13-10. Section through the palatine tonsil of man. ×9.

lymphatic tissue in which are embedded *nodules* of compact lymphatic tissue similar to those of the lymph nodes. The nodules are frequently more or less fused together. The nodules, like those of lymph nodes, may contain *germinal centers* that consist of a lighter-staining central area and a surrounding zone of more closely packed cells.

There is a *capsule* of connective tissue over the attached or basal surface of the lymphatic tissue which is firmly adherent on the one side to the tonsillar tissue and on the other to the surrounding structures from which it separates the tonsils. From the capsule there are *septa* of loose connective tissue that separate the various crypts with their surrounding zones of lymphatic tissue from one another. Infiltrated into this connective tissue are various-sized lymphocytes, plasma cells, mast cells, and frequently, neutrophilic leukocytes.

At various points on the surface of the tonsil, and especially in the crypts, there occurs what is known as *lymphocytic infiltration of the epithelium* (Fig. 13-11). This

consists of an invasion of the epithelium by the underlying lymphocytes. It varies from only a few lymphocytes scattered in the epithelium to an almost complete replacement of epithelium by lymphocytes. In this way, the lymphocytes reach the surface and are discharged into the crypts. These cells probably form the bulk of the so-called salivary corpuscles. In inflammation, the tonsillar tissue also contains numerous polymorphonuclear neutrophilic leukocytes which emigrate from the blood.

Small mucous glands, similar to those found in other parts of the pharynx, are numerous in the connective tissue adjacent to the tonsil. The bodies of these glands are separated from the tonsils by the capsule. Their excretory ducts usually open on the free surface, but occasionally they may open into the tonsillar crypts.

The Lingual Tonsils

These are spherical aggregations of lymphatic tissue situated on the dorsum and sides of the back part of the tongue between

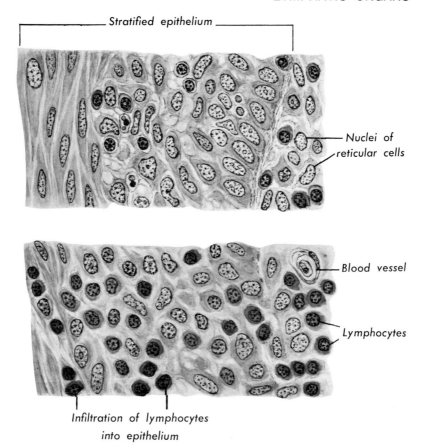

Stratified epithelium

Nuclei of reticular cells

Blood vessel

Lymphocytes

Infiltration of lymphocytes into epithelium

Fig. 13-11. Two fields from different depths along the crypts of a human tonsil. The squamous epithelial cells, facing the lumen of the crypt, are toward the *left*. The *upper figure* shows only slight lymphocytic infiltration of the epithelium. The *lower figure* shows an extensive infiltration that makes it difficult to distinguish the junction of epithelium and underlying connective tissue. ×1000.

the circumvallate papillae and the epiglottis (Fig. 16-4). They contain rather wide-mouthed, deep crypts, which may be branched and which are lined with a continuation of the surface stratified squamous epithelium. As in the palatine tonsile, each crypt is surrounded by an aggregation of lymph nodules containing germinal centers. In most crypts, there is marked lymphoid infiltration of the epithelium (Fig. 13-11). Ducts of some of the mucous glands of the tongue frequently open into the crypts (Fig. 16-5).

The Pharyngeal Tonsil

There is a median aggregation of lymphatic tissue in the posterior wall of the nasopharynx which forms the pharyngeal tonsil. The lymphatic tissue is similar to that of the palatine tonsils. The epithelium over the free surface, as is characteristic for the nasopharynx and other respiratory passages, is largely pseudostratified columnar ciliated epithelium. There are patches of stratified squamous epithelium, which become more numerous in the adult. Hypertrophy of the pharyngeal tonsil, with consequent obstruction of the nasal openings, is common, especially in children, constituting what are known as adenoids.

Blood Vessels of Tonsils

These have a distribution similar to that of the blood vessels of the lymph nodes, but they enter the organ along its entire attached side and not at a definite hilus.

Lymphatic Vessels

The tonsils have no afferent lymphatic vessels and no lymph sinuses. At the peripheral surface of the lymphatic tissue, there are plexuses of lymph capillaries which form the beginnings of efferent lymphatic vessels. The tonsils, therefore, unlike the lymph nodes, which are situated in the course of lymphatc vessels, are situated at the beginnings of lymphatic vessels.

Nerves

The nerves of the palatine tonsils are derived from the glossopharyngeal nerve and from the sphenopalatine ganglion, and they enter the organ along its attached side.

Functions

Fairly numerous mitoses in the germinal centers show that the tonsils participate in lymphocyte development. The presence of plasma cells indicates that the tonsils also participate in antigen-antibody reactions. The tonsils are situated strategically for protecting the body against invasion by bacteria and foreign proteins. On the other hand, the lack of a complete epithelial lining in the deep tonsillar crypts may be a factor leading to general infections that sometimes develop after invasion and proliferation of foreign microorganisms.

Development

The palatine tonsils make their appearance during the 3rd month of development. Evaginations of endoderm grow into the underlying mesenchyme at the site of the second pharyngeal pouch and, at the same time, there is a subepithelial condensation of mesenchyme. The cells of the inner part of the mesenchymal condensation become arranged around the epithelium of the evaginations and gradually develop the reticulum and lymphocytes of the lymphatic tissue, whereas the endodermal evaginations become the crypts. At the outer part of the mesenchymal condensation, fibrous connective tissue develops into the capsule.

The lingual and pharyngeal tonsils begin their development during the later months of fetal life. In the pharyngeal tonsil, definite nodules appear at about the time of birth or during the 1st or 2nd year. In the lingual tonsil, the nodules are not fully formed until the 5th or 6th year.

The Thymus

The thymus has a very important role in the immune mechanism of the body, and it becomes occupied with lymphocytes early in fetal development. It is a relatively large organ at the time of birth, weighing approximately 12 to 15 g, and its growth continues at a rapid rate until the end of the 2nd year. After that time it grows at a somewhat slower rate until puberty, when it reaches a weight of 30 to 40 g. It subsequently becomes smaller in proportion to most other organs and eventually shows an actual decrease in size; i.e., it undergoes "age involution" and is partially replaced by fat and connective tissue (compare Figs. 13-12 and 13-13).

The human thymus consists of two lobes which are closely applied to each other and joined in the midline by connective tissue. The lobes are surrounded by a connective tissue *capsule* which gives off relatively coarse *septa* or *trabeculae;* these partially subdivide each lobe into groups of lobules that are partially subdivided further into individual lobules by slender trabeculae (Fig. 13-12). Each lobule consists of a *cortex* and a *medulla*. In random sections, groups of lobules often appear to be completely separated from each other and individual lobules may also appear to be completely separated. However, serial sections show that at least until involution is well advanced, the medullary tissue is continuous from one lobule to another throughout each of the two lobes.

The thymus, like other lymphatic organs, is composed of lymphocytes and reticular cells. However, the latter differ in origin and structure from those of other lymphatic organs. They are derived from the endoderm of the third pair of pharyngeal pouches; hence they are designated as endodermal reticular cells or thymic *epithelial reticular* cells (see discussion in chapter 4). The earliest lymphocytes associated with the thymus appear in the mesenchyme just outside the endodermal rudiment by the end of the 2nd fetal month and are present within the organ shortly thereafter.

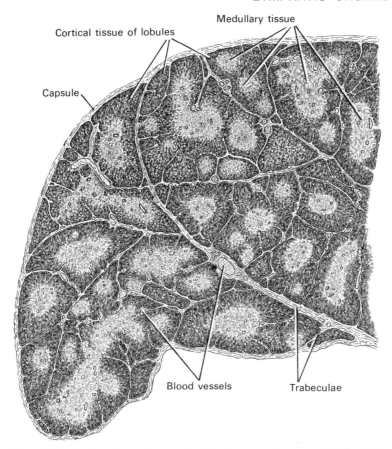

Cortical tissue of lobules

Medullary tissue

Capsule

Blood vessels

Trabeculae

Fig. 13-12. Section through a part of the human thymus at birth. ×12.

These earliest lymphocytes are derivatives of stem cells of yolk sac origin which circulate to the thymus through the blood vessels via the liver and bone marrow. The epithelial reticular cells are close together and have relatively short processes before the initial entrance of lymphocytes into the organ. During the establishment of the lymphocyte population, the cell bodies of the reticular cells are pushed apart and are left in contact with each other by long cytoplasmic processes.

The cortex consists of an abundance of lymphocytes which partially obscure the reticular cells. The lymphocytes, unlike those of lymph nodes, are not arranged in nodules, and, although mitoses occur, there are no germinal centers. The lymphocytes vary in size and cytological characteristics, with the largest cells often located in the subcapsular region of the lobule. They proliferate at a rapid rate, and some of them, known as T lymphocytes, enter the blood

circulation and function in cell-mediated immunity. However, the vast majority of the newly formed lymphocytes degenerate within the thymus; the functional significance of this extensive degeneration is not fully understood.

The thymic cortex is unusual in that its blood vessels consist of capillaries only. The arteries to the thymus follow the connective tissue septa to the junction of cortex and medulla, where they send branches into the cortical and medullary tissues. The medulla receives small arteries and arterioles, which divide into capillaries, whereas the cortex receives capillaries only. The cortical capillaries constitute an important part of a *blood-thymic barrier,* which prevents circulating macromolecules and particulate matter from entering the cortex. This allows the cortical lymphocytes to proliferate and differentiate in an environment free of circulating antigens. Studies of thymic tissues from rodents transfused with labeled

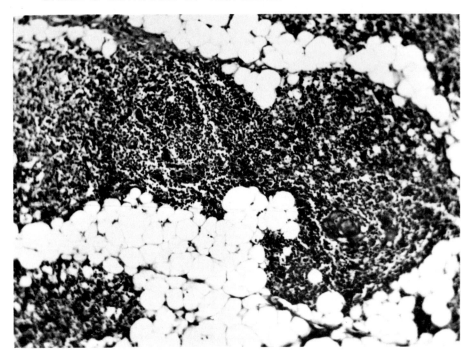

Fig. 13-13. Photomicrograph of a portion of thymus from a man 36 years of age. Note that portions of the organ have undergone involution and have been replaced by fat. ×110.

macromolecules (cytochrome, peroxidase, catalase, and ferritin) show that none of these substances leave the vessels in the cortex, whereas ferritin, with a molecular weight of 462,000, and catalase, with a weight of 240,000, approximately that of IgG, readily leave the vessels in the medulla. The structures separating the blood from the cortical tissues are as follows: endothelial cells joined by occluding junctions, basal lamina of the capillary endothelium, a thin compartment of connective tissue, basal lamina beneath a continuous border of the epithelial reticular cells, and the epithelial reticular cells which have intercellular clefts of 100 to 200 Å. The cytoplasmic processes of the reticular cells, as noted above, are joined by desmosomes.

The medulla resembles the cortex in that it is composed of lymphocytes and epithelial reticular cells, but the lymphocytes are less numerous and therefore the reticular cells are more obvious. The reticular cells of the medulla, like those of the cortex, have oblong-shaped pale-staining nuclei that are much larger than the lymphocyte nuclei (Fig. 13-14). Electron micrographs show that the reticular cells contain tono-

filaments much like those of stratified squamous epithelium and that the filaments extend into the cell processes which are in contact by desmosomes. The cytoplasm contains a relatively small Golgi apparatus, some free ribosomes, and some rough endoplasmic reticulum.

The medulla also contains a number of spherical or oval bodies composed of concentrically arranged cells known as *thymic corpuscles* or Hassall's corpuscles (Fig. 13-14). They are characteristic of the thymus and begin to appear during the first half of fetal life. Their average diameter in the fully developed organ is 20 to 50 μm, but they vary considerably, and much larger corpuscles are often found. The cells are concentrically arranged in the corpuscle and range in shape from polygonal at the surface to flattened at the center. They take a bright red stain with hematoxylin and eosin. Some of the central cells may be completely degenerated. The cellular changes from periphery to center have been likened to the stages in cornification of stratified squamous epithelium.

Because the thymic epithelial reticular cells are endodermal in origin, it is not

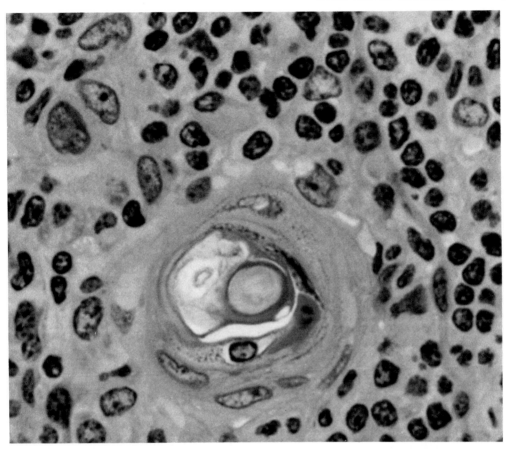

Fig. 13-14. Light micrograph of thymic medulla from monkey showing Hassall's corpuscle, lymphocytes, and large, pale nuclei of thymic epithelial reticular cells. Note the flattened peripheral cells, some containing cytoplasmic granules resembling keratohyaline granules, in the Hassall's corpuscle. ×1000.

surprising to find that they are not generally associated with reticular fibers. The latter are sparse except in the connective tissue around blood vessels. In keeping with their origin, the endodermally derived reticular cells exhibit epithelial characteristics when grown in tissue culture. They also behave like epithelial cells in that they do not show much phagocytic activity for colloidal dyes (e.g., trypan blue), but this may be due at least in part to a failure of the colloidal dyes to penetrate the blood-thymic barrier.

In addition to lymphocytes and epithelial-derived reticular cells, the thymus contains macrophages, particularly in the region of the corticomedullary junction. Plasma cells are not present within the cortex, but a few may be present in the medulla. The connective tissue of the septa and capsule contains fibroblasts plus some plasma cells and mast cells.

Blood Vessels

The thymus is supplied by branches of the internal mammary and inferior thyroidal arteries. The arterial branches give off some vessels to the connective tissue of the septa and continue in the septa around the lobules to the corticomedullary junctions, where they send small arteries into the medulla and capillaries into the cortex. As noted above, the cortical capillaries are impermeable to macromolecules. On the other hand, the postcapillary venules of the medulla are readily traversed by macromolecules and by lymphocytes. This is the route by which the lymphocytes proliferating in the thymic cortex enter the blood vessels.

However, the endothelial cells of the postcapillary venules are not thickened like those of postcapillary venules of lymph nodes. The venules of the thymus converge in the medullary tissue to form larger veins that course in the connective tissue septa to accompany the arteries. They drain into the left innominate and thyroidal veins.

Lymphatics

There are no lymph sinuses in the thymus and no afferent lymphatic vessels; this condition is in contrast with that of lymph nodes but is similar to that of all other organs of the body. Lymphatic capillaries arise around the lymphatic tissue of the lobules and join to form larger lymphatic vessels that accompany the arteries in the connective tissue septa.

Nerves

Branches of the vagus and cervical sympathetics are distributed to the walls of blood vessels. A few fibers have been described as terminating freely in the cortex and medulla.

Functions

It has been known for many years that the thymus is active in lymphocyte proliferation, but the functional significance of this was not recognized before recent experimental studies. A better understanding of thymic function has been achieved by studies on the effects of thymectomy and by transfusions of labeled cells. It has been found that mice thymectomized on the 1st day after birth develop a wasting disease within a few months and die at an early age. There is also a marked deficiency in the deveopment of other lymphatic organs, with few or no germinal centers appearing. The thymectomized mice also accept skin grafts from other strains of mice and rats, whereas normal mice reject foreign grafts. When thymectomized animals are given injections of lymphatic tissue from other strains and species, the injected cells react against the host, whereas normal animals reject the foreign cells. It is known that the rejection of foreign grafts (a part of cell-mediated immunity) is by thymus-derived

germinal centers are not affected

lymphocytes (T lymphocytes) and that the formation of antibodies by plasma cells derived from B lymphocytes occurs with the help (or collaboration) of T cells (chapter 7). As noted earlier, the thymus itself does not form antibodies and its cortex is impermeable to antigens.

Some studies have indicated that the implantation of thymic tissue (lymphocytes and epithelial reticular cells) into thymectomized mice restores the animal's ability to form antibodies. Furthermore, this is described as occurring when the implants are enclosed in Millipore filters, which should prevent the escape of cells. On this evidence, it has been proposed that the thymus may exert an influence on other lymphocytic tissues through a humoral factor, presumably produced by the epithelial reticular cells. The existence of a thymic humoral factor is still controversial. However, some investigators claim that injection of a "purified" thymic product into individuals lacking normal immunological responses can result in establishment of nearly normal immunological function.

Development

The thymus arises as a paired endodermal outgrowth from the median and ventral portions of the third pair of pharyngeal pouches. Each outgrowth contains a narrow, cleft-like lumen at first, but this is soon obliterated by proliferation of the epithelial cells. In the thymus, the reticular cells are derived from epithelial cells and not from mesenchyme as in the other lymphatic organs. Transformation of epithelial cells into a reticulum begins at about the end of the 2nd month in the central portion of the outgrowth. Studies of thymic glands fixed at successive stages of development show that lymphocytes are present in the mesenchyme around the gland earlier than in the epithelial reticulum. In embryos 50 to 60 mm in length, the medulla begins to become differentiated from the cortex as the lymphocytes become more densely aggregated in the peripheral regions of the gland and less numerous at the center. At about this same time, the lobules begin to form and become separated by the septa of connective tissue. As already stated, the connective tissue septa subdivide the cortical tissue but do not completely subdivide the medullary tissue.

Hassall's corpuscles make their first appearance during the first half of fetal life. At first they are few in number and small in size, but they increase rapidly in diameter, and new ones continue to form until the time when thymic involution begins.

The Spleen

The spleen is the largest lymphatic organ in the body. Unlike the lymph nodes, however, it has no afferent lymphatic vessels and no lymph sinuses.

Except at the hilus, the spleen is covered by a serous membrane, the peritoneum. Beneath this is a *capsule* of fibrous tissue containing numerous elastic fibers and some smooth muscle. From the capsule (Figs. 13-15 and 13-16), dense connective tissue trabeculae extend into the interior of the organ. These branch and unite with one another to form very incomplete anastomosing chambers. At one point on the surface of the spleen a deep indentation occurs, which is known as the *hilus*. This marks the entrance and exit of the splenic vessels. Accompanying the vessels, broad strands of capsular tissue extend deep into the organ where they radiate and subdivide to form, with the smaller trabeculae which extend in from other parts of the capsule, the connective tissue framework of the organ. Because of the abundance of elastic tissue, along with some smooth muscle, and because of the arrangement of fibrous connective tissue in wavy bundles, the spleen is distensible and capable of considerable change in volume.

The spaces within the connective tissue framework are filled with a soft, sponge-like tissue known as the *splenic pulp*. On the basis of color differences seen in fresh preparations, different regions of the splenic pulp have been named *red pulp* and *white pulp*. Both types consist of lymphatic tissue (that is, reticular connective tissue and lymphocytes), together with other cell types described below under "The Splenic Pulp."

The red pulp is traversed by a plexus of *venous sinuses* (Figs. 13-16 through 13-20),

by which it is subdivided into anastomosing cords known as *pulp cords* (*cords of Billroth*). The lymphatic tissue of the pulp cords is infiltrated with erythrocytes, the number of which varies under different conditions. The venous sinuses contain erythrocytes which are packed particularly close together when the sinuses are in a storage phase (see below). Thus, the red pulp (venous sinuses plus pulp cords) contains large numbers of erythrocytes which are responsible for its color in fresh preparations.

The white pulp is composed of compact lymphatic tissue arranged around certain divisions of the arteries in the form of a *periarterial sheath,* with ovoid enlargements at intervals which are known as *lymphatic nodules, splenic nodules,* or *Malpighian corpuscles.* The junction of a lymphatic nodule with the surrounding red pulp has characteristic features in the pattern of its vessels and reticulum and is known as the *marginal zone* (Fig. 13-15). Except for their larger blood vessels, the lymphatic nodules of the spleen are very similar to those found in lymph nodes and, like the latter, they may contain germinal centers. In children, a germinal center is usually found in each nodule, but in the adult spleen the germinal centers are less numerous.

The structure of the spleen depends largely upon the characteristic arrangement of the blood vessels, which are described before considering further the minute structure of the organ.

Blood Vessels

The arteries enter the spleen at the hilus and divide into branches which enter the trabeculae to become the *trabecular* or *interlobular arteries* (Fig. 13-20). These are accompanied by the trabecular branches of the splenic veins. After following the trabeculae for a short distance, the arteries leave the veins and the septa and pursue an entirely separate course through the splenic pulp. The adventitial coat of these smaller arteries takes on the character of reticular tissue and becomes infiltrated with lymphocytes, forming a thin periarterial sheath. At various points along the course of the vessels, the lymphatic tissue

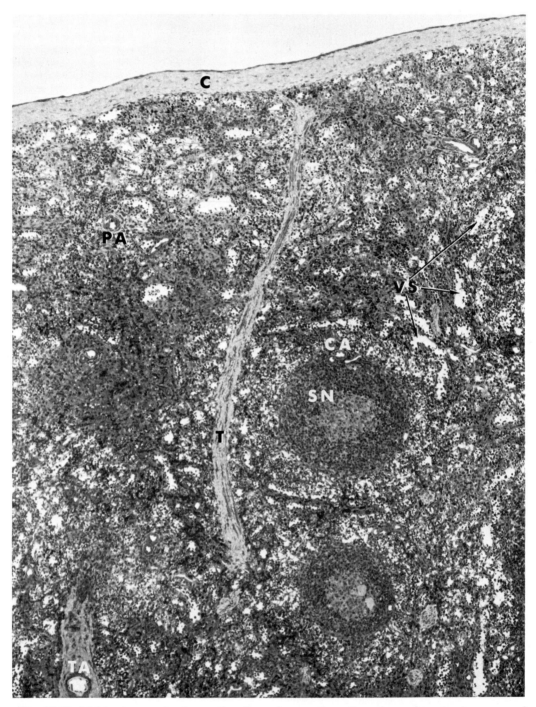

Fig. 13-15. Light micrograph of a section through a portion of monkey spleen to show general topography. *C*, capsule; *CA*, central artery; *PA*, pulp artery; *SN*, splenic nodule; *T*, trabecula; *TA*, trabecular artery; *VS*, venous sinuses. ×165.

is increased in amount and forms the splenic nodules already mentioned. These arteries are called the *central arteries,* although they are eccentrically located with reference to the splenic nodules. When a nodule is located at a point where the artery divides, as frequently happens, two or more arteries are seen in a cross section of the

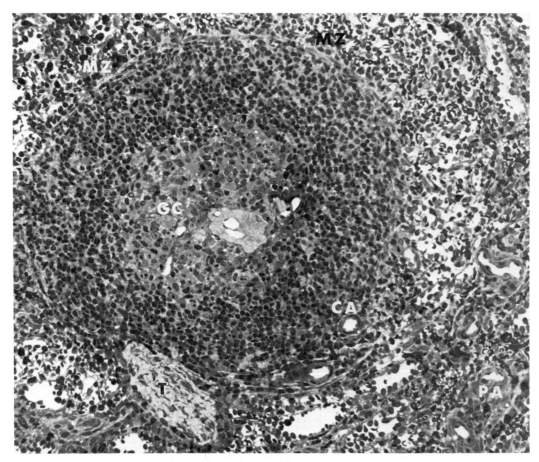

Fig. 13-16. Light micrograph of a section of monkey spleen showing a splenic nodule and its marginal zone. *CA,* central artery; *GC,* germinal center; *PA,* pulp artery; *T,* trabecula; *MZ,* marginal zone. ×420.

nodule. In their passage through the white pulp, the central arteries give off capillaries which nourish the white pulp and continue as capillaries into the red pulp. In other words, [there is no venous return directly from the white pulp.] The central arteries are lined by a *cuboidal* endothelium, and the capillaries given off to the white pulp also have cuboidal endothelium for a part of their course.

After a number of divisions within the white pulp, the central arteries reach the marginal zone, where their sheaths of white pulp become reduced to only a thin layer of scattered lymphocytes. Within the marginal zone, each artery divides into a number of branches which are close together like the bristles of a brush or *penicillus.* These vessels consist of three successive portions: *pulp arteries, sheathed arteries* (or *sheathed capillaries*), and *terminal ar-*

terial capillaries. The pulp arteries are the longest of these segments; they qualify as arterioles, because their wall contains one or two layers of smooth muscle cells. The pulp arteries divide into several "sheathed arteries" that are actually capillaries because they no longer contain any smooth muscle. Their lumen is only about 8 μm in diameter, but their wall is thickened by the presence of concentric layers of reticular fibers and a number of interspersed cells which consist largely of macrophages. The sheath is not prominent in humans, as it is in some of the lower animals such as the dog and pig. On the other hand, some animals, such as rodents, lack this sheath.

Each of the sheathed arteries divides into two or more arterial capillaries, which may have conical enlargements (ampullae) at their terminations. The exact manner in which these vessels terminate has been a

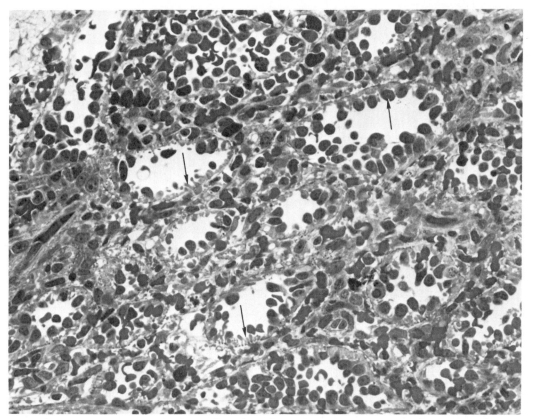

Fig. 13-17. Light micrograph of a section of monkey spleen showing transverse sections of venous sinuses. Note the arrangement of endothelial cells (*arrows*). Compare with Figures 13-19 and 13-23. ×825.

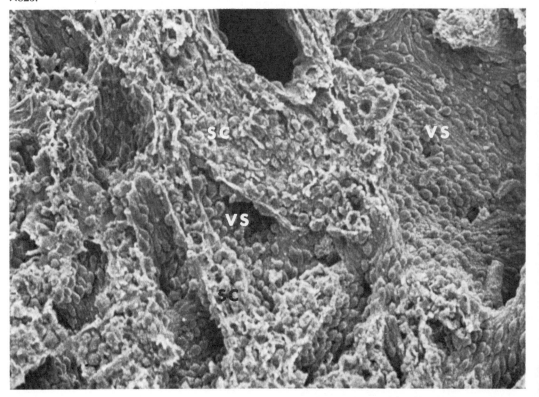

Fig. 13-18. Scanning electron micrograph of red pulp of human spleen showing venous sinuses (*VS*) and splenic cords (*SC*). Courtesy of Dr. Masayuki Miyoshi. ×480.

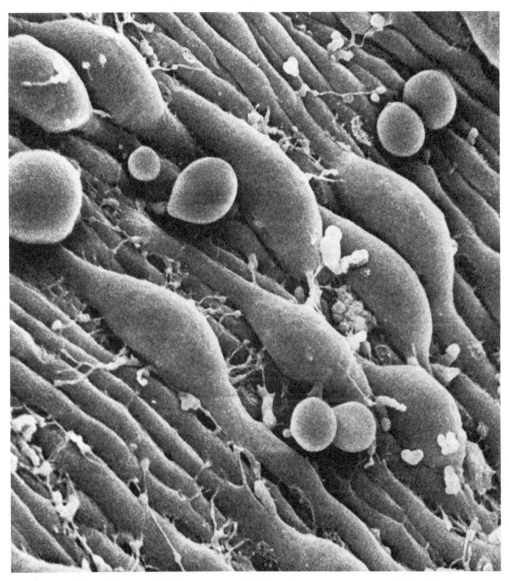

Fig. 13-19. High magnification scanning electron micrograph of the internal surface of a venous sinus in human spleen. The elongate endothelial cells with bulging nuclei run diagonally in the field. Courtesy of Dr. Masayuki Miyoshi. ×4800.

controversial subject. Some authors believe that the capillaries empty into intercellular spaces of the red pulp reticulum and that the blood finds its way from the pulp spaces into the venous sinuses through perforations in the walls of the sinuses. Other authors believe that the capillaries empty directly into the venous sinuses. However, openings of terminal arterioles into the intercellular spaces of the red pulp can be seen in electron micrographs, and it is evi-

dent that at least some of the arterioles terminate in this manner.

The *venous sinuses* form an anastomosing plexus throughout the red pulp, dividing it into pulp cords. The endothelial cells of the venous sinuses differ from ordinary endothelial cells in that they are cuboidal in shape, are more elongated than ordinary endothelial cells, and are arranged paralleling each other in a rather uniform pattern (Figs. 13-17, 13-19, and 13-21). Electron mi-

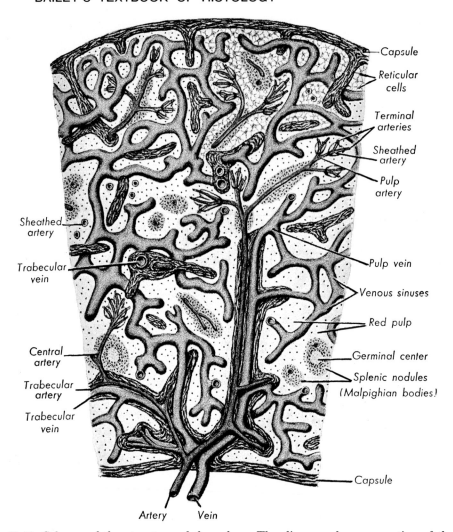

Fig. 13-20. Schema of the structure of the spleen. The diagram shows a portion of the organ extending from the hilus to the opposite (convex) surface. The structural components (vessels, nodules, etc.) that would be contained in such a large section have not been drawn to scale, but have been increased in size and decreased in numbers for clearer illustration. (Redrawn and modified from Hartmann.)

crographs show an incomplete basement membrane of variable thickness beneath the cells (Figs. 13-22 and 13-23).

The outer part of the sinus wall contains relatively coarse, circularly arranged reticular fibers, which are quite obvious in silver-stained preparations under the light microscope (Fig. 13-21). Electron micrographs show that these fibers are embedded in a perforated layer of ground substance. Although the perforations of the basement membrane and the intercellular clefts between the endothelial cells seen with the

light microscope (Fig. 13-21) are exaggerated by shrinkage of cells during standard light microscope preparation of tissues, their presence has been confirmed by electron microscope studies (Figs. 13-19, 13-22 and 13-23).

The terminal veins or venous sinuses unite to form larger *pulp veins,* or *collecting venules.* They enter the trabeculae to become the *trabecular* or *interlobular veins,* which follow the trabeculae toward the hilus, where they unite to form the splenic veins.

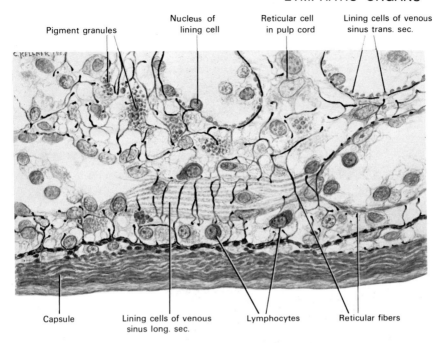

Fig. 13-21. Section of spleen of rhesus monkey stained with silver to show reticular fibers and with hematoxylin-eosin-azure to show cell types. The venous sinus in the *lower part* of the field is cut longitudinally and tangentially so that the section gives a surface view of part of the sinus wall. The two *upper* sinuses are cut transversely. Granules of hemosiderin pigment are unusually abundant in this particular field. ×1045.

Union of Arteries and Veins

The relationship between the arterial capillaries and venous sinuses has been a subject of considerable controversy, with some investigators holding to the view that capillaries open into intercellular spaces in the red pulp (Fig. 13-24) and others believing that all of the capillaries open directly into venous sinuses (Fig. 13-25).

The view that the splenic circulation is closed received its strongest support from studies of blood flow in living animals. Using a quartz rod method of transillumination, Knisely observed arterial capillaries emptying directly into the venous sinuses and also into the collecting venules of the red pulp (Fig. 13-25). He observed cyclic activity in the venous sinuses with conducting and storage phases. Although the method made significant contributions to an understanding of splenic function, it could not provide the resolution obtained later by electron microscopy. Electron microscopic studies indicate that most of the terminal capillaries open into intercellular

spaces in the red pulp and that relatively few vessels open directly into venous sinuses. The endothelial cells of the terminal capillaries apparently make contact with processes of reticular cells, and the latter, in turn, make contact with the lining cells of the sinuses, as diagramatically illustrated in Figure 13-24, except that the intercellular spaces are exaggerated in the diagram. The actual appearance of the intercellular gaps and clefts between the lining cells as seen in electron micrographs is shown in Figures 13-22 and 13-23.

The Splenic Pulp

As already stated, the splenic pulp fills in all of the spaces between the connective tissue trabeculae; it has been subdivided into white pulp, consisting of compact lymphatic tissue surrounding the central arteries, and red pulp, containing an abundance of erythrocytes.

A meshwork of reticular connective tissue extends throughout both the red and white pulp, although its density and ar-

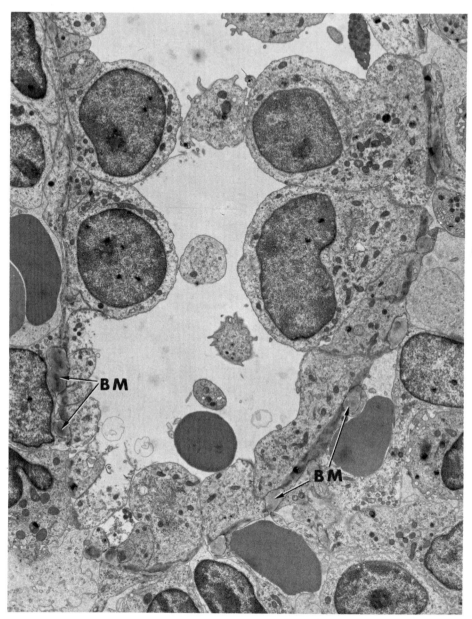

Fig. 13-22. Electron micrograph of a venous sinus of monkey spleen showing the cuboidal appearance of endothelial cells, incomplete basement membrane (*BM*), and filamentous condensations in the bases of endothelial cells. ×4300.

rangement vary in different parts. The reticular cells (Fig. 13-26) and also the fibers (Fig. 13-27) are more numerous and more closely arranged around the arteries and at the marginal zone of the lymphatic nodule than they are elsewhere.

The *reticular cells* resemble those described for lymph nodes. For example, their nuclei are relatively pale-staining in comparison with the densely chromatic nuclei of small lymphocytes, and their cytoplasm stains lightly in most techniques. Electron micrographs show that the processes of reticular cells form a covering for the reticular fibers, as they do in lymph nodes. Although the reticular cells of the spleen were once

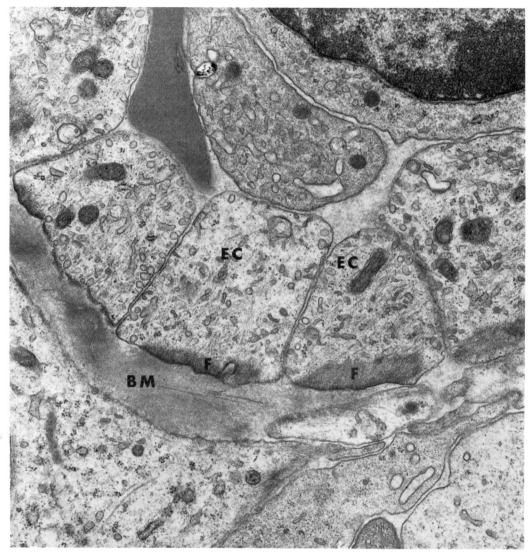

Fig. 13-23. Electron micrograph of a portion of the wall of a venous sinus of monkey spleen showing processes of endothelial cells (*EC*) containing dense basal filaments (*F*) and part of the discontinuous basement membrane (*BM*). ×19,000.

thought to be very phagocytic, more recent studies using transfused labeled cells and electron microscopy indicate that most of the splenic macrophages are derivatives of promonocytes.

Lymphocytes of large, medium, and small sizes are closely packed in the white pulp, with the first two types particularly numerous in the germinal centers. The lymphocytes are much less numerous and more randomly dispersed in the red pulp. A high percentage of the lymphocytes of the spleen belong to the recirculating type, which probably enter the spleen by migrating between the lining cells of the venous sinuses. They tend to localize in specific regions of the white pulp, with T lymphocytes aggregated around the central arteries and B lymphocytes aggregated in the periarterial lymphatic sheaths at the periphery of the nodule.

Monocytes, macrophages, and *plasma cells* are also fairly numerous. Monocytes are brought into the spleen by the blood

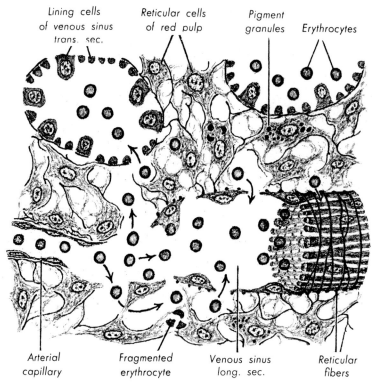

Fig. 13-24. Schema of union of arteries and veins in splenic pulp, showing an "open" type of circulation. The venous sinus at *lower right* is drawn to give a three-dimensional view to show the longitudinal orientation of the lining cells surrounded by circularly arranged reticular fibers. Granules in the reticular cells represent hemosiderin resulting from the phagocytosis of senile erythrocytes.

vessels and also form by proliferation and differentiation of promonocytes within the organ. The macrophages of the spleen are generally similar to those found in other parts of the body. However, they more frequently contain reddish or brownish pigment granules of hemosiderin that are derived from the hemoglobin of phagocytosed erythrocytes (Fig. 13-21).

The red pulp also contains the various types of *granular leukocytes* and a variable number of *erythrocytes.* Because of the thinness of the walls of the sinuses and the presence of some erythrocytes outside the sinuses, it is frequently difficult in ordinary sections to distinguish between the sinuses and pulp cords.

Giant cells or *megakaryocytes,* similar to those of bone marrow, are found in the splenic pulp of a number of animals (e.g., cat, rat). They are present in man during fetal life but are usually absent in the adult.

Lymphatics

Efferent lymphatic vessels are present in the connective tissue of the capsule and trabeculae. Deep efferent lymphatic vessels are also present in the white pulp, coursing parallel with the arteries.

Nerves

These are mainly nonmyelinated, although a few myelinated fibers are present. The latter are probably sensory in function. The nonmyelinated fibers—axons of sympathetic neurons—accompany the arteries, around which they form plexuses. From these plexuses, terminals pass to the muscle cells of the arteries, to the septa, to the capsule, and to the splenic pulp.

Functions of the Spleen

The spleen is not essential for life and can be removed because various other organs, particularly the bone marrow, readily take over its functions.

The spleen acts as a filtering organ for the blood in much the same way as the lymph nodes function as organs of lymph

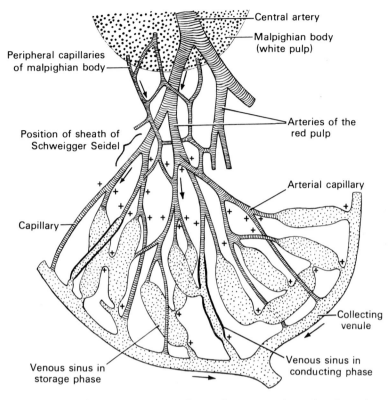

Central artery

Malpighian body
(white pulp)

Peripheral capillaries
of malpighian body

Arteries of the
red pulp

Position of sheath of
Schweigger Seidel

Arterial capillary

Capillary

Collecting
venule

Venous sinus in
storage phase

Venous sinus in
conducting phase

Fig. 13-25. Diagram of the different types of vascular connections that have been observed in the spleens of living animals. *Plus signs* indicate positions of physiological sphincters. (Redrawn and slightly modified from Knisely.)

filtration. The phagocytic cells of the spleen remove foreign particles, including bacteria, degenerating leukocytes, etc., from the circulating blood.

The macrophages also remove fragmented and whole erythrocytes, and in this way the spleen functions as an organ for blood destruction. Many of the engulfed cells have already begun to fragment in the peripheral circulation, but the spleen is thought to play a role in making the cells more fragile. Regardless of what initiates the fragmentation or determines which erythrocytes are to be destroyed, the spleen is of importance as an organ for the removal and phagocytosis of the cells.

Engulfed erythrocytes are digested by the phagocytic cells, and iron is recovered from the hemoglobin and temporarily stored in the cells. In this way the spleen plays a part in the iron metabolism of the body. The stored iron is given up as needed and is utilized by the body in the formation of new hemoglobin.

The spleen functions as an organ for blood development during a part of fetal life, but after birth the only blood cells normally formed in the spleen are lymphocytes and monocytes. In certain pathological conditions, the splenic pulp reassumes its earlier function as a blood-forming organ for all types of cells and becomes similar to bone marrow in appearance, containing all types of myelocytes, erythroblasts, and megakaryocytes.

As already described, the framework of the spleen includes elastic fibers and smooth muscle, and it is able to make rapid changes in volume. Contraction of the spleen expels erythrocytes and increases the number of these corpuscles in the general circulation. Contraction and decrease in volume occurs under many different conditions (e.g., during exercise, after hemorrhage), and, although this reservoir function of the spleen is not necessary for life, there are a great variety of conditions, both normal and pathological, in which it may

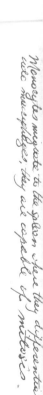

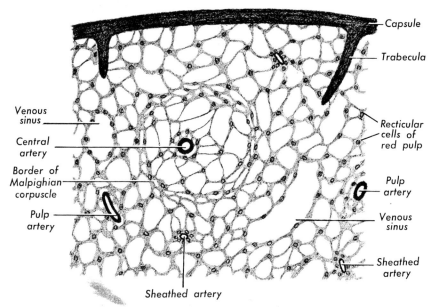

Fig. 13-26. Schema of the arrangement of the reticular cells of the spleen. Reticular fibers are omitted. No structural details are shown for the capsule, trabeculae and walls of arteries, but the positions of these structures are shown as the darkest parts of the schema. (Redrawn from Hartmann.)

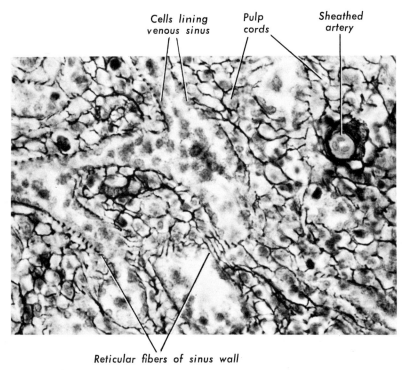

Fig. 13-27. Photomicrograph of spleen of rhesus monkey. Stained with Bielschowsky-Foot silver for reticular fibers and with hematoxylin-eosin-azure for cell types. ×540.

be of considerable value.

The white pulp of the spleen has an important role in the formation of antibodies and in the immune reaction. In response to an antigen entering the body for the first time, i.e., a primary response, lymphoblasts proliferate in numerous portions of the spleen. After 4 or 5 days, there is also an obvious increase in the numbers of plasma cells associated with the lymphatic sheaths along the periarterial vessels of the nodules and along those of the penicilli. Slightly later, changes are seen in the germinal centers, with an increased proliferation of lymphoblasts and with macrophages containing ingested lymphocytes. In the case of the primary response, the centers continue to show some evidence of an increased activity for about 1 month. In a subsequent or secondary response to the same antigen, the germinal centers respond more rapidly.

Development

The spleen arises as a thickening in the mesenchyme in the left side of the dorsal mesogastrium during the 5th or 6th week of fetal development (10-mm embryo). With continued growth, the primordium becomes elevated from the mesentery and the attachment is reduced to a narrow band of tissue surrounding the splenic vessels. The primordium is composed of reticular cells of mesenchymal origin and is invaded by lymphocytes which apparently differentiate from stem cells of yolk sac origin before their transportation via the blood vessels to the liver, bone marrow, and spleen.

The fetal spleen participates in the development of lymphocytes, monocytes, granular leukocytes, erythrocytes, and megakaryocytes. However, erythropoiesis decreases at about the 8th month and generally ceases at about the time of birth. Granular leukocyte development usually ceases soon after birth. The spleen remains active in lymphocyte and monocyte development throughout life and has the ability to revert to erythrocyte development in young individuals when there is an unusual demand.

The enlargements of white pulp to form definite nodules does not occur until late in fetal life, and germinal centers usually do not appear until after birth and after stimulation by foreign antigens.

References

ACKERMAN, G. A. The lymphocyte: its morphology and embryological origin. In Bristol Symposium: The Lymphocyte in Immunology and Haemopoiesis (Yoffey, J. M., editor), pp. 11–20. Williams & Wilkins, Baltimore, 1967.

ACKERMAN, G. A., AND HOSTETLER, J. R. Morphological studies of the embryonic rabbit thymus. Anat. Rec. 166:27–46, 1970.

ALEXANDER, J. W., AND GOOD, R. A. Immunology for Surgeons. W. B. Saunders Company, Philadelphia, 1970.

AUERBACH, R. 1961. Experimental analysis of the origin of cell types of the development of the mouse thymus. Dev. Biol. 3:336–354, 1961.

BARCROFT, J., AND STEPHENS, J. G. Observations on the size of the spleen. J. Physiol. 64:1–22, 1927.

BRADFIELD, J. W. B., AND BORN, G. V. R. The migration of rat thoracic duct lymphocytes through spleen. Br. J. Exp. Pathol. 54:509–517, 1973.

BURNET, F. M. The thymus gland. Sci. Amer. 207:50–57, 1962.

CHEN, L. T., AND WEISS, L. The role of the sinus wall in the passage of erythrocytes through the spleen. Blood 41:529–538, 1973.

CLARK, S. L., JR. The reticulum of lymph nodes in mice studied with the electron microscope. Am. J. Anat. 110:217–257, 1962.

CLARK, S. L., JR. The penetration of proteins and colloidal materials into the thymus from the blood stream. In The Thymus (Defendi, V., and Metcalf, D., editors), Wistar Institute Symposium Monograph 2, pp. 9–32. Wistar Institute Press, Philadelphia, 1964.

CLARK, S. L., JR. The synthesis and storage of protein by isolated lymphoid cells, examined by autoradiography with the electron microscope. Am. J. Anat. 119:375–404, 1966.

COONS, A. H., LEDUC, E. H., AND CONNOLLY, J. M. Studies on antibody formation. J. Exp. Med. 102:49–60, 1955.

EVERETT, N. B., AND TYLER (CAFFREY), R. W. Lymphopoiesis in the thymus and other tissues: functional implications. Int. Rev. Cytol. 22:205–237, 1967.

FORD, C. E., MICKLEM, H. S., EVANS, E. P., GRAY, J. G., AND OGDEN, D. A. The inflow of bone marrow cells to the thymus. Studies with part-body irradiated mice injected with chromosome marked bone marrow and subjected to antigen stimulation. Ann. N. Y. Acad. Sci. 129:283–296, 1966.

GOOD, R. A., AND GABRIELSON, A. E. (editors) The Thymus in Immunology. Hoeber Medical Division, Harper & Row, New York, 1964.

HARTMANN, A. Die Milz. In Handb. mikr. Anat. Menschen (v. Möllendorff, editor), vol. 6, pt. 1, pp. 397–563. Springer-Verlag, Berlin, 1930.

HAYES, T. G. The marginal zone and marginal sinus in the spleen of the gerbil. A light and electron microscopy study. J. Morphol. 141:205–216, 1973.

HELMANN, T. Die Lymphknötchen und die Lymphknoten. In Handb. mikr. Anat. Menschen (v.

Möllendorff, editor), vol. 6, pt. 1, pp. 233–396. Springer-Verlag, Berlin, 1930.

HOSTETLER, J. R., AND ACKERMAN, G. A. Lymphopoiesis and lymph node histogenesis in the embryonic and neonatal rabbit. Am. J. Anat. 124:57–76, 1969.

KALPAKTSOGLOU, P. K., YUNIS, E. J., AND GOOD, R. A. The role of the thymus in development of lympho-hemopoietic tissues. The effect of thymectomy on development of blood cells, bone marrow, spleen and lymph nodes. Anat. Rec. 164:267–282, 1969.

KINGSBURY, B. F. Lymphatic tissue and regressive structure, with particular reference to degeneration of glands. Am. J. Anat. 77:159–188, 1945.

KLEMPERER, P. The spleen. In Handbook of Hematology (Downey, H., editor), vol. 3, pp. 1587–1754. Paul B. Hoeber, New York, 1938.

KNISELY, M. H. Spleen studies. Anat. Rec. 65:23–50, 131–148, 1936.

MACKENZIE, D. W., WHIPPLE, A. O., AND WINTERSTEINER, M. P. Studies on the microscopic anatomy and physiology of living transilluminated mammalian spleens. Am. J. Anat. 68:397–456, 1941.

MCMASTER, P. D. Antibody formation. In The Cell; Biochemistry, Physiology, Morphology (Brachet, J., and Mirksy, A. E., editors), vol. 5, pp. 323–404. Academic Press, New York, 1966.

MILLER, J. F. A. P., MARSHALL, A. H. E., AND WHITE, R. G. The immunological significance of the thymus. Advan. Immunol. 2:111–162, 1962.

NOSSAL, G. J. V. The cellular basis of immunity. Harvey Lect. 63:179–211, 1968.

PECK, H. M., AND HOERR, N. L. The intermediary circulation in the red pulp of the mouse spleen. Anat. Rec. 109:447–478, 1951.

PETTERSEN, J. C., AND ROSE, R. J. Marginal zone and germinal center development in the spleens of neonatally thymectomized and non-thymectomized young rats. Am. J. Anat. 123:489–500, 1968.

RAVIOLA, E., AND KARNOWSKY, M. J. Evidence for a blood-thymus barrier using electron opaque tracers. J. Exp. Med. 136:466, 1972.

ROBERTS, D. K., AND LATTA, J. S. Electron microscopic studies of the red pulp of the rabbit spleen. Anat. Rec. 148:81–101, 1964.

SANEL, F. T. Ultrastructure of differentiating cells during thymus histogenesis. Z. Zellforsch. 83:8–29, 1967.

SNOOK, T. Deep lymphatics of the spleen. Anat. Rec. 94:43–56, 1946.

SNOOK, T. The histology of the vascular terminations in the rabbit spleen. Anat. Rec. 130:711–729, 1958.

SONG, S. H., AND GROOM, A. C. Scanning electron microscopic study of the splenic red pulp in relation to the sequestration of immature red cells. J. Morphol. 149:437–450, 1974.

WAKSMAN, B. H., ARNASON, B. G., AND JANKOVIĆ, B. D. Role of the thymus in immune reactions in rats. III. Changes in the lymphoid organs of thymectomized rats. J. Exp. Med. 116:187–206, 1962.

WEISS, L. Electron microscopic observations on the vascular barrier in the cortex of the thymus of the mouse. Anat. Rec. 145:413–438, 1963.

WEISS, L. The structure of the intermediate vascular pathways in the spleen of rabbits. Am. J. Anat. 113:51–92, 1963.

YOFFEY, J., AND COURTICE, F. Lymphatics, Lymph, and Lymphoid Tissue. Harvard University Press, Cambridge, 1956.

YOFFEY, J. M. (editor). Bristol Symposium: The Lymphocyte in Immunology and Haemopoiesis. Williams & Wilkins, Baltimore, 1967.

CHAPTER 14

The Integument

The integument comprises the skin that covers the entire body, together with certain accessory organs which are derivatives of the skin, such as nails, hair, and glands of various kinds.

The skin performs many important functions. It protects the body from injurious substances and desiccation, helps in the regulation of the body temperature, excretes water, fat, and some other substances, and constitutes the most extensive sense organ of the body for the reception of tactile, thermal, and painful stimuli.

The Skin

The skin or cutis consists of two main parts: (1) the *epidermis,* a stratified epithelial layer derived from the ectoderm, and (2) the *dermis, corium,* or cutis vera, a connective tissue derivative of the mesoderm. Below the dermis is a layer of loose connective tissue, the *subcutaneous tissue* (superficial fascia), which attaches the skin to the underlying organs (Fig. 14-1). In certain places this layer is so richly infiltrated with fat as to be called the *panniculus adiposus.* The subcutaneous tissue makes possible an easy movement of the skin, and where such mobility is slight or absent, as for instance in the soles, palms, and fingertips, this tissue is more dense.

The thickness of the skin varies considerably in different parts of the body. The relative proportions of epidermis and dermis vary also, and a thick skin is found in regions where there is a thickening of either or both layers. On the interscapular region of the back, where the dermis is particularly thick, the skin may be more than 5 mm in thickness, whereas on the eyelids it may be less than 0.5 mm; the usual thickness is 1 to 2 mm. The skin is generally thicker on the dorsal or extensor surfaces of the body than on the ventral or flexor surfaces, but this is not true for the hands and feet; the skin of the palms and soles is thicker than on any dorsal surface except the interscapular region. The palms and soles have a characteristically thickened epidermis, in addition to a thick dermis (Fig. 14-1). The epidermis of these regions is not only thicker than that of other regions but also differs structurally from the thin epidermis present elsewhere.

The whole surface of the skin is traversed by numerous fine furrows which run in definite directions and cross each other to bound small fields of a rhomboid or rectangular form. These furrows correspond to similar ones on the surface of the dermis so that, in section, the boundary line between epidermis and dermis appears wavy. On the thick skin of the palms and soles, the fields form long, narrow ridges separated by parallel coursing furrows, and in the fingertips these ridges are arranged in the complicated loops, whorls, and spirals that give the fingerprints characteristic for each individual. In those regions where the epidermis is thickest, these ridges are more prominent.

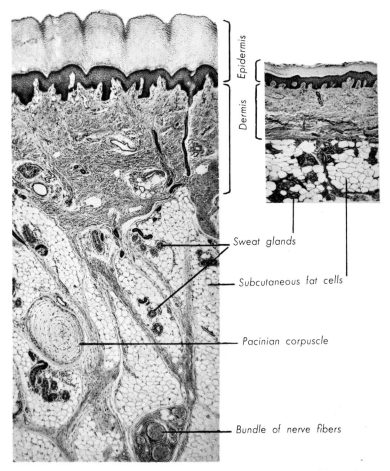

Fig. 14-1. Low power photomicrographs of vertical sections of skin. Thick skin from fingertip at *left*; skin of medium thickness from dorsal surface of finger at *right*. The fields shown do not include the total thickness of the subcutaneous tissue. ×30.

Each of the epidermal ridges of the palms and soles has an underlying ridge of connective tissue known as the *primary dermal ridge*. Each primary ridge is divided into *secondary* dermal ridges by a downward projection of epidermis known as a *rete peg* because it appears peglike in sections (Fig. 14-1). The secondary dermal ridges appear as papillary-like elevations in sections and are known as *papillae* (Figs. 14-1 and 14-2). In the palms and soles, the dermal papillae are numerous, tall, and often branched, varying in height from 0.05 to 0.2 mm. They are likewise numerous and tall in the lips, clitoris, penis, labia minora, and nipples. Where the mechanical demands are slight and the epidermis is thinner, as in the skin of the abdomen, chin, and face, the papillae are low and few in number.

The Epidermis

The epidermis is composed of stratified squamous epithelium the thickness of which varies in different parts of the body.

Epidermis of Palms and Soles. The epidermis of the palms, soles, and volar surfaces of the digits is particularly thick and highly differentiated. In these regions, several components can be identified: (1) the *stratum basale* (*stratum cylindricum*), (2) *stratum spinosum*, (3) *stratum granulosum*, (4) *stratum lucidum*, and (5) *stratum corneum* (Figs. 14-2 and 14-3). The stratum basale and stratum spinosum together compose the *stratum Malpighii*. Mitoses occur chiefly in the basal cells and only occasionally in the spinous layer. When a cell of the basal layer divides, one daughter cell moves upward and begins to

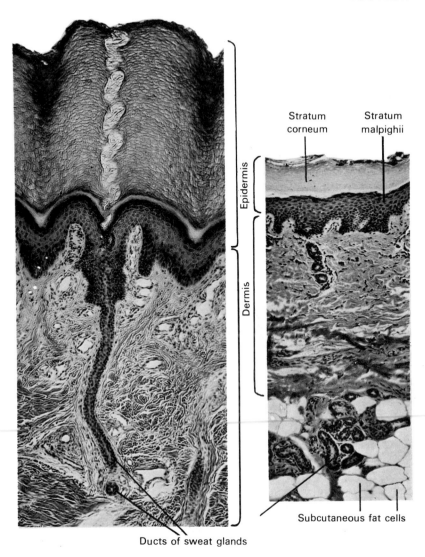

Fig. 14-2. Photomicrographs of vertical sections of skin, showing thick epidermis from fingertip, at *left,* and thinner epidermis from dorsal surface of finger, at *right.* ×94.

differentiate while the other remains undifferentiated. The time occupied from the beginning of differentiation to the loss of the cell at the surface is a matter of weeks (or months) and is quite different for different regions of the body. The process is greatly accelerated after injury. The turnover time is more rapid in rodents and can occur in about 20 days.

The *stratum basale* consists of columnar or high cuboidal cells arranged in a single layer (*stratum cylindricum*) which rests on a basement membrane composed of a basal lamina and lamina reticularis, as described in chapter 4. The lamina reticularis portion

of the basement membrane of light microscopy is relatively thin in mammals but is thicker and more complex in some of the lower animals. Electron micrographs show that the border of the cell and of its underlying basement membrane follows an irregular course. They show slender strands of connective tissue penetrating spaces between infoldings of the cell membrane, and they show hemidesmosomes at the base of the cells. Adherence between the epithelium and its underlying connective tissue is aided by the irregularity of the boundary between the two tissues and by the hemidesmosomes.

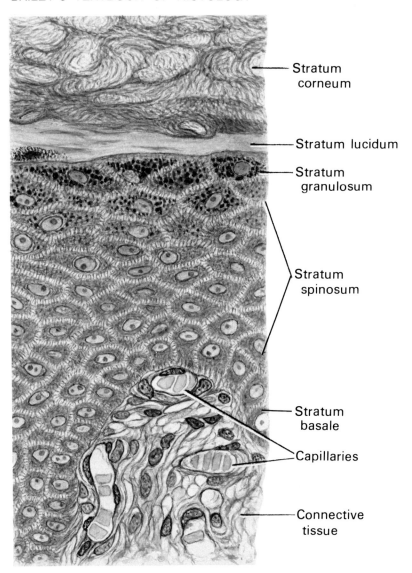

Stratum corneum

Stratum lucidum

Stratum granulosum

Stratum spinosum

Stratum basale

Capillaries

Connective tissue

Fig. 14-3. Vertical section of thick epidermis of fingertip as seen under the oil immersion objective. The field includes only a small fraction of the total thickness of the stratum corneum and does not include all of the stratum spinosum at the sides of the connective tissue papilla. ×700.

The *stratum spinosum* is composed of cells of polygonal shape. The plasma membranes of adjacent cells are normally in close apposition throughout most of their extent, but they tend to pull apart, except in the region of the desmosomes (Figs. 4-4 and 4-5), when the cells shrink during technical procedures used in the preparation of routine sections. Thus, the cells seen in sections have an irregular outline, with delicate processes or spines projecting from their surface. For this reason, these cells are often called "prickle cells" and the whole region is known as the *stratum spinosum*. Before electron microscope studies, it was thought by some histologists that the spinous processes formed protoplasmic connections between cells, the so-called intercellular bridges. Electron micrographs show that the points of apposition between epidermal cells do not represent bridges of protoplasmic continuity but typical *maculae adherens* or *desmosomes* (Chapter 4, Fig. 4-4).

The nuclei of the cells of the stratum Malpighii are deeply chromatic. Their shape varies with that of the cells, being ovoid in the stratum basale and round in the stratum spinosum. The cytoplasm of the cells of the stratum Malpighii is basophilic in its staining reaction, particularly in the deeper cell layers. There is evidence that this is correlated with the ribosomal content of the cytoplasm and hence with active protein synthesis. Electron micrographs show that the cytoplasm of the cells contains numerous fine filaments of about 60 to 80 Å in diameter. Bundles of the filaments are randomly distributed throughout the cytoplasm, and they are found consistently in the cytoplasm adjacent to the desmosomes, often coursing toward these points of cell adhesion (Fig. 4-5). Aggregates of the filaments are visible with the light microscope and, as such, they were originally described by light microscopists as *tonofibrils*. In keeping with this terminology, the individual filaments seen with the electron microscope are often called *tonofilaments*. The epidermal filaments of the deeper cells become the fibrous elements of the filament-matrix complex of the stratum corneum.

Electron micrographs show that the cells of the stratum spinosum contain a variable number of rounded or ovoid granules that are membrane-bounded; these are relatively small and are known as membrane-coating granules. It is thought that they are partially secreted into the intercellular material and that they also contribute to a thickening of the inner surface of the cell membrane that occurs by the time the cells reach the stratum lucidum.

The stratum Malpighii also contains pigment granules that are more readily seen in black than in white races. The cells that form the pigment, known as melanocytes, are described below under "Color of the Skin." Another cell type, known as the Langerhan's cell, can be demonstrated by a gold chloride technique. It was once thought to represent worn-out melanocytes, but this is apparently incorrect; its function remains controversial. Still another type, known as the *Merkel cell*, is present. It stains somewhat differently but is not readily identified in routine preparations. It is associated with the nerve endings of the tactile corpuscle of Merkel, (chapter 10).

The *stratum granulosum* consists of two to five rows of flattened, rhombic cells with their long axes parallel with the surface of the skin (Figs. 14-3 and 14-4). The cytoplasm contains numerous *keratohyalin* granules that stain intensely with hematoxylin. These should not be mistaken for pigment granules, which have color in the natural, unstained state. Electron micrographs show that the keratohyalin granules which appear so well defined under the light microscope are actually irregularly shaped masses of electron-dense material in close association with bundles of filaments. Chemical studies have shown that the keratohyalin granules are relatively rich in proline and in sulfur-containing amino acids. These granules are the precursors of the amorphous portion of the filament-matrix complex of stratum corneum.

The *stratum lucidum* is a thin, lightly staining zone located between the stratum granulosum and the cornified surface layer. The lucidum is readily seen in the epidermis of the palms and soles but is usually not identifiable in most parts of the body. The nuclei begin to degenerate in the outer cells of the granulosa layer and disappear in the lucidum. The cytoplasm of the cells is said to contain a refractile substance known as eleidin, but little is known about this. Electron micrographs show that the tonofilaments are more aggregated and arranged in a more orderly fashion than in the granulosum cells and that the cell membranes are increased in thickness. There is also an increased amount of intercellular material.

The *stratum corneum* is very thick in the palms and soles and is composed of clear, dead, scalelike cells which become more and more flattened as the surface is approached, the most peripheral layer containing flat, horny plates which are constantly desquamated. The cells have a thickened membrane, as noted above, and they are closely interdigitated. The nuclei have disappeared, but some of the spaces that they occupied can be seen.

The cytoplasm has been replaced by keratin proteins. Electron micrographs show

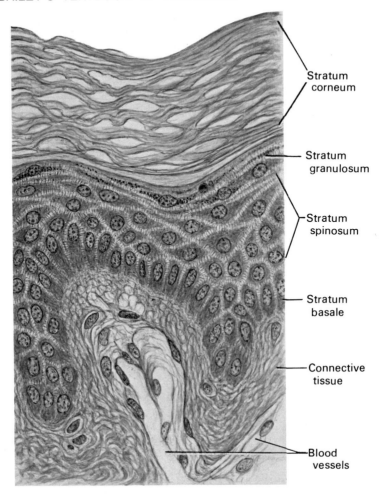

Fig. 14-4. Vertical section of relatively thin epidermis from the median side of the lower extremity. The field includes the total thickness of the stratum corneum. The stratum corneum is very much thinner than that of the fingertip. The stratum granulosum is also thinner than that of thick epidermis and the stratum lucidum is barely discernible. Compare with Figure 14-3. ×700.

that these dead cells are composed of filaments tightly packed in orthogonal arrays that lie parallel to the skin surface and embedded in an opaque, electron-dense, interfilamentous material. Desmosomes, although modified, persist and are thought to play a role in the spatial arrangement. The structural changes in the keratinization process involve changes in the aggregation and arrangement of filaments, the formation of keratohyalin granules as the precursors of the interfilamentous material of keratin, and the loss of cell organelles after the keratohyalin granules have reached their maximal size. The structural changes in the cells as they move from the stratum basale to the cornified layer are

correlated with chemical changes. These include the formation of disulfide groups in keratin from sulfhydryl groups in the filaments of the deeper layers.

The thickened membranes or husks which envelop the horny cells are resistant to keratinolytic agents and provide integrity for the filament-matrix complex within the cell. The filamentous portion of the complex, derived from protein synthesis with the basal epidermal cells, provides for flexibility and elastic recovery of the cell content. The amorphous portion of the filament-matrix complex, derived from keratohyalin granules, is primarily responsible for the chemical resistance of the horny cells.

The cornified layer of the epidermis is composed of *"soft keratin,"* as contrasted with *"hard keratin,"* found in the nails and in the cortex of the hairs. Hard keratin contains relatively more sulfur, is less elastic, and is more permanent, in the sense that it does not desquamate, as does the epidermis.

The peripheral region of the stratum corneum which is constantly being desquamated is often referred to as the *stratum disjunctum.* The desquamated cells are replaced by new cells that formed by mitosis in the germinative layers and moved toward the surface during the process of keratinization.

Epidermis of the General Body Surface. The epidermis of the rest of the body is considerably thinner than that of the palms, soles, and volar surfaces of the digits. All layers of the epidermis are reduced, and the stratum corneum and stratum Malpighii are the only layers that are constantly present in all parts of the body. A thin stratum granulosum, composed of only one or two cell rows, is frequently present, but a definite stratum lucidum is generally absent. The structure varies with the region studied. On the leg, for example (Fig. 14-4), where the epidermis is thicker than that of abdominal or pubic skin yet much thinner than that of the fingertip, a faint stratum lucidum may be found. The reduction in the thickness of layers in thin epidermis is probably due to the fact that keratinization is far less marked and occurs not as a continuous process, but only at certain times.

Color of the Skin. The color of the skin is dependent upon the blood in the capillaries of the connective tissue beneath the epidermis and on the presence of varying amounts of *melanin* pigment. Certain patches of skin, such as the circumanal region, the areolae and nipples, the axilla, the labia majora, the penis, and the scrotum, are especially rich in pigment, whereas practically no pigment is present in the palms and soles. The pigment is stored in the form of granules dispersed chiefly within the cells of the Malpighian layer.

Melanin is formed in specialized cells known as *melanocytes,* which differentiate from *melanoblasts* that migrate from the neutral crest to the dermoepidermal junction during embryonic development. The melanoblasts and melanocytes both lack tonofilaments and desmosomes, and melanoblasts also lack pigment granules. Several intermediate stages can be recognized in the differentiation of a melanocyte from a melanoblast. Morphological differentiation involves a change from the relatively round melanoblasts and premelanocytes to the melanocytes which have numerous long processes. In the cytological and cytochemical differentiation, the polypeptides, which eventually become tyrosinase, are synthesized in association with ribosomes and are transferred to the region of the Golgi complex, where they are condensed and packaged into units surrounded by membranes. Next, the protyrosinase molecules become arranged in an orderly manner in the membrane-bounded units, giving the latter a lamellar pattern in electron micrographs. The units at this stage of differentiation have dimensions of about 0.7 by 0.3 μm and are known as premelanosomes. When the protyrosinase becomes activated as tyrosinase, melanin biosynthesis begins, and the units which now contain melanin in addition to tyrosinase are known as *melanosomes.* The melanin continues to increase in the melanosomes until the latter are transformed into amorphous melanin granules that lack the lamellar pattern seen in electron micrographs of melanosomes; they also lack demonstrable tyrosinase. The differentiation of melanosomes is accompanied by a change in their intracellular position: the premelanosomes appear in the region of the Golgi complex, the melanosomes appear in the basal portion of the cytoplasmic cell processes, and the melanin granules are chiefly in the peripheral portions of the processes. Thus, the body or perikaryon of the melanocyte is relatively free of melanin and appears relatively clear in routine preparations, whereas the processes contain melanin granules. From the melanocyte processes, the melanin granules are distributed to the cytoplasm of the epidermal cells of the Malpighian layer.

The African and Mongoloid races have a somewhat higher number of melanocytes than the white race has, but the difference in color is due chiefly to the manner in which the pigment is dispersed. In the white race, the total amount of melanin is concentrated chiefly within the deepest portion of the Malpighian layer, whereas it is dispersed in numerous granules spread throughout the Malpighian layer in the black race.

The melanocytes can be identified by their reaction to the "dopa" reagent, dihydroxyphenylalanine: they oxidize the solution and stain black. The intracellular substance responsible for the reaction is tyrosinase, the oxidative enzyme responsible for synthesis of melanin from tyrosine. It should be noted that the dopa reaction does not occur for the fully formed melanin granules present in the epidermal cells of the Malpighian layer, or in dermal chromatophores which have obtained their pigment by phagocytosis of melanin synthesized by melanogenic cells. As noted earlier, the mature melanin granules lack tyrosinase, which is presumably the oxidase responsible for the dopa reaction.

The cell bodies of the melanocytes are normally confined to the basal layer of the epidermis, near their place of origin from the primitive melanoblasts. However, melanocyte processes extend for some distance between epidermal cells. When melanin formation is stimulated, e.g., by ultraviolet radiation, or by X-irradiation, the cell bodies of the melanocytes also appear in the suprabasal layers of the epidermis.

The melanocytes supposedly wear out and slough off with the epidermal scales, but their number is maintained by proliferation of cells which are presumably melanocytes in an active phase of melanogenesis.

The Dermis or Corium

The dermis varies from 0.2 to 4 mm in thickness and is composed of dense, irregularly arranged connective tissue. It contains the three types of connective tissue fibers and fibroblasts and histiocytes. Two layers can be distinguished, although they blend without distinct demarcation. The deeper one is relatively thick and is known as the reticular layer. The superficial layer is thinner and is named the subepithelial or papillary layer.

The *reticular layer* is characterized by coarse collagenous fibers and fiber bundles which often unite to form secondary bundles of considerable thickness (nearly 100 μm in diameter). The fibers cross each other to form an extensive feltwork with rhomboid meshes, the direction of the fibers generally being parallel to the surface of the skin. The elastic fibers form complex elastic nets permeating the entire dermis. Here too the course of the main fibers is parallel with the surface, although vertical and oblique fibers are present in considerable number. The elastic fibers form basket-like, capsular condensations around the hair bulbs, and sweat and sebaceous glands.

The *papillary* or *subepithelial layer* is similar in structure to the reticular layer, but the fibers are finer and more closely arranged.

Although the connective tissue fibers of the dermis form complex nets and meshes, those bundles which course parallel with the lines of tension of the skin are more numerous and better developed than the others. The lines of skin tension, which are caused by the direction of the predominant fibers, are known as *Langer's lines*. These lines have different directions in the various parts of the body. Their direction is of surgical importance because incisions made parallel with the lines gape less and heal with less scar tissue than do incisions made across the lines.

As has been mentioned, the surface of the dermis is studded by numerous papillae that indent the underside of the epidermis. These papillae vary in structure and content. Some are simple; others are branched. Some contain loops of capillary blood vessels (vascular papillae); others contain special nerve terminations (nervous papillae) (Fig. 10-51).

In addition to the usual types of connective tissue cells, the dermis of certain regions may contain a few branched, pigmented connective tissue cells, the *dermal chromatophores,* which resemble the pigmented cells of the choroid coat of the eye. The dermal chromatophores are normally scarce in the white race. They occur chiefly in regions where the epidermis itself is richly pigmented, and their pigment is apparently obtained from melanogenic cells of neural crest origin.

Smooth muscle is found in the skin in

connection with the hair (*arrector pili* muscles). Smooth muscle fibers also occur in considerable number in the skin of the nipple, prepuce, glans penis, scrotum (tunica dartos), and parts of the perineum. The fibers are arranged in a network parallel to the surface, and contraction of the fibers gives the skin of these regions its wrinkled appearance. In the face and neck, skeletal muscle fibers from the mimic musculature likewise penetrate the dermis. Both smooth and skeletal fibers end in delicate, elastic bands that are continuous with the general elastic network of the dermis.

Glands of the Skin

Two kinds of glands occur in the skin: sweat glands and sebaceous glands.

Sweat Glands (Glandulae Sudoriferae)

Most of the sweat glands are of the eccrine (merocrine) type; i.e., the product of the cell is secreted without destruction of any part of the cell. Eccrine sweat glands are found over the entire body surface, excepting the margin of the lips, the ear drum, the inner surface of the prepuce, and the glans penis. They are most numerous in the palms and soles and are the only glands found in these places. They are simple, coiled, tubular glands. The deepest portion of the sweat gland is secretory and hence is known as the *secretory tubule*. It is quite coiled and it frequently, but not invariably, begins in the subcutaneous tissue. The secretory tubule drains into the *coiled duct* which continues into a *straight* or *oblique duct* that passes through the dermis to contact the epidermis between two dermal papillae (Fig. 14-2). The *intraepidermal channel* takes a spiral course to the surface, where it opens via a minute pit just barely visible to the naked eye.

Although the nuclei of the cells of the secretory portion of the sweat gland are located at different levels (Figs. 14-5, 14-6*A*, and 14-7), the epithelium is classified as simple columnar because all cells extend from the basal lamina to the lumen or to intercellular canaliculi continuous with the lumen (Fig. 14-6*A*). Two types of cells have been described: *clear* and *dark*. The *clear*

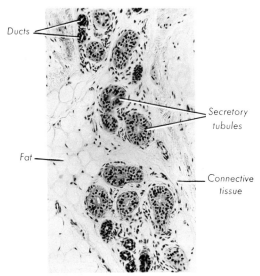

Fig. 14-5. Section of sweat glands of human fingertip. Field shown is at junction of dermis and subcutaneous tissue. Photomicrograph. ×110.

cells are somewhat pyramidal in shape, with a broad base on the basal lamina, whereas the *dark cells* are broader at the luminal surface and slender toward the basal lamina. Electron micrographs show that both types of cells have irregularly arranged and short cytoplasmic processes at the luminal surface and around the cell, including the basal portion that rests on the basal lamina. Electron micrographs also show that the cytoplasm of the *clear cells* contains a considerable amount of smooth endoplasmic reticulum, numerous mitochondria, and an abundance of glycogen, but very few ribosomes. On the other hand, the cytoplasm of the *dark cells* has very few mitochondria but numerous ribosomes and a number of secretory vacuoles which contain protein polysaccharides.

The secretory portion also contains *myoepithelial cells*. These cells are stellate in shape, are contractile, and have processes which bear some ultrastructural resemblance to smooth muscle cells. They differ from smooth muscle in being ectodermal in origin and in not being surrounded completely by an external lamina. It is assumed that their contractions aid in movement of secretions toward the duct.

The chief components of the sweat released by the secretory tubule are water

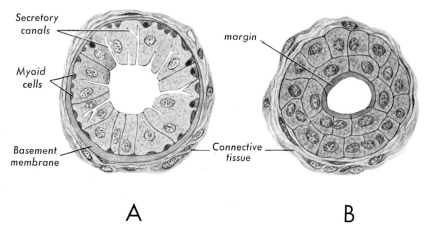

Fig. 14-6. Sections through a terminal secretory tubule (*A*) and a duct (*B*) of a sweat gland. Myoepithelial (*myoid*) cells are seen between the secretory cells and the basement membrane in *A*. ×650. (Redrawn and slightly modified from Schaffer.)

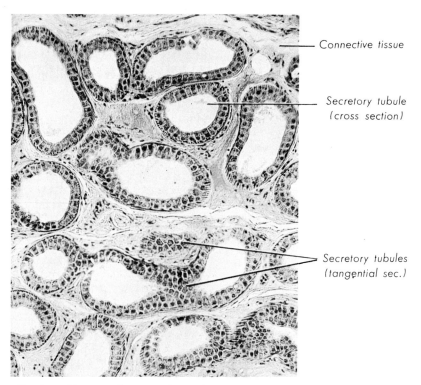

Fig. 14-7. Section of human circumanal glands. Note that these glands are much larger than the typical sweat glands illustrated in Figure 14-5. ×110.

and sodium chloride plus urea, ammonia, uric acid, and protein polysaccharides. The clear cells apparently function in releasing water, sodium chloride, urea, etc., whereas the dark cells apparently secrete protein polysaccharides.

The *duct* of the sweat gland has a wall composed of a two-layered stratified cuboidal epithelium resting on a basal lamina surrounded by connective tissue cells and fibers (Fig. 14-6*B*). It does not have myoepithelial cells. The cells of the inner layer of the duct have a refractile apical border which is acidophilic. Electron micrographs show that the border is composed of irregularly shaped microvilli that are particularly numerous in the coiled portion of the duct. The microvilli contain closely packed microfilaments that project downward in the cytoplasm, where they become aggregated in a manner similar to that of the terminal web of many other types of epithelial cells (chapter 4). After the duct reaches the epidermis, it loses its own wall and becomes a channel through the epidermis (Fig. 14-2). The ducts have an important function in addition to that of conduction: they resorb sodium without water following. Thus, sweat becomes hypotonic as it passes through the duct.

Particularly large sweat glands of a special type are located in the axilla, mammary areola, labia majora, and circumanal regions. These are known as *apocrine* or *odoriferous* glands (Figs. 14-7 and 14-8). The ceruminous glands of the external auditory meatus and the glands of Moll in the margins of the eyelid also belong to this general type. The apocrine glands received their name because some light microscope studies gave the erroneous impression that some of the secretion is produced by the apical ends of the cells breaking off. These results were probably artifacts of poor fixation.

The *apocrine gland secretory tubules* differ from those of merocrine glands in a number of respects. They are wider, they branch, and their myoepithelial cells are more prominent (compare Figs. 14-5 and 14-7). Electron micrographs indicate that there is probably only one parenchymal cell type in the apocrine glands and that it differs from both the light and dark cells of merocrine glands but resembles the dark cells more than the light ones. Its microvilli are more numerous and more prominent than those of merocrine glands; it has nu-

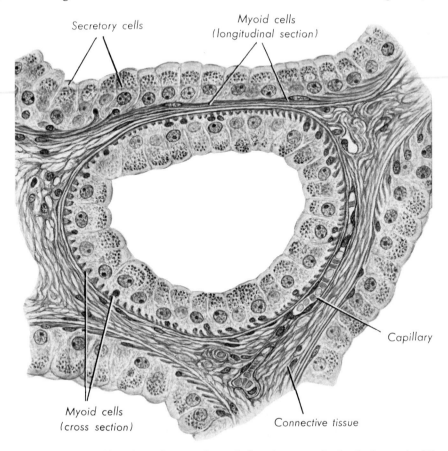

Fig. 14-8. Higher magnification of a portion of the circumanal gland shown in Figure 14-7, showing prominent secretory granules. ×420.

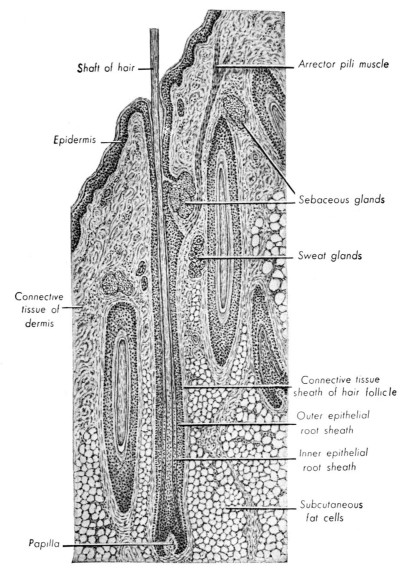

Shaft of hair

Arrector pili muscle

Epidermis

Sebaceous glands

Sweat glands

Connective
tissue of
dermis

Connective tissue
sheath of hair follicle

Outer epithelial
root sheath

Inner epithelial
root sheath

Subcutaneous
fat cells

Papilla

Fig. 14-9. Vertical section of human scalp, showing a longitudinal section of a hair and its follicle. Reconstructed from serial sections to show a complete follicle cut through its longitudinal axis. ×36.

merous mitochondria, lysosomes that contain lipofuscin, and vacuoles which contain considerable protein polysaccharide. The *ducts* of the apocrine glands resemble those of the merocrine glands in that they lack myoepithelial cells, but they differ in that they open into the cavity of the hair follicle rather than by an intraepidermal channel. Their secretion is also more viscous than that of the ordinary sweat glands.

The apocrine glands become functional at about the time of puberty, apparently as a result of the influence of sex hormones.

Their secretion is odorless when it is released but quickly develops a characteristic odor after contamination by bacteria. The apocrine glands respond to adrenergic stimuli, whereas the merocrine glands respond chiefly to cholinergic stimuli.

Sebaceous Glands

These are usually associated with the hair follicles and are described in that connection.

The Hair

The hairs are elastic, horny threads developed from the epidermis. They are placed in deep narrow pits or pockets that traverse the dermis to varying depths and usually extend into the subcutaneous tissue (Fig. 14-9). Each hair consists of a *shaft* that projects above the surface and a *root* that is imbedded within the skin. At its lower end, the root of the hair is expanded into a knoblike structure known as the *hair bulb* which is composed of a *matrix* of epithelial cells that are beginning to differentiate along different lines. The hair bulb is indented on its undersurface by a *papilla* of connective tissue. The hair root, i.e., all of the hair embedded within the skin, is enclosed by the *hair follicle,* which consists of an epidermal (epithelial) portion and an outer, dermal (connective tissue) portion.

Structure of the Hair

The hair is composed entirely of epithelial cells, which are arranged in three definite layers: the medulla, cortex, and cuticle.

The *medulla* forms the central axis of the hair, varying in thickness from 16 to 20 μm. It consists of two or three layers of cells which vary in appearance in different parts of the hair. In the lower portion of the root of the hair, the cells are cuboidal and have rounded nuclei (Fig. 14-10). In the shaft, the cells of the medulla are cornified and shrunken and the nuclei are rudimentary or absent (Fig. 14-11, *A* and *B*). The intercellular spaces are usually filled with air. The medulla is absent from the finer, shorter (lanugo) hairs and also from some of the hairs of the scalp. It frequently fails to extend the whole length of the hair.

The *cortex* makes up the main bulk of the hair and consists of several layers of cells. In the lower part of the root of the hair, the cortex is composed of cuboidal cells with nuclei of normal appearance (Fig. 14-10). The cells become progressively flattened and modified at higher levels. In the upper part of the root of the hair and in the shaft, the cortex is composed of cornified, elongated cells with longitudinally striated cytoplasm and shrunken, degenerated nuclei (Fig. 14-11). In colored hair, pigment granules are found in and between the cells. Air also accumulates in the intercellular spaces and modifies the hair color.

The *cuticle* of the hair is exceedingly thin and is composed of a single layer of clear cells. In the deeper part of the hair root, the cuticular cells are nucleated (Fig. 14-10). In the upper part of the root and on the shaft, the cuticular cells are clear, scalelike, and nonnucleated (Fig. 14-11). The cells overlap like shingles on a roof, giving the surface of the hair a serrated appearance.

The color of the hair is determined primarily by the amount and distribution of pigment but to some extent also by the presence of air, because the latter appears white in reflected light. Hair in which the pigment has faded and the medulla has become filled with air appears silvery white.

Hair Follicle

The hair follicle consists of the inner and outer epithelial root sheaths, derived from the epidermis, and the connective tissue sheaths, derived from the dermis.

The *inner epithelial root sheath* is composed of three distinct layers: the cuticle of the root sheath, Huxley's layer, and Henle's layer.

The *cuticle of the root sheath* lies against the cuticle of the hair and is similar to the latter in structure (Fig. 14-10). It consists of thin, scalelike, overlapping cells, nucleated in the deeper parts of the sheath and nonnucleated nearer the surface. The free edges of the scales project downward and interdigitate with the upward projecting edges of the hair cuticle.

Huxley's layer lies immediately outside the cuticle of the root sheath and consists of several rows of elongated cells whose protoplasm contains eleidin-like granules (trichohyalin). In the deeper portion of the hair follicle, these cells contain nuclei (Fig. 14-12). Nearer the surface the nuclei are rudimentary or absent (Fig. 14-11C).

Henle's layer is a row of rectangular, somewhat flattened, clear cells. The cytoplasm contains longitudinal horny fibrils, and nuclei are present only in the deepest portions of the follicle (Figs. 14-10 and 14-12). Between the cells are sometimes seen short, wedgelike processes which extend from the cells of Huxley's layer.

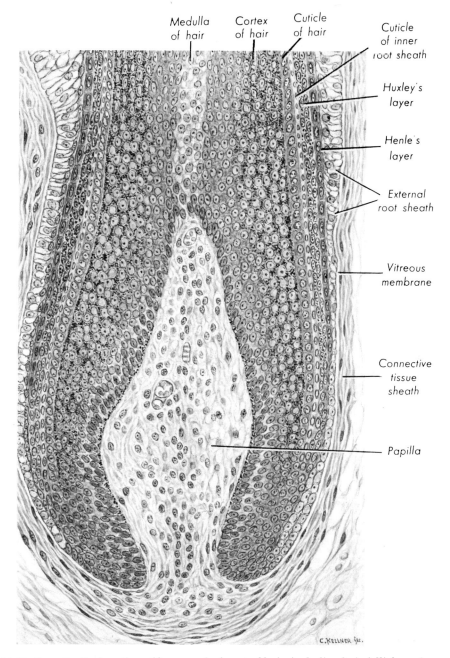

Fig. 14-10. Longitudinal section of lower end of root of hair, including hair follicle and connective tissue papilla. ×310.

The *outer epithelial root sheath* is a direct continuation of the Malpighian layer of the epidermis, to which it corresponds in structure. The outermost cells, adjacent to the connective tissue, are tall and arranged in a single row (the stratum cylindricum). The rest of the cells are more polygonal in shape. They have spinous processes and resemble the prickle cells already described for the stratum spinosum of the skin.

The *connective tissue sheath* is derived from the dermis and consists of an inner, a middle, and an outer layer.

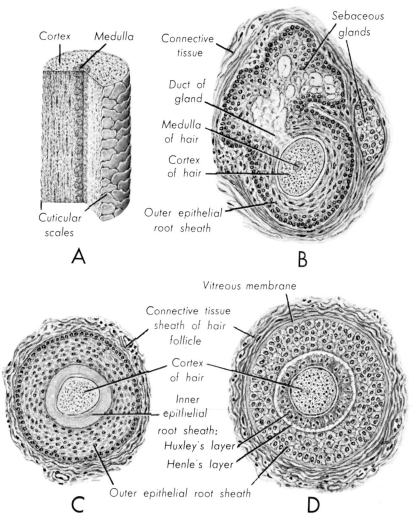

Fig. 14-11. Structure of hair and hair follicles from human scalp. *A*, a portion of the shaft of a hair reconstructed from a surface view and from longitudinal sections. *B, C*, and *D*, cross sections of hairs and their follicles at various levels: *B*, at the level of the sebaceous glands; *C*, midway between epidermis of scalp and papilla of hair root; *D*, through the lower one-third of follicle. No medulla was present in the hairs illustrated in *C* and *D*. *A*, ×280; *B, C*, and *D*, ×175.

The inner layer is a homogeneous, narrow band, the hyaline or *vitreous membrane,* and is closely applied to the cylindrical cells of the outer root sheath. The middle layer is thickest and is composed of fine connective tissue fibers which are arranged circularly. The outer layer is poorly defined and consists of rather coarse, loosely woven bundles of white fibers which run in a longitudinal direction.

In the deeper portion of the root, some little distance above the bulb, all of the layers of the hair and its follicles can be distinctly seen. The differentiation of the layers becomes less marked as one passes in either direction. At the level of entrance of the ducts of the sebaceous glands (Fig. 14-9), the inner epithelial root sheath disappears and the outer root sheath passes over into the Malpighian layer of the epidermis. The connective tissue follicle ceases as a distinct structure at about the level of insertion of the *arrector pili* muscles.

Marked changes are also noted as the bulb is approached. The outer root sheath thins down to two and finally to one layer

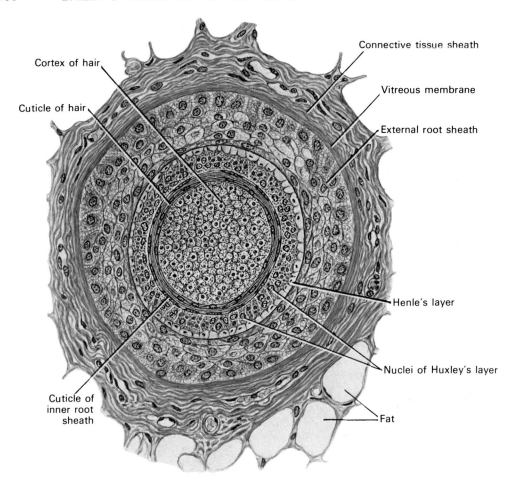

Cortex of hair

Connective tissue sheath

Cuticle of hair

Vitreous membrane

External root sheath

Henle's layer

Nuclei of Huxley's layer

Cuticle of inner root sheath

Fat

Fig. 14-12. Transverse section through root of hair and hair follicle. ×334.

of rather flat cells and then disappears. The layers of the inner root sheath retain their identity until the neck of the papilla is reached, at which point the different layers coalesce.

The bulbous thickening of the hair root which surrounds the papilla is not organized into layers but constitutes a matrix of growing, multiplying cells that superficially become transformed into the horny cells of the hair and the inner root sheath. Laterally, the cells of the bulb become continuous with the outer root sheath, which, like the Malpighian layer of the epidermis, grows by mitosis of cells in the deeper layers, i.e., the external layers of the root sheath. Thus, the growth of the outer root sheath is radial, whereas the hair and inner root sheath grow upward from the thickened base of the follicle. The hair papilla, although much larger, is similar in structure to other dermal papillae and contains delicate elastic and collagenous fibrils, cellular elements, blood vessels, and nerves.

Muscles and Glands of the Hair Follicle

The erectors of the hairs (*arrectores pilorum*) are oblique bands of smooth muscle fibers, from 50 to 220 μm in diameter, which arise in the subepithelial tissue and are usually inserted in the connective tissue follicle of the hair, about the middle of the follicle or a little above. Each muscle, at its origin, is attached to several delicate connective tissue strands, runs for a distance as a compact bundle, and then divides into several bundles that go to the individual hairs of a hair group. The muscles usually arch around the sebaceous glands which fill the angle between the muscle and hair, although large sebaceous glands occasionally penetrate the muscle. The thickness of the muscle bands corresponds roughly to the thickness and length of the hair. They are poorly developed in the hairs of the axilla and in certain parts of the face, where the muscles of facial expression apparently take over the function of erectors. The eyebrows, eyelids, and lashes have no erectors.

The hairs and hair follicles are not perpendicular to the skin but slope distinctly. The *arrector pili* muscle is situated in the obtuse angle between the hair follicle and surface. When the muscle contracts, the hair becomes more vertical to the surface and, at the same time, a small groove appears in the skin at the place where the muscle is attached. This gives rise to the so-called "goose flesh."

The *sebaceous* glands are with few exceptions connected with the hair follicles (Fig. 14-13). They are simple or branched alveolar glands. Their size varies considerably and bears no relation to the size of the hair, the largest glands being frequently connected with the smallest hairs. The glands are spherical or ovoid in shape, and each is encapsulated in connective tissue. The excretory duct is wide and empties into the neck of the follicle. It is lined with stratified squamous epithelium continuous with the outer root sheath and the Malpighian layer of the epidermis. The lower end of the duct opens into several simple or branched alveoli, at the mouths of which the epithelium becomes thinner. The alveoli themselves are completely filled with a stratified epithelium.

The most peripheral cells are rather small and cubical in shape and occasionally show mitotic figures. Toward the interior the polyhedral or spheroidal cells become progressively larger as a result of the accumulation of numerous fat droplets in their cytoplasm. Their secretion, an oily substance called *sebum,* appears to be the direct product of disintegration of the alveolar cells (holocrine mode of secretion), and

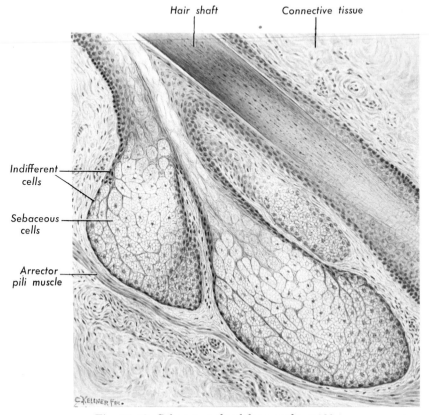

Fig. 14-13. Sebaceous gland from scalp. ×130.

all of the stages of the process are seen in the various layers of cells. The smaller peripheral cells contain only a few small fat droplets or none at all. The most central ones and those in the lumen of the duct show the most marked changes. Their cytoplasm is almost wholly converted into fat, and their nuclei are shrunken or disintegrated. In the middle zone are cells showing intermediate stages.

The replacement of cells lost in secretion is accomplished chiefly by mitotic divisions of the indifferent cells at the periphery of the gland (Fig. 14-13). The stages in this process, as well as the proliferation of new alveoli from the cells of the excretory ducts, can be demonstrated in animals in which the growth of the sebaceous glands is stimulated experimentally. In fetal development, the glands and their ducts arise by proliferation and differentiation from the outer epithelial root sheath of the hair follicle (see Fig. 14-18).

Sebaceous glands unconnected with hair follicles occur along the margin of the lips, in the nipple, in the glans and prepuce of the penis, and in the labia minora.

Replacement of Hairs

Shedding of hair takes place in most mammals at regularly recurring periods. In man there is constant although gradual loss and replacement of hairs. The scalp hairs have the longest duration of life, from 2 to 5 years, whereas those of the eyebrows and ears last only from 3 to 5 months. Even shorter is the age of the eyelashes.

When a hair is about to shed, proliferation of cells above the papilla slows down and finally ceases. The bulb develops into a solid, club-shaped mass and becomes completely keratinized; its lower end splits brushlike into numerous fibers. The club-shaped bulb, firmly fused with the lower ends of the inner root sheath, which likewise cornifies, becomes detached from the papilla and is slowly shifted toward the surface of the skin to about the level of the entrance of the sebaceous ducts. There it may remain for some time, until pulled out or shed or pushed out by a replacing hair. Such hairs are called *club hairs* to distinguish them from hairs that possess papillae.

The papilla atrophies and may completely disappear. The outer root sheath collapses and forms a cord of cells extending between the atrophied papilla and the lower end of the shedding hair.

The formation of a new hair starts with the proliferation of cells of the outer root sheath in the region of the old papilla. The papilla becomes larger and invaginates the cell mass or, according to some authors, a new papilla is formed. From this new matrix or "hair germ," the new hair develops in a manner similar to embryonal hair formation. The new hair grows toward the surface, under or to one side of the dead hair, which it finally replaces.

The Nails

The nails are composed of flat, horny scales which form protective coverings for the distal phalanges of the fingers and toes. Each nail consists of (1) a *body,* the attached uncovered portion of the nail, (2) a *free edge,* the anterior unattached extension of the body, and (3) the *nail root,* the posterior or proximal part of the nail which lies beneath a fold of the skin (Fig. 14-14). Most of the body of the nail is pink because it is sufficiently translucent to transmit the color from the underlying vascular tissue. The proximal part of the nail is whitish and is called the *lunula* because of its shape.

The fold of skin which extends around the proximal and lateral borders of the nail constitutes the *nail fold,* and the skin which lies beneath the nail forms the *nail bed.* The furrow between the nail bed and nail fold is the *nail groove* (Figs. 14-14 and 14-15).

The nail itself is hard and horny and consists of several layers of clear, flat cells that contain shrunken and degenerated nuclei. The striated appearance observed in sections cut perpendicular to the surface is produced by the arrangement of the cells in layers.

The nail bed consists of epithelium and dermis continuous with the epidermis and dermis of the skin of the nail folds. The epidermis of the nail folds usually has the zones characteristic of palmar skin, although the stratum lucidum may be thin

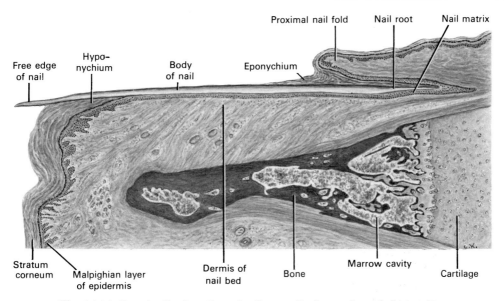

Fig. 14-14. Longitudinal section of a fingernail of a newborn infant. ×22.

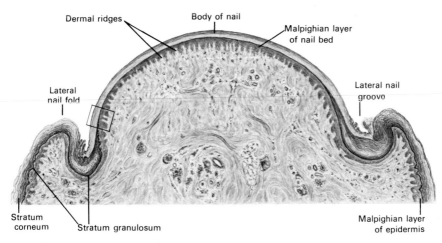

Fig. 14-15. Transverse section of nail and nail bed. Human adult. The area marked by the *square* is enlarged in Figure 14-16. ×20.

or absent in some cases. The stratum corneum of the proximal nail fold turns into the nail groove, spreads over the upper surface of the nail root, and continues for a short distance onto the surface of the body of the nail as the *eponychium* (Fig. 14-14). The stratum corneum of the lateral folds ends in the lateral grooves in contact with the borders of the nail (Figs. 14-15 and 14-16). The stratum granulosum and lucidum terminate in the lower part of the grooves.

The epithelium of the nail bed corresponds to the Malpighian layer of the skin and, like the latter, consists of polygonal prickle cells and a stratum cylindricum resting upon a basement membrane. The epithelium of the posterior part of the nail bed, the part that lies beneath the root and the proximal portion of the body corresponding to the lunula, is thicker than elsewhere and is called the *matrix* because it functions for nail growth. Growth of the nail takes place by a transformation of the more superficial cells of the matrix into true nail cells. In this process, the outer, harder layer is pushed forward over the Malpighian layer, the latter remaining al-

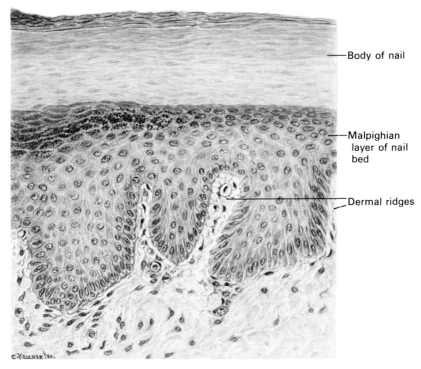

Fig. 14-16. Transverse section through the lateral part of a nail, near the lateral nail groove, as outlined in Figure 14-15. ×365.

ways in the same position. The nails generally increase in length by about 0.5 mm/week.

Under the distal free edge of the nail, the epithelium of the nail bed becomes continuous with the Malpighian layer of the skin, and the other layers characteristic of the epidermis begin. The stratum corneum of the skin beneath the free edge of the nail is thickened and is known as the *hyponychium* (Fig. 14-14).

The dermis of the nail bed differs somewhat from that of ordinary skin. Its connective tissue fibers are arranged partly longitudinal to the long axis of the nail and partly in a vertical plane extending from the periosteum to the nail. Dermal papillae are found beneath the proximal part of the nail root but disappear beneath the distal part of the root, to be replaced by longitudinal dermal ridges which, increasing in height as they pass forward, continue to the distal end of the nail bed. Because the dermal ridges run longitudinally, the boundary between the epithelium and connective tissue appears smooth in longitudinal sections and irregular and papillalike in cross sections (Fig. 14-15).

Blood Vessels, Lymphatics, and Nerves of the Skin

Blood Vessels

From the larger arteries in the subcutaneous tissue, branches penetrate the reticular layer of the dermis, where they anastomose to form cutaneous networks. The latter give off branches that pass to the papillary layer of the dermis and there form a second series of networks, the subpapillary, just beneath the papillae. From the cutaneous networks arise two sets of capillaries, one supplying the fat lobules, the other supplying the region of the sweat glands. From the subpapillary networks are given off small arteries that break up into capillary networks for the supply of the papillae, sebaceous glands, and hair follicles. The return blood from these capillaries first enters a horizontal plexus of veins just under the papillae. This communicates with a second plexus just beneath the first. Small veins from this second plexus pass alongside the arteries of the deeper part of the dermis, where they form a third plexus with larger, more irregular meshes. Into this plexus pass most of the veins from the fat lobules and sweat glands, although one or two small veins from the sweat glands usually follow the duct and empty into the subpapillary plexus. The blood next passes into a fourth plexus in the subcutaneous tissue, from which arise veins of considerable size. These accompany the arteries.

As noted in chapter 12, arteriovenous anastomoses are especially numerous in the dermis of the fingers and toes. In these areas, the arterial part of the anastomosis often forms a part of a specific organ known as a glomus. The artery is coiled or ball-like and its media contains epitheloid cells (Fig. 14-17). The internal diameter of the narrowest part of the anastomosis is usually 20 to 40 μm; thus, the anastomoses convey much more blood than capillaries do. By contraction or relaxation, they influence the amount of blood flowing through localized regions. They play an important role in conserving heat and in regulating the temperature of peripheral areas. In this respect, their high degree of development in the feet of penguins is noteworthy.

Small arteries from the plexuses of the skin and subcutis pass to the hair follicle. The larger arterioles run longitudinally in the outer layer of the follicle. From these are given off branches which form a rich plexus of small arterioles and capillaries in the middle vascular layer of the follicle. Capillaries from this plexus also pass to the sebaceous glands, the arrectores pilorum muscles, and the papillae.

Lymphatics

The lymphatics of the skin begin as capillaries within the dermal papillae and continue into a horizontal network of capillaries and small lymphatic vessels within the papillary layer of connective tissue. The lymphatics from the dermis join larger lymphatic vessels that accompany the blood vessels within the subcutaneous tissue. These become afferent lymphatic channels to lymph nodes, as described in chapter 13.

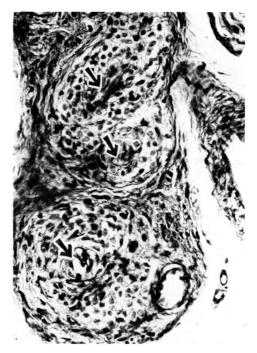

Fig. 14-17. Photomicrograph of a glomus from the dermis of thick skin. A small artery is seen at the *right* of the glomus in longitudinal and tangential section. The artery coils in the glomus and is cut at different levels (*arrows*); its wall is thickened by epithelioid cells. ×290. (From a preparation contributed by Dr. T. E. Hunt.)

For details on the course of the lymphatic vessels in different regions, reference should be made to textbooks of gross anatomy.

Nerves

The nerves of the skin are mainly sensory. Efferent sympathetic axons supply the smooth muscle of the walls of the blood vessels, the arrectores pilorum, and the secretory cells of the sweat glands. The sensory nerves are peripheral processes of somatic ganglion cells. The larger trunks lie in the subcutis, giving off branches which pass to the dermis, where they form a rich subpapillary plexus of both myelinated and nonmyelinated fibers. From the subcutaneous nerve trunks and from the subpapillary plexus are given off fibers which terminate in more or less elaborate special nerve endings (chapter 10). Their location is as follows. (1) *In the subcutaneous tissue*: Vater-Pacinian corpuscles. They are most numerous in the palms and soles. (2) *In the dermis*: tactile corpuscles of Meissner are found in the papillae, especially of the fingertip, palm, and sole. Krause's end bulbs are usually in the dermis just beneath the papillae, more rarely in the papillae themselves. (3) *In the epithelium*: free nerve endings among the epithelial cells.

Branches of the cutaneous nerves supply the hair follicles, which are important in sensory reception. As a rule, only one nerve passes to each follicle, entering it just below the entrance of the duct of the sebaceous gland. As it enters the follicle, the nerve fiber loses its myelin sheath and divides into two branches, which further subdivide to form a ringlike plexus of fine fibers encircling the follicle. From this ring, small varicose fibrils run for a short distance up the follicle, terminating mainly in slight expansions on the vitreous membrane.

Development of the Skin and its Appendages

The *epidermis* develops from the ectoderm and consists at first of a single row of cuboidal cells. By the 2nd month it has

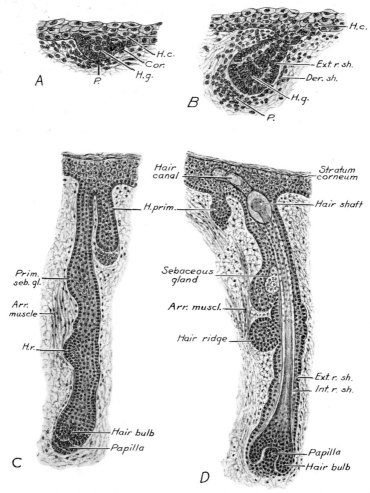

Fig. 14-18. Four stages in the development of a human hair. *A* and *B*, early stages from a frontal skin of a 3-month embryo. *C* and *D*, later stages from chin of a 5-month embryo. *Arr.muscl.*, primordium of arrector muscle; *Cor.*, border of the corium; *Der.sh.*, primordium of dermal sheath (connective tissue follicle); *Ext.r.sh.*, external root sheath; *H.c.*, hair canal cells; *H.g.*, hair germ; *H.prim.*, primordia of young hairs; *H.r.*, hair ridge for attachment of arrector muscle; *Int.r.sh.*, internal root sheath; *P.*, primordium of papilla; *Prim.seb.gl.*, primordium of sebaceous gland. (Redrawn after Shaffer.)

differentiated into two layers. The outer layer, the periderm or epitrichium, consisting of flattened cells, is a transient structure and is lost shortly before or after birth. The inner layer, composed of irregular cells with large nuclei and abundant cytoplasm, gives rise to the entire epidermis. The cells multiply by mitosis and soon form a stratified epithelium. True keratinization, however, begins only in the 5th month.

The *dermis* develops from the parietal mesoderm and consists at first of typical mesenchyme. In the 2nd month, cell differentiation begins, some of the cells becoming fibroblasts. Toward the end of the 2nd month, fibrils make their appearance, at first reticular and collagenous, and, soon after, elastic as well. Some time later the whole mass shows a differentiation into two layers, an upper, denser one, giving rise to the dermis proper, and a deeper, looser one that forms the subcutaneous tissue.

Hair appears in human embryos at the end of the 2nd month, the first places being the brows, upper lips, and chin. By the 7th month, lanugo hairs are distributed all over the body.

Each hair develops as a thickening of the germinative layer that grows down obliquely into the dermis, forming a slender solid cord of cells, the *hair germ* or *hair plug* (Fig. 14-18). The connective tissue cells of the dermis surrounding the cord condense to form the dermal follicle, and an invagination of connective tissue into the lower end of the hair germ forms the papilla.

The cells surrounding the papilla become differentiated into two zones, a central conical mass whose apex is directed toward the surface (the hair bulb) and an outer layer of epithelial cells which becomes the outer root sheath. The cells of the hair bulb grow toward the skin, the axial cells forming the hair and the peripheral cells giving rise to the inner root sheath. The various sublayers are formed from these by subsequent differentiation. Above the apex of the cone, the axial cells of the hair plug cornify and disintegrate, and a channel is formed that penetrates the epidermis. The hair grows into this channel and, when first formed, lies wholly beneath the surface. As the hair reaches the surface, its pointed extremity pierces the surface epithelium and emerges as the hair shaft.

The *sebaceous* gland develops from the outer root sheath and appears first as a thickening in the upper portion of the hair germ (see above). It soon develops into a flask-shaped, solid mass of cells which later differentiate to form the ducts and alveoli of the gland.

The *sweat* glands first appear as solid ingrowths of the epithelium into the underlying dermis. The lower end of the ingrowth becomes thickened and convoluted to form the coiled portion of the gland, and somewhat later the central portion becomes channeled out to form the lumen. The myoepithelial cells, which lie within the epithelium and rest on the basal lamina, are derived from the ectodermal cells of the ingrowth and not from mesoderm.

References

BRAVERMAN, I. N., AND YEN, A. Ultrastructure of the human dermal microcirculation. II. The capillary loops of the dermal papillae. Invest. Dermatol. 68:53–60, 1977.

BREATHNACH, A. S. Identification of keratohyalin in freeze-fracture replicas of rat buccal epithelium. J. Pathol. 123:203–212, 1977.

BREATHNACH, A. S. The cell of Langerhans. Int. Rev. Cytol. 18:1–28, 1965.

BREATHNACH, A. S., BIRBECK, M. S. C., AND EVERALL, J. D. Observations bearing on the relationship between Langerhans cells and melanocytes. Ann. N. Y. Acad. Sci., 100:223–238, 1963.

CAIRNS, J. Mutation selection and the natural history of cancer. Nature 255:197–199, 1975.

CUMMINS, H. Dermatoglyphics; a brief review. In The Epidermis (Montagna, W., and Lobitz, W. C., Jr., editors), pp. 375–386. Academic Press, New York, 1964.

ELLIS, R. A. Fine structure of the myoepithelium of the eccrine sweat glands of man. J. Cell Biol. 27:551–563, 1965.

GIACOMETTI, L. Behavior of Langerhans cells in wound healing. Anat. Rec. 163:188–189, 1969.

GIROUD, A., AND LEBLOND, C. P. The keratinization of epidermis and its derivatives, especially the hair, as shown by x-ray diffraction and histochemical studies. Ann. N. Y. Acad. Sci. 53:613–626, 1951.

HUTCHINSON, C., AND KOOP, C. E. Lines of cleavage in the skin of the newborn infant. Anat. Rec. 126:299–310, 1956.

LAIDLAW, G. F. The dopa reaction in normal histology. Anat. Rec. 53:399–413, 1932.

LERNER, A. B., AND FITZPATRICK, T. B. Biochemistry of melanin formation. Physiol. Rev. 30:91–126, 1950.

LEWIS, T. The Blood Vessels of the Human Skin and Their Responses. Shaw and Sons Ltd., London, 1937.

MACKENZIE, I. C. Spatial distribution of mitosis in mouse epithelium. Anat. Rec. 181:705–710, 1975.

MASSON, P. Pigment cells in man. The Biology of

Melanomas. N. Y. Acad. Sci. (special publ.) 4:15–51, 1948.

MATOLTSY, A. G., AND MATOLTSY, M. N. The chemical nature of keratohyalin granules of the epidermis. J. Cell Biol. 47:593–603, 1970.

MENTON, D. N. The effects of essential fatty acid deficiency on the fine structure of mouse skin. J. Morphol. 132:181–206, 1970.

MENTON, D. N., AND EISEN, A. Z. Structure and organization of mammalian stratum corneum. J. Ultrastruct. Res. 35:247–264, 1971.

MONTAGNA, W. The Structure and Function of Skin. Academic Press, New York, 1962.

MONTAGNA, W., AND KENYON, P. Growth potentials and mitotic division in the sebaceous glands of the rabbit. Anat. Rec. 103:365–380, 1949.

MONTAGNA, W., AND LOBITZ, W. C. (editors). The Epidermis. Academic Press, New York, 1964.

MOYER, F. H. Genetic effects on melanosome fine structure and ontogeny in normal and malignant cells. Ann. N. Y. Acad. Sci. 100:584–606, 1963.

MUNGER, B. L. The ultrastructure and histophysiology of human eccrine sweat glands. J. Biophys. Biochem. Cytol. 11:385–402, 1961.

ODLAND, G. F. Tonofilaments and keratohyalin. In The Epidermis (Montagna, W., and Lobitz, W. C., Jr., editors), pp. 237–249. Academic Press, New York, 1964.

RAWLES, M. E. Origin of melanophores and their role in development of color pattern in vertebrates. Physiol. Rev. 28:383–408, 1948.

ROGERS, G. E. Structural and biochemical features

of the hair follicle. In The Epidermis (Montagna, W., and Lobitz, W. C., Jr., editors), pp. 179–236. Academic Press, New York, 1964.

ROTHMAN, S. Physiology and Biochemistry of the Skin. University of Chicago Press, Chicago, 1954.

ROTHMAN, S. Keratinization in historical perspective. In The Epidermis (Montagna, W., and Lobitz, W. C., Jr., editors), pp. 1–14. Academic Press, New York, 1964.

ROWDEN, G., AND LEWIS, M. G. Langerhans cells: involvement in the pathogenesis of mycosis fungoides. Br. J. Dermatol. 95:665–672, 1976.

SEIJI, M., SHIMAO, K., BIRBECK, M. S. C., AND FITZPATRICK, T. B. Subcellular localization of melanin biosynthesis. Ann. N. Y. Acad. Sci. 100:497–533, 1963.

SELBY, C. C. An electron microscope study of the epidermis of mammalian skin in thin section. J. Biophys. Biochem. Cytol. 1:429–444, 1955.

STARICO, R. G. Amelanotic melanocytes in the outer sheath of the human hair follicle and their role in the repigmentation of regenerated epidermis. Ann. N. Y. Acad. Sci. 100:239–255, 1963.

TROTTER, M. Classification of hair color. Am. J. Physiol. Anthropol. 25:237–260, 1939.

WILLIER, B. H., AND RAWLES, M. E. The control of feather color pattern by melanophores grafted from one embryo to another of a different breed of fowl. Physiol. Zool. 13:177–199, 1940.

ZELICKSON, A. H. (Editor) Ultrastructure of Normal and Abnormal Skin. Lea and Febiger, Philadelphia, 1967.

CHAPTER 15

Glands

Structure and Classification

All cells of the body take up oxygen and nutritive substances from the blood, via intercellular fluid, and give off waste products. In this sense, all cells secrete and excrete. Certain cells of the body, in addition to carrying on these metabolic processes necessary for their own existence, also manufacture specific substances not for their own use but to be extruded from the cells and used elsewhere in the body (secretions, e.g., gastric juice) or discarded (excretions, e.g., urine). Such cells are known as *gland cells* or *glandular epithelium,* and an aggregation of these cells into a definite structure for the purpose of carrying on secretion or excretion is known as a *gland.*

A gland may consist of a single cell, as, for example, the goblet cell (see chapter 4) or the *unicellular glands* of invertebrates. Such a cell produces within itself a substance which is to be used outside the cell. The appearance which this cell presents depends upon the stage of secretion. It is thus possible to differentiate between a "resting" and an "active" cell or between an "empty" and a "loaded" cell.

Most glands are composed of more than one cell (*multicellular glands*). Usually there is a large number of cells, and these cells, instead of lying directly upon the surface, line more or less extensive invaginations into which they pour their secretions.

General Structure and Function of Secretory Cells

The goblet cell of the intestine is one of the simple columnar cells that constitute the surface epithelium of the mucous membrane. It is distinguishable as a mucous cell only after the formation of secretion has begun. When filled with secretion, the apical portion of the cell becomes dilated and the basal portion remains slender, giving the cell a goblet shape. The swollen apical portion in the living cell contains droplets of premucin or mucigen. The mucigen droplets are not generally visible in sections prepared by routine methods because the commonly used fixatives dissolve the mucigen, leaving a loose filamentous network in the cytoplasm. However, the mucigen droplets can be seen readily under the light microscope in sections prepared by appropriate technical procedure (Fig. 15-1).

At the height of the "active" phase of secretion, the mucigen droplets are released at the apical end of the cell (Figs. 15-1 and 15-2) and are dissolved and immediately converted into mucin. In some cases, the droplets are released gradually while new droplets are formed, and the goblet shape of the cell is retained for a considerable length of time. In other cases, the droplets are released rapidly and the cell quickly loses the goblet shape and reverts to a more slender form. After a period of rest, the

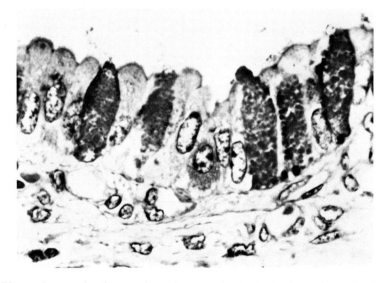

Fig. 15-1. Photomicrograph of a portion of a pancreatic duct of a guinea pig showing several goblet cells interspersed among the columnar lining cells. The mucigen is preserved in droplet form but the resolution of the light microscope is not sufficient to show whether the plasmalemma is complete at the apical end of the cell. Compare with electron micrograph in Figure 15-2. Chrome hematoxylin and phloxine stain. ×1125.

same cell may become active again and pass through the same stages of secretion.

Our knowledge of the processes involved in the synthesis and release of secretory materials by gland cells is based on biochemical studies and on a combination of electron microscopy and radioautography. Biochemical studies show that three classes of RNA are involved in the secretory process: ribosomal RNA, messenger RNA, and transfer RNA. The ribosomes of the cytoplasm are composed of protein combined with ribonucleic acid of nuclear origin. Messenger RNA, formed in association with DNA of the chromosomes, migrates to the cytoplasm, where it becomes associated with ribosomes, usually aggregated into polyribosomes (polysomes on endoplasmic reticulum membranes). The messenger RNA carries information from the DNA of the nucleus to the polysomes of the cytoplasm to direct the particular sequence of amino acids necessary for the formation of a particular protein. Transfer RNA picks up the amino acids (building materials) taken into the cell from the blood via the intercellular fluid and transports them to the region of the polysomes. There is biochemical evidence for a specific transfer RNA for each of the amino acids. In association with the polysomes, the amino acids

are assembled to form molecules and macromolecules of proteins. (see chapter 1 and Fig. 1-18.)

The intracellular transport of secretory proteins from their site of synthesis to their exit from the cell has been studied by cell fractionation methods and by electron microscopic radioautography (see Figs. 1-19 to 1-22).

Secretory proteins of most cells have a carbohydrate moiety, and those of some cells (e.g., goblet cells) have an appreciable amount of carbohydrate. Hence, goblet cells are advantageous for studies on the synthesis of carbohydrates and their conjugation with proteins. Radioautographic studies of goblet cells of tissues taken from animals at intervals after injection of labeled glucose, galactose, or fucose show that sugars are transported to saccules of the Golgi complex, where they are conjugated with the secretory proteins. (For further details on secretion, see "Granular Endoplasmic Reticulum" and "Golgi Apparatus," chapter 1.)

Classification of Glands

As has been mentioned, a gland may consist of a single secretory cell (unicellular gland), or it may be composed of many

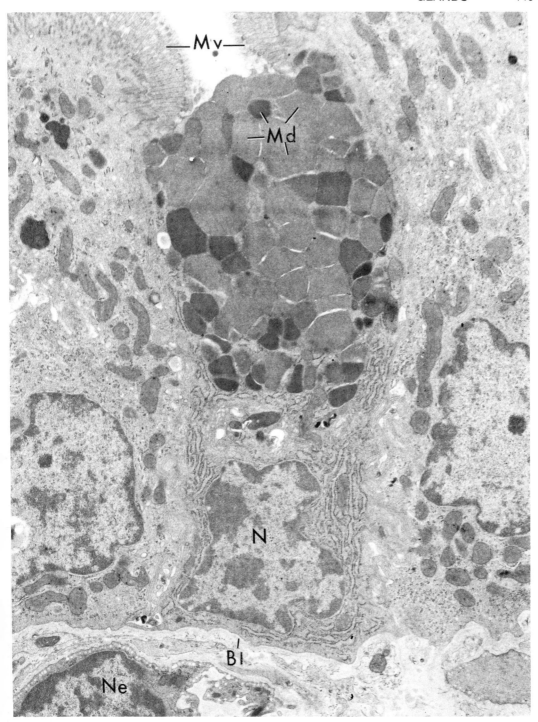

Fig. 15-2. Electron micrograph of a section of the small intestine of a bat showing a goblet cell between two columnar absorbing cells. Mucigen droplets (*Md*) fill most of the cell above the nucleus (*N*). An intact plasmalemma, with a few microvilli, is seen at the adluminal surface of the goblet cell. Numerous microvilli (*Mv*) are present on the adluminal surface of the absorbing cells. *Bl*, basal lamina beneath the intestinal epithelium; *Ne*, nucleus of an endothelial cell of a capillary blood vessel within the connective tissue of the lamina propria. ×11,440. (Courtesy of Drs. Keith Porter and Mary Bonneville.)

cells (multicellular gland); the secretory cells usually line an invagination from the free surface. In the simplest form of a glandular invagination, all of the cells lining the lumen are secreting cells. In more highly developed glands, secretion is primarily by the deeper cells and the remainder of the gland serves to carry the secretion to the surface. This latter part is then known as the *duct,* in contradistinction to the deeper *secreting portion.* In both the duct portion and the secreting portion of a gland, the epithelium rests upon a more or less definite *basement membrane.* Beneath the basement membrane, separating and supporting the glandular elements, is a fine vascular connective tissue.

Glands are sometimes classified, according to the nature of their secretion, into *mucous* (producing a viscous, slimy secretion), *serous* (producing a thin, watery secretion), and *mixed glands* (producing both types of secretion). Although this classification is particularly useful for some of the glands, such as those of the oral cavity, it cannot be satisfactorily used for all glands of the body, such as the sebaceous and mammary glands and the kidney.

The cells of mucous and serous glands differ in structure. The structure of the unicellular mucous gland or goblet cell has already been described. In the multicellular mucous glands or *mucous alveoli* (e.g., of the palatine glands) the cells are usually more or less pyramidal in shape as a result of their arrangement around the lumen of the terminal tubule. When the cell is filled with secretion, the nucleus is flattened against the basal part of the cell. As already described for the goblet cell, the mucigen of these cells is not well preserved with ordinary techniques and is dissolved, leaving a loose network that, with hematoxylin and eosin, remains unstained or stains very faintly with hematoxylin.

The cells of *serous alveoli* secrete a clear, watery, proteinaceous product. The secretion of many serous glands (e.g., pancreas and parotid gland) contains digestive enzymes. In these cells, the secretory granules are the enzyme precursors or *zymogen granules* (Figs. 15-3 and 15-4), and the cells are therefore known as *serozymogenic cells.* Serous cells are usually pyramidal, with rounded nuclei lying in the basal one-

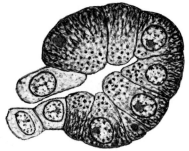

Fig. 15-3. Acinus of human pancreas. Acinar enlargement is produced by the increase in height of the secretory cells, while the lumen remains narrow. All secretory cells are in same functional stage. Zymogen granules appear in apical portion of cells; chromophilic material is in basal portion of cells. Chrome hematoxylin and phloxine stain. ×1100.

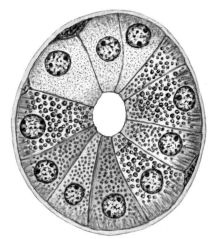

Fig. 15-4. Serous alveolus of human submandibular gland. Cells are shown in different functional stages; the cells containing zymogen granules are taller than those without. Myoepithelial cells are seen between the secretory cells and the basement membrane. Hemalum-mucicarmine-aurantia. (Redrawn after Zimmerman.)

half of the cells. The cells pass through active and resting phases of secretion, like mucous cells. During the resting phase, the secretory granules may become so numerous as to almost fill the cell, but the nucleus does not become flattened as in the mucous cell. The secretory granules, if they are preserved, are acidophilic. Basophilic material (RNA) is found in high concentration in the basal portion of serozymogenic cells, giving that part of the cell a strongly basophilic, striated appearance (Fig. 15-3).

The alveoli of mixed glands (e.g., submandibular and sublingual) contain both mucous and serous cells.

According to whether the secretion is merely a product of the cell or whether it consists of gland cells, the glands may be classified as *eccrine* (merocrine), *apocrine*, or *holocrine*. The majority of the glands are eccrine. The secretion is a product of the cell, extruded without loss of other cellular components. In the sebaceous glands, entire cells laden with secretory material are extruded as the secretion. This is the holocrine type of secretion. An intermediate type of secretion known as apocrine may be found in axillary and circumanal modified sweat glands. In these glands, a microscopic portion of the cell apex may be released along with the secretory material. The gonads (ovary and testis) produce very highly specialized secretions consisting

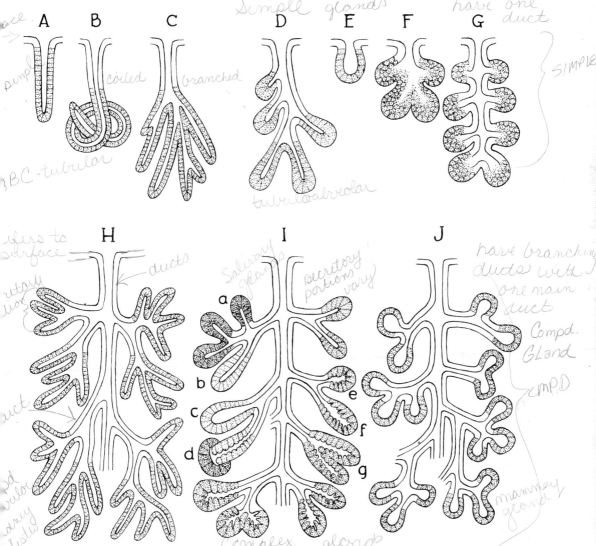

Fig. 15-5. Schema of various types of exocrine glands. *A* to *G*, simple glands; *H* to *J*, compound glands. *A*, simple nonbranched tubular; *B*, simple coiled tubular; *C*, branched tubular; *D*, branched tubuloacinar (tubuloalveolar); *E*, simple nonbranched alveolar; *F* and *G*, branched alveolar as in sebaceous glands; *H*, compound tubular; *I*, compound tubuloacinar, showing some of the various types of terminations. *a*, serous acinus with simple nonbranched canal; *b* and *c*, variations in size of lumen of mucous terminations, as in sublingual, etc.; *d*, tubuloalveolus of mucous tubule and serous demilune; *e, f*, and *g*, serous terminations with branched canals, or intercellular secretory canaliculi as in parotid, etc.; *J*, compound alveolar gland.

of living cells (ova and sperm) that continue to develop after extrusion from the gland. Because they secrete living cells, the ovary and testis are sometimes called *cytogenic glands.*

Glands may also be classified according to whether they possess ducts which carry their secretions to an epithelial surface (*exocrine glands, glands of external secretion*) or whether they are ductless and pour their secretions into the blood or lymph (*endocrine glands, glands of internal secretion*).

The exocrine glands may further be subdivided and classified in accordance with the type of duct system contained. When a gland consists of a single secretory passage or a single system of secretory passages opening into an unbranched duct, it is called a *simple gland* (Fig. 15-5, *A* to *G*). When a gland contains a duct system that is elaborate and branched, it is called a *compound gland* (Fig. 15-5, *H* to *J*). Both the simple and compound glands may be subdivided in accordance with the form of the terminal secretory portions. When the secreting portion is a tubule, the lumen of which is of fairly uniform diameter, the gland is known as a *tubular gland* (Fig. 15-5, *A* to *C*). When the secreting portion is dilated in the form of a sac or alveolus, the gland is known as a *saccular, alveolar,* or *acinar gland* (Fig. 15-5, *E, F, G, J*). In many glands, the secretory passages are neither typically tubular nor alveolar but intermediate in type, combining certain characteristics of both; such glands are called *tubuloalveolar* or *tubuloacinar* (Fig. 15-5, *D, I*). The serous salivary glands and pancreas are typical examples of this type; they have acinar enlargements which are produced by an increase in the height of the secretory epithelium while the lumen remains undilated and tubular (Figs. 15-3 and 15-5, *I, a, e, f,* and *g*). In some of the glands usually included in this group, such as the mucous salivary glands, mucous portions of the mixed salivary glands, and Brunner's glands of the duodenum, the secretory passages vary in type of lumen from tubular forms to dilations resembling elongated alveoli (Fig. 15-5, *I, b, c*).

Glands may thus be classified as follows:

A. Exocrine glands (or glands with ducts)
    1. Simple glands
        (a) Tubular { straight, coiled, branched }
        (b) Tubuloalveolar (tubuloacinar)
        (c) Alveolar (acinar, saccular)
    2. Compound glands
        (a) Tubular
        (b) Tubuloalveolar (tubuloacinar)
        (c) Alveolar
B. Endocrine glands (or glands without ducts)

Exocrine Glands

Simple Tubular Glands

These glands consist of simple, epithelia-lined tubules which open to the surface. All of the cells may be secretory, or only the more deeply situated ones may be. In the more highly developed of the simple tubular glands, we distinguish a mouth opening upon the surface, a neck which is usually somewhat constricted, and a fundus, or deep secreting portion of the gland.

Simple tubular glands are divided according to the appearance of the fundus into (1) straight, (2) coiled, or (3) branched.

Straight Tubular Gland. This is one in which the entire tubule runs a straight unbranched course, e.g., the crypts of the large intestine (Fig. 15-5 *A*).

Coiled Tubular Gland. This is one in which the deeper portion of the tubule is coiled or convoluted (Fig. 15-5 *B*). The sweat glands of the skin are the most typical examples.

Branched Tubular Gland. This is a simple tubular gland in which the deeper portion of the tubule divides into branches that are lined with secreting cells and that open into a superficial portion which serves as a duct (Fig. 15-5 *C*). Examples of branched tubular glands are the glands of the stomach and the glands of the endometrium of the uterus. Many of the pyloric glands of the stomach are also slightly enlarged and coiled at their terminations, so that they resemble to some extent both the convoluted tubular and the tubuloalveolar glands.

Simple Tubuloalveolar Glands

Simple tubuloalveolar or tubuloacinar glands are found only in the branched form (Fig. 15-5D). Included in this group are the smaller glands of the following types: salivary glands of the oral cavity, seromucous glands of the respiratory tract, mucous glands of the esophagus, and submucosal glands of the duodenum. Many of these, such as the esophageal and the duodenal submucosal glands, are classified by some authors as branched tubular, but, because they are frequently enlarged at their terminations, they may be included in the branched tubuloalveolar group.

Simple Alveolar Glands

The simplest form of alveolar gland, consisting of a single sac with a dilated lumen and connected with the surface by a constricted portion, the neck, is shown in Figure 15-5*E*. This simple form of alveolar gland is found in the skin of certain amphibians but does not occur in man. Simple alveolar glands in which there are several saccules are represented by the smaller sebaceous glands (Fig. 15-5*F*). In the sebaceous glands, as pointed out in chapter 14, the secreting cells undergo fatty degeneration, are pushed centrally by new cells, and are finally extruded as the secretion. Consequently, there are a number of layers of cells filling the space that would otherwise represent the lumen of the alveolus. Simple branched alveolar glands (Fig. 15-5*G*), in which a common duct gives rise to a number of saccules, are seen in the larger sebaceous glands and in the Meibomian glands.

Compound Tubular Glands

The compound tubular glands consist of a number of distinct duct systems, which open into a common or main excretory duct (Fig. 15-5*H*). The kidney and testis are examples of compound tubular glands. Some authors, as already stated, classify the smaller mucous glands of the esophagus, etc., as branched tubular glands; accordingly, the larger of the mucous glands of the esophagus, mucous terminations of the salivary glands, and submucosal glands of the duodenum are then classified as compound tubular, but because these glands frequently terminate in enlargements they are usually classified as compound tubuloalveolar.

Compound Tubuloalveolar Glands

The glands of this type (Fig. 15-5*I*) are numerous and widely distributed; they include the parotid, pancreas, mandibular, sublingual, the larger of the mucous glands of the esophagus and seromucous glands of the respiratory tract, many of the duodenal submucosal glands, etc. The structure of the terminal tubules and duct systems varies somewhat in the different glands, and for the finer structure, reference may be made to the special sections dealing with some of the more typical glands of the group, such as the parotid and the pancreas, in chapter 16.

Compound Alveolar Glands

The compound alveolar glands resemble the compound tubular and compound tubuloalveolar glands in having a large number of duct systems, but the terminal ducts, instead of ending in tubular and tubuloacinar secreting passages, end in alveoli with dilated, saclike lumina (Fig. 15-5*J*). The mammary gland is the best example of a compound alveolar gland.

Architecture of Compound Glands

All compound glands are surrounded by connective tissue which forms a more or less definite *capsule*. From the capsule, connective tissue *septa* or *trabeculae* extend into the gland. The broadest septa usually divide the gland into a number of compartments or *lobes*. Smaller septa from the capsule and from the interlobar septa divide the lobes into smaller compartments, usually microscopic in size, the *lobules*. A lobule not only is a definite portion of the gland separated from the rest of the gland by connective tissue but also represents a definite grouping of tubules or alveoli with reference to one or more terminal ducts. The glandular (epithelial) tissue is often referred to as the *parenchyma* of the gland, in contradistinction to the connective tissue or *stroma*.

Development of Glands

The relations of the glandular epithelium to the connective tissue are best understood by reference to development. As a general pattern, glands originate as ingrowths from a surface covered with epithelium. The epithelial invagination grows into the underlying mesenchymal tissue. As the invagination grows and subdivides, the main portion, which is connected with the epithelium at the original point of outgrowth, becomes the excretory duct, while the subdivisions form the larger and smaller ducts and finally the secreting tubules or alveoli. During the development of the gland tubules, the connective tissue is also developing but proportionately less than the more rapidly growing tubules (see discussion of patterns in chapter 4). The gland tubules do not develop irregularly but in definite groups, each group being dependent upon the tubule (duct) from which it originates. Thus the main excretory duct gives rise to a few large branches which may lie either between or within the developing lobes (interlobar and intralobar ducts, respectively); a lobe is formed by all of the subdivisions of one of the lobar branches. From each intralobar duct there arise within the lobe a large number of smaller branches, each of which gives rise to subdivisions which make up a lobule of the gland. These branches lie first between lobules (interlobular ducts) and finally within the lobules to which they give rise (intralobular ducts). As groups of tubules develop into lobes and lobules, the largest strands of connective tissue are left between adjacent lobes (interlobar connective tissue), smaller strands between lobules (interlobular connective tissue), and the finest connective tissue between the tubules or alveoli within the lobule (intralobular connective tissue). The liver and kidney are notable exceptions to this developmental pattern; details of their development are found in chapters 16 and 20.

Endocrine Glands

Certain glands, as already stated, are lacking in ducts; they are called *endocrine glands* or glands of internal secretion, in contrast to those glands with ducts, the exocrine or external secreting glands. Some glands, such as the pancreas and testis, secrete both externally, by way of ducts, and internally, by way of the bloodstream. The endocrine glands secrete specific substances called *hormones* which have spe-cific effects on the other tissues or organs of the body. The endocrine glands include the thyroid, parathyroid, adrenal, hypophysis, islands of Langerhans of the pancreas, and parts of the ovary and testis. The pineal gland is also usually included in this group. For a detailed description of the endocrine glands, see chapter 21.

References

GABE, M., AND ARVY, L. Gland cells. Physiology Morphology (Brachet, J., and Mirsky, A. E., editors), vol. 5, pp. 1–88. Academic Press, New York, 1961.

JAMIESON, J. D., AND PALADE, G. E. Intracellular transport of secretory proteins in the pancreatic exocrine cell. I. Role of the peripheral elements of the Golgi complex. J. Cell Biol. 34:577–596, 1967.

JAMIESON, J. D., AND PALADE, G. E. Intracellular transport of secretory proteins in the pancreatic cell. II, Transport to condensing vacuoles and zymogen granules. J. Cell Biol. 34:597–615, 1967.

NEUTRA, M., AND LEBLOND, C. P. The Golgi apparatus. Sci. Am. 220:100–107, 1969.

PALADE, G. E. The endoplasmic reticulum. J. Biophys. Biochem. Cytol. 2(Suppl.):85–98, 1956.

PALADE, G. E., SIEKEVITZ, P., AND CARO, L. G. Structure, chemistry and function of the pancreatic exocrine cell. In The Exocrine Pancreas (deReuck, A. V. S., and Cameron, M. P., editors), pp. 23–99. Little, Brown and Company, Boston, 1962.

PALAY, S. L. Morphology of secretion. In Frontiers in Cytology. Yale University Press, New Haven, 1958.

PETERSON, M., AND LEBLOND, C. P. Synthesis of complex carbohydrates in the Golgi region as shown by radioautography after injection of labeled glucose. J. Cell Biol. 21:143–148, 1964.

PORTER, K. R., AND BONNEVILLE, M. A. Fine Structure of Cells and Tissues. 3rd Edition, Lea & Febiger, Philadelphia, 1968.

SCHAFFER, J. Das Epithelgewebe. Die Drusen, Handb. mikr. Anat. (v. Möllendorff, editor), vol. 2, pt. 1, pp. 132–231. Springer-Verlag, Berlin, 1927.

SCHARRER, E. Principles of neuroendocrine integration. In Endocrines and the Central Nervous System. Williams & Wilkins, Baltimore, 1966.

SJÖSTRAND, F. S., AND HANZON, V. Ultrastructure of Golgi apparatus of exocrine cells of mouse pancreas. Exp. Cell Res. 7:415–429, 1954.

TURNER, C. D. General Endocrinology. W. B. Saunders, Philadelphia, 1966.

WARSHAWSKY, H., LEBLOND, C. P., AND DROZ, B. Synthesis and migration of proteins in the cells of the exocrine pancreas as revealed by specific activity determination from radioautography. J. Cell Biol. 16:1–23, 1963.

ZIMMERMAN, K. W. Die Speicheldrusen der Mundhöle und die Bauchspeicheldruse. Handb. mikr. Anat. Menschen (v. Möllendorff, editor), vol. 5, pt. 1, pp. 61–244. Springer-Verlag, Berlin, 1927.

CHAPTER 16

The Digestive System

The *digestive system* consists of the alimentary tract and such structures as the tongue, teeth, and accessory glands which are associated with it. The alimentary tract is conveniently divided by structural variations and topographical locations into a series of regions: mouth, pharynx, esophagus, stomach, small intestine, and large intestine, including the rectum and anal canal. The structural modifications of the various regions are associated with the function of the tract, namely, the forwarding of the food through the tube, where in transit it can be mechanically altered and acted on by enzymes, a portion of it absorbed, and the residue eliminated as feces.

General Features of the Alimentary Canal

The innermost layer of the digestive tract is a *mucous membrane* or *mucosa*. This has two constantly occurring components, an *epithelial lining* and a stratum of connective tissue, the *lamina propria*. The lamina propria is formed of interlacing connective tissue fibers, which are usually fine. It contains fibroblasts and macrophages, is frequently infiltrated with lymphocytes, and may also contain plasma cells and eosinophils. Beginning with the esophagus, a thin stratum of smooth muscle (*muscularis mucosae*) appears subjacent to the lamina propria and forms a third component of the mucosa.

A *submucosa,* formed of loose connective tissue, is invariably present beneath the mucosa from the beginning of the esophagus to the lower end of the anal canal. This layer is absent from parts of the mouth and pharynx. It contains rather coarse collagenous fibers which are usually loosely interwoven and among which are elastic and reticular fibers and connective tissue cells. The submucosa attaches the mucosa to the underlying firm structures but allows considerable movement in much the same way that superficial fascia allows movement of the skin. In regions where no definite submucosa is present, the mucosa attaches directly to the firm underlying structures, as, for example, in the gums.

Throughout most of the alimentary canal, there is a rather thick layer of muscle (*muscularis externa*) which has a very regular arrangement. In the mouth the muscle layer has no uniform arrangement and is absent in certain regions.

Beginning with the pharynx, there is an external layer composed of connective tissue (*fibrosa*) or of connective tissue and mesothelium (*serosa, serous membrane*).

During embryonic development, the epithelial lining of the digestive system and its numerous attached glands have originated from the endoderm or, in the oral region, from stomodeal ectoderm. All of the surrounding connective tissue and muscular and vascular investments have arisen from splanchnic mesoderm or mesenchyme of the head.

The Mouth

The *mouth* or oral cavity is an irregularly shaped structure which is bounded by and contains a number of different parts, such as the lips, cheeks, teeth, gums, tongue, and palate. Except over the surface of the teeth, the mouth is lined throughout by stratified squamous epithelium; the lamina propria is rather dense, and a submucosa is present only in certain regions.

Lips and Cheeks. The lips may be divided into three rather distinct regions: the cutaneous area, the red area, and the oral mucosa (Fig. 16-1). The cutaneous area of the lips is covered by typical thin skin with cornified epithelium, hair follicles, and sebaceous and sweat glands. The red area is covered by noncornified, relatively translucent stratified squamous epithelium which is indented by tall vascular connective tissue papillae (Figs. 16-1 and 16-2). The red color of the lip is due to the blood in the vessels of the tall papillae and the translucency of the epithelium. Glands are absent in the red area, except for an occasional sebaceous gland. The red area is continuous with the skin externally and with the mucous membrane of the lips internally.

The inner surfaces of the lips and cheeks are similar in structure. However, the epithelium is not cornified, and connective tissue papillae of moderate length indent it. The lamina propria is rather compact and is connected by a submucosa to the underlying skeletal muscle (orbicularis oris in the lips, buccinator in the cheeks). The submucosal fibers are thick and are so arranged that they closely bind the mucosa to the underlying structures, preventing the formation of folds and thus reducing the chance of biting the mucous membrane during mastication. In the area where the mucosa of the lips and cheeks becomes continuous with that of the gums (fornix vestibuli), the submucosa is very loose, allowing movement.

Numerous glands of a mixed (mucous and serous) type and a mucous type are present in the submucosa of the lips and cheeks, and they also penetrate into the buccinator muscle.

Gums. The epithelium of the *gums* or

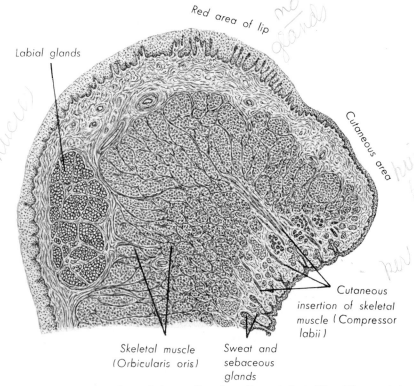

Fig. 16-1. Transverse section through lower lip of newborn infant. Van Gieson stain. The oral surface of the lip is at the *left.* ×12.

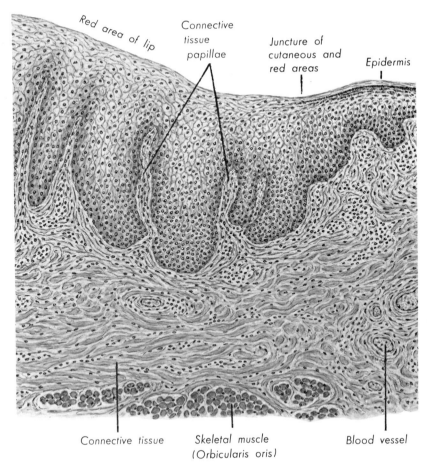

Fig. 16-2. Transverse section through the contiguous cutaneous and red areas of lip of newborn infant. ×110.

gingivae is cornified to a variable degree. Cornification is most pronounced in those areas which are subject to the greatest amount of abrasion from mastication or brushing, i.e., on the free margin of the gums. Numerous long vascular papillae deeply indent the epithelium and are responsible for its pink color. At the gingival sulcus, the epithelium of the gums is continuous with the epithelial attachment of the tooth (see "The Teeth" and Fig. 16-9). The lamina propria of the gums is formed of coarse, interweaving collagenous fibers which bind it closely to the periosteum of the alveolar processes of the maxillae and mandible. The lamina propria is also attached to the gingival fibers of the periodontal membrane. No submucosa and no glands are present in the gingiva.

Hard Palate. The epithelium of the *hard palate* is much like that of the gums.

It has a cornified layer in which the cells are hard and scalelike (Fig. 16-3), and it usually has a stratum granulosum. Long vascular papillae deeply indent it, giving a pinkish color. Except in the area adjacent to the gums and in the midline, a submucosa is present. Its fibers are coarse and run largely in a vertical direction, thus binding the lamina propria firmly to the periosteum of the hard palate. In the anterior region of the hard palate, a considerable amount of fat is present in the submucosa (the fatty zone); in the posterior two-thirds are many mucous glands (the glandular zone). In the narrow longitudinal zone of the raphe, glands are absent. Spherical or ovoid aggregations of flattened, concentrically arranged epithelial cells occasionally occur near the midline. They are remnants of the embryonic fusion of the palatine processes. Structures of this type are called

Cornified layer of stratified squamous epithelium

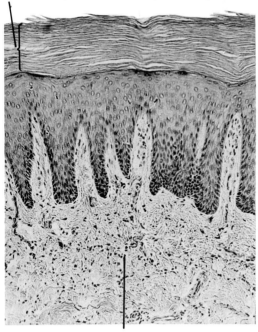

Lamina propria

Fig. 16-3. Mucous membrane from anterior region of hard palate. Human. Photomicrograph by Mr. L. Koster. ×110.

epithelial pearls.

Soft Palate. The oral surface of the *soft palate* and *uvula* is lined by noncornified stratified squamous epithelium. This type of epithelium extends over the free margin and for a variable distance onto the pharyngeal surface, where it becomes continuous with pseudostratified ciliated columnar epithelium. The submucosa is loose and contains many glands: mucous on the oral side and mixed (mucous and serous) on the upper (respiratory) side. A number of small skeletal muscles enter into the formation of the soft palate and uvula.

Floor of the Mouth. The *floor* of the *mouth* is lined by a noncornified epithelium. The submucosa is loose and contains the sublingual glands.

The Tongue

The main bulk of the tongue, particularly of the anterior two-thirds, is skeletal muscle. The interlacing muscle fibers course chiefly in three directions, longitudinally, transversely, and vertically, an arrange-

ment which gives maximal mobility and physical control. In the posterior one-third of the tongue, there are aggregations of lymphatic tissue, the lingual tonsils (Figs. 16-4 and 16-5).

The *lower surface* of the tongue is covered by a stratified squamous epithelium which is not cornified. The lamina propria is thin and closely bound down to the underlying muscle.

The *dorsal surface* of the tongue is divided into an anterior two-thirds and a posterior one-third by a V-shaped row of circumvallate papillae (Fig. 16-4). Some structural features are very different in the two regions. On the *anterior two-thirds,* there are numerous projections, the *lingual papillae.* These papillae are virtually small organs and should not be confused with the connective tissue papillae which indent stratified squamous epithelium. The lingual papillae are formed of a central core of connective tissue and a covering layer of stratified squamous epithelium (Figs. 16-5 to 16-7). The connective tissue core may give rise to small (connective tissue) papillae which indent the epithelium. According to their shape, the lingual papillae are divided into three types: *filiform, fungiform,* and *circumvallate (vallate).*

The *filiform papillae* are by far the most numerous and are quite evenly distributed over the dorsal surface of the anterior two-thirds of the tongue. Each consists of a slender vascular core of connective tissue covered by stratified squamous epithelium which is cornified. The epithelium forms one or more secondary projections which taper into threadlike points (Fig. 16-7).

The *fungiform papillae* are relatively few in number and are interspersed among the filiform papillae. Their summits are rounded and are broader than the bases. They are covered by noncornified epithelium which is indented with connective tissue papillae. The connective tissue core is highly vascular. This and the thinness of the epithelium are responsible for their red color.

The *circumvallate papillae,* usually 9 to 12 in number, are arranged along a V-shaped line, the apex of the V pointing posteriorly. They resemble the fungiform papillae but are much larger and are surrounded by a trench and a wall; hence their name, vallate or circumvallate. The wall is

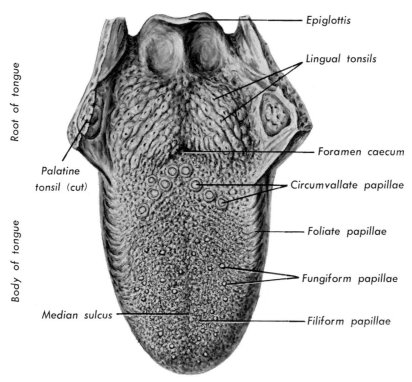

Fig. 16-4. Dorsum of human tongue. (Redrawn after Spalteholz.)

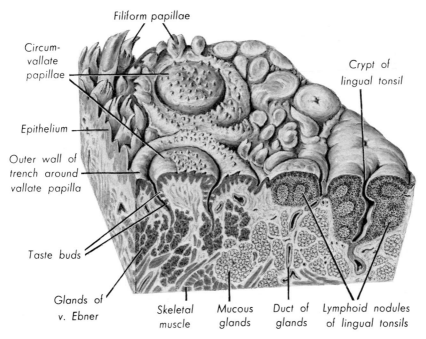

Fig. 16-5. Reconstruction of the surface of the tongue at the juncture of the dorsum and root. ×13. (Redrawn from Braus.)

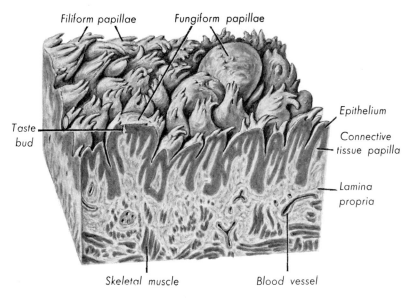

Fig. 16-6. Reconstruction of the surface of the dorsum of the tongue. The *front* surface represents a sagittal section, with the root of the tongue at *right*. ×16. (Redrawn from Braus.)

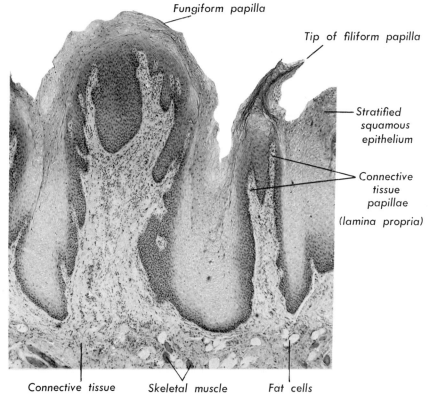

Fig. 16-7. Section of human tongue showing a fungiform papilla (*left*) and a filiform papilla (*right*). Photomicrograph. ×56.

somewhat lower than the papilla, thus allowing the latter to project slightly above the surface. Connective tissue papillae indenting the epithelium are limited to the upper surface; the sides are devoid of them. The circumvallate papillae, the trench, and the wall are covered by noncornified stratified squamous epithelium. In the epithelium of the lateral wall and sometimes in that of the trench also, are small oval bodies, *taste buds* (Figs. 16-5 and 16-8), which serve as receptor organs of taste (see chapter 22).

Along the posterolateral border of the tongue there are folds of the mucous membrane, sometimes called the foliate papillae (Fig. 16-4). They are not well developed in man.

The *dorsal surface* of the *posterior third* of the tongue is free of papillae but has mucosal ridges and *lingual tonsils*. The latter appear as low eminences caused by the underlying aggregations of lymphatic nodules (Figs. 16-4 and 16-5). Each tonsil usually has a centrally placed pit or crypt lined by stratified squamous epithelium. The epithelium is infiltrated with lymphocytes.

No submucosa is distinguishable on the dorsum of the tongue.

Glands of the Tongue. The glands of the tongue can be divided into three main groups according to their structure and location.

A paired group of mixed mucous and serous glands (*glands of Nühn*) are located in the anterior part of the tongue near the apex. They are embedded in the muscle but are closer to the ventral than to the dorsal surface. They have several ducts which open on the ventral surface.

A group of serous glands located in the region of the vallate papillae are known as the *glands of von Ebner*. They extend into the muscle. Their ducts open into the trenches of the vallate papillae (Fig. 16-5).

Mucous glands of the root of the tongue are the most numerous. They lie in the posterior third of the tongue and extend far enough forward to mingle with the serous (von Ebner's) glands. Their ducts open into the crypts of the lingual tonsils and into depressions between the tonsils.

Nerve Supply. The *nerve supply* of the oral cavity is complex. The skeletal muscle of the lips and cheeks is supplied by the seventh cranial nerve (having arisen embryonically from mesenchyme of the second branchial arches—the hyoid arches). Skeletal muscle of the tongue originates from somitic myotomes of the embryonic cervical region, hence receives its innervation from the 12th cranial nerve. The fibers carrying ordinary sensation are from the lingual branch of the fifth nerve and from the ninth nerve, which serve derivatives of the first and third branchial arches, respectively. The fibers carrying the special sense of taste are from the seventh nerve (through the chorda tympani) and from the ninth nerve.

The Teeth

A *tooth* has three anatomic divisions, *crown, root,* and *neck* or *cervix* (Fig. 16-9).

The *clinical crown* refers to that part which is visible with the tooth in situ. In early life the gums cover a part of the enamel so that the clinical crown consists of only a part of the anatomical crown. More of the enamel normally becomes exposed with the aging process, so that later in life the clinical crown includes all of the anatomical crown and even a part of the anatomical root.

The root is embedded in a cavity (the *alveolus* or *socket*) in the alveolar process of either the mandible or the maxilla, and is firmly attached to the bony wall of its socket by connective tissue, the *periodontal membrane* or *ligament*.

Structurally, a tooth has four components: *enamel, dentin, cementum,* and *pulp*.

Enamel. Enamel is the hardest substance in the body and, by weight, is composed largely (96%) of inorganic salts, of which the greater part (about 90%) is calcium phosphate. By volume, however, the organic component of enamel is very considerable, nearly equaling the inorganic element. Enamel is somewhat brittle but, because of the support of the underlying dentin and also because of its internal structural arrangement, it does not fracture from the amount of stress produced by the contact relation (occlusion) of opposing maxillary and mandibular teeth during normal mastication. Enamel is present in greatest amounts on the cusps of the permanent

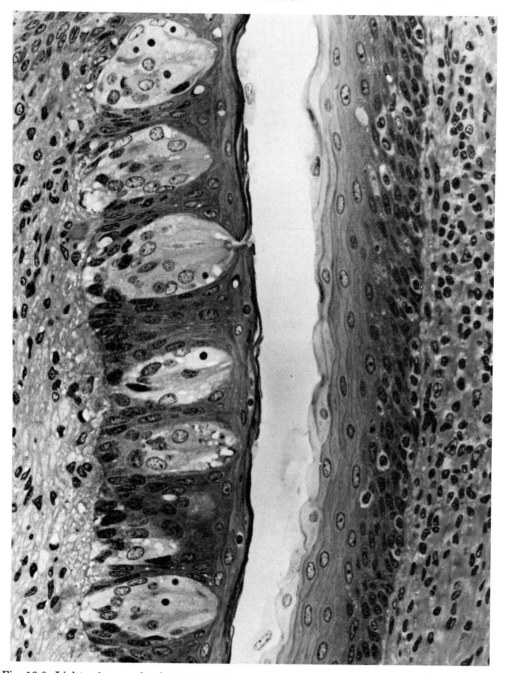

Fig. 16-8. Light micrograph of taste buds in the wall of a vallate papilla from Rhesus monkey. The taste bud at the *upper center* shows a taste pore. At least three types of nuclei can be seen within the taste buds, suggesting at least three different cell types. Lymphocytes can be seen within the stratified squamous epithelium. ×400.

bicuspids and molars, where it is 2 to 2.5 mm in thickness.

Structurally, enamel is composed of *enamel rods* or *prisms* and *interprismatic substance.*

The *enamel rods* are elongated columns, each of which extends throughout the thickness of the enamel layer from the dentinoenamel juncture to the surface of the anatomical crown. They have been depos-

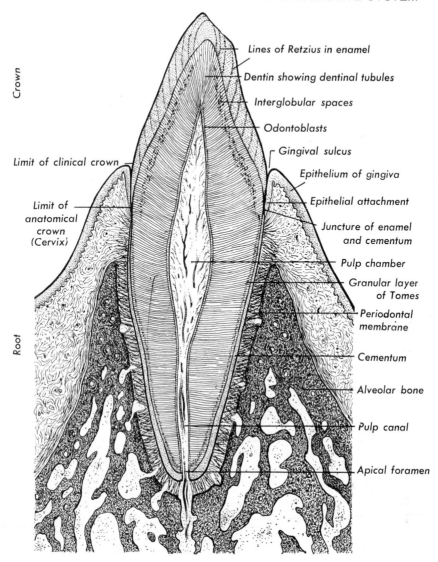

Crown

Lines of Retzius in enamel

Dentin showing dentinal tubules

Interglobular spaces

Odontoblasts

Gingival sulcus

Limit of clinical crown

Epithelium of gingiva

Epithelial attachment

Limit of anatomical crown (Cervix)

Juncture of enamel and cementum

Pulp chamber

Granular layer of Tomes

Periodontal membrane

Cementum

Alveolar bone

Root

Pulp canal

Apical foramen

Fig. 16-9. Diagram of a section through an incisor tooth and surrounding structures. The enamel at the tip of the crown shows some abrasion.

ited, and gradually built up in length, during tooth development before eruption, by the activity of an ectodermally derived epithelium, the *ameloblast layer* (see discussion below). When seen in cross section, some rods are hexagonal, oval, or polygonal, but most are arcade or scale-shaped with a depression on one side (Fig. 16-10). The average diameter of the enamel rods is about 5 μm, i.e., about one-half that of a red blood cell. The diameter of the rods increases as they course toward the periphery, because the area of the outer surface of the enamel is greater than that at the dentinoenamel juncture.

Each enamel rod is composed of submicroscopic crystals of inorganic substance embedded in a sparse framework of organic material. A thin peripheral region, the *rod sheath,* contains a higher proportion of organic material than does the bulk of the rod (Fig. 16-11). Between the rods is a small amount of a calcified organic substance, the *interprismatic* or *interrod substance,* which appears to act as a cementing substance.

Enamel rods are transversely striated, the striations being evenly spaced at intervals of about 4 μm (Fig. 16-12). This is due

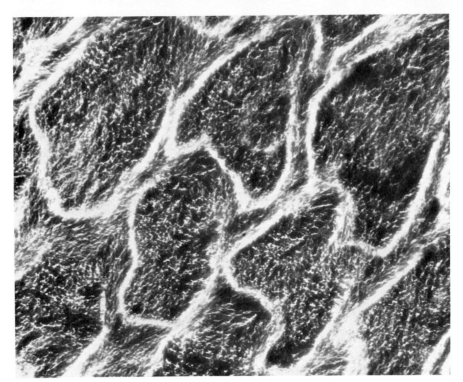

Fig. 16-10. Electron micrograph of demineralized enamel. The field includes cross sections of several enamel rods. Note the submicroscopic fibrillar network of the organic matrix and the more dense peripheral rod sheaths. Human. ×5000. (Courtesy of Dr. D. B. Scott.)

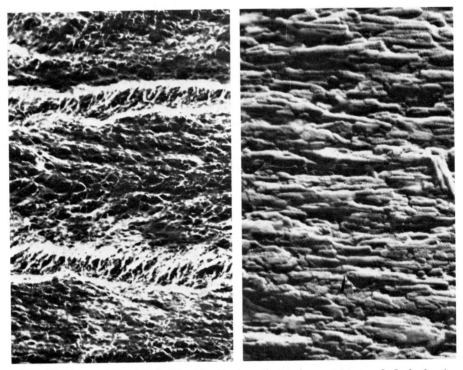

Fig. 16-11. Electron micrographs of longitudinal sections of mature enamel. *Left,* demineralized enamel. The field shows the entire width of one enamel rod and parts of two adjacent rods. Note the submicroscopic fibrillar network of enamel rods and rod sheaths. Extending crosswise between the rods (prisms) are interprismatic fibrils. ×10,000. *Right,* pseudoreplica of acid-etched, ground longitudinal section of mature enamel. The field shows the surface layers of crystallites and the crystalline pattern within a single enamel rod. ×21,000. (Courtesy of Dr. D. B. Scott.)

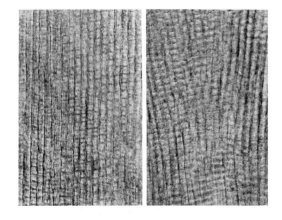

A   B

Fig. 16-12. Photomicrographs of ground section through enamel of human bicuspid tooth. *A*, lateral area in which the prisms are regularly arranged. *B*, cuspal area in which the prisms entwine. ×380.

to the rhythmic longitudinal growth of the rods during development. In addition to the closely spaced striations on the individual rods, there are more widely and somewhat more variably spaced continuous lines in the enamel, the *incremental lines of Retzius* (Fig. 16-9). In coronal sections through the crown, these appear as concentric circles. In longitudinal sections, they form arches over the apex of the dentin. In the deciduous teeth and in the first permanent molar, an especially prominent line, the *neonatal line,* marks the boundary between the enamel formed before and after birth. The incremental lines are due to variations in the rate of enamel deposition and are roughly analogous to the growth rings of a tree. The neonatal line is an accentuated incremental line resulting from a disturbance in the deposition of enamel at the time of birth.

The course of the enamel rods is usually wavy, or, especially on the occlusal surfaces, the rods may entwine, forming *gnarled enamel.* This is a functional adaptation which adds strength to the enamel by reducing the danger of cleavage between the rods.

An awareness of the direction and course of the enamel rods in different regions of a tooth is important in preparation of fillings from the standpoint both of ease in remov-

ing portions of the enamel and of maintaining the strength of the surrounding wall.

A membrane, *Nasmyth's membrane* or *enamel cuticle,* covers the exposed surface of the crown for a short time after eruption (see p. 473).

Dentin. Dentin is hard, yellowish, and elastic. It forms the bulk of a tooth and also gives the main strength to it. Chemically, it contains more mineral than bone but less than enamel (69% by weight, as compared with 46 and 96%, respectively). Morphologically, it resembles bone in that it is composed of collagenous fibers in a calcified ground substance. It differs from bone in that it contains no cells but has only processes of cells (odontoblasts) whose bodies lie adjacent to the dentin in the pulp cavity.

Mesenchymally derived cells responsible for the deposition of dentin, the *odontoblasts,* are arranged in an epithelium-like layer on the inner surface of the forming dentin. Unlike osteoblasts, the odontoblasts do not become imprisoned but retreat progressively as the layers of dentin are deposited, each one leaving a single branching process embedded in the dentin matrix. These *odontoblastic processes* or *dentinal fibers* (of Tomes) become increasingly elongated as the odontoblasts recede with the formation of successive layers of dentin. The dentinal fibers thus occupy narrow, tubular channels within the dentin, the *dentinal tubules.* The dentinal fibers branch and anastomose somewhat, but in general they run parallel to one another in a slightly wavy course through the dentin. This is well shown in ground sections of dentin in which the dentinal canals are filled with air and thus appear dark in transmitted light (Fig. 16-13). The odontoblastic processes probably completely fill the dentinal tubules in the living tooth; the spaces which appear between the processes and the walls of the tubules in fixed sections are probably artifacts (Fig. 16-14). The rim of dentin matrix bordering on the tubule stains darker than the remainder of the dentin and is known as *Neumann's sheath.*

In each layer of dentin, the meshwork of collagenous fibers in the matrix runs perpendicular to the long axis of the tubules, i.e., parallel or tangential to the outer surface of the tooth. The mineral salts are in

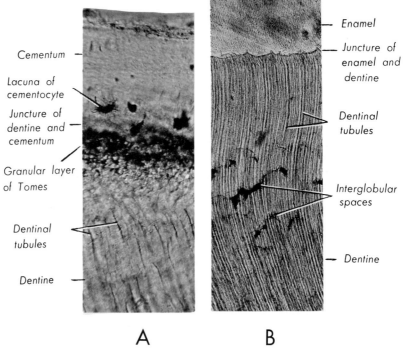

A   B

Fig. 16-13. Photomicrographs of ground section of human bicuspid tooth; *A*, through root, showing dentin and adjoining cementum; *B*, through crown, showing dentin and adjoining enamel. The dark areas in the enamel are not due to pigment or discoloration but to refraction of the rods. ×265.

the form of crystals and have two types of arrangement: (1) the long axes of the crystals are parallel to the collagenous fibers, and (2) the crystals radiate out from a center in spherulitic arrangement. The ground substance of dentin is composed of glycosaminoglycans.

In certain regions of the tooth, there are areas which have less inorganic material than elsewhere, as a result of a failure of the individual areas of calcification to meet and fuse. The matrix in such regions shrinks in ground (dried) sections, and a space is formed which becomes filled with air and so appears dark in transmitted light. One such constantly occurring region is in the root of the tooth close to the dentinocementum juncture. It has a granular appearance and is known as the *granular layer of Tomes* (Figs. 16-13*A* and 16-9). A second location, the *interglobular spaces* (Fig. 16-13*B*), occurs chiefly in the crown (Fig. 16-9) but may be present in the root also. It lies a short distance from the dentinoenamel (or dentinocementum) juncture. Each area is irregular in shape and much larger than

the areas forming the granular layer of Tomes.

Parallel incremental growth lines (*contour lines of Owen, imbrication lines of von Ebner*) which are due to the deposition of dentin in successive lamella-like layers are present. In cross sections of a tooth, they appear like annual rings of a tree.

Dentin, unlike enamel, forms throughout life. The dentin that forms before the completion of root development is known as *primary dentin* in contrast with that which arises subsequently, the so-called *secondary dentin*. The former consists of relatively straight dentinal tubules, whereas the latter has tubules which follow a more wavy course. The distinction between the two types is somewhat arbitrary. The dentin that arises after severe stimuli, such as caries or erosion, is composed of elements that are very irregularly arranged; it is known as *reparative dentin*. The deposition of dentin induced by stress may be so extensive that it obliterates the pulp chamber and even part of the root canal. It is an important protective response.

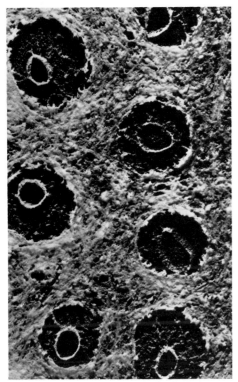

Fig. 16-14. Electron micrograph of thin section of demineralized dentin, showing organic matrix and cross sections of dentinal tubules with their enclosed odontoblastic processes (dentinal fibers). The space between each process and the rim of organic matrix (Neumann's sheath) is probably largely artifact. Human. ×5500. (Courtesy of D. B. Scott.)

Dentin is sensitive to a number of painful stimuli. Despite this well known fact, nerve fibers have not been demonstrated penetrating its matrix to any appreciable extent. The odontoblastic processes presumably convey impulses to the pulp, where many nerve endings are located.

Cementum. Cementum is similar to bone both in morphology and in composition. It is darker than enamel but lighter in color than dentin. It forms a thin sheath on the surface of the dentin of the anatomical root of the tooth (Fig. 16-9). It is usually somewhat thicker at the apex of the root, and sometimes it covers the inner surface of the dentin for a short distance at the apical foramen.

Cementum may either be free from cells, *acellular cementum,* or it may be *cellular,* containing cells similar to osteocytes (*ce-mentocytes*) which lie in irregularly shaped lacunae in the matrix (Fig. 16-13*A*). Except at the apex of the root, the acellular type is usually adjacent to the dentin. The ground substance of cementum resembles that of bone. Collagenous fibers of the matrix extend into the surrounding connective tissue (periodontal membrane) and, as in bone, are known as *Sharpey's fibers.* Cementoblasts on the surface continue to form cementum throughout life. The added layers are irregular in thickness and may be either cellular or acellular. Hypertrophy of cementum frequently occurs in response to ususual stress or movement of a tooth.

Although the bond between dentin and cementum is a firm one, the mode of attachment is not clear. Cementum forms a protective covering over the dentin and serves to attach the tooth to the surrounding structures. Movement of teeth without injury to the tooth structures is possible in orthodontic procedures because cementum is more resistant to resorption than is the alveolar bone.

Periodontal Membrane. The *periodontal membrane* or *ligament* is composed of connective tissue which surrounds the root of the tooth. It attaches the root to: (1) the wall of its alveolus, (2) the gingival connective tissue, (3) the more superficial parts of the roots of adjacent teeth. Fibers extending into the cementum of the tooth interweave with those extending into the alveolar bone, thus binding the tooth to the bone. The fibers do not course in the same direction at different levels (Fig. 16-9) but are arranged in a way that makes them most effective in maintaining the tooth in position and in serving as a suspensory ligament. The fibers are collagenous, but, because of their waviness, some temporary physiological movement of a tooth is possible without morphological alterations in its root and socket.

In the periodontal membrane are fibroblasts, osteoblasts, and cementoblasts. There are also groups of cells which are remnants of Hertwig's epithelial root sheath, a derivative of the enamel organ. Blood vessels and nerve fibers, particularly proprioceptive endings, are present.

The density and strength of a periodontal ligament varies with the stress to which a tooth has been subjected. Thus, if there is no opposing tooth, the fibers of the membrane become more delicate, a change which is accompanied by a rarefaction of the bone of the alveolus. When this is allowed to occur, restorative measures become more difficult.

Pulp Cavity and Dental Pulp. The shape of the *pulp cavity* is quite similar (in miniature) to that of the tooth in which it occurs. It consists of an expanded *pulp chamber,* which lies in the crown portion and adjacent part of the root, and a narrow *pulp canal* or *root canal* in each root (Fig. 16-9). The pulp cavity is much larger in teeth of young than of old individuals, for there is a continuous deposition of dentin throughout life. A root canal communicates with the periodontal tissues through one or more foramina at or near the apex the *apical foramina.*

The *dental pulp* is essential to the nourishment and vitality of the tooth. It consists of fine connective tissue, which fills the pulp cavity. In addition to fibroblasts and histiocytes, it contains the specialized connective tissue cells, odontoblasts, which are responsible for dentin formation.

The pulp is richly vascular. An arteriole entering at the apical foramen forms a profuse capillary network close to the odontoblast layer, the blood being returned by one or more venules.

The dental pulp contains both myelinated and unmyelinated nerve fibers. The sensory fibers terminate as free nerve endings among the odontoblasts. They are pain receptors (eliciting a sensation of pain regardless of the type of stimulus).

Attachment of Gingiva to Teeth. The gums are attached to the teeth in two ways. One, the attachment of the subepithelial connective tissue to the cementum, has been described under "Periodontal Membrane." The other is a direct attachment of the gingival epithelium to the tooth, the *epithelial attachment* (Figs. 16-9 and 16-21). At the gum line the epithelium turns inward and follows along the surface of the tooth, to which it is attached. Although the structural features of this attachment are not clear, it is certain that there is a definite adhesion of the epithelium to the tooth. In contrast with the epithelium of the exposed part of the gums, the epithelium of this zone of attachment is not indented by connective tissue papillae.

With advancing age, an increasing proportion of a tooth becomes exposed; i.e., the clinical crown increases in size. This is due to a continued but slow rate of eruption and also to a normal recession of the gums. As more of the crown becomes exposed, the epithelial attachment gradually grows apically for a short distance over the surface of the anatomical root. Thus, in young individuals, the epithelial attachment is on the enamel only; with increased exposure of the crown, it is partly on the cementum; late in life, it may attach to the cementum only. Mild mechanical stimulation, such as massage and brushing, strengthens the epithelium at its attachment by increasing keratinization of its surface layers.

Development of the Teeth. In man there are normally two sets of natural teeth, the *primary dentition* or deciduous teeth and the *secondary dentition* or permanent teeth. Each tooth develops from a *tooth germ* which is derived from ectoderm and mesoderm. The enamel organ, derived from the ectodermal oral epithelium, forms the enamel. The dental papilla, a condensation of mesenchyme which becomes partially enclosed by the enamel organ, gives rise to the dentin and pulp. The sac of connective tissue that surrounds the enamel organ and papilla, the dental follicle, produces the cementum and periodontal membrane.

The first indication of tooth development in man occurs during the 6th or 7th week of intrauterine life, at which time the embryo measures slightly over 1 cm in length. Tooth development appears to be initiated by an inductive influence of the mesenchyme on the overlying epithelium. The evidence indicates that this mesenchyme is of neural crest origin. The epithelium folds into the underlying mesenchyme as the *dental lamina* along the future dental arch of each jaw. Slightly external to this lamina, but in close association with it, a second epithelial ingrowth occurs, the labiogingival lamina, in which a groove (Fig. 16-15) and then a deep separation will form (Fig. 16-16). This will divide the dental arch from the lips and cheeks. The dental lamina is of nearly uniform thickness at first, but

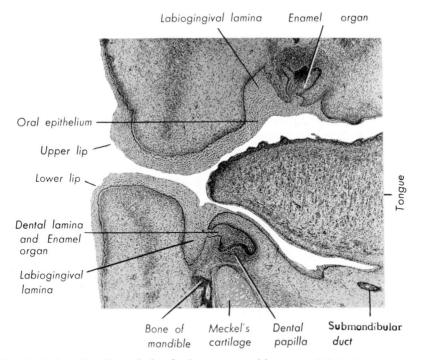

Labiogingival lamina   Enamel   organ

Oral epithelium

Upper lip

Lower lip

Tongue

Dental lamina
and Enamel
organ

Labiogingival
lamina

Bone of   Meckel's   Dental   Submandibular
mandible   cartilage   papilla   duct

Fig. 16-15. Sagittal section through developing upper and lower medial deciduous incisor teeth of a 50-mm human embryo. Age about 10 weeks. Photomicrograph. ×34.

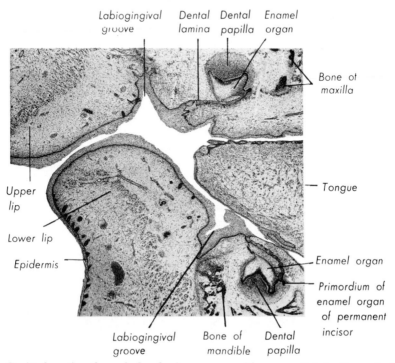

Labiogingival   Dental   Dental   Enamel
groove   lamina   papilla   organ

Bone of
maxilla

Tongue

Upper
lip

Lower lip

Epidermis

Enamel organ

Primordium of
enamel organ
of permanent
incisor

Labiogingival   Bone of   Dental
groove   mandible   papilla

Fig. 16-16. Sagittal section through developing upper and lower medial deciduous incisor teeth of an 86-mm human embryo. Age about 3 months. Photomicrograph. ×34.

proliferations soon form at intervals on its outer side close to the oral epithelium. These proliferations are the primordia of the *enamel organs* of the deciduous teeth. They develop into cap-shaped and then into bell-shaped structures (Figs. 16-15 and 16-16). Within and beneath the concavity of an enamel organ, a proliferation and condensation of the mesenchyme take place, forming the *dental papilla*. It is the primordium of the pulp. Its peripheral cells, i.e., those adjacent to the enamel organ, will become odontoblasts. The mesenchymal differentiation is dependent on the presence of the epithelial component. Experiments with lower organisms have shown that epithelium transplanted from other areas of the embryo are induced to form enamel organs by the jaw mesenchyme. In reciprocal experiments, however, it was found that only the jaw mesenchyme differentiates into dental papillae, and it is this mesenchyme that specifies the type of tooth (molar, incisor, etc.) that will develop.

Somewhat later in development, there appear the primordia of the enamel organs of those permanent teeth that correspond to the milk teeth. Each primordium arises as an inner or lingual growth from the dental lamina at a point coexistent with the enamel organ of a milk tooth. Later, as the dental arch lengthens, the dental lamina also grows dorsally, and from this dorsal extension arise the primordia of the enamel organs of the molars. The primordium of the last molar (wisdom tooth) does not form until the 4th or 5th year. The developmental pattern of the permanent teeth is the same as that of the deciduous teeth.

During the development of an enamel organ, the dental lamina, which connected the enamel organ with the oral epithelium, disintegrates. The developing tooth thus becomes entirely separated from the oral epithelium and does not again come into relationship with it until eruption.

The mesenchyme surrounding the enamel organ and dental papilla plays a role in tooth development. It thickens and forms a capsule-like structure named the *dental sac* or *dental follicle*. From the relationship in the developing tooth, it is evident that the segment of the dental sac adjacent to the papilla has the position of the future periodontal membrane. From it arise the cells associated with the deposition of cementum. Its peripheral part serves as the periosteum of the wall of the future alveolus.

All of the teeth do not show the same degree of development at any one time. The most anterior ones are usually the most advanced in development. In any one tooth, the future occlusal area develops more rapidly than do the more apically situated regions. Thus, at the time of eruption, the crown is fully formed but the root is still in the process of development.

Formation of Dentin. Dentin is the first hard substance formed in a developing tooth. Preceding its actual deposition, several changes occur in the dental papilla. Reticular fibers form in the papilla, particularly in the peripheral zone adjacent to the enamel organ. The outer portions of these fibers (Korff's fibers) fuse with the delicate basal lamina which separates the papilla from the enamel organ, and the thickened membrane thus formed is known as the *membrane preformativa*. The mesenchymal cells closest to the membrane enlarge and form a continuous layer of columnar cells, *odontoblasts*. The Korff's fibers which lie between the odontoblasts enlarge and change their direction so that they become largely parallel to the membrana preformativa. Around them is deposited a gel-like ground substance. The organic matrix of collagen and ground substance is referred to as *predentin*. The final stage in the formation of dentin is the deposition of lime salts in the organic matrix. The organization of the organic matrix controls the deposition of inorganic salts so that fully formed dentin appears to be deposited in lamellae. The incremental or growth lines are known as *contour lines of Owen* or *imbrication lines of von Ebner*.

The odontoblast is an extremely active cell metabolically. It synthesizes and secretes both the collagen and ground substance components of the organic matrix of dentin. The synthesis of these products is carried out in an orderly sequence involving well developed rough endoplasmic reticulum and Golgi material. The secretion of collagen by odontoblasts has been studied extensively by radioautography, and this system has provided some of the best evidence for the mechanism of collagen release from cells that is currently available. The work of Weinstock and Leblond demonstrates that odontoblasts secrete collagen in the form of procollagen by means of small Golgi-derived granules which fuse with the cell surface in much the same manner by which zymogen granules are produced and released by pancreatic acinar cells (see chapter 1). There is increasing evidence now that this is the usual, if not the only, process of collagen secretion by a wide variety of cell types. The apical ends of the odontoblasts prior to the deposition of dentin were in contact with the membrana preformativa. As dentin is deposited, the odontoblasts are not imprisoned but remain on the advancing surface of the dentin. Each, however, leaves a process, the *odontoblastic process* (fiber of Tomes), in the path of its retreat. As more and more dentin is deposited, these processes increase in length, for they extend through the entire thickness of the dentin. The processes branch and contact each other. Communicating junctions have been seen at some of these contact points. The odontoblasts remain functionally active throughout the life of a tooth and, as a consequence, secondary dentin can be formed.

Enamel Organ and Deposition of Enamel. Developing as a continuous epithelial sac which has invaginated basally upon itself, the enamel organ* becomes structurally rather complex (Figs. 16-17 to 16-21). Four layers are usually described which, from its concavity outward, are as follows: (1) The *inner enamel epithelium* is a single layer of columnar cells, the future *ameloblasts*. A basal lamina separates these from the dental papilla. (2) The *stratum intermedium* is composed of two or more layers of squamous or cuboidal cells. (3) The *stellate reticulum* (*enamel pulp*) is composed of loosely arranged branching cells. (4) The

---

* Some authors prefer to substitute the term *epithelial dental organ* for enamel organ, since this structure, although primarily concerned with enamel formation, does contribute to the form and development of the entire tooth, particularly in the formation of root dentin by means of Hertwig's epithelial root sheath. Similarly, there is some justification for the use of the terms *inner* and *outer dental epithelium* in place of inner and outer enamel epithelium.

outer enamel epithelium is a single layer of cuboidal cells, adjacent to which is a rich vascular plexus in the connective tissue. Each of these layers retains many of its epithelial characteristics.

The margin of the bell-shaped enamel organ is called the *cervical loop* (Fig. 16-18). After completion of the crown, the inner and outer enamel epithelial layers of the cervical loop grow apically to form *Hertwig's epithelial root sheath*. This structure determines the shape of the future root or roots and stimulates the differentiation of odontoblasts from the underlying mesoderm. The root sheath later disintegrates, leaving nests of cells in the periodontal membrane.

Deposition of enamel begins only after a layer of dentin is formed. At this time, the cells of the inner enamel epithelium elongate and differentiate into *ameloblasts*. Enamel is elaborated in the form of rods or prisms cemented together by an interprismatic substance. A short segment at the dentinal end of each ameloblast becomes more granular. This part of the cell is then known as *Tomes' process*. This part of the cell is where the organic material produced by the ameloblast is released from the cell surface to form enamel rod matrix. The deposition of the organic matrix by ameloblasts appears to be more precisely controlled than is the deposition of predentin by odontoblasts. The process also differs significantly in that the ameloblast recedes synchronously with matrix deposition so nothing comparable to odontoblastic processes occurs in enamel. The organic matrix forms the framework of enamel prisms. As the enamel prisms increase in length, there is a progressive mineralization, an uncalcified segment always remaining next to the ameloblast. The interprismatic substance between the processes also becomes calcified. The amount of mineral deposited at this time, however, is only about one-fourth that of mature enamel. Complete calcification takes place after the rods have reached full length. At that time, *maturation* of the enamel matrix takes place, water is withdrawn and there is a crystallization and further deposition of salts. Maturation always begins at the occlusal region and progresses toward the gingival attachment.

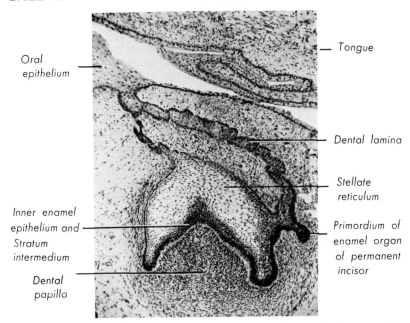

Fig. 16-17. Higher magnification of the developing lower incisor tooth shown in Fig. 16-16 (86-mm human embryo). Photomicrograph. ×73.

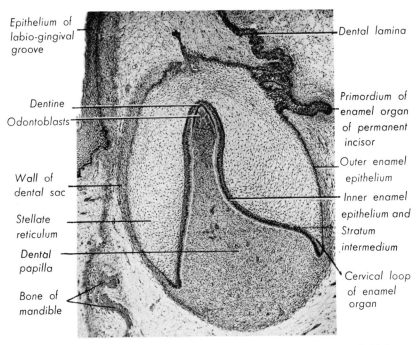

Fig. 16-18. Sagittal section of medial deciduous incisor tooth of an 111-mm (C-R) human embryo. Age about 14½ weeks. Photomicrograph. ×57.

After completion of enamel formation, the ameloblasts deposit on its surface a thin (0.2 μm), homogeneous, protective covering, the *primary enamel cuticle*. The enamel organ then regresses but remains as a few layers of cuboidal cells, the *reduced enamel epithelium*. As the tooth erupts, it is covered by a thicker (up to 10 μm) keratinous layer, the *secondary enamel cuticle,* produced by the reduced enamel epi-

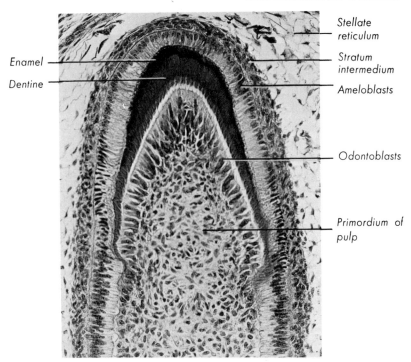

Enamel

Dentine

Stellate reticulum

Stratum intermedium

Ameloblasts

Odontoblasts

Primordium of pulp

Fig. 16-19. Sagittal section through the developing crown of a medial deciduous incisor tooth of a 170-mm human fetus. Age about 5 months. Photomicrograph. ×180.

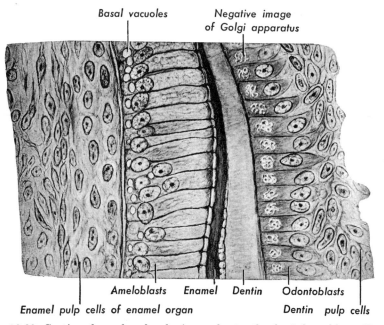

Basal vacuoles

Negative image of Golgi apparatus

Ameloblasts   Enamel   Dentin   Odontoblasts

Enamel pulp cells of enamel organ

Dentin pulp cells

Fig. 16-20. Section through a developing molar tooth of a 5-day-old rat (Beams).

thelium. These two cuticles together form *Nasmyth's membrane,* which covers the surface of the enamel until it is worn off by mastication or brushing. When the tooth erupts, the reduced enamel epithelium fuses with the oral epithelium at the gingival margin and forms the *epithelial attachment* or *attached epithelial cuff.* As the tooth continues to erupt and more of the crown becomes exposed, the epithelial at-

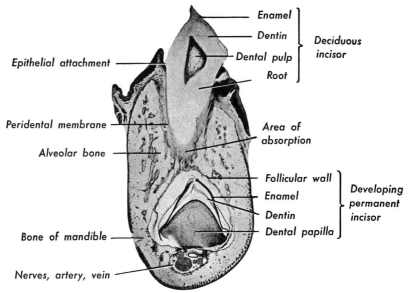

Fig. 16-21. Section through the mandible of a kitten, showing deciduous tooth and developing permanent tooth germ.

tachment gradually separates from the exposed enamel. Concomitantly, the epithelial attachment grows apically on the tooth so that the extent of the attachment does not materially decrease.

Deposition of Cementum. The developing tooth is surrounded by a condensation of embryonal connective tissue which forms the *dental follicle* or *dental sac.* That portion of the follicle adjacent to the dental papilla occupies the position of the future periodontal membrane. It is separated, however, from the papilla by the apically directed extension of the enamel organ, Hertwig's epithelial root sheath. Following the first deposition of dentin of the root, the epithelial root sheath disintegrates. At this time, cells of the dental sac differentiate into *cementoblasts,* following which cementum is deposited on the surface of the root. Mesenchymal cells in the outermost zone of the dental sac differentiate into osteoblasts of the periosteum of the alveolus. Collagenous fibers also develop in the follicular tissue. Some are attached to the cementum, others to the alveolar bone or gingival connective tissue. Together they form the fibrous component of the *periodontal membrane* or *ligament.*

The Pharynx

The *pharynx* extends from the level of the base of the skull to the level of the cricoid cartilage, where it becomes continuous with the esophagus. It is 5 to 6 inches in length. Its cavity is continuous with the cavities of the nose, mouth and larynx. Superiorly and laterally, the Eustachian tubes open into it. The cavity of the pharynx is incompletely divided by the soft palate and uvula into upper (pars nasalis) and lower (pars oralis and pars laryngea) regions.

The *wall of the pharynx* consists of three coats: mucosa, muscularis and fibrosa. There is no submucosa except in the superior lateral region and near the juncture with the esophagus.

The *epithelium* lining the pharynx is not the same throughout. That lining the nasopharynx is the ciliated pseudostratified columnar type, except near the juncture with the oropharynx where the soft palate and uvula come in contact with the posterior wall. There the epithelium changes to a stratified squamous type which continues through the lower region. The *lamina propria* of the pharynx is a tough, fibroelastic layer, subjacent to which is a strongly developed layer of elastic fibers which course mainly in a longitudinal direction. Fibers from it penetrate between the skeletal muscle bundles and thus bind the lamina propria to the muscularis.

The *muscle* of the pharynx, having originated from mesenchyme of the embryonic branchial arches, is skeletal and is quite irregularly arranged. The *fibrosa* is a tough, fibroelastic layer which, with varying degrees of firmness, attaches the pharynx to the surrounding structures.

In the *nasopharynx,* lymphatic tissue is abundant, being arranged both diffusely and as aggregations. These aggregations, the *pharyngeal tonsils,* frequently become enlarged and are then known as adenoids. Mixed glands which often penetrate deeply into the muscular layer are present. (See also chapter 17, under "Nasopharynx.")

In the *oral* and in the *laryngeal pharynx,* scattered nodules of lymphatic tissue occur. The glands are a mucous type and are few in number.

Plan of the Esophagus, Stomach and Intestines

Except for the mucosa, no layer is constantly present throughout the mouth and pharynx. Beginning with the esophagus, however, four layers are constantly present through the remainder of the alimentary tract (Fig. 16-22): *mucosa, submucosa, muscularis externa* and *fibrosa* or *serosa*

(peritoneum). The chief structural modifications in the different segments of the tract occur in the mucosa, and these modifications are closely correlated with differences in function. An additional component, the *muscularis mucosae,* appears for the first time at the beginning of the esophagus. This is composed of smooth muscle, most of the fibers running in a longitudinal direction. The submucosa differs somewhat in successive segments of the alimentary tract, chiefly as regards the presence or absence of glands. The muscularis externa (so named in contradistinction to the muscularis mucosae) is formed of two very regularly arranged layers, an *inner circular* and an *outer longitudinal,* except in the stomach. As in other saccular organs, the muscle of the stomach is irregularly arranged, especially in the upper, more saccular part. Three rather indistinct layers have been distinguished, largely by exposing the muscle through dissection.

Two nerve plexuses from the autonomic nervous system are present, beginning with the esophagus. One of these, the *myenteric (Auerbach's) plexus,* is readily seen in most

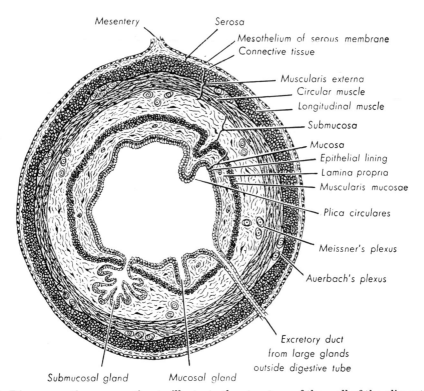

Fig. 16-22. Diagrammatic cross section to illustrate the structure of the wall of the alimentary tract.

sections of the tract. It is located between the two layers of the muscularis externa. The other, the *submucous* (*Meissner's*) plexus, is in the submucosa. It is more difficult to find.

A knowledge of these general features will be helpful in the more detailed descriptions which follow.

The Esophagus

The *esophagus* begins at the level of the cricoid cartilage and extends to slightly below the diaphragm where it becomes continuous with the stomach, a distance of 10 to 12 inches.

There is no sharp structural demarcation between the esophagus and pharynx, although a greater regularity in the muscularis externa and also the beginning of the muscularis mucosae soon become evident. The esophagus is the most muscular segment of the alimentary tract. Except during the passage of food or water, the lumen is small and irregular in shape as a result of the contraction of the inner layer of the muscularis externa, with a consequent formation of longitudinal folds (Fig. 16-23).

Mucosa. The *mucous membrane* (Figs. 16-23 to 16-25) is lined with a stratified squamous epithelium and, as in the pharynx, it is not cornified in man. The lamina propria is formed of fine interlacing connective tissue fibers with fibroblasts and histiocytes, and it may have areas of infiltration with lymphocytes (Fig. 16-24). The *muscularis mucosae* is formed of smooth muscle running in a longitudinal direction but with some inner circular fibers. It occupies a position corresponding to that of the elastic stratum of the pharynx, with which it is continuous. The muscularis mucosae is thicker in the esophagus than in any other segment of the digestive tube.

Submucosa. The *submucosa* is composed mainly of coarse, loosely interweaving collagenous fibers which permit the formation of extensive folds of the mucous membrane. It contains a plexus of the larger blood vessels, lymphatics and occasional autonomic (parasympathetic) ganglion cells and nerve fibers.

Muscularis. The *muscularis externa* of the first quarter or even less of the esophagus is composed of skeletal muscle and, from the juncture with the pharynx, it be-

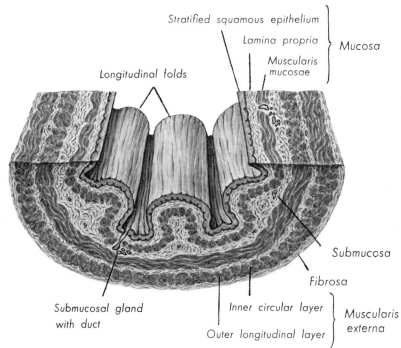

Fig. 16-23. Camera lucida drawing of a segment of the dorsal half of human esophagus. The entire esophagus had been in fixing solution before being cut open, thus preserving the internal longitudinal folds normally present. ×8.

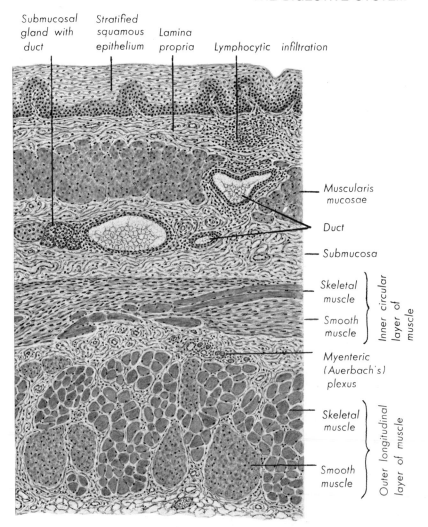

Submucosal   Stratified
gland with   squamous   Lamina
duct   epithelium   propria   Lymphocytic   infiltration

Muscularis
mucosae

Duct

Submucosa

Skeletal
muscle   } Inner circular
                layer of muscle
Smooth
muscle

Myenteric
(Auerbach's)
plexus

Skeletal
muscle   } Outer longitudinal
                layer of muscle
Smooth
muscle

Fig. 16-24. Transverse section through wall of the upper third of human esophagus. ×65.

comes progressively more regularly arranged into inner circular and outer longitudinal layers. This muscle is of branchiomeric origin and its contraction is involuntary. Some smooth muscle soon appears in each of the layers (Fig. 16-24) and gradually increases in amount. Skeletal fibers extend for a variable distance, but in the human they are rarely present below the juncture of the upper and lower halves of the organ and may be entirely replaced by smooth muscle at a higher level. Small groups of autonomic ganglion cells, part of Auerbach's plexus, are frequently found in the connective tissue between the inner and outer layers of muscle.

Fibrosa. The *fibrosa* is composed of loosely arranged connective tissue which binds the esophagus to surrounding structures. The short segment of esophagus that extends below the diaphragm lies in the peritoneal cavity and is covered by a *serosa*.

Glands of the Esophagus. Glands occur in the submucosa (*submucosal glands*) and in the mucosa (*mucosal* or *cardiac glands*). The number of *submucosal glands* is extremely variable in man. In some animals, e.g., the dog, they are numerous. The submucosal glands are composed of typical mucous alveoli such as those in the tongue. Several alveoli may open by short ducts into a main duct which, in its course through the submucosa and muscularis mucosae, may be dilated, forming an ampulla. In the lamina propria, the walls of the duct change from a simple

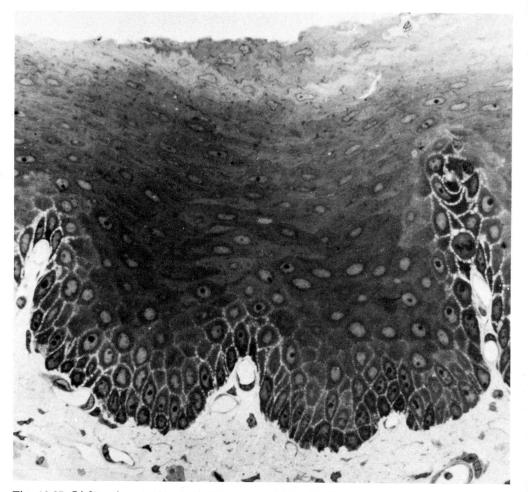

Fig. 16-25. Light micrograph of stratified squamous epithelium of the esophagus of monkey. ×475.

cuboidal to a stratified epithelium, the surface cells being either squamous or columnar (Fig. 16-24).

The *mucosal glands* (*cardiac*) of the esophagus occur in its uppermost and lowermost regions and lie in the lamina propria. The upper group is frequently absent. The cardiac glands are structurally similar to the glands in the upper or cardiac region of the stomach (Fig. 16-26). They are branched tubular glands which secrete a mucous substance.

The Stomach

The stomach extends from the esophagus to the duodenum. In the empty state, it is almost tubular in shape except for the upper part, which has a pear-shaped bulge superiorly and to the left. A frequently assumed shape when the organ is moderately distended is shown in Figure 16-27. As regards motor activity, the stomach is divisible into upper and lower halves. The upper half acts as a reservoir and has no—or only slight—peristaltic contractions. The lower half has peristaltic contractions which increase in intensity toward the pylorus. It is in this part that the various constituents of the food are thoroughly mixed with each other and with the secretions of the glands of the stomach. Associated with this motor activity is an increase in musculature, especially in the pyloric canal.

At the junction of the esophagus and stomach, the epithelium changes abruptly from stratified squamous to simple columnar. The transition is seen strikingly in

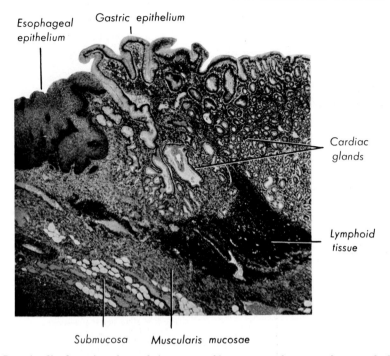

Fig. 16-26. Longitudinal section through juncture of human esophagus and stomach. Photomicrograph. ×26.

fresh specimens where the smooth, whitish mucosa of the esophagus gives way to the more irregular, pinkish mucosa of the stomach. The pink color of the stomach mucosa is due to the thinness of the epithelium and the proximity of the richly vascular lamina propria to the surface.

In the deeper structures, the line of demarcation is not as clear; the muscularis mucosae of the esophagus is continuous with that of the stomach, and glands of the stomach type extend up under the stratified epithelium of the esophagus.

Mucosa. The *mucous membrane* of the stomach has numerous ridges or *folds,* also known as *rugae* (Fig. 16-27), which vary in height and number with the degree of distention of the organ. When the stomach is fully distended, they almost disappear. The epithelial surface is also divided by grooves into small irregular areas, 1 to 5 mm in diameter, the *mamillated* or *gastric areas* (Fig. 16-28).

The entire surface of the mamillated or gastric areas is studded with minute depressions, the *gastric pits* or foveolae (Fig. 16-28). In the fundus, they are comparatively shallow, extending through about

one-fifth the thickness of the mucosa; in the pyloric region, the pits are much deeper, extending through one-half or more of the thickness of the mucous membrane. The glands open into the bottoms of the gastric pits.

The Surface Epithelium. The epithelium that lines the inner surface of the stomach and gastric pits is made up of columnar cells which differ structurally and functionally from the cells of the gastric glands. The characteristics of the stomach lining cells also differentiate them from the lining cells of all other parts of the digestive tract. The apical end of every surface cell has a deep, cup-shaped zone filled with mucigen. Since the mucigen is not preserved and stained in ordinary histological preparations, the cells show a deep, clear distal zone (Fig. 16-29). The nucleus is oval or spheroidal, depending on the shape of the cell and the amount of mucigen in the cytoplasm. These mucous lining cells differ from goblet cells in shape and in the chemical constitution of their mucigen. Electron micrographs show that the mucinogen droplets of the stomach lining cells are smaller, more discrete and more electron-

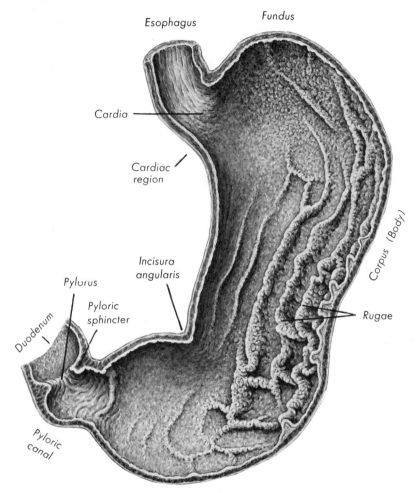

Fig. 16-27. Drawing of a cast of human stomach. The organ had been moderately distended in situ with formalin. Preparation and drawing made by Mr. Kellner. ×4/9.

dense than are those of the goblet cells.

The epithelium lining the stomach, in contrast with that of the intestine, has no striated free border as seen with the light microscope. However, electron micrographs do show microvilli on the free surface of these cells. The absence of an obvious striated border aids in delimiting the epithelium of the stomach from that of the intestine at the stomach-duodenal junction.

As the epithelium extends progressively deeper into the gastric pits, the cells become progressively shorter and have a narrower apical zone of mucigen. This gradual transition correlates with evidence that desquamated cells of the surface of the stomach are replaced by a migration of cells

up the walls of the foveolae. Radioautographic studies using tritium-labeled thymidine, which is incorporated into nuclei only during DNA replication, show that the surface cells arise by differentiation from cells which multiply in the isthmus or neck region of the glands. From the latter regions some cells move upward to replace the worn-out surface cells, whereas others may move downward to differentiate into parietal and zymogenic cells in the gastric glands.

Lamina Propria. The lamina propria (Figs. 16-29 and 16-30), in which the glands are located, consists of delicate, interweaving connective tissue fibers plus connective tissue cells and occasional smooth muscle

Opening of gastric pit   Mamillated area

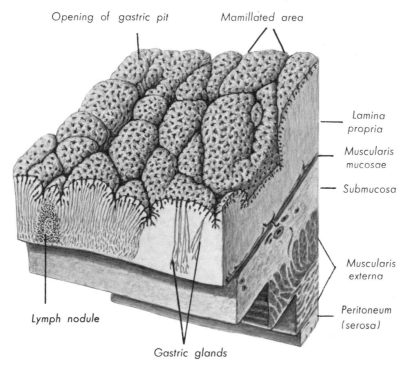

Lamina
propria

Muscularis
mucosae

Submucosa

Muscularis
externa

Peritoneum
(serosa)

Lymph nodule

Gastric glands

Fig. 16-28. Reconstruction of a portion of wall of stomach, semidiagrammatic. (Slightly modified after Braus.) ×17.

cells. In most regions the glands are so numerous that connective tissue fibers are reduced to thin strands. There is a diffuse infiltration of lymphocytes throughout the lamina propria; in addition, there are scattered lymphatic nodules, or "solitary follicles," which occur most frequently in the pyloric region (Fig. 16-35).

Muscularis Mucosae. The muscularis mucosae consists of a thin layer of smooth muscle in which the fibers usually course in both the circular and longitudinal directions. Strands of smooth muscle extend into the lamina propria between the glands.

Glands of the Stomach. The glands extend from the bottoms of the gastric pits, and their epithelium is continuous with that of the pits (Fig. 16-29). There are three types of glands: (1) *gastric* or *fundic glands,** distributed through the greater

part of the gastric mucosa, (2) *pyloric glands,* confined to the region immediately above the pylorus and (3) *cardiac glands,* found in the cardiac region of the stomach near its junction with the esophagus.

The gastric glands produce the essential digestive elements of the gastric juice, and the pyloric and cardiac glands function largely as mucous glands.

The Gastric Glands. The gastric glands (Fig. 16-29) are simple, sometimes branched, tubular glands, of which from three to seven open into each gastric pit. They extend downward through the entire thickness of the lamina propria to the muscularis mucosae.

Each gland consists of (1) a *mouth* opening into the pit, (2) a constricted portion, the *neck,* (3) the *body* or main portion of the tubule and (4) a slightly dilated and bent blind extremity, the *base* (Fig. 16-30).

In the glands proper, one can distinguish three types of cells in most preparations.

*The terminology is not entirely satisfactory. For example, the term *gastric glands* might be thought to indicate that these glands occur throughout the stomach, whereas they are absent from a narrow zone around the cardia and from the lower part of the pyloric region. A synonym, *fundic glands,* is even

more misleading for it indicates that these glands are limited to the fundic region of the stomach, whereas they are much more widely distributed.

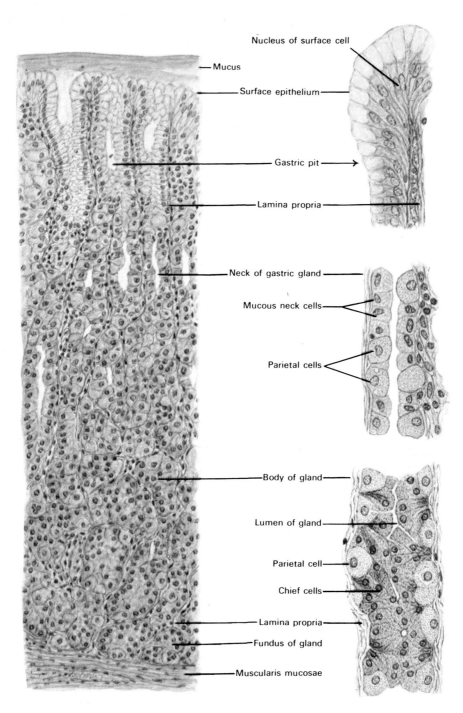

Fig. 16-29. Vertical section through mucous membrane of body of human stomach, showing surface epithelium, gastric pits and gastric glands. Hematoxylin-eosin stain. Figure at *left,* ×250; figures at *right,* ×500.

These are: (a) *chief cells,* (b) *parietal cells* and (c) *mucous neck cells* (Fig. 16-29). A fourth type, the enteroendocrine cell* is present but is difficult to identify except in special preparations.

The *chief cells* (zymogenic cells), as the name indicates, are the most numerous cells of the gastric glands.

They are large squarish or pyramidal shaped cells (Figs. 16-30 through 16-32) whose bases lie against the basal lamina and whose apical borders face the lumen of the gland. The nucleus lies in the basal half of the cell. In the usual histological preparations, the apical region appears as a delicate cytoplasmic meshwork enclosing clear, vacuolated spaces, which represent the position of the unpreserved zymogen granules. With proper fixatives and stains, these zymogen granules can be preserved and stained in situ.

In the base of the cell, below and lateral to the nucleus, there is an accumulation of basophilic substance that consists of granular endoplasmic reticulum and free ribosomes. The high concentration of rough surfaced endoplasmic reticulum in the gastric chief cell is correlated with the function of the cell in synthesizing the proteins of the zymogen granules, in this case, predominantly *pepsinogen.*

Mitochondria tend to be concentrated in the basal region of the cell also, and they are largest and most numerous when the cell is active in replenishing its secretory granules. The Golgi complex occupies a position between the nucleus and the apical border of the cell as is typical for secretory cells.

The stages in the formation of secretions by exocrine glands have been outlined in chapter 15 and described in detail in chapter 1. The same processes occur in the chief cells. The pepsinogen becomes activated

---

* Several names have been applied to these cells reflecting their stainability with silver or dichromate-containing solutions. It is clear from recent studies that there is a population of cells involved rather than one or two types as implied by the names argentaffin and enterochromaffin. Present information indicates that these cells are responsible for secreting a number of endocrine products. The term enteroendocrine seems appropriate and will be employed in this text although some authors prefer the term "basal granule cells."

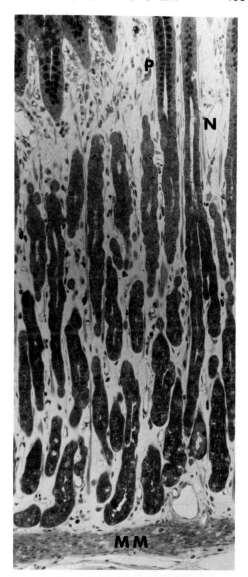

Fig. 16-30. One micrometer section of gastric glands from the monkey stomach. The lumen of the stomach is just out of view at the top and the muscularis mucosae is seen at the bottom (*MM*). A gastric pit lined with mucous surface cells is seen at *P*, and the neck of a branched tubular gland is seen at *N*. ×110.

after release and is converted into *pepsin.*

In addition to forming pepsinogen, in some animals the chief cells appear to be responsible for forming *intrinsic factor* which enhances the absorption of vitamin B_{12} by the lower portion of the small intestine. Recent studies show conclusively that

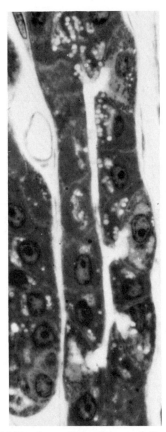

Fig. 16-31. A portion of one of the gastric glands shown in Figure 16-30 showing the continuity of intracellular canaliculi of parietal cells with the gland lumen. ×750.

in the human it is the parietal cell that elaborates intrinsic factor.

The *parietal cells* were the earliest described cells of the gastric glands and have retained their nondistinctive name. They are often spoken of as the HCl cells because they secrete the hydrochloric acid of the gastric juice. The cells are often larger than the chief cells and are oval or polygonal in shape (Figs. 16-29 and 16-31). The nuclei are spherical and centrally located. Binucleate or multinucleate cells are occasionally seen. Unlike the chief cells, the parietal cells have frequently been reported to divide. The cytoplasm of the parietal cells is finely granular throughout. It stains intensely with acid aniline dyes, with the result that, in stained specimens, these cells contrast sharply with the chief cells. In fresh, unstained preparations, the cytoplasm appears clearer than that of the chief

cells. In electron micrographs, it is seen that the cytoplasm contains an abundance of large mitochondria with numerous cristae (Fig. 16-32). These are apparently responsible for the acidophilia and granular appearance of the cytoplasm seen with the light microscope.

The parietal cells are numerous in the neck region of the gland, where they are interspersed among the neck mucous cells. Here their inner margins reach the glandular lumen. In the body and especially in the base of the gland, the parietal cells are pushed away from the lumen by the crowding chief cells, so that they come to lie peripherally against the basal lamina. However, they actually maintain a connection with the lumen of the gland (Figs. 16-31 and 16-32). Good cytological preparations and electron micrographs show that the luminal surface of parietal cells is in fact quite extensive because of the presence of baylike involutions, the so-called *intracellular canaliculi*. The plasmalemma lining the intracellular canals and that covering the remainder of the apical surface of the cell have numerous microvilli which further increase the membrane surface.

The mechanism of acid secretion in the stomach remains somewhat obscure. Since free acid is not found within the parietal cells, investigators have presumed that it must either be present in the form of bound acid or be formed in the vicinity of the cell membrane. In microdissection studies of living gastric mucosa, using a variety of indicator dyes, it has been found that, although the cytoplasm of the parietal cell gives a somewhat alkaline reaction, the intracellular canaliculi and the lumen of the gastric gland contain free acid. It appears, therefore, that the membrane of these cells is a highly selective structure which plays an important part in segregating and secreting both H^+ and Cl^- ions. Present evidence indicates that although the two ions are secreted simultaneously, they are transported independently.

There is considerable evidence that the total chemical change between the blood of the underlying connective tissue and the constituents of the parietal cell concerned with HCl secretion may be expressed by an equation in which sodium chloride and carbonic acid are converted into bicarbon-

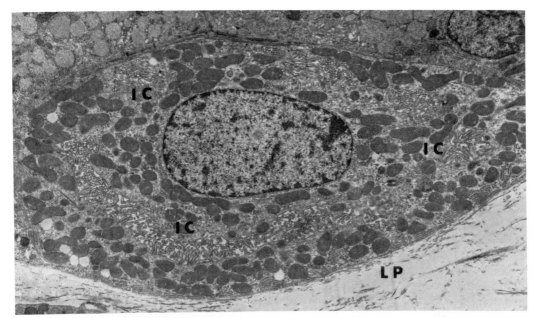

Fig. 16-32. Electron micrograph of a parietal cell from a gastric gland of the monkey. Intracellular canaliculi (*IC*) and numerous mitochondria are obvious. Portions of chief cells are seen at the top of the micrograph and a part of the lamina propria is seen at the bottom (*LP*). ×5000.

ate and hydrochloric acid. In this proposed equation of the changes involved in secretion of HCl, the reaction will go spontaneously toward sodium chloride and carbonic acid, whereas energy will be needed to reverse the reaction in the direction toward bicarbonate and hydrochloric acid. Presumably, the large population of mitochondria supplies the necessary energy. In support of this equation of the changes concerned with secretion, it has been found that the secretion of HCl into the lumen of the stomach is accompanied by an equivalent release of bicarbonate into the blood draining from the stomach. *Carbonic anhydrase,* an enzyme present in the parietal cell, apparently plays an important role by bringing about the formation of carbonic acid from water and carbon dioxide.

Certain cells which differ from the pepsinogen cells are found mainly in the neck region of the gland, where they occur in groups interspersed among the parietal cells. The *mucous neck cells* are cuboidal or low columnar in shape, with a finely granular cytoplasm which, in routine preparations, is paler than that of the chief cells but not as pale as the mucous surface cells. With special fixation and staining, it may be seen that the cells contain many small mucigen granules. The nucleus is situated basally and is frequently oval, with its long axis perpendicular to the long axis of the cell. The upper surface of the nucleus is sometimes indented (Fig. 16-29).

The mucus of the neck cells differs in several respects from that of the surface cells. Histochemical staining reactions indicate that the mucigen in the neck cells is an acid mucopolysaccharide, whereas that in the surface cells is a neutral polysaccharide. The droplets of mucigen are distributed differently, being dispersed throughout the cytoplasm in the neck cells and confined to the apical region of the surface cell. The mucus produced by the two types differs in consistency, that of the neck cells being less viscous. The mucus secreted by the neck cells, however, is apparently similar to that formed by the cardiac and pyloric glands. It has been suggested that the secretion of the mucous neck cell has a role in protecting the gastric gland itself from attack by HCl and proteolytic enzymes released from the other cell types. It is also possible that these cells are capable of transforming into surface mucous cells in the normal sequence of cell turnover.

The *enteroendocrine cells* are not easily recognizable in routine histological preparations but frequently they can be identified by their basal location in the epithelium and by their clear cytoplasm. The classical methods of silver and chromate staining that first delineated these cells and gave rise to the names argentaffin, argyrophil and enterochromaffin have provided an additional source of confusion for the modern histologist. Cell types recognizable by electron microscopy and immunocytology must now be equated with those described by the nonspecific earlier techniques (Figs. 16-33 and 16-34). Evidence is mounting that as many as 8 to 10 different endocrine cell types may exist in the epithelium of the human gastrointestinal tract, and as many as 6 have been described in the stomach alone by some investigators. Four endocrine secretions are known to be produced in the stomach: *serotonin, hista-*

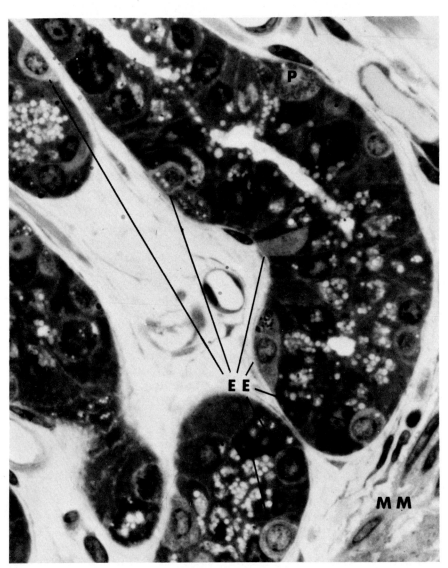

Fig. 16-33. Deep portion of one of the gastric glands seen in Figure 16-30 showing a number of enteroendocrine cells (*EE*). A portion of a parietal cell is at *P* and the cells with prominent secretory granules are chief cells. Smooth muscle of the muscularus mucosae is at the lower right (*MM*). ×900.

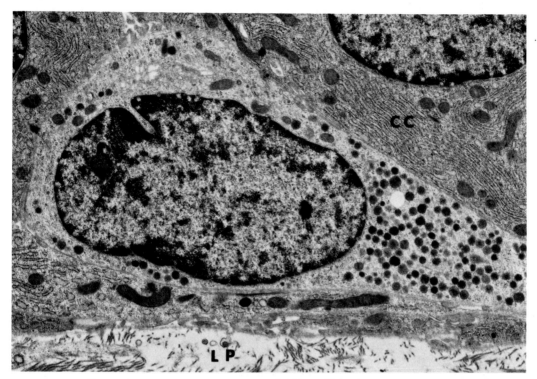

Fig. 16-34. Electron micrograph of an enteroendocrine cell in the wall of the gastric gland of the monkey. This cell lies near the base of the epithelium wedged between chief cells (*CC*). The lamina propria (*LP*) with collagenous fibers is at the bottom. ×8500.

mine, gastrin and *enteroglucagon*. It appears that each may be produced by a morphologically distinct enteroendocrine cell type. Electron microscopy shows that some of the enteroendocrine cells reach the epithelial lumenal surface but all contain granules concentrated basally and their secretion products are released toward the blood vessels of the lamina propria rather than into the gut lumen.

The Pyloric Glands. These are simple, branched, tubular glands, several of which open into each of the deep *pyloric pits*. These pits occupy a much greater proportion of the thickness of the mucous membrane than do the pits of the gastric glands (compare Figs. 16-29 and 16-35), and the proportionate depth occupied by the glands themselves is correspondingly less. The pyloric glands, although short, are quite tortuous, so that in section the tubules are seen cut mainly transversely or obliquely. Most of the pyloric gland cells resemble the mucous neck cells of the gastric glands in that their secretion protects against au-

todigestion. They differ morphologically from the neck cells in that they are taller and their ovoid nuclei are generally oriented parallel with the long axes of the cells. Parietal cells are found only occasionally in the pyloric glands.

The transition from the gastric to the pyloric type of stomach gland is not abrupt but is marked by a "transitional border zone" in which gastric and pyloric glands are intermingled and in which are also found single glands which combine the characteristics of both types.

Cardiac Glands. The transition zone between esophagus and stomach contains glands that resemble those in the lamina propria of the lower end of the esophagus (Fig. 16-26). Because of their location they have been designated *cardiac glands*. Those nearest the esophagus are lined with clear cells which resemble closely the cells of the pyloric glands and the mucous neck cells of the gastric glands. As one passes farther from the gastroesophageal junction, parietal cells and chief cells make their

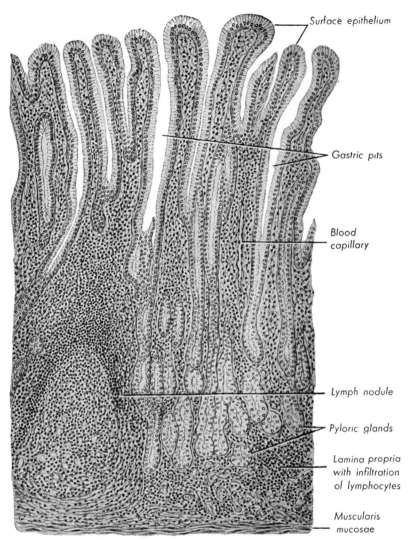

Fig. 16-35. Vertical section through mucous membrane of pyloric canal. ×110.

appearance and become more and more numerous. The glands thus pass over by gradual transition into typical gastric glands. It should be noted that on occasion there may be patches of gastric mucosa in the esophagus or patches of intestinal mucosa in the stomach of normal individuals.

Submucosa. The *submucosa* consists of coarse, loosely arranged connective tissue. It contains the larger blood vessels and nerves, including the plexus of Meissner.

Muscularis. The *muscular coat* of the stomach is usually described as consisting of three layers, an inner oblique, a middle circular and an outer longitudinal. In the fundus, however, the muscle bundles run

in various directions, so that a separation of the muscular coat into layers having definite directions is difficult. The inner and middle layers of the pylorus are thickened to form the sphincter pylori. In the connective tissue which separates the longitudinal and circular muscles, there are groups of parasympathetic nerve cells and fibers which, while much less distinct, are homologous to Auerbach's plexus of the intestine.

Serosa. The *serous coat* consists of a layer of loosely arranged connective tissue which is covered by mesothelium.

Blood vessels, lymphatics and nerves are so similar throughout the stomach and intestines that they are described together at the close of the sections on the intestines.

The Small Intestine

The small intestine, which extends from the pylorus of the stomach to the colon, is commonly divided into three regions, an upper, the *duodenum*; a middle, the *jejunum*; and a lower, the *ileum*. The subdivisions of the small intestine are not demarcated by abrupt structural changes as is the case where the duodenum joins the stomach and where the ileum joins the colon. Changes occur gradually along the small intestine and the differences between different divisions are not as obvious as are the similarities. Therefore the divisions will be described together, pointing out the general characteristics first, and directing attention to certain distinctive features as they occur. However, it may be helpful to understand at the outset that some areas are readily differentiated in routine histological preparations. For example, the first part of the duodenum is easily identified by the presence of Brunner's glands in the submucosa, and the lower part of the ileum is characterized by aggregates of lymphatic tissue known as Peyer's patches. Structural changes along the remainder of the tract (lower duodenum, jejunum, and upper ileum) occur gradually and are more obscure.

If the small intestine is opened by a longitudinal incision through its wall, a series of definite folds will be seen on its inner surface. They are in general parallel to one another and pass in a circular or oblique manner partly around the lumen of the tube. These folds are known as *plicae circulares* (*circular folds*) or *valves of Kerckring*. They are absent in the upper region of the duodenum, tallest in the jejunum and much less prominent in the ileum as it nears the colon. These folds involve the entire mucosa, and a portion of the submucosa (Fig. 16-36). Unlike the folds of the stomach, the plicae cannot be completely flattened out by distention of the intestine.

The mucosa is further carried up into finger-like projections, the *villi,* which cover not only the surface of the plicae but the entire surface of the small intestine (Fig. 16-36). The villi differ in shape in the different parts of the small intestine, being leaf-shaped in the duodenum, rounded in the jejunum and club-shaped in the ileum. The plicae and the villi are characteristic of the small intestine. It is important to note that, while the pits of the stomach are *depressions in* the mucous membrane, the intestinal villi are *projections above* the general intestinal surface. By means of its folds and projections, the absorbing and secreting surface of the intestinal mucosa is enormously increased. Opening between

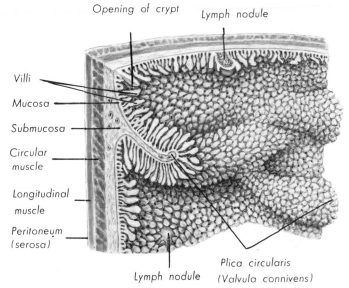

Fig. 16-36. Reconstruction of a portion of the wall of small intestine. (After Braus.) ×17.

the villi and extending into the mucosa as far as the muscularis mucosae are simple glandular pits, the crypts (of Lieberkühn) or *intestinal glands.* All of the above modifications are treated in detail in a discussion of the mucosa.

The wall of the intestine consists of the same four coats that constituted the wall of the stomach: *mucosa, submucosa, muscularis externa* and *serosa.*

Mucosa. The mucosa is composed of its lining *epithelium,* a *lamina propria* with its connective tissue and glands, and a limiting *muscularis mucosae* below. The most characteristic feature of the small intestinal mucosa is the *villus* (Figs. 16-36 to 16-39).

The villi are mucosal projections barely visible to the naked eye. Situated close together and covering the entire mucosal surface, they give the interior of the intestine a soft, velvety appearance grossly.

Each villus consists of a core of delicate, loose connective tissue and an epithelial covering. The connective tissue, the lamina propria of the mucosa, is infiltrated with lymphocytes to a variable extent. In addition to these and the cells of the connective tissue, occasional isolated smooth muscle cells from the muscularis mucosae are present.

A single small lymphatic vessel (lacteal) with definite endothelial lining traverses

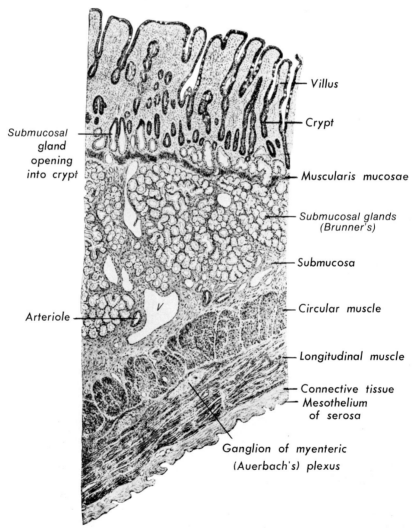

Fig. 16-37. Longitudinal section through upper duodenum of man. (After Schaffer.) ×30.

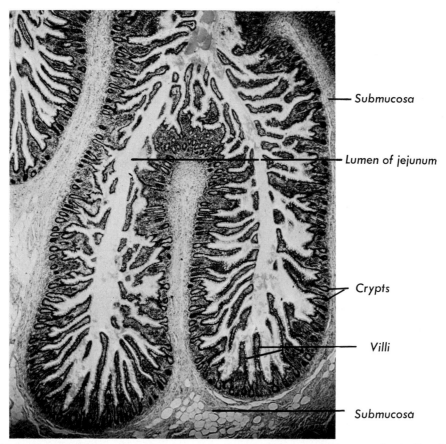

Fig. 16-38. Longitudinal section of mucosa of jejunum. The section shows a short plica circularis in the *center* of the field, and on either side of it part of a taller plica. The entire luminal surface is covered with villi; submucosal connective tissue forms the core of each plica. Hematoxylin-eosin stain. Photomicrograph. ×32.

the center of each villus, beginning at the tip in a slightly dilated, blind extremity. Since this *central lacteal* is usually collapsed in ordinary preparations, it is often difficult to see. It appears most frequently as two closely approximated rows of flat cells with bulging nuclei. During absorption of fat from the intestinal lumen, the lacteals become distended with fat droplets and are then clearly visible (Fig. 16-48). The blood capillaries of the villus form a network which lies, for the most part, away from the lacteal, just beneath the basal lamina of the intestinal epithelium (Fig. 16-40).

Observations of the villi in the living condition have revealed that they continually change in length and undergo waving motions. This is possible because of the presence of smooth muscle in them. These movements bring the villi into contact with new material to be absorbed and aid in the circulation of the villus, particularly in the movement of fluid in the lymph vessels (lacteals).

Epithelium. The *epithelium* covering the villi is a single layer of columnar cells attached to a delicate basement membrane (i.e., basal lamina plus lamina reticularis). The epithelium consists mainly of two quite different kinds of cells, *columnar absorbing cells* and *goblet cells*. Enteroendocrine cells are also present in small numbers. The columnar absorbing cells are quite plastic and, although generally long and narrow, they vary in length and breadth as they adapt themselves to movements of the intestine. Their various shapes can best be studied in dissociated (macerated) epithe-

Goblet cells   Striated border

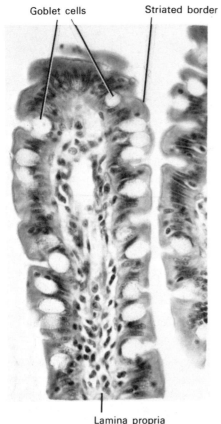

Lamina propria

Fig. 16-39. Light micrograph of a longitudinal section of the upper portion of a villus of the jejunum of a cat. The double border appearance at the tip of the villus is caused by the relationship between the plane of the section and irregularities in the contour of the surface of the villus. The central lacteal is dilated somewhat because the animal was actively absorbing fat prior to the time of autopsy. ×390.

lium. The cytoplasm is finely granular; its appearance changes somewhat in different phases of absorption. It frequently contains fat droplets. The nucleus is ovoid and is usually situated in the lower half of the cell (Fig. 16-41).

One of the most striking and distinguishing features of the columnar absorbing cells is their *striated free border* (brush border). With low magnification, this is seen as a nearly homogeneous, refractile layer (Figs. 1-9, *C*, and 16-41) covering the apical surface of the cell but, with greater magnification, it appears finely striated. By means of phase contrast and electron microscopy, it is seen that the striated free border is ac-

tually composed of a great many very fine, closely packed *microvilli* (Figs. 16-42 and 16-43). The length of the microvilli varies in cells of different regions, being greatest (1 to 1.5 μm) on cells at the tips of the villi. High resolution electron micrographs show that the outer leaflet of the plasmalemma over the microvilli has very slender branching filaments which form a coat of fuzzy appearance. This surface coat gives staining reactions of acid mucopolysaccharides and ranges in thickness from 0.1 to 0.5 μm. The central portion of each microvillus contains fine filaments oriented longitudinally and extending into a feltwork of filaments, the *terminal web,* in the cytoplasm just beneath the level of the microvilli. It has been presumed for some time that the filaments in the microvilli serve a structural function, but their size and reactivity with heavy meromyosin suggest that they are actin-like and probably contractile in nature. The terminal web zone is free of cell organelles and is rich in filaments which course chiefly in a direction perpendicular to the long axis of the cell. The filaments of the web connect laterally with electron-dense material in the subplasmalemmal region of the intermediate junctions and appear to be structural or contractile.

The striated border region contains a number of enzymes, including alkaline phosphatase, maltase, adenosine triphosphatase and aminopeptidase. At least some of these enzymes appear to be integral components of the plasma membrane itself. Thus, the border not only provides an increase in the luminal surface of the cell for absorption but also contains enzymes of importance for the final stages of the digestive process.

The *mitochondria* (Fig. 1-9, *C*) are distributed above and below the nucleus. In both regions they are rod-shaped or filamentous. Those in the basal portion of the cell are particularly numerous.

The *Golgi apparatus* lies between the nucleus and the free surface of the cell. Its possible significance in the absorption of foodstuffs is discussed below under "Cytological Changes During Absorption."

The *endoplasmic reticulum* is chiefly of the smooth variety in the apical part of the cell and mostly of the rough surfaced variety in the deeper portion. Free ribosomes

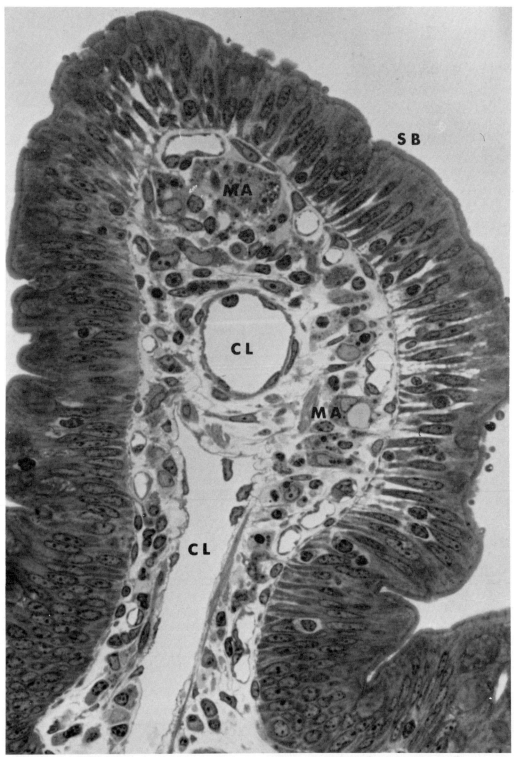

Fig. 16-40. Light micrograph of a 1 μm section of an intestinal villus from the monkey. The epithelium shows numerous goblet cells and a prominent striated border (*SB*). The villar core shows profiles of the central lacteal (*CL*) and numerous cells, including macrophages (*MA*). Blood capillaries are distributed peripherally immediately beneath the basal lamina of the epithelium. ×550.

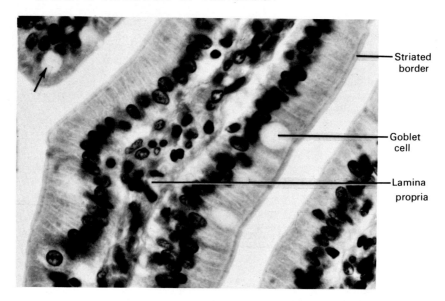

Striated border

Goblet cell

Lamina propria

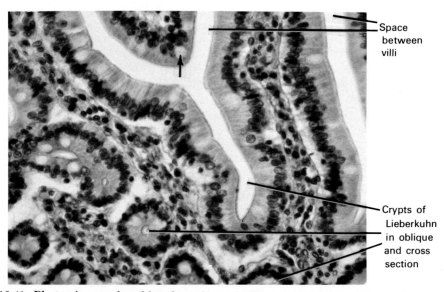

Space between villi

Crypts of Lieberkuhn in oblique and cross section

Fig. 16-41. Photomicrographs of basal portions of villi and subjacent portions of crypts from a section of human jejunum. Some of the crypts are seen in transverse section. The *upper* figure is a higher magnification micrograph that includes the upper portion of the field shown in the *lower* figure. As an aid in orientation, an *arrow* is directed to the same goblet cell in each photograph. *Upper,* ×650; *lower,* ×390.

are also fairly numerous in the basal part of the cell.

The *intercellular junctions* at the adluminal ends of the cells are typical junctional complexes as described in chapter 4 (Fig. 4-9). Maculae adherentes, or desmosomes, are found at deeper levels. It will be recalled that potential intercellular space is sealed around the adluminal ends of the cells by zonular occluding junctions and that the width of the intercellular space in most other regions is about 100 to 200 Å. In the deeper regions of intestinal epithelium, however, the intercellular space may reach a width of 2000 Å.

Goblet cells, unicellular mucous glands,

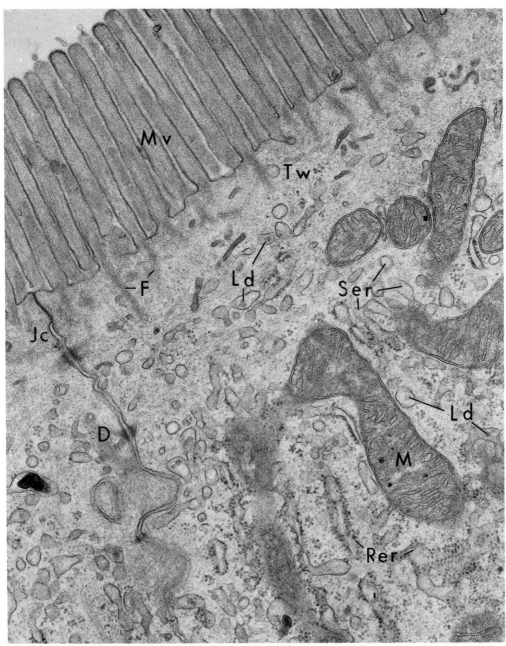

Fig. 16-42. Electron micrograph of a portion of the apical region of a columnar absorptive cell from the jejunum of a rat. The area of the adluminal surface of the cell is increased by microvilli (*Mv*). Fine filaments in the core of each microvillus are continuous with filaments (*F*) in the subjacent cytoplasm, in a region known as the terminal web (*Tw*). Filaments of the terminal web also loop into portions of the juctional complex (*Jc*). The complex consists, from above downward, of a xonula occludens, a zonula adherens and a macula adherens (desmosome) as described in chapter 4. Other desmosomes (*D*) are seen at irregular intervals along the course of apposing membranes of adjacent cells. Tubules of smooth endoplasmic reticulum (*Ser*) become continuous with rough endoplasmic reticulum (*Rer*). Some small lipid droplets (*Ld*) are seen within tubules of the *Ser*. This is explained by the fact that the animal was given fat by stomach tube 45 min before autopsy. *M*, mitochondrion. ×35,000. (Courtesy of Drs. R. R. Cardell, Jr., S. Badenhausen, and K. R. Porter, J. Cell Biol., vol. 34, 1967.)

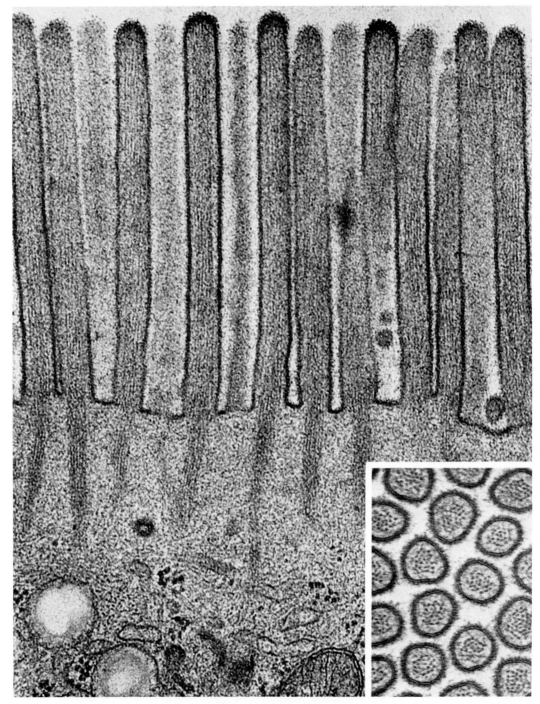

Fig. 16-43. Electron micrograph of the apical region of a columnar absorbing cell, showing the microvilli and the terminal web region of the cytoplasm at higher magnification than in the preceding figure. Note the prominent core of filaments in each microvillus. The adluminal surface of the plasmalemma of each microvillus is covered with a fuzzy coat (see chapter 1, Fig. 1-34). The *inset at lower right* shows the microvilli in transverse section. Small intestine of a rat. ×75,000. (Courtesy of Drs. Mary Bonneville and Keith Porter.)

are dispersed among the columnar absorbing cells. In the early stages of the secretory process, only a few mucigen droplets are present in the cytoplasm adjacent to the Golgi region. As more droplets form, the apical portion of the cell becomes distended to the typical goblet shape, and the nucleus, together with most of the remaining cytoplasm, is displaced into the narrow basal region or stem. These cells differ from the absorbing cells in a number of respects, including shape and staining. The mucigen droplets are dissolved by routine methods of preparing sections for light microscopy; thus, the upper portion of the goblet cell appears relatively empty. When the mucigen droplets are preserved by special methods, they are found to be basophilic, metachromatic and periodic acid-Schiff-positive. Electron micrographs show that microvilli are short and sparse on goblet cells. Because of the regular cellular turnover in the epithelium, it is likely that the goblet cells normally secrete continuously during their brief life span. More details on the goblet cells are given in chapters 4 and 15.

The number of goblet cells is small in the duodenum and becomes progressively greater in the jejunum, ileum and colon.

Crypts or *intestinal glands* occur throughout the small intestine. They are simple tubular glands located in the mucous membrane. They open between the villi and extend down through the lamina propria as far as the muscularis mucosae. The epithelium of the crypt is continuous at its opening with the surface epithelium of the villi. In general, the columnar cells which lie near the base of the gland are less differentiated and somewhat shorter than the columnar absorbing cells of the villi. The striated border of the cells deep in the glands is poorly developed (with microvilli of less than 0.5 μm in length). There is a gradual increase in the height of the microvilli of the striated border on the columnar cells from the base toward the mouth of the crypt. This fact, together with the presence of numerous mitoses in the crypts (Figs. 16-44 and 16-52), correlates well with the results obtained by thymidine labeling studies which show conclusively that the intestinal surface cells arise from cells in the crypts.

Recent studies have elucidated the interrelationships of the various cell types in the crypts and on the villi. *Primitive cells* (undifferentiated) located in the bases of the crypts differentiate to form all of the other cell types. Thymidine labeling indicates that intermediate stages in formation of *goblet cells* (*oligomucous cells*) and the villar *absorptive cells* lie in the midcrypt region. Both of these cell types are still capable of mitosis, but their progeny are committed to their respective cell lines. On the other hand, there are also coarsely granular cells in the bases of the crypts, the *cells of Paneth,* that differentiate from the primitive cells but do not migrate from the bases of the crypts. It appears that Paneth cells do not divide, but they degenerate and are replaced at about the same rate as the other cell types. Paneth cells have prominent acidophilic granules and appear secretory in organization but their precise function is not understood. There is some evidence that they may contain bacteriocidal enzymes and may be phagocytic (Fig. 16-45). The earlier speculation that they elaborate important digestive enzymes has not been confirmed. Their failure to migrate out of the crypts with other differentiating cells has not been explained. Paneth cells occur mainly in the crypts of the small intestine but occasionally they may be present in the large intestine as well.

Enteroendocrine cells also arise in the intestinal crypts. The suggestion by some investigators that these cells may be of neural crest origin has not been verified. In fact, thymidine labeling studies provide strong evidence that these cells also differentiate from the basal primitive cells. The enteroendocrine cells do not appear to be capable of division once they are clearly recognizable morphologically. They are most numerous in the proximal duodenum and the appendix, although they are present throughout the small intestine and colon. Again, the reader is reminded that several cell types are actually represented. These cells are thought to produce the intestinal hormones important in controlling gastric and intestinal motility, release of stomach contents, release of bile from the gall bladder, and release of pancreatic secretions. In addition, as in the gastric mu-

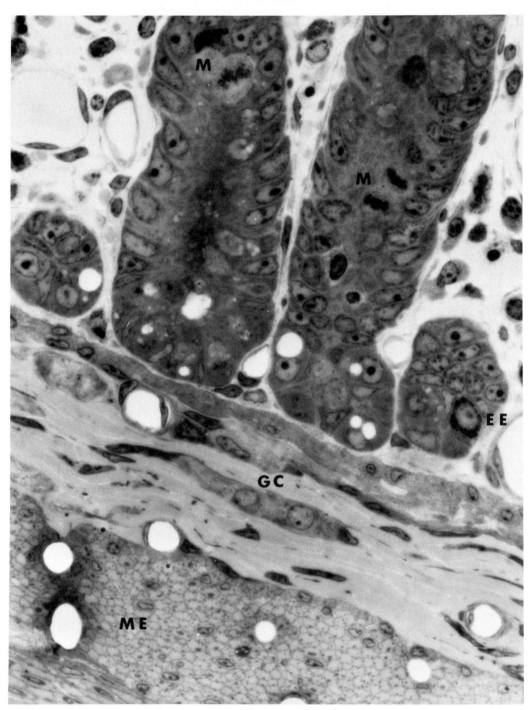

Fig. 16-44. Light micrograph of a 1 μm section of intestinal crypts from the monkey. This is a longitudinal section and the smooth muscle of the internal layer of the muscularis externa appears in cross section (*ME*). Mitotic figures (*M*) and an enteroendocrine cell (*EE*) are apparent in this view. The collagen bundles of the submucosa appear nearly homogeneous in this preparation and two nuclei of ganglion cells from the submucosal plexus are seen at *GC*. Capillaries are expanded because the animal was fixed by vascular perfusion. ×800.

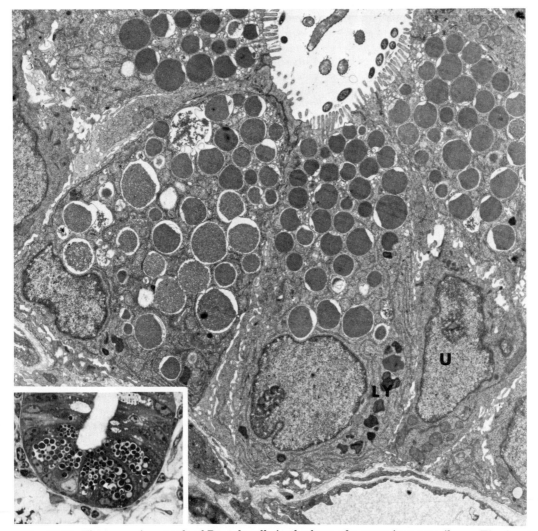

Fig. 16-45. Electron micrograph of Paneth cells in the base of a crypt in mouse ileum. The *inset* shows a comparable area by light microscopy. The lumen of the crypt contains bacteria. *Ly,* lysosomes; *U,* undifferentiated crypt cell. ×5100. Inset, ×400. (Courtesy of Dr. David Chase.)

cosa, one of these cell types produces serotonin and another is thought to secrete enteroglucagon. Enteroendocrine cells migrate out onto the villi with the goblet and columnar absorptive cells. Because of their sporadic appearance with light microscopic techniques their total numbers have not been appreciated until recently.

All of the intestinal epithelial cells turn over at about the same rate, the total life span in humans being 2 to 4 days. Thus, millions of cells are lost daily and minor disruptions in the normal proliferative events can have profound consequences on intestinal function. *It is clear that the major importance of the crypts in the small intestine is not that they represent conventional glands, but that they are responsible for continual renewal of the epithelial cell population.*

Cytological Changes During Absorption. The epithelium of the gastrointestinal tract has two main functions: (1) The *secretion* of substances necessary in digestion (dealt with in connection with the description of the various secretory cells) and (2) the *absorption* of the products of digestion. With regard to the latter function, the epithelium of the intestines is involved in uptake of all three classes of food—carbohydrates, proteins and fats.

The absorption of fats has been studied extensively by biochemical methods and by electron microscopy. Breakdown of dietary fats in the intestine is effected by pancreatic lipase with the aid of bile salts. There have been some questions concerning the amount of hydrolysis which is prerequisite for fat absorption. About one-fourth of the ingested fat is hydrolyzed completely to fatty acids and glycerol, and the remainder is hydrolyzed to monoglycerides and diglycerides. It seems clear that most of the fat is absorbed in the form of fatty acids and monoglycerides and that these are recombined to form triglycerides within the intestinal mucosa.

In order to follow absorption cytologically, the substance being studied must be marked for identification. This is readily achieved for fat, since lipids are blackened by the osmium tetroxide generally used for tissue fixation in electron microscopy. The pathway of fat can be deduced from electron microscope studies of tissue fixed at different time intervals subsequent to introduction of fat into the digestive tube. Within a relatively short time, small lipid droplets are present within the tubules of the smooth endoplasmic reticulum (SER) of the apical portions of the absorbing cells (Fig. 16-42). Lipid droplets are also found within bulbous expansions of the SER and within isolated vesicles of the SER (Fig. 16-46). The vesicles are apparently derived from the SER and some of them may be derived from the Golgi complex with which they are often associated. By this stage of fat absorption, the lipid droplets range up to 500 Å in diameter and aggregates of them are visible under the light microscope (Fig. 16-48). In the process of droplet formation some protein, synthesized in rough endoplasmic reticulum, and some carbohydrate materials are added (the latter probably by the Golgi apparatus). The vesicles, containing the lipid droplets, migrate to the lateral surface of the cell where the droplets are released, free of enveloping membranes, into extracellular space (Fig. 16-47). At this stage they are referred to as *chylomicrons*. The chylomicrons pass through the basal

lamina and into the intercellular connective tissue spaces and thence to lymphatic capillaries. Diagrammatic summaries of the sequence of events in fat absorption, as revealed by electron microscopic and histochemical studies, are shown in Figure 16-49. It is thought that monoglycerides and fatty acids pass from the intestinal lumen into the cytoplasm of the columnar absorbing cell by diffusion through the cell membrane. The monoglycerides and fatty acids then must pass into the tubules of the SER where they are resynthesized to triglycerides that are released into the intercellular spaces.

The pathway from the epithelial cells to the vascular system proceeds primarily by the lymphatics. Neutral fats (triglycerides) pass from the connective tissue underlying the epithelial cells into lymphatic capillaries and eventually reach the blood vessels via the thoracic duct. Most of the absorbed fatty acids which are more than 10 carbon chains in length are resynthesized with glycerol to form triglycerides and enter the lymphatics. Fatty acids with short carbon chains (less than 10 or 12 carbons) pass directly into the blood capillaries of the intestine and thence to the portal vein. The bile salts which were combined with the fatty acids during the absorptive process become free and they are absorbed directly into the blood to return by the portal vein to the liver where they are excreted into the bile for a role in another cycle of fat absorption.

Lamina Propria. The loose connective tissue, besides forming the centers of the villi, fills in the spaces between the crypts and between the latter and the muscularis mucosae. It is composed of interweaving reticular and delicate collagenous fibers, with a considerable number of elastic fibrils. It also contains connective tissue cells: fibroblasts, eosinophils, plasma cells, mast cells and some smooth muscle cells. Lymphocytes are abundant everywhere and in many places they are so numerous as to give the appearance of diffuse lymphatic tissue. Here and there the lymphatic cells are more closely packed together to form distinct lymph nodules. These are known as *solitary nodules* to distinguish them from groups of lymph nodules which occur

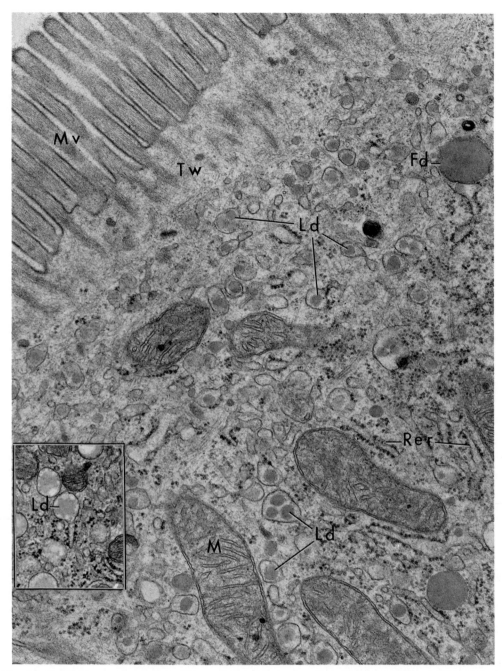

Fig. 16-46. Electron micrograph of the apical portion of an intestinal absorptive cell fixed during active fat absorption. Numerous lipid droplets (*Ld*) are present within tubules of the smooth endoplasmic reticulum. The latter is hypertrophied and is often seen in continuity with the rough endoplasmic reticulum (*Rer*). Lipid droplets are often seen in bulbous expansions of the reticulum (*Ld* of *inset*). Free lipid droplets (*Fd*) within the cell can be distinguished from the droplets in stages of absorption by their diameter and by the absence of an enveloping membrane. *M*, mitochondrion; *Mv*, microvilli; *Tw*, terminal web area. From rat jejunum fixed 40 min after intubation of corn oil; *inset,* from rat jejunum fixed at 60 min after intubation of corn oil. ×31,500. (Courtesy of Drs. R. R. Cardell, Jr., S. Badenhausen, and K. R. Porter, J. Cell Biol., vol. 34, 1967.)

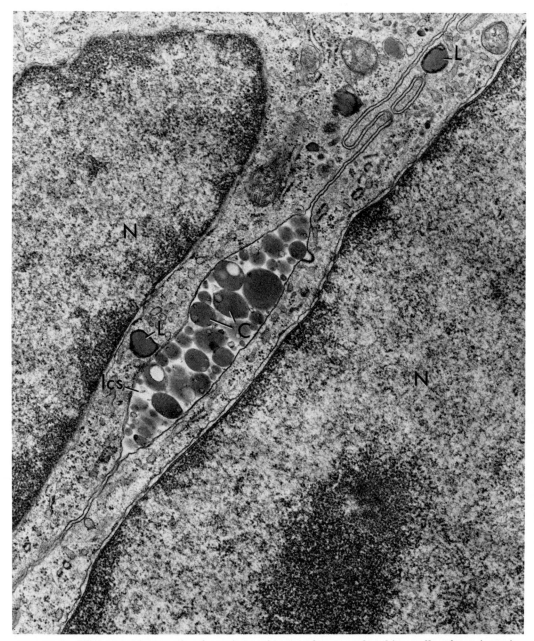

Fig. 16-47. Electron micrograph of portions of two columnar absorbing cells of rat intestine subsequent to the intubation of corn oil. Intercellular spaces (*Ics*) are generally enlarged during fat absorption and they contain chylomicra (*C*) which are similar to the largest lipid droplets (*L*) in the cytoplasm except that the latter are membrane-bounded whereas the former are not. The chylomicra pass downward through the intercellular spaces and through the basal lamina of the epithelium to reach the subepithelial connective tissue where they enter lymphatic capillaries. *N*, nuclei. ×23,225. (Courtesy of Drs. R. R. Cardell, Jr., S. Badenhausen, and K. R. Porter, J. Cell Biol. vol. 34, 1967.)

in the lower sections of the small intestine and are known as Peyer's patches (see below). Solitary nodules are much more nu-

merous in the small intestine than in the stomach. They are identical in structure with those of the stomach. The connective

Fat droplets in   Central lacteal   Lamina propria of villus
columnar absorbing cell

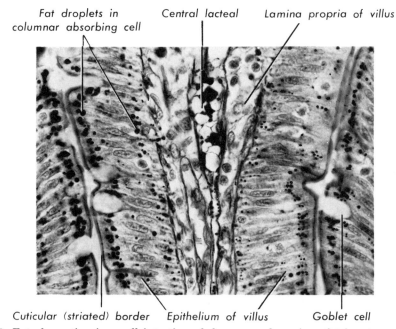

Cuticular (striated) border   Epithelium of villus   Goblet cell

Fig. 16-48. Fat absorption in small intestine of rhesus monkey given fat by stomach tube 4 hr before autopsy. Parts of three villi and two intervillous (luminal) spaces are shown. Fat droplets are seen in the cytoplasm of the apical regions of the columnar cells and also within the central lacteal. On the basis of electron microscopic studies, it can be concluded that the droplets which appear to be in the basal part of the cell, as seen here in a 10 μm thick section under the light microscope, are actually within relatively narrow intercellular spaces. Osmium tetroxide fixation; azocarmine stain. ×480.

tissue of the lamina propria contains a rich capillary bed in addition to the lymphatic vessels (lacteals).

Aggregated Lymph Nodules (Peyer's Patches). These are aggregations of lymph nodules found mainly in the ileum, especially near its junction with the colon. They always occur on the side of the gut opposite the attachment of the mesentery. Each patch consists of from 10 to 70 nodules, which lie side by side and are so arranged that the entire patch has an oval shape, its long diameter lying lengthwise of the intestine. The pear-shaped apices of the nodules are directed toward the lumen and project almost through the mucosa. They are not covered by villi; a single layer of columnar epithelium alone separates them from the lumen of the gut, where their smooth surfaces can readily be seen in gross dissection (Figs. 16-50 and 16-51).

The bases of the nodules are not confined to the lamina propria but extend into the submucosa. The relation of the patch to the mucosa and submucosa can be best appreciated by following the course of the muscularis mucosae. This is seen to stop abruptly at the circumference of the patch, appearing throughout the patch as isolated groups of smooth muscle cells. Sometimes the individual nodules that make up a Peyer's patch are quite discrete and well defined. More frequently, however, the nodules tend to coalesce except at their apices, so that the individual nodules can be definitely outlined only at their apices and identified to some extent by their germinal centers. Peyer's patches are most prominent in children. In the adult and in old age, the lymphatic tissue gradually undergoes regression and involution. This correlates with a gradual decrease in efficiency of the immune response with aging.

Muscularis Mucosae. The muscularis mucosae is thin, consisting of an inner circular and an outer longitudinal layer of smooth muscle. Small groups of muscle fibers extend from the muscularis mucosae into the cores of the villi.

Submucosa. The *submucosa* (Figs. 16-

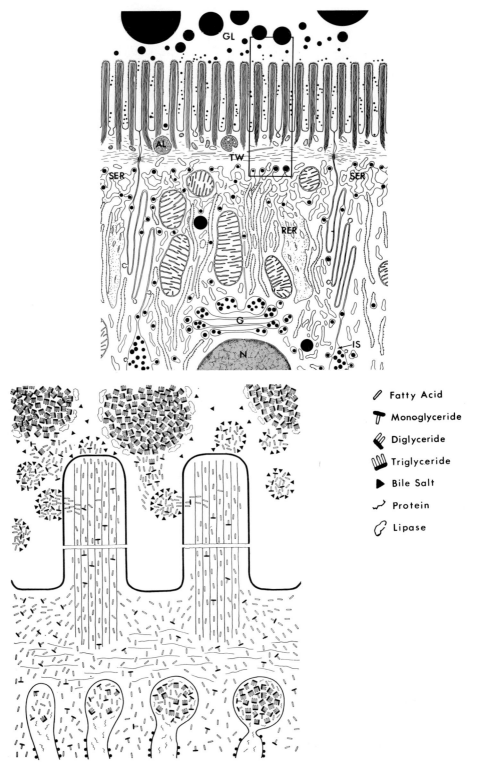

Fig. 16-49. The *upper* figure gives a diagrammatic summary of fat absorption by intestinal epithelial cells as interpreted from results of electron microscopic and biochemical studies. Fat in the gut lumen (*GL*) is broken down to small lipid droplets seen above and between the microvilli.

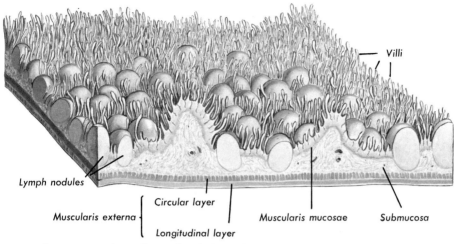

Fig. 16-50. Low power, three dimensional view of a segment of human ileum, showing part of an aggregate of lymph nodules. ×15.

37 and 16-50) consists, as in the stomach, of loosely arranged connective tissue, and it contains the larger blood vessels and lymphatics. Autonomic nerve fibers and parasympathetic ganglion cells are present in scattered groups. They form a plexus (*Meissner's*) that interconnects with the *myenteric* (*Auerbach's*) plexus of the muscularis externa. The submucosa is free from glands except in the duodenum, where it contains *duodenal glands* (*of Brunner*) (Fig. 16-37).

Duodenal glands are the most distinguishing characteristic of the *upper* duodenum and are absent in its inferior part. Duodenal glands are generally classified as branched and compound tubular glands, although the lumen of the terminal portion of the tubule is frequently enlarged to approach a tubuloalveolar form (Fig. 16-37). They are lined with a columnar epithelium similar to that of the pyloric glands. The ducts are also lined with simple columnar epithelium and pass up through the muscularis mucosae and lamina propria and empty usually into a crypt. Occasionally they empty on the surface between the villi. In the region of the juncture between the pylorus and duodenum, there is a zone in which the glands of the two segments merge imperceptibly. Glands of similar structure lie partly in the lamina propria and partly in the submucosa, with strands of the muscularis mucosae present among the alveoli. The juncture of the stomach and duodenum thus is not sharply demarcated by the position of the glands. Duodenal glands, like the pyloric glands, secrete an alkaline mucoid substance.

Muscularis. The *muscular coat* (Figs. 16-37 and 16-50) consists of two well defined layers of smooth muscle, an inner circular

Fat diffuses through the cell membrane in the form of monoglycerides and fatty acids. These enter the tubules of the smooth endoplasmic reticulum (*SER*) where they are resynthesized to form droplets of triglycerides. The membrane-bounded droplets are transported either directly or via the Golgi complex (*G*) to intercellular spaces (*IS*) at the level of the nucleus (*N*). *Al*, apical lysosomes; *RER*, rough endoplasmic reticulum; *TW*, terminal web. The enclosed area is enlarged in the *lower* figure to show the biochemical events in the initial phases of fat absorption. Triglycerides and diglycerides, in the presence of bile salts in the gut lumen, are hydrolyzed by pancreatic lipase to form micelles of monoglycerides and fatty acids. The monoglycerides and fatty acids diffuse from the micelles into and through the cell membrane to enter the cell cytoplasm where they encounter a network of smooth endoplasmic reticulum. Within the tubules of SER, they are resynthesized to triglycerides that form droplets, along with phospholipids and cholesterol, in a protein solution. By the synthesis and sequestration of triglycerides within the cell, an inward diffusion gradient of monoglycerides and fatty acids is maintained. (Both figures, courtesy of Drs. R. R. Cardell, Jr., S. Badenhausen, and K. R. Porter, J. Cell Biol., vol. 34, 1967.)

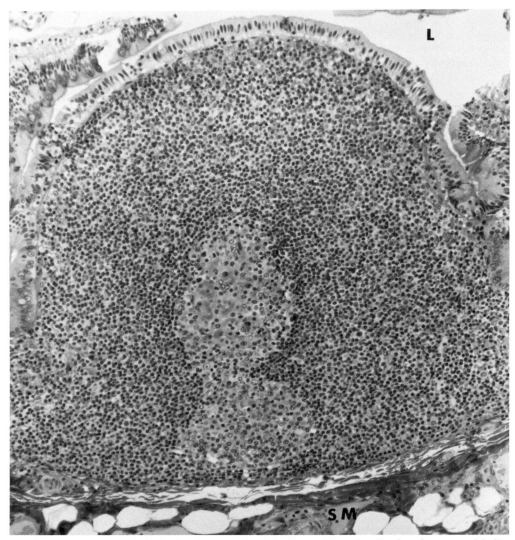

Fig. 16-51. Lymph nodule in the lamina propria of the ileum. Note the simple columnar epithelium covering the luminal surface (L) and the prominent germinal center in the nodule. SM, submucosa. ×160.

and an outer longitudinal. Connective tissue septa divide the muscle cells into groups or bundles, while between the two layers of muscle is a connective tissue septum which varies greatly in thickness at different places and contains the myenteric plexus of nerve fibers and parasympathetic ganglion cells.

Serosa. The *serous coat,* as in the stomach, consists of loose connective tissue covered by a layer of mesothelium.

The Large Intestine

The large intestine is divided topograph-ically and to some extent structurally into three main segments: colon, rectum and anal canal. Throughout the length of the large intestine, the wall consists of the same four coats that have been described for the stomach and small intestine, viz., mucosa, submucosa, muscularis and serosa (or fibrosa).

The Colon. There is an abrupt change at the ileocecal juncture from the small intestine to the *colon.* The greater diameter of the colon is perhaps the most striking difference grossly. Other differences of structure are noted in the description of the various coats.

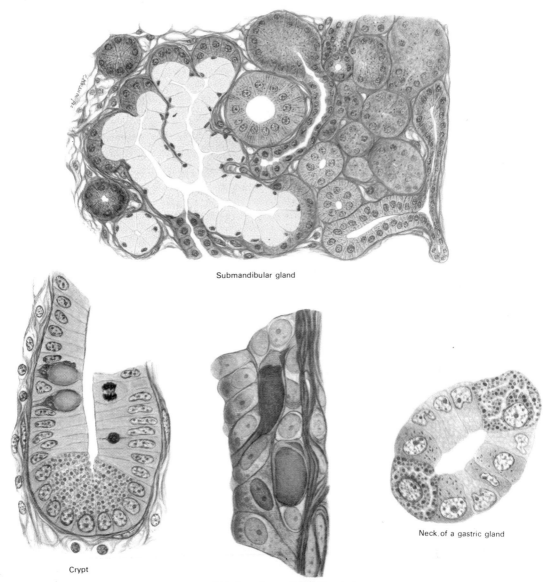

Submandibular gland

Crypt

Epithelium of a parotid interlobar duct

Neck of a gastric gland

Fig. 16-52. Camera lucida drawings of human tissues (except epithelium of interlobar duct, which is from the parotid gland of a rhesus monkey). Stains: hematoxylin, Altmann's acid fuchsin and aniline blue.

Submandibular Gland. At the *left* of the gland, three mucous alveoli (light blue), capped with serous demilunes, empty into the intercalated duct below. At *lower left* are cross sections through serous and mucous alveoli, respectively. At *lower right,* two intercalated ducts join a secretory (salivary) duct, whose cells have a reddish stained (fushsin) granular cytoplasm with blue (aniline blue) basal striations. An intercalated duct from a serous alveolus curves around the *right* side of the large central salivary duct.

Epithelium of Parotid Interlobar Duct. Note that the blue goblet cell at the *right,* although greatly distorted, reaches the surface. The one to the *left* does so also, but it is cut off in this section. The large surface epithelial cell (*second from left*) stretches around the goblet cell to reach the basement membrane at separate places. Adjacent sections show that the four cells at *upper right* likewise reach the basement membrane. Thus, the epithelium, stratified in appearance, is actually pseudostratified.

Crypt. The basal cells, full of large, red secretory granules, are Paneth cells. At *upper left* are two blue goblet cells. One of the columnar epithelial cells on the *right* is dividing. The dark round nucleus of a lymphocyte, migrating between two columnar cells, is also shown.

Neck of Gastric Gland. This cross section shows two large red parietal (HCl) cells with their clear intracellular canals. The light blue cells with indented basal nuclei are mucous neck cells. The darker blue cells are chief cells.

Mucosa. The *mucous membrane* of the colon has a comparatively smooth surface, for *there are no plicae or villi* as in the small intestine. Long, straight, tubular glands extend from the surface down through the entire thickness of the mucosa. These glands are *crypts* as in the small intestine (Figs. 16-53 and 16-54).

The surface *epithelium* is tall columnar. The absorbing cells have a striated border which is thinner than that on the cells of the small intestine. Goblet cells are interspersed among the columnar absorbing cells. As the epithelium continues down into the tubular glands, the columnar cells become lower and goblet cells become exceedingly numerous. In fact, the walls of the glands frequently appear to be composed almost entirely of goblet cells. Primitive cells at the base of the crypts differentiate into goblet, absorptive, enteroendocrine and occasionally Paneth cells in a manner similar to that in the small intestine. Enteroendocrine cells are normally rare but one type may become numerous and form a carcinoid tumor. This tumor is characterized by production of excessive amounts of serotonin.

The mucous membrane of the colon has two chief functions which are attributed to the columnar absorbing and goblet cells, respectively: namely, the absorption of water and the copious production of mucus. This mucous secretion lubricates the surface of the colon and facilitates the forwarding of the gradually dehydrated feces.

The connective tissue of the *lamina propria* extends up between the glands but is reduced to a minimum because the tubules are close together. Solitary lymph nodules are present in the mucosa and push through the muscularis mucosae into the submucosa. The lamina propria of the colon contains numerous lymphocytes, plasma cells and eosinophils.

The *muscularis mucosae* consists of an inner circular and an outer longitudinal layer of smooth muscle.

Submucosa. The *submucosa* is composed of loosely arranged connective tissue. It contains large blood vessels and the submucosal nerve plexus (of Meissner). Soli-

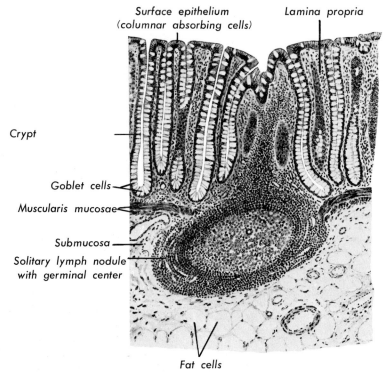

Surface epithelium (columnar absorbing cells)   Lamina propria

Crypt

Goblet cells

Muscularis mucosae

Submucosa

Solitary lymph nodule with germinal center

Fat cells

Fig. 16-53. Transverse section through mucosa and submucosa of colon of man. ×70. (After Braus.)

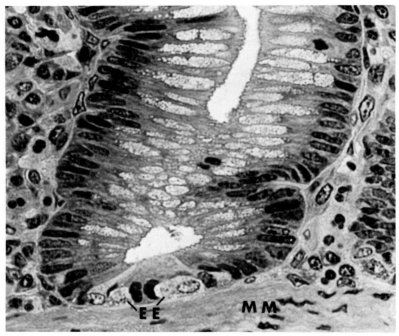

Fig. 16-54. Light micrograph of the base of a crypt in the colon showing enteroendocrine cells (*EE*), *MM*, muscularis mucosae. ×600.

tary lymph nodules, although properly considered as structures of the lamina propria from which they originate, lie mainly in the submucosa.

Muscularis. The *muscularis externa* in the colon shows some variation from its usual structure. The inner circular layer is complete and prominent, but the longitudinal muscles become arranged into three strong, flat, equidistant, longitudinal bands, the *lineae coli* (taenia coli). Between these thick strands the longitudinal muscle coat becomes thinned but is rarely entirely absent. Nerve cell and fiber components of the myentric plexus lie as usual in the connective tissue just external to the circular muscle layer.

Serosa. The *serous coat* is composed of a thin connective tissue layer covered by mesothelium. In certain regions, the mesothelial covering is absent. Here the connective tissue *fibrosa* binds the colon firmly to adjacent structures.

The Vermiform Appendix. The *vermiform appendix* is a diverticulum from the cecum. Its walls are continuous with those of the latter and closely resemble them in general structure. There are the

same four coats: mucous, submucous, muscular and serous.

The *mucous membrane* has its usual characteristic structures: the epithelium, crypts, lamina propria and the muscularis mucosae. The surface epithelium is simple columnar with a striated apical border. It continues into the glands or crypts where the border gradually becomes thinner. The glands frequently have many goblet cells, some Paneth cells and a number of enteroendocrine cells. In the embryo, the mucosal surface is lined with villi, but these disappear early in life. The lumen is often thrown into deep, pocketed folds, and in many adults it is nearly or completely obliterated.

The most characteristic histological feature of the appendix is the lymphatic tissue. Not only is the lamina propria infiltrated with lymphocytes, but it is often conspicuously occupied by a complete ring of solitary lymphatic nodules. These closely resemble the nodules that surround the crypts of the palatine tonsils. The nodules do not remain confined to the mucosa but push through the muscularis mucosae and invade the submucosa. In fact, the lymphatic development frequently makes it difficult to follow the muscularis mucosae and to separate the mucosa from the submucosa (Fig. 16-55). The *submucosa* contains numerous fat cells. It should be mentioned that, in some instances, more commonly after middle age, the mucosa and portions of the submucosa are largely replaced by fibrous connective tissue.

The *muscularis externa* varies greatly, both in thickness and in the amount of admixture of fibrous tissue. The inner circular layer is usually thick and well developed. The outer longitudinal layer differs from that of the large intestine in having no arrangement into lineae, the muscle tissue forming a continuous layer. The muscular layers are covered as usual by the *serosa*.

The Rectum. The *rectum* is usually divided into two parts. The *upper part* (the rectum proper), measuring 5 to 7 inches in length, is structurally similar to the colon. The crypts are longer than in the colon, however, and are lined almost entirely by goblet cells. The longitudinal layer of the muscularis externa is thicker on the front and back than it is on the sides. This retroperitoneal segment of the gut has no mesentery, and the serous coat is incomplete.

The *lower part* (*anal canal*) is 1 to 1½ inches in length. It pierces the pelvic floor and is closed except during defecation. Its mucous membrane has a number of permanent longitudinal folds, the *rectal columns* (*anal columns, columns of Morgagni*) which terminate distally about ½ inch from the anal orifice. These contain strands of smooth muscle and usually an artery and a vein. The bases (distal ends) of these columns are connected by transverse folds of the mucosa, the *anal valves* (Fig. 16-56).

Above the anal valves, the mucosa is lined by simple columnar epithelium like

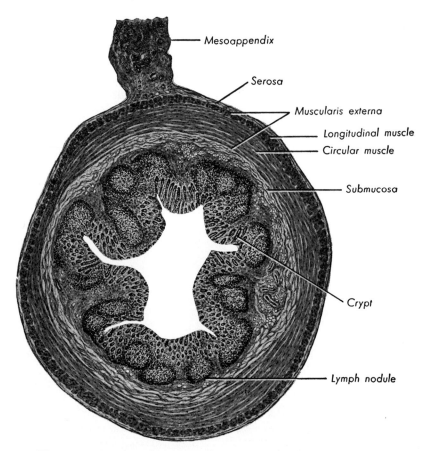

Fig. 16-55. Transverse section of human vermiform appendix. ×14.

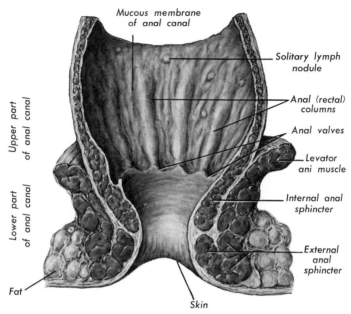

Fig. 16-56. Mucous surface of anal canal. Redrawn. (Courtesy of Wyeth Laboratories, Philadelphia, Pa.)

that of the rectum proper, composed of columnar absorbing cells, interspersed with many goblets cells. Crypts are present.

At the level of the anal valves, the epithelium becomes a stratified squamous type, the surface cells of which are not cornified. No crypts are present below the juncture. The noncornified stratified squamous epithelium extends nearly to the anal orifice, where it changes to epidermis. Hairs, sebaceous glands and sweat glands appear at the anal orifice.

The sweat glands are of two types. One type has the characteristic structure of the general body sweat glands (chapter 14, "Sweat Glands," and Figs. 14-5 and 14-6). The other type (*circumanal glands*) are very large and are structurally similar to the axillary sweat glands. Their secretory cells contain granules, and inside the basal lamina are prominent myoepithelial cells (Figs. 14-7 and 14-8).

At about the level of the anal valves, the muscularis mucosae subdivides into diverging strands which soon disappear.

The submucous coat of the anal canal has a rich plexus of blood vessels. The veins are often tortuous. Their size and arrangement and the absence of valves are conducive to the formation of hemorrhoids.

The circular layer of smooth muscle of the anal canal is thick and forms the *internal anal sphincter*. The longitudinal layer of smooth muscle continues over the sphincter and attaches to connective tissue. The *external anal sphincter* is formed of skeletal muscle. It lies just inside the levator ani muscles which also act as a sphincter (Fig. 16-56).

The Peritoneum

The *peritoneum* is a serous membrane which lines the walls of the abdomen (parietal peritoneum) and is reflected over the contained viscera (visceral peritoneum). It consists of two layers, a loose connective tissue and a mesothelium. The connective tissue is arranged into loose bundles which interlace in a plane parallel to the surface. There are numerous elastic fibers, especially in the deeper layer of the parietal peritoneum, and comparatively few connective tissue cells. The mesothelium consists of a single layer of flat, polygonal cells with bulging nuclei. The cells have irregular, wavy outlines which are easily demonstrated with silver preparations. The shapes of the cells vary considerably according to the direction in which the tissues are stretched.

Over some parts, e.g., the liver and intestine, the peritoneum or serosa is thin and very closely attached. In places where the peritoneum is freely movable, a considerable amount of loose connective tissue, rich in elastic fibers and containing varying numbers of fat cells, connects the peritoneum with the underlying tissue. This is known as the "subserous tissue." The peritoneum is well supplied with blood vessels and lymphatics. The former give rise to a rich capillary network.

The *mesentery* is a sheet-like attachment between the visceral organs and the posterior abdominal wall. Its surfaces are covered by a mesothelium which is continuous with that of the parietal peritoneum lining the abdominal cavity, and the visceral peritoneum enclosing or covering each visceral organ. Between its two mesothelial layers, the mesentery also contains a layer of loosely arranged connective tissue. Here may be found numerous lymph nodes and adipose cells. The connective tissue core of the mesentery also houses the blood vessels, lymphatic channels and nerves which serve each visceral organ. Portions of the mesentery are quite long, allowing freedom of visceral organ movement. Other parts are short, firmly fixing certain organs into position. In some cases (e.g., rectum) a mesentery is nonexistent, the organ being so intimately applied to the posterior abdominal wall, that peritoneum covers only a small portion of its surfaces. Such organs or segments of them are said to be "retroperitoneal."

Mesenteric attachments to the anterior body wall have disappeared during embryonic development, except in a few isolated regions such as the falciform ligament of the liver. Other tough mesenteric continuities (*visceral ligaments*) are also found interconnecting many of the visceral organs and the intestine. In embryonic and fetal life, certain parts of the mesentery and visceral ligaments fuse or expand disproportionately, adding greatly to the complexity of the mesenteric "system." The *greater omentum* is an enormously expanded sacculation of the dorsal mesentery of the stomach (*dorsal mesogaster*). During development its surfaces fuse with each other and enshroud the anterior aspect of most of the coiled intestine. Its connective tissue may become the respository of considerable amounts of stored fat.

Blood Vessels of the Stomach and Intestines

The arteries reach the gastrointestinal tract through the mesentery, give off small branches to the serosa and pass through the muscular coats to the submucosa, where they form an extensive plexus of large vessels (Heller's plexus). Within the muscular coats, the main arteries give off small branches to the muscle tissue. From the plexus of the submucosa, two main sets of vessels arise, one passing outward to form the main supply of the muscular coats, the other inward to supply the mucous membrane (Fig. 16-57). Of the former, the larger vessels pass directly to the intermuscular septum, where they form a plexus from which branches are given off to the two muscular tunics. Of the branches of the submucous plexus which pass to the mucous membrane, the shorter supply the muscularis mucosae, while the longer branches pierce the latter to form a capillary plexus among the glands of the lamina propria. These capillaries are most numerous around the bodies and necks of the glands. They pass over into a dense network of capillaries just beneath the surface epithelium. From the capillaries, small veins take origin which pierce the muscularis mucosae and form a close-meshed venous plexus in the submucosa. These in turn give rise to larger veins, which accompany the arteries into the mesentery. A significant portion of the venous return from the intestine is into the vessels of the hepatic portal system for distribution to the sinusoids of the liver (see below).

In the small intestine, the distribution of the blood vessels is modified by the presence of villi (Fig. 16-58). Each villus receives one small artery or, in the case of the large villi, two or three small arteries. The artery passes through the long axis of the villus close under the epithelium to its summit, giving off a network of fine capillaries which for the most part lie just beneath the epithelium. From these, one or two small veins arise which usually lie on the opposite side of the villus from the artery.

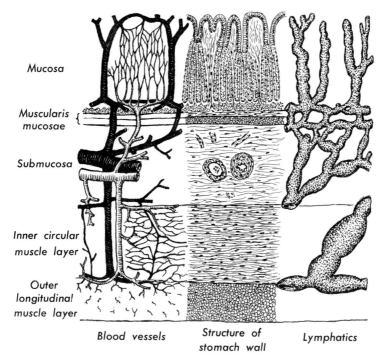

Mucosa

Muscularis
mucosae

Submucosa

Inner circular
muscle layer

Outer
longitudinal
muscle layer

Blood vessels

Structure of
stomach wall

Lymphatics

Fig. 16-57. Three sections of stomach wall placed side by side to show relationship of blood vessels and lymphatics to the different layers. (Redrawn after Mall.)

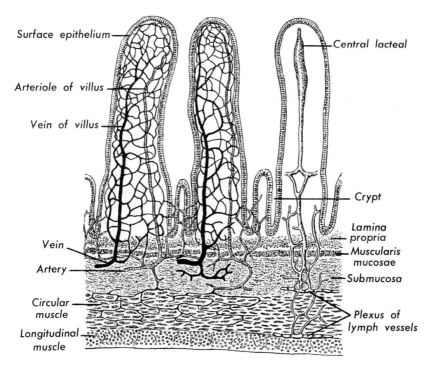

Surface epithelium

Arteriole of villus

Vein of villus

Central lacteal

Crypt

Lamina propria

Muscularis mucosae

Submucosa

Vein

Artery

Circular muscle

Longitudinal muscle

Plexus of lymph vessels

Fig. 16-58. Scheme of blood vessels and lymphatics of human small intestine. (Redrawn from Böhm and von Davidoff, after Mall.)

Lymphatics of the Stomach and Intestines

Small lymph or chyle capillaries begin as blind canals in the lamina propria of the mucous membrane among the tubular glands (Fig. 16-57). In the small intestine, a lymph capillary (lacteal) occupies the center of the long axis of each villus, ending in a blind extremity beneath the epithelium of its summit (Fig. 16-58). The walls of the lymph capillaries are made up of a single layer of large endothelial cells. Although the lymph capillaries are considerably larger than the blood capillaries, they are usually collapsed and inconspicuous. These vessels unite to form a narrow-meshed plexus of lymph capillaries in the deeper part of the lamina propria, lying parallel to the muscularis mucosae. Vessels from this plexus pass through the muscularis mucosae and form a wider meshed plexus of larger lymph vessels in the submucosa. In this region they often expand into sinuses surrounding the lymphatic nodules. A third lymphatic plexus lies in the connective tissue which separates the two layers of muscle. From the plexus in the submucosa, branches pass through the inner muscular layer, receive vessels from the intermuscular plexus and then pierce the outer muscular layer to pass into the mesentery in company with the arteries and veins. The larger lymph vessels are provided with definite valves, and their walls are also supported by a thin tunic of smooth muscle cells. In their course through the mesenteries, they are associated with numerous mesenteric lymph nodes. These relations are well demonstrated in the cat by the injection of 1% Berlin blue into the intestinal wall.

Although the primary function of the lymphatic system is the return of tissue fluids to the blood stream, the vessels of the small intestine form channels through which absorbed fats are drained. During digestion, the lymph fluid, carrying a rich emulsion of fat (chyle), gives to the vessels a white appearance and renders them clearly visible.

Nerves of the Stomach and Intestines

The nerves to the stomach consist of preganglionic parasympathetic fibers (branches of the vagus nerve) and postganglionic sympathetic fibers. They reach the intestinal walls through the mesentery. In the connective tissue between the two layers of muscle, these fibers are associated with groups of parasympathetic ganglion cells to form the *myenteric plexus (of Auerbach)*. Within this plexus, the preganglionic parasympathetic fibers synapse with the ganglion cells. The axons are grouped together in small nonmyelinated bundles which pass, together with the sympathetic fibers, into the muscular coats. There they form intricate plexuses, from which are given off club-shaped terminals to the smooth muscle cells. From the myenteric plexus, fibers pass to the submucosa, where they form a similar but finer meshed and more delicate plexus which is also associated with other groups of parasympathetic ganglion cells, the *submucosal plexus (of Meissner;* see Fig. 16-44). Both fibers and cells are smaller than those of the myenteric plexus. From the submucosal plexus, delicate nerve fibers pass to their terminations in submucosa, muscularis mucosae and mucous membrane. Some fibers appear to end within the epithelium itself, but their functional role in that location is not fully understood.

Extrinsic Digestive Glands

The smaller tubular and tubuloalveolar glands which form a part of the mucous membrane and submucosa of the alimentary tract have been described. There remain to be considered certain larger compound tubuloalveolar glands, the development of which is similar to that of the smaller glands but which come to lie wholly outside the alimentary tract, connected with it by their main excretory ducts. Functionally, they are an important part of the digestive system. These structures are: (1) the *salivary glands,* (2) the *pancreas* and (3) the *liver.*

The Salivary Glands

The salivary glands include a number of glandular structures which secrete a liquid, the *saliva.* The smaller of these glands are situated in the oral mucous membrane, which their secretions serve constantly to lubricate and moisten. The larger of the glands are some distance removed from the oral cavity, to which their products are conveyed through excretory ducts. These glands, which are paired structures and may be spoken of as the salivary glands proper, are the *parotid, submandibular* and the *sublingual glands*. Their secretions contain enzymes which aid in preparing the food for the digestive processes that ensue in the stomach and intestines. Their secretions, together with those from the numerous smaller glands of the oral cavity, are very important in moistening and softening each bolus.

In the following account, only the salivary glands proper—the parotid, submandibular and sublingual—are considered. These three are compound tubuloalveolar glands. In man, the parotid has only serous alveoli; the submandibular and sublingual have serous and mucous alveoli. Hence the latter are known as mixed glands, in contradistinction to the purely serous glands (parotid, von Ebner's glands) and the purely mucous (palatine) glands.

Structure of the Salivary Glands. Each gland consists of a glandular epithelium (*parenchyma*) and a supporting connective tissue framework (*interstitial tissue, stroma*). In the parotid and subman-

dibular, there is a definite connective tissue capsule which encloses the gland and blends with the connective tissue of surrounding structures. The sublingual has no distinct capsule. Connective tissue septa divide each gland into *lobes* and *lobules*. In these septa are found the larger ducts, the blood vessels and occasional ganglion cells. For a description of the development of the duct system, see chapter 15 under "Architecture of Compound Glands."

Some of the larger divisions of the *intralobular ducts* are lined by simple columnar epithelium similar to that of the interlobular ducts, into which they open. Most of the intralobular ducts of the salivary glands, however, are lined with columnar cells which have a contributory role in the secretory process. They are known as *striated ducts* (salivary ducts). In the parotid and submandibular glands these ducts are continuous with small terminal ducts with narrow lumina lined with low cuboidal or flat epithelium. Since they lie between the striated ducts and the alveoli (Figs. 16-59 and 16-60), they are known as *intercalated* ducts (intermediate tubules, necks, isthmuses). In the embryo the secretory epithelium of salivary glands is derived from oral ectoderm. The ducts develop first

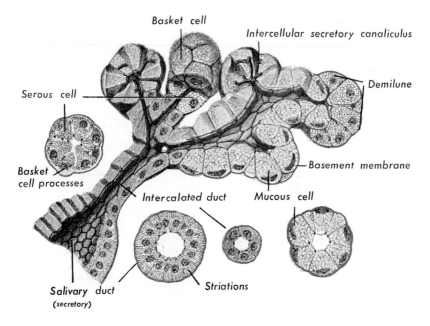

Fig. 16-59. Reconstruction of terminal ramification of human submandibular gland, showing salivary and intercalated ducts and several alveoli. (From Braus, after a reconstruction by A. Vierling.)

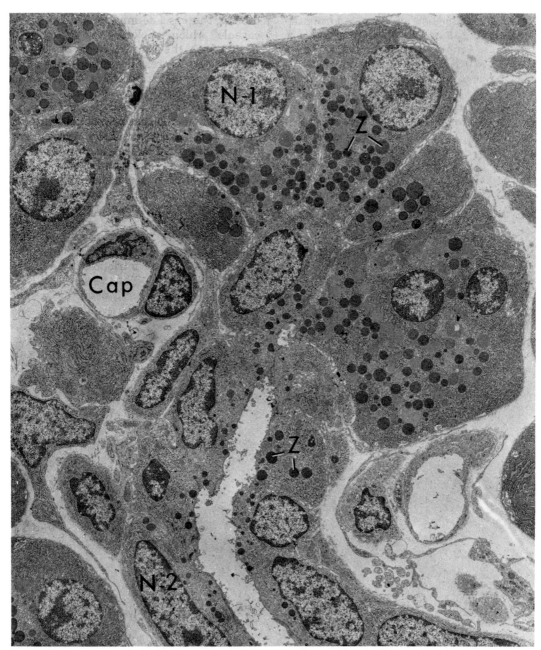

Fig. 16-60. Electron micrograph of a rat parotid gland showing the junction of an intralobular intercalated duct with an acinus composed of parenchymal cells. The cells lining the junctional region of the duct have ultrastructural characteristics that are intermediate between those of acinar and duct cells. They have some zymogen granules and they also have more rough endoplasmic reticulum than do typical duct cells. *Cap*, capillary; *N-1*, nucleus of acinar parenchymal cell; *N-2*, nucleus of duct cell; *Z*, zymogen granules. ×2250. (Courtesy of Dr. I. Joel Leeb.)

and give rise secondarily to the alveoli. In the adult the ducts may still proliferate mitotically and give rise to new alveoli. However, alveolar cells can also divide in the adult.

The Serous Alveoli. The serous alveoli are lined with pyramidal epithelial cells which rest upon a basal lamina and surround a narrow lumen. The cell boundaries are likely to be indistinct. The appearance of these cells varies according to their particular phase of activity as well as the mode of preservation (see Fig. 15-4). In a "resting" condition, the cytoplasm is filled with a number of small, highly refractile secretory droplets, the zymogen granules.

There is an abundance of *basophilic material* (rough endoplasmic reticulum) in the basal portion of the cells. This region may have a striated appearance in the light microscope, as a result of the parallel arrangement of rod-shaped mitochondria and the configuration of the endoplasmic reticulum. The ribosomes are sites for synthesis of the protein molecules of the enzymes. The protein is combined with polysaccharides in the Golgi region to form membrane-bounded glycoprotein secretory droplets. The latter move into the apical region of the cell for storage as zymogen granules until the time of secretion.

By employing the Golgi silver technique, using thin plastic embedded sections, or by electron microscopy, one can demonstrate fine *intercellular secretory canaliculi* between adjacent cells of the serous alveoli.

Although not apparent in routine histological preparations, peculiar stellate-shaped cells may be demonstrated by special techniques in the region between the secreting cells and the basal lamina. They lie in close contact with the secreting cells, and their processes form a sort of basket-work around the alveolus. These are the *basal* or *basket cells* (Fig. 16-61), and they are similar to the *myoepithelial cells* of the sweat glands and circumanal glands (Figs. 14-6 and 14-8). They also occur in intercalated and striated ducts. By their contraction, they assist in the discharge of the secretion products into the excretory ducts.

The Mucous Alveoli. In ordinary hematoxylin-eosin preparations, the purely mucous alveoli present a light bluish purple appearance, in contrast with the deep reddish purple of the serous alveoli (Fig. 16-59). Usually the lumen is fairly large and may contain masses of mucin. The mucous cells rest on a basal lamina, and their boundaries are usually quite distinct. When the cell becomes filled with secretory droplets, the nucleus becomes flattened in the basal part of the cell. Most of the cell is occupied by a network of cytoplasm with spaces that, in the living state, were occupied by secretory droplets. The mucigen droplets are dissolved out by most of the routine methods used in preparing sections for light microscopy, leaving only a network of cytoplasm and remnants of some of the precipitated secretory droplets. After the cell discharges its secretion, the nucleus resumes a spherical or oval shape. Mitochondria are present, but rough endoplasmic reticulum is sparse. There is also a well developed Golgi apparatus. Intercellular canaliculi are not seen in the mucous alveoli.

In the mixed glands, several types of terminal alveoli may be seen. Some alveoli may be composed entirely of serous cells, others entirely of mucous cells. An alveolus may contain both kinds of cells, in which case the serous cells are more likely to occupy the blind end of the alveolus, with the mucous cells nearer the exit (Fig. 16-59). In many instances, at the base of the mucous alveolus or along its sides, there occur crescent-shaped groups of serous cells, the *demilunes* (*of Heidenhain*) (Fig. 16-59). These may have direct access to the lumen of the alveolus, but more often they communicate with it by means of intercellular secretory canaliculi which pass between the mucous cells and branch among the serous cells of the demilune.

Consideration is now given to the more important characteristics of the particular glands.

The Parotid Gland. The *parotid gland* is the largest of the salivary glands and, in man, dog, cat and rabbit, it is entirely *serous* (Figs. 16-62 and 16-63). Its duct system is complex. The main excretory duct (Stenson's) opens into the oral cavity opposite the second upper molar tooth. It is lined with pseudostratified or stratified columnar epithelium, with occasional goblet cells. The main duct divides into interlobar ducts which, in turn, divide to form interlobular ducts, the various branches following the connective tissue septa. Except in the larger of these ducts (Fig. 16-52), the epithelium becomes reduced to a' simple columnar type. All of these ducts are often referred to as excretory ducts. From the interlobular ducts, branches are given off which penetrate the lobules.

Most of the large intralobular ducts are of the striated variety (*salivary* or *secretory* ·

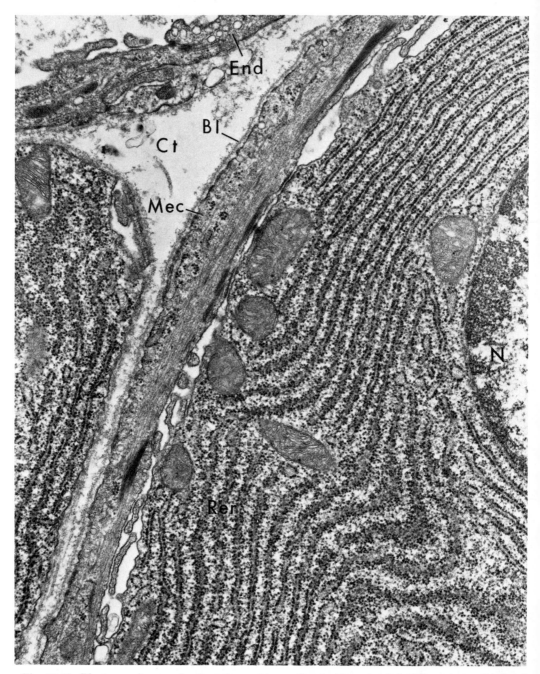

Fig. 16-61. Electron micrograph of portions of two cells of adjacent acini of the rat parotid gland. A portion of a basket cell (*Mec*) is seen between the basal end of an acinar cell and the basal lamina (*Bl*) of the acinar cells. The basket cells resemble the smooth muscle cells of other parts of the body in that they have a number of fine filaments and are contractile. *Ct,* connective tissue space; *End,* endothelium lining a small blood vessel; *N,* nucleus of acinar cell; *Rer,* rough endoplasmic reticulum. ×22,500.

ducts). They are lined by a single layer of columnar cells in which the nucleus is spheroidal and centrally located. The cytoplasm is acidophilic. The basal portion of the cell presents a characteristic striated appearance (Figs. 16-59 and 16-63). The rodlike

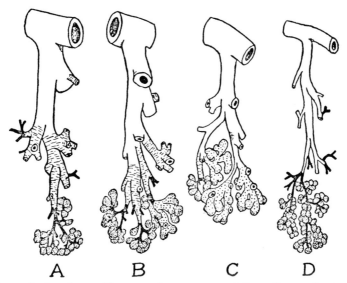

Fig. 16-62. Schematic drawing to illustrate the structure of the salivary glands and pancreas. *A*, parotid; *B*, submandibular; *C*, sublingual; *D*, pancreas. Excretory ducts, white; salivary ducts, cross striped; intercalated ducts, black; mucous alveoli, coarse stipple; serous alveoli, fine stipple. (Redrawn, slightly modified, after Braus.)

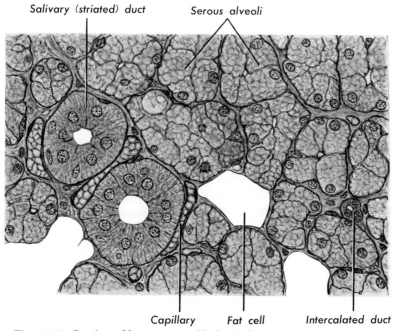

Fig. 16-63. Section of human parotid gland. Surgical specimen. ×465.

mitochondria are oriented perpendicular to the base of the cell, and electron micrographs show deep infoldings of the basal plasma membrane into the cytoplasm, a configuration somewhat like that in the proximal convoluted tubules of the kidney. This arrangement is characteristic of re-

gions active in transport of sodium and fluids. The *intercalated ducts,* connecting the salivary ducts and the terminal alveoli are of small diameter (Figs. 16-59 and 16-60) and are lined by low cuboidal epithelium. In the parotid, they are fairly long.

The gland is covered by a thick connective tissue capsule, from which branches extend inward around subdivisions of glandular tissue known as lobes and lobules. Fine connective tissue fibers also envelop each alveolus. Fat cells are frequent in the connective tissue of the parotid, and they tend to increase in number with age.

The Submandibular Gland. The *submandibular* (submaxillary) in man and most mammals is a *mixed gland,* but the proportion of serous and mucous alveoli varies. In man, it is preponderantly serous (Fig. 16-64). The main duct (Wharton's) opens into the mouth beneath the tongue. It is lined by pseudostratified columnar epithelium and has, in addition, a richly cellular stroma and longitudinally disposed smooth muscle cells. The main duct branches in the manner described for the parotid, the pseudostratified epithelium continuing into the larger interlobular ducts. The intralobular ducts are of the same types as in the parotid gland. The striated ducts are longer and more numerous than in the parotid; the intercalated ducts are short and narrow.

The serous alveoli greatly outnumber the mucous ones. The latter frequently are capped by serous demilunes. Some mucous alveoli have serous cells lining their terminal portions. The connective tissue within the lobules and in the capsule is well developed.

The Sublingual Gland. The *sublingual gland* is also a *mixed gland* in man, dog, cat, rabbit and sheep. It is the smallest of the large salivary glands and in man is preponderantly mucous. A series of ducts opens into the mouth at the side of the frenulum of the tongue, near the opening of Wharton's duct. The pseudostratified epithelium that lines the larger ducts is replaced by simple columnar in the smaller ones. There are relatively few intralobular ducts. Typical striated ducts are rare. However, patches of striated cells may occur in the walls of intralobular ducts with an otherwise unmodified simple columnar epithelial lining. Intercalated ducts are likewise reduced in number so that most of the terminal alveoli, which are often quite elongated, either open directly into the larger

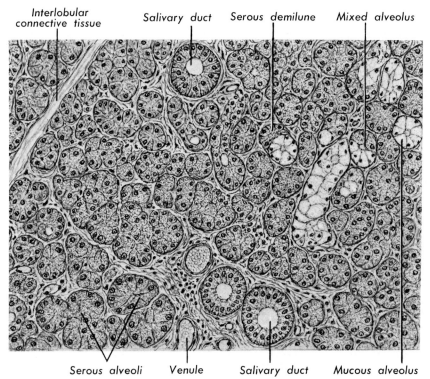

Fig. 16-64. Section of human submandibular gland. ×216.

intralobular ducts (Fig. 16-65) or into the interlobular ducts at the periphery of the lobule. Some investigators believe that typical intercalated ducts are entirely lacking.

The terminal alveoli are mostly of the mucous type. Serous cells occur mostly in the form of demilunes around mucous alveoli. Such demilunes are numerous and large (Fig. 16-59).

The connective tissue septa are well developed in the sublingual, but the gland does not have a distinct capsule, as do the parotid and submandibular glands.

Blood Supply. The salivary glands have a relatively rich blood supply. The larger arteries run in the connective tissue septa with the ducts, giving off branches which accompany the divisions of the ducts to the lobules, where they break up into capillary networks surrounding the alveoli. These give rise to veins which follow the course of the arteries.

Lymphatics. Relatively few in number, the lymphatics begin as minute vessels in the smaller connective tissue septa and empty into lymph vessels which accompany the arteries.

Nerve Supply. The sensory innervation of the salivary glands is by the trigeminal nerve. The motor innervation is derived form both sympathetic and parasympathetic systems. Preganglionic sympathetic fibers run in the thoracocervical trunk to terminate in the superior cervical ganglion. Here they form synapses with postganglionic fibers which course in the walls of the branches of the carotid artery to the respective glands.

The parasympathetic supply to the parotid is by way of preganglionic fibers of the ninth cranical nerve to the otic ganglion, from which postganglionic fibers pass to the gland. The parasympathetic innervation of the submandibular and sublingual glands is by way of preganglionic fibers in the chorda tympani nerve to the mandibular ganglion, which usually lies within the glands. Short postganglionic fibers pass to the elements of the gland. Nerve endings are seen to penetrate the basal lamina and lie within the epithelium itself.

The Pancreas

The pancreas is a compound tubuloacinar gland, lying behind the stomach and

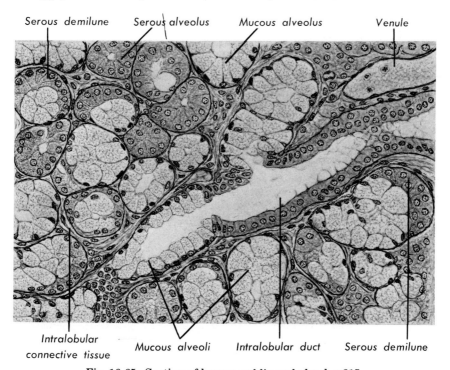

Fig. 16-65. Section of human sublingual gland. ×315.

extending transversely from the spleen to the loop of the duodenum. The broader portion of it, the *head,* lies in the concavity of the latter organ. The head is joined to the *body* of the gland by a slightly constricted portion, the *neck.* The body tapers gradually into an extremity, the *tail.*

The pancreas is both a gland of *external secretion,* furnishing the pancreatic juice which is conveyed to the duodenum and which contains several digestive enzymes, and a gland of *internal secretion,* elaborating substances which, circulating in the blood, play an essential role in the regulation of the carbohydrate metabolism of the body. Serving the former function, it has a system of excretory ducts and terminal secreting acini, the arrangement of which somewhat resembles that of the parotid gland. For the performance of its endocrine function, there are highly vascularized aggregations of secreting cells, the *islands* (or *islets*) *of Langerhans* (Fig. 16-66).

The pancreas has no distinct connective tissue capsule but is covered with a thin layer of loose tissue from which septa pass into the gland, subdividing it into many small lobules. In some of the lower animals (as, for instance, the cat), these lobules are well defined, being completely separated from one another by connective tissue. A number of these *primary lobules* are grouped together and surrounded by connective tissue which is considerably broader and looser in structure than that separating the primary lobules. These constitute a *lobule group* or secondary lobule. It is difficult to distinguish lobes and lobules in sections of human pancreas because the connective tissue septa are incomplete.

The main excretory duct of the pancreas, the *pancreatic duct* or *duct of Wirsung,* extends almost the entire length of the gland, giving off short lateral branches, one of which courses to each lobule. As the ducts enter the lobules, their epithelium becomes low cuboidal. They have characteristics similar to intercalated ducts of other glands, and it should be noted that these ducts of narrow caliber are the only intralobular ducts present in the pancreas; there are no striated ducts as in the salivary glands. The intralobular intercalated ducts are long, and they branch many times be-

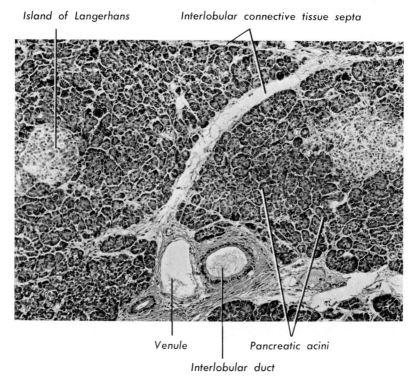

Island of Langerhans   Interlobular connective tissue septa

Venule   Pancreatic acini

Interlobular duct

Fig. 16-66. Section of human pancreas. Surgical specimen. Photomicrograph. ×100.

fore terminating in the serous acini. The terminal cells of the duct system are usually surrounded by acinar cells and are referred to as centroacinar cells (Figs. 16-67 and 16-68). It is to be noted that intercalated duct cells of the pancreas do not contain secretory granules as they do in some of the duct cells of the salivary glands.

In addition to the main excretory duct, there is also a secondary excretory duct, the *accessory pancreatic duct* or *duct of Santorini*. It may have an independent opening into the duodenum; otherwise, it communicates with the duct of Wirsung.

The interlobular and main ducts are lined with a simple high columnar epithelium which rests upon a basal lamina. Occasional goblet cells and enteroendocrine cells are present in this epithelium. Outside of the epithelium is a connective tissue coat, the thickness of which is directly proportional to the size of the duct. In the accompanying connective tissue of the main duct and its larger branches, there are small mucous glands. As the ducts decrease in size, the epithelium becomes lower until, in the intercalated ducts, it is low cuboidal.

The *acini* are all of the serous (serozymogenic) type. They are lined by irregu-

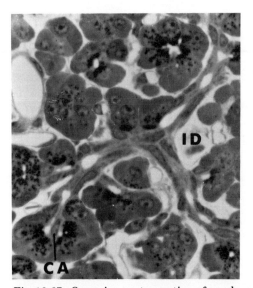

Fig. 16-67. One micrometer section of monkey pancreas showing branching of intercalated ducts (*ID*) to several acini. The acinus at the lower left shows a prominent centroacinar cell (*CA*). ×300.

larly pyramidal epithelial cells resting on a basal lamina. Delicate intercellular secretory canaliculi extend between the acinar cells. In each cell, there may be distinguished a juxtalumenal zone and an intensely staining zone toward the basal lamina. The first contains numerous *zymogen granules* (Figs. 16-67 and 16-68). These granules vary in number with the functional activity of the cell, and they are the intracellular antecedents of the enzymes.

The nucleus lies in the basal zone of the cell. It is spherical and characteristically contains one or more distinct nucleoli. Binucleate cells may occur, but this is infrequent in man.

The basal zone is *basophilic* (see above under "Serous Alveoli") and usually appears striated. Electron micrographs show this region to contain a highly developed rough endoplasmic reticulum (Fig. 16-68). The surfaces of its membranes are studded with ribosomes, which accounts for the basophilic staining. The striated appearance in the basal region of the cell is accentuated by the presence of numerous elongated mitochondria between the lamellae of endoplasmic reticulum.

Pancreatic Islets. As mentioned earlier in this discussion, the pancreas also has an *endocrine* function, which is carried on by cellular aggregations interspersed irregularly among the acini or along the ducts. These cell groups are the *pancreatic islets* ("islands" of Langerhans); their secretion is poured directly into the bloodstream, and they have no functional communication with the duct system of the gland.

In ordinary hematoxylin-eosin preparations, the islets appear as more or less spheroidal masses of pale staining cells, arranged in the form of irregular anastomosing cords (Fig. 16-69). Between the cords, closely applied to the epithelial cells, are numerous blood capillaries. Only a few fine connective tissue fibers are present within the islets. The islets may be more or less closely surrounded by pancreatic acini (Fig. 16-69), or they may lie in the interlobular connective tissue septa.

The size of the islets varies from those having only a few cells to islets which are macroscopically visible. Isolated islet cells are also found occasionally among the cells

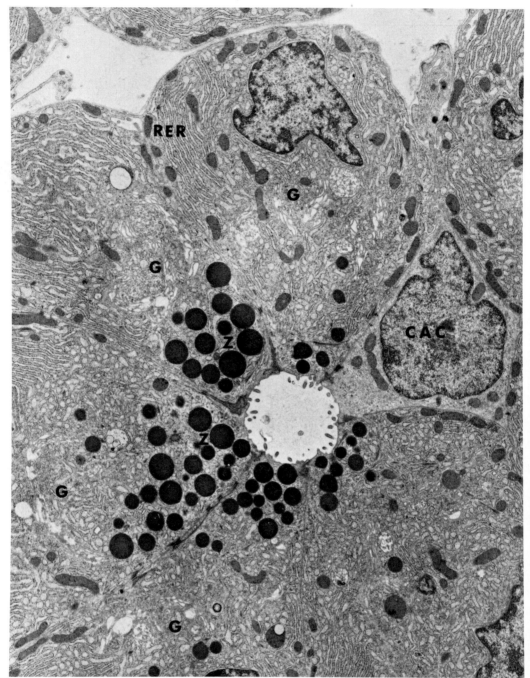

Fig. 16-68. Part of pancreatic acinus from monkey. The prominent rough endoplasmic reticulum (*RER*), Golgi complexes (*G*) and zymogen granules (*Z*) are seen. A centroacinar cell (*CAC*) also borders the secretory lumen of the acinus. ×6,250.

lining the ducts of the exocrine pancreas. The number of islets varies in different portions of the gland as well as in different individuals. They are more abundant in the tail of the pancreas than in the head.

In routine histological preparations, all of the islet cells appear to be similar (Fig. 16-69); by special methods, however, three types of cells have been distinguished in the human pancreas, namely, A or *alpha*

Zymogen granules

Pancreatic acinus

Centro-acinar cells

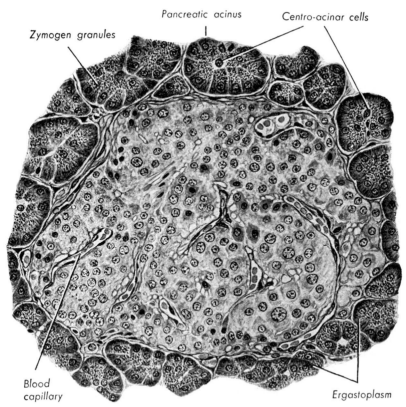

Blood
capillary

Ergastoplasm

Fig. 16-69. A section through an islet of Langerhans and surrounding acini. Human pancreas. Hematoxylin-eosin. ×450.

cells, B or *beta* cells and D cells. The A and B cells are by far the most numerous, the D cells being relatively few in number.

The granules of the A and B cells differ from each other in solubility and in staining reactions. The A cell granules are preserved by alcohol, whereas those of the B cells are soluble in alcohol. Of the various staining methods used for differentiating the cells (e.g., Masson's trichrome, chrome hematoxylin-phloxine, aldehyde fuchsin), the chrome hematoxylin and phloxine method is the one most commonly used. With this technique (Fig. 16-70) the A cells are seen to contain numerous fine, red-staining granules in contrast with blue-staining granules of B cells. Electron micrographs show that the granules are enclosed by membranes. The A cell granules are highly opaque (electron-dense), relatively uniform in size and distributed evenly in the cytoplasm. The granules of the B cells are less opaque than those of the A cell, they are more variable in cytoplasmic distribution, and each granule is characteristically separated from its

enclosing membrane by a prominent clear space. The B cell granules vary in shape in different species; in man, dog, and cat, they appear as crystalloids.

Although the relative numbers of A and B cells vary in different islets, the B cells are generally more numerous. B cells may also occur outside the islets, either singly or as small groups, in association with fully developed ducts or with acini. Estimates of the percentages of the various cell types indicate that the B cells comprise 60 to 90% of all of the islet cells in the human pancreas.

The D cells are differentiated by Masson's triple stain (Fig. 1-9, *B*), which also selectively colors the A cells. There are few D cells in the human, and their significance is not clearly understood.

Another type of cell has also been described in the pancreas of the guinea pig. Its cytoplasm contains no granules. It has been suggested that this type, the C cell, represents the progenitor of the A cells.

The question of the source of new islet

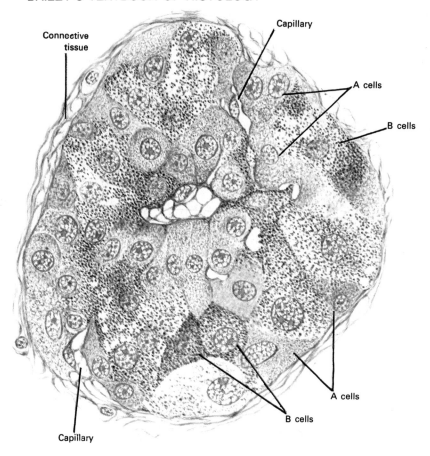

Fig. 16-70. A section of an islet of Langerhans of human pancreas showing A and B cells. A 3 μm section of a surgical specimen. The relative proportions and distributions of the A and B cells are unusual in the particular section illustrated. The B cells are generally about 3 times as numerous as the A cells and the latter are usually found toward the periphery of the islet. Chrome hematoxylin and phloxine stain (Gomori). ×113.

cells in the adult, particularly whether acinar cells may be transformed into islet cells, has frequently been raised. In study of the pancreas of the guinea pig, Bensley described a system of fine, anastomosing tubules which originate from the intralobular ducts and branch freely in the connective tissue surrounding these ducts. Bensley regarded these branching tubules as tissue of a low order of differentiation, capable, under proper conditions, of producing by differentiation and mitotic division new islets or acini. Recent studies indicate that duct cells can undergo mitosis independently so the validity of this concept seems questionable. During embryonic development, both islet and acinar cells are of endodermal epithelial origin, the islets having become detached from the presumptive pancreatic duct system.

Secretions of the Pancreas. The *external secretion* of the pancreas is an alkaline liquid, the pancreatic juice, the important constituents of which are certain enzymes. Among these are *trypsin,* a powerful proteolytic enzyme which breaks down proteins into amino acids, *amylase,* which converts starches into maltose, and *lipase,* which splits fats into glycerol and fatty acids. It is interesting to note that, although these several chemically dissimilar enzymes are elaborated by the pancreatic acini, the acinar cells are apparently cytologically similar.

Secretory pathways have been studied extensively in pancreatic acinar cells. These are described in some detail in the sections on "Granular Endoplasmic Reticulum" and the "Golgi Apparatus" in chapter 1 and they are reviewed in chapter 15.

The pancreas may be stimulated to activity either by nervous impulses from the vagus or by the action of the hormones, *secretin* and *pancreozymin*, formed in the duodenal mucosa probably by separate types of enteroendocrine cells and carried to the pancreas in the bloodstream. Secretin appears to be formed whenever acid substances, such as the acid contents of the stomach or acid bile, come in contact with the duodenal mucosa. It stimulates intercalated duct cells to secrete bicarbonate. Pancreozymin stimulates release of zymogen granules from the acinar cells.

The *internal secretion* of the pancreas includes two hormones. One of these, *insulin*, is known to play an important role in carbohydrate metabolism. Without this hormone, the cells of the body are unable to utilize the available glucose and allow formation of glycogen stores. The clinical condition resulting from a deficiency of insulin, *diabetes mellitus*, is thus marked by hyperglycemia and glycosuria of variable severity.

Insulin is produced in the islets, specifically by the B cells. Evidence for this is available from various sources, both clinical and experimental. Impaired sugar assimilation results from removal of the entire pancreas but not from ligation of the pancreatic duct, which destroys the acinar tissue but leaves the islets intact. Furthermore, it has been amply demonstrated, as in the first successful extractions of insulin by Banting and Best, that insulin is present in such a duct-ligated pancreas. In man, functional tumors of the B cells produce hypoglycemia, the effect being comparable to that caused by the administration of insulin. Removal of the tumor restores the patient to a normal condition. Experimentally, diabetes can be produced in many animals by the selective destruction of the B cells by injection of the drug alloxan. Also, in certain species the repeated injection of crude extracts of the anterior pituitary gland results in B cell injury and diabetes.

The islets also secrete another hormone known as *glucagon*, a hyperglycemic-glycogenolytic factor. This hormone is formed by the A cells and it has an effect which is, in some respects, antagonistic to that of insulin. It causes an elevation of blood sugar. Like insulin, it is present in pancreatic tissue following duct ligation. Unlike insulin, it is present in the pancreas of a duct-ligated, alloxan-treated animal.

Blood Supply. The pancreas receives its blood supply from the superior and inferior pancreaticoduodenal arteries and from pancreatic rami of the splenic artery. The vessels course in the interlobular connective tissue and give off branches which enter the lobules. These form capillary networks among the acini and in the islets. The islets have an extremely rich vascular network, a characteristic which they share with other endocrine tissues. Also in common with other endocrine tissues, the capillaries have a fenestrated endothelium with diaphragms spanning the pores. The extensiveness of the capillary network within the islets is not usually appreciated in sections but can be demonstrated in injected specimens. The blood leaves the pancreas by the pancreaticoduodenal veins to the superior mesenteric and portal veins and by several small pancreatic veins to the splenic vein.

Lymphatics. The lymph vessels lie mainly in the interlobular connective tissue. They drain chiefly into the celiac lymph nodes.

Nerve Supply. The nerves to the pancreas are from the splanchnic (sympathetic) and the vagus (parasympathetic). The former are nonmyelinated. The latter are myelinated preganglionic fibers; the cell bodies of their postganglionic fibers lie within the substance of the gland. The terminal fibers of the nerves are distributed about the secreting acini, some penetrating the basal lamina to lie within the epithelium, on the walls of blood vessels and within the islets in close association with both vessels and endocrine cells. Pacinian corpuscles are occasionally found in the interlobular connective tissue of the gland.

The Liver

The liver is the largest gland of the body. Its organization differs from that of the other major digestive glands because most of its functions relate to producing chemical and morphological changes in the blood rather than exocrine secretion. The liver does secrete bile, which is conveyed to the intestine by a system of ducts, but even this function is as much excretory as digestive in nature. The liver is involved in processing or storage of all the major categories of food materials, fats, carbohydrates, proteins and vitamins, performs an essential function in the removal of waste products from the blood and synthesizes serum proteins, lipoproteins and clotting factors. Because of its role in releasing products directly into the blood stream it has been considered an endocrine organ, by broad definition of the term endocrine. Current concepts of endocrine function center around the elaboration of hormones, however, and the liver does not produce true hormones. Despite the multiplicity and diversity of its functions, the liver has no groups of cells cytologically specialized for the performance of one function or the other, as is the case, for example, in the pancreas.

The unique organization of the liver has its origins in its mode of development. Rather than forming from a branching primary duct system as do typical exocrine glands, the liver arises from an initial diverticulation of the foregut and a secondary mass of proliferating endodermal epithelial cells that invade the mesenchyme of the embryonic septum transversum. These latter cells interdigitate with mesenchymally derived primary vascular spaces (vitelline venous channels). They form cords or sheets that help to subdivide the vascular channels into endothelium-lined sinusoids and the epithelial cells remain intimately associated with these sinusoids throughout life. Intrahepatic bile ducts arise secondarily by dedifferentiation of partially differentiated hepatic parenchymal cells and these ducts then join the extrahepatic duct system. The latter, along with the gall bladder, develops from the original gut diverticulum.

The adult liver is situated in the upper and right part of the abdominal cavity, immediately below the diaphragm to which it is attached. Several fissures partially divide it into four *lobes*. It is incompletely invested by an outer *tunica serosa*, derived from the peritoneum, within which is a delicate connective tissue capsule, the *capsule of Glisson*. This capsule, which contains a fair abundance of elastic fibers, covers the entire surface of the organ. At the *porta hepatis* (transverse fissure, hilus), it surrounds the entering blood vessels and follows into the gland, forming a framework and dividing it into innumerable small *lobules*. In some animals, e.g., the pig and camel, each lobule is completely invested by connective tissue. In man, the connective tissue is sparse and the lobular investment is incomplete. It is apparent mainly at points where three or more lobules meet (Fig. 16-71). The lobules are cylindrical or irregularly prismatic in shape and approximately 1 mm in breadth and 2 mm in length. Except just beneath the capsule, where they are frequently arranged with their apices directed toward the surface, the lobules are irregularly arranged.

The *hepatic lobule*, which may be considered the anatomical unit of structure of the liver, has two main constituents: an epithelial parenchyma and a system of anastomosing blood sinusoids. The parenchyma is made up of hepatic cells arranged in irregular, branching, interconnected plates. Since in sections the sheets of cells often give the appearance of cell cords (Fig. 16-71), they have frequently been called the *hepatic cords*. However, reconstructions which portray the interrelationships of the cells in three dimensions clearly show that the cells are aligned in broad plates or sheets (Fig. 16-72). The plates tend to be arranged in a radiating manner around the central blood vessel of the lobule.

The hepatic plates or laminae form the secretory portions of the gland and are thus analogous to the secretory tubules of other glands. The hepatic plates are arranged in a definite manner relative to the blood channels, forming partitions between them. The blood vessels may therefore conveniently be considered first.

Blood Supply. The blood supply of the liver is peculiar in that, in addition to the ordinary arterial supply and venous return which all organs possess, the liver receives venous blood in large quantities through the portal vein. There are thus *two afferent vessels*, the *hepatic artery* and the *portal*

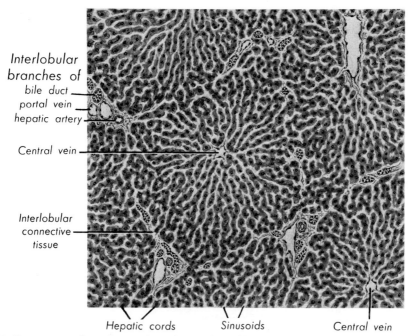

Interlobular
branches of
  bile duct
  portal vein
  hepatic artery

Central vein

Interlobular
connective
tissue

Hepatic cords   Sinusoids   Central vein

Fig. 16-71. Low power view of a portion of a section of human liver, showing one complete lobule
and portions of adjacent lobules. ×60.

vein, the former carrying arterial blood, the latter venous blood from the intestines and spleen. Both vessels enter the liver at the porta and divide into large *interlobar branches* which follow the connective tissue septa between the lobes. From these are given off *interlobular branches* which run in the smaller connective tissue septa between the lobules.

From the interlobular branches of the portal vein arise veins which are still interlobular. These send branches into the lobule, where they subdivide to form a specialized capillary bed, the hepatic *sinusoids* (Figs. 16-72 to 16-74). The sinusoids all converge toward the center of the lobule, where they empty into the *central vein.* The central veins are the smallest radicles of the *hepatic veins*, the efferent vessels of the liver. As it passes through the center of the long axis of the lobule, the central vein constantly receives sinusoids from all sides and, increasing in size, leaves the lobule at its base. Here it unites with the central veins of other lobules to form a *sublobular vein*, which is a branch of a hepatic vein.

The hepatic artery accompanies the por-

tal vein, following the branchings of the latter through the interlobar and interlobular connective tissue. Some of the interlobular arterioles break up into capillary networks which supply the interlobular structures and then empty into the smaller branches of the portal veins. Other arterioles empty peripherally into the hepatic sinusoids.

Intrahepatic Ducts. The duct system of the liver serves to convey the external secretion, the *bile*, to the duodenum. The smallest branches of the duct system are the narrow, intralobular *bile canaliculi* which form a ramifying network of channels between the parenchymal cells of the hepatic plates (Fig. 16-72). Like the plates in which they lie, the canaliculi radiate outward from the central axis of the lobule. Most of the canaliculi drain into small *interlobular bile ducts* found at the periphery of a lobule. The short connections between the hepatic cells and the interlobular bile ducts are called *terminal ductules, cholangioles* or ducts of Hering. They are lined by cuboidal cells which are smaller and paler staining than the hepatic cells. The lumen is little if at all larger than that of a

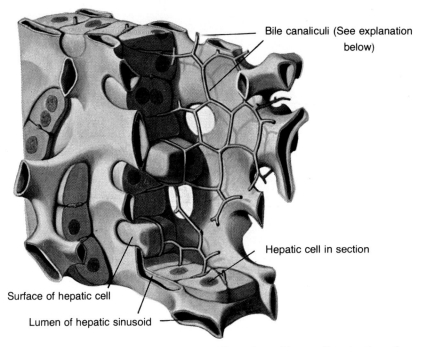

Bile canaliculi (See explanation
below)

Hepatic cell in section

Surface of hepatic cell

Lumen of hepatic sinusoid

Fig. 16-72. Diagrammatic reconstruction of a small portion of human liver to show the relationship of the anastomosing plates of hepatic cells to the blood sinusoids and to the network of bile canaliculi. For the purposes of the diagram, both the sinusoids and the bile canaliculi are shown as independent structures, particularly at *right,* where the hepatic cells have been "dissected away." It should be recalled, however, that the bile canaliculi, being formed by the modified cell membranes of adjacent hepatic cells, are always surrounded by hepatic cells. Therefore, the green network in the diagram represents the contents of the biliary canaliculi, not a separate lining. The lining of the sinusoids is not smooth and homogeneous as shown, but is perforated and made up of endothelial cells, Kupffer cells and fine reticular fibers. (Redrawn and modified from Braus.)

bile canaliculus (Fig. 16-75). A few of the terminal ductules extend to variable depths within the lobule.

Each interlobular duct joins with others, forming progressively larger ducts lined by cuboidal or columnar epithelium. As the ducts increase in size toward the porta of the liver, the epithelium becomes high columnar and the connective tissue layer becomes thicker, with many elastic fibers and a few scattered smooth muscle cells.

In their ramifications through the connective tissue septa, the interlobular bile ducts always accompany the branches of the portal vein and the hepatic artery. These three structures are often referred to as the *portal triad.* Together with the interlobular connective tissue which marks the point of separation of three or more lobules, they occupy the *portal canal* or *portal area* (Fig. 16-74). A network of lym-

phatic vessels accompanies the branches of the portal vein in the portal area and in the interlobular connective tissue. However, the lymphatic vessels tend to collapse and are not obvious in sections prepared by routine methods.

Extrahepatic Ducts. The right and left hepatic ducts join to form the *hepatic duct* which, after its juncture with the cystic duct, becomes the *common bile duct* (ductus choledochus) and conveys the bile to the duodenum. The hepatic ducts, the cystic duct and the common bile duct are referred to as the *extrahepatic ducts* of the liver, in contrast with the intrahepatic system of ducts. The extrahepatic ducts are lined by high columnar epithelium which rests on a connective tissue lamina propria containing smooth muscle and elastic fibers. The epithelium and underlying lamina propria are thrown into numerous folds.

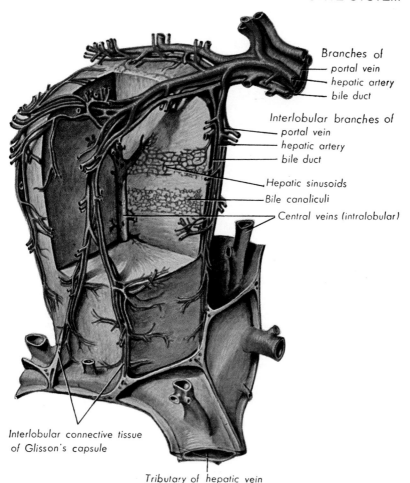

Branches of
— portal vein
— hepatic artery
— bile duct

Interlobular branches of
— portal vein
— hepatic artery
— bile duct

Hepatic sinusoids
Bile canaliculi
Central veins (intralobular)

Interlobular connective tissue
of Glisson's capsule

Tributary of hepatic vein

Fig. 16-73. Reconstruction of a lobule from the liver of a pig. A portion of the lobule is cut away to show the hepatic sinusoids and bile canaliculi. (Redrawn and slightly modified from Braus, after a reconstruction by A. Vierling.)

Goblet cells occur in the epithelium, more abundantly in the lower portion of the common bile duct. Small multicellular glands may be seen extending into the lamina propria. In the cystic duct, the smooth muscle fibers are disposed in transverse, longitudinal and diagonal directions. They are less abundant in the hepatic ducts and the common duct, except in the duodenal end of the latter, where they form a sphincter.

The Hepatic Lobule. It is apparent that the hepatic lobule, the *anatomical unit* of structure of the liver, differs markedly from the lobules of glands such as the pancreas or salivary glands. In the latter, the lobule is surrounded by interlobular connective tissue and comprises a group of secreting tubules drained by the terminal branch of an interlobular duct. Thus, the unit of

structure and the unit of function are identical.

In the liver, the parenchyma comprising one hepatic lobule is drained of its secretion by several interlobular bile ducts lying in the adjacent portal canals. As a result, a single interlobular bile duct carries off the secretions of portions of several adjacent hepatic lobules. This area of hepatic tissue, drained by a single interlobular bile duct lying in the axis of the area, has been designated a *portal lobule*. According to another interpretation, a *functional unit* of liver tissue is defined as a small parenchymal mass (*acinar unit*) that surrounds a terminal branch of a portal vein, accompanied by a hepatic arteriole and a bile ductule (Rappaport et al., 1954). A diagrammatic representation of this unit is shown

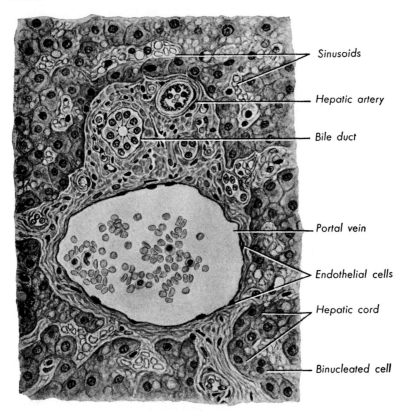

Sinusoids

Hepatic artery

Bile duct

Portal vein

Endothelial cells

Hepatic cord

Binucleated cell

Fig. 16-74. The juncture of three lobules of the human liver, showing interlobular branches of the portal vein, hepatic artery and bile duct. The region occupied by this aggregation of structures is frequently designated as a portal canal. Hematoxylin-eosin. ×455.

in Figure 16-76. It can be seen that this interpretation differs from the portal lobule in that it includes only the parenchymal tissue around a terminal branch of a portal vein rather than all of the parenchyma around all branches of a portal vein located at an axis. The diagram of acinar units also calls attention to the fact that triads (composed of portal veins, hepatic arteries and bile ducts), are present in only two or three of the portal canal areas of hexagonal shaped lobules. The hexagonal lobule is readily identified in the liver of the pig and a few other mammals, but this is not the case in man and in most other mammals. Acinar units are of particular interest in relation to certain pathological lesions. In many cases the pathological changes occur in a pattern corresponding to the units of parenchyma around terminal branches of the portal venules. In some cases, however, the changes appear in patterns corresponding more to the classically described hepatic

lobule. Therefore, the concepts of lobulation should be considered as complementary, not mutually exclusive. It is also important to realize that lobulation is only found in mammals and does not appear until after birth.

The Hepatic Plates or Laminae. The parenchymal cells of the liver were described in the older literature as being arranged in elongated, anastomosing cords made up of two rows of cells, with the main channel of the bile canaliculus extending throughout the length of the cord and its branches. This interpretation was based largely on studies of the liver of lower vertebrates. In sections of liver of man and other mammals, the cord appears to be either one cell thick or two or more cells thick, depending on the plane of the section. Since the cords radiate from the periphery of the lobule to the center with the cells of a row frequently arranged in a vertical relationship to each other (i.e., in a plane

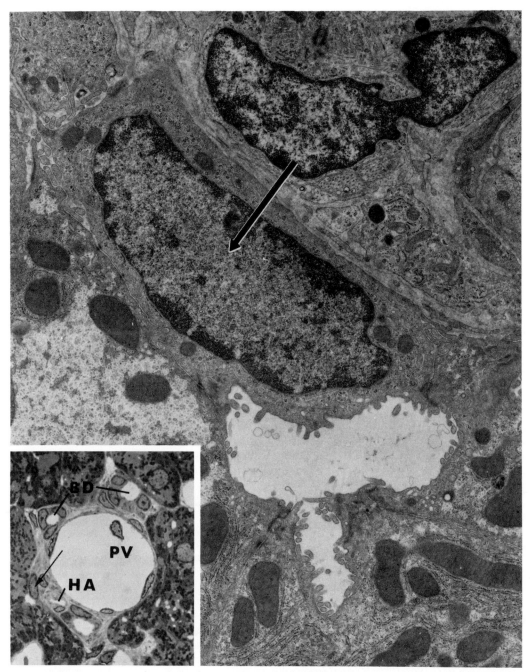

Fig. 16-75. Transition between bile canaliculi and terminal ductules in rat liver. The *inset* shows a 1 μm section of a portal area with branches of the portal vein (*PV*), bile ducts (*BD*) and the hepatic artery (*HA*). The *arrow* indicates a region of transition between a bile ductule and a bile canaliculus. The electron micrograph is from an adjacent thin section. The *large arrow* is on the nucleus of the transition ductule cell. Electron micrograph ×10,500, Inset ×980.

parallel to the course of the central vein), cross sections of a lobule often show the cord as a single row of cells. Cords of two rows of cells, as outlined above, are found in some embryonic livers and in livers of some of the lower vertebrates. However, a

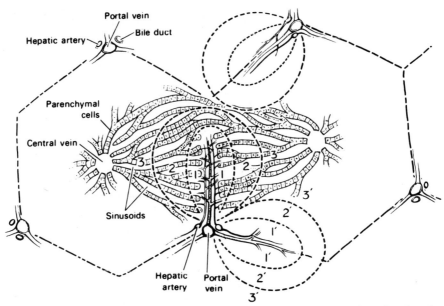

Fig. 16-76. Diagram of the arrangement of liver parenchymal cells in functional units (acinar units) around terminal afferent blood vessels and terminal bile ductules. The oxygen tension and nutrient level of the blood is highest in zone 1 and lowest in zone 3. Zones labeled as 1', 2', and 3' represent corresponding regions of an adjacent acinar unit. (Adapted from A. M. Rappaport, Z. J. Borowy, W. M. Lougheed, and W. N. Lotto, Anat. Rec., vol. 119, 1954.)

modified arrangement is present in man and other mammals where the cells are arranged in sheets known as *hepatic plates* or *hepatic laminae*. This understanding of the cell arrangement resulted from a study of reconstructions showing the structure of the liver lobule in three dimensions.

Bile Canaliculi. Between the hepatic cells are minute intercellular channels, the *bile canaliculi*. These branch and have a very irregular course (Fig. 16-72). Short side branches of the canaliculi frequently extend between the liver cells toward the surface of a plate. They ramify throughout the hepatic parenchyma, anastomosing with the canaliculi of adjacent anastomosing plates (Fig. 16-73), but they seldom approach the surface of a plate.

Each canaliculus lies midway along the interface between adjacent hepatic cells and is formed by the somewhat modified cell membranes of the two opposing cells. They can be demonstrated in light microscope preparations particularly well by the Golgi silver impregnation method or histochemical staining for certain phosphatase enzymes. They are difficult to distinguish in ordinary preparations. Electron micro-

graphs show that the membranes of the hepatic cells which form the canaliculi have short microvilli projecting into the lumen (Figs. 16-77 and 16-78). The canalicular space is separated from the remaining intercellular space by a junctional complex. However, the occluding junction close to the lumen is not highly developed and resembles those of other areas in the body that are only moderately tight. Their organization is especially well seen in freeze-fracture preparations (Fig. 16-79).

Hepatic Cells. The hepatic cells which make up the hepatic plates are polyhedral in form and, under normal conditions, their boundaries are quite sharply defined. Each cell has a central nucleus with a distinct nuclear membrane and one or more prominent nucleoli. Multinucleate hepatic cells are occasionally seen, the usual variation being the binucleate condition.

Binucleate cells result from mitotic division of the nucleus of a mononucleate cell without accompanying division of the cytoplasm. Each of the two nuclei is of approximately normal size and possesses the normal (diploid) number of chromosomes; the cytoplasmic portion of the cell may be

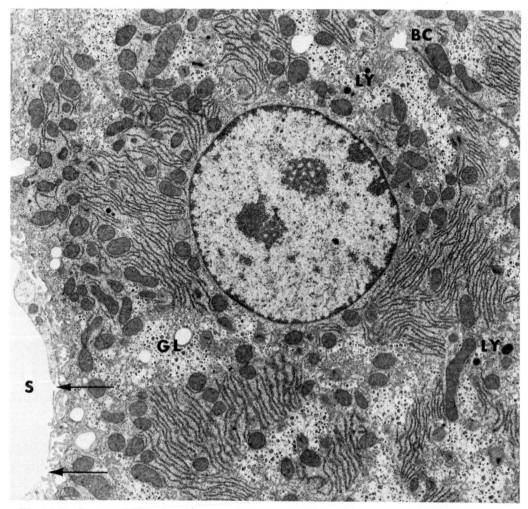

Fig. 16-77. Low magnification electron micrograph of a liver cell of mouse showing relationships to bile canaliculus (*BC*) and the blood sinusoid (*S*). Gaps in the sinusoidal endothelium are shown at the arrows. *LY*, lysosomes; *GL*, glycogen. Clumps of rough edoplasmic reticulum characteristic of liver cells are seen. ×5500.

large. Large hepatic cells with either one or two unusually large nuclei also occur. These result from mitotic division of the above mentioned binucleate cells in which all of the chromosomes merge on one spindle, with the formation of either (1) two large mononucleate cells, each with an unusually large nucleus containing a tetraploid number of chromosomes, or (2) one large cell with two large tetraploid nuclei. Further divisions of this type may produce mononucleate cells with still larger nuclei having a further increase in chromosome number.

The mitochondria of the hepatic cells are spherical, rod-shaped, or filamentous, depending on the location of the cell within the lobule and on the functional state. The Golgi apparatus lies either near the edge of the cell beneath the bile canaliculus, or close to the nucleus. The cytoplasm contains angular clumps of *basophilic material* which is found by histochemical methods to consist chiefly of nucleoproteins. Electron micrographs show that this material is in the form of clusters of free ribosomes plus ribosomes attached to the cisternae of the endoplasmic reticulum (rough endoplasmic reticulum). Electron micrographs show that there are also numerous areas

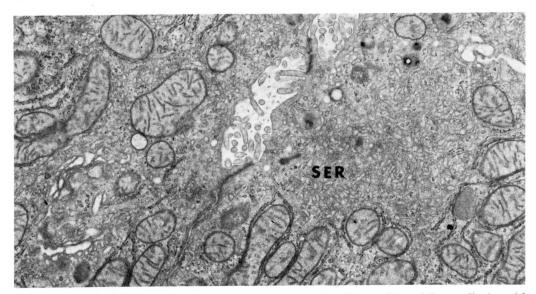

Fig. 16-78. Electron micrograph of portions of two hepatic cells bounding a bile canaliculus with a prominent Golgi zone in the cell at the left. This animal had been treated experimentally and smooth endoplasmic reticulum (SRE) is increased in amount. ×10,850.

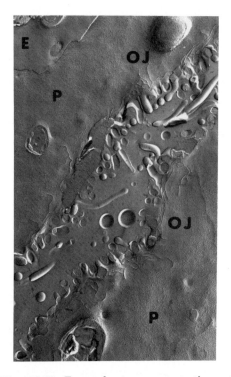

Fig. 16-79. Freeze-fracture preparation of mouse liver showing a bile canaliculus and adjacent structures. Strands of occluding junctions (*OJ*) are apparent on the *P*-faces of adjacent cells. A portion of the *E* fracture face of an overlying cell is seen at the *upper left*. ×17,500.

of smooth endoplasmic reticulum which becomes continuous in places with the rough reticulum (Fig. 16-80). Lysosomes are present, and another organelle known as a *microbody* or *peroxisome* is present. The peroxisomes vary somewhat in morphology in different species. In most species, but not in man, they have a dense core or nucleoid (Figs. 16-80 and 16-81). They contain oxidative enzymes, including urate oxidase and catalase. The urate oxidase is localized to the nucleoid and the absence of this component of the peroxisome in man is correlated with a lack of liver urate oxidase. These organelles appear to arise from the endoplasmic reticulum and are thought to be involved in some manner with lipid metabolism. They are not lysosomes, as was once believed, but their exact function is not known.

Scattered throughout the cytoplasm in ordinary preparations are small clear areas. These represent areas of *glycogen* which can be seen with the light microscope only after appropriate methods of fixation and staining. Electron micrographs show glycogen in liver cells in the form of rosettes of dense granules (Figs. 16-77, 16-80 and 16-81). *Fat droplets* may also appear as inclusions in the cytoplasm, particularly after fasting or after ingestion of an excess

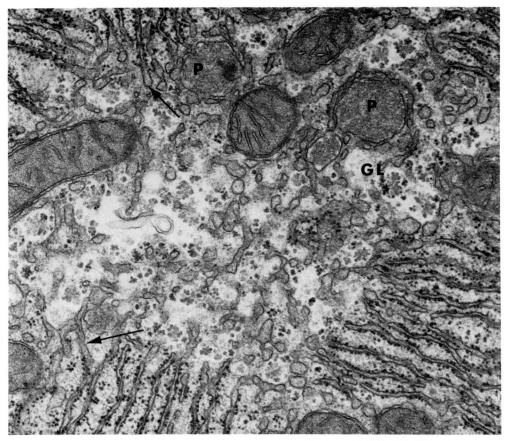

Fig. 16-80. Electron micrograph of a portion of the cytoplasm of an hepatic cell in the rat showing continuity between rough endoplasmic reticulum and smooth endoplasmic reticulum (*arrows*). *P*, peroxisomes; *GL*, glycogen. ×34,000.

of fats. The amount of fat which may be demonstrated in the hepatic cells varies inversely with the amount of glycogen. Pigment granules (bile pigments) are occasionally seen in the cytoplasm.

As in other gland cells, the appearance of the cytoplasm varies with the functional state of the cell. Both glycogen and the basophilic material are markedly reduced after a prolonged period of fasting, and they reaccumulate in the cytoplasm with refeeding. Glycogen is more abundant in the hepatic cells after digestion of a carbohydrate meal. It represents stored carbohydrate, which is returned to the blood as glucose when the needs of the body demand it.

In addition to the cell junctions associated with bile canaliculi already described, apposed liver cell membranes frequently have desmosomes and gap junctions. The latter are correlated with physiological evidence that hepatic cells are electrically coupled.

The liver lobule may be divided into three zones on the basis of structural and functional differences: an inner, hepatic zone around the central vein, an outer, portal zone at the periphery of the lobule and an intermediate zone between the central and peripheral regions. The mitochondria differ in appearance in the different zones, probably in relation to functional activity. The basophilic substance also differs in the different zones. The zones differ, particularly in relation to their storage and release of glycogen. When the livers of rats and mice are depleted of glycogen by prolonged fasting, feeding results in the deposition of glycogen in the peripheral region first, progressing centrally until the lobule is filled.

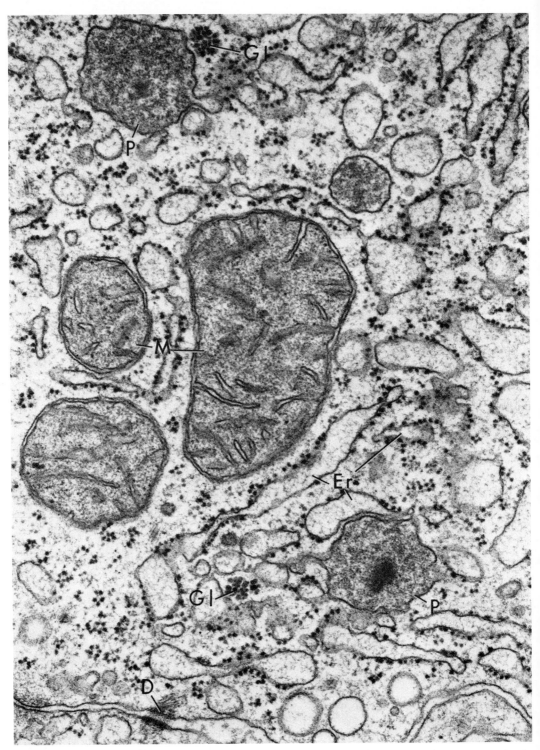

Fig. 16-81. Electron micrograph showing peroxisomes (microbodies) in a liver parenchymal cell of a fetal rat. The peroxisomes (*P*) of the rat liver (and of most mammals other than man) contain electron dense cores (nucleoids) in which liver urate oxidase is localized. Outpouchings are seen at the surface of two of the peroxisomes present in the field illustrated. This suggests that new peroxisomes form either as buds from other peroxisomes or as vesicles derived from the smooth endoplasmic reticulum, consisting of a mixture of smooth and rough varieties. *Gl*, glycogen; *M*, mitochondria. ×50,000.

After completion of the period of digestion, glycogen is usually given up from the peripheral region of the lobule first, leaving a central region with stored glycogen. Zonation is also described for Rappaport's liver acinus. In either case, the areas most closely associated with the blood supply are the most active metabolically.

The membranes of the hepatic cells which border on the sinusoids show a surface modification similar to that on the free surfaces of cells in many other locations. Short, irregular microvilli which can be seen only with the electron microscope project from the cells (Fig. 16-77); in most areas the processes are covered by the lining cells of the sinusoids.

Hepatic Sinusoids. The hepatic sinusoids make up the intralobular system of blood capillaries which course centripetally through the lobule and convey the blood from the interlobular branches of the portal vein and the hepatic artery to the central vein. They have relatively wide lumina,

they anastomose irregularly and everywhere they separate the hepatic plates one from another. It thus follows that the hepatic cells have one or more surfaces abutting on bile canaliculi and one or more surfaces always adjacent to blood sinusoids (Fig. 16-82).

The sinusoids appear to be lined by two morphologically recognizeable types of cells. It has long been debated whether these constitute two separate cell types or are merely functional states of a single cell. The evidence now indicates that the sinusoids are lined primarily by *endothelial cells* similar to those of other blood vessels (Fig. 16-82). The nucleus is dark and the cytoplasm is attenuated. In most mammals, including man, the lining cells form a discontinuous layer which is remarkable in that it is not underlain by a complete basal lamina (Fig. 16-77). The other principal sinusoidal cell has branching pseudopodial processes and is highly phagocytic. It is commonly called a *Kupffer cell* (Figs. 16-

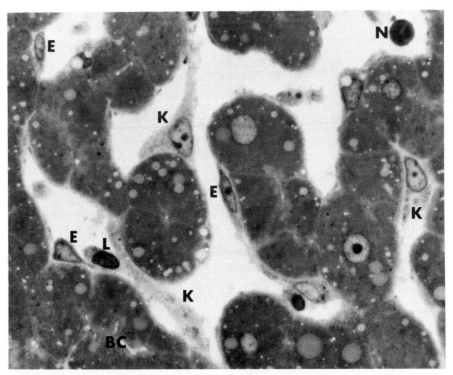

Fig. 16-82. Light micrograph of a 1 μm section of monkey liver showing liver plates and sinusoids. The difference in morphology between endothelial cells (*E*) and Kupffer cells (*K*) can be seen. A lymphocyte (*L*) and a neutrophil (*N*) are also present in the sinusoidal lumen. A bile canaliculus is at lower left (*BC*). ×800.

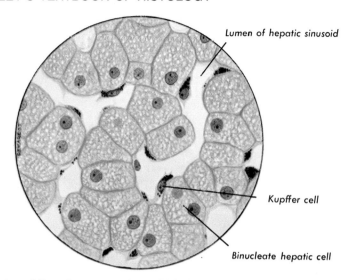

Fig. 16-83. Section of liver from a monkey which had received several intraperitoneal injections of trypan blue. Most of the sinusoidal lining (Kupffer) cells have taken in some of the dye by phagocytosis. Azocarmine and metanil yellow stain. ×720.

82 and 16-83). Kupffer cells normally lie on the lumenal side of the endothelial cells and may extend processes through some of the endothelial discontinuities. However, they occasionally appear to be interposed between endothelial cells and thus may form a minor portion of the sinusoidal wall. Even more frequently they are seen to span the sinusoidal lumen, appearing stellate in shape (Fig. 16-82). Neither endothelial cells nor Kupffer cells develop obvious junctional complexes at their points of intercellular contact. The porosity of the sinusoidal lining is also enhanced by fenestrations in the endothelial cells (Figs. 16-84 and 16-85). Intercellular gaps, cellular fenestrations and the lack of a complete basal lamina permit blood plasma to have direct access to the hepatic parenchymal cell surfaces. This has obvious advantages for efficiency in nutrient uptake and the release of synthesized products directly into the blood stream.

Perisinusoidal Space. Between the sinusoidal lining cells and the hepatic cells is a connective tissue space of variable dimensions. In early light microscopy this space was frequently exaggerated by the preparation techniques and it was termed the *space of Disse.* It is now recognized that the space is normally rather small, but nonetheless real. Besides the microvilli of

hepatic cells it contains reticular fibers and occasional perisinusoidal cells differing from either the endothelial or the Kupffer cells. The perisinusoidal cells often contain lipid droplets and have been referred to as *fat storage cells.* Their function is not well understood. Typical fibroblasts are not present in the perisinusoidal space, and it is believed that the endothelial cells are responsible for synthesis of the collagen that is deposited as reticular fibers in this space.

Connective Tissue. Ordinary sections of the human liver reveal scant amounts of connective tissue. The interlobular connective tissue concentrated in the portal areas has already been described. Silver stains and electron micrographs show that there is a framework of reticular (argyrophilic) fibers within each lobule (Fig. 16-86). They form a network which envelops each sinusoid and radiates outward from the region of the central vein. As mentioned previously these reticular fibers lie in the perisinusoidal space.

Lymphatics. The lymph vessels of the liver form a rich plexus in the capsule of Glisson and in its connective tissue septa within the gland. Lymph vessels enmesh the larger blood vessels and ducts, and there are anastomoses between lymphatics which surround the portal veins and those

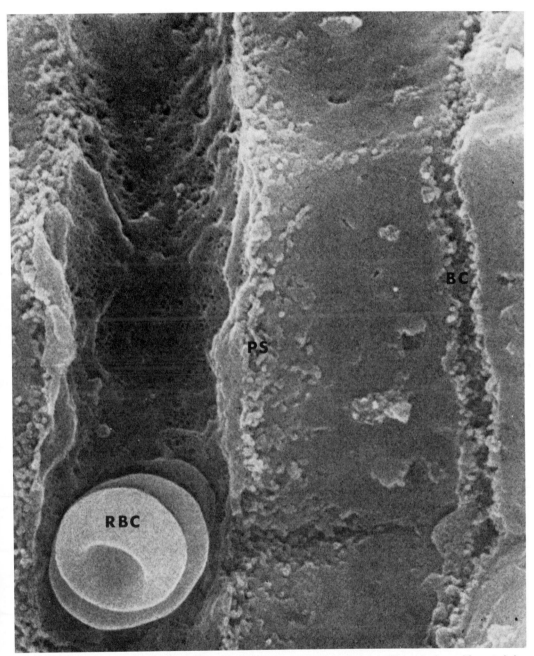

Fig. 16-84. Scanning electron micrograph of a portion of cleaved mouse liver. A sinusoid containing red blood cells (*RBC*) is seen at the *left* and the perisinusoidal space (of Disse) (*PS*) and a bile canaliculus (*BC*) are also apparent. The sinusoidal wall shows fenestrations. ×8,250.

which surround hepatic veins. Anastomoses between lymphatics of neighboring portal canals enclose the hepatic lobules in a network of small lymph vessels but, so far as can be determined, no lymphatic vessels penetrate the lobules themselves. Since the lobules comprise the bulk of the liver tissue, it is puzzling that more lymph flows from the liver than from any other organ of the body. It has been postulated that the lymph is formed in the perisinusoidal space; this space should not, however, be confused

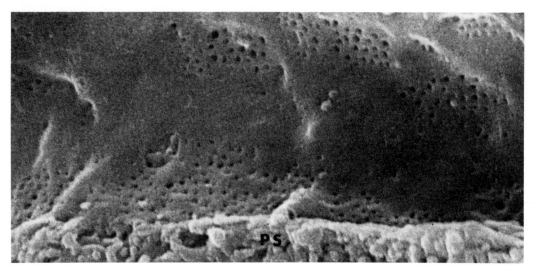

Fig. 16-85. Scanning electron micrograph of a portion of a sinusoidal wall from the same animal as shown in Figure 16-84. Endothelial fenestrations are apparent. *PS,* perisinusoidal space. ×14,500.

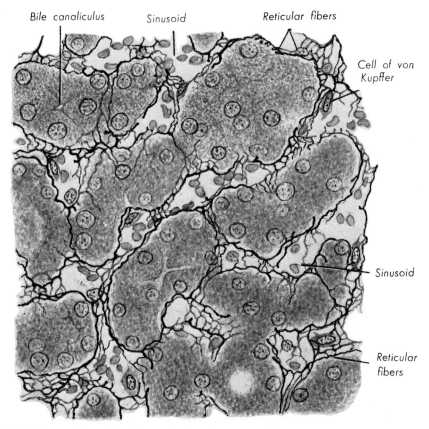

Fig. 16-86. Human liver, showing reticular tissue in a lobule. Reticular fibers do not extend through the lumen of the sinusoid, although tangential sections through the wall of the sinusoid may give this impression. Foot's silver technique. ×700.

with a lymphatic vessel as it is not an endothelium-lined space.

Nerve Supply. The nerves of the liver are mainly nonmyelinated fibers of the sympathetic system. They accompany the blood vessels and bile ducts, around which they form plexuses. These plexuses give off fibers which terminate on the blood vessels and bile ducts but do not appear to penetrate the lobule.

Functions of the Liver. The exocrine function of the liver is concerned with the production of bile, which is carried by the system of bile ducts into the duodenum.

Bile is a product of the hepatic cells and is partly a secretion important in the absorption of fats and partly an excretion carrying off waste products which are eliminated with the feces. Among the constituents of bile are: bile acids, bile pigments, cholesterol, lecithin, neutral fats and soaps, traces of urea, and water and bile salts. The bile salts, as emulsifying agents, facilitate the absorption of fats in the intestine. They are themselves reabsorbed in part from the intestine and are again secreted by the hepatic cells. The bile pigments are derived from the breakdown of hemoglobin; this apparently does not take place in the liver, although the Kupffer cells may play a part. The bile pigments are removed from the blood by the liver and excreted in the bile as a waste product. Cholesterol is also excreted in the bile.

Claude Bernard was the first to show that the liver stores glycogen and gives it up as glucose. The liver not only stores reserve sugars, but it is essential for the transformations which are necessary before some of the sugars can be utilized by the body. Conversion of fats and perhaps also of proteins to carbohydrates is accomplished in the liver (gluconeogenesis). Through its diversified chemical processes, the liver is able to maintain a constant blood sugar level under widely different dietary conditions.

The liver has other important functions. It is involved in protein metabolism and is the chief site of deaminization of amino acids, with the production of urea as a by-product. Fats are likewise metabolized and stored in the liver. Some of the plasma proteins (fibrinogen, prothrombin, albumin) are synthesized in the liver. The liver is also an important place of storage for many vitamins, chiefly A, D, B_2, B_3, B_4, B_{12} and K, which are essential to the body. The liver also plays an important role in the detoxification of a number of lipid soluble drugs, e.g., barbiturates. The enzymes which perform the detoxification are in smooth endoplasmic reticulum (Fig. 16-78). This organelle increases markedly on challenge of the liver with such drugs. The increased amount of smooth reticulum makes drug metabolism more efficient and is responsible for the development of drug tolerance. The same basic set of enzymes is involved with alcohol degradation and this overlap in function accounts for the potential danger of combining alcohol imbibition with certain kinds of drug therapy.

Regeneration of Liver. When a part of the liver is removed by operation or when there is partial destruction by toxic agents (chloroform, etc.), the organ regains its normal weight within a relatively short time. In the rat, surgical removal of as much as 75% of the gland is followed by complete weight restitution within 1 month. The repair is accomplished by mitotic multiplication of parenchymal cells throughout the remaining portion of the organ and by cell enlargement. Differentiation of new liver cells from budding interlobular bile ducts may also play a part. In restored liver tissue, there is an increased number of the mononucleated cells which have large nuclei containing a multiple number of chromosomes. These are produced by division of binucleated cells. There is also a general increase in nuclear size of all of the parenchymal cells.

The liver also variably regenerates after toxic injury. If the injury is singular and not immediately fatal, complete regeneration may be possible. If the toxic condition is chronic, the regeneration is only partial and gradual impairment of function usually ensues. Under these conditions normal lobulation is lost, there is an increase in fibrous tissue (fibrosis) and cirrhosis of the liver may eventually develop.

The Gall Bladder

The gall bladder is a hollow, pear-shaped organ lying obliquely on the inferior surface of the liver. It may be regarded as a diverticulum of the bile duct. It consists of a *fundus*, which is the blind end, a *body* and a *neck* which passes into the cystic duct. In the neck, folds of the mucosa form the *spiral valve of Heister*.

The wall of the gall bladder is composed of three layers: *mucosa, muscularis* and an *adventitia* or *serosa*. The mucosa is thrown into numerous folds which divide the surface roughly into irregular polygonal areas (Fig. 16-87). The epithelium is composed of tall columnar cells with oval nuclei situated in the middle or the basal zones (Figs. 16-88 and 4-10, *B*). A thin, striated border can be seen on the apical surface of the cells. It is less prominent than that of the intestinal cells, so that is is seen well only with special preparation (Fig. 16-89) or by electron microscopy (Fig. 16-90). Intercellular spaces occur between the epithelial cells. These change in dimension in re-

sponse to physiological activity in water absorption (Figs. 16-89 and 16-91). The tunica propria consists of connective tissue containing extensive vascular plexuses and a few scattered smooth muscle cells derived from the muscularis. Near the neck of the gall bladder, small tubuloalveolar glands occur in the mucosa.

Small diverticula of the mucosa which extend down into the muscular and perimuscular layers are known as the *Rokitansky-Aschoff sinuses*. Their epithelium is a continuation of the surface epithelium.

The muscular layer of the gall bladder is formed of interlacing bundles of smooth muscle fibers. Bundles of longitudinal fibers occur nearer the lamina propria, coursing the length of the bladder and curving over the fundus. The remainder of the muscle bundles, which form the greater part of the muscularis, are circularly disposed. Connective tissue, with an abundance of elastic

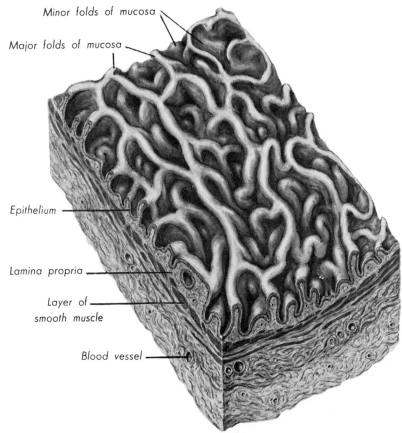

Minor folds of mucosa

Major folds of mucosa

Epithelium

Lamina propria

Layer of smooth muscle

Blood vessel

Fig. 16-87. Low power, three dimensional view of a portion of the wall of a human gall bladder. ×24.

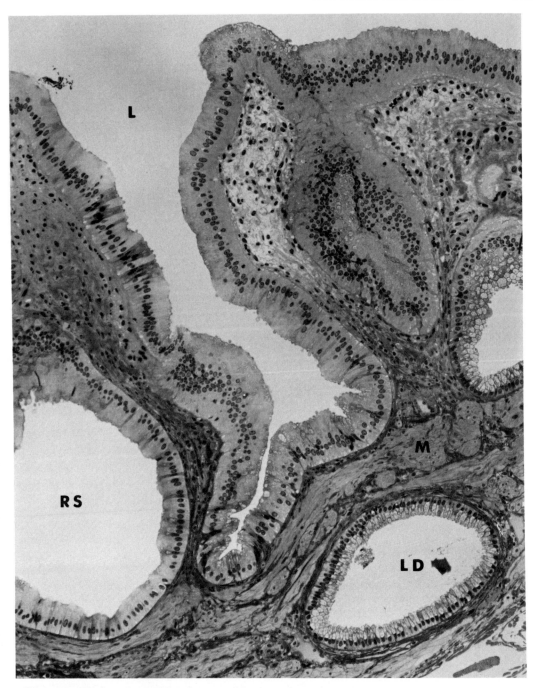

Fig. 16-88. Light micrograph of a 1.5 μm section from gall bladder of the monkey. The lumenal surface is lined with tall columnar epithelium. A mucosal diverticulum appears at the *lower left* (*RS*). The space at the *lower right* lies in the muscular wall (*M*) and may represent a portion of a duct of Luschka. *L*, lumen; *M*, muscularis; *RS*, sinus of Rokitansky-Aschoff; *LD*, Luschka duct. ×140.

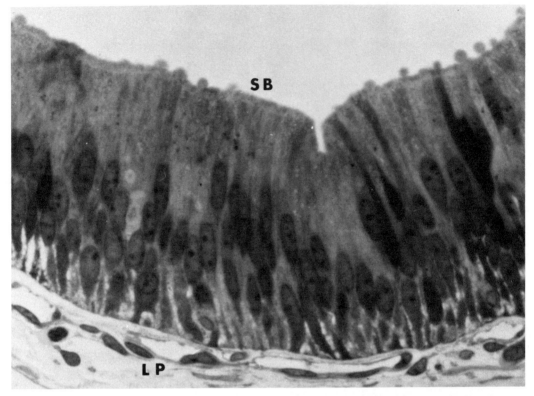

Fig. 16-89. Light micrograph of a 1 μm section of monkey gall bladder. The tall columnar epithelium shows intercellular spaces basally and a striated border at the apex. *SB,* striated border; *LP,* lamina propria. ×1,100.

fibers, occurs between the muscle bundles.

The external connective tissue layer is usually thick but shows wide individual differences. Just external to the muscularis, it consists of fibrous connective tissue sufficiently distinct to be designated the *perimuscular layer.* Outside this is a subserous layer of connective tissue containing blood and lymph vessels and nerves. On its free surface, the gall bladder is covered by the peritoneum; the connective tissue of its attached surface merges with that of the liver.

Lymph nodules occur in the wall of the gall bladder. One may also find ductlike structures, lined with epithelium, which have no connection with the lumen of the bladder, although they have occasionally been described as having connections with the bile ducts. These are known as *Luschka ducts* (Fig. 16-88). They are interpreted as aberrant embryonic bile ducts.

The gall bladder functions as a reservoir for the bile produced by the liver. By the reabsorption of large quantities of water and mineral salts through its mucosal layer, it also serves to concentrate the bile.

The Bile Ducts

There are three main ducts associated with the gall bladder. These are (1) the cystic duct, (2) the hepatic duct and (3) the common bile duct (*ductus choledochus*). The hepatic duct conducts bile from the liver to a point where the cystic duct from the gall bladder meets the common bile duct leading to the duodenum. The bile then passes through the cystic duct into the gall bladder for concentration and storage. Contraction of the gall bladder forces the bile back through the cystic duct and thence through the common bile duct to the intestine. As the ductus choledochus passes obliquely through the wall of the duodenum, it lies side by side with the ductus pancreaticus. In their course through

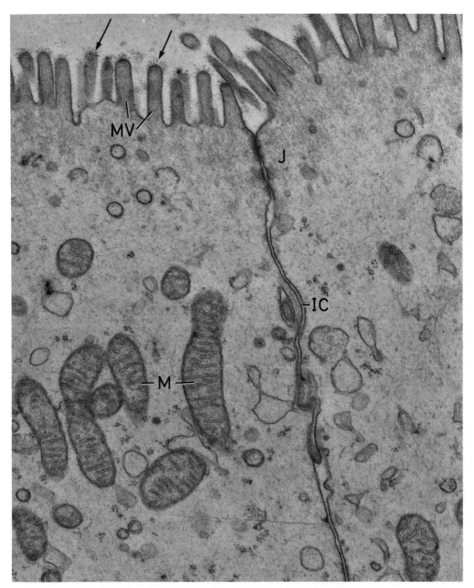

Fig. 16-90. Electron micrograph of the apical portion of two epithelial cells from the gall bladder of a rabbit. The microvilli (*MV*) are covered by hairlike projections or "fuzz." A typical junctional complex (*J*) is present at the adluminal end of the intercellular space (*IC*). *M*, mitochondria. ×27,000. (Courtesy of Drs. G. I. Kaye, H. O. Wheeler, R. T. Whitlock, and N. Lane. J. Cell Biol., vol. 30, 1966.)

the submucosa of the duodenum, the associated pancreatic and bile ducts are surrounded by layers of smooth muscle which form the *sphincter of Oddi*. A portion of this muscular sheath which encircles only the bile duct is known as the *sphincter choledochus*. While this sphincter remains contracted (as for example during fasting), pressure is maintained in the duct system, and bile from the liver is forced into the gall bladder for storage. Upon the ingestion of food, especially fats or proteins, the sphincter of Oddi relaxes, the gall bladder is stimulated to contract and bile traverses the cystic duct and common bile duct to the duodenum.

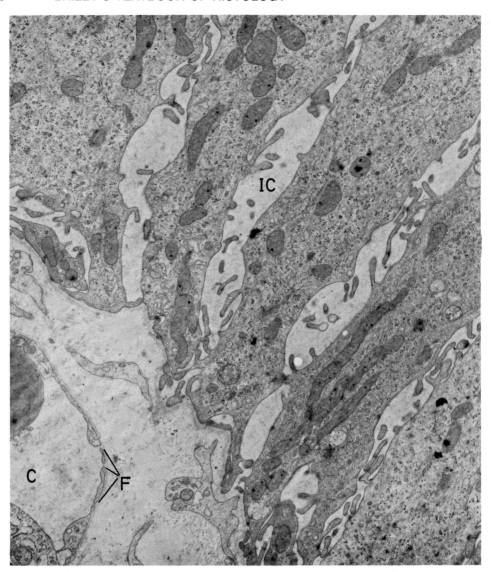

Fig. 16-91. Electron micrograph of the basal portion of several epithelial cells from a gall bladder that has been stimulated to absorb water at an accelerated rate. The contents of a surgically exposed gall bladder from an anesthetized rabbit were aspirated and replaced with a Krebs-Henseleit bicarbonate solution for a period of 1 h before fixation of the tissue. Note that the width of the intercellular space (*IC*) in the basal portion of the epithelium is increased in correlation with increased absorption. A capillary (*C*) with fenestrated endothelium (*F*) is seen within the connective tissue lamina propria. ×15,000. (Courtesy of Drs. G. I. Kaye, H. O. Wheeler, R. T. Whitlock, and N. Lane. J. Cell Biol., vol. 30, 1966).

The ducts are lined with a columnar epithelium similar to that of the gall bladder. Most of the bile ducts have epithelial-lined outpouchings which simulate irregularly distributed glands. Mitosis of epithelial cells occurs chiefly in these outpouchings, and the cells move upward to replace worn-out cells of the luminal surface much like the replacement cells in the intestine by mitosis of cells in the crypts. Near the neck of the gall bladder, the mucosa of the cystic duct has a series of relatively high folds which are continuous with those of the spiral valve of Heister. After removal of the gall bladder surgically, the common bile duct expands and assumes some of the storage functions of the gall bladder. The muscularis of the ducts is not as prominent as in the gall bladder. The arrangement of muscle fibers into layers is not definite, but they tend to be circularly arranged in the hepatic duct and longitudinally disposed in the cystic and in the common bile duct preceding its entry into the duodenum.

Development of the Digestive System

In the development of the digestive system, all of the layers of the blastoderm are involved. Mesoderm and endoderm are the layers most involved, however, as the ectoderm forms the lining of only a part of the mouth, the epithelium of some of the salivary glands and a part of the anal canal.

The primary gut, composed of endoderm and its surrounding mesoderm, is at first a *blind tube,* except for its temporary opening to the yolk stalk. Connections to the exterior occur later by oral and anal invaginations of ectoderm which extend inward and open into the ends of the hitherto imperforate gut. The epithelial lining of the gut and the parenchyma of all glands connected with it are derived from endoderm. The muscle, the connective tissue and the mesothelium of the serosa are developed from mesoderm.

The mesodermal elements show little variation throughout the gut, the peculiarities of the several anatomical divisions being dependent mainly on special differentiation of the endoderm (epithelium). Beneath the endodermal cells is a narrow layer of loosely arranged tissue which later separates into lamina propria, muscularis, mucosae and submucosa. Outside this, a broader mesodermal band of firmer structure represents the future muscularis.

The *stomach* first appears as a spindle-shaped dilation about the end of the first month. Its endodermal cells, which had consisted of a single layer, increase in number and arrange themselves in short, cylindrical groups. These are the first traces of tubular glands. They increase in length and extend downward into the mesodermal tissue. The cells lining the gastric glands are apparently alike, before about the fourth month when differentiation into chief cells and parietal cells takes place.

In the *intestines* a proliferation of the epithelium and of the underlying connective tissue results in the formation of *villi.* These appear about the 10th week, in both small and large intestines. In the former they increase in size, while in the latter they atrophy and ultimately disappear. The simple tubular glands of the intestines develop in a manner similar to those of the stomach.

The mesothelium of the serosa is derived from the mesodermal cells of the primitive body cavity.

The *development of the larger glands* connected with the digestive tract takes place in a manner similar to the formation of the simple tubular glands. All originate as extensions of endodermal cords into the underlying mesodermal tissue. From the lower ends of these cords, branches extend in all directions to form the complex systems of tubules found in the compound glands.

The *salivary glands,* being developed from the oral cavity, originate as similar invaginations of ectodermal tissue.

The *pancreas* arises as two separate outgrowths from the embryonic duodenum. The dorsal outgrowth forms a part of the head and all of the body and tail of the adult pancreas. The ventral outgrowth forms the remainder of the head of the pancreas. The endodermal evaginations grow into the underlying mesenchyme which forms the connective tissue and vascular framework of the organ. The endodermal outgrowths differentiate into ducts and acini. The duct of the ventral outgrowth enlarges to form the main pancreatic duct (duct of Wirsung) which drains the acini derived from both outgrowths. A small accessory duct often persists at the site of the dorsal outgrowth. The islets of Langerhans develop as buds from a system of fine tubules which are derived from the ducts and which form a network around the ducts. Many of the islets become secondarily detached, but some of them retain their attachment to the tubules in the adult.

References

BEAMS, H. W., AND KING, R. L. The origin of binucleate and large monoucleate cells in the liver of the rat. Anat. Rec. 83:281–297, 1942.

BENSLEY, R. R. The gastric glands. Special Cytology (Cowdry, editor), vol. 1, pp. 199–320. Paul B. Hoeber, New York, 1932.

BOAS, A., AND WILSON, T. H. Cellular localization of gastric intrinsic factor in the rat. Am. J. Physiol. 206:783–786, 1963.

CARDELL, R. R., JR., BADENHAUSEN, S., AND PORTER, K. R. Intestinal triglyceride absorption in the rat. An electron microscopical study. J. Cell Biol. 34:123–155, 1967.

CARO, L. G., AND PALADE, G. E. Protein synthesis, storage and discharge in the pancreatic exocrine cell. J. Cell Biol. 20:473–495, 1964.

CHENG, H. AND LEBLOND, C. P. Origin, differentiation and renewal of the four main epithelial cell types in the mouse small intestine. V. Unitarian theory of the origin of the four epithelial cell types. Am. J. Anat. 141:537–562, 1974.

CLARA, M. Der Gallenkapillaren unter physiologischen und experimentellen Bedingungen; morphologische und experimentelle Untersuchungen an der Kaninchenleber. Z. Mikr. Anat. Forsch 35:1–56, 1934.

CLARK, S. L., JR. The ingestion of proteins and colloidal materials by columnar absorptive cells of the small intestine in rats and mice. J. Biophys. Biochem. Cytol. 5:41–49, 1959.

COHEN, P. J. The renewal areas of the common bile duct epithelium. Anat. Rec. 150:237–242, 1964.

DE DUVE, C. Glucagon. The hyperglycemic-glycogenolytic factor of the pancreas. Lancet 2:99–104, 1953.

DUKES, H. H. The Physiology of Domestic Animals. Comstock Publishing Associates, Cornell University Press, Ithaca, 1955.

ECKMAN, C. A., AND HOLMGREN, H. The effect of alimentary factors on liver glycogen rhythm and the distribution of glycogen in the liver lobule. Anat. Rec. 104:189–216, 1949.

ELIAS, H. A re-examination of the structure of the mammalian liver. I. Parenchymal architecture. Am. J. Anat. 84:311–333; II. The hepatic lobule and its relation to the vascular and biliary system. Am. J. Anat. 85:379–456, 1949.

FORSMANN, W. G., ORCI, L., PICTET, R., RENOLD, A. E., AND ROUILLER, C. The endocrine cells in the epithelium of the gastrointestinal mucosa of the rat. An electron microscope study. J. Cell Biol. 40:692–715, 1969.

FRAZER, A. C. The absorption of triglyceride fat from the intestine. Physiol. Rev. 26:104–120, 1940.

FRIEND, D. S. The fine structure of Brunner's glands in the mouse. J. Cell Biol. 25:563–576, 1965.

HIGGINS, G. M., AND ANDERSON, R. M. Experimental pathology of the liver. I. Restoration of the liver of the white rat following partial surgical removal. Arch. Pathol 12:186–202, 1931.

HOEDEMAKER, P. J., ABELS, J., WACHTERS, J. J., ARENDS, A., AND NIEWEG, H. O. Investigations about the site of production of Castle's gastric intrinsic factor. Lab. Invest. 13:1394–1399, 1964.

HOEDEMAKER, P. J., AND ITO, S. Ultrastructural localization of gastric parietal cell antigen with peroxidase-coupled antibody. Lab. Invest. 22:184–188, 1970.

HUNT, T. E., AND HUNT, E. A. Radioautographic study of proliferation in the stomach of the rat using thymidine-H^3 and compound 48/80[1,2]. Anat. Rec. 142:505–517, 1962.

ITO, S. The enteric surface coat on intestinal microvilli. J. Cell Biol. 27:475–491, 1965.

ITO, T., AND NEMOTO, M. Über die Kupfferschen Sternzellen und die "Fettspeicherungszellen" ("fat storing cells") in der Blutkapillarenwand der menschlichen Leber. Fol. Anat. Jap. 24:243–258, 1952.

JONES, A. L., AND FAWCETT, D. W. Hypertrophy of the agranular endoplasmic reticulum in hamster liver induced by phenobarbital (with a review of the functions of this organelle in liver). J. Histochem. Cytochem. 14:215–232, 1966.

KAYE, G. I., WHEELER, H. O., WHITLOCK, R. T., AND LANE, N. Fluid transport in rabbit gall bladder. A combined physiological and electron microscope study. J. Cell Biol. 30:237–268, 1966.

KRAEHENBUHL, J. P., AND CAMPICHE, M. A. Early stages of intestinal absorption of specific antibodies in the newborn. J. Cell Biol. 42:345–365, 1969.

LADMAN, A. J., PADYKULA, H. A., AND STRAUSS, E. W. A morphological study of fat transport in the normal human jejunum. Am. J. Anat. 112:389–419, 1963.

LECHAGO, J., AND BENCOSME, S. The endocrine elements of the digestive system. Int. Rev. Exp. Pathol. 12:119–201, 1973.

LEGG, P. G., AND WOOD, R. L. New observations on microbodies. A cytochemical study on CPIB-treated rat liver. J. Cell Biol. 45:118–129, 1970.

LINDERSTRØM-LANG, K. Distribution of enzymes in tissues and cells. Harvey Lectures, Ser. 34, pp. 214–245, 1939.

MALL, F. The vessels and walls of the dog's stomach. Johns Hopkins Hosp. Rep. 1:1–36, 1896.

PALADE, G. E. The endoplasmic reticulum. J. Biophys. Biochem. Cytol. 2: no. 4 (suppl.) 85–97, 1956.

PALADE, G. E., AND SIEKEVITZ, P. Pancreatic microsomes. J. Biophys. Biochem. Cytol. 2:671–690, 1958.

PALAY, S. L., AND KARLIN, L. An electron microscope study of the intestinal villus. I. The fasting animal. J. Biophys. Biochem. Cytol. 5:363–384, 1959.

PALAY, S. L., AND REVEL, J. P. The morphology of fat absorption. In Lipid Transport (Meng, H. C., editor). Charles C Thomas, Publisher, Springfeld, Ill., 1964.

PORTER, K. R., AND BRUNI, C. An electron microscope study of the early effects of 3-Me-DAB on rat liver cells. Cancer Res. 19:997–1009, 1959.

RALPH, P. H. The surface structure of the gall bladder and intestinal epithelium of man and monkey. Anat. Rec. 108:217–225, 1950.

RAPPAPORT, A. M., BOROWY, Z. J., LOUGHEED, W. M., AND LOTTI, W. N. Subdivision of hexagonal liver lobules into a structural and functional unit. Role in hepatic physiology and pathology. Anat. Rec. 119:11–34, 1954.

RAPPAPORT, A. M. Acinar units and the pathophysiology of liver. In The Liver; Morphology, Biochemistry, Physiology (Rouiller, Ch., editor), vol. 1, pp. 265–328. Academic Press, New York, 1963.

REISER, R., BRYSON, M. J., CARR, M. J., AND KUIKER, K. A. The intestinal absorption of triglycerides. J. Biol. Chem. 194:131–138, 1952.

SCOTT, D. B. Recent contributions in dental histology

by use of the electron microscope. Int. Dent. J. 4:64–95, 1953.

SELZMAN, H. M., AND LIEBELT, R. A. Paneth cell granules of mouse intestine. J. Cell Biol. 15:136–139, 1962.

SENIOR, J. R. Intestinal absorption of fats. J. Lipid Res. 5:495–521, 1964.

SINGH, I. On argyrophile and argentaffin reactions in individual granules of enterochromaffin cells of the human gastro-intestinal tract. J. Anat. 98:497–500, 1964.

SOLCIA, E., CAPELLA, C., VASSALLO, G., AND BUFFA, R. Endocrine cells of the gastric mucosa. Int. Rev. Cytol. 42:223–286, 1975.

SPICER, S. S., STALEY, M. W., WETZEL, M. G., AND WETZEL, B. K. Acid mucosubstance and basic protein in mouse Paneth cells. J. Histochem. Cytochem. 15:225–242, 1967.

STRAUSS, E. W. Electron microscopic study of intestinal fat absorption in vitro from mixed micelles containing monoolein, and bile salt. J. Lipid Res. 7:307–323, 1966.

SULKIN, N. M. A study of the nucleus in the normal and hyperplastic liver of the rat. Am. J. Anat. 73:107–125, 1943.

TROTTER, N. Electron opaque, lipid-containing bodies

in mouse liver at early intervals after partial hepatectomy and sham operation. J. Cell Biol. 25: no. 3, pt. 2, 41–55, 1965.

WEINSTOCK, M., AND LEBLOND, C. P. Synthesis, migration and release of precursor collagen by odontoblasts as visualized by radioautography after H^3-proline administration. J. Cell Biol. 60:92–127, 1974.

WILSON, J. W., AND LEDUC, E. H. Role of cholangioles in restoration of the liver of the mouse after dietary injury. J. Pathol. Bacteriol. 76:441–450, 1958.

WILSON, J. W., AND LEDUC, E. H. Mitochondrial changes in the liver of essential fatty acid-deficient mice. J. Cell Biol. 16:281–313, 1963.

WISSE, E. Observations on the fine structure and peroxidase cytochemistry of normal rat liver Kupffer cells. J. Ultrastruct. Res. 46:393–426, 1974.

WISSE, E. Kupffer cell reactions in rat liver under various conditions as observed in the electron microscope. J. Ultrastruct. Res. 46:499–520, 1974.

YAMADA, E. The fine structure of the gall bladder epithelium of the mouse. J. Biophys. Biochem. Cytol. 1:445–458, 1955.

ZETTERQVIST, H. The ultrastructural organization of the columnar absorbing cells of the mouse jejunum. Aktïebolage Godvil, Karolinska Institutet, Stockholm, 1956.

CHAPTER 17

The Respiratory System

The respiratory system consists of the lungs and a series of passages leading to them. On the basis of their primary functions, the different parts of the system can be classified in two categories: (1) an *air conducting division* composed, in sequence, of the nasal cavity, nasopharynx, oropharynx (which serves for conduction of air as well as food), larynx, trachea, bronchi and bronchioles, and (2) a *respiratory division* specialized for the exchanges of gases between air and blood. The latter is composed of respiratory bronchioles, alveolar ducts, alveolar sacs and alveoli. These divisions of the respiratory system perform their functions with the aid of a ventilation mechanism that includes the rib cage, the intercostal muscles, the disphragm and the elastic tissue of the lungs.

The Nasal Cavity and Nasopharynx

Nasal Cavity

The nasal cavity extends from the nares (nostrils) to the choanae, through which it opens into the nasopharynx. The cavity of the nose is divided into lateral halves or *fossae* by a median cartilaginous and bony septum. The inferior region of each fossa is somewhat expanded and is named the *vestibule* (Fig. 17-1). This leads into the major cavity, which is named the respiratory region in contrast with the olfactory region in the upper part of each fossa, which has receptor cells for the sense of smell.

The medial wall of each fossa (the septum) is smooth, but the lateral wall has an irregular contour because of the presence of horizontal scroll-shaped structures, the *conchae* (Figs. 17-1 and 17-2). Each concha is attached along its upper margin to the lateral wall, and the space beneath each concha is known as a *meatus*. The lacrimal duct and some of the nasal sinuses open into the meatuses.

The main current of air passing through the nose comes in contact with the mucosa of the septum and the medial surfaces of the conchae. Therefore, these surfaces are subjected to more cooling and drying than are the less exposed surfaces of the meatuses and the even less exposed mucous membranes of the sinuses. The mucous membranes of different parts of the nasal cavity have histological differences that appear to be correlated with differences in exposure.

The nasal passages function for the conduction of air and also as efficient air conditioning and filtering units. By the numerous blood vessels beneath the epithelium of some areas, the inhaled air is warmed before being transmitted to the lungs. By the mucous and serous glands, the moisture content of the air is maintained at a proper value and the epithelium itself is protected from excessive drying. The mucous coat over the epithelium, combined with ciliary

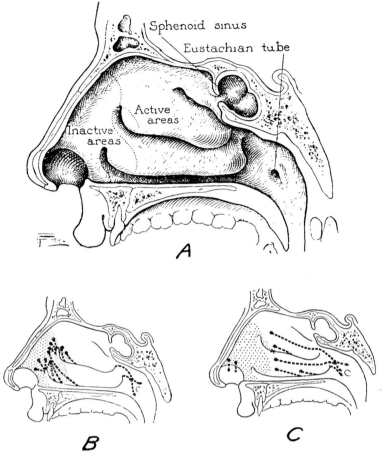

Fig. 17-1. Lateral wall of right nasal fossa and nasal pharynx. The superior, middle and inferior nasal conchae are seen, together with the opening of the sphenoid sinus into the sphenoethmoidal recess above the superior nasal concha. The right frontal sinus opening, which opens usually into the middle meatus in back of the middle concha, is not seen. A, the areas of the lateral wall where ciliary movements are active and relatively inactive. B, the course of mucous drainage of the inactive area. C, the course of mucous drainage of the active area. (After Hilding.)

action, traps a portion of the particulate matter of the inspired air and moves it to the oropharynx to be expectorated or swallowed into the digestive tract.

The lining of the anterior part of the vestibule is quite similar to the epidermis of the nose. However, it has long thick hairs or vibrissae and associated sebaceous glands. Sweat glands are also present. The junction of the anterior part of the vestibule with the major or respiratory region of the nasal cavity is known as a transitional zone. The latter has stratified squamous epithelium like that of the anterior part of the vestibule, but it lacks sweat glands, sebaceous glands and hair follicles. It has mixed mucous and serous glands like those of the respiratory region.

The *respiratory region* is lined by a ciliated pseudostratified columnar epithelium which is the characteristic type of the conducting division of the respiratory system. In the more exposed areas, the epithelium is thick, goblet cells are numerous and the basement membrane (basal lamina plus lamina reticularis) is prominent (Fig. 17-3) by reason of a relatively thick lamina reticularis. In the meatuses, the epithelium is thinner, goblet cells are fewer and the basement membrane is not prominent. Intraepithelial glands (mucous crypts) are present in a few individuals. These glands are

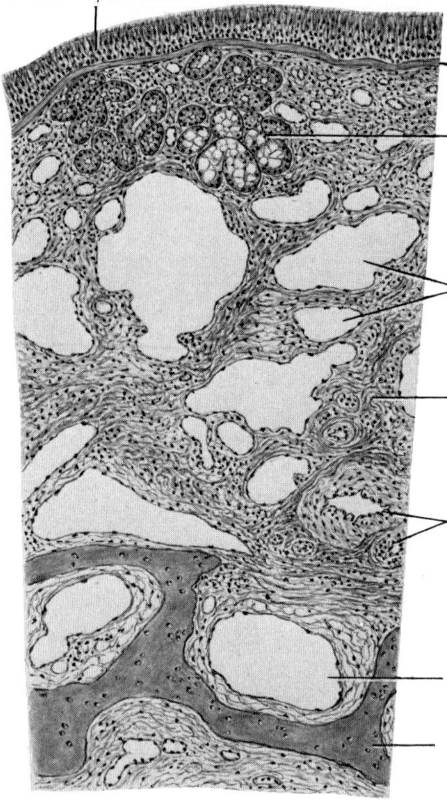

Ciliated pseudostratified
columnar epithelium

Basement membrane

Mixed serous and
mucous glands

Veins

Connective tissue

Arteries

Vein

Bone

Fig. 17-2. Section through the medial portion of an inferior nasal concha of a woman 47 years of age. Blood which filled the veins is not shown. ×67.

depressions in the epithelium and are lined by a continuous layer of goblet cells.

The *olfactory mucosa* occupies a small area in the upper part of the respiratory region. For details of the structure of the olfactory region, see chapter 22.

Experimental work shows that the nasal epithelium will change its character with increased ventilation. If all of the air is made to pass through one side of the nose by occluding the other nostril, the epithelium of the side subjected to the increased ventilation at first hypertrophies and then changes to a stratified squamous type (metaplasia).

The lamina propria contains numerous mucous and serous glands, particularly in the more exposed regions. Lymphocytes are usually present in both the epithelium and the lamina propria (Fig. 17-3).

The lamina propria of the nasal mucosa is quite vascular everywhere, but on the

medial surfaces of the middle and inferior conchae, and to a degree on the apposed surface of the septum, it is so vascular as to be distinctive. There are many large veins (Fig. 17-2) which may become engorged with surprising rapidity. With their engorgement, the mucosa becomes swollen and turgid, obstructing the flow of air through the nasal cavities, e.g., in allergic reactions.

The *paranasal sinuses*—maxillary, ethmoid, frontal, sphenoid—are lined by an epithelium which is continuous with that of the nasal passages. It is a pseudostratified columnar ciliated epithelium (Fig. 17-4), but is only about half as thick as that which lines the nose, having two or three rows of nuclei instead of four or five as in the nasal epithelium. Goblet cells and glands are also less numerous. In contrast with the nasal and tracheal epithelium, the basement membrane is very thin. The lam-

Ciliated pseudostratified columnar epithelium   Goblet cells

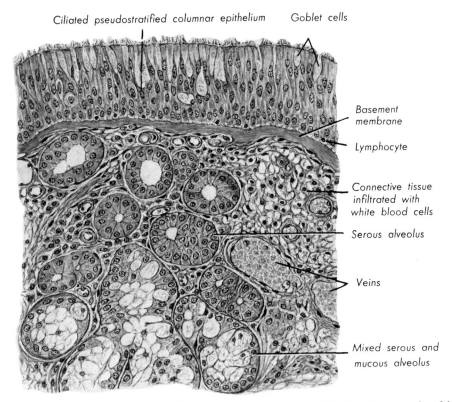

Basement
membrane

Lymphocyte

Connective tissue
infiltrated with
white blood cells

Serous alveolus

Veins

Mixed serous and
mucous alveolus

Fig. 17-3. Section through the epithelium and subjacent part of the lamina propria of inferior nasal concha. Human, 49 years old, with no history of nasal inflammation. ×286.

Lymphocyte

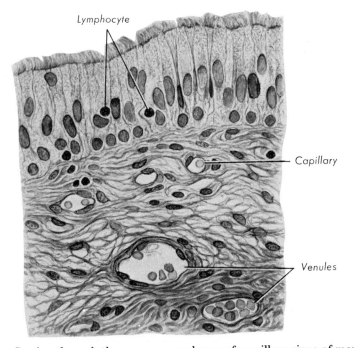

Capillary

Venules

Fig. 17-4. Section through the mucous membrane of maxillary sinus of man. ×665.

ina propria is thin and is attached to the periosteum.

Nasopharynx

In the *nasopharynx,* both stratified squamous and pseudostratified ciliated columnar epithelia are found. The distribution of these two types here and in the other respiratory passages is correlated with the attrition to which the surface is subjected. When surfaces are frequently brought in contact with each other, they are lined by stratified squamous epithelium. Those passages which usually remain open are lined by pseudostratified epithelium. Since, in the occlusion of the upper part of the naso- from the oropharynx, the soft palate and its appendage (the uvula) are brought in contact with the posterior wall of the nasopharynx, these surfaces are lined by stratified squamous epithelium. Other areas of the nasopharynx are lined by pseudostratified columnar epithelium.

In the deeper stratum of the subepithelial connective tissue of the posterior and lateral walls of the pharynx, there is a layer of elastic tissue whose fibers course largely in a longitudinal direction. It is closely applied to the subjacent muscle layer, into which it sends fibers. Near the juncture with the esophagus, the elastic layer disappears. In the superior lateral region, but not elsewhere in the pharynx, a submucosa which lies beneath the elastic stratum can be distinguished.

Glands are present throughout the nasopharynx. In the regions covered by stratified squamous epithelium, they are mucous and lie beneath the elastic layer. In the other areas, they are mixed serous and mucous, as in the other parts of the respiratory passages, and they lie more superficially.

Lymphatic tissue is especially abundant in the superior part of the nasopharynx. In addition to the general lymphatic infiltration of the connective tissue, there are, in the posterior wall, aggregations of lymph nodules known as the pharyngeal tonsils. Lymphatic aggregations also occur behind the openings of the Eustachian tubes, forming the tubal tonsils.

The *muscle* of the pharynx, which is striated, is deficient near the base of the skull. External to it there is a fibrosa.

Ciliary Action. The epithelium lining the paranasal sinuses, nasal passages and nasopharynx is coated with a mucous film. The cilia lie mostly underneath the mucous film. The viscosity of the mucous coat would greatly hinder the movement of cilia if it were to fill the interstices between them. In fact, the watery proteinaceous secretions of serous glands provide the medium that enables the cilia to remain motile. Since the cilia of the paranasal sinuses beat toward the openings of these cavities into the nose, and since the cilia on the epithelium lining the nose and nasopharynx beat toward the oropharynx, there is a continuous movement of this mucous coat toward the oropharynx. The surfaces are thus freed of particulate matter that has impinged on and adhered to the mucous covering. In the posterior three-fourths of the nose, the movement is more rapid than it is in the anterior part, which has led to the characterization of these two portions as active and inactive parts. The path of movement of the mucus is shown in Figure 17-1.

The Larynx

The wall of the larynx consists essentially of a mucosa, a poorly defined submucosa, a series of irregularly shaped cartilages connected by joints of fibroelastic membranes and a group of intrinsic skeletal muscles which act upon the cartilages.

Each lateral wall of the larynx has two prominent folds, between which is a deep recess or *ventricle.* The superior pairs of folds, the *ventricular folds,* are also known as the false vocal cords; the inferior pair, the *vocal folds,* are the true vocal cords. The *epiglottis* is a broad, flat structure projecting upward from the anterior wall of the larynx. During swallowing, there is active constriction of the pharyngeal wall, with a depression of the epiglottis and an upward movement of the larynx, trachea and pharynx. The latter movement plays an important role in closure of the glottis, preventing food from entering the larynx and trachea. The lidlike action of the epiglottis appears relatively unimportant, inasmuch as surgical removal of the tip of the epiglottis does not interfere with swallowing.

Two types of epithelium line the walls of the larynx, pseudostratified ciliated columnar and stratified squamous. These are distributed in accordance with the principle discussed in connection with the nasopharynx. At the juncture of these two types of epithelium, a third type—ciliated stratified columnar—is frequently present (Fig. 17-5). The wall of the aperture of the larynx, including the epiglottis down nearly as far as its tubercle or cushion, is lined by stratified squamous epithelium. This is succeeded by the ciliated pseudostratified type that lines the remainder of the laryngeal wall, except for the vocal folds, which have the stratified squamous variety.

The lamina propria is rich in elastic fibers. It is infiltrated with lymphocytes, and lymphatic nodules occur in the stroma of the ventricles. There is no sharp demarcation between the mucosa and the submucosa. The latter is structurally less dense and more cellular than the lamina propria. Over the vocal folds and epiglottis, the mucosa is more closely adherent to the underlying framework than it is in the other parts of the larynx. Mixed glands are present except in the vocal folds and are especially numerous in the ventricular folds (false vocal cords).

Most of the cartilages composing the framework of the larynx are hyaline. The epiglottic, the corniculate and the cuneiform cartilages are elastic, and this variety of cartilage is said also to occur inconstantly

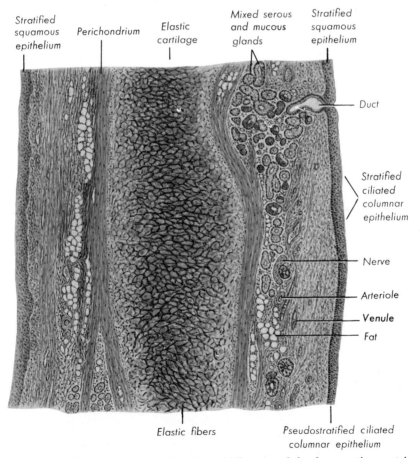

Fig. 17-5. Epiglottis of a boy 13 years old. The middle part of the free portion, cut in a sagittal plane is illustrated. The lingual surface is at *left*. Stained with elastin H, Delafield's hematoxylin and eosin. ×45.

in the apex and vocal process of each arytenoid cartilage. Calcification in the thyroid and cricoid cartilages begins in males during the second decade of life and at a somewhat later period in females.

The Trachea and Chief Bronchi

The layers composing the larynx continue, with certain modifications, into the trachea and bronchi. The chief changes are in the cartilaginous framework and musculature (Fig. 17-6).

The trachea and chief bronchi are lined by pseudostratified columnar ciliated epithelium which rests on a distinct basement membrane (Figs. 4-23, 17-7, 17-8 and 17-9). Several types of cells can be identified. The tall *ciliated columnar* cells are the most numerous. *Goblet cells* are fairly numerous and exhibit the characteristics already described in chapter 15 (Fig. 15-1). There are nonciliated columnar cells (brush cells) which have microvilli as seen under the electron microscope. It has been suggested that they represent an inactive stage of the goblet cell. There are a number of *short*

cells, more or less pyramidal in shape, which rest on the basal lamina but do not extend to the lumen as the other cell types do. The lamina propria contains many elastic fibers, which are especially numerous in the deeper zone of the lamina (membrana elastica interna). The submucosa consists of loose connective tissue and contains fat and mixed glands, the latter often penetrating into or even through the muscle layer (Fig. 17-6).

The framework of the trachea and chief bronchi consists of a series of regularly spaced, C-shaped hyaline cartilages. The open segment points posteriorly. The cartilages vary in width and thickness; their ends may bifurcate, and they may have bars that fuse with an adjoining cartilage. The lowest tracheal cartilage (carinal cartilage) especially varies in shape.

A fibroelastic membrane, which blends with the perichondrium of the cartilages, extends across their open segments and connects adjacent cartilages to each other, thus forming a tube. Posteriorly, in the cartilage-free zone, smooth muscle is imbedded in the fibroelastic membrane.

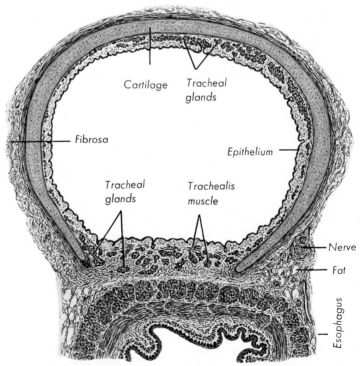

Fig. 17-6. Transverse section through midregion of trachea and adjacent part of esophagus. The section is through a cartilage ring. Woman, 35 years old. ×5.

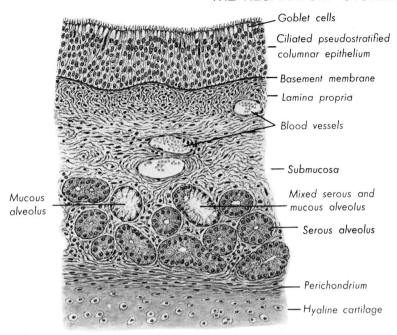

Fig. 17-7. Transverse section through anterior wall of trachea. Woman, 39 years old. ×165.

Most of these muscle fibers run transversely. Some, however, run longitudinally and obliquely. The transverse fibers attach largely to the inner surface of the ends of the cartilage rings and to a lesser extent to the intervening membrane. This is often called the "trachealis" muscle.

Localized areas of stratified squamous epithelium have been described in the trachea and bronchi of individuals suffering from chronic coughs. This change to a stratified squamous type of epithelium is possible because of the capacity of the pseudostratified epithelium of the respiratory passages to undergo metaplasia and to change to the more resistant type when subjected to attrition, as has been pointed out in the description of the nasopharynx.

The Lungs

The lungs are paired structures which, together with the mediastinum, fill the thoracic cavity. On the right side, the lung is divided by two deep clefts into three lobes; on the left side, it is divided by a single deep cleft into two lobes. Entering the hilus, and forming the root of each lung, are a bronchus, a pulmonary artery and vein, bronchial arteries and veins, lymphatics and nerves. These structures are embedded in connective tissue.

The surface of the lungs is covered by a serous membrane, the visceral pleura, which dips into the interlobar fissures and covers the interlobar surfaces. At the hilus, the visceral pleura becomes continuous with the parietal pleura.

The surface of the lungs is pinkish in early life but later becomes grayish in color as a result of the inspired particulate matter which is in the pulmonary tissue. On the surface of the lungs, small, irregularly shaped areas (1 to 2 cm) are delineated by dark lines. Each of these areas is the base of a lobule (Fig. 17-10), the apex of which points toward the hilus of the lung. The dark lines are due to deposits of inspired particulate matter in the delicate interlobular connective tissue. Each of these units is designated a *secondary lobule,* to distinguish it from smaller *primary lobules.* Each of the latter is made up of a respiratory bronchiole and its branches.

Plan of the Lungs

A main bronchus, the primary division from the trachea, enters the root of each lung. There it divides, one secondary bron-

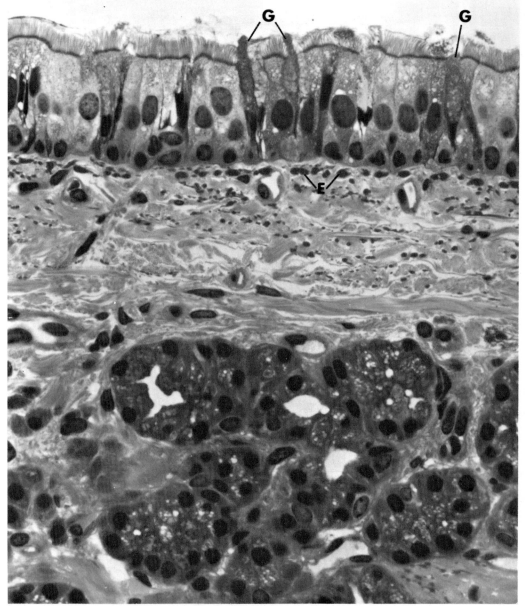

Fig. 17-8. Light micrograph of transverse section through mucosa and submucosa of monkey trachea. The pseudostratified epithelium with cilia and goblet cells (*G*) is underlain by a basement membrane, elastic fibers (*E*) and bundles of collagen. A mixed gland lies in the submucosa at the bottom of the field. ×610.

chus going to each lobe. Thus there are three branches to the right and two to the left lung. Each lobar (secondary) bronchus divides, the number of branches varying from two to five in the different lobes. Each of these bronchi supplies a portion of a lobe known as a *segment* or bronchopulmonary segment. There are 10 segments in the right lung and eight in the left lung. These segments are of considerable importance from a surgical standpoint. The segmental bronchi divide a number of times within the lung, with a progressive reduction in diameter and a gradual decrease in cartilage (Fig. 17-11). When the tubes reach a caliber of about 1 mm, the cartilage disappears

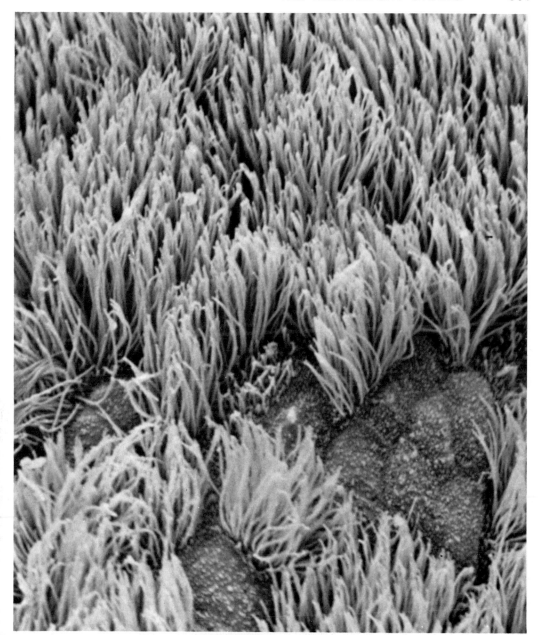

Fig. 17-9. Scanning electron micrograph of lumenal surface of human tracheal epithelium. Most of the surface cells are ciliated. Nonciliated cells with short microvilli presumably represent goblet cells. ×4500. (Courtesy of Drs. A. Zaitsu and M. Miyoshi.)

completely and the tubes are known as *bronchioles*. The bronchioles continue to divide and, when their branches have been reduced to a caliber of about 0.5 mm (or less), they become devoid of glands and goblet cells and are known as *terminal bronchioles* (Figs. 17-12, 17-13 and 17-14).

There are a number of terminal bronchioles within a secondary lung lobule. The terminal bronchioles, as their name implies, are the terminal segments of the purely conducting division of the respiratory system. Each of them terminates by branching into two or more *respiratory bronchioles* (Figs.

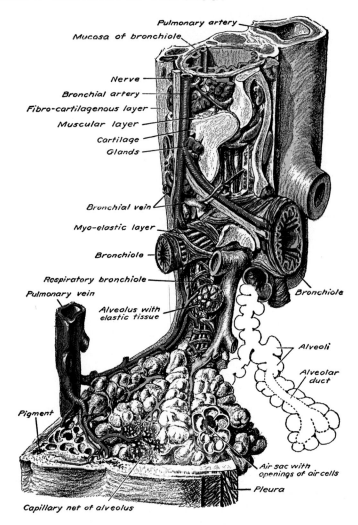

Fig. 17-10. A portion of a lung lobule. (After Braus, from a reconstruction by A. Vierling.)

17-12, 17-13 and 17-14). As noted earlier, each respiratory bronchiole and its subsidiary divisions make up a functional unit known as the *primary lobule*. Each respiratory bronchiole undergoes further divisions into *alveolar ducts* (ductuli alveolares). These in turn may further branch, terminating after a relatively long course in *alveolar sacs* (sacculi alveolares, air sacs). The smallest units or subdivisions are the *pulmonary alveoli* (air cells), small outpocketings that form the lining of the alveolar ducts and alveolar sacs and in whose walls the interchange of gases between air and blood takes place.

Pulmonary alveoli are confined to the respiratory division of the lung. They first appear, in the branching system outlined above, in the respiratory bronchioles, which have characteristics of both the conducting and respiratory divisions. The alveolar ducts and alveolar sacs have continuous pulmonary alveoli forming their walls. The pulmonary alveoli of one system interdigitate with those of neighboring systems, so that two adjacent alveoli have a common capillary bed, an arrangement which gives a maximal surface area for the exchange of gases.

Changes in the Lungs during Respiration

An understanding of the changes that occur during respiration gives a better ap-

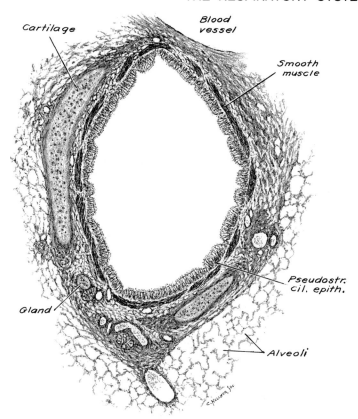

Fig. 17-11. Section through a bronchus approximately 2 mm in diameter.

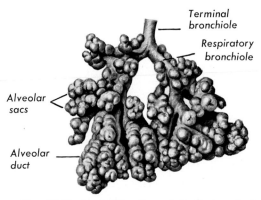

Fig. 17-12. Cast (Wood's metal) of a terminal bronchiole and its branches. (Braus, after Loeschcke.)

preciation of the distribution of elastic tissue, smooth muscle and cartilage within different parts of the respiratory system. Since the existence of a negative (subatmospheric) pressure within the pleural cavities is an important factor in respiration, it is one of the first items to consider. It should be noted that the lungs fill the pleural cavities in early embryos and that a negative pressure is not present at first. However, as the pleural cavities enlarge and as elastic tissue and smooth muscle develop within each lung, tending to contract each toward its hilus, a negative intrathoracic pressure develops. This exerts an expanding or stretching action on the lungs. The presence of an elastic recoil mechanism is clearly demonstrated by the fact that the lung collapses and retracts toward its hilus when air is allowed to enter the pleural cavity through a hole in the chest wall, producing *pneumothorax,* and when fluid increases in the cavity, producing *hydrothorax.* The retraction of the lung tissue is brought about by the recoil of the stretched elastic tissue and by contraction of the spirally arranged smooth muscle fibers in the walls of the conducting divisions and parts of the respiratory divisions of the lungs.

In respiration, the volume of the lung changes in correlation with changes in intrathoracic pressure, and the latter in turn varies in association with changes in intra-

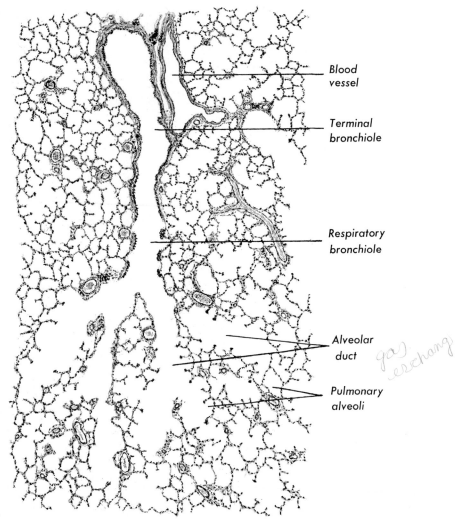

Blood vessel

Terminal bronchiole

Respiratory bronchiole

Alveolar duct

gas exchange

Pulmonary alveoli

Fig. 17-13. Section through a terminal bronchiole, together with part of the system arising from it. Camera lucida drawing. Human lung. ×19.

thoracic volume. In inspiration, the volume of the thoracic cavity is increased by muscular movements which elevate the ribs to increase the cross sectional area of the thoracic cavity and by contraction of the diaphragm to increase the cephalocaudal dimension. This increases the negative pressure, and the lungs expand. In expiration, the elastic forces of the lungs are usually sufficient to expel the air and allow the chest to return passively from its expanded state in a person at rest. Muscular movements play a greater part in expiration during strenuous exercise, when there is an increase in rate and amplitude of respiration.

We can now outline some of the ways in which the microscopic structures of the several parts of the conducting and respiratory divisions of the lungs are adapted to perform particular functions. The presence of hyaline cartilage in the form of separate plates in the walls of the bronchi (Fig. 17-11) gives strength to these divisions without hindering changes in their length and diameter. The presence of smooth muscle, coursing in a spiral direction around the bronchi and bronchioles and onto the alveolar ducts, provides for reducing the length and breadth of these passages by muscular contraction. Elastic tissue is present in the form of a dense feltwork of lon-

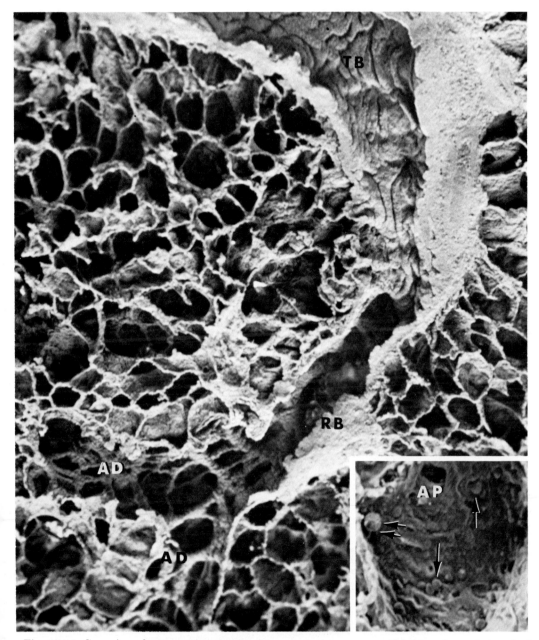

Fig. 17-14. Scanning electron micrograph of terminal air passages of human lung. A terminal bronchiole (*TB*) opens into a respiratory bronchiole (*RB*) which in turn opens into two alveolar ducts (*AD*). The inset shows the internal surface of a pulmonary alveolus with an alveolar pore (*AP*) and protruding type II alveolar cells (*arrows*). The larger cell at the double arrow probably represents a dust cell. ×120. Inset, ×550. (Courtesy of Drs. A. Zaitsu and M. Miyoshi.)

gitudinally oriented fibers in the lamina propria of the conducting divisions and as a network around all of the respiratory divisions. This permits expansion of lung tissue when the negative intrathoracic pres-

sure is increased during inspiration. The elastic recoil plays an important part in the contraction of the lung tissue during expiration. The epithelium lining the conducting and respiratory divisions shows particularly important functional adaptations. These can best be considered in connection with a more detailed description of structure.

Structure of the Lungs

The Conducting Division. Modifications in the structure of the bronchi appear with the first branching in the root of the lungs and continue to take place with each subsequent branching. A comparison of a terminal segment (terminal bronchiole) with a main bronchus reveals how great these changes have been. The series of changes, however, is gradual, and therefore our discussion focuses on the nature of the modifications that occur, rather than describing bronchi of different diameters.

The epithelium, although continuing as a pseudostratified columnar type through most of the conducting division, nevertheless decreases in height as the tubes become progressively smaller. In the terminal bronchiole, it becomes a single layer of columnar or cuboidal cells which, however, still bear cilia (Fig. 17-15). Both goblet cells and glands (seromucous) become fewer, and both cease to be present before the terminal bronchioles are reached.

The lamina propria also decreases in thickness as the conducting divisions decrease in caliber, and elastic fibers become relatively more numerous. The elastic fibers form a feltwork, with the majority of them coursing in a longitudinal direction. Smooth muscle increases in relative amounts along the conducting divisions and is arranged in bundles that follow a spiral course around the bronchi, interior to the cartilage plates (Fig. 17-11). This contrasts with the trachea, in which the smooth muscle is found primarily in the posterior wall, in the region between the ends of the C-shaped cartilages. The smooth muscle is relatively most abundant in the terminal bronchioles, where it forms a prominent component of the wall (Fig. 17-15).

The outer layer of the bronchi and bronchioles also shows pronounced changes. With the first branching of the primary bronchi, the cartilage ceases to occur as C-shaped rings and becomes distributed in irregularly shaped plates. As the bronchi continue to branch and decrease in diameter, the cartilaginous plates are replaced by islands of cartilage (insulae cartilagineae). As noted earlier, cartilage disappears completely when the bronchioles are reached, at a diameter of about 1 mm. The mucosa of the bronchioles usually has longitudinal folds as a result of the absence of cartilage and the proportional increase in muscle and elastic tissue.

Terminal bronchioles (0.5 mm or less in caliber) are lined by simple columnar or cuboidal cells, both ciliated and nonciliated. There are no goblet cells or glands. Elastic tissue and smooth muscle are closely associated, and the amount of muscle in proportion to the diameter of the tubule is proportionally higher than in the other divisions of the system.

It is significant that the cilia extend far-

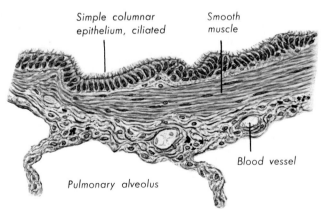

Fig. 17-15. Transverse section through a portion of the wall of a terminal bronchiole and adjacent pulmonary alveoli. Human lung. ×320.

ther down the tubes than do the mucous secreting elements. If the reverse were the case, accumulations of mucus might occlude the tubules.

The Respiratory Division. Each terminal bronchiole divides into two or more respiratory bronchioles (Fig. 17-12) which may further branch so that respiratory bronchioles of the first (I) and second (II) order are formed. The *respiratory bronchioles* bear pulmonary alveoli on those portions of their walls which are not in contact with the accompanying pulmonary artery. The alveoli are few in number proximally but become more numerous distally. Between the alveoli, the wall of the respiratory bronchiole is lined by cuboidal epithelium; cilia are present in the proximal part but not distally. The nonciliated cells are secretory in appearance and have been referred to as Clara cells or bronchiolar epithelial cells. Smooth muscle and elastic fibers are well developed in the respiratory bronchiole, although they do not form as thick a layer as in the terminal bronchiole.

Collagenous and reticular fibers are also present. The smooth muscle bundles and the elastic fibers course obliquely, i.e., in a spiral direction, but they branch and anastomose, thus forming a loose elastic and contractile network. In sections through the opening of an alveolus into a respiratory bronchiole, the muscle fibers are seen to be cut obliquely or transversely. The walls of the alveolar ducts are formed by pulmonary sacs and alveoli without intervening patches of cuboidal epithelium. Small smooth muscle bundles which branch and anastomose are present. They are concentrated around the openings of the alveoli so that, in a transverse section through an alveolar duct, the muscle bundles mark the circular extent of the lumen (Fig. 17-16). Reticular, elastic and delicate collagenous fibers are also present (Figs. 17-17 and 17-18). The alveolar ducts terminate in a variable number of alveolar sacs.

The *alveolar sacs* are thin-walled structures which are closely studded with pulmonary alveoli. The walls of the alveolar

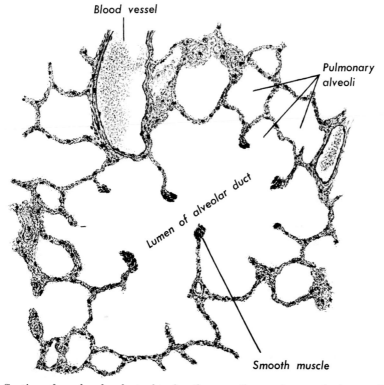

Fig. 17-16. Section of an alveolar duct, showing the smooth muscle near the lumen. Human lung. ×78.

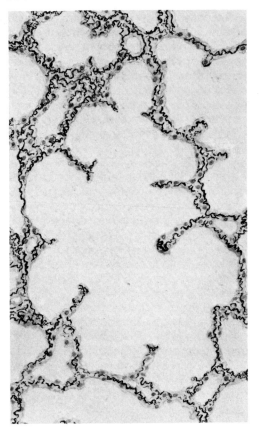

Fig. 17-17. Section through an alveolar duct, showing the reticular fibers (*black*). Lung of rhesus monkey. Foot-Hortega silver carbonate method and Orth's carmine. ×240.

sacs contain little smooth muscle but have elastic and reticular fibers. Some authorities do not distinguish alveolar sacs, as their walls cannot be distinguished from those of the pulmonary alveoli.

The Pulmonary Alveoli. Pulmonary alveoli (air cells) are cup-shaped structures through whose thin walls the interchange of gas between the blood and air takes place. The open end or mouth of each alveolus opens into the lumen of a respiratory bronchiole, an alveolar duct or an alveolar sac (Figs. 17-10 and 17-13). Because of the interdigitating arrangement of the alveoli, a single wall, or *interalveolar septum,* is usually formed between adjacent alveoli (Figs. 17-16 and 17-18).

An *interalveolar septum* is composed of the lining cells of adjacent alveoli and the structures interposed between the alveoli.

Capillaries occupy a major portion of the septum, and they are shared by the lining cells of the adjacent alveoli (Figs. 17-19 and 17-21). It should be noted that the capillaries have wide lumina and that they anastomose so freely that the total area of the vascular network exceeds that of the intervening spaces (Fig. 17-20). The meshes of the capillary network contain reticular and elastic fibers arranged in a manner to permit expansion and contraction of the alveolar wall. The intercapillary spaces also contain a few fibroblasts, some wandering leukocytes, histiocytes and occasional smooth muscle cells (Fig. 17-19).

The interalveolar septa are interrupted in places where adjacent alveoli not only make contact but open to each other to form *alveolar pores* (Figs. 17-14 and 17-19). The pores are about 10 to 15 μm in diameter in the expanded lung. In certain pathological conditions, they become more prominent and contain strands of fibrin extending from one alveolus to another. With regard to their functional significance, it has been suggested that, by providing intercommunication, they prevent the overdistention of some alveoli and the collapse of others when small bronchioles of a functional unit are occluded.

The alveolar lining cells have been studied extensively. Prior to the advent of electron microscopy, there was considerable controversy as to whether the alveoli were completely lined by epithelium. It was known from light microscope studies that the entire pulmonary system is lined by epithelium in early stages of fetal development, but this was questionable as applied to late fetal life and postnatal life when the walls of the alveoli thinned out. The problem was clarified by electron microscope studies which showed that the alveoli are completely lined by epithelium but that the cells have regions which are so attenuated that they lie at the limits of resolution provided by the light microscope.

The alveolar lining consists of *type I alveolar cells* (small alveolar cells) and *type II alveolar cells* (great alveolar cells).

The *type I alveolar cells* have low or flat nuclei, much like those of the cells of mesothelium. The cytoplasm becomes very thin or attenuated beyond the perinuclear

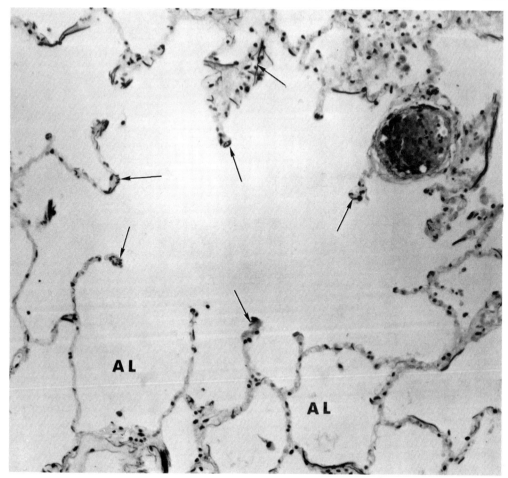

Fig. 17-18. Light micrograph of an alveolar duct. Elastic fibers (*black*) are obvious in alveolar septa, especially in the expanded terminations (*arrows*). Red blood cells are also stained black. AL, pulmonary alveoli. Human lung, Verhoeffs stain. ×195.

region (Figs. 17-19 and 17-21). The squamous cells have junctional attachments laterally with each other and with the type II alveolar cells.

The *type II alveolar cells* have an irregular, cuboidal shape. They are fairly numerous, they are taller than the squamous cells (Fig. 17-14, inset), and can be seen more readily with the electron microscope. They have characteristic cytoplasmic structures which look like vacuoles under the light microscope (Fig. 17-22), but which are seen in electron micrographs as osmiophilic bodies with internal concentric lamellae. These bodies, which are 0.2 to 1.0 μm in diameter, are known as *cytosomes*. They are periodic acid-Schiff-positive, and they also stain with Sudan black. Although it

has been suggested that the cytosomes arise from mitochondria, transitional forms between multivesicular bodies and cytosomes have been reported. The cytosomal contents are ultimately secreted onto the alveolar surface, and it is this material that is believed to form the pulmonary surfactant that coats alveolar cells and lowers surface tension. Early investigations provided some confusion between bronchiolar Clara cells and type II alveolar cells, but more recent studies indicate that the two cell types are probably unrelated. There is no evidence that Clara cells form surfactant. Infants born prematurely may fail to produce adequate surfactant material and exhibit respiratory distress syndrome. These individuals do not have normally

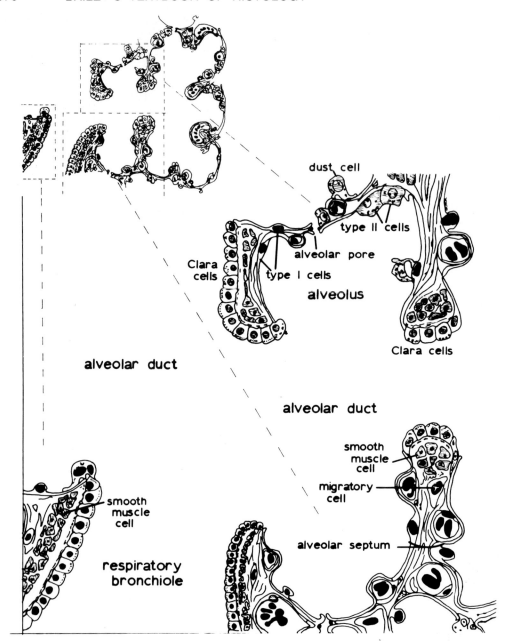

Fig. 17-19. Diagram showing relationships of components of terminal air passages.

developed type II alveolar cells but have normal appearing Clara cells.

The *alveolar membrane* may be defined as the barrier through which gases must pass in exchange between air and blood. This membrane consists of the *type I alveolar cell* together with its underlying *basal lamina* and the *capillary endothelial cell* with its *basal lamina*. The basal laminae

of epithelium and endothelium are fused in some areas and are separated in many other areas only by a few elastic or reticular fibers. The endothelium of the capillaries is relatively thin, is not fenestrated, but has numerous caveolae. Besides the exchange of gases, the capillary bed of the lungs is involved in the metabolism of certain vasoactive substances, such as angiotensin and

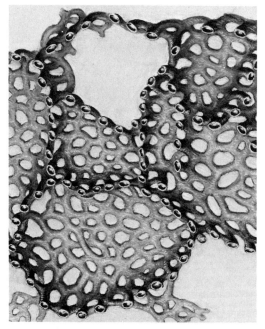

Fig. 17-20. Injected lung, showing capillaries in walls of pulmonary alveoli. Dog. Preparation by Mr. Kellner. ×400.

prostaglandins. There is evidence suggesting that activation of angiotensin by peptidase activity may occur in association with the caveolae of the endothelial cells.

Alveolar macrophages or *dust cells* are found within the alveolar wall and also in the alveoli resting on the alveolar surface. They are highly phagocytic cells and received the name dust cells because they remove inspired particles that reach the alveoli. In clinical disorders in which the pulmonary vessels become congested with blood, the macrophages ingest some of the erythrocytes and become filled with brownish granules of hemosiderin.

Dust cells may arise from several sources. They may develop from mononuclear leukocytes which migrate into the alveolar lining, or they may arise from connective tissue cells of the septa. Earlier studies suggesting that they are also related to the type II alveolar cells have not been substantiated by more recent work.

Inspired Particulate Matter

Many particles of dust are present in the air which is inspired, and the number of particles is greatly increased in smoky regions and in industries or regions in which the air is laden with dust. Many of the inspired particles are removed by their adherence to the vibrissae in the nasal vestibule and by lodging on the mucous film of the respiratory portion of the nose, nasopharynx, larynx and trachea. The mucous film and adherent particles are constantly being moved by ciliary action to the oropharynx, from which they are either expectorated or swallowed. The upper portion of the respiratory tract thus serves not only to humidify and warm the air but also to remove particulate matter.

The bronchi and bronchioles in the lung also play a very important role in the removal of particulate matter. As repeated branchings take place, with only a slight increase in cross section area (volume), the surface of the walls is greatly increased. Because of the increased area, particles would be more likely to impinge on the mucous coat than in the upper, larger passages. For this lower part of the conducting system, Hilding has proposed the name "bronchiolar filter." As in the trachea and nasal passages, ciliary action carries the particles lodged on the mucous film to the oropharynx.

Many of the smaller particles, however, reach the alveoli of the lungs, and their removal by ciliary action is not possible. A different mechanism operates to dispose of them. The particles are removed by alveolar macrophages or dust cells.

The dust cells phagocytize the particles on the alveolar walls and deposit them, perhaps after passage through several cells, in the connective tissue of the lungs or in the lymphatic tissue. In this transport of the particles, the lymph vessels play an important role. The connective tissue may increase greatly in amount (fibrosis) and may encapsulate masses of the particles. The degree of connective tissue overgrowth is influenced by the type of the inhaled dust. Siliceous dust and asbestos, for instance, cause a marked fibrosis, whereas coal dust, even when present in large amounts, induces a very slight reaction, or none at all, of the connective tissue. The condition which results from the dust is termed pneumoconiosis, special names (an-

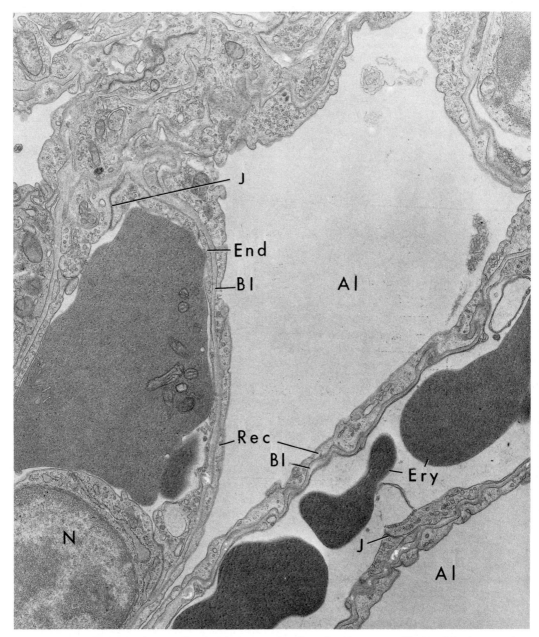

Fig. 17-21. Electron micrograph of pulmonary alveoli and adjacent capillaries. The lumen of an alveolus (*Al*) is separated from the lumen of the capillaries by a thin layer of tissue composed of: 1) small alveolar cells (*Rec*) that line the alveolus; 2) a basal lamina (or laminae, *Bl*); and 3) endothelial cells (*End*) that line the capillaries. The basal lamina of the endothelium appears to be fused with that of the squamous respiratory cells along a considerable portion of the interalveolar septum. The respiratory cells are very attenuated in regions where they are apposed to the endothelial cells, but they form a continuous layer. Likewise, the endothelial cell is attenuated except in the region around the nucleus (*N*). *Ery,* erythrocytes in the capillaries; *J,* intercellular junctions of endothelial cells. From the lung of a mouse. ×16,000. (Courtesy of Drs. K. R. Porter and M. A. Bonneville.)

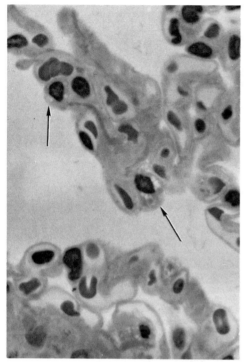

Fig. 17-22. Light micrograph of monkey lung showing vacuolated type II alveolar cells (*arrows*). The thinness of the wall between alveolar space and capillary lumina is well shown. There are no obvious cell bodies of type I alveolar cells in this field. ×765.

thracosis, silicosis, asbestosis, etc.) being used to designate the reactions to the various types of dust.

The Pleura

The pleura is a mesothelial serous membrane which completely lines the pleural cavity. The visceral portion invests and is closely adherent to the lungs. It is continuous with the parietal pleura at the root of the lungs. Beneath the mesothelial lining of the pleura is a fibroelastic connective tissue which contains smooth muscle. In the connective tissue are blood capillaries and a rich plexus of lymph vessels.

Continuous with the connective tissue of the pleura are delicate septa that extend between the lobules, anastomosing with each other and with the peribronchial connective tissue. The septa are composed of fibrous and elastic connective tissue, and

they contain smooth muscle, lymph and blood vessels and macrophages.

The Blood and Lymph Circulation of the Lungs

Blood Vessels. The lungs receive blood from two sources: venous blood, to be purified, through the *pulmonary arteries,* and arterial blood, for the nutrition of the walls of the conducting system and blood vessels, through the *bronchial arteries.* This blood is returned to the systemic circulation through the pulmonary and bronchial veins. The former, in contrast with the latter, are devoid of valves.

The pulmonary artery enters the lung with the corresponding chief bronchus. It branches with and follows the bronchial tree to the termination of the respiratory bronchioles. As the alveolar duct is reached, the artery gives rise to the capillary plexus in the walls of the alveoli (Figs. 17-20 and 17-23). Veins arise from these capillaries. They do not immediately join the bronchioles but course in the septa. Later they join the bronchioles and course along them to the root of the lung.

The bronchial arteries likewise accompany the bronchi. Along their course they give origin to capillaries which supply the walls of the bronchi, arteries, veins and the peribronchial and septal connective tissue. The bronchial arteries do not extend beyond the respiratory bronchioles. The capillaries arising from them in that segment anastomose with the pulmonary capillary plexus. Part of the blood carried by the bronchial arteries passes into the pulmonary veins through this anastomosis. The remainder returns through the bronchial veins.

The pleura, in man, is supplied by the bronchial arteries. This blood returns through the pulmonary veins.

Lymphatics. There are two sets of lymphatic vessels in the lung: a superficial set in the pleura and a deep set in the substance of the lung. The superficial (pleural) lymph vessels are particularly numerous near the juncture of the interlobular septa with the pleura, and thus they outline the lobules (Figs. 17-23 and 17-24). There are numerous anastomoses between the vessels of the su-

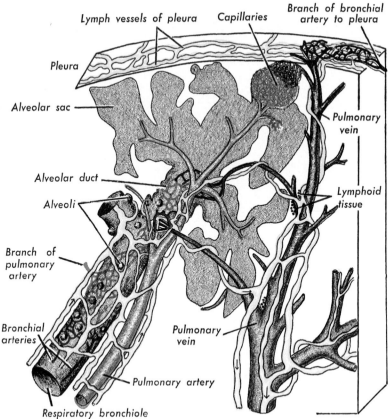

Fig. 17-23. The blood supply and lymph drainage of a portion of a lung lobule and the pleura. (From Miller, The Lung. Charles C Thomas.)

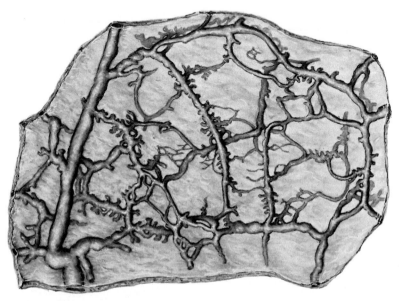

Fig. 17-24. Lymphatics of pleura; the area outlined by the large (peripheral) vessel is the base of a lung lobule. ×8. (Miller.)

perficial and deep plexuses at the surface of the lung. These serve as afferents to the superficial vessels; numerous valves in the latter prevent the backflow of lymph. The efferents of the superficial plexus course first in the pleura and then in the connective tissue along the larger bronchi to the root of the lung.

The vessels of the deep plexus are found chiefly in the following locations: around the bronchi and bronchioles, around the branches of the pulmonary artery and in the interlobular connective tissue associated with the branches of the pulmonary veins. There are no lymphatics in the interalveolar septa; they begin in the connective tissue around the respiratory bronchioles and blood vessels. Although some of the lymph from the deep plexus enters the superficial vessels by channels of anastomosis over the lung surface, a considerable portion of the lymph of the deep plexus is carried by larger vessels which follow the bronchi and blood vessels to the hilus, where the main vessels of the two sets of lymphatics join. There are no valves in the deep lymphatics, except in a few of the larger trunks.

Lymphatic tissue in the form of lymph nodes or solitary nodules with germinal centers occurs along the larger bronchial branches. The amount of lymphatic tissue is said to increase with age. It becomes infiltrated with the inspired particulate matter. There is also a lymphocytic infiltration of the walls of the bronchi.

Nerves. The bronchi are accompanied by sympathetic and parasympathetic nerves. The latter come from the vagus. Ganglion cells are present in the walls of the bronchi. The vagus fibers cause constriction of the air tubes; the sympathetic fibers cause dilation.

Development of the Respiratory System

The epithelium of the respiratory system develops from entoderm. The rudiment of the larynx, trachea and lungs appears as a ventral, groove-like evagination in the floor of the primitive pharynx. This evagination grows caudally and becomes cut off by constriction from the digestive tube except in its superior part, and its apex bifurcates. The portion which does not bifurcate, together with the surrounding mesenchyme, forms the larynx and trachea. The bifurcated part is the anlage of the epithelium and epithelial derivatives of the bronchial system and lungs, the mesenchyme forming the other portions of the walls. The right branch subdivides into three branches corresponding to the three lobes of the future right lung, and the left divides into two branches corresponding to two lobes of the left lung. By repeated branching of these tubules, the entire bronchial system of the lungs is formed. This process is similar to the development of a compound gland. The last to develop are the respiratory bronchioles and the alveolar ducts and sacs, structures that are characteristic of the lung. During fetal life, the alveoli are lined by a cuboidal epithelium. At the time of birth, these cells become extremely thin, so thin in fact that filmlike peripheral portions of the cells are masked by the underlying denser tissue.

Following birth, as well as during gestation, there is a continued growth of the lung. The bronchioles increase in length, and new respiratory units are formed. The increase in the length of the bronchioles, while to a small degree caused by an interstitial growth of the existing bronchioles, is mainly due to the transformation of the repiratory bronchioles, alveolar ducts and alveolar sacs into bronchioles. The lengthening of the respiratory division takes place by a terminal budding and growth of the air sacs. Their growth is thus much like that which occurs in a tree.

References

ADAMS, F. H. Fetal and neonatal cardiovascular and pulmonary function. Annu. Rev. Physiol. 27:257–284, 1965.

AVERY, M. E. The alveolar lining layer. A review of studies of its role in pulmonary mechanisms and in pathogenesis of atelectasis. Pediatrics 30:324–330, 1962.

BERTALANFFY, F. D., AND LEBLOND, C. P. The continuous renewal of the two types of alveolar cells in the lung of the rat. Anat. Rec. 115:515–542, 1953.

BOYDEN, E. A. Segmental Anatomy of the Lungs. A study of the patterns of the segmental bronchi and related pulmonary vessels. The Blakiston Division, McGraw-Hill Book Company, New York, 1955.

BOYDEN, E. A., AND TOMPSETT, D. H. The changing

patterns in the developing lungs of infants. Acta Anat. 61:164–192, 1965.

DEREUCK, A. V. S., AND M. O'CONNOR (editors) Ciba Foundation Symposium on Pulmonary Structure and Function. Little, Brown and Company, Boston, 1961.

ELEFTMAN, A. G. The afferent and parasympathetic innervation of the lungs and trachea of the dog. Am. J. Anat. 72:1–27, 1943.

ENGEL, S. Lung Structure. Charles C Thomas, Publisher, Springfield, Ill., 1962.

HAYEK, H. VON (translated by V. E. Krahl) The Human Lung. Hafner Publishing Company, New York, 1960.

HILDING, A. C. The physiology of drainage of nasal mucus. Arch. Otolaryngol. 15:92–100; 16:9–17, 1932.

HILDING, A. C., AND HILDING, D. The volume of the bronchial tree at various levels and its possible physiological significance. Ann. Otol. 57:324–342, 1948.

JACKSON, C. L., AND HUBER, J. F. Correlated applied anatomy of the bronchial tree and lungs with a system of nomenclature. Dis. Chest 9:319–326, 1943.

KING, R. J. The surfactant system of the lung. Fed. Proc. 33:2238–2247, 1974.

KRAHL, V. E. Anatomy of the mammalian lung. In American Physiological Society Handbook of Physiology. Section 3, vol. 1, p. 213. American Physiological Society, Washington, D.C., 1964.

LARSEL, O., AND DOW, R. S. The innervation of the human lung. Am. J. Anat. 52:125–146, 1933.

LATTA, J. S., AND SCHALL, R. F. The histology of the epithelium of the paranasal sinuses under various conditions. Ann. Otol. 43:945–972, 1934.

LOOSLI, C. G. Interalveolar communications in normal and pathological mammalian lungs. Arch. Path.

(Chicago) 24:743–776, 1937. See also: Am. J. Anat. 62:375–425, 1938.

LOW, F. N. The pulmonary alveolar epithelium of laboratory mammals and man. Anat. Rec. 117:241–264, 1953.

LOW, F. N. The extracellular portion of the blood-air barrier and its relation to tissue space. Anat. Rec. 139:105–123, 1961.

MACKLIN, C. C. The musculature of the bronchi and lungs. Physiol. Rev. 9:1–60, 1929.

MACKLIN, C. C. Alveolar pores and their significance in the human lung. Arch. Pathol. 21:202–216, 1935.

MILLER, W. S. The Lung. Charles C Thomas, Publisher, Springfield, Ill., 1947.

PRATT, S. A., FINLEY, T. N., SMITH, M. H., AND LADMAN, A. J. A comparison of alveolar macrophages and pulmonary surfactant (?) obtained from the lungs of human smokers and nonsmokers by endobronchial lavage. Anat. Rec. 163:497–508, 1969.

ROBERTSON, O. H. Phagocytosis of foreign material in the lung. Physiol. Rev. 21:112–139, 1941.

SAID, S. The lung in relation to vasoactive hormones. Fed. Proc. 32:1972–1976, 1973.

SMITH, U., AND RYAN, J. Electron microscopy of endothelial and epithelial components of the lungs: correlations of structure and function. Fed. Proc. 32:1957–1966, 1973.

SOROKIN, S. P. A morphologic and cytochemical study of the great alveolar cell. J. Histochem. Cytochem. 14:884–897, 1966.

TOBIN, C. E. Lymphatics of the pulmonary alveoli. Anat. Rec. 120:625–636, 1954.

WEIBEL, E. R. Morphogenetics of the lung. In American Physiological Society Handbook of Physiology. American Physiological Society, Washington, D.C., 1964.

CHAPTER 18

The Urinary System

The Kidney

The kidney is a compound tubular gland which separates urea and other nitrogenous waste products from the blood. It also maintains the constituents of blood plasma at proper levels, and, in so doing, it has an important role in regulating the chemical composition of the extracellular fluid which bathes the cells and tissues of the body. It is enclosed by a firm connective tissue capsule composed of collagenous fibers and a few elastic fibers. In many of the lower animals and in the human fetus, septa extend from the capsule into the gland dividing it into a number of lobes. In human adults, the lobated character is obliterated by the great reduction of the interstitial connective tissue and the apparent blending of the peripheral parts of the different lobes. Rarely, the fetal divisions persist in adult life, such a kidney being known as a "lobated kidney." In some animals, such as the guinea pig and rabbit, the entire kidney consists of a single lobe.

On the mesially directed border of the kidney is a depression known as the *hilus*. This serves as the point of entrance for the *renal artery* and of exit for the *renal vein* and *ureter*.

On section, the kidney is seen to consist of *cortex* and *medulla* partially surrounding a cavity—the *renal sinus*—which opens at the hilus (Fig. 18-1). The renal sinus contains: (1) the upper, expanded portion of the ureter which is known as the *renal pelvis*, (2) subdivisions of the pelvis that form two or three *major calyces* and about eight *minor calyces*, (3) branches of the renal arteries, veins and nerves, and (4) loose connective tissue and fat. In fresh, unfixed kidneys, the outer or cortical zone of the kidney is dark brown in color and granular in appearance. It contains many convoluted tubules and numerous round, reddish bodies, the *renal* or *Malpighian corpuscles*, which are barely visible to the unaided eye. The inner, medullary zone of the kidney is radially striated in appearance because its tubular and vascular elements run in parallel radial lines.

The cortex not only forms the outer zone of the kidney but, at intervals, plugs of cortical tissue, the *columns of Bertini* or *renal columns*, penetrate the whole depth of the medulla. The main medullary mass consists of 8 to 18 *medullary* or *Malpighian pyramids*, the number corresponding to the number of lobes in the fetal kidney. The broad base of each pyramid is in contact with the cortex, and the rounded apex projects into a minor calyx (Fig. 18-1). As a rule, two or sometimes three pyramids unite to form a single *papilla*; hence, the number of papillae is less than that of the pyramids. The tip of the papillary surface presents a sieve-like appearance, *area cribrosa*, as a result of the presence of 10 to 25 pores or *foramina papillaria*, which are the openings of the uriniferous ducts. Even

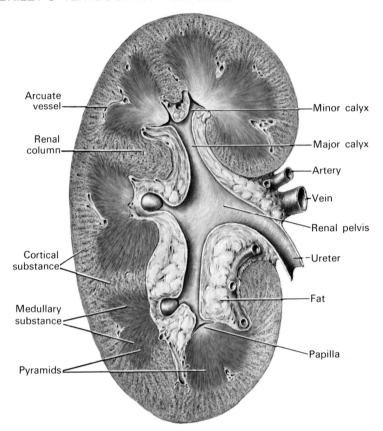

Arcuate vessel

Renal column

Cortical substance

Medullary substance

Pyramids

Minor calyx

Major calyx

Artery

Vein

Renal pelvis

Ureter

Fat

Papilla

Fig. 18-1. Longitudinal section of a human kidney. Natural size.

in gross preparations, two zones may be distinguished in the medulla: an outer, more deeply colored zone in contact with the cortex, and an inner, somewhat paler papillary zone.

The cortical region is subdivided into many radiating, slender columns composed of straight tubules alternating with regions containing glomeruli and convoluted tubules (Figs. 18-2 and 18-3). The columns of straight tubules radiate outward from the medulla and hence are named *pars radiata* or *medullary rays*. The regions between the rays contain glomeruli and convoluted tubules and are called *pars convoluta* or *cortical labyrinths*. A medullary ray and the portions of the adjacent labyrinths whose tubules drain into the collecting tubules constitute a *lobule*.

The Uriniferous Tubules

The parenchyma of the kidney consists of closely packed uriniferous tubules, be-

tween which are blood vessels and a scanty amount of interstitial connective tissue. As in any other gland, two types of tubules are distinguished: the terminal or "secretory" tubules, which function in the formation of the urine, and the collecting tubules, which are the ducts conveying the urine to the pelvis and ureter. The terminal tubule constitutes a structural and functional unit known as the *nephron*. Each nephron is long (30 to 40 mm) and unbranched and, for the greater part of its course, it is highly tortuous, forming compact convoluted masses (Fig. 18-4). Each nephron begins as a double walled, cup-shaped expansion known as *Bowman's capsule*, which encloses a tuft of capillaries, the *glomerulus*. Bowman's capsule and the glomerulus together form the *renal* or *Malpighian corpuscle* (Fig. 18-5).

The Renal Corpuscle. The renal corpuscles are spheroidal, slightly flattened bodies that occur in large numbers in the cortical labyrinths (Fig. 18-2). Their diam-

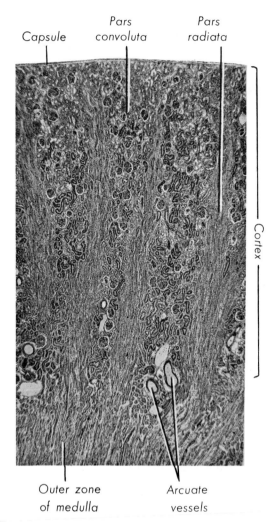

Capsule | Pars convoluta | Pars radiata

Cortex

Outer zone of medulla | Arcuate vessels

Fig. 18-2. Low power photomicrograph of a section of a kidney from an infant of 8 months, showing topography of the cortex and a part of the outer zone of the medulla. ×28.

eter in the adult is about 200 μm, although there are considerable variations in size. As a rule, the larger ones are found near the border of the medulla. Their structure is best understood by a brief reference to their development (chapter 20 and Fig. 20-46). During development, the rounded, blind end of a tubule grows around a blood vessel, giving the impression that the tubule is being invaginated by the blood vessel. By this growth and differentiation, the end of the tubule becomes transformed into a two-layered capsule, the capsule of Bowman, which encloses the glomerulus.

The glomerulus consists of a number of capillary loops connecting an afferent arteriole with an efferent arteriole; in other words, *the entire vascular system of the glomerulus is arterial.* The afferent vessel is named the *afferent glomerular arteriole*; the efferent vessel is known as the *efferent glomerular arteriole.* These vessels usually lie close together at the point where they enter and leave the glomerulus (Fig. 18-6), and the region where they enter and exit is spoken of as the *vascular pole* of the renal corpuscle.

As it enters the glomerulus, the afferent arteriole divides into four or five relatively large capillaries. Each of the latter vessels subdivides into a number of smaller capillaries that follow an irregularly looped course in their pathway from the afferent to the efferent arteriole. The looped capillaries arising from each main branch of the afferent arteriole tend to be grouped together, giving the glomerulus a lobulated appearance. Carefully injected preparations show that there are numerous anastomoses between the capillaries within each lobule, as well as occasional anastomoses between those of different lobules. All of the capillaries of the different lobules eventually reunite to form the efferent arteriole, which is always smaller in caliber than is the afferent arteriole. The difference in size correlates with a functional condition: the efferent vessel carries less fluid than the afferent vessel because a considerable quantity of fluid is filtered from the blood while it flows through the glomerular capillaries. A small amount of connective tissue accompanies the arterioles into the renal corpuscle for a short distance at the vascular pole, but connective tissue fibers and the different types of connective tissue cells do not follow the capillaries throughout their course as they do in most other parts of the body. Electron micrographs, however, show a third type of cell (i.e., in addition to endothelium and epithelium) deep within the renal corpuscle. These are known as *mesangial cells* (Gr. *mesos*, between, and *angeion*, vessel). They are mesenchymally derived cells that are structurally similar to pericytes on vessels in other locations (chapter 12) and they are similarly enveloped by a glycoprotein layer that is fused with the basal lamina of the endothelium. They are not very numerous and

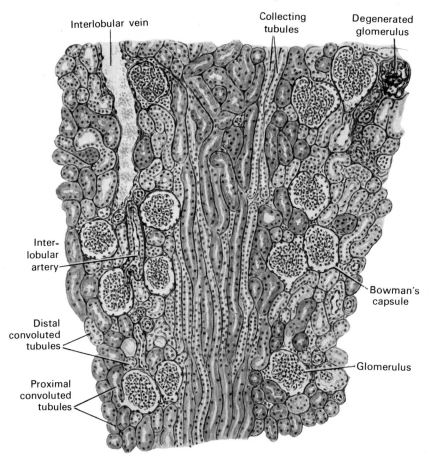

Fig. 18-3. Section through a part of the cortex of a human kidney, showing the structure of a pars radiata (*central part of figure*) and of adjacent cortical labyrinths (*lateral parts of figure*). ×55.

their nuclei are generally located at a level opposite to that of the endothelial cell nuclei. They are phagocytic and they apparently have a role in the removal of material that piles up at the basal lamina during filtration.

Bowman's capsule consists of an inner or "visceral" layer covering the glomerulus and an outer or "parietal" layer (Figs. 18-5 through 18-7). The visceral layer follows an irregular course as it closely invests the glomerulus and dips down between the lobules of glomerular capillaries. It is composed of a single layer of epithelial cells resting on a basal lamina which is fused with the basal lamina beneath the endothelium of the capillaries; i.e., visceral epithelium and endothelium are separated merely by a single thin layer (Fig. 18-8). This layer

between endothelium and visceral epithelium is often referred to as a basement membrane, but it lacks the lamina reticularis component of basement membranes of most other types of epithelium (chapter 4). It is more correctly designated *basal lamina* or *basement lamina*. It is also known as a *lamina densa* because it is relatively electron-dense in electron micrographs. The lamina varies in thickness from 0.08 to 0.12 μm, and is observable under the light microscope in sections stained with the periodic acid-Schiff (PAS) technique. It is difficult to identify in hematoxylin-eosin preparations.

The *endothelial cells of the glomerular capillaries* are extremely thin, with the exception of the regions where the nuclei are located. Most of the endothelial cell cyto-

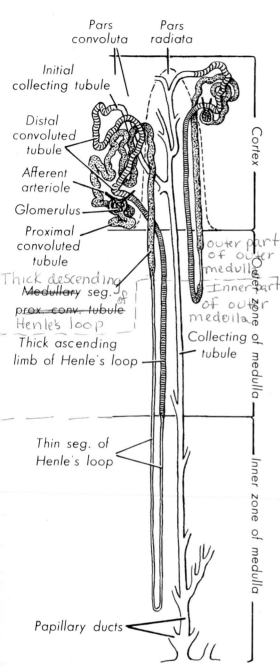

Pars convoluta Pars radiata

Initial collecting tubule

Distal convoluted tubule

Afferent arteriole

Glomerulus

Proximal convoluted tubule

Thick descending Medullary seg. of prox. conv. tubule Henle's loop

Thick ascending limb of Henle's loop

Thin seg. of Henle's loop

Papillary ducts

Cortex

Outer part of outer medulla

Inner part of outer medulla

Collecting tubule

Outer zone of medulla

Inner zone of medulla

Fig. 18-4. Diagram of the subdivisions of the uriniferous tubules to show their relations and locations in a section extending from the capsule to the tip of a renal pyramid. (Redrawn and modified from Peter.)

plasm extends along the basal lamina in the form of a cribriform plate (lamina fenestra), with pores that have an average diameter of about 800 Å (Figs. 18-9 and 18-

10). Electron micrographs show that most of these pores lack diaphragms and thus they differ from the pores of fenestrated capillaries in other parts of the body (Fig. 18-10). This ultrastructural feature correlates with results obtained from studies with tracers which show that relatively large molecules such as ferritin (molecular weight of 600,000 and a diameter of about 100 Å) readily pass through the glomerular endothelium.

The cells of the *visceral layer* of Bowman's capsule are relatively large and their nuclei bulge into the capsular space (Figs. 18-7 and 18-8). Electron micrographs show that these cells contain the usual organelles including microtubules and microfilaments. The cells also have trabecular-like extensions (primary processes) that divide into numerous foot-like secondary processes or pedicels that rest on the basal lamina (Figs. 18-8, 18-9 and 18-11). The entire epithelial cell with its little feet is known as a *podocyte* and the pedicels of neighboring podocytes interdigitate along the basal lamina (Figs. 18-11 and 18-12). The spaces between the pedicels range in width from about 0.02 to 0.04 μm and they are spanned by an electron dense membrane known as the *slit diaphragm* (slit membrane) that is only about 50 Å thick (Fig. 18-10). High resolution electron micrographs of renal tissue preserved by vascular transfusion of particular fixatives (e.g., tannic acid and glutaraldehyde) show that the slit diaphragm contains an axial filament coursing lengthwise at a position equidistant from the membranes of the adjacent podocyte processes. Furthermore, there are regularly spaced cross bridges between the axial filament and the cell membranes of the podocyte pedicels. As a result of this axial filament and cross bridge pattern, the slit diaphragm has a regular arrangement of pores, with each pore having a dimension of about 40 × 140 Å.

As outlined above, the layer of tissue through which substances must pass in moving from blood to provisional urine consists of an endothelium with pores, a relatively thick basal lamina and a visceral epithelium containing slits that are spanned by diaphragms with pores. The endothelium normally prevents the escape of blood

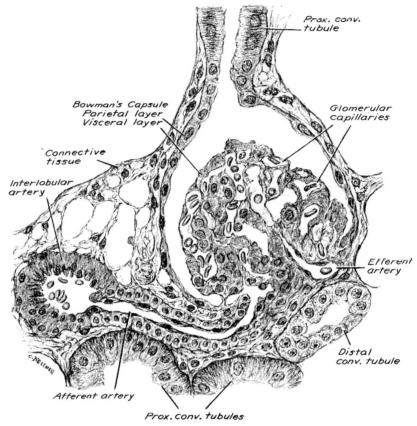

Fig. 18-5. Renal corpuscle from kidney of mouse. ×1320.

cells but allows passage of relatively large molecules such as ferritin. The latter piles up at the basal lamina which was once thought to be the ultimate barrier. However, further studies with tracers of different molecular weight have shown that myeloperoxidase (molecular weight of about 160,000) readily passes through the basal lamina and piles up at the slit membranes which apparently constitute the ultimate barrier. Serum albumin with a molecular weight of about 68,000 and an estimated dimension of about 150 × 38 Å is about at the limit of substances that can pass. Substances with a weight of less than 60,000 readily pass through the final barrier to enter the lumen of the expanded end of the uriniferous tubule.

The *parietal layer of Bowman's capsule* begins where the visceral layer is reflected at the vascular pole (Figs. 18-6 and 18-7). At the urinary pole, usually opposite the vascular pole, the parietal layer becomes continuous with the wall of the proximal segment of the renal tubule through a short transitional zone which is called the "neck." At this point, the capsular space (Bowman's space) becomes continuous with the lumen of the proximal tubule. The wall of the parietal layer is composed of simple squamous epithelium resting on a thin basal lamina, surrounded by a thin layer of connective tissue. The epithelial cells are more uniform in thickness than those of the visceral layer. The cells increase in height and become cuboidal in the neck region.

Terminal Uriniferous Tubule. The terminal tubule or nephron consists of an expanded portion, described above as Bowman's capsule, and an elongated tubular portion composed of a proximal thick segment, an intermediate thin segment and a distal thick segment. The proximal thick and distal thick segments can both be sub-

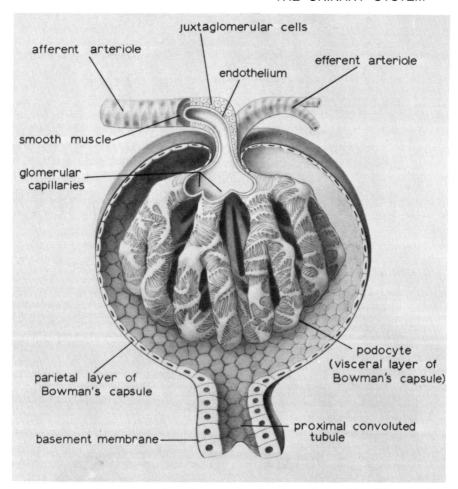

Fig. 18-6. Diagram of structure of renal corpuscle, showing relationship of Bowman's capsule to glomerular capillaries. (Redrawn and modified from Bargmann.)

divided into convoluted and straight portions. Hence, the tubular portion of the nephron is composed of the following segments: (1) the proximal convoluted tubule, (2) the straight or medullary segment of the proximal tubule (this part forms the thick *descending* proximal segment of Henle's loop), (3) the thin segment of Henle's loop, (4) the thick distal (ascending) segment of Henle's loop, and (5) the distal convoluted tubule. The latter joins the arched (initial) collecting tubule which begins the system of ducts or collecting tubules.

(1) *The proximal convoluted tubule* is the longest and most convoluted segment of the nephron, and it forms a major portion of the cortical substance. It has a length of about 14 mm, an overall diameter of about

50 to 60 μm, and a lumen whose diameter varies in proportion to the amount of provisional urine formed by its renal corpuscle. It follows a winding, looped course in the vicinity of the glomerulus and eventually turns toward the nearest medullary ray (pars radiata of cortex), where it continues as the straight segment of the proximal tubule.

The proximal convoluted tubule is lined by a single layer of low columnar or pyramidal cells with round nuclei and granular cytoplasm which stains deeply with eosin (Fig. 18-13). The cell boundaries are difficult to make out in ordinary preparations. In silver impregnations, they appear irregularly serrated, with processes which interdigitate with those of adjacent cells.

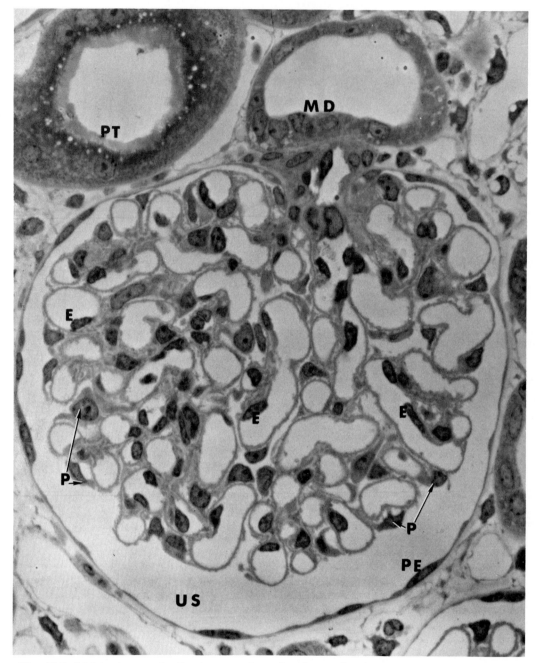

Fig. 18-7. Light micrograph of a 1 μm section of a glomerulus from perfused monkey kidney. *MD*, macula densa; *PT*, proximal tubule; *PE*, parietal epithelium of Bowman's capsule; *P*, podocytes (visceral epithelium of Bowman's capsule); *E*, endothelial cell nuclei; *US*, urinary space. ×700.

An important characteristic of the proximal convoluted tubule is the *brush border* at the apical surface of the cells (Fig. 18-13). Because this region undergoes rapid postmortem change, it often has a ragged appearance in routine histological preparations. Electon micrographs of well fixed material show that the brush border is composed of microvilli about 1.2 μm in length and about 0.03 μm in width (Fig. 18-14).

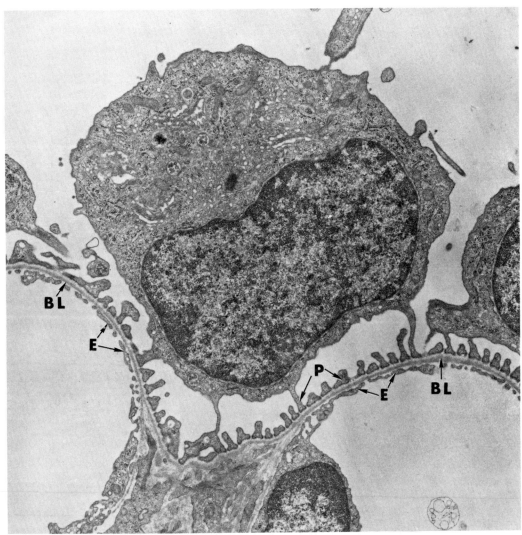

Fig. 18-8. Electron micrograph of mouse kidney glomerulus showing podocyte processes (*P*), fenestrated endothelium (*E*) and the interposed thick basal lamina (*BL*). ×10,800.

The cell surface available for resorption is thus greatly increased. Histochemical studies show that the border has a high concentration of alkaline phosphatase and oxidative enzymes. The border also contains protein-polysaccharides, as indicated by its intense staining with the PAS reagent. In electron micrographs, invaginations are often seen between the bases of the microvilli, and vesicles are present in the apical cytoplasm. An increase in the number of vesicles during diuresis indicates that micropinocytosis has a role in tubular resorption as discussed in more detail below under "The Excretion of Urine." The supranu-clear cytoplasm also contains mitochondria of variable shape and size (Fig. 18-14) and the usual organelles such as ribosomes. Peroxisomes and lysosomes are present and the latter apparently have a role in the breakdown of resorbed proteins into amino acids which are released into the peritubular connective tissue to subsequently enter the peritubular venous capillaries. The Golgi complex of the proximal convoluted tubule cells is usually on the adluminal side of the nucleus, but it sometimes becomes infranuclear during compensatory hypertrophy of the kidney.

The subnuclear portions of the cytoplasm

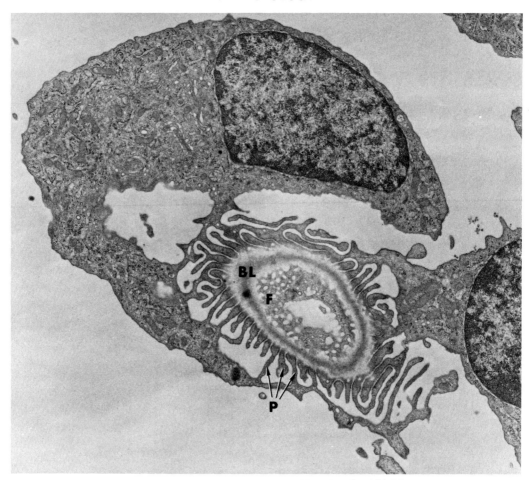

Fig. 18-9. Electron micrograph of mouse kidney glomerulus showing interdigitated podocyte processes on the surface of a capillary in tangential section. *P*, podocyte processes; *F*, fenestrated endothelium; *BL*, basal lamina. ×9200.

of the proximal tubule cells appears striated in light microscope preparations. Electron micrographs show that this appearance is due to deep infoldings of the plasmalemma at the base of the cell (Fig. 18-15) and to the longitudinal arrangement of numerous rod-shaped mitochondria. There are also irregular infoldings and interdigitations of the lateral cell borders and this explains why the intercellular boundaries cannot be followed in ordinary preparations under the light microscope. It is to be noted that the cell interdigitations are extensive and that processes of different cells alternate along the basal lamina in a manner somewhat like that described above for the pedicels of podocytes.

(2) *The straight or medullary portion of the proximal tubule* is a direct continuation of the convoluted portion of the proximal tubule and is not sharply delimited from it. As the proximal tubule leaves the cortical labyrinth and enters the medullary ray, it assumes first a spiral and then a straight course. This segment is known as the *straight portion* of the proximal tubule because of its course, and it is also named the *medullary segment* of the proximal tubule because it is located in the medullary ray and in the outer, subcortical zone of the medulla (Fig. 18-4). It is lined by cells that appear structurally similar with those of the convoluted portion of the proximal tubule as seen in preparations stained with

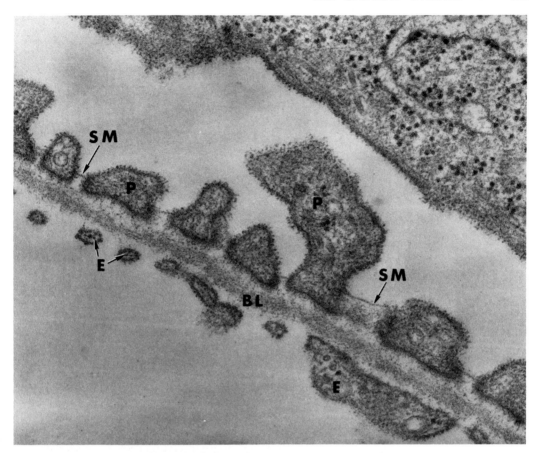

Fig. 18-10. Mouse kidney glomerulus showing podocyte processes (*P*), basal lamina (*BL*), fenestrated endothelium (*E*) and filtration slit membranes (*SM*). Part of a podocyte cell body is at the upper right. ×57,500.

hematoxylin and eosin; that is, the cells have a brush border, an acidophilic granular cytoplasm and the other characteristics described for the convoluted segment. However, high resolution electron micrographs show that the cells of the straight segment, in comparison with the convoluted segment, have fewer intercellular interdigitations, less mitochondria and fewer lysosomes. These findings indicate that the straight portion of the proximal segment does not participate in transcellular transport to the same extent that the convoluted segment does.

The straight segment of the proximal tubule forms the proximal portion of the descending arm of Henle's loop (Fig. 18-4). It should be noted that this loop is composed of three parts: a proximal thick segment, a thin segment and a distal thick segment.

(3) *The thin segment of Henle's loop* is about 15 μm in diameter and is lined by a single layer of flattened epithelial cells with nuclei that bulge into the lumen (Fig. 18-16). In the primate kidney, the cells of the thin segment are somewhat less flattened than are the endothelial cells of the adjacent blood vessels (Fig. 18-17). The nuclei also differ from those of the endothelium in shape and they stain less intensely in routine hematoxylin and eosin preparations. Electron micrographs show the presence of a few very short microvilli. Thin segment cells display abundant perinuclear cytoplasm and extremely attenuated regions elsewhere (Fig. 18-17). The cells have fewer mitochondria than those of other seg-

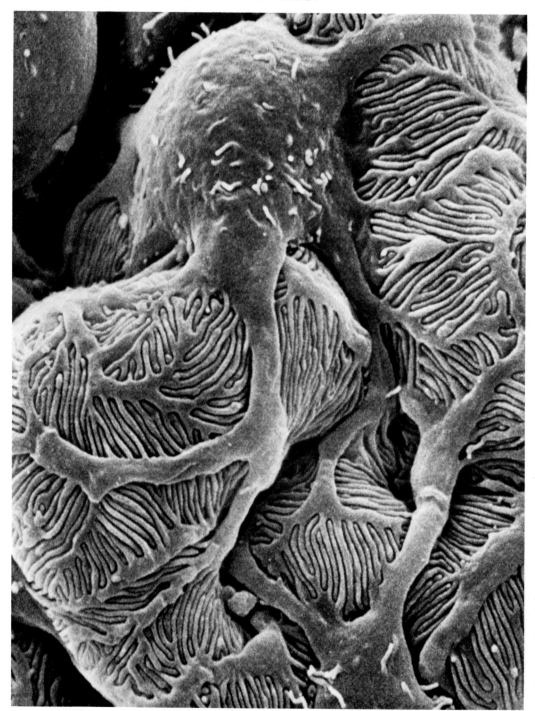

Fig. 18-11. Scanning electron micrograph of a portion of a glomerulus of human kidney showing the interdigitation of podocyte cell processes over the surfaces of capillary loops. ×9800. (Courtesy of Dr. Masayuki Miyoshi.)

ments of the nephron. Electron micrographs of thin sections cut approximately parallel with the basement membrane show

that the cells have an irregular starfish outline, with processes of one cell interdigitating with those of another. Consequently,

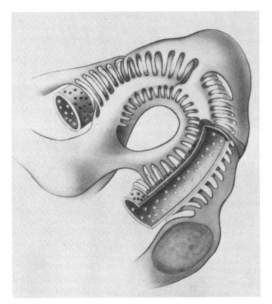

Fig. 18-12. Diagram of a portion of a capillary loop of the glomerulus summarizing the relationship of podocyte processes to the capillary wall. (Based on a diagram from Pease, 1955.)

electron micrographs show numerous membrane-bounded nonnucleated regions of cytoplasm. Electron micrographs also show some cytological differences between the thin descending and thin ascending limbs of the loop that are particularly obvious in rodents.

The extent of the thin segment, the level at which it is located, and the length of the entire loop, all vary with the location of the renal corpuscle (Figs. 18-4 and 18-18). As a rule, the tubules whose renal corpuscles are located near the corticomedullary junctions have long thin segments that begin in the outer (subcortical region) of the medulla, descend deep into the inner zone of the medulla and then continue up the ascending limb to the junction of the outer and inner zone of the medulla (Figs. 18-4 and 18-18). On the other hand, the thin segments of the uriniferous tubules that are associated with glomeruli that are located within the outer part of the cortex have short loops with the thin segment confined to a small part of the descending limb (1 to 2 mm or even less). The shorter loops with short thin sements outnumber the long ones by about seven to one.

(4) *The thick distal (ascending) segment of Henle's loop* is about 9 mm long and 30 μm in diameter. In the short loops, it may begin in the lower part of the proximal limb (Fig. 18-4). It ascends to the cortex and closely approaches the vascular pole of the glomerulus from which the nephron began. At this point, it becomes continuous with the distal convoluted tubule. It is lined by cuboidal cells which are lower than are those of the thick segment of the proximal limb of the loop. In comparison with the proximal segment, the cells of the distal segment are narrower and therefore their nuclei appear closer to each other in sections. No brush border is observable under the light microscope, although a few short microvilli can be seen in electron micrographs. There are numerous infoldings of the plasma membrane at the basal part of the cell and the mitochondria are more numerous in the cells of the distal limb than in those of the proximal limb. These are characteristics of cells which function in pumping sodium and they also account for the basal striations seen with the light microscope. Electron micrographs also show numerous infoldings of cell membranes and complex interdigitations along the lower portions of the lateral borders of the cells. This correlates with the fact that the basal portions of the intercellular boundaries are not as apparent under the light microscope as are the apical (adluminal) portions.

(5) The *distal convoluted tubule* begins near the vascular pole of the glomerulus and terminates by becoming continuous with the arched collecting tubule (Fig. 18-4). At one point, it comes in direct contact with the afferent glomerular arteriole (Figs. 18-5 and 18-7). It is much less convoluted than the proximal tubule and is only 4½ to 5 mm in length. It has an irregular outline, and its diameter varies from 22 to 50 μm. It is lined by cuboidal cells containing a granular cytoplasm which stains less intensely with acid dyes than does the cytoplasm of the proximal convoluted tubules. The basal striations are less pronounced than those of the distal ascending limb, and no brush border is observable under the light microscope. Electron micrographs show fewer mitochondria and less basal infoldings in the cells of the distal convoluted tubule than in the distal ascending limb. The distal convoluted segment resem-

Distal convoluted tubule   Proximal convoluted tubule

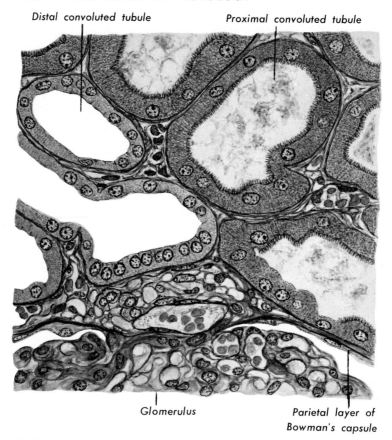

Glomerulus   Parietal layer of
                                  Bowman's capsule

Fig. 18-13. Portion of a glomerulus and adjacent tubules from the cortex of a human kidney. One of the segments of a distal convoluted tubule shows a modification, known as the macula densa, where it borders on the vascular pole of the glomerulus. In this region, there is an increase in the height and number of cells with a concentration of nuclei. ×635. (The slide from which this drawing was made was kindly supplied by Dr. T. E. Hunt.)

bles the distal ascending limb in that its cells are not as broad as those which line the proximal convoluted tubules, and therefore the nuclei are closer together and more numerous in sections of distal tubules than they are in sections of proximal tubules (Fig. 18-13).

The cells of the distal tubules show special cytological characteristics where the tubule comes in contact with the glomerular arterioles. This is also the approximate point at which the distal ascending segment becomes continuous with the distal convoluted portion. In this region, the cells on the side of the tubule adjacent to the afferent arteriole and a portion of the efferent arteriole are taller and more slender than elsewhere in the distal tubules. The nuclei

are closer together and the region appears darker under the light microscope; hence, it is named the *macula densa* (Figs. 18-7 and 18-13). The Golgi complex of these cells is in a subnuclear position, in contrast with its supranuclear position in other portions of the tubules. A thin basement membrane is the only structure separating the macula densa cells from the *juxtaglomerular cells* of the afferent arteriole (Fig. 18-19).

Collecting Tubules. The *arched* (initial) *collecting tubules* are still in the cortical labyrinth and empty into the *straight collecting tubules*. The straight tubules receive a number of arched tubules (7 to 10) as they pass down through the medullary rays of the cortex, but they receive no branches in the outer zone of the medulla

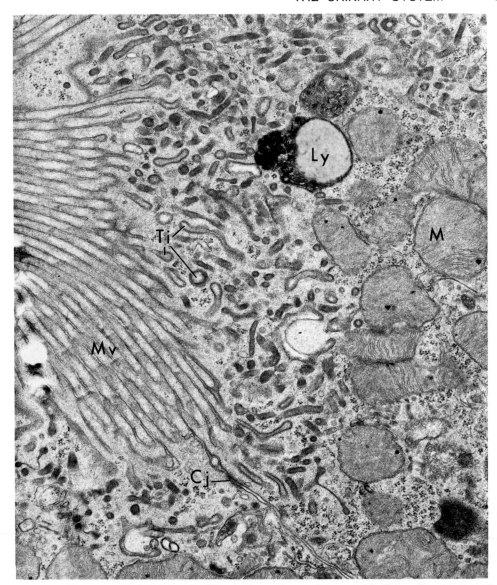

Fig. 18-14. Electron micrograph of adluminal portions of two epithelial cells of a proximal convoluted tubule of a mouse kidney. The adluminal surface of each cell is increased in area by numerous microvilli (*Mv*). Invaginations, arising from clefts between the basal portions of the microvilli, penetrate downward into the cell to form tubular invaginations (*Ti*) that are also known as apical canaliculi. The invaginations become continuous with vesicles in the cytoplasm and they apparently function in the resorption of large molecules, such as proteins. *Cj*, junction of apposing cells; *Ly*, lysosomes; and *M*, mitochondrion. ×23,250. (Courtesy of Drs. K. R. Porter and M. A. Bonneville.)

(Fig. 18-4). In the inner zone of the medulla, they unite with other straight tubules, and after a number of fusions the *papillary ducts* or *ducts of Bellini* are formed, which open on the area cribrosa of the papilla. It appears that about seven successive fusions occur before the papillary ducts are formed.

The caliber of the collecting tubules ranges from about 40 μm for those located in the medullary rays to over 200 μm for the papillary ducts of the medullary pyramids. The lining cells range in height from

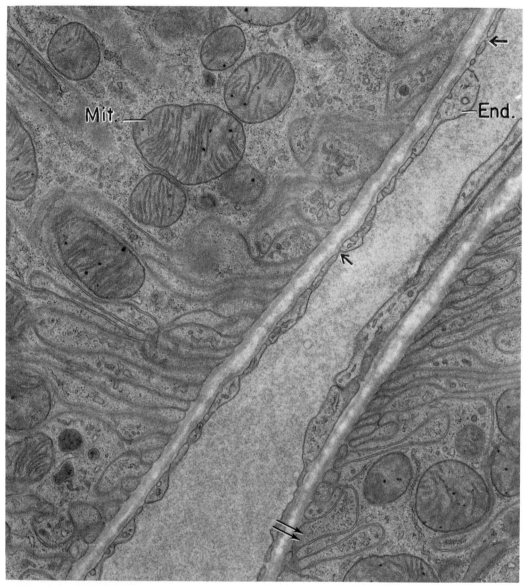

Fig. 18-15. Electron micrograph of the basal portions of epithelial cells of two proximal convoluted tubules and a blood capillary within the connective tissue between the tubules. The plasmalemma of the basal surface of each proximal tubule cell has numerous infoldings which partially partition the cytoplasm of the basal region into cylindrical columns around the mitochondria (*Mit*). Isolated cell processes (*double arrows*) are seen along the basal lamina of each tubule. Processes of different epithelial cells apparently interdigitate along the basal lamina in a manner somewhat like that of podocytes of glomerular epithelium. The endothelial cells (*End*) of the capillaries around the tubules are attenuated and have "pores" or fenestrae (*arrows*). The basal lamina of the endothelium is separated from the basal lamina of the proximal tubule by only a narrow space. Section of a kidney of a bat. ×27,000. (Courtesy of Dr. Keith Porter.)

cuboidal in the initial collecting tubule to tall columnar in the papillary ducts. The intercellular borders are more distinct than in any of the other portions of the urinifer-

ous tubule and this correlates with electron microscope studies which show only a few or no intercellular projections and invaginations. Microvilli are very short and often

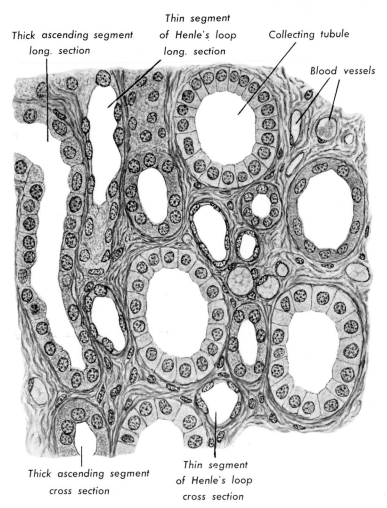

Fig. 18-16. Section from the medulla of a human kidney. ×575.

absent. The cytoplasm stains lightly and is less acidophilic than in any other segments of the tubules; this correlates with electron microscopic studies which show only a few mitochondria and numerous ribosomes.

Light microscope studies of well stained preparations often show some dark staining cells interspersed with the more numerous light staining cells in the initial part of the collecting tubule. Electron micrographs show that the dark staining cells of light microscopy have numerous mitochondria whereas the light staining cells have relatively few mitochondria and only a few invaginations along their basal surface. Since this mixture of cells occurs in the region where tubules of metanephrogenic origin join with tubules that arise as out-

growths from the ureteric bud (Fig. 20-46) it has been suggested that the mixture of dark and light cells is related to differences in embryonic origin, with the dark cells arising from metanephrogenic tissue.

The length of the collecting tubule from its beginning in the medullary ray to its opening on the papilla is 20 to 22 mm; that of the terminal tubule (nephron) is 30 to 38 mm. The entire uriniferous tubule thus measures from 50 to 60 mm, the variations depending mainly on the length of Henle's loop.

A summary of the locations of the various portions of the uriniferous tubules is given in Table 18-1, p 597. The epithelium of all parts of the uriniferous tubule rests on a basement membrane. The interstitial con-

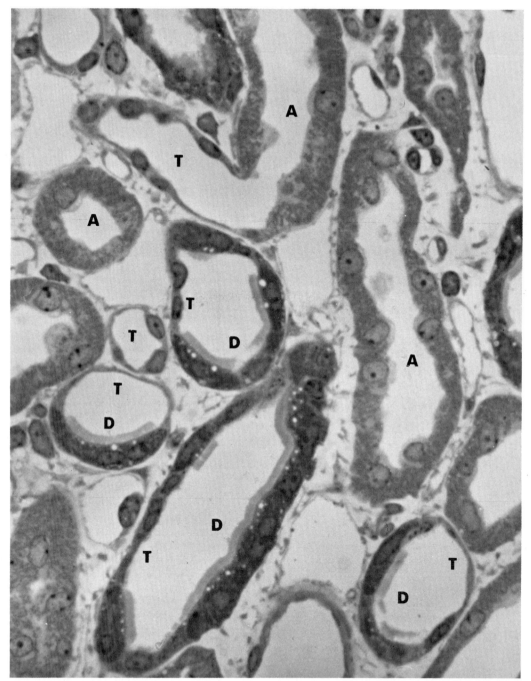

Fig. 18-17. Light micrograph of monkey kidney medulla showing transition in morphology of the tubule epithelium in the loop of Henle. Descending thick limbs with brush border (*D*) grade into thin limbs (*T*) which in turn grade into ascending thick limbs with a morphology characteristic of the distal tubule (*A*). ×740.

nective tissue is scanty in the cortical region but more developed in the medulla (Figs. 18-13 and 18-16). It consists of a fine network of fibers, together with the usual connective tissue cells, chiefly fibroblasts.

Blood Vessels (Fig. 18-18)

The *renal* artery enters the kidney at the hilus and splits into a number of large branches, the *interlobar arteries*. These

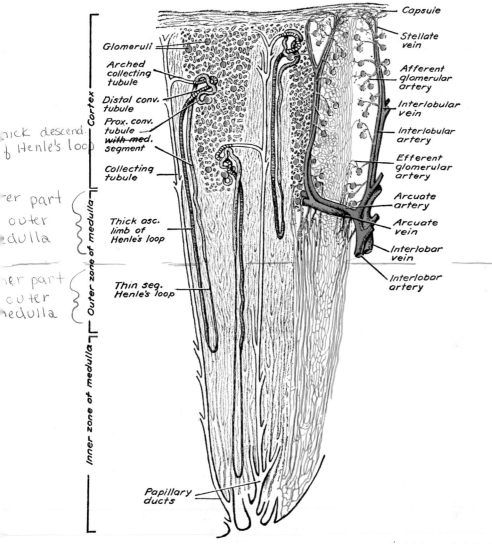

Labels on the figure:

Glomeruli

Arched collecting tubule

Distal conv. tubule

Prox. conv. tubule with med. segment

Collecting tubule

Cortex

nick descend. f Henle's loop

er part outer dulla

Outer zone of medulla

er part outer edulla

Inner zone of medulla

Thick asc. limb of Henle's loop

Thin seg. Henle's loop

Papillary ducts

Capsule

Stellate vein

Afferent glomerular artery

Interlobular vein

Interlobular artery

Efferent glomerular artery

Arcuate artery

Arcuate vein

Interlobar vein

Interlobar artery

Fig. 18-18. Diagram of the structure of the human kidney. The cortical labyrinth is indicated by the presence of convoluted tubules and glomeruli, and the medullary ray is marked by the parallel arrangement of tubules. The medullary ray with adjacent regions of cortical labyrinths represents the lobule. Note that the straight medullary (*med.*) segment of the proximal tubule forms the upper part of Henle's loop and that these loops extend varying distances into the medulla. The thick ascending (*asc.*) limb of the loop is sometimes subdivided into a proximal opaque portion (stippled) and a distal more clear portion (closely cross-lined). Electron microscope studies show that the portion described by light microscopists as opaque has more mitochondria and more basal infoldings. For clearer illustration, the convoluted tubules are simplified and all segments of the tubules are magnified more in width than in length. (Blood vessels are redrawn and modified from Braus and tubules are modified from Peter.)

give off fine twigs to the pelvis and to the capsule; then without further branching they pass between the pyramids to the boundary zone of medulla and cortex. Here they bend sharply and form short arches, the *arcuate* or *arciform arteries,* which run parallel to the surface. The arches do not communicate with one another as was formerly believed; each represents merely the curved terminal portion of an interlobar artery. The arcuate arteries divide into a large number of finer branches, the *interlobular arteries,* which ascend perpendicularly through the cortical labyrinths to the

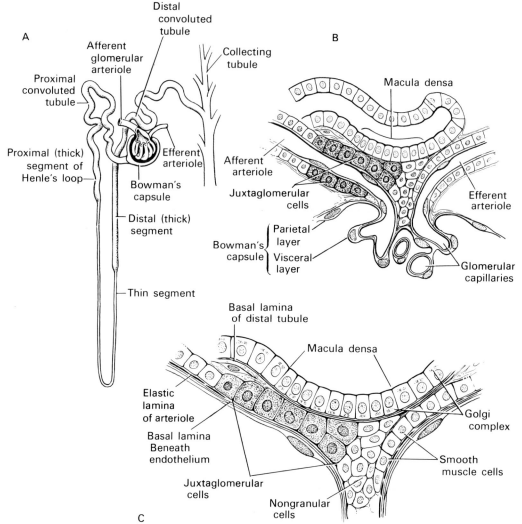

Fig. 18-19. Diagrams of a uriniferous tubule and its glomerular arterioles to show the location and structure of the juxtaglomerular cells and macula densa. *A*, a diagram of the relationship between the glomerular arterioles and the uriniferous tubule at the point where the distal segment of Henle's loop continues into the distal convoluted tubule. *B*, a portion of the region at higher magnification. The *macula densa* in the wall of the distal tubule is apposed to portions of the afferent and efferent glomerular arterioles and is particularly close to the *granular juxtaglomerular cells*. *C*, an enlargement of a portion of *B* showing that the internal elastic lamina of the arteriole and most other connective tissue elements are absent from the region where the macula densa cells and granular juxtaglomerular cells are apposed.

surface, about midway between adjacent medullary rays. The interlobular arteries give off numerous short lateral branches, each of which enters a renal corpuscle as the afferent glomerular vessel and subdivides as described above under "Renal Corpuscle." Often the short branches subdivide and supply a cluster of glomeruli. On reaching the periphery of the cortex, the terminal

portions of most interlobular arteries themselves become afferent glomerular vessels.

As the afferent glomerular arteriole approaches the glomerulus, some of its muscle cells are replaced by *myoepithelioid* cells that form part of a juxtaglomerular complex. The *juxtaglomerular complex* consists of (1) *juxtaglomerular (JG) cells* (granular and nongranular) in the wall of

TABLE 18-1

Locations of portions of uriniferous tubules

Location of kidney	Portion of tubule
CORTEX	
Cortical labyrinth	Malpighian corpuscles Proximal convoluted tubules Distal convoluted tubules Arched collecting tubules
Medullary ray	Straight portions (medullary segments) of proximal tubules Thick segments of ascending arms of Henle's loops Straight collecting tubules
MEDULLA	
Outer zone	Straight portions (medullary segments) of proximal tubules Thick segments of ascending arms of Henle's loops Thin segments of Henle's loops Crests of shorter loops Straight collecting tubules
Inner zone	Thin segments of Henle's loops Crests of long loops Straight collecting tubules Fusions of straight collecting tubules Papillary ducts

the afferent arteriole, (2) a group of so-called *polkissen cells,* between the afferent and efferent arterioles at the vascular pole of the renal corpuscle and (3) the *macula densa* of the distal tubule. The polkissen cells have an agranular, pale staining cytoplasm and they resemble the *nongranular juxtaglomerular cells* in the wall of the arteriole. The *granular juxtaglomerular cells,* together with a few nongranular cells, form a collar or *juxtaglomerular cushion* on the afferent arteriole that replaces the smooth muscle cells of the tunica media in this part of the vessel (Fig. 18-19). The JG cells are separated from the blood in the afferent arterioles only by an endothelium and basal lamina, and their opposite poles are separated from the macula densa of the distal tubule only by a thin basal lamina. The close anatomical relationship of the JG and macula densa cells lends support to the view that they are in functional intercommunication. The granular JG cells have cytoplasmic granules which are readily seen under the light microscope in preparations treated with PAS or with Bowie's

ethyl violet. Electron micrographs show the granules as electron-dense and membrane-bounded.

It has been known for many years that the kidney secretes a proteolytic enzyme known as *renin.* Recent evidence from the use of fluorescent antibody techniques shows that renin is secreted by the granular JG cells. Renin acts on a specific substrate in the bloodstream known as *angiotensinogen,* causing the latter to change into *angiotensin I* which is converted into *angiotensin II* through the action of an enzyme produced in the capillaries of the lungs. Since angiotensin II is a vasoconstrictor, it has a direct effect on blood pressure. An increase in renin also increases blood pressure by stimulating aldosterone secretion by the adrenal cortex; the latter secretion decreases the rate of sodium and water resorption by the distal tubules. Under normal conditions, the combined responses of the afferent arterioles to pressure changes and of the JG cells to sodium concentrations maintain a normal blood pressure. The JG cells apparently have an additional

function in that they secrete a renal erythropoietic factor (REF) which stimulates
stem cells of hemopoietic tissue to differentiate into proerythroblasts (chapter 7).

The efferent glomerular arteriole divides
into a *second* system of capillaries, the *peritubular plexus,* which forms a dense network around the tubules of the cortex (Fig.
18-18). So densely are the capillaries arranged that the tubules seem bathed in
blood.

Nonglomerular arterioles may be found
extending directly from an afferent arteriole
to the peritubular plexus. Known as Lud-
wig's arterioles, they are infrequent in normal kidneys and are said to arise from a
continuity of afferent and efferent vessels
following glomerular degeneration.

*The arterial supply of the medulla is
furnished by the efferent glomerular vessels of those renal corpuscles which lie
close to the medulla (Fig. 18-18).* These
vessels, the *arteriolae rectae spuriae,* pursue a straight course into the outer layer
of the medulla and give rise to long-meshed
capillary nets that extend to the apex of
the pyramids. The *arteriolae rectae* and
venae rectae together with their capillary
loops are known as the *vasa recta.* Although the vessels which form the loops
have a wider lumen than that of ordinary
capillaries, they have thin walls. The hair-

pin vascular loops are closely associated
with the loops of Henle and they are arranged in patterns seen best in sections cut
perpendicular to the long axis of the pyramids (Figs. 18-20 through 18-22). The endothelium of the venae rectae is of the
attenuated (fenestrated) type. The vasae
rectae not only provide the main blood
supply to the medulla, but by their arrangement have an important role in maintaining
the osmotic gradient responsible for concentrating the urine.

The blood from the peripheral portion
of the cortex is collected into small venules
that unite beneath the capsule to form the
stellate veins of Verheyen. From these arise
the *interlobular veins,* which accompany
the corresponding arteries and empty into
the arcuate veins. The latter also receive
short interlobular veins from the deeper
portions of the cortex. Straight veins, the
venae rectae, collect the blood from the
capillary nets of the medulla and accompany the straight arteries, to terminate in
the *arcuate veins.* The venous arches, unlike the arterial ones, combine with one
another to form venous arcades. From the
arcuate veins the large *interlobar veins*
pass down between the medullary pyramids
and unite to form the renal vein.

In addition to the distribution just described, some interlobular arteries on

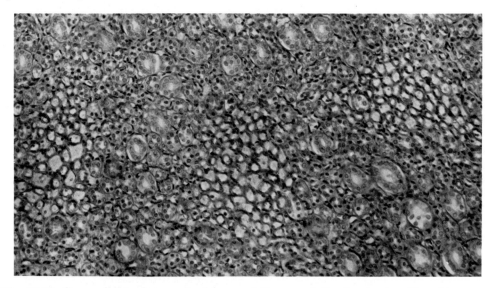

Fig. 18-20. Survey light micrograph of human kidney medulla showing bundles of transversely
sectioned vasa recta surrounded by transversely sectioned tubules. (See Fig. 18-21 for higher
magnification of part of this field.) ×150.

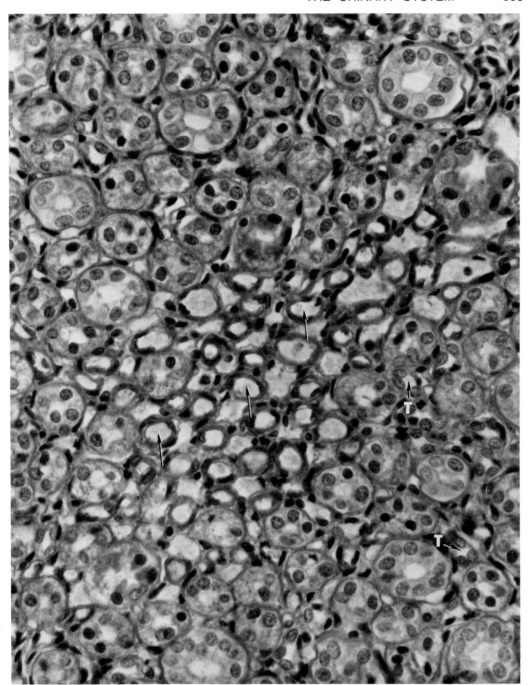

Fig. 18-21. Light micrograph of human kidney medulla showing vasa recta. Thicker-walled vessels (*arrows*) are descending (arterial) segments and thinner-walled vessels are ascending (venous) segments. Thin limbs of Henle's loop are difficult to distinguish among the vasa recta in this preparation, but some are seen close by (*T*). ×475.

reaching the periphery of the cortex break up into capillaries that supply the fibrous capsule of the kidney. These anastomose with capillaries from the suprarenal, lum- bar and phrenic arteries and with those of the capsular twigs which arise directly from the renal artery or its interlobar branches.

Arteriovenous anastomoses have been

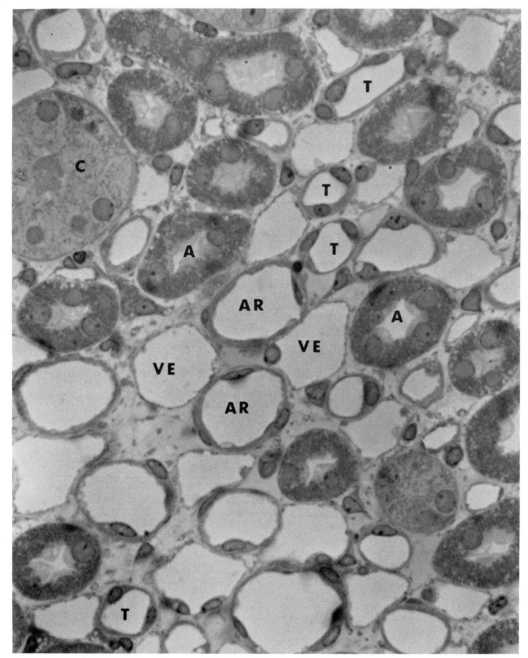

Fig. 18-22. One micrometer section of kidney medulla from a monkey fixed by vascular perfusion. The thicker-walled arterial segments (*AR*) of the vasae rectae are clearly distinguished from the thinner-walled venous segments (*VE*) and the thin limbs of Henle's loop (*T*). *A*, ascending thick segment of Henle's loop; *C*, collecting duct. ×800.

described at various levels: between inter-lobar arteries and veins, between arcuate arteries and veins and between interlobular arteries and veins.

Lymphatics

The lymph capillaries are arranged in two systems: a superficial system which ramifies in the capsule, and a deeper system which lies in the glandular tissue. The capsular lymph is collected by superficial lymph vessels that communicate with the lymphatics of adjacent organs. The lymph from the parenchyma is collected by a number of lymphatic trunks which accompany the blood vessels. They leave the kidney at the hilus to enter lymph nodes that are situated on both sides of the aorta.

Nerves

The kidneys are richly supplied with nerves, the majority of which are unmyelinated. They are derived from the celiac plexus and from the 10th to the 12th thoracic nerves. It is probable that branches from the vagus also supply the kidney. The nonmyelinated fibers follow the blood vessels and terminate by numerous endings in the vascular wall, particularly in the glomerular arterioles. Delicate terminals have been described as ramifying in the basement membrane of the tubules or even between the epithelial cells. Sensory myelinated fibers go to the capsule, the smooth muscle of the pelvis and the adventitia of the renal vessels.

The Excretion of Urine

The kidney has several important functions. It excretes urea and other nitrogenous waste products, it eliminates substances foreign to the body and it maintains the constant volume of the blood by the elimination of excess water. It is important to note that water and other substances needed by the body are eliminated only to the extent that they exceed the needs; in other words, the kidneys conserve the proper amounts of water, electrolytes and other chemicals of value to the body.

By maintaining the constituents of blood plasma at normal values, the kidneys play an important role in regulating the chemical composition of the extracellular fluid which is the internal environment for the cells and tissues of the body. The kidneys share the regulation of the internal environment with the lungs, which control the levels of oxygen and carbon dioxide.

The kidneys perform their functions by (1) filtration of blood plasma in the glomeruli, (2) selective reabsorption by the tubules of substances which the body needs to retain, (3) active excretion by the tubules of certain substances to be added to the urine and (4) exchange of hydrogen ions and formation of ammonia as part of the process of acid base regulation.

The renal corpuscles have a number of structural features that facilitate filtration. The presence of glomerular capillaries between afferent and efferent arterioles rather than between arterioles and venules provides for a glomerular capillary blood pressure of about 75 mm Hg. This is higher than the pressure in other capillaries, and it is more than sufficient to overcome the factors which oppose filtration (osmotic pressure of the blood plasma, renal interstitial pressure and resistance to flow in the tubule). A large surface area for filtration is provided by the number of tortuous capillary loops in each glomerulus and by the large number of glomeruli (over 2,000,000 for the two kidneys). The filtration surface has been estimated as 5200 to 5860 mm^2 per g of human kidney. The layer of tissue between the blood and the lumen of the upper, expanded end of the nephron consists of a fenestrated endothelium, a basal lamina and the processes of the podocytes (Fig. 18-8). Filtration through this layer is a physical process and depends on the pressure within the glomerular capillaries, the condition of the filtering membrane and the nature of the blood plasma.

The *capsular* or *provisional* urine is an ultrafiltrate of plasma and contains unchanged all of the constituents of plasma with the exception of all but a trace of the plasma proteins, fat droplets and blood cells, which are unable to pass through the normal filtration barrier because of their molecular weight or size. Direct evidence that the provisional urine is a filtrate of plasma was established by chemical analysis of capsular urine withdrawn by micropipette from the renal corpuscles of amphibians. Although it is more difficult to apply the micropipette method to the mammalian kidney, studies of this type have been made, with results essentially similar to those obtained on amphibians.

Procedures for determining the rates at

which different substances are "cleared" from the blood by excretion into the urine have contributed greatly to our knowledge of the function of the human kidney. *para*-Aminohippuric acid (PAH) and the polysaccharide inulin are particularly useful chemicals for clearance studies. PAH is filtered in the glomeruli and is eliminated in addition by tubular excretion. It is cleared completely from the plasma in one passage through the kidney when injected in low concentrations. Therefore, by measuring the amount of PAH in the urine in a unit of time and knowing the initial concentration in the plasma, one can readily calculate the renal blood flow. By this method, it has been found that the average normal flow through the two kidneys is about 1220 cc per min, or about 1750 liters of whole blood in a 24-h period.

Inulin is eliminated solely by glomerular filtration, and none is reabsorbed in the tubules. Therefore, by simultaneous measurements of the plasma level of inulin and the amount of inulin excreted in the urine in a unit of time, one can calculate the glomerular filtration rate. Studies of this type show that about 175 liters of fluid are filtered daily through the two kidneys under normal conditions.

The 175 liters of capsular or provisional urine become concentrated to 1 liter or less of actual urine and become altered in composition by the resorption of water and other constituents during passage through the uriniferous tubule. In the process of resorption, substances pass through the tubular epithelium to the surrounding connective tissue and thence to the peritubular capillaries and venules. The proximal tubules and their capillaries come into close association at many points where only a minimal amount of connective tissue separates the basal lamina of the tubular epithelium from that of the capillary endothelium (Fig. 18-15). Although some resorption occurs by diffusion through the tubular epithelium, the resorption of most substances is dependent upon work done by the cells.

Resorption has been studied by a variety of methods. One of the earliest methods consisted of a chemical analysis of urine samples withdrawn by micropipettes. Another method for studying resorption is to

compare the rate of clearance of any given substance with that of inulin which is almost completely cleared in one passage. For example, the clearance of a substance at a rate higher than that for inulin indicates tubular excretion in addition to glomerular filtration, whereas clearance at a lower rate indicates tubular resorption. Another method consists of stop-flow experiments. In this case, the ureter is blocked for several minutes and then opened for the collection of urine samples in series. It is assumed that the first samples come from the more distal portions of the nephron and the later samples from more proximal portions. The study of the functional activity of thin slices from different regions of the kidney in solutions of known composition has been a valuable method for analyzing factors involved in active transport.

Resorption in the proximal convoluted tubules is facilitated by the extensive surface area provided by the convolutions of the tubule and by the multitude of closely packed, slender processes that form the brush border. Surface area is only one of many factors affecting resorption, however. A partial list of other factors includes the types of enzymes at the cell borders as well as within the cells, the complexity and arrangement of mitochondria, infoldings at the basal ends of the cells, the relations of the resorbing cells to the capillaries, the osmotic pressures within the peritubular connective tissue, the presence of certain hormones within the blood and the concentration of the substance in question within the blood plasma. For example, glucose is completely resorbed in the proximal tubule under normal conditions and is maintained in the blood plasma at a definite level which is known as its threshold value. When the plasma glucose level exceeds its threshold value, as in diabetes mellitus, the amount of glucose filtered by the renal corpuscle exceeds the resorptive capacity of the tubule, and glucose appears in the urine. A comparison of the resorption of glucose with that of urea illustrates the selectivity involved. Urea and other protein wastes are destined to be completely eliminated. They have no threshold values in the blood and are resorbed only passively or not at all.

About 80% of the sodium and water filtered from the blood in the renal corpuscle is resorbed in the proximal tubule. Sodium, like glucose, is moved from the lumen of the tubule to the peritubular capillaries by an active process, i.e., by work on the part of the cells. This establishes an osmotic force favoring the passive diffusion of water, chlorides and bicarbonates in the same direction. Since salts and water are resorbed together in the proximal convoluted tubules, the provisional urine is reduced in volume in this segment of the nephron without any change in osmolality. The urine entering the descending limb of Henle's loop is isosmotic with the surrounding connective tissue and with blood plasma.

The appearance of thin segments in birds and mammals during phylogenesis allows these forms to secrete hypertonic urine and conserve water. In the process of conserving water, there are marked changes in the osmolality of the provisional urine along the course of Henle's loops in correlation with differences in the osmolality of the interstitial connective tissue at different levels of the medulla. There is a progressive increase in the hypertonicity of the urine as it passes down the thin segment of the descending limb, and a progressive decrease in hypertonicity as it passses up the ascending limb, becoming hypotonic in the upper part of the ascending limb and hypertonic again in the collecting tubules. The intertubular connective tissue of the medulla also becomes progressively more hypertonic toward the papilla of the pyramids, in contrast with renal cortical tissue, which is isosmotic. Likewise, blood collected from capillaries of the papillary regions of the medulla is hypertonic to systemic blood. The progressive loss of hypertonicity as the urine passes up the ascending limb results from the active pumping of sodium out of the thick ascending segment through an epithelium impermeable to water. By the pumping of sodium without water, the intertubular tissue becomes hypertonic. Some of the sodium reenters the thin descending limb of Henle's loop, probably by diffusion, and recirculates through the loop, to be pumped out again without water in the ascending limb. This provides a *countercurrent multiplier effect*. The increased osmolality of the connective tissue also provides for resorption of water by diffusion from the collecting tubules when the epithelium of these segments becomes water-permeable under the influence of the antidiuretic hormone (ADH) from the neurohypophysis. Although solutes and fluids pass from the connective tissue to the blood vessels, the hypertonic state of the connective tissue is maintained by the countercurrent multiplier effect in Henle's loops as noted above and also by a countercurrent exchange between the ascending and descending limbs of the neighboring capillary loops of the vasae rectae.

In the distal convoluted tubule there is further resorption of sodium, accompanied in this case by water. The permeability of the epithelium of the distal convoluted tubule and of the collecting tubule is controlled by ADH. A deficiency or lack of ADH produces a type of diuresis known as *diabetes insipidus*. In this condition, water cannot diffuse from the collecting tubules into the hypertonic connective tissue of the medulla. This differs from diabetes mellitus, in which diuresis may occur as an accompaniment to an increase of solute (glucose) in the urine. Resorption of sodium from the distal convoluted tubule is under the influence of the mineralocorticoid, aldosterone, which is formed in the adrenal cortex.

For further details on countercurrent factors in kidney function, reference may be made to textbooks of physiology and to an excellent account by Pitts.

The Renal Pelvis and Ureter

The renal pelvis with its subdivisions (the calyces) and the ureter constitute the *main excretory duct* of the kidney. The walls of the renal pelvis and ureter consist of three coats: an inner mucous, a middle muscular and an outer fibrous.

The *mucosa* of the calyces and ureter is lined by transitional epithelium which varies in thickness, depending on the state of distension of the ureter (Figs. 18-23 and 4-30). In the collapsed state, the cells of the basal layers are cuboidal, almost columnar. The superficial layer consists of large cuboidal cells with lighter cytoplasm, often

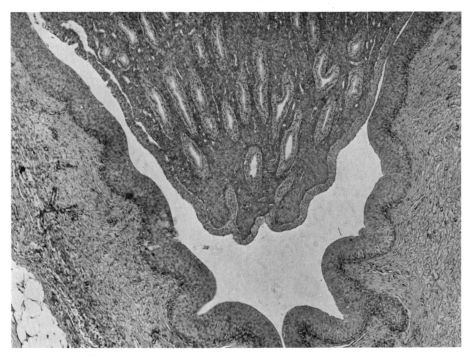

Fig. 18-23. Survey light micrograph of a minor calyx and renal papilla of monkey kidney. Papillary ducts open at the tip of the papilla with their lining epithelium becoming continuous with that on the surface of the papilla. This columnar epithelium grades into transitional epithelium that lines the calyx and continues into the ureter and bladder. ×60.

containing two or more nuclei. A basement membrane is not discernible with the light microscope, but a basal lamina and a thin lamina reticularis can be seen in electron micrographs. Diffuse lymphatic tissue frequently occurs in the lamina propria, especially of the pelvis. Occasionally the lymphatic tissue takes the form of small nodules. There is no distinct submucosa, although the outer part of the stroma is sometimes referred to as such.

The *muscularis* consists of an inner longitudinal and an outer circular layer (Fig. 18-24). In the lower part of the ureter, a discontinuous outer longitudinal layer is added.

The *fibrosa* consists of loosely arranged connective tissue and contains many large blood vessels. It is not sharply limited externally but blends with the connective tissue of surrounding structures and serves to attach the ureter to the latter.

The larger *blood vessels* run in the fibrous coat. From these, branches pierce the muscular layer, give rise to a capillary network among the muscle cells and then pass to the mucosa, in the stroma of which they break up into a rich network of capillaries. The veins follow the arteries.

The *lymphatics* follow the blood vessels, being especially numerous in the stroma of the mucosa.

Plexuses of both myelinated and nonmyelinated *nerve fibers* occur in the walls of the ureter and pelvis. The nonmyelinated fibers pass mainly to the cells of the muscularis. Myelinated fibers enter the mucosa, where they lose their myelin sheaths. Terminals of these fibers have been traced to the lining epithelium.

The Urinary Bladder

Except for the increased thickness of the muscular coat, the walls of the bladder are similar in structure to those of the ureter. The mucous membrane is thrown up into folds or is comparatively smooth, according to the degree of distention of the organ. The epithelium is of the same general type—transitional—as that of the ureter and, as already described for the ureter,

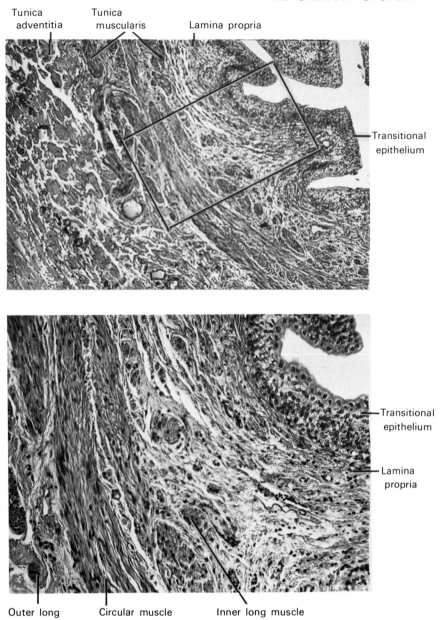

Tunica adventitia

Tunica muscularis

Lamina propria

Transitional epithelium

Transitional epithelium

Lamina propria

Outer long muscle

Circular muscle

Inner long muscle

Fig. 18-24. Portions of a transverse section of a human ureter. The area outlined in the *upper* figure is shown at higher magnification in the *lower* figure. The inner and outer longitudinally (long) oriented smooth muscle fibers do not form continuous layers. *Upper figure*, ×60; *lower figure*, ×145.

the surface cells may have two or more nuclei. The ultrastructural characteristics of transitional epithelium are shown in Fig. 18-25 and they are discussed in some detail under "Transitional Epithelium" in chapter 4. The number of layers of cells and the shapes of the cells depend largely upon whether the bladder is full or empty. In the moderately distended bladder, the superficial cells become flatter and the entire epithelium thinner than in the contracted organ. In the distended organ, there is still further flattening of the superficial cells, and the entire epithelium may have a thick-

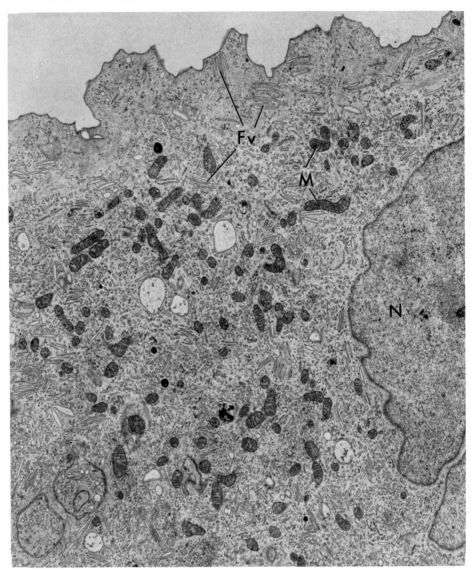

Fig. 18-25. Electron micrograph of a portion of a surface cell of transitional epithelium of the urinary bladder. The inner surface has an irregular contour, showing a number of crests and hollows. The cytoplasm just beneath the adluminal surface contains a meshwork of fine filaments but is generally free of mitochondria (*M*). Fusiform vesicles (*Fv*) are found throughout the cytoplasm of the surface cells. They are lined by trilaminar membranes similar to the plasmalemma. Electron micrographs of sections of bladders fixed after intraluminal injection of marker substances (e.g., ferritin) show the marker within the fusiform vesicles. The latter apparently form by a pinching off of trough-like depressions from the surface into the underlying cytoplasm. *N*, nucleus. From a section of the urinary bladder of a mouse. ×8650. (Courtesy of Drs. K. R. Porter and M. A. Bonneville.)

ness of only two or three cells. The stroma consists of fine, loosely arranged connective tissue containing many lymphocytes and sometimes small lymph nodules. There is no distinct submucosa and, as in the ureter, there are no glands.

The three muscular layers of the lower part of the ureter continue onto the bladder, where the muscle bundles of the different layers anastomose but still retain some indication of three layers—inner longitudinal, middle circular and outer longitudinal.

The fibrous layer, which is similar to that of the ureter, attaches the organ to the surrounding structures.

The blood and lymph vessels have a distribution similar to that in the ureter.

Sensory myelinated nerve fibers pierce the muscularis, branch repeatedly in the stroma, lose their myelin sheaths and terminate among the cells of the lining epithelium. Sympathetic fibers form plexuses in the fibrous coat, where they are interspersed with numerous small groups of ganglion cells. Axons of these sympathetic neurons penetrate the muscularis. Here they form plexuses, from which terminals are given off to the individual muscle cells.

The Urethra

The male and female urethrae differ from each other in many respects. The short female urethra is merely the terminal urinary passage conducting urine from the bladder to the vestibule. The relatively long male urethra constitutes a urogenital duct conducting both urine and seminal fluid to the exterior.

The Male Urethra. The male urethra has a length of about 20 cm and is divisible into three portions, prostatic, membranous and cavernous. The *prostatic portion*, about 3 to 4 cm in length, is surrounded by the prostate gland. From the dorsal wall of this portion a conical elevation, the *colliculus seminalis*, extends into the lumen. On the apex of the colliculus is the small opening of a blind tubule, the *utriculus prostaticus* or *uterus masculinus*, a remnant of the Müllerian duct. On either side of the utricle are the slitlike openings of the ejaculatory ducts, the terminal portions of the ductus deferens (see chapter 19 on the male reproductive system). Also in this part of the urethra are the numerous small openings of the ducts of the prostate gland.

The *membranous* portion is the narrowest and shortest, measuring about 1 cm in length.

The *cavernous* portion is about 15 cm long and extends through the penis to open on the end of the glans. At its beginning, the lumen is enlarged to form the *bulb* of the urethra. Then it continues with a uniform diameter to the glans penis, where the lumen is again enlarged in a dorsoventral direction and is known as the *fossa navicularis*. Throughout its course this portion is surrounded by a cylindrical mass of erectile tissue, the *corpus spongiosum* or *corpus cavernosum urethrae* (Figs. 18-26 and 19-29).

The structure of the mucous membrane varies in the different portions. The prostatic urethra is lined by a transitional epithelium similar to that of the bladder. In the membranous and cavernous portions, the epithelium is stratified columnar or pseudostratified, up to the fossa navicularis. There it changes to stratified squamous which, at the external urethral opening, becomes continuous with the epidermis of the skin. More or less extensive areas of stratified squamous epithelium are often seen throughout the whole course of the urethra.

The epithelium rests on a thin basement membrane, beneath which is a stroma of loose connective tissue rich in elastic fibers and containing in its deeper portion a plexus of capillaries and thin walled veins. Smooth muscle fibers, both longitudinally and circularly disposed, are found in the prostatic and membranous portions. A definite submucosa cannot be distinguished.

The prostatic urethra is surrounded by the fibromuscular tissue of the prostate which, under ordinary conditions, keeps the urethral lumen closed. The membranous portion is encircled by a sphincter of skeletal muscle fibers from the deep transverse perineal muscle.

The mucosa of the cavernous portion contains very little muscle and is surrounded by a cylindrical mass of erectile tissue, the corpus spongiosum. The latter consists of a network of large, irregular, venous spaces, or lacunae, which are lined by endothelium and are separated from each other by trabeculae of fibroelastic tissue containing numerous smooth muscle fibers running both longitudinally and circularly. These lacunae connect with the plexus of veins in the mucosal stroma. The corpus spongiosum is enclosed in a connective tissue capsule containing numerous elastic fibers and, on its inner surface, smooth muscle cells.

The lumen of the urethra shows a num-

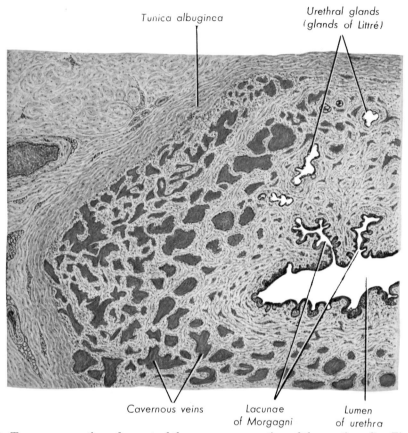

Fig. 18-26. Transverse section of a part of the cavernous portion of the urethra. See Figure 19-29 for lower magnification, showing complete section of penis. ×19.

ber of deep, irregular outpocketings, the *lacunae of Morgagni*. The lacunae continue into branched tubular glands, the *glands of Littré*, which extend deep into the stroma and may even penetrate into the corpus spongiosum. They are most numerous in the dorsal part of the cavernous portion of the urethra (Figs. 18-26 and 18-27). Most of the cells lining the gland tubules are clear staining, mucous secreting cells. Isolated mucous cells or groups of them (intraepithelial glands) are likewise found interspersed in the epithelium lining the lacunae of Morgagni.

The Female Urethra. The female urethra is a short tube 3 to 5 cm long. The epithelium varies considerably in different individuals. Near the bladder it is usually transitional. The remainder of the urethra is lined mainly by stratified squamous epithelium, with areas of stratified columnar or pseudostratified epithelium. The mucosa

is thrown into longitudinal folds. Glands of Littré, although fewer in number than in the male, open into the lacunae between the folds.

The abundant stroma is rich in elastic fibers and contains a plexus of numerous thin walled veins.

The rather indefinite muscularis contains both longitudinal and circular smooth muscle fibers, many of which penetrate into the stroma between the veins. An outer layer of skeletal muscle fibers forms a urethral sphincter.

A definite fibrosa is absent, the outer connective tissue fusing with that of the vagina.

Development of the Urinary System

The development of the urinary system is closely associated with that of the repro-

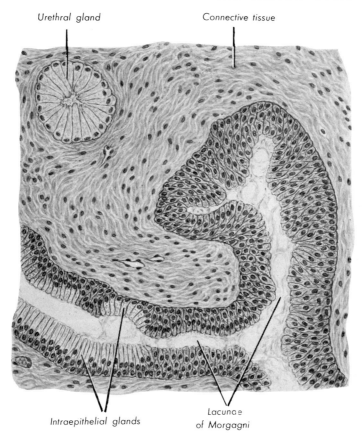

Urethral gland   Connective tissue

Intraepithelial glands   Lacunae of Morgagni

Fig. 18-27. Section through the dorsal portion of the corpus cavernosum urethrae, showing clear, mucous-secreting cells in a tubule of the urethral glands (glands of Littré) and groups of similar cells (intraepithelial glands) in the lacunae of Morgagni. ×294.

ductive system. The formation of these systems is given at the end of chapter 20.

References

AJZEN, H., SIMMONS, J. L., AND WOODS, J. W. Renal vein renin and juxtaglomerular activity in sodium-depleted subjects. Circ. Res. 17:130–134, 1965.

ANDREWS, P. M., AND PORTER, K. R. A scanning electron microscope study of the nephron. Am. J. Anat. 140:81–116, 1974.

BARAJAS, L., AND LATTA, H. Structure of the juxtaglomerular apparatus. Circ. Res. 21: suppl. 2, 15–28, 1967.

BULGER, R. E. The shape of rat kidney tubular cells. Am. J. Anat. 116:237–255, 1965.

BULGER, R. E. Rat renal capsule: presence of layers of unique squamous cells. Anat. Rec. 177:393–408, 1973.

BULGER, R. E., AND NAGLE, R. B. Ultrastructure of the interstitium in the rabbit kidney. Am. J. Anat. 136:183–204, 1973.

BURG, M., AND GREEN, N. Effect of ethacrynic acid on the thick ascending limb of Henle's loop. Kidney Int. 4:301–308, 1975.

EDWARDS, J. G. Studies of aglomerular and glomerular kidneys. Am. J. Anat. 42:75–108, 1928.

EVAN, A. P., AND DAIL, W. G., JR. Efferent arterioles in the cortex of the rat kidney. Am. J. Anat. 187:135–146, 1977.

FARQUHAR, M. G., AND PALADE, G. E. Functional evidence for the existence of a third cell type in the renal glomerulus. Phagocytosis of filtration residues by a distinctive "third" cell type. J. Cell Biol. 13:55–87, 1962.

FARQUHAR, M. G., WISSIG, S. L., AND PALADE, G. E. Glomerular permeability. I. Ferritin transfer across the normal glomerular capillary wall. J. Exp. Med. 113: pt. 1, 47–66, 1961.

FISHER, E. R. Lysosomal nature of juxtaglomerular granules. Science 152: 1752–1753, 1966.

FOOTE, J. J., AND GRAFFLIN, A. L. Cell contours in the two segments of the proximal tubule in the cat and dog nephron. Am. J. Anat. 70:1–20, 1942.

FORSTER, R. P. Kidney cells. In The Cell; Biochemistry, Physiology, Morphology (Brachet, J. and Mirsky, A. E., editors), vol. 5, pp. 89–161. Academic Press, New York, 1961.

FORSTER, R. P., AND TAGGART, J. V. Use of isolated renal tubules for the examination of metabolic processes associated with active cellular transport. J.

Cell. Comp. Physiol. 36:251–270, 1958.

GERSH, I. Histochemical studies on the mammalian kidney. II. The glomerular elimination of uric acid in the rabbit. Anat. Rec. 58:369–385, 1934.

GOTTSCHALK, C. W., AND MYLLE, M. Micropuncture study on the mammalian urinary concentrating mechanism: evidence for the countercurrent hypothesis. Am. J. Physiol. 196:927–936, 1959.

GRAHAM, R. C., AND KARNOVSKY, M. J. The early stage of absorption of injected horseradish peroxidase in the proximal convoluted tubules of mouse kidney: ultrastructural cytochemistry by a new technique. J. Histochem. Cytochem. 14:291–302, 1966.

HATT, P.-Y. The juxtaglomerular apparatus. In Ultrastructure of the Kidney (Dalton, A. J., and Haguenau, F., editors), pp. 101–141. Academic Press, New York, 1967.

HICKS, R. M. The fine structure of the transitional epithelium of rat ureter. J. Cell Biol. 26:25–48, 1965.

KARNOVSKY, M. J., AND RYAN, G. B. Substructure of the glomerular slit diaphragm in freeze-fractured normal rat kidney. J. Cell Biol. 65:233–236, 1975.

KIRKMAN, H., AND STOWELL, R. E. Renal filtration surface in the albino rat. Anat. Rec. 82:373–392, 1942.

LATTA, H., JOHNSTON, W. H., AND STANLEY, T. M. Sialoglycoproteins and filtration barriers in the glomerular capillary wall. J. Ultrastruct. Res. 51:354–376, 1975.

LATTA, H., MAUNSBACH, A. B., AND OSVALDO, L. The fine structure of renal tubules in cortex and medulla. In Ultrastructure of the Kidney (Dalton, A. J., and Haguenau, F., editors), pp. 2–56. Academic Press, New York, 1967.

MACCALLUM, D. B. The bearing of degenerating glomeruli on the problem of the vascular supply of the mammalian kidney. Am. J. Anat. 65:69–93, 1939.

MALVIN, R. L., WILDE, W. S., AND SULLIVAN, L. P. Localization of nephron transport by stop flow analysis. Am. J. Physiol. 194:135–142, 1958.

MOLLENDORFF, W. v. Der Exkretions-apparat. Handb. mikr. Anat. Menschen. (v. Möllendorff, editor), vol. 7, pt. 1, pp. 1–328. Springer-Verlag, Berlin, 1930.

7, pt. 1, pp. 1–328. Springer-Verlag, Berlin, 1930.

MONIS, B., AND DORFMAN, H. D. Some histochemical observations on transitional epithelium of man. J. Histochem. Cytochem. 15:475–481, 1967.

MONIS, B., AND ZAMBRANO, D. Ultrastructure of transitional epithelium of man. Z. Zellforsch. 87:101–117, 1968.

PEASE, D. C. Fine structure of the kidney seen by electron microscopy. J. Histochem. Cytochem.

3:295–308, 1955.

PETER, K. Untersuchungen über Bau und Entwicklung der Niere. Fischer, Jena, 1927.

PITTS, R. F. Physiology of the Kidney and Body Fluids; an Introductory Text. Year Book Medical Publishers, Chicago, 1968.

RHODIN, J. A. G. Electron microscopy of the kidney. In Renal Disease (Black, D. A. K., editor). Blackwell Scientific Publications, Ltd., Oxford, 1962.

RHODIN, J. A. G. The diaphragm of capillary endothelial fenestrations. J. Ultrastruct. Res. 6:171–185, 1962.

RICHARDS, A. N. Urine formation in the amphibian kidney. Harvey Lectures, Ser. 30, pp. 93–118, 1935.

RODEWALD, R., AND KARNOVSKY, M. J. Porous substructure of the glomerular slit diaphragm in the rat and mouse. J. Cell Biol. 60:423–433, 1974.

SMITH, H. W. The Kidney: Structure and Function in Health and Disease. Oxford University Press, New York, 1951.

SMITH, H. W. Principles of Renal Physiology. Oxford University Press, New York, 1956.

STRAUS, W. Cytochemical observations on the relationship between lysosomes and phagosomes in kidney and liver by combined staining for acid phosphatase and intravenously injected horseradish peroxidase. J. Cell Biol. 20:497–507, 1964.

STRUM, J. M., AND DANON, D. Fine structure of the urinary bladder of the bullfrog. Anat. Rec. 178:15–40, 1974.

TRUETA, R. J. Studies of the Renal Circulation. Charles C Thomas, Publisher, Springfield, Ill., 1948.

TRUMP, B. F., AND BULGER, R. E. Morphology of the Kidney. In Structural Basis of Renal Disease (Becker, E. L., editor), pp. 1–92. Hoeber Medical Division, Harper & Row, New York, 1968.

WAGERMARK, J., UNGERSTEDT, U., AND LJUNGGVIST, A. Sympathetic innervation of the juxtaglomerular cells of the kidney. Circ. Res. 22:149–153, 1968.

WALKER, F. The origin, turnover and removal of glomerular basement membrane. J. Pathol. 110:233–244, 1973.

WALKER, A. M., BOTT, P. A., OLIVER, J., AND MAC-DOWELL, M. C. The collection and analysis of fluid from nephrons of the mammalian kidney. Am. J. Physiol. 134:580–595, 1941.

WEBER, W. A., AND WONG, W. T. The function of the basal filaments in the parietal layer of Bowman's capsule. Can. J. Physiol. Pharmacol. 51:53–60, 1973.

WIRZ, H. Der osmotische Druck in den corticalen Tubuli der Rattenniere. Helv. Physiol. Acta 14:353–362, 1956.

CHAPTER 19

The Male Reproductive System

The reproductive system of the male consists of the testes, the various excretory ducts, the accessory reproductive glands—seminal vesicles, prostate and bulbourethral glands—and the penis (Fig. 19-1).

The essential constituents of the seminal fluid, the spermatozoa, are not products of cellular secretion but are themselves cellular elements that are formed in the tubules of the testis and leave the body through the genital ducts. For this reason, the testes, and the ovaries as well, are known as *cytogenic* organs. The other constituents of the semen are not formed in the testis but are secreted by the genital ducts, seminal vesicles, prostate and bulbourethral glands. Besides forming the cellular sex elements, the testes and ovaries secrete physiologically important substances directly into the blood, and hence they are endocrine glands.

The *testes* are ovoid or walnut-shaped bodies that have the organization of compound tubular glands. Each testis is enclosed in a dense fibrous capsule, the *tunica albuginea*, underneath which there is a looser layer of connective tissue rich in blood vessels, the *tunica vasculosa*. A closed serous sac, the *tunica vaginalis*, surrounds the anterior and lateral surfaces of the testis. This cleftlike sac is a detached diverticulum from the peritoneal cavity. The testes have approximately the same relationship with this sac as they had with the peritoneal cavity before their descent into the scrotum. The visceral layer of the

tunica vaginalis adheres as a smooth, glistening membrane to the tunica albuginea; the parietal layer lines the inner surface of the scrotum. Both layers are lined by mesothelial cells. Posteriorly the serous sac is lacking, the testis lying behind and outside the tunica vaginalis.

The tunica albuginea of the posterior portion of the testis is greatly thickened to form the *mediastinum testis* or *corpus Highmori*, from which connective tissue septa, the *septula testis*, radiate into the organ and blend with the tunica albuginea at various points (Fig. 19-1). In this way, the interior of the testis is subdivided into a number of pyramidal lobules, with bases directed toward the periphery and apices at the mediastinum. The septula do not form complete partitions; the lobules anastomose with each other in numerous places.

Behind the testis and outside of its tunica albuginea is an elongated body, the *epididymis*. Three regions may be distinguished in it: (1) an upper expanded portion, the *head* or *globus major*, which projects above the upper pole of the testis, (2) a narrower middle portion or *body*, and (3) a somewhat thickened lower portion, the *tail* or *globus minor*. At the lower pole of the testis, the tail of the epididymis turns sharply upon itself and becomes continuous with the main excretory duct, the *ductus deferens*.

Each lobule of the testis contains several intricately coiled tubules, the *seminiferous tubules*, surrounded and supported by in-

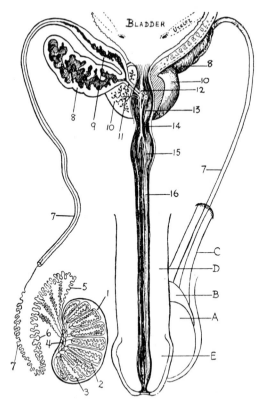

Fig. 19-1. Sketch of male genital organs. *A*, testis; *B*, head of epididymis; *C*, spermatic cord; *D*, penis, *E*, glans penis; *1*, tunica albuginea; *2*, septum of testis; *3*, seminiferous tubule; *4*, mediastinum with rete testis; *5*, ductulus efferens; *6*, ductus epididymis; *7*, ductus deferens; *8*, seminal vesicle; *9*, ampulla of ductus deferens; *10*, prostate gland; *11*, ejaculatory duct; *12*, colliculus seminalis with opening of utriculus prostaticus; *13*, *14* and *16*, prostatic, membranous and penile portions of urethra; *15*, bulb of urethra. (After Dickinson.)

tertubular connective tissue. They have a length of 30 to 70 cm and a caliber varying in different individuals from 150 to 300 μm. In the same individual, the diameter is relatively constant.

The tubules do not end blindly but form single, double or even triple arches. Both limbs of an arch are not always in the same lobule. Communication between the tubules of adjacent lobules is established by lateral branches that pass through the incomplete interlobular septa. The course of the seminiferous tubules, which has been determined in laboratory mammals by teasing out the tubules after maceration and

by reconstructions, forms the basis of the description given here. Toward the apex of a lobule, the convoluted tubules unite with the narrow *straight tubules*, which are about 30 μm in diameter. The straight tubules pass into the mediastinum and there empty into an irregular network of thin walled channels, the *rete testis* (Fig. 19-15). The straight tubules and rete testis form the beginning of the genital duct system.

From the rete testis arise 8 to 15 tubules, the *ductuli efferentes*, which pass into the head of the epididymis and there converge to form the *duct of the epididymis* (Fig. 19-1). The efferent ductules start as straight tubules but, soon after leaving the mediastinum, they pursue a tortuous spiral course, each tubule with its surrounding connective tissue forming a conical lobule or *conus vasculosus* of the head of the epididymis. The length of the efferent tubules is about 6 to 10 cm. The most anterior ductule becomes directly continuous with the duct of the epididymis, which then receives the remaining efferent ductules at shorter or longer intervals.

The duct of the epididymis is an enormously convoluted tubule having a length of about 4 m. It begins in the head, where it receives the ductuli efferentes, and winds in a most intricate manner through the body and tail of the epididymis. At the caudal pole, it turns sharply upon itself and passes without any definite demarcation into the *ductus deferens*.

The Testis

The Seminiferous Tubule

The wall of a seminiferous tubule consists of (a) an outer capsule or tunica propria of fibroelastic connective tissue and flattened fibroblastic cells, which closely invest the tubule, (b) a basal lamina and (c) a lining of a complex stratified epithelium (Fig. 19-2).

The flattened cells of the tunica propria are in multiple layers in primates. The layer closest to the epithelium usually assumes characteristics of smooth muscle and these cells are referred to as *myoid cells*. There is evidence that such cells in lower animals may assist the transport of sperm out of

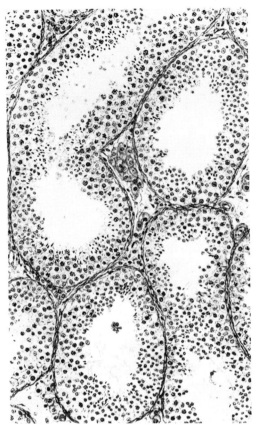

Fig. 19-2. Section through the right testis of a healthy man, 34 years of age. ×150. (After Stieve.)

the tubules by their contractions, but this function has not been documented for the human.

A basal lamina separates the epithelium from the tunica propria. Actually, the myoid cells are completely enclosed by a basal lamina-like layer (external lamina) as are typical smooth muscle cells.

The epithelium consists of two kinds of cells, the supporting cells or cells of Sertoli and the spermatogenic cells.

(1) The *cells of Sertoli* (Figs. 19-3 and 19-5) are tall, irregularly columnar cells that extend from the basal lamina to the lumen. Their sides are markedly uneven, showing pits and depressions into which fit the adjoining germ cells. The nucleus is ovoid and pale staining with finely dispersed chromatin, and it usually contains one or more prominent nucleoli. The nuclear membrane often shows a characteristic longitudinal

groove. The location of the nucleus varies in different Sertoli cells from the basal position to positions located at a considerable distance from the basal lamina. Electron micrographs show that the mitochondria, described as filamentous from light microscope studies, are unusually long and slender. In addition to the usual organelles, the cytoplasm contains lipid droplets, glycogen and, in man, a spindle-shaped crystalloid. The cell border is difficult to distinguish in routinely stained preparations, but the entire cell and its borders can be defined by silver methods.

The Sertoli cells are the only ones that extend from the basal lamina to the lumen, and thus they give structural organization to the tubule. They rest on the basal lamina in a patterned array that is readily seen in silver preparations of tangential sections of the tubule. Following the Sertoli cell from the basal lamina to the lumen, one finds that it is surrounded first by spermatogonia and then by different stages of spermatocytes and spermatids. The pattern of arrangement is seen best at the level of the primary spermatocytes, which are arranged in rings around the Sertoli cell. In ordinary preparations it frequently appears that the spermatogenic cells are contained within the cytoplasm of the Sertoli cells.

Electron micrographs show the presence of occluding junctions between the basal portions of apposing Sertoli cells. Studies with tracers indicate that these junctions are mainly responsible for a blood-testis barrier at the level of the preleptotene primary spermatocytes (Fig. 19-3).

Freeze-fracture studies have revealed even more strikingly the extensiveness of the occluding junctions (Fig. 19-4). In effect these specializations establish two intercellular compartments within the seminiferous tubule. The basal compartment permits fairly free exchange of nutrients and waste products between the interstitial vasculature and the more primitive spermatogenic cells. The more apical compartment, beyond the level of the occluding junctions, is isolated from such direct exchanges. Thus, the Sertoli cells control the availability of substances presented to the more differentiated stages of the developing germ cells.

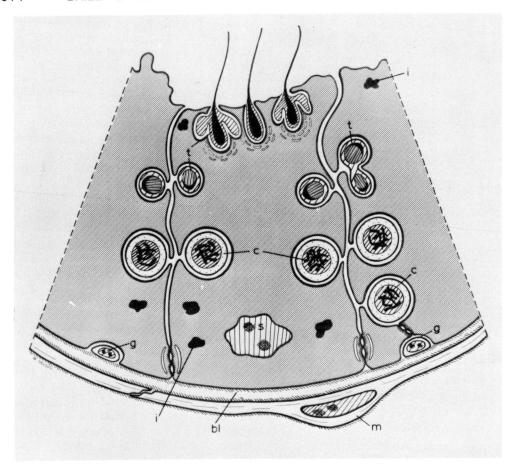

Fig. 19-3. Diagram of cellular relationships in the seminiferous tubule. Sertoli cells extend from the basal lamina to the tubule lumen. Invaginations of their surface membranes surround the developing germ cells throughout maturation. Early spermatogonia are exposed to the basal lamina but by the time they have differentiated into spermatocytes they have lost this relationship and have migrated luminally past a series of occluding junctions. The occluding junctions isolate the maturing germ cells from direct influence of substances present in the intertubular connective tissue spaces, thus providing a blood-testis barrier. *g*, spermatogonia; *c*, spermatocytes; *t*, spermatids; *s*, Sertoli cell nucleus; *i*, inclusion bodies in Sertoli cell cytoplasm; *bl*, basal lamina; *m*, myoid cell.

The Sertoli cells are also responsible for phagocytosis of residual cytoplasm cast off during maturation of spermatocytes and for the synthesis of androgen-binding protein that helps to maintain the high androgen levels within the seminiferous tubule essential for proper germ cell differentiation.

Special staining methods show that the cytoplasmic processes of the Sertoli cells increase in number and size when the spermatids are maturing. Thus, the Sertoli cells exhibit a cyclic activity that is correlated with the stage of spermatogenesis in any given region of the seminiferous tubule.

(2) The *spermatogenic cells* lie between the cells of Sertoli in an orderly manner, with four to eight layers occupying the space between the basal lamina and the lumen. In the undeveloped testis, only the primitive germ cells or spermatogonia are present. With the onset of sexual maturity, the spermatogenic cells are represented in all stages of differentiation and are arranged in several more or less distinct layers (Fig. 19-5).

The primitive germ cells, or *spermatogonia*, from which all of the spermatozoa are ultimately derived, are located directly

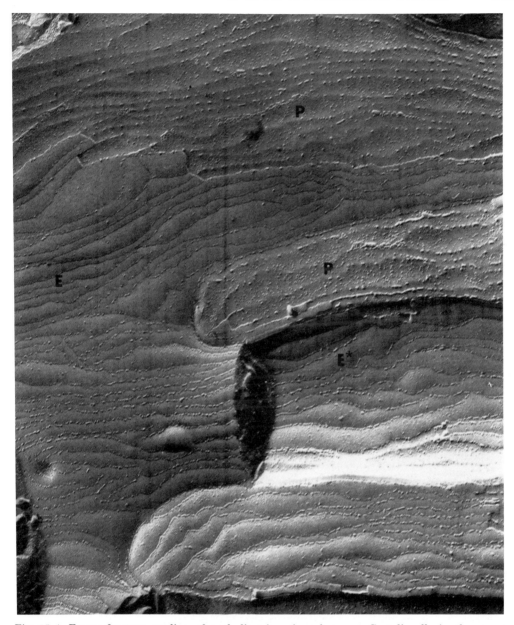

Fig. 19-4. Freeze-fracture replica of occluding junctions between Sertoli cells in the mouse. Granular material occurs on the ridges and in the grooves of the fractured membrane surfaces. *E*, fracture face adjacent to cell exterior; *P*, fracture faces adjacent to cell cytoplasm; *E**, E fracture face of a second cell process. ×47,000. (Courtesy of Dr. Toshio Nagano.)

inside the basal lamina. They are spherical or cuboidal in shape, with a diameter of about 12 μm. They have a spherical nucleus with granular chromatin. They divide to maintain their own number and to provide the cells that differentiate into spermatocytes. Two main types of spermatogonia can be identified by special stains, namely, the *A* and the *B* spermatogonia. They differ in the intensity of cytoplasmic staining, and the A cells usually have one or two nucleoli at the inner surface of the nuclear envelope, whereas the B cells usually have a centrally located nucleolus. An A cell may divide either into two new stem cells or into two derivatives. The latter divide further before differentiating into spermatocytes. Electron micrographs show that the majority of divisions of the spermatogonia are incomplete regarding the cytoplasm, and that spermatogonia, spermatocytes and spermatids remain connected by cytoplasmic bridges until maturation into spermatozoa is nearly finished (Fig. 19-6). Only a small number of primitive type A spermatogonia have complete cytoplasmic divisions and thereby maintain a stem cell population of spermatogonia.

The *primary spermatocytes* lie next to the spermatogonia on their inner side. They are large cells with a diameter of 17 to 19 μm and are formed from the innermost layer of the spermatogonia (Fig. 19-7). The chromatin of the large vesicular nuclei has

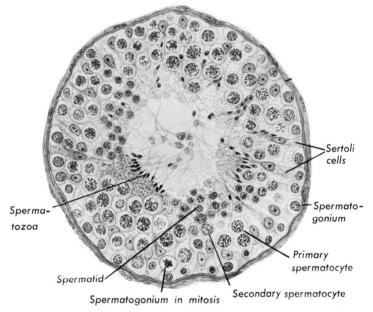

Fig. 19-5. Section through a seminiferous tubule of a man 19 years old showing the basic organization. ×360. (After Stieve.)

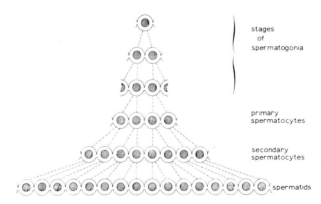

Fig. 19-6. Diagram illustrating germ cell interconnection beginning with spermatogonia and continuing through successive divisions and the formation of spermatids. The interconnections are a result of incomplete cytokinesis. Because of the interconnections among spermatogonia, the final number of interconnected spermatids can be considerably greater than the 16 cells shown here. During spermiogenesis the sloughing cytoplasm remains interconnected as residual bodies are formed.

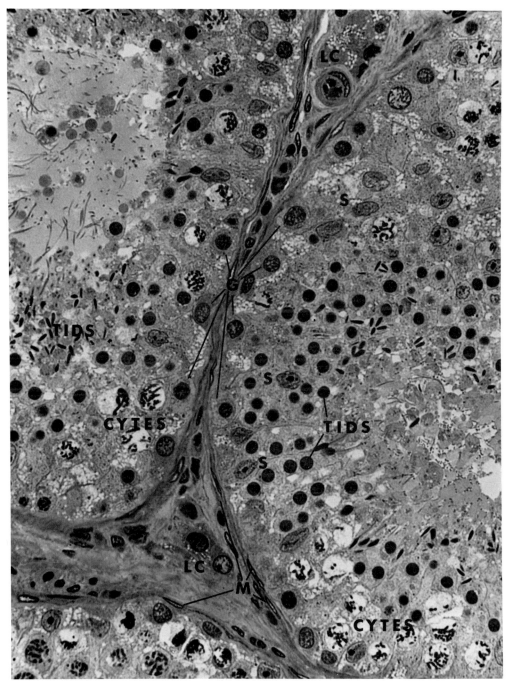

Fig. 19-7. Light micrograph of seminiferous tubules of the monkey testis. The progression of maturation of the germ cells is from gonial cells (*G*) to spermatocytes (*CYTES*) to spermatids (*TIDS*). Early spermatids are indicated in the tubule to the *right* and late spermatids in the tubule to the *left*. Myoid cells (*M*) are seen at the surfaces of the tubules and Leydig cells (*LC*) appear in the interstitial regions. ×1300.

a variable appearance, depending on the stage of meiotic prophase. This stage of spermatogenesis is a lengthy one in which the critical events of genetic exchange between replicated strands of DNA occur prior to reduction in genetic content which is characteristic of germ cell development (details below).

Each primary spermatocyte gives rise to two smaller *secondary spermatocytes* that lie internal to the primary spermatocytes. Almost as soon as it is formed, each secondary spermatocyte divides to form two spermatids. As noted above, the progeny of these spermatocyte divisions remain interconnected by cytoplasmic bridges resulting in clusters of 16 or more interconnected spermatids. The clusters of developing spermatids may be associated with more than one Sertoli cell. The Sertoli cells, in turn, are joined to each other by gap (communicating) junctions (Fig. 19-8). It is thought that these relationships are important in synchronizing the development of groups of spermatozoa.

The *spermatids* adjoin the lumen of the

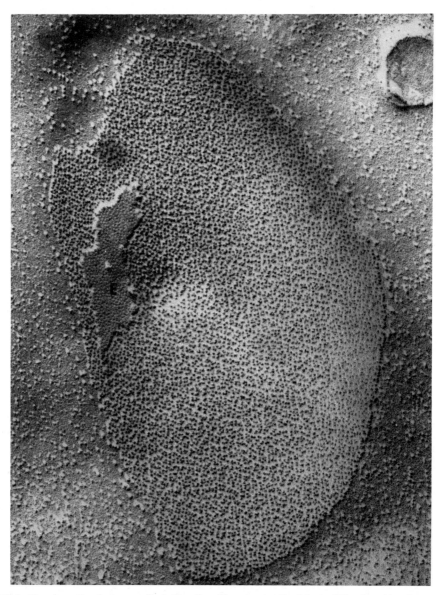

Fig. 19-8. Gap junction between Sertoli cells of human testis. Most of the junction is seen on the P fracture face but a small fragment of fracture face E of the adjacent cell is visible at *E*. ×90,000. (Courtesy of Dr. Toshio Nagano.)

tubule. They are easily recognized by their small size (about 9 μm) and location. These cells form the last generation in the spermatogenic process. They undergo no further division but, by profound changes in their structure, they become directly transformed into the mature *spermatozoa*. The process of transformation of spermatids into spermatozoa is referred to as *spermiogenesis*.

As the spermatids mature their flagellated tails extend out into the lumen of the tubule. When they are released from the Sertoli cell to become free in the lumen they are called spermatozoa. Actually, free spermatozoa in the lumen of the tubule are relatively rare, for as soon as they are detached from the Sertoli cells they pass into the epididymis for storage and a variable amount of additional maturation.

In lower animals that have a continuous reproductive activity the histological appearance of the seminiferous tubules varies along its length. This is a reflection of the fact that the process of germ cell maturation requires a finite period of time. This total maturation time is referred to as *spermatogenesis*. A confusing terminology has arisen in reference to the process of spermatogenesis and the cytological changes within the seminiferous tubule. The timing for spermatogenesis was worked out by noting that certain patterns of cellular relationships occur and, after radioactive labeling, determining the time necessary for a similar pattern to reappear at the same location in the tubule. The time so measured is related to the total maturation time for the germ cells but is not identical. The cycle of reestablishing identical cellular relationship patterns in the seminiferous epithelium has been termed the *spermatogenic cycle,* a misleading term, for one would tend to consider the total maturation time as the spermatogenic cycle. In the rat the spermatogenic cycle is 12 days and there are four cycles between the earliest differentiation of a spermatogium into a spermatocyte and the development of mature spermatozoa; the total time of spermatogenesis then is 48 days. In human the spermatogenic cycle is 16 days and spermatogenesis takes a total of 64 days. (70)

In addition to the confusion in terminol-

ogy with regard to spermatogenesis, adjacent regions of the tubule appear to be influenced by their neighbors in such a way that release of spermatozoa proceeds sequentially down the tubule toward the rete testis. This sequential release is called the *spermatogenic wave.*

The precise timing for the maturation and release of spermatozoa is difficult to appreciate for human testis because cellular relationships and germ cell maturation occur in a mosaic pattern along the tubule rather than being uniform at any specific level of the tubule. The picture is further complicated in human seminiferous tubules by the fact that active areas of germ cell proliferation appear to be intermingled with inactive areas. Despite these complications, careful studies have shown that spermatogenesis in human proceeds under the same precise controls as in lower animals; both a spermatogenic cycle and a semblance of a spermatogenic wave have been described.

In animals with periodic rutting seasons, transverse sections through several seminiferous tubules during the rutting season show all stages of spermatogenesis. During the long intermissions between breeding seasons, the tubules revert to a prepubertal condition and contain only spermatogonia and Sertoli cells.

In many human testes secured at autopsy, there are regions in which spermatogenesis is greatly reduced or entirely absent, the seminiferous epithelium either reverting to a prepubertal condition or occasionally showing an entire absence of germ cells. After prolonged sickness and in senility, the degenerative changes may be very pronounced. Fairly extensive degenerative changes in the testes may also occur in medically normal men during the reproductive period of life. In studies of medically normal men ranging in age from 20 to 50 years, Sand and Okkels found that only 17 of their 72 cases showed a structural condition of the testes that is usually depicted in textbooks as normal. In the remainder, the basement membrane and capsule of the seminiferous tubules and often the intertubular connective tissue were thickened either diffusely or in localized areas. Hyalinization of the connective tissue was not infrequent. In about one-third of their cases, spermatogenesis was severely reduced. They noted that the illustrations of seminiferous tubules in textbooks of histology must have been obtained from carefully selected material. Figure 19-9 illustrates pronounced degenerative changes in the testes of a healthy middle aged individual.

The mechanism causing the sperm to pass from the seminiferous tubules into the rete and hence into the efferent ductules, a very considerable journey, is of particular interest. The sperm do not become motile until they leave the testes and the duct system of the reproductive tract and, consequently, their migration cannot be caused

by an intrinsic movement. Experimental studies on laboratory animals show that a considerable quantity of fluid is "secreted" by the seminiferous tubules and resorbed by the rete tubules, efferent tubules and the duct of the epididymis. The current thus produced may be an important factor in moving the sperm from the seminiferous tubules. As mentioned previously, the movement of sperm out of the tubules also may be aided by contraction of myoid cells in the walls of the tubules. Beginning with the efferent tubules, the walls of the ducts have appreciable amounts of typical smooth muscle.

The testes of sexually mature mammals

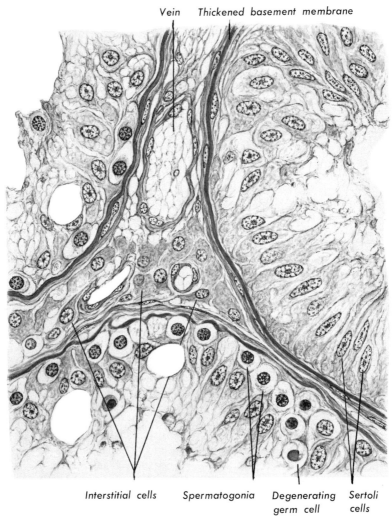

Vein   Thickened basement membrane

Interstitial cells   Spermatogonia   Degenerating germ cell   Sertoli cells

Fig. 19-9. Parts of three seminiferous tubules, showing pronounced degeneration. The tissue was from a healthy middle aged man. Camera lucida drawing. ×565.

are rich in hyaluronidase. This enzyme is present elsewhere (chapter 1), but the testes of slaughterhouse animals are the main source of the hyaluronidase used experimentally and clinically. There is more than one hyaluronidase; that derived from testes is designated as "testicular hyaluronidase."

Spermatozoa are the source (or carriers) of testicular hyaluronidase. The latter is not present in the testes before sexual maturity or in those devoid of sperm. It is still present in sperm that have been washed several times. If sperm are autolyzed, a large amount of the enzyme is found. Hyaluronidase is present in semen, being localized chiefly in the sperm.

Spermatogenesis

The cytological details and genetic significance of spermatogenesis are fully discussed in textbooks of genetics. Only a brief sketch can be given here of the various changes through which the primitive germ cells are transformed into mature sperm (Fig. 19-10).

It is convenient to distinguish several successive periods or stages in spermatogenesis as outlined above, even though the stages merge into one another as parts of a continuous process.

The nucleus of each spermatogonium, the stem cell from which all sperm are eventually derived, contains the somatic or diploid number of chromosomes. This number in man is 46, consisting of 23 pairs; one member of each pair is of maternal and the other of paternal origin. After a number of ordinary mitotic divisions, by which each daughter cell receives the diploid number of chromosomes, the last generation of spermatogonia enters an intermitotic period characterized by growth and by nuclear change leading to differentiation of the cells to primary spermatocytes.

At the close of the growth period of the primary spermatocyte, long thread-like chromosomes can be seen in the nucleus that seem to be like those present in early prophase stages of spermatogonia. As the threads shorten and thicken, however, it can be seen that they are not single as in mitotic prophase, but double as the result of synapsis (pairing) of homologous chromosomes. Instead of 46 single chromosomes, there are 23 double threads. Next, each member of the pair, having replicated DNA prior to prophase, partially divides and a tetrad is formed. The tetrads have individual differences in size and form by which they may be identified. Even after they thicken and go on to the spindle, they retain individual characteristics.

In the *first maturation division,* the chromosomes that paired during synapsis become separated, one member from each pair going to each of the resulting two secondary spermatocytes. This division differs from ordinary mitosis in that it does not consist of the longitudinal splitting of individual chromosomes after DNA replication,

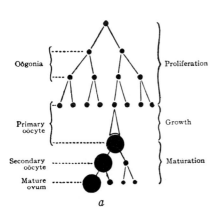

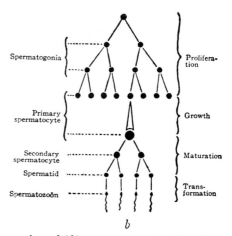

Fig. 19-10. Diagrams comparing stages of (*a*) oogenesis and (*b*)spermatogenesis. (Modified from Boveri.)

but whole, previously paired chromosomes are separated from each other, the daughter cells actually receiving only half the somatic number. It is a *reductional* or *heterotypic* division, in contrast to the ordinary *equational* or *homeotypic* division. It is the first nuclear division in the process known as *meiosis,* in contrast to *mitosis.* Each tetrad separates into two dyads, each dyad representing an original single chromosome whose DNA was replicated precociously for the second maturation division. The result of meiosis is the production of germ cells with a haploid number of chromosomes. Of equal importance is the exchange of segments of homologous chromosomes, a process known as *crossing over,* during the prolonged meiotic prophase. Thus, the maturing spermatids have a different genetic composition from typical somatic diploid cells. The importance of the dual compartments of the seminiferous epithelium should now become apparent. Cells of different genetic composition have the potential of eliciting an immune response by the rest of the body; the Sertoli cell occluding junctions provide a barrier that normally prevents such an undesirable interaction from occurring.

The two secondary spermatocytes, which are smaller than the primary spermatocyte, pass through a short interphase period and then enter the second maturation division to form four spermatids. The dyads are separated into single elements or monads, and one monad from each dyad goes to each daughter cell. Each spermatid is about half the size of the secondary spermatocytes.

By spermatogenesis, every primary spermatocyte, the tetrad spermatocyte, gives rise to four spermatids, each containing the haploid number of chromosomes. Likewise, each spermatid nucleus contains only half as much DNA as those of the spermatogonia.

It is important to keep in mind that the terms haploid and diploid were first introduced to describe chromosome numbers. During spermatogenesis the DNA content has been replicated to a tetraploid condition prior to the first meiotic prophase, exactly as occurs in the interphase preceding an ordinary mitosis. Because of the pairing of homologous chromosomes and their separation in the first meiotic division, the chromosome number has been reduced to haploid in the secondary spermatocyte but the DNA is still present in diploid amount. The second meiotic division results in the haploid content of DNA in each definitive spermatid.

A similar reduction in number of chromosomes and in DNA content occurs during the maturation of the oocytes. Fertilization restores the diploid number of chromosomes with the characteristic amount of DNA.

The members of one pair of chromosomes (the sex chromosomes) are dissimilar in the male. One is known as the X chromosome and is of maternal origin. The other is the Y chromosome, of paternal origin. When the members of homologous pairs of chromosomes separate during the meiotic division of the primary spermatocytes, one half of the secondary spermatocytes receive an X chromosome, whereas the other half receive a Y chromosome. This differs from the condition in the female, in which each ovum contains an X chromosome. Consequently, when a sperm carrying an X chromosome fertilizes an ovum, an XX combination is established and a female develops. On the other hand, when a sperm bearing a Y chromosome fertilizes an ovum, an XY combination is produced and the embryo develops as a male.

Spermiogenesis

The spermatids do not divide but mature to form the spermatozoa by a process known as spermiogenesis. During most of their maturation, the spermatids are enveloped by the cytoplasmic processes of the Sertoli cells, from which they apparently receive nourishment. A specialized attachment region occurs at the surface of the Sertoli cell where the spermatids are present. The mechanism by which the mature spermatids are released from their special relationship to the Sertoli cell is not understood.

The spermatids are small cells, about half the size of the secondary spermatocytes. They have round and rather dark staining nuclei. The stages of their transformation into mature sperm have been clarified by the use of electron microscopy.

One of the earliest changes is in the Golgi complex where small granules, known as *proacrosomal granules,* appear in some of the Golgi vacuoles. Fusion of these leads to the formation of a larger vacuole with a relatively large granule, the *acrosomal granule,* visible with the light microscope. Continued growth of the acrosomal complex occurs by incorporation of other newly formed vesicles and granules. In the meantime, the acrosomal system of the Golgi complex moves closer to the nucleus, thereby marking the anterior pole of the cell. The acrosomal vesicle increases its zone of contact with the nucleus, and then the vesicle, with its enclosed acrosomal material, forms a caplike structure over the anterior two-thirds of the nucleus that is known as the *acrosomal cap,* or head cap. The cap can be identified as a distinct structure in the mature sperm of many species, but in man it becomes closely flattened against the nucleus.

Concurrently with the changes outlined above, the centrioles move toward the caudal portion of the cell, where the distal centriole functions as a basal body for the development of the flagellum. Then the centrioles and the base of the flagellum move back toward the nucleus. The proximal centriole becomes closely applied to the caudal pole of the nucleus and maintains its ultrastructural characteristics in the mature sperm. While these changes have been occurring, a ring appears around the nucleus at about the level of the caudal end of the acrosomal cap. Microtubules project caudally from the ring, forming a cylindrical *caudal sheath* or *manchette.* This is followed by a rapid elongation of the cell, accompanied by a redistribution of cytoplasm caudally, and the mitochondria move to a position in the proximal portion of the developing tail of the sperm.

While the changes in centrioles are occurring, another structure known as an *annulus* arises in a region near the distal centriole. It was once named a ring centriole, although it has none of the structural features of a centriole. The annulus eventually moves to a position at the caudal end of the middle piece of the tail (Fig. 19-11).

In summary, spermiogenesis produces a slender motile cell retaining only the essentials for fertilization and for transmitting hereditary material. It retains its nucleus, the Golgi-derived acrosomal cap, a proximal centriole and mitochondria; the remainder of the cytoplasm is extruded.

The Mature Spermatozoa

The spermatozoa are slender, motile, flagellate bodies having a total length of 55 to 65 μm. They are formed in enormous numbers. It has been estimated that about 60,000 spermatozoa are contained in 1 mm^3 seminal fluid, or 200 to 600 million in a single ejaculation. By the undulatory motion of the tail, they can move independently, and when fully active they can cover a distance of 1 to 3 mm/min. In the seminiferous tubules and ducts of the testis, they are sluggish or entirely quiescent. When expelled by the peristaltic action of the ductus deferens and duct of the epididymis, they are activated into movement by the secretion of the accessory genital glands, especially the prostate. In the favorable environment of the male genital tract, the spermatozoa remain alive for some time after leaving the testis. Living spermatozoa have been found in the epididymis several weeks after the experimental ligation of the ductuli efferentes. In the female reproductive tract, their life is short.

The mature spermatozoan consists of a *head* and a *tail.* The latter is composed of the following parts in sequence: *middle piece, principal piece* and *end piece.* The junction between the head and tail is known as the *neck.*

The *head* of the human spermatozoan is a flattened, oval body with a length of 4 to 5 μm and a maximal width of about 3 μm. The anterior portion is thinner than the posterior so that in profile it is pear-shaped (Fig. 19-11). It consists chiefly of a nucleus with compact, deep staining chromatin enclosed within the nuclear envelope. The anterior two-thirds of the nuclear envelope is covered by the acrosomal cap, and the entire cell is covered by the cell membrane or plasmalemma. The different membranes

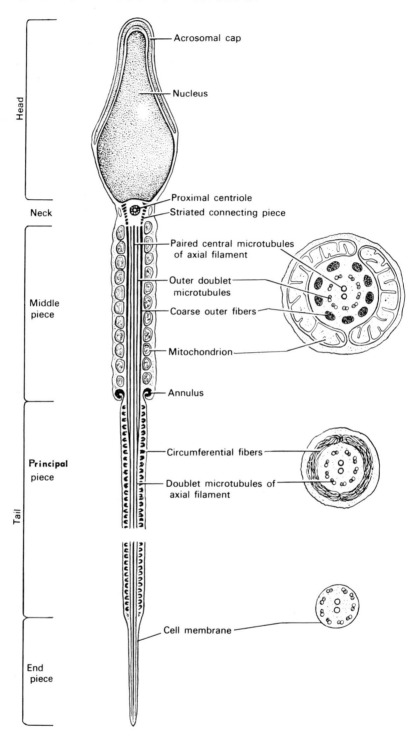

Fig. 19-11. Diagrammatic representation of the structure of a mature spermatozoon as determined by light and electron microscopic studies. At the *left*, a longitudinal section; at the *right*, transverse sections of the tail at levels of the middle piece, principal piece, and end piece, respectively. (Diagrams based on descriptions and electron micrographs by Dr. Don W. Fawcett.)

cannot be identified by light microscopy. An understanding of their structure and arrangement has evolved from electron microscope studies of developing sperm.

The *neck* is a short region connecting the head of the sperm with the middle piece. The proximal centriole is located against the basal end of the nucleus (or head) at an angle of about 45° to the axis of the tail. The peripheral portion of the neck region contains coarse fibers that are continuous with the longitudinally oriented fibers of the middle piece. Electron micrographs show that some of the coarse fibers are fused in the neck region, and they also appear cross banded due to electron-lucent segments. The central pair of microtubules of the flagellum continues farther into the neck and closer to the proximal centriole than do the nine outer doublets.

The *middle piece* is about 5 to 9 μm in length and about 1 μm in width. It has a core with the typical structure of a flagellum or elongated cilium, i.e., a central pair of single microtubules surrounded by nine doublets (Figs. 19-11 and 19-12). Peripheral to the axial complex, there is a ring of nine longitudinally oriented, dense fibers. These are large and well defined in the proximal part of the middle piece, but they gradually taper and become more irregular during their course caudally in the middle piece. A sheath of longitudinally oriented mitochondria is a characteristic feature of the middle piece.

The *principal piece* is the longest portion of the tail, being 40 to 45 μm in length. It lacks the mitochondrial sheath of the middle piece, and the outer coarse fibers continue only a short distance into this segment in human sperm. A characteristic feature of the principal piece is a fibrous sheath shown by electron micrographs to consist of a large number of circumferentially oriented, riblike bundles that pass halfway around the axial filament complex

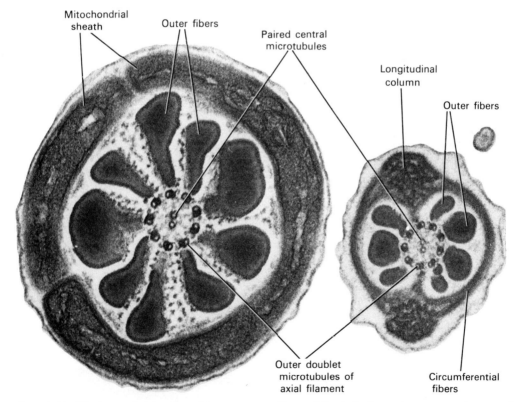

Fig. 19-12. Electron micrographs of transverse sections of the tail of a mature spermatozoon of a Chinese hamster. At the *left*, micrograph of a section through the middle piece; at the *right*, through the principal piece. (Courtesy of Dr. Don W. Fawcett.)

to fuse with two longitudinal columns of fibers (Fig. 19-12).

The *tail piece* is relatively short and slender, being about 5 to 10 μm in length. It has the typical appearance of a flagellum, with two single microtubules surrounded by nine doublets.

The significance of the different parts of the spermatozoon has been brought out in the description of its development. It is seen that the spermatozoon, like the mature ovum, is a sex cell containing one-half the somatic number of chromosomes. In spite of its small size and modified form, it contains all of the elements important for fertilization and heredity. The head carries the genetic material, a Golgi-derived acrosomal cap important in penetrating the ovum, and a centriole. The tail is a temporary accessory that enables the spermatozoon to reach the ovum by active movement. However, the exact functional roles of the specialized structural features of the middle piece and principal piece are not fully understood.

Tunica Albuginea

The *tunica albuginea testis* is a tough, fibrous membrane that encapsulates the testis (Fig. 19-13). It is about 0.5 mm in thickness. Externally it is covered by mesothelium. During the early development of the testis, this covering layer of epithelium is cuboidal and is the germinal epithelium.

Beneath the basal lamina of the simple squamous epithelium there is a layer of rather fine, closely woven collagenous fibers that blends with a deeper layer of interweaving, coarse collagenous fibers. This deeper layer forms the main component of the tunica albuginea. The inner part of the tunic is composed of looser connective tissue, the innermost part of which is highly vascular and is called the *tunica vasculosa*. Just beneath the tunica vasculosa are seminiferous tubules and delicate connective tissue, the latter forming the interlobular septa of the testis which are continuous with the tissue of the tunica vasculosa.

The surface epithelium of the testis and the subjacent connective tissue is often called the *visceral layer* of the *tunica vaginalis*. At the posterior part of the testis, this layer is continuous with the parietal layer of the tunica vaginalis. Between the visceral and parietal layers ia a cavity which is a remnant of the peritoneal cavity.

The tunica vasculosa contains numerous quite large blood vessels. Branches of these penetrate the denser part of the tunica albuginea.

Interstitial Cells

Besides the usual connective tissue elements, the stroma contains characteristic cells known as the *interstitial cells* or *cells of Leydig*. These cells form the internal secretion known as testosterone (see below under "Internal Secretion of the Testis").

The interstitial cells occur in groups of various sizes and are quite distinct in the

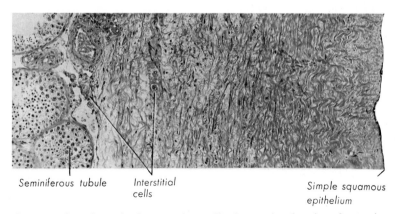

Seminiferous tubule   Interstitial cells   Simple squamous epithelium

Fig. 19-13. Cross section through the anterior wall of a testis, showing the tunics of the organ and subjacent seminiferous tubules. Masson's trichrome stain. ×104.

human testis (Figs. 19-7, 19-13 and 19-14). Small blood vessels are usually present in the groups. The interstitial cells are large and are ovoid or polygonal in shape. They have a large nucleus which is frequently eccentrically located. The cytoplasm of the interstitial cells is granular and fairly dense near the nucleus but peripherally it is vacuolated, and in usual preparations it stains quite lightly. This is largely due to the dissolving out of lipid granules and droplets. Most of the endoplasmic reticulum is of the smooth-surfaced type, and the mitochondria have tubular rather than shelflike cristae. These are characteristic but not universal features of cells that secrete steroid hormones. The interstitial cells also contain lipochrome pigment granules and crystalloids. The pigment granules increase in number in older men, and ultrastructural studies indicate that they may represent autophagic vacuoles. The crystalloids are rod-shaped structures and in cross section are oval or round. Their number and size vary greatly. They are formed of an albuminous substance and are quite resistant to solvents. Fixation soon after death is necessary to preserve them.

Electron micrographs show two types of Leydig cells: fusiform cells with relatively

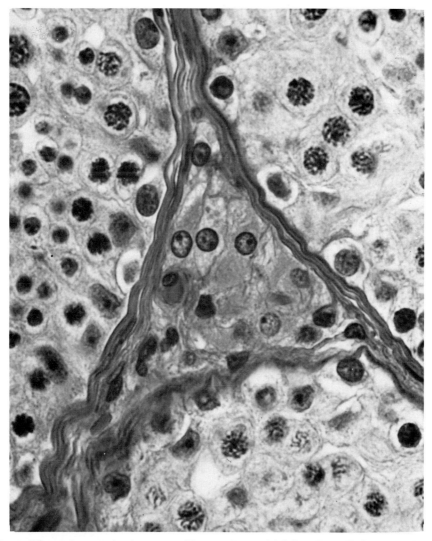

Fig. 19-14. Photomicrograph of a group of human interstitial (Leydig) cells between three contiguous seminiferous tubules. (Courtesy of Dr. Don W. Fawcett.)

few organelles, and large cells that have the usual organelles plus many small membrane-bounded vesicles, granules, lipid droplets, osmiophilic pigment and large protein crystals. The presence of cells with intermediate characteristics indicates that the fusiform cell is probably a precursor stage of the mature interstitial cell.

The Leydig cells arise from fibroblasts and may revert to cells that are indistinguishable from fibroblasts.

There are also numerous macrophages in the interstitial tissue interposed among the Leydig cells. In fact, many of the cells identified by light microscopy as Leydig cells are seen by electron microscopy to be macrophages. The significance of the numerous macrophages in this location is not yet understood.

Blood Vessels

Branches of the spermatic artery ramify in the mediastinum and tunica vasculosa. These send branches into the septa of the testis which give rise to a capillary network around the seminiferous tubules. The blood is collected by veins that accompany the arteries.

Lymphatics

In the intertubular tissue are numerous lymphatics, appearing as clefts lined by endothelium. These connect with lymph vessels in the mediastinum. Relatively few lymphatics are found in the tunica albuginea.

Nerves

Nerve fibers accompany the blood vessels and enter the interior of the testes through the mediastinum. Some fibers go to blood vessels; the termination of other fibers is not known.

The Genital Ducts

Straight Tubules and Rete Testis

At the juncture of a seminiferous tubule with a straight tubule, there is an abrupt change in structure. The junctures occur at varying distances from the rete, the straight tubules thus varying in length. Close to a juncture, the developing sex cells of a seminiferous tubule decrease in number and then finally disappear. The Sertoli cells change somewhat in structure, their cytoplasm becoming more vacuolated and their nuclei more dense. They increase in number and finally form a continuous epithelial layer. This protrudes into the enlarged end of the straight tubule (Figs. 19-15 and 19-16). The epithelial lining then changes abruptly into the columnar type characteristic of the straight tubules; subsequently there is a transition to the cuboidal cells lining the rete.

The rete testis is composed of wide, anastomosing channels, the general course of which is upward toward the ductuli efferentes. The spaces of the rete are lined by a simple epithelium that varies somewhat in height but is characteristically cuboidal (Fig. 19-15). Some of the cells have a single cilium (flagellum) that is connected to a basal body. No secretion droplets are present. In contrast with Sertoli cells, the nuclei stain deeply and the cell membrane is well defined. The tubules of the rete have no definite lamina propria that is distinct from the connective tissue comprising the mediastinum. No smooth muscle is present around the straight tubules or rete testis.

Ductuli Efferentes

The epithelium of the efferent ductules consists mainly of groups of high columnar cells alternating with groups of cuboidal cells. This gives the inner surface of the tubule a characteristic irregular contour, with the low cells lining cryptlike depressions or pockets (Fig. 19-17). The basal border of the tubule is not affected by the alternating height of the cells and has a relatively smooth contour. In addition to the columnar and cuboidal cells, rounded cells that do not extend to the lumen occasionally occur at intervals along the basal lamina; hence, the epithelium, strictly speaking, belongs to the pseudostratified type.

Cilia are present on many of the tall cells and generally absent from the cuboidal cells, but the distribution is variable. Most of the low cells have microvilli. Bleblike

Vein   Artery   Connective tissue of mediastinum

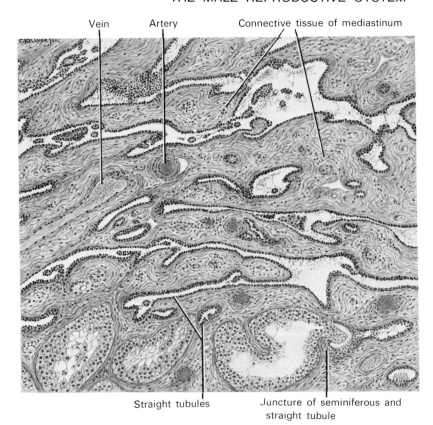

Straight tubules   Juncture of seminiferous and
                        straight tubule

Fig. 19-15. From a longitudinal section through a testis, showing a part of the mediastinum and
rete testis and the adjacent seminiferous tubules. The juncture of a seminiferous with a straight
tubule is shown in the *lower right quadrant* of the figure. The separation between the rete and the
straight tubules is topographical, not structural. The upper pole of the testis is to the *right*. Human,
accident case, 54 years old. ×65.

apical projections, generally interpreted as
secretory material, are seen on some cells
of both types. In addition to the usual organelles, the cytoplasm often contains fat
droplets and pigment granules. The cytoplasm of the cells with the higher content
of lipid takes a lighter stain in routine preparations.

The epithelial cells of the efferent ductules are generally described as secretory,
but studies of the pathway of injected dyes
show that the tubules also absorb some
substances. Beating of cilia, chiefly of the
tall columnar cells, aids in the transport of
sperm.

The epithelium rests on a distinct basement membrane, surrounded by a lamina
propria of connective tissue containing
many capillaries and some circular smooth
muscle fibers.

Ductus Epididymidis (Duct of the Epidid-
ymis)

The epididymis is a single elongated duct,
but its extreme tortuosity gives the impression in sectioned material that there are
several ducts making up the organ. Each
profile of the duct shows an even contour
of both the external and internal surfaces,
for the lining epithelial cells all end at the
same level and the underlying smooth muscle does not ordinarily contract sufficiently
to cause a folding of the mucosa. The lining
epithelium of the epididymis is composed
of two types of cells: very narrow, tall columnar cells and rounded or angular basal
cells (Figs. 19-18 and 19-19). Although it
cannot be determined with certainty, even
in very thin sections, that all of the columnar cells overlying the basal ones reach the

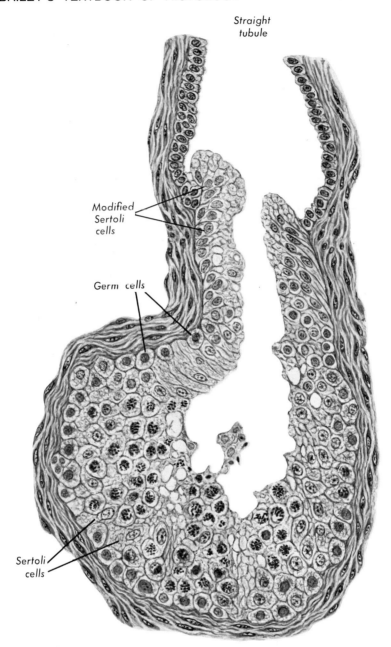

*Straight
tubule*

*Modified
Sertoli
cells*

Germ cells

*Sertoli
cells*

Seminiferous tubule

Fig. 19-16. A juncture of a seminiferous tubule and a straight tubule. The seminiferous tubule is cut somewhat obliquely. From the same testis shown in Figure 19-15. ×445.

basal lamina, many of them certainly do and presumably all of them reach the basal lamina. The epithelium is thus pseudostratified.

The columnar cells bear nonmotile processes originally called stereocilia. Electron micrographs show that these structures lack the axial complex characteristic of cilia and that they are merely long, branching cell processes. They differ from typical microvilli by their greater length and by their branching. Nevertheless, they are usually

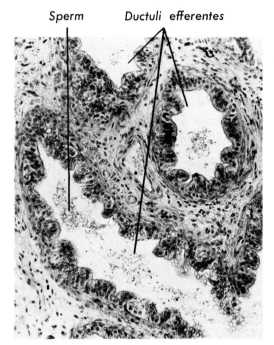

Sperm   Ductuli efferentes

Fig. 19-17. Sections of ductuli efferentes from the head of the epididymis. Adult man. Photomicrograph. ×130.

regarded as modified microvilli. The cytoplasm of columnar cells contains fairly numerous lysosomes and some pigment granules. The nuclei of the columnar cells are elongate and lie at somewhat different levels. The basal cells are similar to those in the efferent tubules but are much more numerous (Fig. 19-19). From ultrastructural studies and from studies of the course of injected dyes, it appears that the epididymis functions predominantly in resorption. As the sperm progress slowly through the epididymis they undergo continued maturation so that motility and fertilizing capacity are increased.

There is a basal lamina and lamina propria. The smooth muscle is circular but is small in amount except near the juncture with the ductus deferens where it increases in amount and longitudinal bundles appear.

Ductus Deferens

The main genital duct is a direct continuation of the duct of the epididymis. Its proximal portion, which runs along the ep-

Sections through ductus epididymis

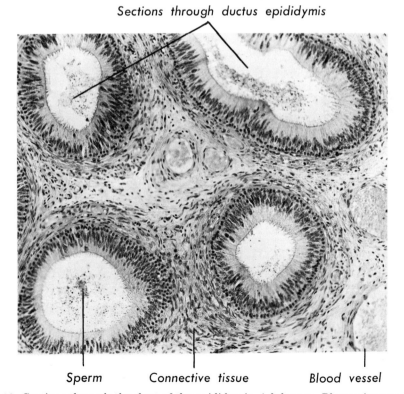

Sperm   Connective tissue   Blood vessel

Fig. 19-18. Sections through the duct of the epididymis. Adult man. Photomicrograph. ×105.

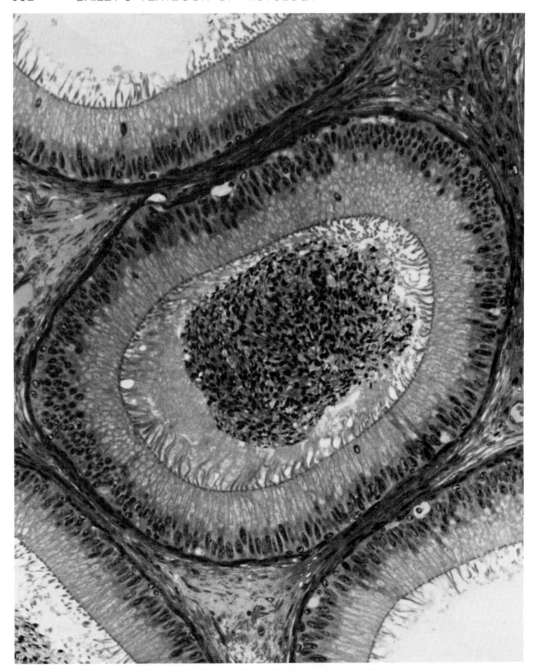

Fig. 19-19. Light micrograph of the epididymis of monkey. Tall, columnar cells with apical stereocilia and intermittent basal cells characterize this epithelium. A clump of spermatozoa appears in the central profile of the tubule. ×300.

ididymis, is coiled. Then it straightens out and, as part of the spermatic cord, passes into the abdominal cavity to terminate in the prostatic portion of the urethra. Shortly before reaching the prostate, the ductus deferens shows a spindle-shaped dilation, the *ampulla,* which gradually narrows to form the thin *ejaculatory duct.* The two ejaculatory ducts penetrate the prostate gland and empty into the urethra on either side of the prostatic utricle. When fully straightened, the duct is about ½ m in length.

The wall of the ductus deferens consists of three coats: mucosa, muscularis and fibrosa (Fig. 19-20).

The *mucosa* is lined by a pseudostratified columnar epithelium somewhat similar to that of the duct of the epididymis. The surface cells are lower, however, and the stereocilia show a variable distribution, being absent on some cells and present on others. Cytoplasmic granules are not as numerous as they are in the epithelium of the epididymis. The epithelium is surrounded by a connective tissue exeedingly rich in elastic fibers and in the deeper portion, numerous blood vessels. Owing to the abundant elastic tissue and strong muscularis, the mucosa is thrown into four or five longitudinal folds, so that in transverse section the lumen appears star-shaped.

The *muscularis* is by far the thickest coat (1 to 1½ mm) and consists of three smooth muscular layers: an inner longitudinal, a middle circular and an outer longi-

tudinal. The middle and outer coats are strongly developed layers. The inner longitudinal layer is relatively thin (Fig. 19-21).

The *fibrosa* consists of fibroelastic tissue containing numerous blood vessels, nerves and often scattered bundles of smooth muscle fibers. It merges without definite demarcation with the surrounding connective tissue.

In the *ampulla,* the mucosa shows numerous folds forming crypts or recesses, many of which extend as tubular structures into the underlying connective tissue (Fig. 19-22). These are glandular structures lined by a cuboidal or columnar epithelium of a secretory character; the cells frequently contain yellow pigment granules.

The *ejaculatory ducts* have a thin mucous membrane thrown into numerous fine folds, with glandular recesses like those of the ampulla. The epithelium is simple columnar or pseudostratified and becomes transitional near the urethral opening. Beneath the epithelium is a rich network of elastic fibers. A distinct muscularis is present only at the beginning. In the prostatic

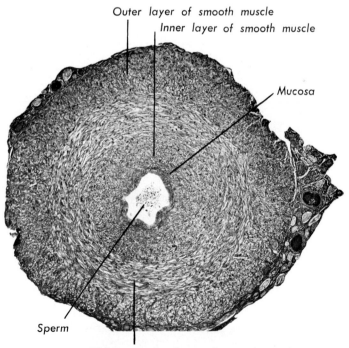

Outer layer of smooth muscle

Inner layer of smooth muscle

Mucosa

Sperm

Middle circular layer of smooth muscle

Fig. 19-20. Transverse section through ductus deferens. Adult man. ×38.

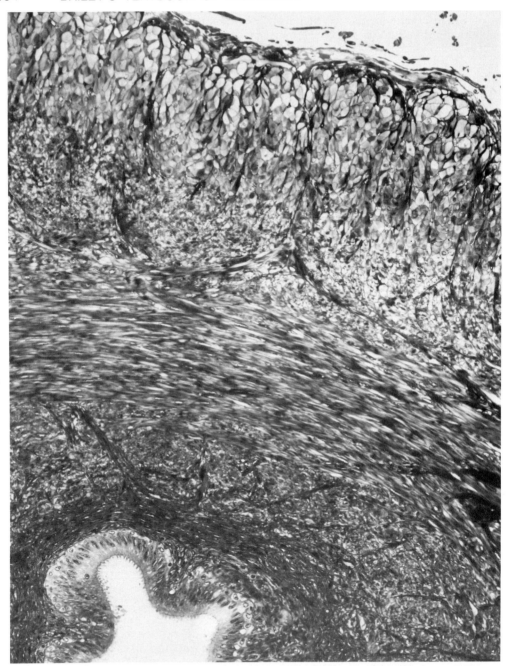

Fig. 19-21. Light micrograph of a cross section of a portion of the wall of the ductus deferens of the monkey. The lumen at the lower left is lined with epithelium similar to that of the epididymis (Fig. 19-19). The layering of smooth muscle in the wall is prominent. Some of the most external muscle cells are considerably swollen in this preparation. ×190.

portion, the muscularis disappears and is replaced by the fibromuscular tissue of the prostate gland.

Storage of Sperm

The ductuli efferentes, epididymis, and the first part of the ductus deferens are the storehouse for the sperm. The passage of the sperm through the straight tubules and rete testis must be relatively rapid, for they are rarely seen in these ducts, although they are numerous in the ductuli efferentes

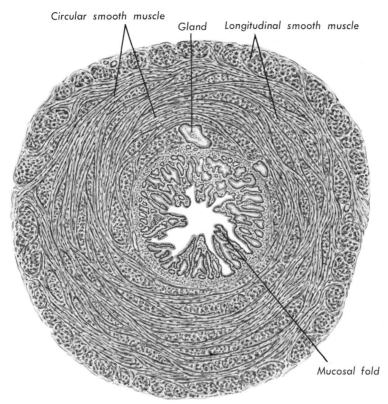

Fig. 19-22. Section through the ampulla of the ductus deferens. Man, 21 years of age. ×30. (After Stieve.)

and the duct of the epididymis. The storage place of the sperm is thus correlated with the regions with wider lumina lined by cells having specialized microvillar processes and intracellular vacuoles. For many years it was thought that these regions of the male duct system were primarily secretory, but current evidence suggests that they are actually more absorptive than secretory. The role of stereocilia is not entirely clear, but it has been suggested that they may be important in preventing the stored sperm from making extensive contact with the cell surfaces, thus reducing the chance of phagocytosis of normal spermatozoa (Fig. 19-19). Ligation experiments in animals have shown that, when the testes are left intact, the sperm retain their capacity of becoming motile for 40 to 60 days, although the period during which they retain the capacity to fertilize the egg is somewhat shorter. During at least a part of their sojourn in these ducts, they are probably undergoing further maturation. It is certain that their survival is aided by a secretion

from the epithelium. If the testes are removed, thus depriving the animal of testosterone, and the ducts are left intact, the epithelium involutes and the life of the sperm is reduced by about one-half.

Vestigial Structures in Testis and Epididymis

Connected with the testis and its ducts are remains of certain fetal structures associated with the development of the genital system.

(1) The *paradidymis* or *organ of Giraldés* is situated between the vessels of the spermatic cord near the testis. It consists of several blind tubules lined with a simple columnar epithelium, part of which is ciliated. The cells may vary in height and the tubule may have the appearance of an efferent duct.

(2) The *ductus aberrans Halleri* or inferior aberrant duct arises from the lower portion of the ductus epididymidis and extends toward the head, where it ends

blindly. It is lined with simple columnar, ciliated epithelium.

A smaller *superior aberrant duct* is often present. It arises from the rete testis and ends blindly in the epididymis.

(3) The *appendix testis* (hydatid of Morgagni) is situated on the cranial pole of the testis near the epididymis. It is a vesicular structure lined by simple columnar epithelium surrounded by vascular connective tissue.

(4) The *appendix epididymidis* (stalked hydatid) is found occasionally on the head of the epididymis near the appendix testis. Its lumen is lined with a single layer of cuboidal or columnar cells.

The paradidymis, aberrant tubules and appendix epididymidis represent vestiges of the fetal mesonephros, while the appendix testis is derived from the Müllerian duct.

Accessory Genital Glands

The Seminal Vesicles

The seminal vesicles are elongated, convoluted sacs which lie closely apposed to the ampullae and open into the ductus deferens at the junction of ampulla and ejaculatory duct. The mucosa is folded in a complicated manner, forming numerous irregular chambers or crypts (Fig. 19-23). The epithelium varies somewhat but is usually pseudostratified, being composed of cuboidal or columnar cells that reach the surface, and irregularly shaped basal cells similar to those described in the genital ducts. The borders of the surface cells are very distinct (Fig. 19-24). The cytoplasm of these cells contains secretion granules and a yellowish lipochrome pigment. The pigment makes

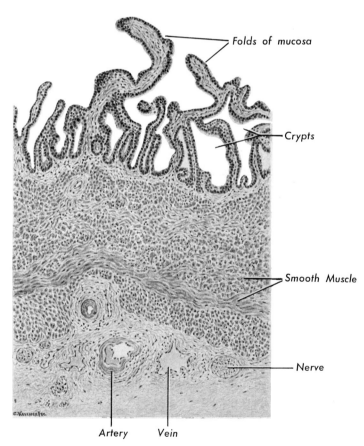

Fig. 19-23. From a section through wall of seminal vesicle. Human, 34 years old. Mallory-azan stain. ×65.

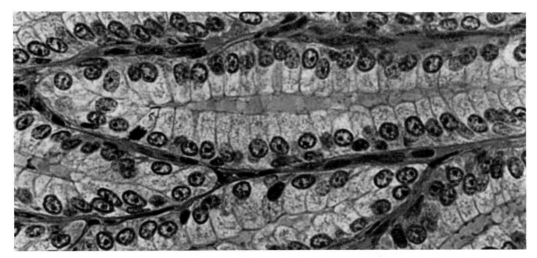

Fig. 19-24. Light micrograph of the seminal vesicle of an immature monkey. The epithelial cells are columnar and contain granular secretory material. Basal cells are also obvious. ×600.

its appearance at sexual maturity and increases with age.

The lamina propria is rich in elastic fibers and forms a continuous layer around the vesicle. The connective tissue of the folds is likewise rich in elastic fibers and contains some smooth muscle cells. Outside of the lamina propria is smooth muscle, which may display indistinct inner circular and outer longitudinal layers, both layers being thinner than in the ductus deferens.

Spermatozoa in varying numbers are often seen in the seminal vesicles. Their presence there is accidental, however. The seminal vesicles are not storehouses for sperm but are glandular structures contributing a slightly alkaline, viscid secretion to the seminal fluid. The secretion is rich in fructose which serves as an energy source for the sperm.

The Prostate Gland

The prostate gland (Figs. 19-25 to 19-27) is in reality an aggregation of many branched tubuloalveolar glands with wide ducts and terminal tubules. The glands number from 30 to 50, and their ducts converge to form 20 or more terminal ducts which open into the urethra.

The gland is surrounded by a vascular capsule of fibroelastic tissue containing numerous smooth muscle fibers in its inner layer. From the capsule, broad septa penetrate into the interior and become continuous with an unusually abundant fibroelastic supportive tissue, which separates scattered tubules or alveoli. This fibromuscular tissue may constitute one-third or even more of the whole mass of the prostate.

The epithelium shows a great variation in different glands and alveoli and even in a single alveolus. It is usually a simple cuboidal or columnar type. Basal cells may be present. The borders of the epithelial cells are usually distinct. Certain cells show apical protrusions. The cytoplasm contains secretion granules and lipid droplets. The epithelium and subjacent connective tissue form folds that project into the cavities of the glands. The ducts are lined by a simple columnar epithelium that changes, near the terminations of the ducts, to the transitional epithelium of the urethra.

Corpora amylacea (concretions) occur normally in some of the alveoli of most prostate glands (Fig. 19-26). Typically, they are spherical bodies about 250 μm in diameter, but there is considerable variation in size. In the fresh condition, they are fairly soft and light yellowish brown in color. In sections, concentric layers that stain with different intensities are evident. They are composed of protein and carbohydrates. Corpora increase in number with age. They may become calcified and then are known as calculi, some of which reach a very large size.

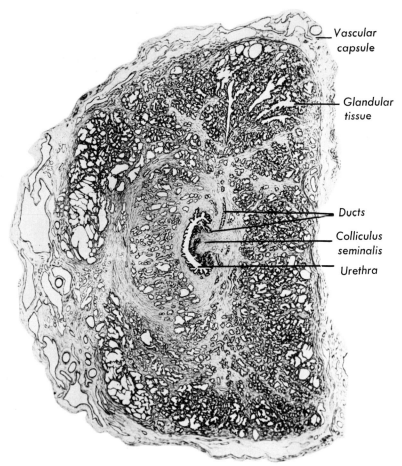

Fig. 19-25. Transverse section through the prostate at the level of the colliculus seminalis. Man, 19 years old. ×4. (After Stieve.)

Prostatic secretion is rich in citric acid and contains lipids. "Lipid bodies" that stain with eosin are frequent. Prostatic secretion also contains large amounts of acid phosphatase which, because of a normal daily discharge of prostatic secretion (0.5 to 2 ml/day), is present also in urine. Normal blood serum also contains acid phosphatase in small amounts. In prostatic carcinoma, however, there is frequently a pronounced discharge of the enzyme from the prostate into the bloodstream. The acid phosphatase content of the blood may be increased sufficiently to make its determination of clinical significance in judging whether metastasis has occurred. It may also be useful in indicating the response to therapy.

Within the prostate is found the *vesicula prostatica* (*utriculus prostaticus, uterus*

masculinus), the remains of the fetal *Müllerian duct*. It consists of a blind tubule with a folded mucous membrane lined by a simple or pseudostratified columnar epithelium that dips down to form short tubular glands.

The *blood vessels* of the prostate ramify in the capsule and trabeculae. The small arteries give rise to a capillary network that surrounds the tubules. From these arise small veins that accompany the arteries in the septa and form venous plexuses in the capsule.

The *lymphatics* begin as clefts in the trabeculae and follow the general course of the blood vessels.

The *nerves* of the prostate are both motor and sensory; the majority are unmyelinated. Many of them come from groups of autonomic ganglion cells which are found

Concretions   Alveolus

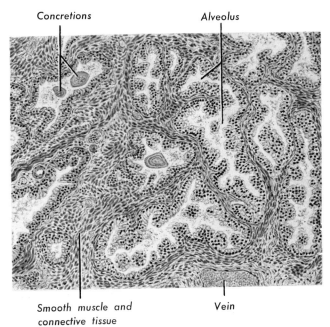

Smooth muscle and   Vein
connective tissue

Fig. 19-26. Section of prostate gland. Human, accident case, 54 years old. Hematoxylin-eosin. ×65.

Secretion granules

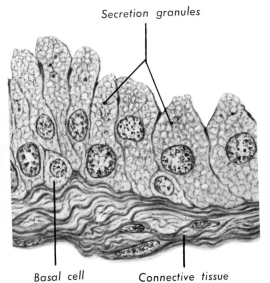

Basal cell   Connective tissue

Fig. 19-27. Epithelium of prostate gland. Human, 54 years old. Accident case. Mallory-azan stain, 3 μm section. ×1660.

underneath the capsule and in the larger trabeculae. Axons of these cells pass to the smooth muscle of the trabeculae and blood vessels and probably also to the epithelium of the tubules.

The Bulbourethral Glands

The bulbourethral glands or *glands of Cowper* (Fig. 19-28) are two small glandular structures placed close to the bulb of the urethra. They are compound tubuloalveolar glands whose tubules and ducts have a very irregular diameter. The terminal portions may be tubular or alveolar or in the form of cystlike dilations. They are lined by a simple epithelium whose height varies from columnar to low cuboidal and which may even be flat in distended alveoli. Most of the columnar cells are of the mucous type, with the nuclei basally placed, and the cytoplasm containing mucinogen droplets. Other cells stain darker with eosin and have a granular appearance, often containing fibrillar or spindle-shaped inclusions. During erotic stimulation, the gland secretes a glairy substance resembling mucus into the urethra. This probably serves as a lubricant for the epithelium.

The smaller ducts are lined by a simple epithelium and seem to be secretory in character. They unite to form two main ducts that run parallel to the urethra for a variable distance and then open into the latter. The main ducts have a stratified columnar epithelium.

The connective tissue between the tubules consists of fibroelastic tissue with only a few muscle fibers. Smooth and skeletal muscle fibers are, however, quite nu-

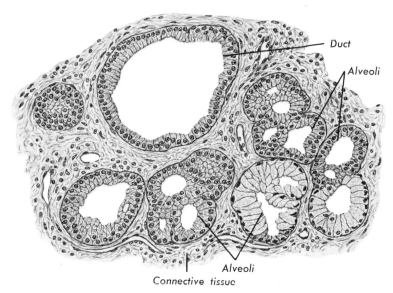

Fig. 19-28. Section through a lobule of the bulbourethral (Cowper's) gland. Human, 23 years old. ×200.

merous in the septa between the lobules. Externally, the glands are enclosed by a layer of skeletal muscle fibers from the deep perineal and bulbocavernosus muscles.

The Penis

The penis (Fig. 19-29) consists largely of three cylindrical masses of erectile tissue, the paired, dorsally placed *corpora cavernosa* and, lying underneath them, the unpaired *corpus spongiosum* (*corpus cavernosum urethrae*). The latter surrounds the urethra and terminates distally in a conical enlargement, the *glans penis*. The three cylindrical bodies are enclosed in a common fascia of loose, irregularly arranged connective tissue rich in elastic fibers, to which the covering skin is loosely attached. In the glans, the loose connective tissue is lacking and the skin adheres firmly to the underlying erectile tissue.

Each corpus cavernosum is surrounded by a dense capsule or *tunica albuginea* composed of collagenous fibers, the inner ones running circularly, the outer ones longitudinally. Elastic fibers are quite numerous. Between the cavernosa, the capsules fuse to form a median septum which is thickest and most complete near the root of the penis. Farther forward it becomes thinner and contains numerous slitlike spaces that permit a communication be-

tween the two bodies (Fig. 19-29). Directly underneath the albuginea is an irregular plexus of small veins.

The interior of each body consists of a network of large spaces or lacunae lined by endothelium (cavernous veins). These are separated by fibrous trabeculae rich in smooth muscle fibers which are disposed both circularly and longitudinally. The lacunae are large and trabeculae are thin in the central portion. At the periphery is a layer of narrower spaces which communicate with the venous plexus on the inner surface of the albuginea. In the flaccid organ, the lacunae are kept closed by the tonus of the trabecular muscle and appear as mere slits.

The corpus spongiosum has a similar structure, but the albuginea is thin and contains many elastic fibers, so that the organ is not highly resistant to expansion. The trabeculae are thin, the lacunae are quite uniform in size and a peripheral layer of smaller lacunae is absent. Toward the urethra the lacunae become continuous with the mucosal plexus of veins; at the periphery they communicate with the venous network of the albuginea.

In the glans, the erectile tissue has the character of a dense, venous plexus. An albuginea is lacking, the skin being firmly attached to the erectile tissue.

The skin of the penis is characterized by

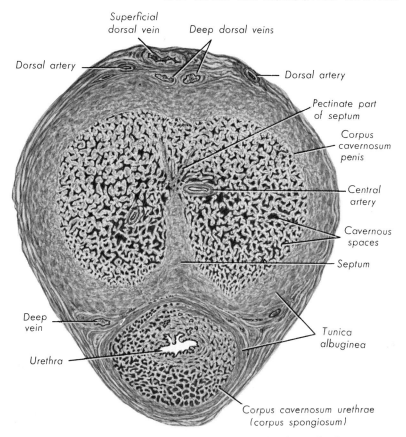

Fig. 19-29. Cross section of penis of adult man. The section is at the juncture of the proximal two-thirds and the distal one-third of the organ. The skin has been removed. ×4.5.

tall dermal papillae and a thin epidermis containing considerable pigment in the basal layer. Coarse hairs are found only at the root, but fine lanugo hairs are distributed over all of the shaft. Only the glans and inner surface of the prepuce are entirely hairless.

The *prepuce* is a fold of skin that overlies the glans. It consists of fibroelastic tissue containing bundles of muscle fibers and is covered by a very thin epidermis. On its inner surface, and on the glans as well, are found a number of modified sebaceous glands, the *glands of Tyson*.

Blood Vessels

The penis has a complicated blood supply that can respond to its varying functional states. The organ is chiefly supplied by the *arteria dorsalis* and the *arteria profunda,* which are branches of the *arteria penis.* The dorsal artery sends twigs to the albu-

ginea and the larger cavernous trabeculae, where they break up into capillaries. Leaving the capillaries, the blood enters the lacunae and is drained by the plexus of albugineal veins. This is the course of most of the blood during the flaccid state.

The principal vessels for filling the lacunae during erection are the deep arteries (*arteriae profundae*), one of which runs lengthwise in each corpus cavernosum. They give off numerous branches that are supported by the trabecular tissue and end in minute arteries that open directly into the cavernous spaces. In the flaccid organ, many of the arterial branches project into the lacunae as looped or spiral vessels, the *helicine arteries.* Similar vessels are found in the corpus spongiosum.

The helicine arteries have an unusually thick media of circular muscle fibers, and in many of them the intima shows valve-like structures in the form of marked longitudinal thickenings or cushions. When the muscle of the arteries contracts, these thickenings plug up the lumen and shut off the blood supply.

During erection, the muscle of the helicine arteries and of the cavernous trabeculae relaxes, and the lacunae are flooded with arterial blood from the helicine vessels, which empty mainly in the central spaces of the cavernous bodies. The sudden filling of the large central spaces tends to compress the narrower peripheral ones, which communicate with the venous plexus of the albuginea. Egress of blood is blocked or at least greatly reduced, and the organ becomes swollen and rigid. At the end of the erectile state, the muscle of the helicine arteries contracts and the inflow of blood is shut off. The trabecular muscle regains its tonus and the blood is slowly driven out into the venous plexus. There are special provisions for emptying the corpora cavernosa. One or perhaps several veins originate directly from the central lacunae. These are equipped with funnel-shaped valves whose small openings permit the passage of only a small stream of blood. When the blood supply of the helicine arteries is cut off, these veins begin to empty the central lacunae. The internal pressure is reduced, the peripheral lacunae open and then the blood is pressed out more rapidly into the peripheral veins, the organ gradually returning to the flaccid condition. Most of the blood from the corpora cavernosa is drained by the *vena profundis penis.*

The corpus spongiosum is filled in a similar manner. However, the albuginea is more elastic, the lacunae are more uniform in size and the outflow of blood is not blocked to the same extent. The spongiosum naturally swells during erection, owing to the increased blood supply, but it always remains compressible and does not assume the rigidity of the paired cavernous bodies.

Lymphatics

Numerous lymphatics are found in the skin of the shaft, prepuce and glans (superficial plexus) and in the mucosal stroma of the urethra. A deeper lymphatic network in the erectile tissues has also been described. The lymphatics drain chiefly into the inguinal lymph nodes.

Nerves

The penis is abundantly supplied with spinal, sympathetic and parasympathetic nerve fibers. The sensory spinal fibers terminate in a variety of end organs: free sensory endings, Meissner's corpuscles in the papillae and Pacinian corpuscles and end bulbs of Krause in the connective tissue.

Sympathetic and parasympathetic motor fibers form extensive networks in the walls of the blood vessels and the smooth muscle of the cavernous trabeculae.

Internal Secretion of the Testes

It has been known for a long time that the testes are in some way responsible for the appearance of the secondary sex characters. When the testes are removed before puberty, these characters remain in an infantile condition or are entirely suppressed. The penis and prostate gland are small, the male type of chest and pelvis fails to develop, the face, chest and limbs are hairless, the larynx remains small and, as a result, the voice maintains its infantile pitch. The bones grow beyond their normal length but are not robust. Sometimes there is considerable deposition of fat, its distribution characteristic of the feminine type.

When castration is performed after puberty, the effects are less pronounced, for the sex characters are already established and the changes are retrogressive.

The most profound and constant effects of castration in mammals, as shown experimentally, are upon the genital ducts and accessory glands. The epithelium of these structures fails to develop to the normal height and does not show secretory activity if the testes are removed before puberty or, if they are removed after maturity, the epithelium of these structures will involute. The effect of the testes on these accessory reproductive structures appears to be due solely to a hormone secreted by the testes called *testosterone.* There are other male sex hormones that are found in the urine, but presumably they are not secreted by the testes but are transformation products of the testis hormone or are secreted by other organs (adrenals), although not in sufficient amounts to substitute for the testis hormone. The response of the various accessory reproductive organs and of the comb of the capon have been used in assays of the male hormone content of extracts.

The evidence is quite conclusive that the interstitial cells of the testes secrete the male sex hormone. In undescended or partially descended testes (cryptorchid), the epithelium of the seminiferous tubules, but not the interstitial tissue, atrophies from continued exposure to the temperature of the body cavity. Extensive degeneration of the spermatogenic cells is likewise produced by treatment with X-rays, the interstitial cells being uninjured when the correct dosage is used. In both cases, the secondary sex characters remain normal. Histochemical studies have shown that compounds with the chemical properties of testosterone are present in the interstitial cells but not elsewhere in the testis. There is a correlation between the testosterone content and amount of interstitial tissue.

Estrogen, the female sex hormone, also occurs in the male. It has been shown that about 80% of the estrogen arises from the Leydig cells and about 20% from the adrenal gland.

Hormones secreted by cells of the anterior hypophysis are essential for the endocrine and spermatogenic function of the testis. The activity of the interstitial cells of Leydig is dependent on the interstitial cell-stimulating hormone (luteinizing hormone), and the development of germ cells is dependent on the follicle-stimulating hormone (chapter 21). The anterior hypophysis has an indirect influence on the accessory reproductive organs through its action on the testis.

Semen

Semen consists of seminal plasma, spermatozoa and usually some cells cast off from the lining of the reproductive ducts and glands. Seminal plasma consists of the secretion of the prostate, seminal vesicles, bulbourethral glands and epididymis, the chief contribution being from the prostate and seminal vesicles. The seminal plasma serves as a food source and vehicle for the spermatozoa.

The volume of semen from a normal ejaculation varies greatly among different individuals and in the same individual, as does also the number of sperm. The usual range in volume is from 2 to 5 or 6 ml. The total number of sperm ranges from a high of 500,000,000, or even more, to a low of a few million or to complete azoospermia. A variable percentage of sperm are malformed or inactive.

Testicular or epididymal sperm are inactive but quickly become active in seminal plasma (or saline). They carry little of the foodstuff for metabolism but acquire this from the carbohydrates, chiefly fructose, in the seminal plasma. The sugar is reduced to lactic acid, glycolysis being best carried out under nearly anaerobic conditions.

The role of the high content of hyaluronidase in sperm is not entirely understood, but histochemical studies indicate that it breaks down the egg coating and aids the sperm in penetrating the egg.

References

ALBERT, A. The mammalian testis. *In* Sex and Internal Secretion (Young, W. C., editor), vol. 1, pp. 305–366. Williams & Wilkins, Baltimore, 1961.

AUSTIN, C. R., AND PERRY, J. S. (editors) Symposium on Agents Affecting Fertility. Little, Brown and Co., Boston, 1965.

BAWA, S. R. The fine structure of the Sertoli cell of the human testis. J. Ultrastruct. Res. 9:459–474, 1963.

BURGOS, M. H. Uptake of colloidal particles by cells of the caput epididymis. Anat. Rec. 148:517–525, 1964.

CHANG, M. C., AND PINCUS, G. Physiology of fertilization in mammals. Physiol. Rev. 31:1–26, 1951.

CHRISTENSEN, A. K. The fine structure of testicular interstitial cells in the guinea pig. J. Cell Biol. 26:911–935, 1965.

CHRISTIANSEN, A. K. Specific contacts between Leydig cells and macrophages in the rat testis. Anat. Rec. 184:377, 1976.

CLERMONT, Y. The cycle of the seminiferous epithelium in man. Am. J. Anat. 112:35–52, 1963.

CLERMONT, Y. Kinetics of spermatogenesis in mammals: seminiferous epithelium cycle and spermatogonial renewal. Physiol. Rev. 52:198–236, 1972.

DEANE, H. W., AND PORTER, K. R. A comparative study of cytoplasmic abasophilia and the population density of ribosomes in the secretory cells of mouse seminal vesicle. Z. Zellforsch. 52:697–711, 1960.

DYM, M., AND FAWCETT, D. W. The blood-testis barrier in the rat and the physiological compartmentation of the seminiferous epithelium. Biol. Reprod. 3:308–326, 1970.

ELFTMAN, H. The Sertoli cell cycle in the mouse. Anat. Rec. 106:381–393, 1950.

ELFTMAN, H. Sertoli cells and testis structure. Am. J. Anat. 113:25–34, 1963.

FAWCETT, D. W., AND BURGOS, M. H. Studies on the

fine structure of the mammalian testis. II. The human interstitial tissue. Am. J. Anat. 107:245–270, 1960.

FAWCETT, D. W., AND ITO, S. The fine structure of bat spermatozoa. Am. J. Anat. 116:567–610, 1965.

FRANK, A. L., AND CHRISTENSEN, A. K. Localization of acid phosphatase in lipofuscin granules and possible autophagic vacuoles in interstitial cells of guinea pig testis. J. Cell Biol. 36:1–13, 1968.

HELLER, C. G., AND CLERMONT, Y. Spermatogenesis in man: an estimate of its duration. Science 140:184–185, 1963.

HELLER, C. G., AND CLERMONT, Y. Kinetics of the germinal epithelium in man. In Recent Progress in Hormone Research (Pincus, G., editor), vol. 20, pp. 545–575. Academic Press, New York, 1964.

HOOKER, C. W. The postnatal history and function of the interstitial cells of the testis of the bull. Am. J. Anat. 74:1–37, 1944.

HUGGINS, C. The prostatic secretion. Harvey Lectures, Ser. 42, pp. 148–193, 1947.

LEBLOND, C. P., AND CLERMONT, Y. Definition of the stages of the cycle of the seminiferous epithelium in the rat. Ann. N.Y. Acad. Sci. 55:548–573, 1952.

MANN, T. Biochemistry of Semen and of the Male Reproductive Tract. John Wiley & Sons, Inc., New York, 1964.

MASON, K. E., AND SHAVER, S. L. Some functions of the caput epididymis. Ann. N.Y. Acad. Sci. 55:585–593, 1952.

MOORE, R. A. The evolution and involution of the prostate gland. Am. J. Pathol. 12:599–624, 1936.

MOORE, R. A. Morphology of prostatic corpora amylacea and calculi. Arch. Pathol. 22:24–40, 1936.

MORITA, I. Some observations on the fine structure of the human ductuli efferentes testis. Arch. Histol. Jap. 26:341–365, 1968.

NAGANO, T., AND SUZUKI, F. Freeze-fracture observations on the intercellular junctions of Sertoli cells and of Leydig cells in the human testis. Cell Tissue Res. 166:37–48, 1976.

ROOSEN-RUNGE, E. C. The process of spermatogenesis in mammals. Biol. Rev. 37:343–377, 1962.

ROOSEN-RUNGE, E. C., AND BARLOW, F. D. Quantitative studies on human spermatogenesis. Am. J. Anat. 93:143–169, 1953.

ROSS, M. H. Contractile cells in human seminiferous tubules. Science 153:1271–1273, 1966.

SAND, K., AND OKKELS, H. The histological variability of the testis from normal and sexual-abnormal, castrated men. Endokrinologie 19:369–374, 1938.

SCHMIDT, F. C. Licht- und elektronemikroskopische Untersuchungen am menschlichen Hoden und Nebenhoden. Z. Zellforsch. 63:707–729, 1964.

STEINBERGER, E. Hormonal control of mammalian spermatogenesis. Physiol. Rev. 51:1–22, 1971.

STIEVE, H. Mannlichen Genitalorgane. Handb. mikr. Anat. Menschen (v. Möllendorff, editor), vol. 2, pt. 2, pp. 1–399, 1930.

YAMADA, E. Some observations on the fine structure of the interstitial cell in the human testis. In Fifth International Conference on Electron Microscopy (Breese, S. S., Jr., editor), vol. 2, pp. LL-1. Academic Press, New York, 1967.

The Female Reproductive System

The female genital organs are comprised of the ovaries in which the egg cells are formed, a system of genital ducts—the Fallopian tubes, uterus and vagina—and the external genitalia, including the labia majora, labia minora and clitoris. The mammary glands, although not one of the genital organs, are important glands of the female reproductive system. The ovaries, like the testes, are also important glands of internal secretion.

The Ovary

The ovaries are somewhat flattened, ovoid bodies, measuring about 4 cm in length, 2 cm in width and 1 cm in thickness. One lies on each side of the uterus in relation to the lateral wall of the pelvis (Fig. 20-1). Each is attached at its hilus to the back of the broad ligament by a peritoneal fold, the mesovarium, and by the ligament of the ovary. The ovary is pinkish gray and does not have the glistening or shiny appearance characteristic of the peritoneum. Its surface is uneven and becomes puckered to an increasing degree with aging.

At the hilus, the connective tissue of the mesovarium and ovarian ligament passes into the ovary and becomes continuous with the ovarian connective tissue. The mesothelial covering of the mesovarium changes at the hilus to a low cuboidal *surface epithelium* which covers the ovary. This is also known as germinal epithelium,

although there is no convincing evidence that it is the site of formation of the germ cells.

In sections of the ovary, two zones may be distinguished, a central deeper portion, the *medulla* or *zona vasculosa*, and a broad outer layer, the *cortex* (Fig. 20-2). The two zones blend into each other without any distinct demarcation.

The medulla is composed of a framework of loose connective tissue rich in elastic fibers and containing numerous large blood vessels, lymphatics and nerves. Bundles of smooth muscle fibers are found near the hilus. In some individuals, vestiges of certain fetal structures, the *rete ovarii*, occur as epithelial strands or tubules in the region of the hilus.

The cortex is a broad peripheral layer interrupted at the hilus where the medulla becomes continuous with the tissues of the mesovarium. It consists of a compact, richly cellular connective tissue in which are scattered the characteristic epithelial structures of the ovary, the *ovarian follicles* (Fig. 20-2). The connective tissue cells are fusiform or spindle-shaped, with elongated vesicular nuclei. They are placed in a feltwork of delicate collagenous fibrils. Elastic tissue, except in the walls of the blood vessels, is practically absent. Directly underneath the surface epithelium, the connective tissue forms a denser fibrous layer, the *tunica albuginea*, composed of fewer cells and more closely packed fibers.

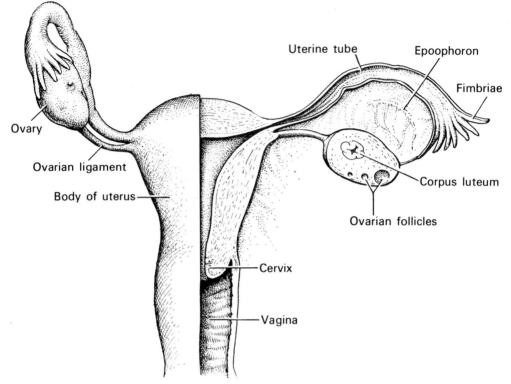

Fig. 20-1. Diagram of the internal organs of the female reproductive system seen from behind. The ovary and uterine tube are shown in approximately normal position at the left and they are drawn apart and away from the uterus at the right.

The Follicles

Each ovarian follicle consists of an ovum surrounded by epithelial cells. A brief outline of the embryonic origin of the follicles is given to facilitate an understanding of their nature in pre- and postnatal stages.

Primordial germ cells appear in the wall of the yolk sac during the 3rd week of human development, and they migrate to the germinal ridges (embryonic gonads) by the 5th week. The primordial germ cells become intermingled with the surface epithelial cells, and cordlike projections of cells extend from the surface into the underlying gonadal tissue during the 2nd and 3rd months. These masses of cells proliferate actively and become subdivided into clusters, each composed of several primordial germ cells and numerous follicular cells. It was once thought that the germ cells as well as the follicular cells arise by differentiation of ovarian surface cells. The evidence is now convincing that the germ cells

arise in the yolk sac and it is generally held that the endoderm is the germ cell layer of origin.

After a relatively short period, the clusters of cells that have invaded the gonadal tissue become subdivided into smaller bodies known as *primordial* and *primary follicles*, each consisting of an oocyte surrounded by a single layer of follicular cells (Fig. 20-3, *A*). A primordial follicle was originally defined as one in which the oocyte is inconstantly and incompletely surrounded by a very low epithelium, whereas the oocyte of a primary follicle is completely surrounded by a cuboidal epithelium. It seems easier to distinguish these two stages on the basis of developmental activity of the oocyte. When the oocyte begins to enlarge, the follicular epithelium increases in prominence and becomes multilaminar. The primordial follicle then is the inactive stage and as maturation begins, it becomes a primary follicle. In late fetal life, the tunica albuginea is formed, and the

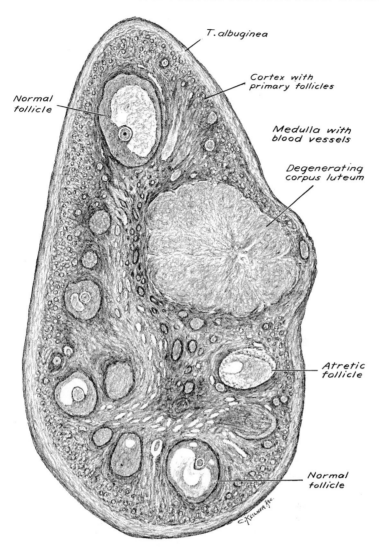

T. albuginea

Cortex with
primary follicles

Normal
follicle

Medulla with
blood vessels

Degenerating
corpus luteum

Atretic
follicle

Normal
follicle

Fig. 20-2. Longitudinal section through the ovary of a normal adult rhesus monkey. The corpus luteum is probably degenerating.

surface epithelium is reduced to a single layer of cells. These cells are columnar in early life and cuboidal in the adult.

There is considerable evidence that multiplication of oogonia in the human generally ceases by about the 6th fetal month. In fact, the most marked proliferation occurs even earlier, and the majority of the cells differentiate to the primary oocyte stage by the 5th fetal month. The primary oocytes spend a long time before completing their differentiation to the first meiotic (chromosomal reduction) division.

Most of the follicles in the ovary of the newborn are of the primordial and primary types, with the former predominating. A few follicles with small antra (vesicular stage) may be present in the ovary at birth for a brief period, apparently through stimulation by maternal hormones during the latter part of fetal life. Estimates of the total number of oocytes present at birth vary within wide limits. Counts made on serial sections show that at least 400,000 primordial and primary follicles are present in the ovaries of the newborn infant.

Of this large number, relatively few are destined to reach full maturity. The repro-

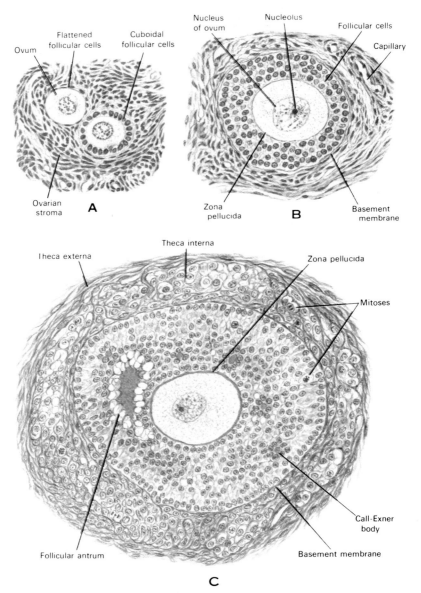

Fig. 20-3. Follicles in various states of development. These were selected from a normal human ovary removed surgically on the 14th day of the cycle and fixed by injection with Bouin's fluid. The patient was 36 years of age. The illustrations are drawn at a uniform magnification, ×289. Sections illustrated in *A* and *B* were stained in hematoxylin and eosin, *C* in Masson's trichrome stain without a preliminary application of hematoxylin. *A*, two follicles in early stages of development: primordial (*left*) and primary (*right*). *B*, an early stage of a growing follicle. *C*, a follicle, showing the beginning of the formation of the antrum (early secondary follicle).

ductive life of a woman, from puberty to menopause, lasts about 30 to 35 years. During this period, even if no disturbing factors appear, one ovum matures normally each month, so that only about 400 eggs actually reach maturity. All of the others ultimately degenerate and, from birth on, the follicles progressively diminish in number. Follicular degeneration occurs most intensely in early life but continues actively throughout the period of sexual maturity. After the menopause, the remaining follicles degenerate within a few years.

In the mature ovary, the follicles are found in all stages of growth. Most numerous are the primary follicles found mainly in the peripheral layer of the cortex. As a follicle grows, it occupies progressively deeper positions.

The primary follicles (Fig. 20-3) are spheroidal bodies measuring 30 to 40 μm. The central oocyte, about 20 μm in diameter, has a large, vesicular nucleus with deeply staining chromatin and a rather indistinct nucleolus. The cytoplasm is finely granular. The follicular cells are either flattened or low cuboidal. A definite connective tissue capsule is lacking.

Growth and Maturation of the Follicles

The growth of the primary follicles is characterized by proliferation of the follicular cells, increase in size of the oocyte and formation of a connective tissue capsule. The follicular cells become cuboidal, divide actively and soon form a stratified layer around the ovum (Fig. 20-3). Irregular small spaces appear in the follicular mass and fuse to form a crescent-shaped cavity, the *antrum* or follicular cavity, filled with a serous fluid, the *liquor folliculi*. Subsequent to the formation of a definite antrum, the structure is known as a *secondary follicle* but may also be referred to as a *vesicular follicle*.

While the follicle is increasing in size, it assumes an ovoid shape and moves to a deeper position. By continual division of follicular cells and by an expansion of the antrum, the oocyte is pressed to one side of the follicle, where it is surrounded by a mound of follicular cells forming the *cumulus oophorous* or germ hill (Fig. 20-4, A). The follicular cells immediately adjacent to the oocyte form a *corona radiata* around the oocyte.

Concurrently with the growth of the oocyte and the multiplication of the follicular cells, the connective tissue around the follicle develops into a follicular sheath, the *theca folliculi*, composed of an inner vascular region, the *theca interna*, and an outer fibrous layer, the *theca externa* (Figs. 20-3 to 20-5). Although the cells of both layers of the theca folliculi are connective tissue derivatives, those of the theca interna have epithelioid characteristics. They are ovoid or polyhedral, have ovoid or rounded nuclei and have lipid droplets in their cytoplasm. Electron micrographs show that the cristae of their mitochondria are tubular rather than shelf-like and that they resemble those of cells known to be active in the secretion of steroid hormones. It seems likely that the theca interna cells form the estrogen secreted by the follicle. The theca externa is composed of connective tissue fibers and spindle-shaped fibroblastic and smooth muscle cells. The interna is separated from the follicle cells by the *follicular basement membrane* (Fig. 20-5). There is no distinct boundary between the theca interna and the theca externa, and the junction of the latter with the surrounding connective tissue is very poorly defined.

The oocyte grows rapidly during the early stages of follicular growth and is already approaching its maximal size by the time the antrum appears in the follicle (Fig. 20-3, C). The nucleus becomes large and vesicular (germinal vesicle), with dispersed chromatin and a large, deeply staining nucleolus (germinal spot). Yolk accumulates in the cytoplasm, particularly in the interior, which becomes coarsely granular in contrast with the finely granular, clearer zone at the periphery. A relatively thick membrane known as the *zona pellucida* is formed around the outer surface of the oocyte (Figs. 20-4 to 20-7). It is rich in polysaccharides, and apparently it is formed partly by the ovum and partly by the follicle cells. It is a resistant membrane which persists during atresia longer than the oocyte. Phase and electron microscope studies show that processes from the corona radiata cells extend through the zona pellucida to make contact with the plasma membrane of the oocyte. Communicating

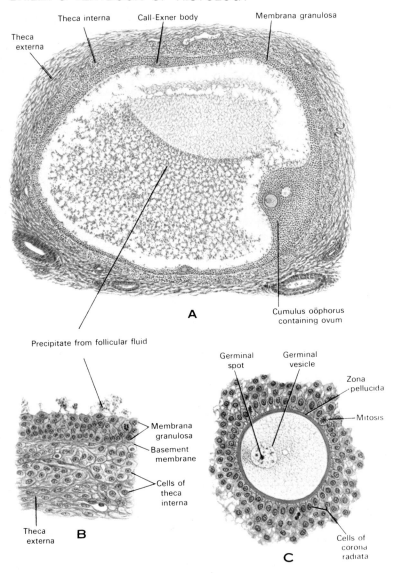

Theca externa

Theca interna

Call-Exner body

Membrana granulosa

Precipitate from follicular fluid

Cumulus oöphorus containing ovum

A

Membrana granulosa

Basement membrane

Cells of theca interna

Theca externa

B

Germinal spot

Germinal vesicle

Zona pellucida

Mitosis

Cells of corona radiata

C

Fig. 20-4. On this plate is illustrated a follicle with a maximal dimension of 4.5 mm. From the same ovary as Figure 20-3. Masson's trichrome stain. *A*, low power view, ×53. *B*, a portion of the wall of this follicle, ×287. *C*, the oocyte of this follicle drawn at the same magnification as the illustrations in Figure 20-3, ×287.

junctions are established at some of these points of contact. It is thought that the processes facilitate the transport of metabolic substances to the developing oocyte. Other processes (microvilli) extend from the oocyte into the zona pellucida (Fig. 20-6). As will be described under oogenesis, the oocyte does not complete its maturation until after ovulation.

The *mature vesicular follicle* (Graafian follicle) attains a diameter of 10 to 12 mm.

It extends through the whole thickness of the cortex and encroaches peripherally upon the tunica albuginea, producing a bulge which is visible on the surface of the ovary. In the latter part of follicular maturation, fluid continues to accumulate in the antrum, and fluid-filled spaces also appear among the cells of the cumulus oophorous, thereby weakening the attachment of the oocyte and its associated cells to the follicular wall.

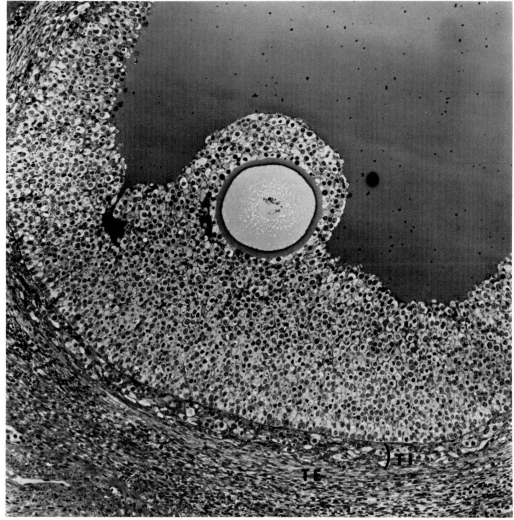

Fig. 20-5. Light micrograph of a secondary follicle from monkey ovary. The oocyte, surrounded by zona pellucida, sits in the cumulus oophorus. The follicle cells are separated from the theca interna (*TI*) by a distinct basement membrane. The theca externa (*TE*) contains spindle-shaped fibroblastic and smooth muscle cells. ×150.

Ovulation

Just prior to ovulation, there is a marked increase of fluid in the antrum, producing greater pressure on the wall of the follicle and on the thin layer of ovarian tissue at the surface. In laboratory animals in which the events of ovulation can be observed, it is seen that blood flow stops in a small area near the center of the translucent bulge on the ovarian surface just prior to ovulation. A small conical projection appears at this spot, known as the *stigma*, and the follicle ruptures. Fluid escapes, and the ovum, together with its corona radiata and a number of cells of the germ hill, also passes through the opening. This process of rupture of the follicle and discharge of the oocyte is known as *ovulation*. The egg and its associated cells enter the peritoneal cavity briefly, then pass into the fimbriated funnel of the oviduct. The fimbriae of the duct are close to the surface of the ovary at this time.

The oocyte must be fertilized soon after ovulation or it will degenerate, fragment and disappear. Although data for the human are difficult to obtain, studies on animals show that the egg does not retain the capacity to be fertilized much longer than 24 hr. In some species fertilization must

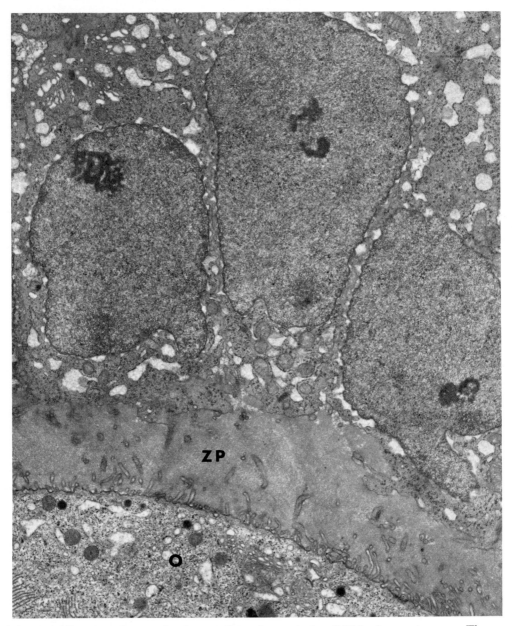

Fig. 20-6. Electron micrograph of a portion of a maturing follicle from rat ovary. The zona pellucida (*ZP*) contains cellular processes of both the oocyte (*O*) and follicle cells. ×7500.

occur within 4 to 6 hr after ovulation. The union of oocyte and sperm takes place either before or immediately after the oocyte enters the fimbriated extremity of the tube. After fertilization, the journey of the egg down the tube to the uterus is a leisurely one. Data from early human embryos secured by Hertig and Rock show that the cleaving ovum reaches the uterus about 3 days after ovulation. It is implanted in the endometrium about 6 days after ovulation.

Atresia

Of the numerous follicles, only a few reach full maturity and discharge the oocyte. The vast majority undergo degeneration either as primary follicles or after a varying period of growth. The degeneration of follicles is known as *atresia*.

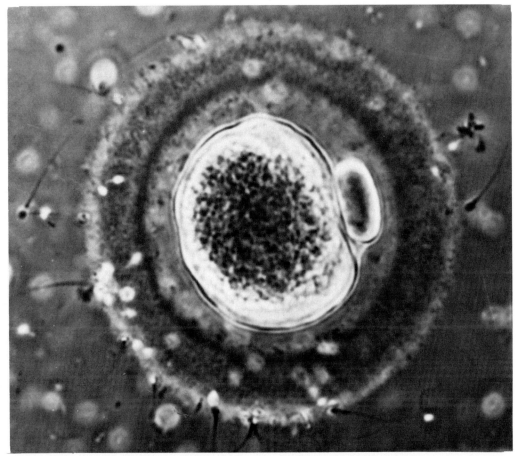

Fig. 20-7. Photomicrograph of living human ovum and its first polar body surrounded by zona pellucida and by cumulus cells. Sperm, which are attempting to reach the oocyte, are seen at the periphery of the cumulus cells. (Courtesy of Dr. L. B. Shettles.)

In atresia of the *primary follicles*, the oocyte undergoes degeneration, and this is followed by similar changes in the follicular cells. The follicle is resorbed and disappears, and the space that it occupied is filled with connective tissue.

Atresia of the *growing* and *maturing follicles* is a more complicated process which varies in details, depending on the size of the follicle and the behavior of the theca interna. Here too the disintegrative changes start in the oocyte and spread to the follicular cells. These changes are in the nature of fatty degeneration, evidenced by the accumulation of fatty granules in the cytoplasm, disintegration of the nuclei and ultimate liquefaction. The zona pellucida swells, becomes folded and may persist for some time after the disappearance of the oocyte and follicular cells. (Fig. 20-8).

The theca interna cells persist for a longer period than do the follicle cells (Figs. 20-8 and 20-9). The former enlarge and show an increase in cytoplasmic lipid droplets, thereby resembling lutein cells. These cells persist for long periods in some animals and form the *ovarian interstitial cells*. They disappear more rapidly in humans, and cells of interstitial type cannot be identified with certainty in the adult human ovary. They can be recognized during childhood when large numbers of follicles are continually undergoing atresia.

In the mature ovary, there are always several antrum-containing follicles of various sizes. Most of these are destined to undergo atresia at some stage in their growth. As a rule, only one follicle matures each month, and the process of transformation from a growing to a mature follicle

Invading blood vessels   Ovarian stroma

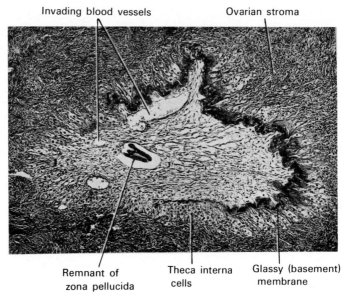

Remnant of   Theca interna   Glassy (basement)
zona pellucida   cells   membrane

Fig. 20-8. Medium stage of follicular atresia. Normal ovary of a woman 36 years old. The ovary was surgically removed at the midcycle. Masson's trichrome stain. Photomicrograph, ×95.

Vein   Arteriole

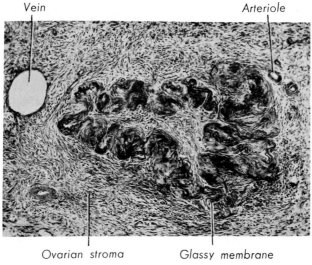

Ovarian stroma   Glassy membrane

Fig. 20-9. Late stage of follicular atresia. Normal ovary of a woman 36 years old. The ovary was surgically removed at the midcycle. Masson's trichrome stain. Photomicrograph. ×95.

is accomplished in about 2 weeks. In rare instances, two or even several follicles may ripen at the same time.

Oogenesis

In preparation for the union with the spermatozoon, the oocyte passes through a series of changes similar to that described for the sperm cells (see under "Spermatogenesis," chapter 19) and with the same end result, namely, the reduction of its chromosomes to one-half the somatic number. The changes differ, however, in one important respect. In the male, each primary spermatocyte gives rise to four functioning spermatozoa. In the female, one primary oocyte gives rise to but one mature ovum, the other three being discarded as abortive minute bodies, the *polar bodies.*

The *oogonia,* or primitive ova which contain the somatic (*diploid*) number of chromosomes, divide mitotically as do the spermatogonia, the daughter cells likewise containing the full number of chromosomes. The mitotic period for oogonia differs, however, from that for spermatogonia, ending at about the 6th month of fetal life for oogonia and continuing to old age for spermatogonia. Replication of DNA in the chromosomes of the primary oocytes is completed during fetal life. During the growth of the primary oocytes, homologous chromosomes become paired (undergo synapsis) as in primary spermatocytes. The primary oocyte then passes through the two *maturation divisions, meiosis*, as a result of which the chromosomes are reduced to the *haploid* number. In these divisions, the chromatin is divided equally between the daughter cells, but the division of the cytoplasm is extremely unequal. The spindle of the first maturation division forms near the periphery of the cell (Fig. 20-10) and, when cleavage occurs, one of the *secondary oocytes* receives most of the cytoplasm, while the other, the *first polar body*, receives practically none and soon degenerates.

The second maturation division is similar to the first. Once more the spindle forms at the periphery, and again two cells of unequal size are formed. One, the *mature ovum*, retains most of the cytoplasm; the other is cast off as the *second polar body*. In some lower forms, the first polar body may also divide, so that altogether three polar bodies are formed, all of which ultimately degenerate. Thus, of the four cells formed from the primary oocyte, only one reaches functional maturity, retaining practically all of the cytoplasm with its nutritive contents. The volume of the mature ovum is about 250,000 times greater than that of the spermatozoon.

The egg cells of the primary follicles are often described as oogonia. DNA replication is completed during fetal life, however, and the oogonia differentiate to early stage oocytes (diplotene stage of the first meiotic prophase) before birth. Thus, the egg cells of the primary follicles are early stage primary oocytes that have entered a long period of rest. The majority of these degenerate before much growth occurs, but degeneration may occur at any stage of follicular growth. In most mammals, including humans, the first polar body is formed in

the ovary just prior to ovulation. Thus, it is a secondary oocyte that is actually ovulated. The chromosomes then line up on the metaphase plate and remain in this condition until fertilization. Sperm penetration activates the oocyte to complete the

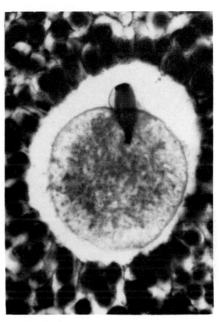

Fig. 20-10. Photomicrograph of oocyte during first maturation division. Corona radiata cells are seen encircling the oocyte. ×700. (From a preparation by Dr. T. E. Hunt.)

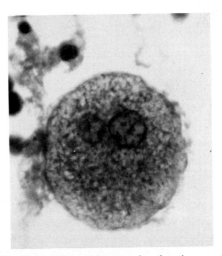

Fig. 20-11. Photomicrograph showing male and female pronuclei in an ovum shortly after sperm penetration. Oocyte was located by sectioning the Fallopian tube. ×700. (From a preparation by Dr. T. E. Hunt.)

second maturation division forming the second polar body. The appearance of the ovum shortly after sperm penetration is shown in Figure 20-11.

The Corpus Luteum

After ovulation, the ruptured follicle does not degenerate at once but is transformed

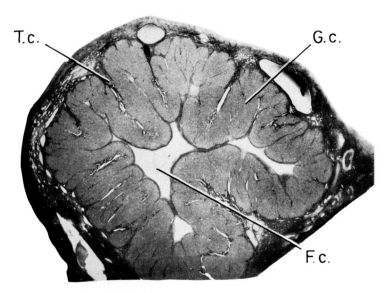

Fig. 20-12. Photomicrograph of a section of a human ovary, showing a fully formed corpus luteum of pregnancy. Granulosa lutein cells (*G.c.*) form the major portion of the corpus; theca lutein cells (*T.c.*) surround it and penetrate between folds of granulosa lutein cells; a remnant of the follicular cavity (*F.c.*) contains loose connective tissue. ×5.

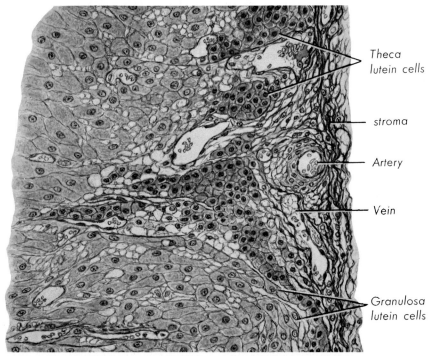

Fig. 20-13. Section through the peripheral part of corpus luteum removed during the progravid stage of the sexual cycle. Masson's trichrome stain. ×200.

temporarily into a glandular structure, the *yellow body* or *corpus luteum* (Figs. 20-12 and 20-13). The follicular cavity closes over by healing of the wound and becomes filled with a serous, fibrin-containing fluid which usually contains some blood. The granulosa cells of the follicle do not proliferate to any significant degree but increase greatly in size. Both granulosa and theca interna cells enlarge and become epithelioid in their characteristics. They can be distinguished from each other, however, on the basis of their location, size and staining reactions. In comparison with the *granulosa lutein cells*, the *theca lutein cells* are peripheral in position, they are smaller and their nuclei stain darker (Fig. 20-13).

The cytoplasm of the lutein cells contains yellowish lipochrome pigment droplets and lipid droplets. Removal of lipids by the routine methods in preparing sections generally gives a finely vacuolated appearance to the cytoplasm as seen under the light microscope. Electron micrographs show that the cytoplasm contains considerable smooth endoplasmic reticulum, some free ribosomes and mitochondria with tubular cristae. Thus, the cells which are known to secrete progesterone have the cytological characteristics of other steroid hormone-secreting cells.

Connective tissue from the theca externa penetrates the lutein mass and forms delicate interlacing septa, in which are numerous capillaries. The connective tissue finally penetrates the entire layer and spreads to form a continuous covering on the inner surface of the lutein cells. In the center, the follicular cavity remains as a greatly reduced space of irregular outline, still filled with a serous fluid or, more rarely, with the disintegrating remains of the blood clot (Figs. 20-12 and 20-14).

If the discharged ovum is not fertilized and dies on its way to the uterus, the corpus luteum reaches its greatest development about 1 week after ovulation and then begins to degenerate. This is the *corpus luteum of menstruation*. The cells of such a corpus luteum gradually decrease in size, show increasing vacuolization and are finally resorbed. The connective tissue between the lutein cells increases in amount, and a loose, gelatinous type of connective tissue, often containing brownish pigment

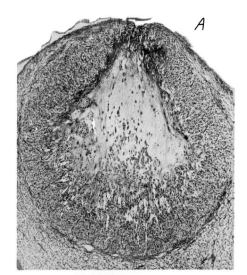

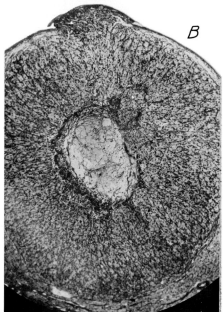

Fig. 20-14. Stages in the formation of the corpus luteum in the rabbit. *A*, corpus luteum from an ovary removed 48 hr after mating (about 36 hr after ovulation). *B*, corpus luteum from the other ovary of the same animal. This ovary was removed 4 days after mating (about 84 h after ovulation).

of the extravasated blood, fills the central cavity. The gland becomes progressively smaller and, several weeks after beginning of involution, is transformed into a whitish scar of microscopic size, the *corpus albicans*.

If the ovum is fertilized, the corpus increases in size for a time and is known as the *corpus luteum of pregnancy*. It attains a size of 20 to 30 mm, and persists until the later months of pregnancy, when it likewise undergoes a slow involution.

Although human corpora lutea are bright yellow, this is not true for all mammals. The corpora lutea of cows have an orange hue. In some animals (dog, cat and some rodents) they contain no pigment and consequently are pale in color.

Interstitial Cells

In many mammals, the cortical stroma contains clusters or strands of epithelioid connective tissue cells whose cytoplasm contains fine lipid granules. These form from the theca interna and are known as *interstitial cells.* In the mature human ovary, the theca interna cells of degenerating follicles form radiating cords which persist for only a short time (Figs. 20-8 and 20-9). There are relatively few cells in the mature human ovum that resemble the interstitial cells of rodents. It is thought that they arise from theca interna cells of atretic follicles.

Hormones of the Ovary

The ovary is under the direct influence of hormones of the anterior hypophysis. These hormones, the gonadotropins, control the maturation of follicles and the formation of corpora lutea. The ovary in turn produces hormones of its own, which affect the accessory reproductive organs such as the uterus, Fallopian tubes and mammary glands, and which also exert a regulatory effect upon the anterior hypophysis.

The ovarian hormones are steroids. One of them, *estrogen* (principally *estradiol*), is secreted by the growing follicles and to a lesser degree by the corpus luteum. The other, *progesterone,* is produced mainly by the corpus luteum but also to some extent by the mature follicle just prior to ovulation. Because there is a wave of follicular maturation during the first half of each month, followed by formation of a corpus luteum immediately after ovulation, the levels of the two hormones normally show regular cyclic fluctuations. Estrogen secretion is high during the preovulatory period and reaches a peak at about the time of ovulation; progesterone secretion increases rapidly as the ruptured follicle becomes luteinized, and it remains at a high level until regression of the corpus luteum. The fluctuations in ovarian hormone levels are reflected, as discussed later, in cyclic variations in other structures, notably in the mucous membrane of the uterus.

Blood Vessels

Branches of the ovarian and uterine arteries enter the medulla at the hilus and divide into a number of spirally coursing vessels. These vessels run to the boundary zone of cortex and medulla, where they ramify and anastomose into plexuses. From these are given off branches that enter the cortex radially and break up into extensive capillary networks in the thecae of the growing and mature follicles. From the capillaries, veins arise that accompany the arteries, form an extensive plexus in the medulla and leave the ovary at the hilus.

Lymphatics

Lymph capillaries begin in the theca externa of the follicles and unite into somewhat larger vessels which pass radially through the medulla and leave at the hilus. There they are collected in a number of lymphatic trunks that drain into the lumbar lymph nodes.

Nerves

Nerve fibers, mostly unmyelinated, enter at the hilus and follow the course of the blood vessels. Many terminate in the muscle fibers of the medullary blood vessels. Others enter the cortex and form delicate plexuses in the thecae but apparently do not penetrate the basement membranes of the follicles. According to some authors, groups of sympathetic ganglion cells are found in the medulla.

Vestigial Structures

As is the case with the testis, certain rudimentary organs, the remains of fetal structures, are associated with the ovary.

The *epoophoron* consists of a number of blind tubules situated in the folds of the broad ligament between the ovary and the oviduct. The tubules open into a longitudinal duct, the canal of Gärtner, which passes along the lateral wall of the uterus and reaches the vagina. The duct is often interrupted and may be altogether absent in some cases.

The *paroophoron* is situated in the connective tissue of the hilus and consists of a few blind tubules or cords. It is rarely found in the adult.

Both epoophoron and paroophoron are remains of the embryonal mesonephros, while Gärtner's canal represents a vestige of the Wolffian (mesonephric) duct.

The Fallopian Tubes

The Fallopian (uterine) tubes are paired structures, each of which is about 15 cm long and 6 to 8 mm in diameter. One end of a tube opens into the peritoneal cavity near the ovary; the other end opens into the superior lateral part of the uterine cavity. The tubes conduct the ova that are discharged at ovulation to the uterine cavity.

Four regions of the tubes are usually distinguished. Beginning with the ovarian end, these are: (a) infundibulum, (b) ampulla, (c) isthmus and (d) uterine or interstitial segment. The *infundibulum* is funnel-shaped and is formed of a number of processes or fimbriae (Fig. 20-1). The *ampulla* is the longest of the segments and, like the fimbriae, is thin walled. It terminates in a relatively short segment which extends to the uterus, the *isthmus*. This segment is smaller in diameter and thicker walled than the ampulla. The last portion, *pars uterina,* is embedded in the wall of the uterus. The mucosa of the infundibulum and ampulla is thrown into many tall folds with correspondingly deep grooves. The lumen thus is very irregular in shape (Fig. 20-15). The folds progressively decrease in height toward the uterus and are low in the isthmus. In the pars uterina, there are only slight folds, and the cavity reaches its smallest diameter, about 1 mm.

The wall of the Fallopian tube consists of three coats: mucosa, muscularis and serosa.

The *epithelium* lining the Fallopian tubes is a simple columnar type, some cells of which are ciliated, whereas others are narrow, peg-shaped and nonciliated (Figs. 20-16 through 20-18). The height of the epithelium and the proportion of ciliated to nonciliated secretory cells, although varying considerably even in neighboring regions of a tube, show changes that correlate with the stages of the menstrual cycle. The epithelium during the first half (follicular phase) of the cycle is taller than it is in the second half, which is under the influence of the corpus luteum. The relative number of nonciliated, peg-shaped cells also increases in the corpus luteum phase of the cycle. During pregnancy, the epithelium is quite low and there is an increased number of "peg" cells. Cyclic changes also occur in numbers and size of cilia on the

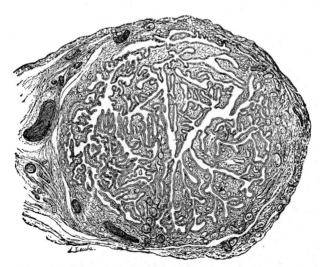

Fig. 20-15. Cross section of Fallopian tube near fimbriated extremity, showing complicated foldings of mucous membrane (Orthmann).

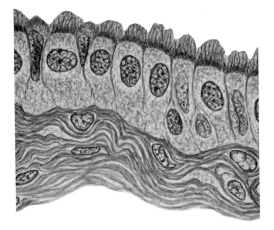

Fig. 20-16. Section of Fallopian tube removed at the middle of the menstrual cycle, showing the characteristic type of epithelium present at that stage. ×1200.

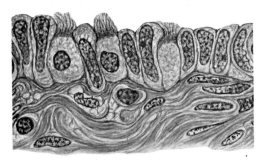

Fig. 20-17. Section of Fallopian tube of a woman 2½ months pregnant, showing the type of epithelium characteristic of pregnancy and of the progravid stage of the menstrual cycle. ×1200.

ciliated cells. This has been most thoroughly studied in monkeys. Ciliogenesis in the uterine tubes is responsive to estrogen levels. Other ciliated epithelia in the body do not respond in a similar way to estrogen hormone levels. The tubal epithelium secretes mucus and probably other substances necessary for the maintenance of the ovum during its journey down the tube.

The cilia beat toward the uterus. The beating of the cilia and the waves of muscular contraction transport the ovum through the tubes. No glands are present in the Fallopian tubes.

The connective tissue of the lamina propria is richly cellular; it is quite compact in the isthmus but more loosely arranged in the high folds of the ampulla.

The *muscularis* is thickest in the isthmus and gradually thins out toward the fimbriated end. It consists of a well developed inner circular layer and a rather thin outer longitudinal layer. The latter is complete only in the isthmus. In the ampulla, the longitudinal muscle bundles are discontinuous and may be absent altogether in the fimbria.

The *serosa* has the usual structure of peritoneum.

The larger *blood vessels* run in the connective tissue along the bases of the folds. They send off branches that give rise to a dense capillary network.

The *lymphatics* arise as relatively large lacunae in the connective tissue of the mucosal folds. These empty into narrower channels that pass through the muscularis and form a rich subserous net. The lymphatics drain into the upper lumbar lymph nodes.

The *nerves* form a rich plexus in the connective tissue, from which fibers pass to the blood vessels and muscular tissue and to the epithelial lining.

The Uterus

The uterus is a thick walled, pear-shaped organ, somewhat flattened dorsoventrally in its upper two-thirds. It varies considerably in size, averaging some 7 cm in length, 5 cm in width at its upper (broadest) part and 2.5 cm in thickness. Its cavity conforms to the general shape of the organ, being very narrow dorsoventrally in the body of the organ and more circular in the lower portion. The uterine tubes open into the superior lateral part of the uterine cavity, one on either side. The lower part of the cavity (the cervical canal) opens into the vagina.

Anatomically, two main regions of the uterus are distinguished: (a) an upper *body* or *corpus* with its rounded, dome-shaped top, the *fundus,* and (b) a narrower, cyclindrical *neck* or *cervix* whose terminal portion projects into the vagina as the *portio vaginalis.* The narrow zone of transition between corpus and cervix is known as the *isthmus.*

The wall of the uterus consists of three coats which, from the outermost inward, are the serosa or *perimetrium,* the muscu-

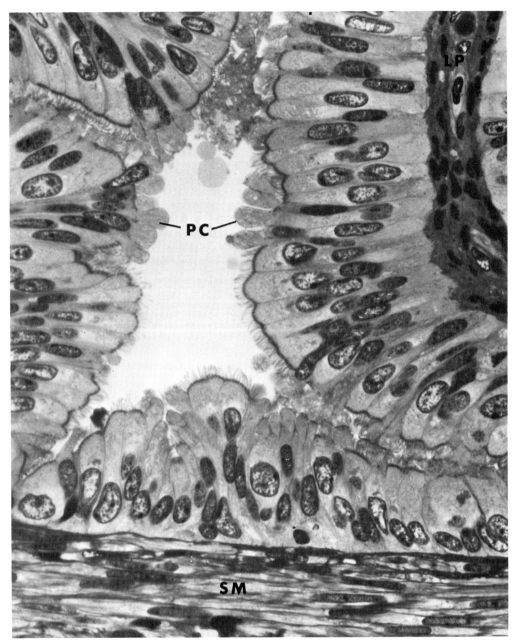

Fig. 20-18. Light micrograph of a portion of the Fallopian tube of a monkey. Peg cells (*PC*) are interspersed with ciliated cells. *SM*, smooth muscle cells of muscularis; *LP*, lamina propria (*upper right*). ×685.

laris or *myometrium* and the mucosa or *endometrium*.

The *perimetrium* is the peritoneal layer of the broad ligament, which covers the corpus and a portion of the cervix. It is firmly attached to the underlying muscularis and has the usual structure of a serous membrane.

Myometrium

The myometrium is a massive muscular coat, about 15 mm in thickness, consisting of bundles of smooth muscle fibers held together by connective tissue. The disposition of the muscle fibers is quite complicated but, in a general way, three layers may be distinguished. The inner, muscular layer, the *stratum subvasculare,* consists of fibers running longitudinally, i.e., parallel to the long axis of the organ. The middle layer, *stratum vasculare,* forms the bulk of the muscularis and is composed mainly of fibers running circularly or spirally. In the interstitial tissue are numerous large blood vessels, especially veins. The outer layer, *stratum supravasculare,* is relatively thin and is composed of both circular and longitudinal fibers. The latter predominate and form a fairly distinct subserous layer which becomes continuous with the longitudinal muscle coat of the vagina. In the cervix, the inner longitudinal layer is absent.

The muscle cells of the virgin uterus have a length of 40 to 90 μm, the variations conforming to definite phases of the menstrual cycle. The fibers are shortest in the 1st week after menstruation and reach their greatest length in the 4th week of the cycle. During pregnancy, the muscle tissue of the uterus is greatly increased. This is due partly to an increase in the number but mainly to the tremendous increase in the size of the muscle fibers, which in the later stages of pregnancy may have a length of over 500 μm.

The interstitial tissue contains numerous blood vessels and consists of loosely arranged collagenous fibers and relatively few connective tissue cells. Elastic fibers are found in considerable amounts in the outer layer of the muscularis and in the subserous connective tissue. The inner portions of the myometrium are relatively poor in elastic tissue. In the cervix, elastic tissue is abundant.

Endometrium

The endometrium is lined by simple columnar epithelium composed of small patches of ciliated cells interspersed with nonciliated cells. Numerous tubular glands are present, and they are lined by columnar cells which resemble those at the surface except that there are fewer ciliated cells. There is no submucosa, and the mucosa is closely attached to the myometrium, the juncture between them being very irregular.

During the childbearing period, the mucosa of the corpus and fundus passes through cyclic changes, each cycle closely related to the maturation of an ovarian follicle, the discharge of the contained oocyte and the subsequent formation of a corpus luteum. In general, these changes are in the nature of a preparation for pregnancy, and they consist of a hypertrophy of the glandular, vascular and interstitial elements of the mucosa. If the egg is fertilized and implantation occurs, the hypertrophy continues. If the egg is not implanted, the hypertrophied layer breaks down, and the tissue debris, together with a certain amount of blood, is discharged as the *menstrual fluid.* With cessation of the flow, regeneration occurs rapidly and a new cycle sets in, determined as before by a new ovarian cycle. A uterine bleeding or *menstruation* occurs typically at intervals of about 28 days and lasts for 3 to 5 days, but there is great variability among different individuals and often in any one individual. The 1st day of menstruation is counted as the 1st day of the uterine or menstrual cycle.

Four stages, each of which has characteristic structural features, are distinguishable in the endometrium during an ovulatory menstrual cycle. It should be kept in mind, however, that the endometrium undergoes a continuous change, and that in each stage the structural features change somewhat, so that one stage does not abruptly pass into the next. The indicated duration of each stage is based on a 28-day cycle. (1) The *menstrual* stage occupies the first 3 to 5 days of the cycle, during which time there is an external menstrual discharge. (2) The *proliferative* (estrogenic) stage begins with the termination of menstruation and extends to about the middle of the cycle, namely, to the 13th or 14th day. (3) The *progravid* or *secretory* (luteal or progestational) stage extends from the middle of the cycle to the 26th or 27th day. (4) The *premenstrual* stage is 1 or 2 days in length and is terminated by the appearance of external bleeding. The length of the proliferative stage is less constant than that of the others, and variations in its duration are chiefly responsible for the varying lengths of the menstrual cycles.

The *proliferative* stage of the cycle (Fig. 20-19, *A*) is characterized by rapid regen-

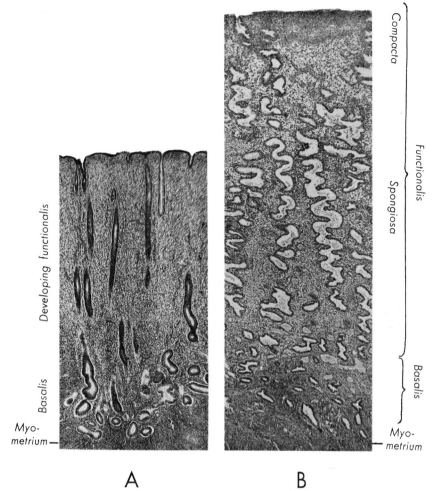

Fig. 20-19. Human endometria. *A*, proliferative stage, about day 10 of menstrual cycle; *B*, late secretory stage, day 25 of cycle. ×30. The tissue of the secretory stage illustrated in this figure and the stages illustrated in Figures 20-20 through 20-23 were supplied by Dr. Arthur Hertig.

eration of the endometrium from the narrow basal zone remaining after menstruation (Fig. 20-20, *B*). Epithelial cells from the remaining portions of the glands migrate and cover the raw surface of the mucosa. Numerous mitoses occur in cells of the glands and of the connective tissue. As the gland cells increase in number, they become tall and closely packed together (Fig. 20-21), and the glands increase in length. Although forked terminations of the glands are frequent, the glands remain relatively straight and uniform in diameter (Fig. 20-19, *A*). Near the close of the proliferative stage, some secretion appears in the basal ends of the gland cells. The connective tissue framework (stroma) contains branching

cells and reticular fibers. Blood vessels (coiled arteries) grow into the regenerating tissue and, toward the end of the proliferative stage, a considerable degree of edema develops, although it is not as pronounced as in the secretory stage. During the proliferative stage, the endometrium increases from a postmenstrual thickness of 0.5 mm or less to 2 or 3 mm.

In the *secretory* stage of the cycle, the endometrium hypertrophies, reaching a thickness of 4 to 5 mm. The increase is due not to mitotic activity but to hypertrophy of the gland cells and to an increase in edema and vascularity. The gland cells remain about the same in height but become broader (Figs. 20-21 and 20-22). The glands

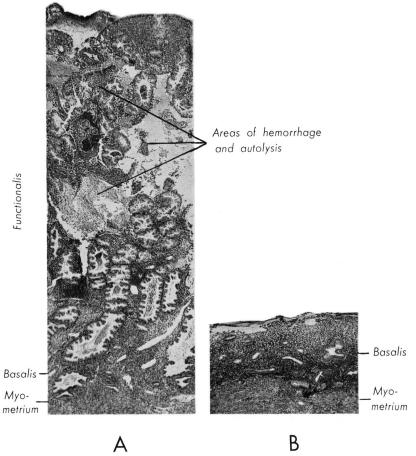

Functionalis

Areas of hemorrhage
and autolysis

Basalis

*Myo-
metrium*

Basalis

*Myo-
metrium*

A   B

Fig. 20-20. Human endometria. *A*, early menstrual phase; *B*, termination of menstruation. ×30.

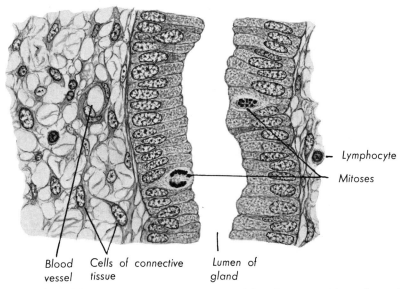

Lymphocyte

Mitoses

*Blood
vessel*   *Cells of connective
tissue*   *Lumen of
gland*

Fig. 20-21. A section of human endometrium in the proliferative stage (about day 11), showing a part of a gland tubule and adjacent stroma. ×650.

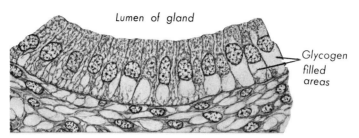

Lumen of gland

Glycogen
filled
areas

Fig. 20-22. A section of human endometrium in the early secretory stage. Day 19 of menstrual cycle. ×650.

assume a corkscrew shape, and their lumina become large and irregular in diameter, giving them a characteristic appearance (Fig. 20-19, *B*). The edema increases, and the coiled arteries grow nearly to the surface.

With the development of the secretory stage, several layers can be distinguished in the endometrium (Fig. 20-19). The *basalis* is the deepest layer and is relatively narrow. Its glands undergo little or no change. This layer is not lost at menstruation or at parturition. The *functionalis* comprises all of the endometrium lying above (superficial to) the basalis. It undergoes periodic changes in the menstrual cycle and is lost at menstruation and at parturition. The functionalis is divided into two layers, a superficial layer, the *compacta,* and a deep layer, the *spongiosa.* The *compacta* is relatively narrow. It has little edema, and the portions of the glands that lie in it are quite straight. The *spongiosa* comprises the bulk of the endometrium. It is edematous, and the glands are tortuous and have large lumina, giving the zone a spongy appearance. It is emphasized that these zones become evident only with the development of the secretory stage.

During the secretory stage, the gland cells undergo certain progressive secretory changes. With the onset of this stage, both glycogen and mucigen increase rapidly in the gland cells of the functionalis, and these secretions are localized at first in the basal portions of the cells. With the usual technical procedures, the secretion is dissolved (Fig. 20-22). During the latter half of the secretory stage, the secretion moves to the apical zone of the gland cells, and the nuclei consequently become basally located (Fig. 20-23). The secretion, composed of glycogen, mucin and some fat, then appears in

the lumina of the glands, thus terminating the secretory cycle of the cells of the glands.

In the *premenstrual* phase of the cycle, important changes occur in the coiled arteries, leading to a breakdown of the functionalis. In studies made on living endometrial transplants in the anterior chamber of the eye in monkeys, Markee observed that a constriction of the coiled arteries and vascular stasis occurred during the premenstrual period, producing a condition of anemia and anoxia. Finally, blood escaped from the vessels. These observations assist in explaining the immediate factor responsible for the areas of hemorrhage and autolysis seen in sections of fixed tissue (Fig. 20-20, *A*). In the premenstrual stage there is also a decrease in edema and an infiltration of the stroma with leukocytes. The glands fragment, the surface of the endometrium breaks down and blood and tissue debris appear in the uterine lumen.

During *menstruation,* the functionalis is lost, although there may be considerable variation in the amount of endometrial destruction. The coiled arteries undergo necrosis and some blood may spurt from them, although most of the menstrual blood comes from veins. To this blood are added the secretion of the glands and the broken down tissue of the functionalis.

Thus, in each uterine cycle a period of growth and proliferation is followed by one of secretory activity. In the first period, a new functional layer is built up, with its glands and interstitial tissue. In the second, the functional layer is tranformed into a swollen nutritive compartment ready for the implantation of the fertilized ovum. If the egg is not implanted, desquamation of the functionalis occurs, rapidly followed by regeneration of the epithelial surface. Men-

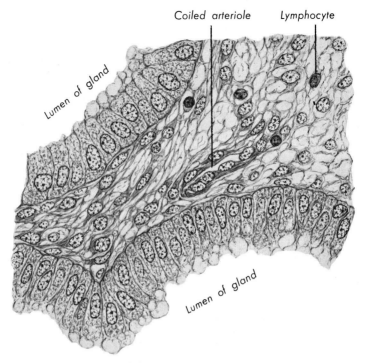

Fig. 20-23. A section of human endometrium in the late secretory stage. Day 25 of cycle. ×650.

struation thus indicates a "biological failure," a failure of the egg to be fertilized and implanted.

The mucosa of the *cervix* (Fig. 20-24) is somewhat thicker than that of the body and fundus of the uterus and shows numerous folds, the *plicae palmatae*. The stroma also is firmer and less cellular.

The lining epithelium consists mainly of high columnar mucous secreting cells, although a few ciliated cells may also be present. The numerous forked glands are much larger than those of the body of the uterus and are lined by tall mucous secreting cells. Closure of the mouths of some of the glands frequently occurs, leading to the formation of cysts of considerable size, the so-called *ovula Nabothi*. Near the external opening of the cervix, the simple columnar epithelium changes abruptly to a stratified squamous epithelium, which likewise covers the external surface of the portio vaginalis. The cervix does not exhibit distinct menstrual changes.

Relation of Menstruation to Ovulation

As already stated, the cyclic uterine changes are closely related to the ovarian cycles associated with ovulation. From the available evidence, it is possible to relate, temporally, the specific phases of the two cycles. The postmenstrual proliferative changes correspond to the preovulatory period of maturation of the follicle. The secretory stage is always associated with the formation and growth of the corpus luteum, and it lasts as long as the latter retains its full function. The beginning involution of the corpus luteum always marks the onset of menstruation. Ovulation occurs normally at the end of the proliferative period, although the estimates of different investigators vary within relatively wide limits (from the 8th to the 20th day of the cycle). Very precise and extensive data have been collected by Hartman on rhesus monkeys. Their sex cycles and reproductive processes are very similar to those of the human. In some 300 observations, Hartman found that ovulation occurred most frequently on days 11, 12 and 13 (dated from the 1st day of the preceding menstruation), although occasional instances of ovulation were found between the 8th and 23rd day of the cycle. A schema of the temporal relations of two cycles is given in Figure 20-25.

Evidence secured from the human as well

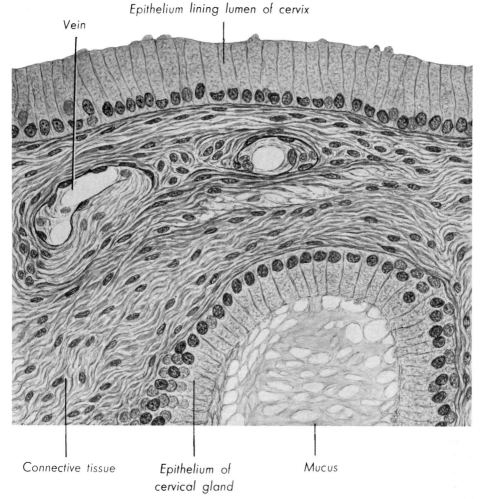

Fig. 20-24. Transverse section through the superficial portion of the cervical mucosa of a woman 31 years old. End of the 2nd month of pregnancy. Therapeutic abortion. Stained with iron hematoxylin. ×625.

as from rhesus monkeys has revealed that the cyclical uterine changes are induced by estrogen, a product of the follicle and perhaps of other parts of the ovary, and of progesterone, a product of the corpus luteum. The endometrium involutes after ovariectomy but can be caused to undergo the proliferative changes by estrogen injections. Continued injections of this hormone will not cause a development of the secretory phases, progesterone administration being necessary to induce the development of this phase, but injection of progesterone must be preceded by estrogen treatments in order for it to act. It is established that the corpora lutea in women secrete estrogen as well as progesterone and that, in the latter half of the cycle, the uterus is under the influence of both of these hormones. A more highly developed secretory type of endometrium can be produced experimentally if the progesterone injections are supplemented by estrogen administration. By the use of these two hormones, the endometrial changes characteristic of the normal cycle can be secured in ovariectomized women, as well as in monkeys. The changes thus induced obviously correlate with the follicular and lutein phases through which the ovary passes in the complete ovulatory cycle.

Experimental work has revealed the role of the hormones in menstruation, although it was confused for a time by the fact that,

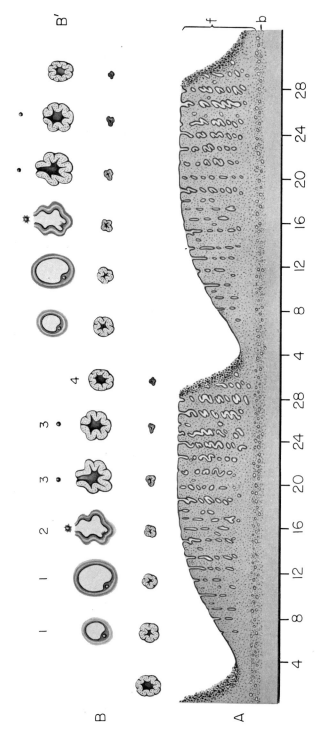

Fig. 20-25. Diagram illustrating relation of menstruation to ovulation. A, cyclic changes in uterine mucosa; B, ovarian cycles; b, basal layer, and f, functional layer of mucosa; 1, 1, maturing follicle; 2, rupture of follicle and discharge of ovum (ovulation); 3, 3, corpus luteum in full function; 4 and remaining figures, degenerating corpus luteum. Numbers at base indicate days of menstrual cycle. (Redrawn after Schroeder.)

during the summer months, rhesus monkeys in captivity do not ovulate or form corpora lutea but still exhibit periodic menstruation. Such cycles are known as *anovulatory cycles*. It has been demonstrated that bleeding will occur from a proliferative endometrium if the estrogen administration that induced this phase is stopped. If progesterone injections are commenced at the time that the estrogen injections are stopped, however, menstruation does not occur but will take place a few days after the progesterone treatment is terminated. The institution of estrogen injections when the progesterone treatment is withdrawn, however, will not inhibit the expected menstruation that results from progesterone withdrawal.

Blood Vessels

Branches from each uterine artery penetrate to the middle (vascular) layer of the uterine muscle and then continue both ventrally and dorsally in this layer to the midline, forming the arcuate arteries. They anastomose with the branches from the other uterine artery. Two sets of branches arise from these arched arteries: (1) small branches that course peripherally and supply the supravascular (outer) part of the uterus, and (2) larger branches that course centrally. Branches from the latter in turn form two systems. One set, which penetrates the endometrium for a variable distance, depending on the stage of the cycle, is extremely coiled (coiled arteries) and terminates in a tuft of arterioles (Fig. 20-26). The other set supplies the inner layer of the uterine muscle and the basal part of the endometrium, where branches from it anastomose with the branches of the coiled arteries. The endometrium is thus supplied by a basal and a superficial set of vessels. The basal set, as would be expected, does not undergo modifications with the stages

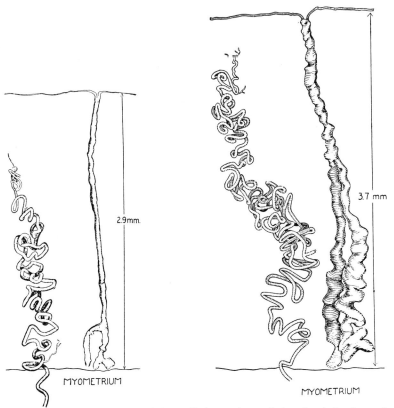

Fig. 20-26. Projection reconstructions of the coiled arteries and the glands in the endometrium of rhesus monkey (Old World monkey). *Left*, early proliferative stage (early postmenstrual); *right*, late progravid stage. (After Daron.)

of the cycle, but the coiled arteries show pronounced changes. During the proliferative stage of the cycle, they penetrate only one-half or two-thirds through the thickness of the endometrium, but during the secretory stage they increase in extent, approach the surface and, with the tissue loss at menstruation, may protrude into the uterine lumen. Their peripheral part then undergoes necrosis. With the reparative postmenstrual process, the vessels again grow. The menstrual blood, however, does not come mainly from the arteries but from the veins. Two mechanisms appear to operate to prevent the bleeding of the coiled arteries. One of these is the tortuosity of the vessels, which would slow the flow. The other and more effective mechanism is arterial constriction, a constriction that is aided by localized thickenings or cushions, composed of longitudinal smooth muscle, on one side of the arterial lumen.

Menstrual fluid is composed of extravasated blood, desquamated tissue and the secretion of the uterine glands. The discharge does not clot, for it is markedly fibrinolytic. It is also toxic, as shown by injection into experimental animals.

Lymphatics

The lymph vessels are larger and more abundant in the uterus than in most other organs of the body. They are enlarged during pregnancy. All layers of the uterine wall have lymph vessels except the superficial part of the endometrium (compacta), which is devoid of them. During its cyclical changes, the endometrium exhibits pronounced changes in its water content, and these changes are probably responsible for the unusually extensive lymph drainage.

Nerves

Both myelinated and unmyelinated nerve fibers occur in the uterus. The latter predominate and are connected with minute ganglia found in the upper vaginal wall near its junction with the cervix. These fibers supply the walls of the blood vessels and the muscle tissue of the myometrium. The myelinated fibers apparently run to the mucosa and form a scanty plexus beneath the epithelium. The distribution and endings of the mucosal nerve fibers have not been fully investigated.

The Uterus during Pregnancy

The ovum, if fertilized, becomes implanted in the endometrium at about the 6th day after ovulation. At this time, the endometrium has reached a highly developed secretory or progravid condition. It is thick and edematous, and the lumina and cells of the glands are large and contain glycogen, mucigen and some lipid. Implantation may take place in any region of the uterine mucosa and even in the tubal epithelium. The uterine changes and correlated events in the ovary and ovum during the early phases of pregnancy in women are shown in Figure 20-27.

From the extensive studies of Hertig et al. on a considerable series of ova and later stages, secured from timed hysterectomies, it appears that the following events occur subsequent to ovulation. Fertilization takes place before or soon after the oocyte enters the uterine tube. The migration down the uterine tube is leisurely, the ovum undergoing cellular division during its migration and arriving in the uterus on the 3rd day after ovulation. An ovum having two normal blastomeres was recovered from the middle third of the uterine tube 2 to 2½ days after the estimated time of ovulation, and one in an eight-cell stage was recovered from the uterus on the 3rd day. A blastula, also lying free in the uterine cavity, was recovered on the 4th day. It was found to consist of a thin epithelial membrane and a small inner cell mass, destined to form the embryo. A blastocyst secured 7 to 7½ days after ovulation was implanted just beneath the surface of the endometrium, and the eroded epithelium had not, as yet, undergone sufficient repair to cover it. The chorionic membrane had proliferated; it is now known because of its nutritive role, as the *trophoblast*. From the evidence summarized above, together with evidence from other fertilized but abnormal ova that have been recovered, it has been concluded that implantation occurs about the 6th day after ovulation (Fig. 3-1).

At somewhat later stages, when the developing ovum is imbedded entirely within the endometrium, the trophoblast over the entire surface is found to have undergone growth (Fig. 20-28). The outer surface of the trophoblast shows irregular processes, between which are irregular spaces or lacunae. In these spaces, maternal blood which comes from the eroded coiled arteries of the endometrium will later flow. This is returned by the maternal veins.

Some of the trophoblast cells differen-tiate into a syncytial layer very early, and two layers can be distinguished in the trophoblast by the 11th day. These are: an inner layer, the *cytotrophoblast,* and an outer layer, the *syntrophoblast* (Fig. 3-2). Beneath these is a stratum of mesenchyme which is destined to form the connective tissue component of the chorion. From the irregularities on the outer surface of the

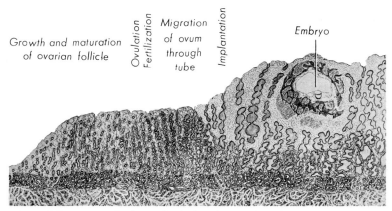

Fig. 20-27. A semidiagrammatic figure depicting the uterine changes and correlated events in the ovary and ovum. (That part of the diagram showing the uterine changes has been taken from Schroeder.)

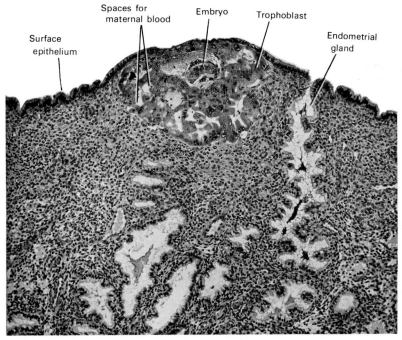

Fig. 20-28. Section through a human embryo 9½ days old. The embryo lies just beneath the epithelial surface of a 26-day secretory endometrium. ×100. (Courtesy of Drs. Rock and Hertig.)

trophoblast, finger-like sprouts or *villi* grow into the surrounding space. These at first are composed only of epithelial cords (primitive villi). Later, a core of embryonal connective tissue, which is connected with the inner stratum of mesenchyme mentioned above, forms within them. They are then designated as secondary (chorionic) villi. In the core of embryonal connective tissue, branches of the fetal blood vessels soon develop.

On the surface of the chorion facing the uterine lumen, the villi do not grow as rapidly as on the deeply embedded surface. They disappear from the luminal surface at about the end of the first third of pregnancy, leaving that surface smooth. It is named the *chorion laeve.* On the deep-lying surface of the chorion, i.e., the surface facing the myometrium, the villi continue to increase and form the fetal component of the placenta. This portion of the chorion is designated the *chorion frondosum.* That part of the chorion to which the villi of this deep surface are attached forms a fairly firm plate-like structure and is called the *chorionic plate.*

The *endometrium* also undergoes important changes in pregnancy. It is called the *decidua graviditatis* because, except for the deepest layer, it is destined to be cast off at parturition. Thus, the process at birth is not unlike menstruation except that it is much more cataclysmic and involves the loss of much more tissue.

In relation to the developing embryo, three regions of the decidua are distinguished: (a) the *decidua basalis* or *serotina,* that part of the mucosa lying beneath the embryo, i.e., between the embryo and the myometrium, (b) the *decidua capsularis,* or *reflexa,* that part of the mucosa which lies between the embryo and the lumen of the uterus, and (c) the *decidua parietalis* or *vera,* which consists of all of the remaining mucosa of the body and fundus of the uterus (Fig. 20-29).

In the early part of pregnancy, the endometrium increases in thickness. The glands enlarge and become more tortuous, and the cells of the endometrial stroma become large and rounded, forming characteristic cellular elements, the *decidual cells.* These are described later. In the latter

half or two-thirds of pregnancy, the parietal decidua gradually becomes thinner and the glands become reduced to slitlike spaces. As the lumen of the uterus is obliterated by the growth of the fetus, the decidua parietalis and capsularis come in contact with each other. The capsularis degenerates, and the parietalis, denuded of epithelium, fuses with the external fetal membrane, the chorion.

The Placenta

The human placenta at term measures about 7 inches in diameter and 1 inch in thickness. It is usually circular but may vary a good deal in shape. The placenta reaches nearly its maximal diameter during the first half of pregnancy but continues to increase in thickness throughout most of gestational period as a result of the growth of the villi.

The placenta consists of two components, a *fetal* and a *maternal,* which develop as described in the preceding section. The *fetal component* consists of a chorionic plate and branching processes or villi which arise from the chorionic plate and lie in the spaces through which the maternal blood circulates.

The *chorionic villi* are usually classified into two types, *anchoring* and *free* or *floating* villi, the structure of the two being similar. The anchoring villi pass from the chorionic plate to the decidua basalis; thus, one of their functions is the anchoring of the chorionic plate to the decidua (Fig. 20-30). They give origin throughout their length to branches that float in the blood-filled lacunar spaces between the fetal portion of the placenta and the decidua basalis, and these are known as free or floating villi. As development proceeds, the villi become very numerous. They also become increasingly irregular in shape, with many protuberances which correspond with the loops and coils of the capillaries that they contain. Their complex pattern is seen particularly well in pictures made by use of the scanning electron microscope (Figs. 20-31 and 20-32). Their total surface area has been estimated to be 6 to 7 m^2. Each villus has a central core of mesenchymal tissue and contains branches of fetal blood vessels. These receive their blood from the umbili-

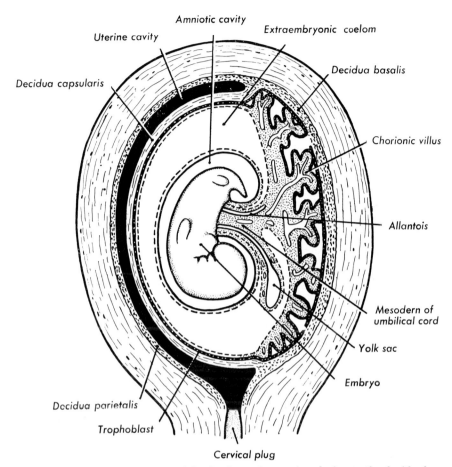

Amniotic cavity

Extraembryonic coelom

Uterine cavity

Decidua basalis

Decidua capsularis

Chorionic villus

Allantois

Mesodern of
umbilical cord

Yolk sac

Embryo

Decidua parietalis

Trophoblast

Cervical plug

Fig. 20-29. Diagram of the formation of the fetal membranes in relation to the decidual membranes. (Redrawn after Hamilton, Boyd and Mossman.)

cal arteries and drain into the umbilical vein. They are covered by trophoblast, as are also the chorionic plate and the chorionic surface of the decidua basalis (Fig. 20-30). The outer (maternal) border of the villus often has adherent fibrin and fibrinoid material, particularly in the later months of pregnancy.

The structure of the trophoblast differs somewhat according to the age of the embryo. A syncytial layer differentiates from some of the trophoblast cells early, and two layers then become distinguishable, an inner cellular and an outer syncytial layer (Figs. 20-33 and 20-34). Because the cells of the inner layer are discrete and well defined, this layer is named the *cellular trophoblast* or *cytotrophoblast*. The cells composing it are frequently called *Langhans cells*. The outer layer of the tropho-

blast, i.e., the layer next to the spaces filled with maternal blood, is plasmodial in nature and is named, therefore, the *syncytial trophoblast* or *syntrophoblast*. These two cell layers persist for approximately the first half of pregnancy. The cells of the cytotrophoblast then gradually decrease in number and, at term, they are inconspicuous.

The cells of the *cytotrophoblast* are irregularly ovoid in shape and vary considerably in size (Fig. 20-33). Their cytoplasm stains lightly and contains some glycogen. Their nuclei are distinct and have a small amount of chromatin and distinct nucleoli. Beneath the cellular trophoblast is a delicate basement membrane composed of a basal lamina and a lamina reticularis of argyrophilic fibers. It is generally accepted that the cytotrophoblastic cells divide and

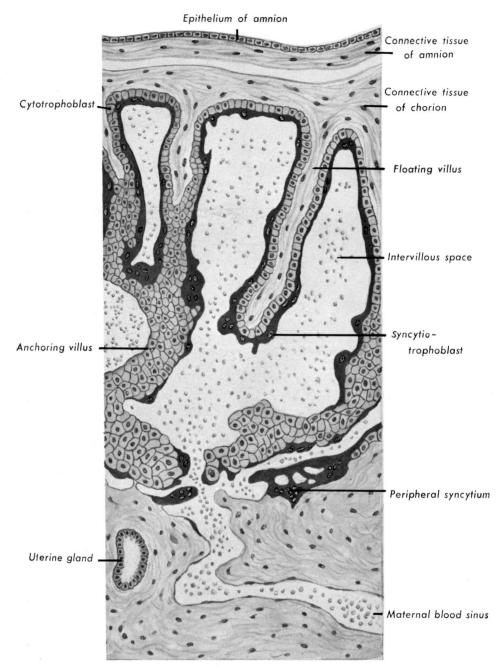

Fig. 20-30. Semischematic diagram of structure of fetal and maternal tissues of the placenta. (Redrawn and modified after Hamilton, Boyd and Mossman.)

give rise to the syncytial cells.

The *syntrophoblast* persists throughout pregnancy. It forms a narrow lamina in which dark staining nuclei are fairly regularly spaced in young placentae (Figs. 20-33 and 20-35); in older placentae, knots or clumps of nuclei occur frequently (Fig. 20-34). No intercellular boundaries can be distinguished. As seen under the light microscope, the syntrophoblast has an irregular brush border at its surface and scattered vacuoles and granules in its cytoplasm.

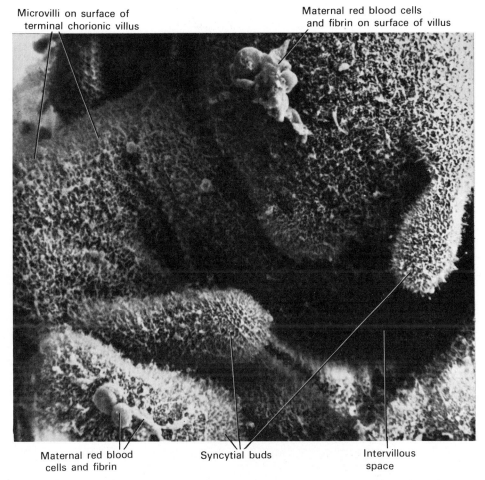

Microvilli on surface of
terminal chorionic villus

Maternal red blood cells
and fibrin on surface of villus

Maternal red blood
cells and fibrin

Syncytial buds

Intervillous
space

Fig. 20-31. Scanning electron microscope micrograph of a portion of the chorion of an 11-week human fetus. The micrograph shows the chorionic surface facing the intervillous spaces and gives a three dimensional effect. ×3000. (Courtesy of Dr. Edward W. Dempsey.)

Electron micrographs reveal that the surface is quite irregular in contour and that it has numerous microvilli (Fig. 20-36). Invaginations of the plasmalemma connect with canaliculi and with vacuoles within the cytoplasm of the apical region, indicating that this zone functions in absorption. The middle zone of the cytoplasm contains an extensive network of rough endoplasmic reticulum, indicating that this region is secretory in function. The ultrastructure of the basal part of the syntrophoblast has many of the characteristics of the cytoplasm of the cytotrophoblast. This correlates with the evidence derived from radioautographic studies that the syntrophoblast is derived from the cytotrophoblast. Many of the blood vessels (fetal) of

the villi, especially in the latter two-thirds of pregnancy, lie close to the surface of the villus (Fig. 20-35), the syntrophoblast over them being attenuated and thin.

The *maternal component of the placenta* is formed by the decidua basalis. This comprises all of the endometrium beneath the fetal portion of the placenta except the deepest part, which is destined to remain after parturition as in normal menstruation. In the decidua basalis, and also in the decidua parietalis, many of the connective tissue cells undergo a pronounced change. They hypertrophy, forming large, ovoid cells of somewhat irregular shape, and are named *decidual cells*. They are one of the most striking features of the endometrium in the first half of pregnancy, for they are

Microvilli on surface
of chorionic villus

Fetal
capillary

Fetal red
blood cells

Maternal
(intervillous) spaces

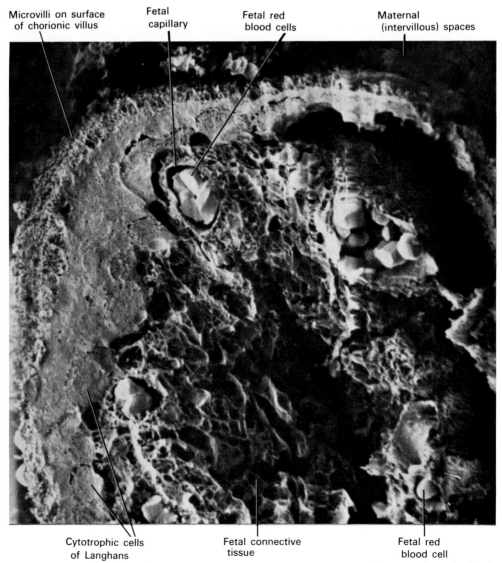

Cytotrophic cells
of Langhans

Fetal connective
tissue

Fetal red
blood cell

Fig. 20-32. Micrograph made with a scanning electron microscope showing a portion of a chorionic villus that is broken in a manner that gives a "sectional" view of the wall of the villus. The micrograph shows the interior of the villus in a three dimensional view. Chorion of an 11-week human fetus. ×3000. (Courtesy of Dr. Edward W. Dempsey.)

very numerous and some become relatively very large (Fig. 20-37). Some of them contain two or more nuclei. The nuclei are large with sparse chromatin and nucleoli. The cytoplasm is vesicular or finely granular. Especially the smaller decidual cells contain large amounts of glycogen.

Some indication of decidual cell formation may be seen even in the terminal phase of a nonfertile menstrual cycle (predecidual reaction). With the onset of pregnancy,

these cells develop rapidly and form a large component of the decidua in early pregnancy, as stated above. They then regress and by the end of pregnancy are rarely present. Their function is obscure.

Function of the Placenta. An obvious function of the placenta is to transfer from the maternal to the fetal circulation the nutritive and other substances necessary for the development of the embryo. It also transfers waste products of fetal metabo-

Blood vessels   Cells of cytotrophoblast

Syncytial trophoblast

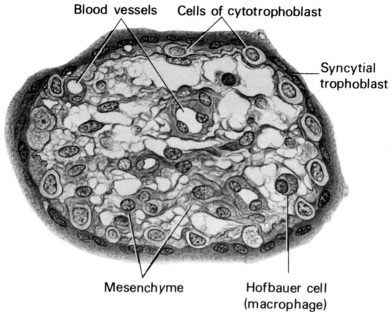

Mesenchyme   Hofbauer cell
(macrophage)

Fig. 20-33. Transverse section of a secondary (free) villus of a human placenta. From a pregnancy of 4½ months duration. Therapeutic abortion. Masson's trichrome stain. ×775.

Group of nuclei of syncytial trophoblast

Blood vessels

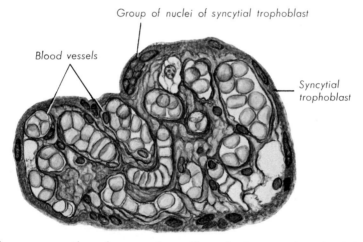

Syncytial trophoblast

Fig. 20-34. Transverse section of a secondary villus of a human placenta at term. The blood vessels are engorged. Masson's trichrome stain. ×775.

lism to the maternal circulation. Although the circulations of the mother and child are entirely separate, they are in close contiguity. The maternal blood circulates through the intervillous spaces, and thus it is separated from the fetal circulation only by the syntrophoblast, the cytotrophoblast (in the first part of pregnancy), a delicate basement membrane and the structures forming the walls of the fetal blood vessels.

The placenta also acts as a selective barrier against the transmission of certain substances from the maternal to the fetal circulation.

Another function of the placenta is the elaboration of hormones. It is known to secrete the steroids *estrogen* and *progesterone*. If the ovaries are removed in women, even early in pregnancy, abortion does not occur and the urinary excretion of estrogen

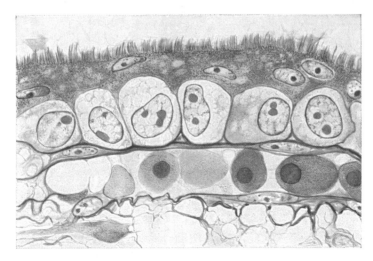

Fig. 20-35. The trophoblast of a secondary villus of a 30-day human placenta. The syncytial layer is faintly vacuolated and has a distinct brush border. The cytotrophoblastic cells form a continuous layer. Subjacent to the basement membrane is a capillary which contains nucleated erythrocytes. Mallory's connective tissue stain. ×1600. (Courtesy of Drs. Wislocki and Bennett.)

and a degradation product of progesterone—pregnandiol—shows only a temporary decrease. Estrogen and progesterone can be extracted from the placenta. The fetal part of the placenta also forms a hormone called *chorionic gonadotrophin,* which differs physiologically from gonadotrophin of hypophyseal origin. This hormone begins to be formed, as judged by urinary assays, shortly after implantation and reaches a maximum in about 2 months, after which it gradually decreases in amount. There is evidence from histochemical and immunochemical studies that the syntrophoblast forms chorionic gonadotrophin, estrogen and progesterone. The cytotrophoblastic cells appear to function chiefly in the formation of the syntrophoblast.

Other Uterine Changes during Pregnancy

The changes described above involve the endometrium of the body and fundus of the uterus. A very pronounced hypertrophy of the smooth muscle of these regions of the uterus also takes place. The muscle fibers increase both in diameter and length. They may reach a length of ½ mm. An increase in the number (hyperplasia) of the muscle fibers also takes place. Although the major uterine changes during pregnancy involve the body and fundus, some

changes in the cervix also occur. The glands become more extensive and secrete copious amounts of mucus which forms a plug that occludes the cervical canal.

The Vagina

The wall of the vagina consists of three coats: mucosa, muscularis and fibrosa (Figs. 20-38 and 20-39).

The *mucosa* shows transverse folds or rugae. It is lined by stratified squamous epithelium which rests on a basement membrane and an underlying lamina propria. Many studies have been made from biopsy specimens in attempts to correlate changes in the epithelium with the menstrual cycle. The findings described, however, are not entirely harmonious, because there are variations in the structure of the epithelium in different parts of the vagina that make it difficult to establish the presence or absence of cyclical changes.

The vaginal epithelium is rich in glycogen which, in the primates, increases with the administration of estrogen. This has also been established in women, and it has been fairly well determined that, in the estrogen phase of the cycle, the vaginal fluid has a lower pH than at other times. This is attributed to the action of the lactic acid-forming bacteria on the carbohydrate from the vaginal epithelium. The effect of estro-

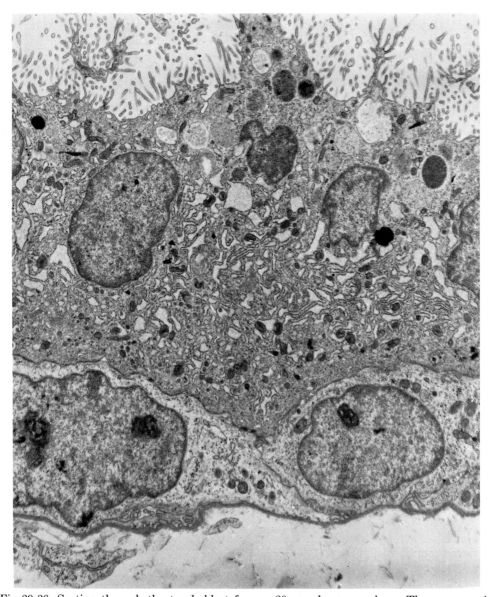

Fig. 20-36. Section through the trophoblast from a 20 mm human embryo. The upper region, facing the intervillous space, has several protrusions and many branched and unbranched microvilli. Indenting the surface, invaginations connect with a canalicular system probably terminating in the small and large apical vacuoles. These structures, and small mitochondria, characterize the apical, *absorptive* zone. Beneath it, occupying approximately the middle third of the figure, is a region rich in rough endoplasmic reticulum. The cisternae are filled with an amorphous substance. The cisternae and the sparse but medium-sized mitochondria distinguish the middle, *secretory* zone. It contains granular cytoplasm, moderately-sized mitochondria and other organelles resembling those of the cytotrophoblast. Dalton's fixation. ×8500. (Figure and legend, Courtesy of Dr. Edward W. Dempsey.)

gen on the formation of glycogen, and the consequent increase of acidity of the vagina, is used clinically in the treatment of gonorrheal vaginitis in children.

In the tissue beneath the epithelium, lymphocytes and polymorphonuclear leukocytes are common. These invade the epithelium especially just before, during and just after menstruation, and they appear as free cells in the lumen of the vagina.

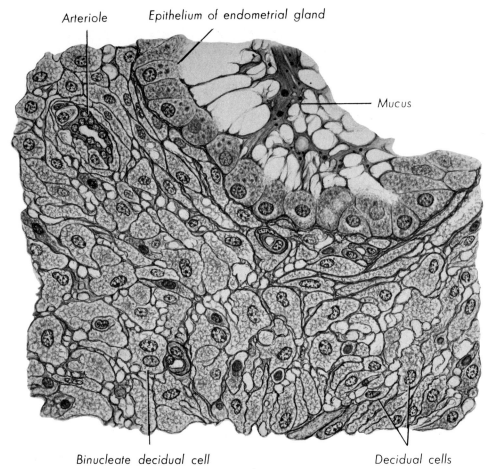

Fig. 20-37. Section through the decidua of a 6-week human pregnancy. The numerous decidual cells and a part of an endometrial gland are illustrated. Therapeutic abortion. Masson's trichrome stain. ×500.

In some lower mammals (e.g., rat), the different types of free cells in the vagina show periodic changes in their proportions which are correlated with the ovarian cycle. The free cells consist of desquamated epithelial cells and leukocytes. The stage of the cycle is thus readily diagnosed by smears. This finding, first established by Stockard and Papanicolaou in 1917, has been of the greatest value in experimental work on reproduction. Although the cyclical changes are not as clear in the human as in some other species, the vaginal smear techniques developed by Papanicolaou are extremely valuable in detecting malignancy at an early stage.

The lamina propria consists of loose connective tissue especially rich in elastic fibers. It also contains polymorphonuclear leukocytes and lymphocytes, as noted above, and it occasionally has aggregations of lymphocytes resembling solitary nodules. A few isolated glands resembling those of the cervix may be found in the uppermost portion of the vagina. Elsewhere the vaginal wall is entirely devoid of glands, and the mucus found in the lumen is derived from the glands of the cervix. In the posterior wall of the vagina, the connective tissue papillae are especially high.

The *muscularis* consists mainly of bundles of longitudinally disposed smooth muscle fibers that become continuous with the myometrium of the uterus. In the inner portion of the muscularis, circular bundles interlace with the longitudinal ones. The muscle bundles are separated by connective tissue rich in elastic fibers. At the entrance

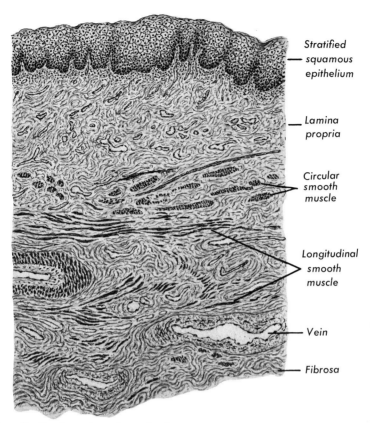

Stratified squamous epithelium

Lamina propria

Circular smooth muscle

Longitudinal smooth muscle

Vein

Fibrosa

Fig. 20-38. Longitudinal section through the posterior wall of vagina. Human, age 50 years. Camera lucida drawing. ×35.

there are skeletal muscle fibers in the vaginal wall.

The *fibrosa* consists of dense connective tissue with many coarse elastic fibers. It serves to connect the vagina with the surrounding structures.

The *hymen* is a thin, transverse semilunar fold at the opening of the vagina into the vestibule. It has the same structure as the vaginal mucosa.

The larger *blood vessels* run in the deeper portion of the mucosa, giving off branches that break up into capillary networks in the stroma and muscularis. These networks have a general direction parallel to the surface. The capillaries empty into the veins that form a plexus of broad venous channels in the muscularis. In the rugae, there are large veins which give the rugae somewhat the character of erectile tissue.

An unusually well developed system of *lymph vessels* is present in the wall of the vagina.

The vagina receives both myelinated and unmyelinated *nerve fibers.* The latter, which are connected with scattered groups of ganglion cells, innervate the muscle tissue and walls of the blood vessels (Fig. 20-40). Sensory myelinated fibers arborize in the mucosa. Their terminals are not fully known.

The External Genitalia

The *vestibule,* into which the vagina and urethra open, is lined by a typical stratified squamous epithelium whose superficial layers are cornified. It contains numerous small mucous glands, the *glandulae vestibulares minores,* placed chiefly near the clitoris and opening of the urethra. They are similar in structure to the glands of Littré of the male reproductive system. The larger *glandulae vestibulares majores* or *glands of Bartholin,* analogous to the bulbourethral glands of the male, are placed in the

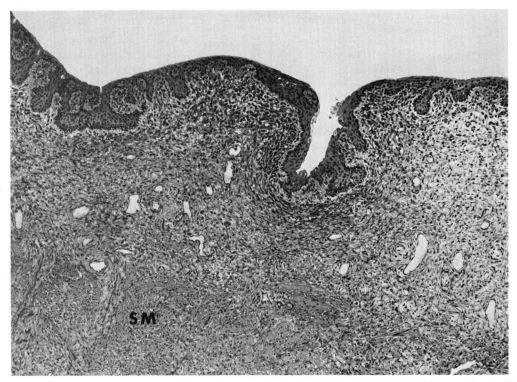

Fig. 20-39. Light micrograph of a portion of the vaginal wall of a monkey. *SM*, smooth muscle. ×170.

lateral wall of the vestibule, their ducts opening close to the base of the hymen.

The *clitoris* consists mainly of erectile tissue similar to that of the corpora cavernosa of the penis. It is covered with a thin stratified squamous epithelium, underneath which is a papillated stroma rich in blood vessels and containing numerous sensory nerve fibers with highly specialized terminations, such as Meissner's corpuscles and Pacinian corpuscles.

The *labia minora,* which flank the vestibule, are covered with a stratified squamous epithelium whose basal layer contains considerable pigment. The underlying, richly vascular connective tissue contains numerous elastic fibers and sends tall slender papillae into the epithelium. In the stroma are found large sebaceous glands, not associated with hairs, and nerve endings similar to those of the clitoris.

The *labia majora* are folds of skin which cover the labia minora. They have the general structure of skin and consist of a stratified squamous epithelium and an underlying dermis of fibroelastic tissue. On the outer side there are numerous hairs, sweat glands and sebaceous glands. On the inner side the epidermis is thinner and hairs are absent. The interior of the labia are filled with fatty tissue.

The Mammary Glands

The mammary glands are cutaneous in origin, developing within the superficial fascia (tela subcutanea). Each gland consists of 15 to 20 lobes, each of which is a compound gland with a separate lobar duct opening at the apex of the nipple.

Connective Tissue Framework (Stroma)

The stroma is both fibrous and fatty in nature. Surrounding or encasing the gland both on the superficial (except at the areola) and deep surface is a layer of fat. Fat is also present within the gland, the amount varying with the functional state. Extending from the dermis into the gland are rather dense fibrous strands (Cooper's ligaments) serving a suspensory function.

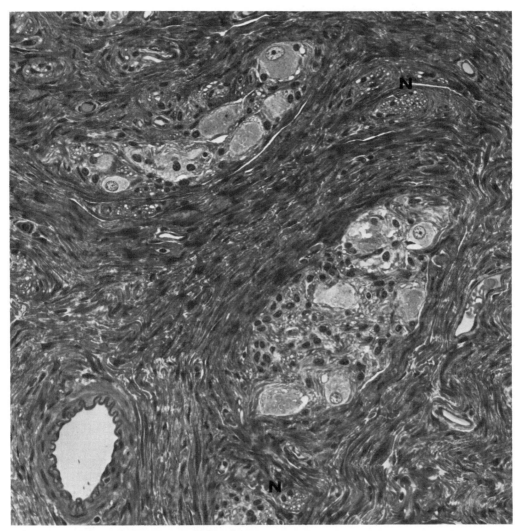

Fig. 20-40. Light micrograph of ganglion cells and nerve fibers (*N*) in the vaginal wall of a monkey. An arteriole is at the *lower left.* ×275.

The interlobar and interlobular connective tissue is also a dense type and forms septa between the subdivisions of the gland. The intralobular connective tissue, on the other hand, is fine and cellular (Fig. 20-41). The amount of connective tissue varies considerably with the functional state of the glands, being reduced in the lactating gland.

Ducts

There is one main duct for each lobe. These lobar ducts course through the nipple and open on the surface. Just beneath the nipple there is a local enlargement (sinus lactiferous). The ducts branch as in any compound gland, a terminal duct finally entering each lobule as an intralobular duct. The epithelium lining an intralobular duct is simple cuboidal. It increases in height as the ducts increase in size, and it becomes stratified squamous near the opening onto the surface. Lying within the epithelium basally are myoepithelial cells. These are more readily observed in the larger ducts.

Nipple and Areola

The skin of the nipple is pigmented and somewhat wrinkled, and it has tall connective tissue papillae. It has many sebaceous

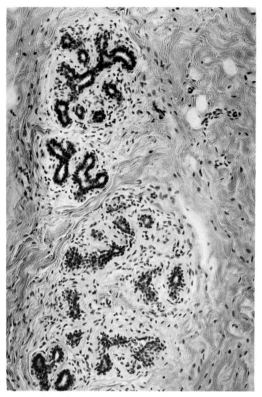

Fig. 20-41. Photomicrograph of a section through two lobules of an inactive mammary gland. Woman, 20 years of age. ×140.

but no sweat glands or hairs. The *areola*, an area extending outward from the nipple for 1 to 2 cm, is also pigmented and has modified mammary glands (glands of Montgomery) whose ducts open through the skin of the areola. These glands, which have some of the features of sweat glands, produce small elevations on the surface. Sweat and sebaceous glands and a variable number of coarse hairs are also present. The subcutaneous tissue of the nipple and areola contains both radially and circularly coursing smooth muscle fibers.

Glandular Epithelium

The epithelium of the mammary gland varies greatly with its functional state and among individuals.

The Inactive Mammary Gland

The glandular tissue in a nonlactating mammary gland of a sexually mature, non-

pregnant woman is sparse and consists of tubules that have the appearance of ducts. These are grouped together in lobules (Figs. 20-41 and 20-42). Many inactive glands show deviations from this normal structure, however, and a considerable percentage has, without any clinical symptoms, some degree of gross or microscopic cystic disease or other abnormalities, as for instance, groups of secretory cells. The examination of many autopsy and surgical specimens is necessary in order to secure "normal" mammary gland tissue.

The Mammary Gland during Lactation

Throughout pregnancy, the mammary gland undergoes extensive changes in preparation for lactation. The tubules characteristic of the inactive gland form buds that enlarge into alveoli. As this growth of glandular tissue proceeds, the fat and the intralobular and interlobular connective tissue decrease in amount, the latter forming septa in which the ducts are embedded (Figs. 20-43 and 20-44). The alveoli at the

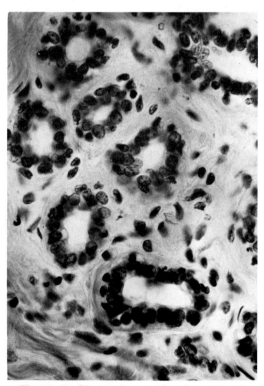

Fig. 20-42. Photomicrograph of an inactive mammary gland. Woman, 20 years of age. ×720.

Inactive lobule   Active lobule

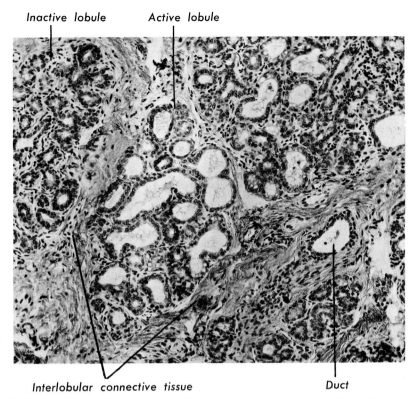

Interlobular connective tissue   Duct

Fig. 20-43. Photomicrograph of a section of mammary gland showing active and inactive glandular tissue. Fourth day postpartum. Woman, 29 years of age. Surgical specimen. ×140.

termination of pregnancy are large and irregular in shape, although there is frequently great variation in the degree of development among the lobules or even within a lobule (Fig. 20-43). The alveoli are lined by a simple cuboidal epithelium that rests on a delicate basement membrane. Electron micrographs show that the cells have randomly distributed microvilli, relatively large mitochondria, a Golgi complex that enlarges during secretory activity and granular endoplasmic reticulum that increases during cell activity. The secretory process for protein constituents of milk resembles that of other cells which synthesize proteins for export.

The proteins are synthesized in association with polyribosomes, packaged in the Golgi complex and then transported in membrane-bounded vesicles to the apical surface, where they are discharged by a merocrine mode of secretion. Lipid droplets appear to arise in the cytoplasm outside the Golgi complex and pass to the apical end of the cell. They project outward and are pinched off into the lumen enclosed by a membrane derived from the cell plasmalemma, along with an ultramicroscopic portion of cytoplasm. The amount of cytoplasm lost is so small that it is questionable whether the process should be classified as an apocrine mode of secretion. With the usual preservation techniques, the fat droplets are dissolved and the spaces that they occupied appear as vacuoles (Figs. 20-44 and 20-45).

After cessation of lactation, the epithelium of the mammary glands involutes, and the alveoli decrease in size until they become no longer recognizable. The connective tissue and fat again become abundant as the structure of an inactive gland is reassumed.

The mammary glands undergo progressive atrophy after the *menopause*. Some of the lobules and ducts may be obliterated; the connective tissue becomes increasingly dense and frequently hyalinized. Cystic dilation of the ducts frequently occurs.

Milk consists of a proteinaceous fluid

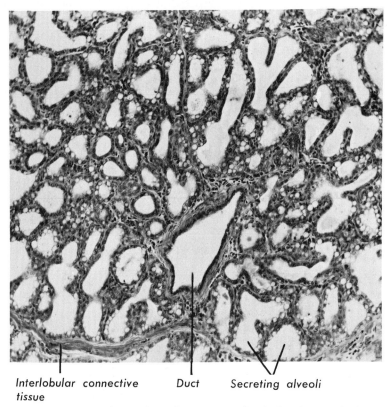

Interlobular connective   Duct   Secreting alveoli
tissue

Fig. 20-44. Photomicrograph of a section of mammary gland, showing marked secretory activity. ×140.

containing casein, milk sugar (lactose) and salts in which fat droplets are suspended. Milk is rich in calcium needed by the growing infant. Some cellular debris is also present.

Colostrum is the secretion formed during the first few days after parturition. It contains colostrum corpuscles, which are large spherical or oval cells filled with fat droplets of varying sizes. They are probably leukocytes or other wandering cells that have migrated into the alveoli and have taken up fat droplets by phagocytosis.

The Mammary Gland of the Male

There is little agreement as to the constitution of the male breast. Some mammary tissue always is present, but it attains its maximal development during early adolescence and then normally undergoes involution. The gland consists of ducts with usually no alveoli or lobulation. Under conditions of abnormal hormonal stimulation,

as in some testicular tumors, the male mammary gland may enlarge and develop extensively, a condition designated as gynecomastia.

Hormonal Control of the Mammary Gland

Although some development of the mammary gland occurs during childhood, growth characteristically is greatly accentuated during adolescence. At this time the gland comes under the influence of estrogen and progesterone secreted cyclically by the ovaries, a secretory process which in turn is dependent on hormones from the anterior hypophysis. During gestation, when there is a continuous and prolonged production of both estrogen and progesterone by the ovaries and placenta, the greatest development of the mammary glands takes place, with alveoli and a presecretory condition being established.

The role of estrogen and progesterone in the development of a secretory condition

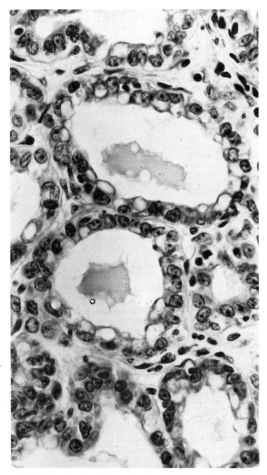

Fig. 20-45. Section of a few of the alveoli of a mammary gland in active secretion. ×720.

of the mammary gland has been extensively investigated experimentally. Both of these hormones are essential, but the degree of response to each is subject to some species variation. In general, estrogen causes duct growth, which is followed by the development of alveoli when progesterone is subsequently administered.

The influence of the anterior hypophysis on the hyperplasia of the mammary gland, aside from its indirect effect through the ovarian hormones, has not been fully clarified. In those animals that do not abort following hypophysectomy during gestation (rats, mice, guinea pigs, rhesus monkeys) the mammary glands will attain a nearly complete gestational development in the absence of the anterior hypophysis and will briefly lactate. Lactation is not maintained

in the absence of the hypophysis, however. Although some fat droplets form in the secretory cells of the mammary gland during the latter part of pregnancy, there is a tremendous increase in secretory activity after parturition. This is brought about by the action of an increased amount of *lactogenic* (*luteotrophic, LTH*) hormone from the anterior hypophysis. The effects attributed to LTH seem well established for rodents and for some other species. It is reported, however, that growth hormone will produce the results ascribed to LTH in some species, including humans (see chapter 21).

The maintenance of lactation, after its initiation by LTH, appears to depend on a number of hormones. Crude extracts from the anterior hypophysis have an effect, and the adrenal cortex is essential.

One of the neurohypophyseal hormones, *oxytocin*, has a definite and pronounced effect on the lactating mammary gland, causing the contraction of the myoepithelial cells that surround the alveoli. This is the "milk ejection" or "milk let-down" effect. The secretion of oxytocin is initiated by nerve impulses reaching the hypothalamus, the most effective stimulus being suckling or similar stimulation of the nipple area. Some investigators also favor the possibility that oxytocin, reaching the anterior hypophysis by way of the bloodstream, may be responsible for the release of anterior pituitary factors necessary for milk secretion.

It is difficult to secure material to determine whether structural changes occur in the human breast during the menstrual cycle. Material must be secured either at autopsy, usually after a debilitating illness, or by surgical removal because of pathological conditions. In an extensive study of rhesus monkeys, which have menstrual cycles similar to humans, it has been found that there is lobular enlargement and dilation of mammary alveoli during the corpus luteum phase of the menstrual cycle. This supplies presumptive evidence that similar changes occur in women.

Blood Vessels

The blood supply of the mammary gland comes from several neighboring vessels: the intercostals, internal mammary and thoracic branches of the axillary arteries. These vessels subdivide and form a rich capillary plexus around the ducts and alveoli. The richness of the blood supply fluctuates with activity, being much greater in the active than in the inactive or the involuted gland. From the capillaries, veins arise which accompany the arteries.

Lymphatics

The lymph vessels of mammary glands are numerous. An understanding of the course of these vessels is facilitated by keeping in mind the fact that the gland arises from the ectoderm and grows into the underlying mesoderm and that in this underlying tissue there is, over the whole body, a plexus of lymph vessels. Thus, as the developing ducts grow deeply into the connective tissue, lymph vessels accompany them and drain toward the surface into the subcutaneous lymph plexus. This plexus is particularly well formed beneath the areola. From the subcutaneous plexus, vessels pass to the axillary lymphatics and nodes along the pectoral muscles. There are accessory paths of drainage. Some vessels cross the midline, others follow the branches of the internal mammary artery and drain through the sternal nodes, and still others may drain into the abdominal lymph nodes. Because of the frequency of mammary carcinoma, the lymph drainage of this gland is of great importance.

Nerves

Cranial, spinal, and sympathetic nerves supply the gland, the larger trunks following the interlobar and interlobular connective tissue septa. The nerve terminals break up into plexuses that surround the alveoli just outside their basal laminae. From these plexuses, delicate fibrils have been described passing through the basal lamina and ending between the secreting cells.

Development of the Urinary and Reproductive Systems

During development, three generations of urinary structures make their appearance. These in order of their succession are known as the *pronephros, mesonephros*

and *metanephros*. The first two, which are present only in the embryo in higher animals, are important in furnishing the efferent duct system of the male reproductive organs. The metanephros, generally known as the kidney, forms the adult urinary organ in all of the higher vertebrates (reptiles, birds and mammals).

All three kidney generations arise from the *intermediate cell mass* or *nephrotome*, a mesodermal mass which connects the primitive somites with the lateral plates. In man, only the cranial portion of the intermediate cell mass shows a definite segmentation corresponding to that of the primitive somites, and it is in this region that the pronephros develops. Below the 10th somite, the segments of the nephrotome are so close together as to form a continuous cord of mesoderm, the nephrogenic strand, extending to the sacral region of the body. The upper, longer portion of the strand (mesonephric strand) furnishes the mesonephros. The uriniferous tubules of the permanent kidneys are formed from the lower portion (metanephric strand).

The *pronephros* in man is a variable and rudimentary structure which has no urinary function whatever. In some embryos it may be entirely missing. It arises in the cranial segments of the nephrotome in the form of ridge-like condensations which may or may not acquire a lumen. The most anterior ridges or tubules are the most rudimentary and soon undergo involution. The caudal ones become somewhat longer and fuse at their lateral ends to form a duct, the pronephric duct, which grows caudally beyond the territory of the pronephros and ultimately empties into the cloacal portion of the intestine. The pronephric duct is placed lateral to the nephrotome, directly underneath the ectoderm. The greatest extent of the pronephros is seen in embryos of about 2.5 mm, while in embryos of 5 mm involution of the tubules has definitely begun. All of the tubules gradually disappear, leaving only the pronephric duct.

The *mesonephros* or Wolffian body begins its development in embryos of 2.5 mm, just caudal to the pronephros. Cellular condensations appear in the mesonephric strand and soon become vesicular by developing lumina. The vesicles elongate and are transformed into S-shaped tubules, which then connect at one end with the pronephric duct. The latter is now called the *mesonephric* or *Wolffian duct*. The distal end of each tubule becomes invaginated to form a two-layered capsule which encloses a tuft of blood vessels, the glomerulus, derived from a branch of the aorta. The capsule, together with the enclosed glomerulus, constitutes a Malpighian corpuscle.

The mesonephric tubules develop progressively from the front backward and finally form a series extending from the cervical to the pelvic region of the embryo. By increase in number and length of the tubules, each mesonephros comes to form a large structure projecting into the dorsal part of the body cavity. The greatest extent is reached during the 5th or 6th week.

From the 6th week on, the mesonephros gradually atrophies, leaving finally only certain parts which differ in the two sexes. In the male, 8 to 15 tubules in the cephalic portion persist as the ductuli efferentes, while a few in the caudal portion remain as the paradidymis and aberrant ducts. The mesonephric duct is transformed into the ductus epididymidis, ductus deferens and ejaculatory duct. In the female, the mesonephric tubules disappear for the most part; only a few remain to form the epoophoron and paroophoron, while the duct persists in part as Gärtner's canal.

Each *metanephros* or kidney begins in embryos of about 5 mm as a hollow bud from the dorsal side of the mesonephric duct near its opening into the cloaca. This bud, the anlage of the ureter, grows dorsally and cranially into the *metanephric blastema*, where it ends in a terminal dilation or ampulla, the primitive pelvis. The pelvis elongates in a cranioventral direction and forms four to six branches that likewise terminate in ampullae. These branches are the primordia of the primary calyces. Each ampulla then divides into two to four secondary ampullae, and this process is repeated again and again until the whole system of collecting tubules is formed.

The nephrons, or uniniferous tubules proper, have an independent origin from the metanephric tissue which forms caplike condensations around the growing ampullae and the collecting tubules (Fig. 20-46).

Portions of the condensations acquire a lumen and detach themselves from the nephrogenic cap. Each vesicle elongates into an S-shaped tubule which secondarily establishes a communication with the collecting tubule. The place of junction becomes the arched or junctional collecting tubule. By further growth and histological differentiation, the S-shaped tubule gives rise to the convoluted tubules and loop of Henle, while the enlarged blind end becomes invaginated as Bowman's capsule to enclose a glomerulus (Fig. 20-46). Thus, the two types of tubules found in the adult kidney have separate origins. The nephrons are derived from the metanephric blastema (metanephric strand). The ureter, pelvis, calyces and all of the collecting tubules are formed from the ureteric bud, an outgrowth from the mesonephric duct.

The *gonads* or sex glands make their first appearance on the mesial surface of the mesonephros as ridge-like thickenings of the celomic epithelium, the *genital ridges*, which at first extend from the midthoracic to the sacral levels. As development proceeds, the anterior portion retrogresses and the gonads become restricted to the lumbar region. The cells of the ridge proliferate and form a band composed of a large number of small cuboidal cells which stain rather intensely. Scattered between these are larger spherical cells with vesicular nuclei and clearer cytoplasm, the primitive germ cells. The primitive germ cells do not arise in situ but migrate in from the yolk sac and are believed to be endodermal in origin. The whole epithelial band is known as the *germinal epithelium.*

As the germinal epithelium continues to proliferate, irregular plugs or strands of epithelial cells, the *medullary* or *sex cords*, extend into the underlying connective tissue. These contain the two types of cells. The deepest portions of the cords, which lie closest to the mesonephric tubules, anastomose with one another to form the anlage of the *rete*.

Up to about the 6th week, development proceeds similarly in both sexes. This is the so-called "indifferent" period. Although sex is determined by the constitution of the fertilized egg, histological differences between the male and female cannot be observed during this period.

Expanded, growing end of collecting tubule

Primordium of uriniferous tubule

Metanephrogenic tissue

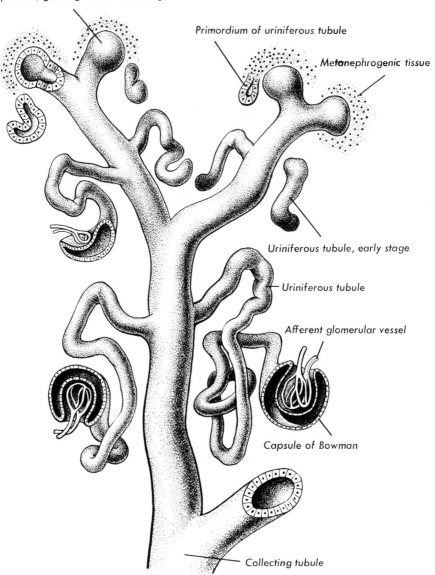

Uriniferous tubule, early stage

Uriniferous tubule

Afferent glomerular vessel

Capsule of Bowman

Collecting tubule

Fig. 20-46. Diagram of development of kidney tubules. Early differentiation of uriniferous tubules from metanephrogenic tissue is shown in the *upper part* of figure; later stages are shown in the *lower portion* of the diagram. (Redrawn and modified from Corning.)

From the 6th week on, histological changes occur that lead to a definite differentiation of the gonads. In the *testis*, a layer of embryonal connective tissue, the future *tunica albuginea*, grows in between the medullary cords and the germinal epithelium, and the latter becomes gradually reduced to a single layer of flat cells, the visceral layer of the tunica vaginalis. The medullary cords become more distinct and elongate to form the convoluted *seminiferous tubules*. The deeper anastomosing portions of the cords unite with a number of mesonephric tubules to form the *rete testis* of the adult. As already stated, the mesonephric tubules with which such union is established become the *ductuli efferentes*, while the mesonephric duct is transformed into the *ductus epididymidis* and *ductus deferens*. The larger sex cells of the cord seem to become smaller temporarily, but the germ cells remain distinct in chromosomal content and eventually give rise to spermatogenic cells. The other cells give rise to the cells of Sertoli.

Differentiation of the *ovary* begins at a later period and differs considerably from the process in the male. The medullary cords and rete formed during the indifferent period gradually disappear, although vestiges of the rete may remain in the adult ovary. On the other hand, the cells at the surface continue to proliferate and form a layered epithelial mass. The masses of cells are subdivided by strands of connective tissue into clusters containing oogonia, derived from primordial germ cells that migrated from the yolk sac and follicular cells derived from the germinal epithelium. At first, the clusters consist of several larger egg cells scattered in a mass of small (follicular) cells. Later, each cluster is broken up by invading connective tissue into several primordial follicles, each containing a single oogonium surrounded by a layer of flattened follicular cells.

Proliferation of oogonia continues until about the 6th month. By the time of birth all of the germ cells in the ovary are primary oocytes and the connective tissue of the ovary forms a dense tunica albuginea beneath the germinal epithelium. The germinal epithelium persists as a layer of cuboidal or columnar cells on the free surface of the ovary.

The primordia of the female genital ducts are the *Müllerian ducts* of the embryo. These begin in both sexes as celomic invaginations into the cranial portions of the mesonephric ridge which then grow backward, running parallel and close to the mesonephric duct. Caudally, the two Müllerian ducts approach each other and fuse to form a terminal unpaired tube which ends in the urogenital sinus between the openings of the mesonephric ducts. In the male, the Müllerian duct degenerates, leaving as vestiges the *appendix testis* and the *colliculus seminalis* (utriculus prostaticus, uterus masculinus). In the female, the paired upper portions become the *Fallopian tubes* or *oviducts*, while the unpaired terminal portion forms the *uterus* and *vagina*.

Development of Mammary Glands

In animals with numerous glands, the beginnings of the mammary glands are represented by two ridges of thickened epithelium, the mammary lines, which extend from the axillary to the inguinal regions. At various points on these ridges, epithelial proliferations form the primordia of future glands, while the intermediate portions of the milk lines ultimately disappear. In the human, the mammary line (ridge) is poorly defined and of brief duration, and normally only one pair of glands develops. Each gland appears in the 2nd month as a broad epidermal thickening in the region of the future nipple, produced by a proliferation and downgrowth of the germinative layer. The thickening spreads laterally to form a hemispherical mass whose convex surface is directed towards the dermis. Externally, the circular patch of skin, or mammary area, corresponding to the thickening sinks below the surface as the mammary pit.

About the 5th month, a varying number of secondary sprouts, the future lactiferous ducts and sinuses, grow down into the dermis and there branch repeatedly with the branches ending in terminal swellings. At first the sprouts are solid but, from the 7th month on, lumina appear in various places and finally become confluent. This process of branching and canalization continues until birth, the histological picture being that of a prepubertal gland. The formation of the glandular alveoli does not take place until adolescence.

Soon after birth, the shallow mammary pit is raised above the surface by the proliferation of connective tissue. The central portion develops into the nipple, which contains the openings of the lactiferous ducts. The remainder of the mammary area forms the areola, which is distinguished from the surrounding skin by its hairlessness, pigmentation and thinness of epidermis.

References

ADAMS, E. C., AND HERTIG, A. T. Studies on the human corpus luteum. I. Observations on the ultrastructure of development and regression of the luteal cells during the menstrual cycle. J. Cell Biol. 41:696–715, 1969.

AGATE, F. J., JR. The growth and secretory activity of the mammary glands of the pregnant rhesus monkey (Macaca mulatta) following hypophysectomy. Am. J. Anat., 90:257–284, 1952.

AMSTERDAM, A., LINDER, H., AND GRÖSCHEL-STEW-
ART, U. Localization of actin and myosin in the rat
oocyte and follicular wall by immunofluorescence.
Anat. Rec. 187:311–327, 1977.

ANDERSON, E., AND ALBERTINI, D. Gap junctions
between the oocyte and companion follicle cells in
the mammalian ovary. J. Cell Biol. 71:680–686, 1976.

BAKER, B. L., HOOK, A., AND SEVERINGHAUS, A. E.
The cytological structure of the human chorionic
villus and decidua parietalis. Am. J. Anat. 74:297–327,
1944.

BARGMAN, W., AND KNOOP, A. Über die Morphologie
der Milchsefkretion: Licht- und Elektronen-mikros-
kopische Studien ab der Milchdrüse der Ratte. Z.
Zellforsch. 49:344, 1959.

CORNER, G. W., JR. The histological dating of the
human corpus luteum of menstruation. Am. J. Anat.
98:377–402, 1956.

CRAWFORD, J. M. The foetal placental circulation. J.
Obstet. Gynaecol. Brit. Emp. 63:542–547, 1956.

DARON, G. H. The arterial pattern of the tunica mucosa of the uterus in Macacus rhesus. Am. J. Anat.
58:349–419, 1936.

DEMPSEY, E. W., AND LUSE, S. A. Electron microscopic observations on fibrinoid and histiotroph in
the junctional zone and villi of the human placenta.
Am. J. Anat. 128:463–484, 1970.

ENDERS, A. C. Fertilization, cleavage and implantation. *In* Reproduction and Breeding Techniques for
Laboratory Animals. (Hafez, E. S. E., editor), pp.
137–156. Lea & Febiger, Philadelphia, 1970.

ENDERS, A. C. The fine structure of the blastocyst.
In The Biology of the Blastocyst (Blandau, R. J.,
editor), pp. 71–94. The University of Chicago Press,
Chicago, 1971.

FRANCHI, L. L., MANDL, A. M., AND ZUCKERMAN, S.
The development of the ovary and the process of
oogenesis. *In* The Ovary (Zuckerman, S., editor),
vol. 1, pp. 1–88. Academic Press, New York, 1962.

GRANDY, H. G., AND SMITH, D. E. (editors) The
Ovary. Williams & Wilkins, Baltimore, 1963.

HARTMAN, C. G. Ovulation, fertilization and the transport and viability of eggs and spermatozoa. *In* Sex
and Internal Secretions (Allen, editor), pp. 630–720.
Williams & Wilkins, Baltimore, 1939.

HERTIG, A. T. Human Trophoblast. Charles C
Thomas, Publisher, Springfield, Ill., 1968.

HERTIG, A. T., AND ADAMS, E. C. Studies on the
human oocyte and its follicle. I. Ultrastructural and
histochemical observations on the primordial follicle
stage. J. Cell Biol. 34:647–675, 1967.

HERTIG, A. T., ROCK, J., AND ADAMS, E. C. A description of 34 human ova within the first 17 days of
development. Am. J. Anat. 98:435–494, 1956.

KEENAN, T. W., MORRÉ, D. J., OLSON, D. E., YUN-
GHANS, W. N., AND PATTON, S. Biochemical and
morphological comparison of plasma membrane and
fat globule membrane from bovine mammary gland.
J. Cell Biol. 44:80–93, 1970.

LUCKETT, W. P. The fine structure of the flattened
villi of the rhesus monkey. Anat. Rec. 167:141–164,
1970.

MARKEE, J. E. Menstruation in endometrial transplants in the rhesus monkey. Carnegie Inst. Wash.
Contrib. Embryol. 28:221–308, 1940.

MIDGLEY, A. R., JR, AND PIERCE, G. B., JR. Immunohistochemical localization of human chorionic go-
nadotropin. J. Exp. Med. 115:289–294, 1962.

MILLS, E. S., AND TOPPER, Y. J. Some ultrastructural
effects of insulin, hydrocortisone, and prolactin on
mammary gland explants. J. Cell Biol. 44:310–328,
1970.

NOYES, R. W., HERTIG, A. T., AND ROCK, J. Dating
the endometrial biopsy. Fertil. Steril. 1:3–25, 1950.

PAPANICOLAOU, G. N. The sexual cycle in the human
female as revealed by vaginal smears. Am. J. Anat.
53:519–637, 1933.

PAPANICOLAOU, G. N., TRAUT, H. F., AND MAR-
CHETTI, A. A. The Epithelia of Woman's Reproductive Tract. Commonwealth Fund, New York, 1948.

RAMSEY, E. M. Circulation in the maternal placenta
of the rhesus monkey and man, with observations
on the marginal lakes. Am. J. Anat. 98:159–190,
1956.

RICHARDSON, G. S. Ovarian Physiology. N. Engl. J.
Med.   274:1008–1015,   1064–1075,   1121–1134,
1184–1194, 1966.

ROCK, J., AND HERTIG, A. T. Some aspects of early
human development. Am. J. Obstet. Gynecol.
44:973–982, 1942.

ROCK, J., AND HERTIG, A. T. The human conceptus
during the first two weeks of gestation. Am. J.
Obstet. Gynecol. 55:6–14, 1948.

SHETTLES, L. B. Studies on living human ova. Ann.
N.Y. Acad. Sci. 17:99–102, 1954.

SHETTLES, L. B. The nourishment of the human
ovum. Bull. Sloane Hosp. Women 4:34–38, 1958.

SIMKINS, C. S. Development of the human ovary from
birth to sexual maturity. Am. J. Anat. 51:465–505,
1932.

TRAUT, H. F., BLOCH, P. W., AND KUDER, A. Cyclical
changes in the human vaginal mucosa. Surg. Gynecol. Obstet. 63:7–15, 1936.

VELARDO, J. T. (editor) The Endocrinology of Reproduction. Oxford University Press, New York, 1958.

VILLEE, D. B. Development of endocrine function in
the human placenta and fetus. N. Engl. J. Med.
281:473–484, 533–542, 1969.

WISLOCKI, G. B., AND DEMPSEY, E. W. Remarks on
the lymphatics of the reproductive tract of the female rhesus monkey. Anat. Rec. 75:341–364, 1939.

WISLOCKI, G. B., AND DEMPSEY, E. W. Electron
microscopy of the human placenta. Anat. Rec.
123:133–168, 1955.

WITSCHI, E. Embryology of the Ovary. *In* The Ovary
(Grady, H. G., and Smith, D. E., editors). Williams
& Wilkins, Baltimore, 1963.

YOUNG, W. C. (editor). Sex and Internal Secretions,
vols. 1 and 2. Williams & Wilkins, Baltimore, 1961.

CHAPTER 21

The Endocrine Glands

The endocrine glands, or glands of internal secretion, include a diverse group of tissues and organs widely scattered in the body. Although physiological criteria are of primary importance in deciding whether any given tissue or organ belongs to the endocrine system, all tissues and organs of this system do have certain anatomical features in common. They have no ducts and they secrete directly into the vascular channels; therefore, they are known as ductless glands. They have a rich supply of blood vessels to provide not only for their own metabolic needs but also for the transport of their secretions to other parts of the body. The functional secretory cells of the endocrine organs are usually, although not invariably, composed of cells of epithelial or epithelioid characteristics (the parenchyma). In other anatomical features, such as arrangement of cells and cytological characteristics, the various endocrine glands differ widely from each other.

Physiologically, the endocrine glands have certain similarities. Each endocrine gland secretes one or more specific substances, called *hormones,* and each hormone has a specific effect upon a particular tissue or organ or on the body as a whole. Since the hormones are secreted into the blood or lymph, they all reach all parts of the body. Only a limited part of the organism may respond, however, as for example, a particular organ. The responsive structure, designated the "target" organ or tissue, selectively utilizes the circulating hor-

mone. This is in contrast with the transmission of nerve impulses, which cause a response in a limited part of the organism because they are carried over definite, discrete pathways to a limited area.

In some cases, it can readily be determined whether or not an organ has an endocrine function. Experimental ablation of the thyroid gland, for example, produces certain effects which are reversed by thyroid hormone administration. Such is also the case, as can be shown both experimentally and clinically, with the anterior hypophysis, neurohypophysis, adrenal cortex, the parathyroids, the testes and ovaries (their endocrine portions only) and the islets of the pancreas. The specific hormones of most of the endocrine glands have been chemically isolated and analyzed and a number of them have been synthesized.

Although the endocrine glands are diverse in their histology and in the exact chemical composition of their secretions, they can be grouped into two general categories on the basis of the chemical nature of their secretions. Since the hypophysis, thyroid, parathyroids and pancreatic islet beta cells secrete substances rich in proteins, glycoproteins or polypeptides, they are often grouped under the heading of *protein* and *polypeptide secreting endocrine glands.* These are glands whose secretory cells are of endodermal or ectodermal origin. On the other hand, the gonads and adrenal cortex secrete substances composed of steroids, and hence they are clas-

sified as *steroid secreting endocrine glands.*
Moreover, their secretory cells originate
from mesoderm.

The cells of the protein and polypeptide
secreting endocrine glands have many cytological characteristics similar to those of
the exocrine glands but with their ultrastructural features less developed. For example, the rough endoplasmic reticulum is
less abundant, and clusters of free ribosomes are often present. The Golgi complex
is smaller than that in exocrine glands and
is located, as one would expect, in the vascular pole of the cell.

The steroid secreting cells of the gonads
and adrenal cortex have little or no rough
endoplasmic reticulum but an abundance
of smooth endoplasmic reticulum that is in
the form of anastomosing tubules. The
Golgi complex is well developed and there
are numerous mitochondria that characteristically have tubular cristae as described
below under the adrenal gland and as described for the gonads in chapters 19 and
20.

Whereas severe disabilities or even death
may result from ablation of certain endocrine glands, this is not true of all. For
example, removal of the adrenal medulla,
whose hormone was the first one to be
chemically analyzed and synthesized, does
not produce severe disabilities.

Hormone, the term applied to the specific
product of an endocrine gland, is used in a
somewhat limited sense. By derivation it
means a chemical excitant. In this sense,
carbon dioxide would be a hormone since
it is an excitant of the respiratory center
of the brain. Carbon dioxide is a general
product of tissue metabolism, however, and
it is usually not spoken of as a true internal
secretion or hormone.

There are some tissues which have an
endocrine function but which are not organized into definite glandular organs. The
mucosa of the gastrointestinal tract, for
instance, secretes hormones that have effects on other structures, such as the exocrine portion of the pancreas and the muscle of the gall bladder.

Although the follicles and corpora lutea
of the ovary, the fetal placenta, the interstitial tissue of the testis and the islets of
the pancreas elaborate hormones, it has
seemed wise to include a description of

them under the organs to which they belong.

The Hypophysis Cerebri

Macroscopic Structure

The *hypophysis* (pituitary gland) is derived in part from oral ectoderm of the
dorsal median region of the *stomodeum*
(*Rathke's pouch*) and in part from the brain,
with which it maintains its connections in
the adult (Fig. 21-1). The major part of the
gland (anterior and posterior lobes) lies in
a bony fossa, the *sella turcica.* This part is
ensheathed by the dura, an extension of
which, the *diaphragma sellae,* roofs over
the sella turcica. There is a small aperture
in the diaphragma through which the *pituitary stalk* passes. The suprasellar portion of the gland includes the pituitary stalk
and that portion of the hypothalamus
known as the *median eminence* of the *tuber
cinereum.* The *infundibular stem* forms the
bulk of the pituitary stalk. The smaller
component, the *pars tuberalis,* surrounds
the infundibular stem and flares out onto
the median eminence.

Table 21-1 gives the various parts of the
gland, their embryological derivation and
the more common synonyms.

The *pars nervosa* and *pars intermedia*
are intimately fused, forming a single main
division, the posterior lobe. However,
spaces lined by epithelial cells are often
present between the intermediate lobe and
the neural lobe. They frequently contain
some colloid, and they are often described
as Rathke's cysts; they should not be confused with remnants of Rathke's pouch
which rarely persist. Some animals (whale,
porpoise, birds, and armadillo) lack a pars
intermedia and Rathke's cysts. In these
species, the neural lobe is encapsulated by
the meninges and consequently is entirely
separated from the anterior lobe.

The human pituitary gland measures
about 1.2 to 1.5 cm in the transverse plane,
about 1 cm in the sagittal plane and about
0.5 cm in height. Its weight varies considerably but correlates better with stature
than with body weight. In the human, the
weight of the anterior lobe increases with
pregnancy and decreases slightly in old age.
The average weight of the hypophysis in

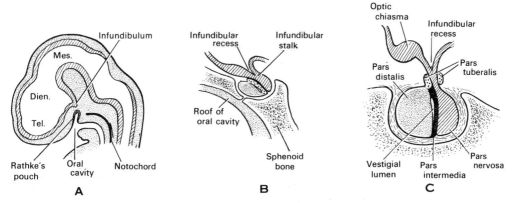

Fig. 21-1. Diagrammatic sagittal sections of the human pituitary gland at different stages of development. *A*, cephalic region of a 6-week embryo showing Rathke's pouch as an outgrowth from the dorsal wall of the oral cavity. The infundibulum is seen as a thickening in the floor of the diencephalon (*Dien.*). *Tel.*, telencephalon and *Mes.*, mesencephalon. *B* and *C*, stages of pituitary development at the end of the 3rd and 4th months, respectively. The interrelationships of the major subdivisions of the gland in the 4-month fetus approximate those of the adult. (Redrawn and modified after Langman.)

TABLE 21-1

Components of hypophysis and their derivation

Derivations	Divisions	Components		Lobes of pituitary gland within sella turcica
Oral ectoderm	Adenohypophysis	Pars tuberalis Pars distalis—pars anterior Pars intermedia		Anterior lobe
Neural ectoderm	Neurohypophysis	Pars nervosa—infundibular process (neural lobe)		Posterior lobe
		Infundibulum (neural stalk)	Infundibular stem Median eminence of tuber cinereum	

the male is about 0.6 g. In multipara it may weigh more than 1 g.

Blood and Nerve Supply

The *blood supply* of the hypophysis has unusual features, and it plays such an important role in pituitary gland function that it seems appropriate to describe it in advance of the microscopic structure.

The hypophysis is supplied by *superior hypophyseal arteries,* which arise from the internal carotids and circle of Willis, and by a pair of *inferior hypophyseal arteries* from the internal carotids. The superior hypophyseal vessels supply the infundibulum and thence the anterior lobe by way of a portal system. The inferior hypophy-

seal vessels serve mainly for the blood supply of the neural lobe, although their interlobar branches do give off some vessels that anastomose with branches from the superior hypophyseal vessels to supply the lower portion of the infundibulum and thence, by a portal system, the anterior lobe. It is to be noted that the anterior lobe usually receives no direct arterial supply and it is dependent upon the portal system from the infundibulum.

Although there are several superior hypophyseal arteries and their pattern is complex due to numerous variations and anastomoses, two main vessels can usually be identified on each side. These are known as the *anterior superior hypophyseal artery,* which enters the anterior portion of the infundibulum, and the *lateral* or *posterior superior hypophyseal artery,* which continues around the stalk to enter the posterior portion of the infundibulum (Fig. 21-2). Within the infundibulum, some branches from both the anterior and posterior hypophyseal arteries ascend to supply the median eminence of the tuber cinereum, while other branches descend to anastomose with vessels projecting upward from the lower part of the stalk. The latter are derivatives from a pair of vessels (loral arteries, trabecular arteries) that arise from the anterior superior hypophyseal arteries, descend in front of the neural stalk to enter the anterior lobe and then swing backward and upward into the stalk (Fig. 21-2). A branch of each loral artery also continues caudally toward the lower portion of the infundibular stem, where it anastomoses with branches from the inferior hypophyseal arteries in supplying parallel arteries to the lower infundibulum. A small, inconstant branch of the loral artery also enters

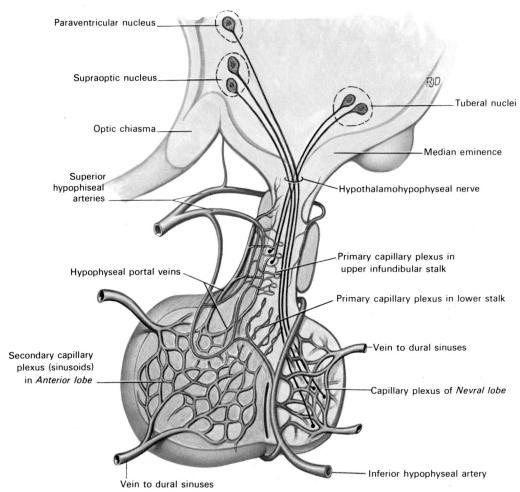

Fig. 21-2. Diagram of the blood supply of the pituitary gland as seen from the left side. The infundibular stalk is shown in sagittal section and portions of the left sides of the anterior and neural lobes have been removed in order to show the vessels that penetrate deeply into the glandular tissue. The left inferior hypophyseal artery is shown in its course at the exterior of the gland, above the cut surface of the glandular tissue. The inferior hypophyseal artery joins with its corresponding vessel of the opposite side (not visible from the left) to form an arterial circle around the junction of the neural lobe with the anterior lobe. Branches from the circle penetrate inward, as shown, to supply the neural lobe and the lower portion of the infundibular stalk. (Based on descriptions and diagrams by Greep, 1963; Xureb et al., 1954; Stanfield, 1960; and others.)

the interlobar fibrous connective tissue core.

The arterioles in the median eminence and upper part of the stalk terminate in characteristic patterns of looped sinusoidal capillaries, (primary set of capillaries), which join to form venules that in turn unite to form long descending veins which course downward in the peripheral portion of the stalk to supply sinusoidal capillaries in the pars distalis (secondary set of capillaries). A characteristic pattern of short venous trunks draining from the capillaries in the upper and lower portions of the infundibulum and ending in the sinusoidal capillaries of the pars distalis constitutes the *hypophyseal portal system*. Thus, a pathway is established by which neurosecretory material released from nerves in the median eminence can pass directly to the pars distalis. It has also been found that the vascular pattern of the neurohypophyseal capillary bed is such that the direction of blood flow in different portions of the bed can be reversed. Thus, hormones released into the vascular bed in the anterior lobe could conceiveably flow directly back to the median eminence and thus provide a short range feedback mechanism not involving the systemic circulation. This possibility is currently under active investigation.

The pars nervosa (neural lobe) receives its blood supply from the *inferior hypophyseal arteries,* which form an arterial circle near the junction of the anterior and posterior lobes. Numerous arterial branches pass into the neural lobe tissue to enter sinusoidal capillaries. Interlobar arteries from the arterial circle also contribute branches which anastomose with vessels from the superior hypophyseal arteries, as outlined above, to supply the lower (intraglandular) portion of the infundibulum and thence to the sinusoidal capillaries of the pars distalis (Fig. 21-2). The sinusoidal capillaries of the neural lobe have an important function in receiving neurosecretory material conveyed to the neural lobe by nerve fibers from the hypothalamus.

The sinusoidal capillaries of the pars distalis form an elaborate plexus of channels which are wider than the sinusoidal capillaries of the neural lobe. Electron micrographs show a fenestrated type of endothelium in the sinusoidal capillaries of both locations with diaphragms spanning the fenestrae as described in chapter 12.

The *innervation* of the hypophysis consists chiefly of the hypothalamico-hypophyseal tracts of nonmyelinated nerve fibers that extend into the neural lobe from their cells of origin in the supraoptic and paraventricular nuclei and of tracts to the upper part of the stalk (Fig. 21-2). They serve to carry neurosecretory substances. There are no nerves to the anterior lobe, other than some vasomotor fibers with blood vessels. Although the parenchymal cells of the pars distalis have no nerve supply, there is substantial evidence that they are under nervous control.

Section of the pituitary stalk in rabbits prevents ovulation after mating. In this species, as in the cat and ferret, ovulation occurs only after copulation. The inhibition of ovulation after stalk section is attributed to the interruption of the *neurohumoral pathway* from the hypothalamus to the anterior lobe. Coitus in the rabbit normally causes the release of certain anterior lobe hormones, the stimulation for this release being a substance produced in the brain and transmitted to the anterior lobe by way of the *hypophyseal portal system*. Other functions of the anterior hypophysis are regulated by the brain through neurohumoral pathways.

Microscopic Structure and Function

Pars Distalis. About 75% of the hypophysis is anterior lobe. The parenchyma of this lobe is formed of anastomosing cords of cells separated from sinusoidal capillaries by only a meager amount of irregularly arranged connective tissue. Small masses of colloid occur within the cell cords only occasionally (Fig. 21-3).

The parenchymal cells fall into two main categories: *chromophobes* and *chromophils*. The latter were subdivided into *acidophils* and *basophils* by the early pituitary cytologists on the basis of some of the staining reactions in routine preparations. In hematoxylin and eosin preparations, the cytoplasmic granules of the acidophils stain well with eosin, although the granules of

Colloid   Acidophiles   Sinusoid

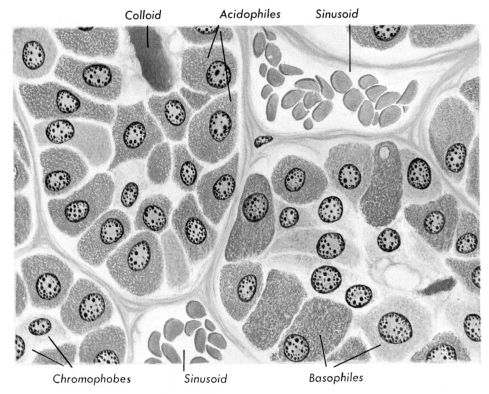

Chromophobes   Sinusoid   Basophiles

Fig. 21-3. Human anterior hypophysis. The section shows parts of several cords of cells containing acidophils (orange), two types of basophils (purple and green) and chromophobes. Fine connective tissue and sinusoids separate the cords. Masses of colloid are seen in the centers of two of the cords. A 4 μm section stained with aldehyde fuchsin-fast green-orange G. Woman, age 26. Camera lucida drawing. ×1200.

the so-called basophils do not stain well with hematoxylin. Moreover, the granules of the basophils stain very well with the aniline blue of the Mallory's and modified Masson's trichrome stains, reacting in this sense like collagen, which is acidophilic (Fig. 21-15, *A*). It is obvious that the terms acidophils and basophils are not particularly appropriate for pituitary cells, but the terms are well established in the literature. The three types of cells identified in trichrome-stained preparations are known as: *chromophobes* (about 50%), *acidophils* (35%) and *basophils* (15%). Additional types within the acidophil and basophil groups can be identified by special staining and by histochemical methods. Electron micrographs also show differential characteristics, such as granules of different sizes in different cells. By the various available techniques, at least six different types of

cells have been identified in the pars distalis.

The *chromophobes* tend to appear in groups near the centers of the cords. Their nuclei are surrounded by a small amount of diffuse, light staining cytoplasm, and cell boundaries are not distinguishable in ordinary preparations. Secretory granules of specific types are usually not seen by light microscopy in cells classified as chromophobes. However, electron microscope studies show relatively few nongranular cells, and it appears that most of the cells counted as chromophobes in routine preparations are acidophils and basophils that have become degranulated following a secretory cycle.

The *acidophils* (*alpha cells*) stain readily and are easily identified in ordinary preparations (Figs. 21-3 and 21-15). These cells are usually larger than the chromophobes, and their cytoplasm contains secretion granules which take the acid dyes such as eosin, acid fuchsin and orange G. They also take certain basic dyes such as safranin. Therefore, some investigators use the name alpha cell in preference to acidophil.

The acidophils can be divided into two groups by the use of special staining methods, using either a modified Heidenhain azan stain or a tetrachrome stain. Some acidophils show a strong affinity for orange G, whether in simple dye mixtures or in the tetrachrome mixture; hence, they are sometimes described as orangeophils, but are more commonly designated *somatotrophs* because they secrete growth hormone. Another group of acidophils show an affinity for the azocarmine in the tetrachrome stain; they are commonly named *mammotrophs (prolactin cells, luteotrophs)* because they stimulate secretory

activity of the mammary gland and corpus luteum.

The evidence for separating the acidophils into two types has been strengthened by results obtained by immunohistohemical studies which utilize labeled antibodies. In this procedure for identifying the location of growth hormone, an enzyme, horseradish peroxidase, is conjugated to the growth hormone. After sections of the gland have been reacted with the enzyme-labeled antibody, the slides containing the sections are chemically treated to visualize the peroxidase at the sites where the antibody has reacted with its specific hormone. Next, the immunochemically stained sections are photographed, then destained and subsequently restained by the trichrome method in order to identify the immunochemically reacting cells in terms of acidophils and kbasophils (Fig. 21-4). The mammotrophs

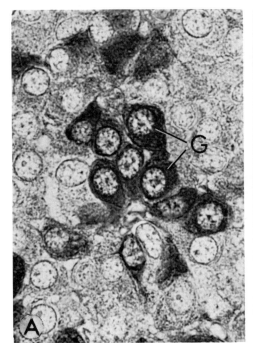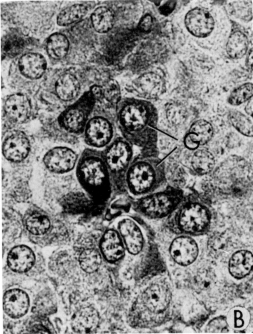

Fig. 21-4. Photomicrographs of a section of rat anterior hypophysis. In *A*, the section has been stained immunochemically, after application of a rabbit antiserum to human growth hormone. This selectively demonstrates the cells (*G*) whose cytoplasm contains growth hormone. In *B*, the section shown in *A* has been destained and subsequently restained by the Masson's trichrome procedure which shows that these cells stain as acidophils. The growth hormone cells shown in *A* have given the characteristic reaction of cells that are identified as acidophils by routine histological methods. Both figures, ×1000 (Courtesy of Dr. Burton L. Baker, J. Histochem. Cytochem., vol. 18, 1970).

have been similarly studied and identified.

Electron micrographs also show two types of acidophils, with the mammotrophs being polyhedral in shape and having coarse cytoplasmic granules ranging up to 700 nm. The somatotroph granules are smaller and only measure up to about 350 nm. Both types of acidophils have rough endoplasmic reticulum, free ribosomes and a Golgi complex that is well developed but smaller than that of exocrine gland cells as noted at the beginning of this chapter. Further details on each cell type are given below under "Functions of the Anterior Hypophysis."

The *basophils* (*beta cells*) show considerable variation in their staining properties, both within an individual gland and from one species to another. The cytoplasmic granules also vary in size in a given cell and in different species. Electron micrographs show that they measure up to about 200 nm in the rat (Figs. 21-5 and 21-6). Thus, the granules are definitely smaller than in the acidophils. The granules stain poorly with hematoxylin, well with the aniline blue of the trichrome methods (Fig. 21-15) and excellently with the periodic acid-Schiff (PAS) technique. It is to be noted that the granules of all of the basophils of the pars distalis stain by the PAS method because of their content of glycoproteins, and that none of the acidophils stain with PAS.

The aldehyde fuchsin technique enables one to distinguish two types of basophils: an aldehyde fuchsin-positive type (beta basophil) and an aldehyde fuchsin-negative type (delta basophil). The *beta basophils* are polyhedral or angular in shape, and they tend to be located centrally in the gland. They show pronounced changes after thyroidectomy, and they apparently secrete thyrotrophic hormone, as shown by immunohistochemical methods using peroxidase-labeled antibody for thyrotrophic hormone.

The *delta basophils* are more rounded in shape than are the beta basophils (thyrotrophs). There is substantial evidence that they secrete the gonadotrophic hormones, i.e., *follicle-stimulating hormone* (FSH) and *luteinizing hormone* (LH). By special staining techniques and experimental procedures, evidence has been obtained that the delta basophils can be divided into two types, one for FSH and one for LH. When separately labeled antibodies, one for FSH and one for LH, are applied to the same sections, however, some of the basophils located peripherally in the gland are seen to have FSH and LH in the same cell, whereas some other basophils located centrally contain only LH. Thus, in this instance, the same cell often contains both FSH and LH.

The proportion of each of the cell types present in the cell cords varies greatly, not only in different regions of the anterior lobe but even in adjacent cords. In the human hypophysis, the basophils are most numerous in the region of the midsagittal plane and anterolateral margin of the gland. The acidophils are most numerous in the central and posterior part of each lateral half of the gland. A survey of much of the gland is necessary in order to determine the percentages of the various cell types.

The *lineage* of the cells of the anterior lobe is important in the interpretation of experimental work and tumor formation. Since mitoses are rare, it is certain that few if any of the cells are destroyed when their secretion is liberated; thus the cells must pass through secretory cycles. The chromophobes apparently represent the nonsecretory stage of a cycle. As the cells pass into an active stage, new granules form that are specific for the cell type, acidophils in some cells and basophils in others. After the secretion is liberated, the cell returns to the chromophobe type. Evidence for this type of cycle was obtained by studies of the Golgi complex in the rat hypophysis; in this species, the Golgi complexes of the acidophils and basophils differ from each other in their morphology and position. Two types of chromophobes can be identified in the rat and different stages of granule formation and discharge can be defined.

No constant differences in the Golgi complexes of acidophils and basophils have been found in species other than the rat. However, there is presumptive evidence for secretory cycles similar to those in the rat. Electron microscope studies have shown progressive stages in the formation and depletion of granules in the different cell

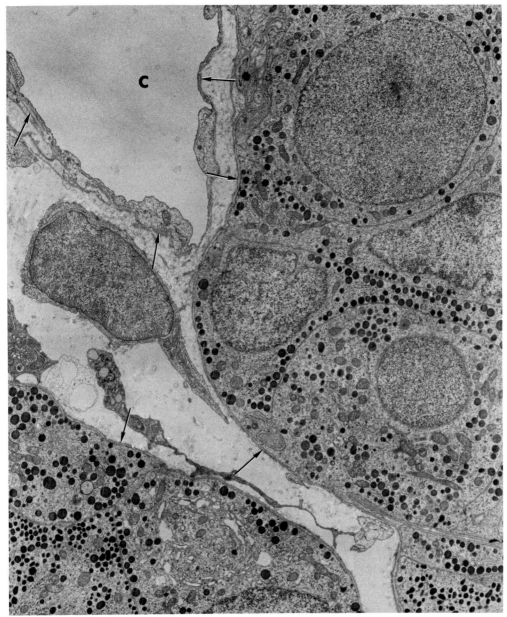

Fig. 21-5. Electron micrograph of a portion of anterior hypophysis from monkey showing granulated secretory cells (those with larger granules are acidophils), a fenestrated sinusoidal capillary (*C*) and intervening connective tissue components. The secretory cells and the vascular endothelium are both separated from the connective tissue by basal laminae (*arrows*). The perivascular cells appear fibroblastic in nature. ×6000.

types. The mature secretory granules are apparently released from the cells by exocytosis, similar to that observed for exocrine glands (Fig. 21-6).

Functions of the Anterior Hypophysis. The multiplicity of the functions of the anterior hypophysis is shown by the disabilities that result from its surgical removal or destruction by disease.

After hypophysectomy, there is a cessation of general body growth and an involution of the gonads, the thyroid and the

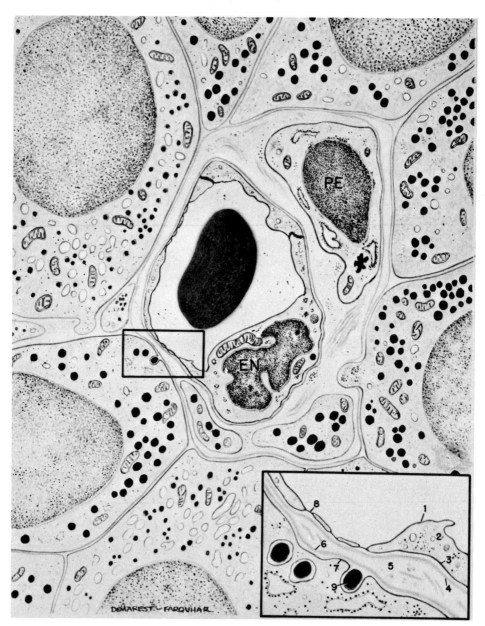

Fig. 21-6. A composite diagram of some of the details observable in electron micrographs of the anterior hypophysis. The cytoplasm of the capillary endothelial cell is generally attenuated except in the region around the nucleus (*EN*). The perivascular space may be narrow as seen at the *left* of the capillary or it may be relatively broad as shown at the *right*. It contains collagen and connective tissue cells; a perivascular macrophage (*PE*) is included in the diagram. The parenchymal cells also rest on a basal lamina. The area enclosed by the rectangle is enlarged at the *lower right*. Structures between the lumen of the capillary and the cytoplasm of a parenchymal cell are numbered in sequence. *1,* plasma membrane of luminal surface of endothelial cell; *2,* endothelial cell cytoplasm; *3,* membrane of basal surface of endothelial cell; *4,* basal lamina of endothelial cell; *5,* perivascular space; *6,* basal lamina of parenchymal cell; and *7,* the plasma membrane of a parenchymal cell. In some areas, *8,* the endothelial cells have fenestrae closed only by thin diaphragms. At *9,* the membrane around a secretion granule is shown in continuity with the parenchymal cell membrane. ×12,000; inset, ×40,000. (Courtesy of Dr. M. G. Farquhar, Angiology, vol. 12, 1961.)

cortex of the adrenal glands. Numerous secondary effects also result. For instance, the inactivation of the gonads with loss of their endocrine function is followed by involution of the accessory reproductive organs. Involution of the thyroid brings about a lowering of the basal metabolic rate. The involution of the adrenal cortex results in a lowering of resistance to stress and a disturbance in carbohydrate metabolism. The anterior hypophysis is well named the master gland of the endocrine system.

The anterior hypophysis secretes at least six different hormones. They are proteins of complex chemical structure, and the exact amino acid composition has not been worked out for all of them. However, six have been prepared from the anterior hypophysis in quite pure form, as judged by their physiological activity and by their molecular homogeneity as shown by electrophoresis and ultracentrifugation.

The hormones receive their names, in most cases, from the name of the target organ plus the suffix *trophic* or *tropic*. The two suffixes are often used interchangeably, although their literal meanings are different. Trophic (to nourish) implies the nourishment of the target organ by the anterior pituitary, whereas tropic (to turn toward) implies that the hormone is "aimed at" the target organ. Used in a broad sense, either suffix can be interpreted to mean that the hypophysis influences the activities of the target organ. The names and chief characteristics of the hormones are as follows.

(1) *Somatotrophin (somatotrophic hormine, STH; growth hormone, GH)*. Somatotrophin stimulates body growth, particularly growth of long bones by promoting the proliferation of cartilage cells in the epiphyses. Hypophysectomy of growing animals brings about a cessation of growth, which can be restored by administration of the hormone. In the human, anterior lobe tumors produce gigantism when they occur before closure of the epiphyses; when they occur after epiphyseal closure, they produce acromegaly, i.e., an increase in thickness of the mandible and of the bones of the calvaria, hands and feet.

The growth hormone was obtained originally from pituitary glands of cattle. More recently, it has been isolated from human and monkey pituitary glands, and it has been synthesized. Its molecular weight and amino acid composition differ for different species. In humans, the growth hormone has a molecular weight of about 21,000 and consists of amino acid residues, arranged in a straight chain structure.

(2) *Lactogenic hormone (prolactin, mammotrophin, luteotrophic hormone, LTH)*. This hormone is a glycoprotein with a molecular weight of about 25,000, and it stimulates the secretion of milk after parturition. Its action is on mammary glands that have hypertrophied during pregnancy under the influence of estrogen and progesterone. The lactogenic hormone also initiates and maintains the secretion of progesterone from the cells of the corpus luteum; hence, the alternate name luteotrophic hormone (LTH).

(3) *Adrenocorticotrophin (adrenocorticotrophic hormone, ACTH; corticotrophin)*. This hormone is a polypeptide with a molecular weight of about 45,000. The atrophy of the adrenal cortex which follows hypophysectomy can be prevented by injections of ACTH. Administration of ACTH to normal animals produces hypertrophy and hyperplasia of the adrenal cortex, particularly of the zona fasciculata and zona reticularis. Hypertrophy and hyperplasia of the cortex also result from hyperfunction of the hypophysis. ACTH has been prepared in a highly purified state from sheep and pig pituitaries, and the hormone has also been synthesized.

(4) *Thyrotrophin (thyrotrophic hormone; thyroid-stimulating hormone, TSH)*. Thyrotrophin is apparently a glycoprotein with a molecular weight of about 25,000. Injections of TSH to normal animals produce all of the symptoms of hyperthyroidism. Injections of TSH into hypophysectomized animals restore the involuted thyroids and relieve the hypothyroid symptoms resulting from hypophysectomy. That the effect is through thyroid stimulation is demonstrated by the fact that it is not produced when TSH is administered to thyroidectomized animals.

(5) *Follicle-stimulating hormone, FSH*. This hormone is a glycoprotein with a molecular weight of about 30,000. It stimulates growth of the follicles in the ovaries and

spermatogenesis in the seminiferous tubules of the testes. Atrophy of the gonads after hypophysectomy can be partially prevented by administration of FSH, but complete maintenance requires some luteinizing hormone in addition to FSH.

(6) *Luteinizing hormone, LH (interstitial cell-stimulating hormone, ICSH).* This hormone is a glycoprotein with a molecular weight of about 26,000. In the female it does the following: (a) stimulates the theca interna cells to secrete estrogen following their prior stimulation by FSH; (b) contributes to the maturation of the ovarian follicle after follicular growth has been stimulated by FSH; (c) brings about ovulation after follicular maturation; and (d) produces luteinization of the granulosa and theca interna cells following ovulation. In the male, LH (ICSH) stimulates the interstitial cells of Leydig to produce testosterone which, in turn, maintains the accessory reproductive organs and the secondary sex characteristics. LH also has an indirect effect on spermatogenesis through testosterone which, in proper amounts, will augment the action of FSH. In excess amounts, testosterone depresses spermatogenic activity through an inhibition of formation of FSH by the hypophysis.

The rate of hormone production by the target organ influences the rate of secretion by the hypophysis itself. For example, administration of the thyroid hormone (or iodide) decreases the output of thyrotrophic hormone by the hypophysis. On the other hand, the administration of an antithyroid drug such as propylthiouracil inhibits the formation of hormone by the thyroid, and the decreased level of circulating thyroid hormone causes an increase in thyrotrophic hormone secreted by the hypophysis. Similarly, administration of adrenal cortical hormones or of sex hormones (estrogen, androgen) decreases the hypophyseal output of adrenocorticotrophic or of gonadotrophic hormones. This is a feedback type of regulation in which the hormones from the end organs modify the secretion of the specific trophic hormones from the controlling organ. In this feedback mechanism, the circulating end organ hormones (e.g., estrogen, progesterone, etc.) act on certain hypothalamic centers which secrete substances known as *releasing hormones* that are carried by way of the hypophyseal portal system to the anterior lobe. There are apparently specific releasing factors for most of the hormones produced in the anterior lobe. This is a complex field that is under active study.

Several lines of evidence associate the secretion of growth hormone with the acidophils. In acromegaly and gigantism, tumors of acidophils are almost invariably present. In a strain of mice showing hereditary dwarfism in a mendelian ratio, the hypophyses of the dwarfs lack acidophils and no growth hormone is shown by the most sensitive tests.

There is good evidence that the acidophils also secrete luteotrophin (prolactin). The acidophils increase in number and size during pregnancy and, at the same time, there is a comparable increase in the luteotrophin content of the hypophysis. As noted above, immunochemical studies with labeled antibodies show the presence of a special type of acidophil for luteotrophin.

A number of facts indicate that the basophils secrete FSH, TSH and LH (ICSH). Chemical analyses show that these hormones are rich in glycoproteins, and cytochemical studies reveal that the granules of the basophils, but not of the acidophils, contain glycoprotein.

After castration, there is an increase in the number of uniformly dispersed delta basophils, and many of these cells become so vacuolated that they have a signet ring appearance (castration cells); these represent a type of delta basophil that secretes LH (ICSH). In the human anterior hypophysis, two types of basophils can be distinguished by their staining reactions under the light microscope and by the size of their granules in electron micrographs; presumably, they are thyrotrophs and gonadotrophs.

Attempts to associate the secretion of ACTH with a particular cell type have given controversial results. Most of the recent evidence, however, including results of immunohistochemical studies, indicates that the adrenocorticotroph is a type of basophil.

Pars Intermedia. The pars intermedia of most mammals consists of several layers of epithelial cells located, as the name implies, between the anterior lobe and the pars nervosa. This lobe is somewhat rudimentary in man and consists of a relatively thin zone of cells that are often grouped around vesicles that contain colloid. The latter contains only a small amount of colloid and differs from that of the thyroid. The zone blends with the pars distalis anteriorly and some of its cells migrate posteriorly into the contiguous neural lobe (Fig. 21-7). Some of the cells stain deeply with basic dyes, whereas others are small and pale staining.

A *melanocyte-stimulating hormone* (MSH) is produced by the pituitary gland, and the evidence indicates that it is present in the intermediate lobe in animals in which this lobe is well demarcated. The hormone is found both in the pars distalis and pars nervosa in man. The cell of origin is controversial, but it is apparently a type of basophil.

In amphibians, MSH controls the dispersal of melanin granules within the cytoplasmic branches of the melanocytes and thus alters skin color. The normal function of this hormone in mammals is obscure, but its injection does increase pigmentation, probably by stimulating melanin synthesis.

Neurohypophysis. The neural lobe of the hypophysis or infundibular process is a downgrowth from the hypothalamic region of the brain. Both anatomically and functionally, it forms a part of a larger unit, the *neurohypophysis*. The neurohypophysis includes the infundibular process (neural lobe) and the infundibulum which, in turn, includes the infundibular stem and the median eminence of the tuber cinereum (Figs. 21-2 and 21-8). These regions are similar in that they possess the same type of cell and the same nerve and blood supply, and they yield the same active substances upon extraction.

The cells of the neural lobe are known as *pituicytes*. In some respects, the pituicytes resemble the neuroglia cells found elsewhere in the central nervous system, i.e., they are small cells with ramifying processes but without the distinctive features of nerve cells. Unlike neuroglia cells, many of the pituicytes contain variable numbers of refractile droplets or granules in their cytoplasm. Some of the pituicytes also contain yellow-brown pigment granules, the number of which increases with age.

The nuclei of the pituicytes (Fig. 21-9) are round or oval with a fine chromatin network. The cytoplasm is drawn out into a variable number of processes which often end either on the walls of blood vessels or on connective tissue septa of the gland. In routine preparations, the cytoplasm surrounding the nucleus is barely discernible, and the processes cannot be followed. Be-

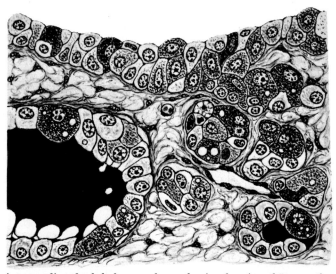

Fig. 21-7. Pars intermedia of adult human hypophysis, showing the growth of cords of cells up into the neural lobe. The formation of vesicles with colloid (black) is shown in two of the ingrowths. The basophilic cells are dark. (Rasmussen.)

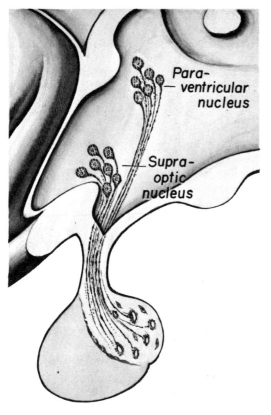

Fig. 21-8. Diagram of the hypothalamico-hypophyseal tract in the human. Nerve fibers from the supraoptic and paraventricular nuclei of the hypothalamus carry the neurosecretion to the blood vessels of the pars nervosa by way of the infundibular stem.

tween the cell bodies, the meshwork of interweaving processes stains faintly. The pituicytes may be blackened by special silver techniques and their form may thus be determined. Romeis, who has made a thorough study of the cytology of the human neural lobe, distinguished several types of pituicytes according to their morphological characteristics in silvered preparations.

The secretory substances released into the blood vessels of the neurohypophysis are formed in cell bodies of the nerve cells of the supraoptic and paraventricular nuclei located in the hypothalamus of the brain, and they pass by way of the unmyelinated fibers of the cell bodies to the neural lobe.

After sectioning of the pituitary stalk in experimental animals, the stainable neurosecretory material accumulates in large masses in relation to the severed nerve

fibers proximal to the cut. Normally, accumulations of stainable neurosecretory material are found also within the nerve fiber terminals of the human posterior lobe; these are known as the Herring bodies (Fig. 21-9).

The neurosecretory material, both in the nerve cells of the supraoptic and paraventricular nuclei and in the nerve fibers of the hypothalamico-hypophyseal tract, is stained by a number of methods, among them chrome hematoxylin (Figs. 21-9 and 21-10). This stainable material of the neurohypophysis is believed to be a protein associated with the actual hormones, perhaps as a carrier. The amount of stainable material corresponds to the amount of hormone that can be extracted from the tissue, although the purified hormones themselves are not stained.

Most of the fibers of the hypothalamico-hypophyseal tract terminate in various regions of the neural lobe, a few going to the pars tuberalis and the pars intermedia. They terminate in close association with the capillaries, often in a palisade arrangement along the wall of the blood vessel. Electron micrographs show that the cell bodies and axon terminals contain membrane bounded electron-dense granules which represent the neurosecretory material (Figs. 21-11 and 21-12). There is a marked increase in the number of granular vesicles in physiological conditions which stimulate secretion. The nerve terminals also contain smaller agranular vesicles (Fig. 21-12). The endothelium of the capillaries of the neurohypophysis is seen in electron micrographs to be fenestrated (Fig. 21-11). This presumably facilitates the passage of the secretion into the lumina of the capillaries.

Extracts of the tissue components of the neurohypophysis yield two hormones, both polypeptides. Both substances have also been synthesized. One of these, *oxytocin*, stimulates the contraction of the uterine musculature during the latter part of pregnancy. It is used clinically in obstetrics for the induction of labor. Oxytocin also has a contractile action on the myoepithelial cells of the alveoli and ducts of the mammary gland and thus brings about the ejection of milk; hence it is also known as the milk let-down factor. The other fraction, *vaso-*

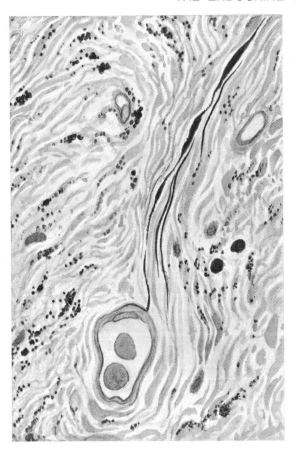

Fig. 21-9. Posterior hypophysis. A section from the para nervosa, human, age 26. Nerve fibers containing neurosecretory material (deep blue) are cut in both cross and longitudinal sections. One of the longitudinal sections shows three bulging masses of neurosecretory material; it appears to terminate on the surface of a small blood vessel (*lower center of field*). Larger accumulations of neurosecretion (Herring bodies) appear at *right*. Nuclei of pituicytes are stained red. A 4 μm section, stained with chrome hematoxylin and phloxine. ×1200.

pressin (*antidiuretic hormone, ADH*), inhibits diuresis by increasing the permeability of the distal and collecting tubules of the kidney for water resorption. Vasopressin also raises blood pressure and, in large doses, causes contraction of the intestinal and bronchial musculature.

Pars Tuberalis. Like the parenchyma of the pars distalis and intermedia, the tuberalis takes its embryonic origin from Rathke's pouch epithelium. It continues to form a layer of cuboidal cells that covers the neural stalk and tuberal area of the brain (Fig. 21-1, *c*). The cytoplasm of the cells is faintly basophilic. In contrast with the pars intermedia, the pars tuberalis is quite vascular. The cells frequently form vesicles which contain colloid. In the pars tuberalis, especially at its upper and lower poles, groups of squamous cells have been described which probably are "remnants" from the craniopharyngeal duct.

Pharyngeal Hypophysis. A small body of tissue which resembles that of the anterior lobe is generally present in the vault of the human nasopharynx, but not in other species. It is located near the position where the anterior lobe develops, and it is described as a structure measuring 3.5 to 7 mm in length by 1 mm or less in width. The cells appear to be structurally identical to those of the anterior lobe by light microscopy but studies in which this tissue has been implanted into animals do not give any evidence that this tissue contains pituitary hormones.

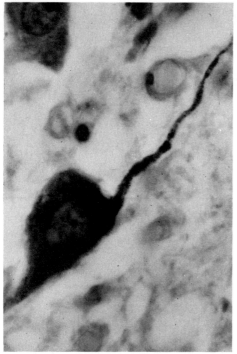

Fig. 21-10. Photomicrograph of a neuron from the human supraoptic nucleus. Both the nerve cell body and its axon contain granular neurosecretory material. Chrome hematoxylin stain. ×1200. (Courtesy of Dr. S. L. Palay.)

The Thyroid Gland

Structure

The adult thyroid gland consists of two lateral lobes and a connecting part, the isthmus. The lobes lie lateral to the superior part of the trachea and the inferior part of the larynx. The isthmus crosses anterior to the trachea at the level of the second to fourth tracheal cartilages. A median process, the pyramidal lobe, is present in a number of individuals, extending upward from the left side of the isthmus. The thyroid has a connective tissue sheath formed by the deep cervical fascia. Beneath this is a delicate stratum of connective tissue, the true capsule of the gland. Delicate trabeculae and septa penetrate the gland substance, indistinctly dividing it into lobes and lobules.

The thyroid is an extremely labile gland and varies in size and structure in response to a large number of factors, among which are sex, nutrition, temperature, age, season and the iodine content of the food, the latter being of great importance.

The structural unit of the thyroid is the *follicle* or acinus (Fig. 21-13). These units are usually of microscopic dimensions but may become sufficiently large, as in colloid goiter, to be visible macroscopically. Follicles vary greatly in shape as well as in size, but they are usually irregularly spheroidal. In highly activated glands they become extremely irregular in shape (Fig. 21-14). A follicle consists of a layer of simple epithelium enclosing a cavity, the follicular cavity, which usually is filled with a gel-like material, *colloid.*

Thyroid follicles are primarily epithelial derivatives of the endodermal lining of the embryonic pharyngeal floor. During early development, a single median evagination proliferates and separates from the pharyngeal floor, sinks into the underlying mesenchymal stroma and continues expansion as it migrates into the stroma of the neck where it bifurcates somewhat in achieving the normal adult shape. The diverticular pattern of epithelial proliferation leads to separation of follicles from the original parent mass (see discussion in chapter 3). Hence, connecting ducts are lost, and the gland becomes crowded with individual follicles, each encased by a highly vascular connective tissue. Occasionally, isolated small masses of active thyroid tissue are left behind along the migratory route.

The *principal thyroid cells, follicle cells,* have their apical ends facing inward, i.e., toward the follicular cavity, and their basal ends resting on the basal lamina. In addition to the principal cells, there are *parafollicular cells* which are found singly or in small groups both within the follicle and within the interfollicular connective tissue. Those within the follicle are wedged between the principal cells and the basal lamina; they generally do not extend to the colloid cavity.

Parafollicular cells are apparently of different embryonic origin than the principal cells. In lower vertebrates it can be demonstrated that they arise by budding from the endodermal epithelium of the lower part of the paired fifth pharyngeal pouches (the so-called ultimobranchial bodies). They too undergo extensive migration, but

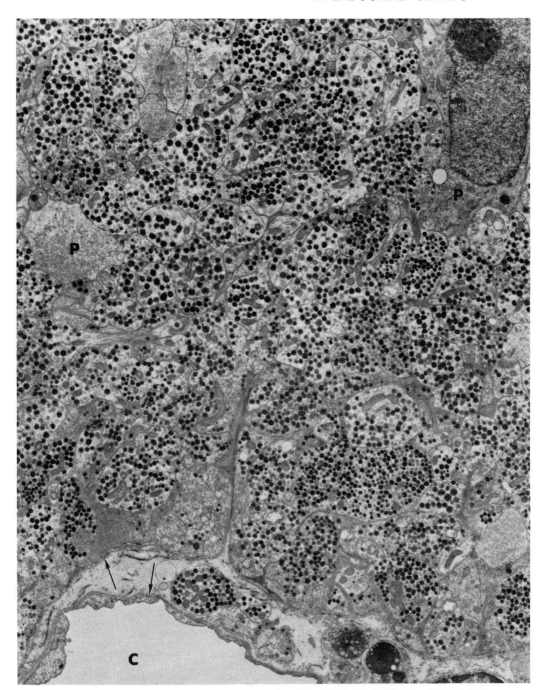

Fig. 21-11. Electron micrograph of a portion of monkey neurohypophysis showing many axons with neurosecretory granules, portions of pituicytes (*P*) and a fenestrated sinusoidal capillary (*C*). The perivascular connective tissue space contains some axons as well as connective tissue cells. The vascular endothelium is surrounded by basal lamina, as is the neuroepithelium (*arrows*). ×6700.

in this case more as individual cells rather than masses, before coming to mingle with the principal cells of thyroid follicles. The parafollicular cells are generally larger than the principal cells, and they have a lighter staining cytoplasm. They apparently form *thyrocalcitonin*, a hormone that lowers blood calcium and thus exerts an effect

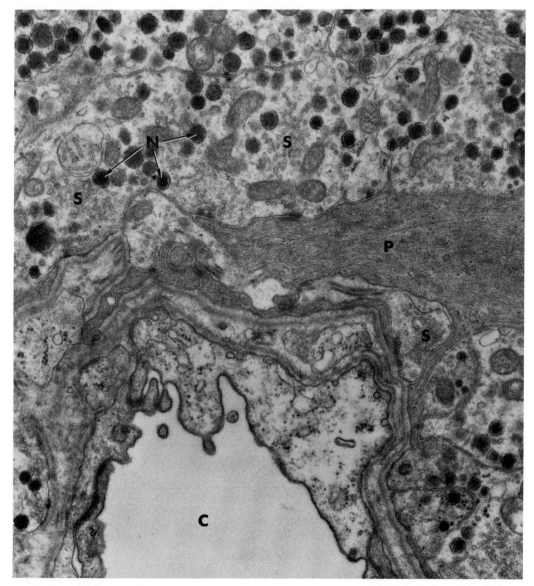

Fig. 21-12. Electron micrograph showing axonal terminations in neurohypophysis of monkey. The axonal terminals contain both dense neurosecretory granules (N) and small clear vesicles (S) resembling synaptic vesicles. C, capillary; P, pituicyte process. The basal laminae are obvious. ×24,000.

opposite to that of the parathyroid hormone.

The principal cells are generally cuboidal in the normal gland (Fig. 21-13) but become low cuboidal or even squamous in the relatively inactive gland. They enlarge and become tall columnar cells during periods of increased activity (Figs. 21-14 and 21-15, D). The intercellular boundaries are distinct and fairly obvious under the light micro-

scope. Electron micrographs show the presence of typical junctional complexes (chapter 4).

The nuclei are generally rounded in shape, and the cytoplasm is lightly basophilic. The mitochondria are rod-shaped or filamentous and vary in number with the activity of the cell. The Golgi complex, which is located on the apical side of the nucleus, becomes enlarged during cell activ-

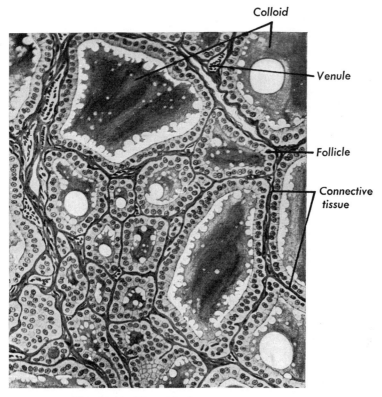

Fig. 21-13. Thyroid of human adult. (Stöhr.)

ity. The cytoplasm also contains lipid droplets and PAS-positive droplets (colloid resorption droplets). An additional type of cell is occasionally seen in the follicle, the colloid cells of Langendorff. They are slender cells with darkly staining cytoplasm that often appears to be filled with colloid, and they have pyknotic nuclei. They are degenerating cells.

Electron micrographs show that the apical end of the principal cell has short, irregularly distributed microvilli which are more numerous on the columnar (hyperactive) cells than on the lower, relatively inactive cells. Electron micrographs also show that there is an increase in rough endoplasmic reticulum in the activated cells. Lysosomes are present, predominantly in the apical region. The basal lamina of the follicle cells is often in close association with the basal lamina of the endothelium of the sinusoidal capillaries. The endothelial cells are of the fenestrated type, a characteristic of many regions in which there is rapid transport.

The cavity of the thyroid follicle is filled with a semifluid or gel-like substance, the thyroid *colloid*. In most preparations for light microscopy, a number of relatively large vacuoles may be seen in the colloid, particularly at the junction of the colloid with the apical ends of the cells. Most of these vacuoles apparently arise as a result of shrinkage of colloid and cells during the ordinary technical procedures used in preparing slides. Nevertheless, the vacuoles tend to occur more frequently in follicles with heightened activity in colloid resorption (Fig. 21-15, *C* and *D*). The colloid also becomes less dense during resorption and takes a lighter, more irregular stain.

Thyroid colloid varies in its chemical composition as well as in its physical properties. It is composed chiefly of nucleoproteins, thyroglobulin and proteolytic enzymes. It also occasionally contains desquamated cells. *Thyroglobulin* is an iodinated glycoprotein in which iodine and tyrosine are important constituents of a macromolecular complex. Both the amount of thyroglobulin in the colloid and the degree of

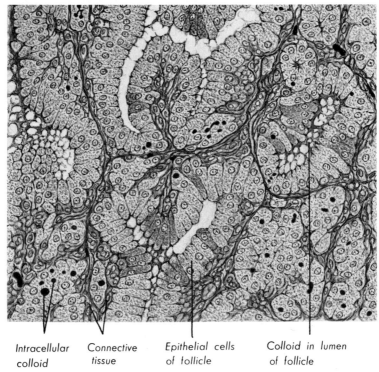

Intracellular   Connective   Epithelial cells   Colloid in lumen
colloid   tissue   of follicle   of follicle

Fig. 21-14. Surgical specimen of human thyroid showing diffuse extreme hyperplasia. The patient was a woman with toxic goiter who had been treated with thiouracil and then operated upon without pretreatment with iodine. A surgical specimen. Heidenhain's azan stain. ×320. (Aranow et al., Surg. Pathol., No. 88452. Ann. Surg. 124:167, 1946.)

iodination may vary. For instance, in colloid goiter, which is associated with hypothyroidism, the iodine content is lower than in the colloid of a normal gland. The iodine content, however, generally does not vary to any significant extent in the follicles of the same individual at any given time.

The *secretory process* of the thyroid involves the synthesis of the thyroid hormone, which is a component of the follicular colloid, and it also involves the transport of the thyroid hormone from the follicular cavity to the perifollicular capillaries. Both the formation of new secretion and the outward transport of the stored hormone may occur at the same time.

The synthesis of thyroid hormone has been studied by techniques of radioautography in combination with light and electron microscopy. By fixing tissues from experimental animals at different intervals after injection of labeled precursors of hormones, one can follow the events in hormone synthesis. Leucine, one of the essen-

tial amino acids, has been used in labeled form to trace the formation of proteins. ^{3}H-labeled leucine appears over the basal portion of thyroid cells in about 10 min after intraperitoneal injection (Fig. 21-16). It is seen first over the cisternae of the rough endoplasmic reticulum, later in the Golgi complex and still later in the colloid. It seems clear that the proteins are synthesized from amino acids in association with the polyribosomes, that they are then transported via the cisternae of the reticulum to the Golgi complex, where they are combined with polysaccharides to form tyrosyl groups, and that they are secreted later into the lumen of the thyroid follicle. In other studies utilizing radioactive iodide (^{125}I), it is found that iodide begins to appear in the thyroid cells about 5 min after an intraperitoneal injection. It appears first at the basal end of the cell, which has a remarkable capacity for taking iodide from the blood and concentrating it. The iodide is oxidized by a peroxidase enzyme within

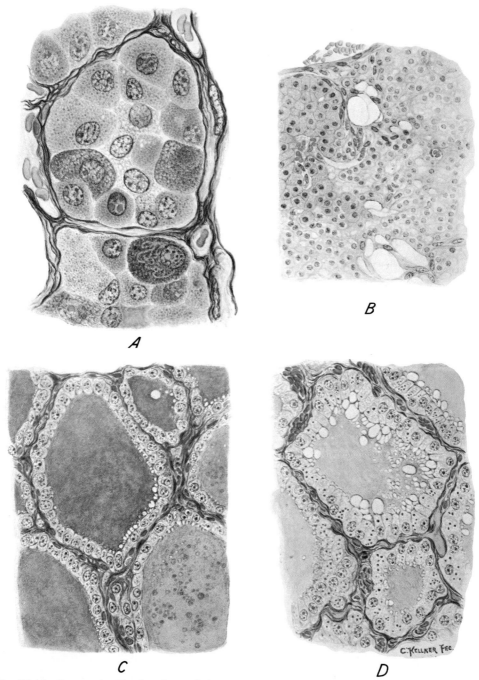

Fig. 21-15. Camera lucida drawings of the normal anterior hypophysis and parathyroid of man (*upper*) and the normal and activated thyroid of the rhesus monkey (*lower*). *A,* anterior hypophysis of an executed man, 38 years old. Cords of cells are from the central part of the gland. In three of the acidophils (pink), the Golgi area is stained bluish. In the basophil in the lower cord, a negative picture of the Golgi apparatus is shown as clear canals. Chromophobes are present in the middle of the central cord. The rather large amount of connective tissue shown in the drawing is characteristic of the human anterior hypophysis. A colloid mass (blue) is shown at the lower part of the inferior cell cord. Modified Masson stain. ×1250. *B,* parathyroid of normal human adult. The oxyphils are pink and the chief cells are bluish purple. The spaces shown were filled with fat. Hematoxylin-eosin stain. ×350. *C,* thyroid of a normal adult rhesus monkey. A few peripheral and central colloid vacuoles are shown. Modified Masson stain. ×570. *D,* activated thyroid of a normal adult rhesus monkey. The thyroid was activated by injections of an anterior hypophysis extract. The epithelium is high and many absorption vacuoles are present. Colloid droplets and vacuoles are present in the thyroid epithelium. Modified Masson stain. ×570.

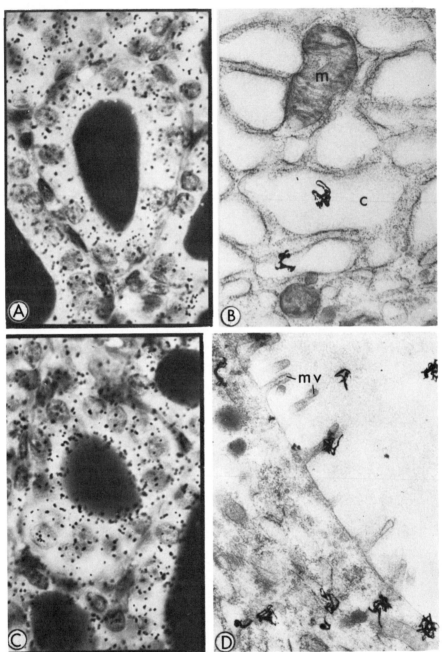

Fig. 21-16. Light and electron micrographs of radioautographic preparations of thyroids from rats sacrificed at different intervals of time after injection of leucine-^{3}H. *A*, radioautograph of a periodic acid-Schiff and hematoxylin stained preparation from an animal sacrificed at 30 minutes after injection of labeled leucine. Radioactivity is seen rather diffusely over the cytoplasm in the light micrograph. *B*, electron micrograph of a radioautographic preparation from an animal sacrificed at 1 hr after injection. Irregularly shaped silver grains, indicating the location of the incorporated leucine, are seen over the cisternae (*c*) of the endoplasmic reticulum. *m*, mitochondrion. *C*, radioautograph of tissue fixed at 4 hr after injection of labeled leucine. The labeled material is present chiefly in the adluminal ends of the cell. *D*, electron micrograph of a radioautograph at 3½ hr after injection of labeled leucine. Silver grains are seen in the adluminal cytoplasm and also in the colloid. *mv*, microvilli. *A* and *C*, ×1200; *B* and *D*, ×30,000. (Courtesy of Drs. N. J. Nadler, B. Young, C. P. Leblond, and B. O. Mitmaker, Endocrinology, vol. 74, 1964.)

the cell to form active iodine. Then, the tyrosol groups are iodinated to form *mon-oiodotyrosine* and *diiodotyrosine*. Although the exact location of this step is obscure, it is generally assumed to occur near the apical end of the cell, either at or just outside the plasmalemma. *Triiodothyronine* and *tetraiodothyronine (thyroxin)* are derived from mono- and diiodotyrosine precursors. Only the thyronines have hormonal activity and they constitute only a small portion of the macromolecular complex known as thyroglobulin. The thyroglobulin is stored for variable periods, depending on the functional activity of the gland. In hyperactive thyroids, the hormone is released into the capillaries almost as soon as it is formed.

The reabsorption of the colloid and release of hormone into the vessels involves hydrolysis of thyroglobulin. Droplets of colloid are taken up by a process resembling pinocytosis and hydrolysis occurs within the cell through lysosomal action (Fig. 21-17). The active principles of the hormone are released into the capillaries as triiodothyronine and tetraiodothyronine, with the latter in much greater proportion. Only a small percentage of the iodine in the thyroid colloid is in the form of tetraiodothyronine. When thyroglobulin is hydrolyzed, the mono- and diiodo-components are liberated, as well as the tri- and tetraiodo-components. The former are deiodinated, and thus their iodine becomes available for use in the formation of new thyroglobulin.

Thyroxin circulating in the blood is carried almost entirely in association with thy-

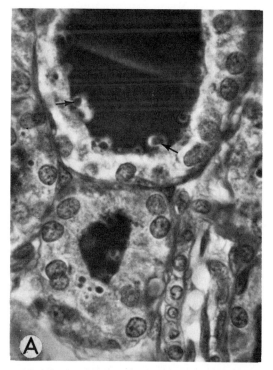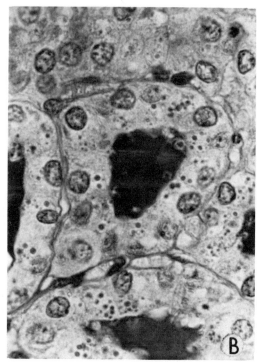

Fig. 21-17. Photomicrographs of periodic acid-Schiff and hematoxylin stained sections of rat thyroid fixed at different intervals of time after an injection of thyroid stimulating hormone (TSH). *A,* from tissue fixed at 8 min after TSH. Colloid droplets in contact with the adluminal ends of the cells are apparently being surrounded by cytoplasmic processes of the cells. (Two of the several droplets in the field are indicated by *arrows.*) *B,* from tissue fixed at 30 min after TSH. Droplets are present chiefly in the adluminal cytoplasm but a few are still being formed at the adluminal surfaces and some have migrated to the basal ends of the cells. The sequence of events indicates that the colloid is taken into the cells by a process resembling pinocytosis and that the droplets are hydrolyzed by lysosomal activity to release the hormone that enters the blood vessels which are closely associated with the basal laminae of the thyroid cells. ×900. (Courtesy of Drs. N. J. Nadler, S. K. Sarkar, and C. P. Leblond, Endocrinology, vol. 71, 1962.)

roxin-binding hormones. Triiodothyronine, which has several times the hormonal potency of thyroxin (tetraiodothyronine), is not as firmly bound. Only a small percentage of the hormone is entirely unbound or "free" as a metabolically active substance within the plasma. The level of the binding proteins in the plasma has an important role in regulating the level of free hormone.

The use of *tracer doses* of radioactive iodine has found clinical application, especially in two ways. The rapidity with which the radioiodine is taken up by the thyroid (as determined by a Geiger counter) is an indication of the activity of the gland of a patient. In thyroid carcinoma, the site of metastases can frequently be determined by their radioactivity. Radioiodine is also extensively used as a therapeutic agent in hyperthyroidism. As a result of the radiation from the ^{131}I taken up, part of the overactive gland tissue is destroyed. This reduction in functioning tissue thus substitutes for surgical removal.

Blood Vessels

The thyroid has a rich plexus of blood and lymph capillaries, which are in intimate relation to the follicular epithelium. The arteries, at the places where they branch, frequently have localized padlike thickenings beneath the intima. These do not encircle the vessels. They probably assist in shunting the blood to different parts of the gland as the arteries contract, and they may also serve to reduce the pulse wave. Arteriovenous anastomoses are common. The architecture of the blood vessels, as well as the fact that all of the follicles do not show the same degree of activity at any one time, indicates that there are fluctuations in the amount of blood received by different parts of the gland.

Nerves

A large number of nonmyelinated nerve fibers are present in the walls of the thyroid arteries. Most of these terminate in plexuses around the blood vessels.

Function

The main effect of the thyroid hormone is on the rate of metabolism of tissues in general. The ramifications of this effect are very extensive, however, extending to activities as diverse as the rate of absorption in the intestine, carbohydrate metabolism, the rate of the heart beat, mental activity, general body growth and many other effects. *Hypothyroidism* in the infant causes *cretinism*; in the adult, it causes *myxedema*. The symptoms in both conditions are attributable to a lowered metabolic rate not only in the general body tissues but in other endocrine glands. Administration of thyroid hormone has a striking therapeutic effect. The opposite condition, *hyperthyroidism*, leads to *overactivity* and sometimes is followed by *exophthalmic goiter* (Grave's disease). Surgical removal of a part of the thyroid, or the use of antithyroid drugs or radioiodine, reduces the metabolic rate but does not alleviate the exophthalmos when this is once established. The thyroid is not essential to life, although in early work the close topographical association of the parathyroids with it caused confusion on this point.

The Parathyroid Glands

Structure

There are normally two pairs of parathyroids in mammals. Because of the origin of their parenchymal cells from the endodermal epithelium of the third and fourth pharyngeal pouches, respectively, they are designated as parathyroids III and IV. In man, a member of each pair lies on the posterior surface of each lateral lobe of the thyroid, near the arterial anastomosis of the inferior and superior thyroid arteries. These glands, which are somewhat flattened, measure some 6 mm in length and about half this in width. In man they are brown, but in some species they are white or only faintly colored. A connective tissue capsule separates them from the thyroid. Delicate connective tissue septa partially divide the gland into poorly defined lobules, and still finer septa tend to separate the epithelial cells into anastomosing cords and groups. The separation of epithelial cell groups by connective tissue becomes particularly obvious in the adult as a result of a marked increase in fat cells.

The epithelial parenchyma is composed

of two types of cells: the *principal* or *chief cells* and the *oxyphil cells* (Fig. 21-15 *B*). The chief cells are of constant occurrence, while the oxyphil cells do not appear in man until near the end of the first decade of life. They have not been observed in many other species, except in monkeys and cattle.

The chief cells are polyhedral in shape and have round nuclei with a loosely arranged chromatin giving a vesicular appearance. They have been subdivided into *light cells* and *dark cells*, primarily on differences in staining of the cytoplasm. The light chief cells are more numerous than the dark ones, and they are usually slightly larger. Their cytoplasm appears nongranular in routine preparations, but PAS-positive granules and a few argyrophilic granules can be demonstrated by appropriate techniques. The dark chief cells have numerous fine cytoplasmic granules which are mostly argyrophilic. Electron micrographs show that the dark cells contain membrane-bounded secretory granules, a relatively large Golgi complex, enlarged filamentous mitochondria and very little glycogen. The membrane-bounded granules apparently correspond to the argyrophilic granules seen with the light microscope. The light cells have a smaller Golgi complex, few or no secretory granules and considerable glycogen. It seems obvious that the dark cells represent an active secretory stage and that the light cells represent a resting or less active stage of the same cell type.

The oxyphil cells are larger than the chief cells, but they usually have smaller and darker staining nuclei. Their cytoplasm stains well with eosin and contains fine granules. Electron micrographs show that the cytoplasm of the oxyphil contains an abundance of mitochondria, a factor that is apparently responsible for their acidophilic staining in light microscopy. The function of these cells is unknown. It has been suggested that they may represent a stage in the life cycle of the chief cells because transitional forms between the cell types are often seen in preparations for light microscopy. This suggestion has not been confirmed experimentally.

Small colloid follicles are of frequent occurrence in the parathyroid. This colloid has no relation functionally to that of the thyroid. In contrast with the thyroid, the parathyroid, contains no more iodine than do other tissues of the body.

Blood Vessels and Nerves

The parathyroids have an abundant blood supply, but in vascular injections the capillaries do not appear to be as numerous as in the thyroid. In man there is said to be a plexus of veins at the periphery of the gland.

Unmyelinated nerves in small numbers occur in the parathyroid. They are probably vasomotor.

Function

The parathyroid glands regulate calcium concentration in bone and in body fluids. Removal of the parathyroids causes a fall in blood calcium, nervous hyperexcitability and spasms, leading to death. Calcium administration relieves these symptoms, and the injection of parathyroid extract or parathyroid hormone maintains the animals in good health. Such injections in normal animals raise the blood calcium, and excessive doses will cause death.

Removal of one or more of the parathyroids does not cause a compensatory hypertrophy of those which remain. In rickets the parathyroids enlarge. The parathyroids readily "take" in autotransplantation.

The Adrenal Glands

The adrenal glands are paired organs, one being situated close to the cranial pole of each kidney in the retroperitoneal tissue. Both are somewhat flattened, the left adrenal gland being crescentic, the right one more triangular in shape. The combined weight of the two glands is some 10 to 12 g, the left usually being somewhat heavier than the right one. In most mammals they are more regular in shape than in the human, being ovoid or spheroid.

The adrenal glands are composite organs consisting functionally and structurally of two distinct parts, the *cortex* (*interrenal tissue*) and the *medulla* (*chromaffin tissue*). The principal secretory cells of medulla and cortex have differing embryogenic origins; those of the medulla are derived from neural crest cells whereas those of the cortex differentiate from mesodermal mesenchyme. In lower vertebrates, the two components are not united into a common organ but are topographically separated. Correlated with the evolution of the higher vertebrates is a progressively closer association of the cortical and medullary components. In mammals, the chromaffin tissue is surrounded by the interrenal tissue.

Gross examination of slices of fresh human adrenal shows that an outer and broader yellowish zone of the cortex can be distinguished from a brownish yellow inner zone. The unstained medulla is white or gray.

The adrenal gland is covered by a thick capsule of connective tissue composed chiefly of collagenous fibers and fibroblasts. Vessels and nerves course in the capsule. Delicate connective tissue trabeculae composed of collagenous and reticular fibers extend inward from the capsule. Arterioles also extend into the gland in a characteristic pattern described below under "Blood Supply."

The hilus is situated ventromedially (toward the vena cava) and is chiefly marked by the emerging thick walled adrenal vein.

The arrangement of the cortex and medulla in the human does not have the uniformity characteristically found in laboratory animals. This may be due in part to the irregularity in shape of the human ad-

renal. The line of separation between the cortex and medulla is frequently very irregular and, in single sections, clumps of cortical cells may appear to be surrounded by medulla, but studies of serial sections show that these clumps are connected with the cortical zone. The distribution of the medulla also varies in different adrenal glands. It often is absent from the "wings" of the glands and then the two sides of the cortex abut against each other, separated only by connective tissue and small veins (Fig. 21-18). A study of sections through the gland near the emergence of the adrenal vein may reveal cortical tissue adjacent to the vein. This cortical tissue may be partly enclosed by medulla, outside of which are the peripheral cortical zones (Fig. 21-18). The cortex surrounding the vein appears to have been inverted into the gland, with the outermost zone of the cortex lying next to the wall of the vein.

In the zonation of the cortex, there is not as much uniformity in the human as in laboratory animals, although the zones are always readily recognizable.

Cortex

The cortex is classically divided into three zones according to differences in the cordlike arrangement of its cells: an outer zone, the *glomerulosa;* a middle zone, the *fasciculata;* and an inner zone, the *reticularis* (Fig. 21-19). The fasciculata is by far

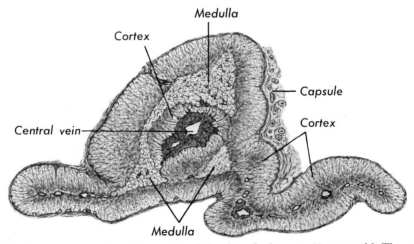

Fig. 21-18. A transverse section through the left adrenal of a man 72 years old. The adrenal was surgically removed in an attempt to give relief in prostatic carcinoma with metastases. The central vein has a thick wall containing bundles of smooth muscle. Camera lucida drawing. ×6.

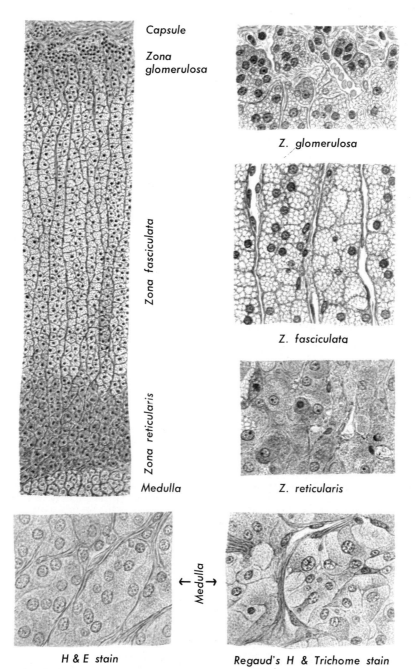

Capsule

Zona glomerulosa

Zona fasciculata

Zona reticularis

Medulla

Z. glomerulosa

Z. fasciculata

Z. reticularis

← Medulla →

H & E stain

Regaud's H & Trichome stain

Fig. 21-19. Sections through the right adrenal of a man 35 years old. The adrenal was removed in an attempt to give relief from a testicular tumor with metastases. The tissue was fixed in Helly's fluid (formol Zenker). The section used for all of the drawings, except the *lower left one,* was stained with Regaud's hematoxylin and Masson's trichrome. The low power (*upper left*) is ×205; the others, ×535.

the broadest of the three but is not uniform in structure throughout. Primarily because of differences in the lipid content of its cells and the consequent differences in staining, the fasciculata may be divided into outer and inner zones (Fig. 21-19), but there is no sharp demarcation between these zones.

The *zona glomerulosa* is a relatively narrow zone in which the arrangement of the cords is such that the cells are in ovoid groups. There is no central cavity within a cell group as in exocrine glands, but there is a rich network of blood vessels just outside. The cells tend to be columnar, and they have spherical nuclei that stain rather heavily. A few lipid droplets may be found in the cytoplasm, but they are sparse in comparison with the droplets in the zona fasciculata. Electron micrographs show that the cytoplasm has a well developed smooth endoplasmic reticulum and that the Golgi complex is often on the side of the nucleus facing toward the blood vessel. The mitochondria of this region generally have shelflike cristae similar to those of most other organs.

The *zona fasciculata,* the broadest zone, is composed of cell cords coursing parallel to one another in a radial direction toward the medulla. As seen in sections, the cords are usually only one or two cells in width. In three-dimensional reconstructions, it is seen that each cord is enclosed by a longitudinally oriented meshwork of sinusoidal capillaries. The secretory cells are generally cuboidal or polyhedral in shape, and they are often binucleate. The nuclei appear more vesicular than those of the glomerulosa, with less dense chromatin. The cells are relatively large, and their cytoplasm contains an abundance of lipid droplets composed of cholesterol, fatty acids and neutral fat. Cholesterol is concentrated chiefly in this zone. Since the lipids are dissolved by the usual technical procedures, the cytoplasm has a spongy appearance, and the cells are often called spongiocytes. Electron micrographs confirm the presence of numerous lipid droplets and show that most of the endoplasmic reticulum is of the smooth-surfaced type. Mitochondria are numerous and are characterized by having tubular rather than shelflike cristae (Fig. 21-20). In the rat adrenal, which has been studied extensively, the cristae are vesicu-

lar-like invaginations from the inner limiting membrane, practically filling the matrix of the mitochondrion. It has been noted that the mitochondria have a close relationship with the lipid droplets.

The *zona reticularis* is composed of a network of cell cords. The cells are generally smaller than those of the fasciculata, and they frequently have deeply staining nuclei. The cytoplasm has relatively few lipid droplets in comparison with the fasciculata, and it takes a darker stain in routine preparations. Toward the inner part of the reticular zone, some of the cells stain particularly darker than others, and "dark" and "light" cells have been described. The former have pyknotic nuclei and often have more lipofuscin pigment in their cytoplasm. The cells of the reticularis, like those of the fasciculata, have a smooth endoplasmic reticulum.

It should be noted that the secretory cells form continuous cords through the zones and that the change in cytology from one zone to the next is gradual rather than abrupt. According to one theory, new cells arise in the glomerulosa, move inward through the fasciculata in correlation with changes in their secretory activity and finally degenerate in the reticularis. This view is based partly on the fact that a complete cortex can regenerate in the rat after removal of all of the cortex except the outer part of the glomerulosa. On the other hand, it is clearly established that mitoses occur in the fasciculata and to some extent in the reticularis. The latter is not merely a zone of degenerating cells. Furthermore, the different zones have functional differences, and they respond differently to hormones from the anterior hypophysis. The fact that the glomerulosa serves as a regenerative zone after the extirpation of the rest of the cortex does not conflict with the view that the glomerulosa also serves for the secretion of particular hormones. Neither does it conflict with the fact that mitoses normally occur in the fasciculata and that the latter serves for secretion of different hormones.

Medulla

The secretory cells of the medulla are found in anastomosing groups in close association with blood vessels. When the tis-

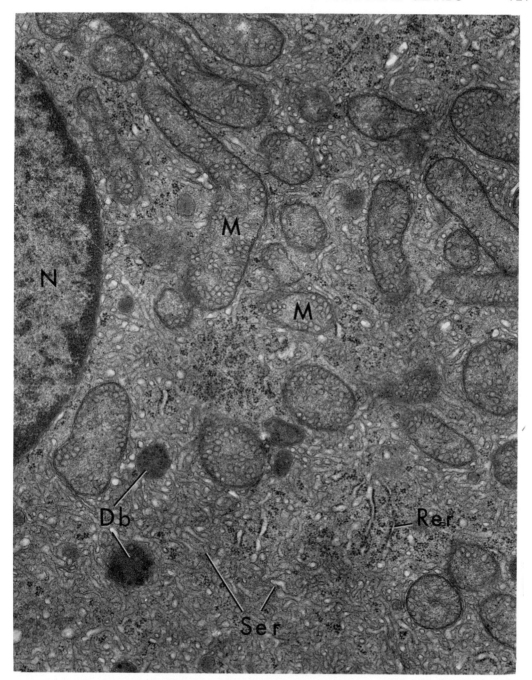

Fig. 21-20. Electron micrograph of a section of the zona fasciculata of the human adrenal cortex. Note that the mitochondria (*M*) have tubular rather than shelflike cristae. Smooth endoplasmic reticulum (*Ser*) is abundant, although some rough endoplasmic reticulum (*Rer*) is present. *Db*, dense bodies, probably lysosomes; *N*, nucleus. ×22,000. (Courtesy of Drs. J. A. Long and A. L. Jones.)

sue is fixed by vascular perfusion, which prevents collapse of blood vessels, it is seen that the cells are arranged as a collar or sleeve around the vessels, each cell with one end in contact with a small venule and the opposite end in contact with a capillary. The cells tend to be columnar in shape, and the Golgi complex and most of the secretory granules are in the advenous end of the cell. The cells contain fine cytoplasmic granules which become brown when oxidized by potassium bichromate, and they are therefore known as *chromaffin cells*. The granules also "stain" by other oxidizing agents. Thus, they become green with ferric chloride, yellow with iodine and brown with osmium tetroxide. The chromaffin reaction of the granules is due to their content of *catecholamines,* derivatives of tyrosine. Two types of catecholamines are present in the medulla: *epinephrine* and *norepinephrine*. In correlation with this, two types of cells can be identified on the basis of their "staining reactions" with solutions of substances such as silver and iodide and on the basis of differences in autofluorescence; the norepinephrine secreting cells give much stronger reactions than the epinephrine secreting cells do (Table 21-2). By electron microscopy the granules of both cell types are similar in size but those of the norepinephrine type are more electron dense. Both types of cells have a well developed Golgi complex, an average number of mitochondria and a granular type of endoplasmic reticulum.

The secretory cells of the adrenal medulla have many similarities to postganglionic neurons: both are derived from neural crest in the embryo, both are innervated by preganglionic sympathetic fibers and both secrete norepinephrine. However, both types of medullary cells differ from postganglionic neurons in that the neurons cannot convert norepinephrine into epinephrine and medullary cells secrete into blood vessels rather than at nerve endings.

Blood Supply

The adrenal glands are highly vascular organs. The arterial supply is subject to great individual variation in the human, but there is always a number of small arteries to each gland. These commonly arise from the inferior phrenic, celiac and renal arteries. The adrenal arteries usually branch before entering the gland so that there are small branches entering the capsule at intervals over most of its surface. From arteries that enter and course in the capsule, three sets of branches arise (Fig. 21-21). One set supplies capillaries to the capsule and the blood from these is collected in the veins of the capsule. The second set supplies sinusoidal capillaries to the cortex which then empty into veins within the medulla. The third set sends arterial branches directly through the cortex to the capillary plexus of the medulla (Fig. 21-21). The venules arising from the second and third sets drain into the vena cava through the medullary vein, which is unusually thick walled for a vein with many longitudinally directed smooth muscle fibers (Fig. 21-18). In both the cortex and medulla, the terminal network from the arterioles is in close relationship to the secretory cells. Electron micrographs show that the sinusoidal capillaries have a fenestrated type of endothelium. Lymph vessels have not been described in the adrenal gland except in relation to the larger blood vessels.

Nerves

The adrenals are abundantly supplied with nerves. Most of these are derived from the sympathetic division of the autonomic nervous system and course through the splanchnic nerves. Some of the fibers are distributed to the cortex. The majority, however, pass to the medulla; these have been described as being preganglionic. A

TABLE 21-2
Characteristics of adrenal medulla cells

Cell types	Color reactions with		Reactions with silver and iodide	Degree of autofluorescence	Granules by electron microscopy	
	Potassium bichromate	Ferric chloride			Size	Density
Epinephrine secreting cells	Brown	Green	Slight	Absent	200 nm (range 50–350)	Light
Norepinephrine secreting cells	Brown	Green	Strong	Moderate	200 nm (range 50–350)	Very dense

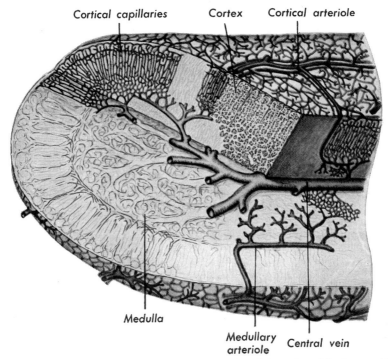

Cortical capillaries   Cortex   Cortical arteriole

Medulla

Medullary arteriole   Central vein

Fig. 21-21. Blood supply of adrenal of dog. One end only of the adrenal is shown. (After Flint.)

few ganglion cells are present in the medulla.

Stimulation of the splanchnic nerves causes an outpouring of epinephrine. Cutting the splanchnics inhibits the secretory activity of the medulla.

Function

Attention was first attracted to the physiological importance of the adrenal glands by Addison in 1855. He described a fatal syndrome, since named Addison's disease, which resulted from a destruction of the adrenals by some disease process. Experimentally, work beginning with that of Brown-Séquard in 1856 has shown that the adrenal cortex, but not the medulla, is essential for life. Destruction of the *cortex* causes a loss of sodium and an accumulation of potassium, so that diets high in sodium and low in potassium are helpful. There is a concentration of the blood, a sluggish circulation and an increase in urea resulting from impaired kidney function. Carbohydrate stores are depleted, and there is hypoglycemia with lowered resistance to insulin. There is a decreased resistance to stress (heat, cold, trauma, fatigue, etc.). Cortical extracts, first successfully

prepared in 1930, are assayed on the basis of their ability to prolong life or to alleviate the other disabilities resulting from adrenalectomy.

Thus far, more than 40 crystalline compounds (steroids) have been isolated from the adrenal cortex. A number of these have been shown to have physiologic effects as evidenced by their substitutive action in survival tests on adrenalectomized animals. In general, the active compounds can be divided into two main categories as judged by their type of activity. Those in one category have an effect on electrolyte and water balance (*mineralocorticoids*); those in the other category have their greatest effect on carbohydrate metabolism (*glucocorticoids*). In addition, there is a third group of steroids which includes the female sex hormones (estrone and progesterone) and several androgenic steroids. Certain adrenal tumors have a feminizing or a masculinizing influence. The cortical hormones (except possibly the estrogens) may be synthesized from cholesterol, in which the adrenal cortex is rich.

There is some evidence that the mineralocorticoids are produced primarily in the zona glomerulosa, the glucocorticoids in the zona fasciculata and the sex hormones in the zona reticularis.

The normal activity of the adrenal cortex is at least partially under the control of a hormone of the anterior hypophysis, the adrenocorticotrophic hormone. Injection of ACTH causes a drop in the cholesterol and ascorbic acid content of the adrenal. This response is commonly used (with hypophysectomized rats) in determining the potency of ACTH extracts. The zona glomerulosa is less under pituitary control than are the other cortical zones. After hypophysectomy the zona glomerulosa shows less atrophy than the remainder of the cortex, and electrolyte metabolism is less affected after hypophysectomy than after adrenalectomy. This is interpreted as evidence for the continued secretion of some mineralocorticoids by the zona glomerulosa after hypophysectomy.

Clinical use of one of the adrenal steroids (cortisone) and also of ACTH is quite extensive in some of the "collagen" diseases, e.g., rheumatoid arthritis and rheumatic fever.

The hormone of the adrenal medulla was the first hormone obtained in crystalline form (1901). It was first thought to be a single compound but it has since been shown that what appeared to be a pure compound is actually two closely related compounds, epinephrine and norepinephrine. The two compounds have different physiological effects. For example, epinephrine increases the heart rate without any significant increase in blood pressure, whereas norepinephrine has little effect on heart rate but markedly increases blood pressure by producing vasoconstriction. Norepinephrine is readily converted to epinephrine and it may serve as a precursor for epinephrine in the synthetic process in the cells of the adrenal medulla.

The adrenal medulla or chromaffin tissue is not essential to life, but lack of its secretions reduces the ability of the body to respond to stress. Its norepinephrine is chemically identical to that secreted by autonomic ganglion cells but adrenal norepinephrine has a prolonged effect in contrast to that of autonomic ganglion cells. Furthermore, the medulla secretes into blood vessels and thus acts on tissues that are widely dispersed in the body. Differences between the epinephrine and norepinephrine adrenal medulla cell types are summarized in Table 21-2.

When an animal is exposed to danger from an adversary, it responds either by fighting or by running away. Man often suppresses this reaction but responds, as other animals, to danger or frustration for a period of time. In this "fight or flight
situation," the [illegible] ase
in the rat [illegible] by
the adrena [illegible] increased rate [illegible] eu-
rons. As a [illegible] in
heart rate and [illegible] also
a marked incre [illegible] etal
and cardiac mu [illegible] ase
in blood flow t [illegible] nal
effects include the [illegible] gen
to glucose in the liver [illegible] ate
of release of the latter i [illegible] ion.

Postnatal Involution of [illegible] *nal Glands*

The adrenal glands at birth in the human are relatively large bodies about one-third the size of the kidneys, whereas in the adult they are about 1/28 the size of the latter organs. Immediately following birth, the adrenals undergo a pronounced involution. In the first 14 days of postnatal life, this decrease amounts to one-third their birth weight, and in the first 4 months it amounts to one-half. The loss in weight is due to the degeneration of the inner part of the cortex. At birth the cortex consists of a narrow, outer zone, which will proliferate and form the cortex of the adult, and a massive inner zone which is destined to degenerate, the so-called "fetal cortex."

The adrenal glands attain their large prenatal size by a steady growth throughout intrauterine life. Their growth in this period is proportionate to general body growth.

The Paraganglia

Under the heading of *paraganglia* are included groups of cells that are closely associated both anatomically and embryologically with the sympathetic nervous system. They are largely retroperitoneal, occurring in association with sympathetic ganglia. In shape, staining reaction, and neural crest origin, the cells are similar to those composing the adrenal medulla. They are clear when unstained, become yellow with chromic acid and its salts and turn dark with osmic acid. The cells are oval or polyhedral and have a cordlike arrangement. They lie in close contact with capillaries. Because they are embryologically and structurally similar to the chromaffin cells composing the medulla of the adrenal and have the same staining reaction, it is assumed that they secrete epinephrine.

The *aortic chromaffin bodies* (lumbar paraganglia, organs of Zuckerkandl) are relatively large, irregularly paired masses formed by a fusion of paraganglia. They are located retroperitoneally and lie ventrolaterally to the aorta at about the level of the origin of the inferior mesenteric artery.

The Pineal Body

The pineal body or pineal gland (epiphysis cerebri) in man is a slightly flattened, cone-shaped appendage of the brain measuring 8 to 12 mm in length and 5 to 8 mm in width. Its base is constricted to form a hollow penduncle by which it is attached to the roof of the third ventricle with a narrow prolongation of the third ventricle extending up into it. Pia mater covers the pineal body except at its attachment and forms a capsule from which connective tissue trabeculae invaginate the epithelially derived parenchyma of the organ, partially dividing it into poorly defined lobules. The capsule and trabeculae carry numerous blood vessels and nerves (Fig. 21-22).

In all vertebrates that have pineal systems, a saccular organ is present during

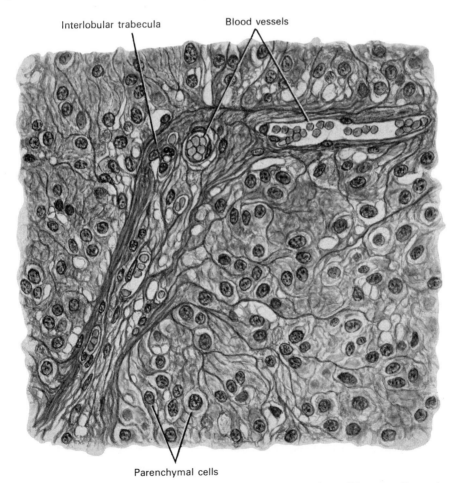

Fig. 21-22. Section through the pineal gland of a woman 37 years of age. Hematoxylin-eosin. ×535.

embryonic stages as the primordium evaginates from the roof of the diencephalon. However, in all mammals, in some reptiles (snakes and turtles) and in some birds, there is a rapid proliferation of secondary, tertiary and subsequent evaginations which converts the sac into cords and follicles of *pinealocytes* (principal pineal cells) interwoven with *glial cells* within the parenchyma of the organ.

The *pinealocytes* have relatively large nuclei with prominent nucleoli, and their nuclei often have an irregular contour because of infoldings of the nuclear envelope. The cytoplasm usually stains lightly in hematoxylin and eosin preparations. The cells have an irregular shape which can be demonstrated after the del Rio-Hortega silver method (Fig. 21-23) or when traced in serial electron micrographs. They have cytoplasmic processes with club-shaped terminations near other principal cells and in the vicinity of perivascular spaces.

Electron micrographs show that the endoplasmic reticulum of the pinealocytes is

mostly smooth surfaced and that ribosomes and polysomes are randomly dispersed. The Golgi complex consists of flattened sacs and rounded vesicles of the usual pattern. The mitochondria are fairly large and have the usual shelflike cristae. The cytoplasm is characterized particularly by numerous microtubules of indefinite length. The cytoplasm also has lipochrome pigment and lysosomes, and most importantly, abundant, dense-cored, membrane-bounded granules, particularly in the pinealocyte processes.

The *glial cells* provide a network surrounding and pervading the cords and follicles (Figs. 21-24 and 21-25). They are less numerous than the pinealocytes, and their nuclei are smaller and darker staining. Their cytoplasm is also more basophilic. The cells are usually elongated, and they have long cytoplasmic processes seen best after special silver techniques. They are often described as a type of astrocyte. Electron micrographs show that microtubules are scarce and that those which may be present lack the beaded appearance seen on microtubules of pinealocytes. The glial cells are characterized by numerous fine

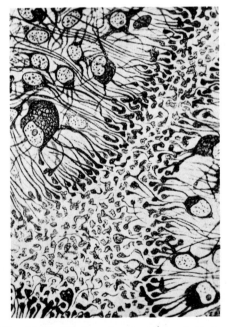

Fig. 21-23. Section of a pineal gland of a boy. The parenchymal cells and their processes were impregnated with silver. The processes are shown extending into an interlobular septum. Collagenous tissue and glia are not shown with this technique. Semidiagrammatic. (After del Rio-Hortega.)

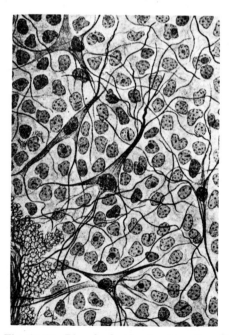

Fig. 21-24. Pineal gland, showing the glial cells and their processes. The nuclei of the parenchymal cells are also shown. Silver preparation. (After del Rio-Hortega.)

Glia   Parenchyma

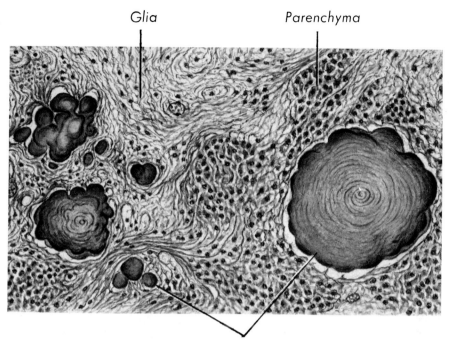

Calcareous granules (acervuli)

Fig. 21-25. Section through a region of the pineal gland of a woman 37 years old, showing calcareous granules (acervuli, brain sand). Hematoxylin-eosin. ×240.

filaments, 50 to 60 Å in diameter, that are not nearly so abundant in pinealocytes, and their mitochondria have unusually electron-dense matrices. The cristae also have a different arrangement, with some oriented longitudinally and some transversely. The endoplasmic reticulum is rough surfaced and is unevenly distributed in compact masses. The cytoplasm also has numerous single membrane-bounded bodies of varying diameter, which are probably responsible for the fine granulation seen under the light microscope; these are probably lysosomes.

Sand granules (corpora arenacea, acervuli) are generally present in the human pineal body and, according to some authors, they tend to increase with age. They are mulberry-shaped concretions which show concentric zones in sections (Fig. 21-25). They are found in the capsule and also within the organ, usually surrounded by or adjacent to areas rich in glia. They are not present in many species, and their significance is not understood.

The pineal body reaches its maximal development in man by the middle of the first decade or shortly thereafter. It shows regressive changes later in life, but these are quite variable in time of appearance.

The mammalian pineal body is supplied by *postganglionic sympathetic nerve fibers* which have their cells of origin in the superior cervical ganglion. This is one of the rare instances in which a portion of the central nervous system receives a sympathetic supply. The pineal also has a *rich vascular supply.* Studies on the rat show that substances such as intravital colloidal dyes diffuse into the pineal body. This is not true of brain tissue in general, in which there is a hematoencephalic or blood-brain barrier. However, the lack of a pineal blood-brain barrier should not be assumed for other mammals until further study.

The pineal system of some of the *lower vertebrates* (e.g., many lizards) consists of two bodies: a *parietal* (or *parapineal*) *organ,* which is placed in or above an opening in the roof of the skull as a "third eye," and a deeper lying intracranial *epiphysis.* Cytological studies show that many of the cells lining the lumina of these structures have characteristics similar to the cones of the retinae. The pineal organs of mammals, birds and some reptiles lack such photoreceptor elements and differ markedly from the pineals of the lower vertebrates. However, there is reason to believe that the mammalian pinealocyte is homologous to the pineal photoreceptor of lower vertebrates because both display synaptic ribbons in their cytoplasm and because pineal photoreceptors in some lower vertebrates also contain dense-cored membrane-bounded vesicles suggestive of secretory activity.

Although there have been a number of divergent opinions regarding the *functions of the pineal body* in mammals, it is generally agreed that it is an endocrine or neuroendocrine organ and not a useless vestige. There is considerable evidence that it has an inhibitory action on the development and maturation of the gonads. This was suggested first by clinical observations that boys having tumors of pineal-supporting elements (which presumably crowd out the pinealocytes) show precocious development of the gonads. This view has been supported by experimental studies which show that pinealectomy of young rats results in early maturation of the gonads in both sexes.

Biochemical and histochemical studies have shown that the pineal organ of the rat has a high phosphate turnover, high amino acid formation and a high level of serotonin. The pineal also contains melatonin (5-hydroxyindole) and an enzyme, hydroxyindole *O*-methyltransferse (HIOMT) that has a role in the synthesis of melatonin from serotonin. It is known that melatonin produces blanching of melanophores in amphibians, having an effect opposite to that of the melanocyte-stimulating hormone of the pituitary gland. Although the functional significance of melatonin in man remains obscure, it is known that it partially counteracts the effects of pinealectomy when injected into experimental animals, and that it is one of the pineal hormones but not the only one.

The rat pineal contains melatonin, serotonin and several of their synthesizing enzymes in amounts which vary according to diurnal rhythms. Such circadian rhythms are governed by periodic release of norepinephrine from the sympathetic fibers which innervate the organ. Hence, serotonin levels fall in the darkness as melatonin levels rise. This circadian rhythm in pineal amine levels appears to be generated by a biological clock in the hypothalamus which is controlled in an inhibitory sense by environmental light perceived by the retina. These responses to light are abolished by extirpation of the superior cervical ganglion, the source of the postganglionic nerve fibers to the pineal. On the basis of the various findings, it has been proposed that the pineal is part of a neuroendocrine mechanism regulating the gonads, and perhaps other organs, in response to light.

Eventually, the pineal organ may be found to have other important products and functions in addition to those suggested by the evidence concerning melatonin and serotonin. Some workers now suggest that non-melatonin peptides are produced and secreted which enter into other pituitary functions; for example, two peptides are suspected of competing for LH and ACTH releasing factor binding sites and hence of controlling the level of these hormones.

Whereas in many lower vertebrates the pineal itself seems to be a photoreceptor, in higher forms the photic input to the organ seems to have been assumed by the lateral eyes. The sensory input is relayed to the pineal via fibers that course in the optic nerves and the median forebrain bundle to make apparent connection with the sympathetic fibers supplying the gland. Pineal function is a subject of active investigation, and additional information is anticipated with further utilization of newer techniques.

References

Hypophysis

BAKER, B. L. Studies on hormone localization with emphasis on the hypophysis. J. Histochem. Cytochem. 18:1–8, 1970.

BAKER, B. L. Functional cytology of the hypophysial pars distalis and pars intermedia. *In* Handbook of Physiology, Section 7: Endocrinology (Knobil, E., and Sawyer, W. H., editors), vol. IV, part 1, pp. 45–80. American Physiological Society, Washington, D.C., 1974.

BARGMANN, W. Relationship between neurohypophysial structure and function. *In* Proc. 8th Symp. Colston Res. Soc. (Heller, H., editor), pp. 11–22. Academic Press, New York, 1957.

BARGMANN, W., HILD, W., ORTMANN, R., AND SCHIE-

BLER, T. H. Morphologische und experimentelle Untersuchungen über das hypothalamischhypophysäre System. Acta Neuroveg. (Wien) 1:233–275, 1950.

BARRNETT, R. J., LADMAN, A. J., McALLASTER, N. J., AND SIPERSTEIN, E. R. The localization of glycoprotein hormones in the anterior pituitary glands of rats investigated by differential protein solubilities, histological stains and bio-assays. Endocrinology 59:398–418, 1956.

COSTOFF, A., AND McSHAN, W. H. Isolation and biological properties of secretory granules from rat anterior pituitary glands. J. Cell Biol. 43:564–574, 1969.

DORFMAN, R. I., AND UNGAR, F. Metabolism of Steroid Hormones. Academic Press, New York, 1965.

DU VIGNEAUD, V. Hormones of the posterior pituitary gland: oxytocin and vasopressin. Harvey Lectures, Ser. 50, pp. 1–26, 1954.

ELFTMAN, H. Combined aldehyde-fuchsin and periodic acid-Schiff staining of the pituitary. Stain Technol. 34:77–80, 1959.

ELFTMAN, H., AND WEGELIUS, O. Anterior pituitary cytology of the dwarf mouse. Anat. Rec. 135:43–49, 1959.

FARQUHAR, M. G. Fine structure and function in capillaries of the anterior pituitary gland. Angiology 12:270–292, 1961.

FARQUHAR, M. G., AND RINEHART, J. F. Electron microscopic studies of the anterior pituitary gland of castrate rats. Endocrinology 54:516–541, 1954.

FARQUHAR, M. G., AND WELLINGS, S. R. Electron microscopic evidence suggesting secretory granule formation within the Golgi apparatus. J. Biophys. Biochem Cytol., 3:319–322, 1957.

FRIEDGOOD, H. B., AND DAWSON, A. B. Physiological significance and morphology of the carmine cell in the cat's anterior pituitary. Endocrinology 26:1022–1031, 1940.

GREEN, J. D. Electron microscopy of the anterior pituitary. In The Pituitary Gland (Harris, G. W., and Donovan, B. T., editors), vol. 1, pp. 233–241. University of California Press, Berkeley, 1966.

GREEP, R. O. Architecture of the final common pathway of the adenohypophysis. Fertil. Steril. 14:153–179, 1963.

HALMI, N. S. Two types of basophils in the rat pituitary: "thyrotrophs" and "gonadotrophs" vs. beta and delta cells. Endocrinology 50:140–142, 1952.

HARRIS, G. W., AND DONOVAN, B. T. (editors) The Pituitary Gland. University of California Press, Berkeley, 1966.

HEIDINGER, C. E., AND FARQUHAR, M. G. Elektronenmikrospische Untersuchungen von zwei Typen acidophiler Hypophysenvorderlappenzellen bei der Ratte. Schweiz. Z. Allg. Pathol. 20:766–768, 1957.

HELLER, H. C. (editor) The Neurohypophysis. Academic Press, New York, 1957.

HERLANT, M. Étude critique de deux techniques nouvelles destinées à mettre en évidence les différentes catégories cellulaires présentes dans la glande pituitaire. Bull. Micr. Appl. Ser. 2 10:37–44, 1960.

HYMER, W. C., AND McSHAN, W. H. Isolation of rat pituitary granules and the study of their biochemical properties and hormonal activities. J. Cell Biol. 17:67–86, 1963.

MORIARTY, G. C., AND GARNER, L. L. Immunochem-

ical studies of cells in the rat adenohypophysis containing both ACTH and FSH. Nature, 265:356–358, 1977.

NAKANE, P. K. Classification of anterior pituitary cell types with immunoenzyme histochemistry. J. Histochem. Cytochem. 18:9–20, 1970.

PAGE, R. B., MUNGER, B. L., AND BERGLAND, R. M. Scanning microscopy of pituitary vascular casts. Am. J. Anat. 146:273–302, 1976.

PALAY, S. L. Fine structure of the neurohypophysis. Prog. Neurobiol. 2:31–44, 1957.

PURVES, H. D. Morphology of the hypophysis related to its function. In Sex and Internal Secretion (Young, W. C., editor), vol. 1, pp. 161–239. Williams & Wilkins, Baltimore, 1961.

PURVES, H. D. Cytology of the adenohypophysis. In The Pituitary Gland (Harris, G. W., and Donovan, B. T., editors), vol. 1, pp. 147–232. University of California Press, Berkeley, 1966.

RINEHART, J. F., AND FARQUHAR, M. Electron microscope studies of the anterior pituitary gland. J. Histochem. Cytochem. 1:93–113, 1953.

ROMEIS, B. Hypophyse. In Handb. mikr. Anat. Menschen (v. Möllendorff, editor), vol. 6, pt. 3. Springer-Verlag, Berlin, 1940.

SCHARRER, E., AND SCHARRER, B. Neurosekretion. In Handb. mikr. Anat. Menschen (v. Möllendorff, editor), vol. 6, pt. 5, pp. 953–1066. Springer-Verlag, Berlin, 1954.

SEVERINGHAUS, A. E. The cytology of the pituitary gland. In The Pituitary Gland, pp. 69–117. Williams & Wilkins, Baltimore, 1938.

SIPERSTEIN, E. R. Identification of the adrenocorticotrophin-producing cells in the rat hypophysis by autoradiography. J. Cell Biol. 17:521–546, 1963.

SMITH, P. E. Hypophysectomy and a replacement therapy in the rat. Am. J. Anat. 45:205–273, 1930.

SMITH, P. E., AND MacDOWELL, E. C. The differential effect of hereditary mouse dwarfism on the anterior-pituitary hormones. Anat. Rec. 50:85–93, 1931.

STANFIELD, J. P. The blood supply of the human pituitary gland. J. Anat. 94:259–273, 1960.

TESAR, J. T., KOENIG, H., AND HUGHES, C. Hormone storage granules in the beef anterior pituitary. I. Isolation, ultrastructure and some biochemical properties. J. Cell Biol. 40:225–235, 1969.

WISLOCKI, G. B. The vascular supply of the hypophysis cerbri of the rhesus monkey and man. In The Pituitary Gland, pp. 48–68. Williams & Wilkins, Baltimore, 1938.

ZUEREB, G. P., PRICHARD, M. M. L., AND DANIEL, P. M. The hypophyseal portal system of vessels in man. Quart. J. Exp. Physiol. 39:219–229, 1954.

Thyroid Gland

ANDROS, G., AND WOLLMAN, S. H. Autoradiographic localization of iodine^{125} in the thyroid epithelial cell. Proc. Soc. Exp. Biol. Med. 115:775–777, 1964.

DEGROOT, L. J. Current views on formation of thyroid hormones. N. Engl. J. Med. 272:243–250, 297–303, 355–362, 1965.

DEMPSEY, E. W. The chemical cytology of the thyroid gland. Ann. N. Y. Acad. Sci. 50:336–357, 1949.

DEROBERTIS, E. Cytological and cytochemical basis of thyroid function. Ann. N.Y. Acad. Sci. 50:317–333, 1949.

GROSS, J., AND PITT-RIVERS, R. Triiodothyronine in relation to thyroid physiology. Recent Prog. Horm. Res. 9:109–128, 1954.

KLINCK, G. H., OERTEL, J. E., AND WINSHIP, I. Ultrastructure of normal human thyroid. Lab. Invest. 22:2–22, 1970.

NADLER, N. J., SARKAR, S. K., AND LEBLOND, C. P. Origin of intracellular colloid droplets in the rat thyroid. Endocrinology 71:120–129, 1962.

NADLER, N. J., YOUNG, B. A., LEBLOND, C. P., AND MITMAKER, B. Elaboration of thyroglobulin in the thyroid follicle. Endocrinology 74:333–354, 1964.

PEARSE, A. G. E., AND CARVALHEIRA, A. F. Cytochemical evidence for an ultimobranchial origin of rodent thyroid cell. Nature 214:929–930, 1967.

PITT-RIVERS, R., AND TROTTER, W. R. (editors) The Thyroid Gland. Butterworth, London, 1964.

ROBINSON, W. L., AND DAVIS, D. Determination of iodine concentration and distribution in rat thyroid follicles by electron-probe analysis. J. Cell Biol. 43:115–121, 1969.

TURNER, C. D. General Endocrinology, ed. 4. Saunders, Philadelphia, 1966.

WISSIG, S. L. Morphology and cytology. In The Thyroid Gland (Pitt-Rivers, R., and Trotter, W. R., editors), pp. 32–70. Butterworth, London, 1964.

Parathyroid Glands

BAKER, B. L. A study of the parathyroid glands of the normal and hypophysectomized monkey (*Macaca mulatta*). Anat. Rec. 83:47–73, 1942.

GAILLARD, P. J., TALMAGE, R. V., AND BUDY, A. M. (editors) The Parathyroid Glands. University of Chicago Press, Chicago, 1965.

GREEP, R. O. Parathyroid glands. In Comparative Endocrinology (von Euler, U. S., and Heller, H., editors), vol. 1, pp. 325–370. Academic Press, New York, 1963.

MUNGER, B. L., AND ROTH, S. I. The cytology of the normal parathyroid glands of man and Virginia deer. A light and electron microscopic study with morphologic evidence of secretory activity. J. Cell Biol. 16:379–400, 1963.

Adrenal Glands

BENNETT, H. S. Cytological manifestations of secretion in the adrenal medulla of the cat. Am. J. Anat. 69:333–383, 1941.

COUPLAND, R. E. The Natural History of the Chromaffin Cell. Longmans, Green and Company, London, 1965.

DEROBERTIS, E. D. P., AND VAZ FERREIRA, A. Electron microscopic study of the excretion of catechol-containing droplets in the adrenal medulla. Exp. Cell Res. 12:568 574, 1958.

GREEP, R. O., AND DEANE, H. W. Histological, cytochemical and physiological observations on the regeneration of the rat's adrenal gland following enucleation. Endocrinology 45:42–67, 1949.

INGLE, D. J., AND BAKER, B. L. Physiological and Therapeutic Effects of Corticotrophin (ACTH) and Cortisone. American Lecture Series, no. 179. Charles C Thomas, Publisher, Springfield, Ill., 1953.

JONES, C. I. The Adrenal Cortex. Cambridge University Press, London, 1957.

LEVER, J. D. Electron microscopic observations on the adrenal cortex. Am. J. Anat. 97:409–430, 1955.

LONG, J. A., AND JONES, A. L. Alterations in fine structure of the opossum adrenal cortex following sodium deprivation. Anat. Rec. 166:1–26, 1970.

MERKLIN, R. J. Suprarenal gland lymphatic drainage. Am. J. Anat. 119:359–374, 1966.

SABATINI, D. D., AND DEROBERTIS, E. D. P. Ultrastructural zonation of adrenal cortex in the rat. J. Biophys. Biochem. Cytol. 9:105–119, 1961.

WASSERMAN, G., AND TRAMEZZANI, J. H. Separate distribution of adrenaline- and noradrenaline-secretory cells in the adrenal of snakes. Gen. Comp. Endocrinol. 3:480–489, 1963.

WOOD, J. G. Identification of and observations on epinephrine and norepinephrine containing cells in the adrenal medulla. Am. J. Anat. 112:285–303, 1963.

WOOD, J. G., AND BARRNETT, R. J. Histochemical demonstration of norepinephrine at a fine structural level. J. Histochem. Cytochem. 12:197–209, 1964.

Pineal Body

ANDERSON, E. The anatomy of bovine and ovine pineals: light and electron microscope studies. J. Ultrastruct. Res. suppl. 8, 1–80, 1965.

AXELROD, J. The pineal gland; a neurochemical transducer. Science 184:1341–1348, 1974.

KELLY, D. E. Pineal organs: photoreception, secretion, and development. Am. Sci. 50:597–625, 1962.

KITAY, J. I., AND ALTSCHULE, M. D. The Pineal Gland. Harvard University Press, Cambridge, 1954.

REITER, R. J., AND FRASCHINI, F. Endocrine aspects of the mammalian pineal gland: a review. Neuroendocrinology 5:219–255, 1969.

WOLSTENHOLME, G. E. W., AND KNIGHT, J. (editors) The pineal gland. A Ciba Foundation Symposium. Churchill-Livingston, Edinburgh, 1971.

WURTMAN, R. J., AXELROD, J., AND KELLY, D. E. The Pineal. Academic Press, New York, 1968.

CHAPTER 22

The Organs of Special Senses

The Eye

The *eyeball* (*bulbus oculi*) is essentially a spherical structure, lightproof except for its transparent anterior surface (the *cornea*), which contains a system of refracting media with convex surfaces. These transmit light rays reflected from outside objects and bring them to a focus on a photosensitive surface (the *neural retina*) in the form of a small inverted image. The photosensitive cells (*rods and cones*) on which the images fall thereby initiate nervous activity which, when amplified, coordinated and integrated by other excitable cells of the retina, is relayed over fibers of the optic nerve to the brain. There the sensation of vision is experienced. Focus is accomplished by changing the curvature of one of the refracting bodies (the *lens*) through alteration of the tension exerted on it by the mechanism from which it is suspended (the *ciliary body*). In front of the lens and perpendicular to the optic axis (direction of light transmission) is an adjustable diaphragm (the *iris*), the adjustable aperture of which (the *pupil*) regulates the amount of light admitted.

The eye is suspended by a series of ligaments in the bony orbit. The orbit also contains the *extrinsic ocular muscles* (which control movements of the eyeball), the *lacrimal gland* (which moistens the anterior surface), the nerves and blood vessels supplying the eye and orbital structures and a considerable amount of connective tissue and fat. Also associated with the eye are the lids and a duct system which drains the tears from the eye into the nasal cavity.

In form, the eyeball (Fig. 22-1) departs slightly from that of a ball; it is more accurately described as consisting of the segments of two spheres, unequal in size. The larger sphere forms the posterior five-sixths of the eyeball. The anterior one-sixth, which is the cornea, constitutes a segment of the smaller sphere and hence is more curved than the posterior part. The two segments are structurally continuous.

A brief insight into the embryonic origins of the component parts of the eye is essential to understanding their interrelationships in the fully developed organ. Basically, there are three sites of origin for these parts: (1) the lateral neuroectodermal walls of the embryonic brain in the region of the diencephalon; (2) the surface ectoderm of the head; and (3) the mesenchyme interposed around and between the above two epithelial components. Shortly after neural tube closure (chapter 3), lateral outpocketings on left and right sides of the diencephalon result in the formation of two neuroepithelial *optic vesicles,* each remaining attached to the brain wall via a hollow *optic stalk.* Each optic vesicle comes to underlie closely the surface ectoderm of the head and at the point of approximation induces that ectoderm to undergo an inward invagination to form a *lens vesicle.* As the lens vesicle pinches off from the surface ectoderm, its basal surface and that of the

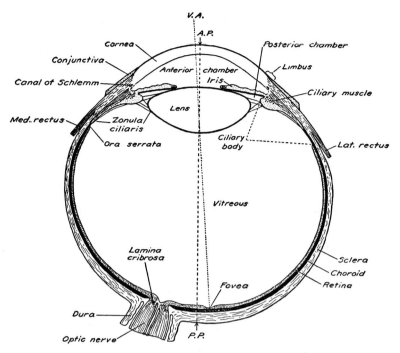

Fig. 22-1. Schematic horizontal meridional section of right eye. *A.P.*, anterior pole; *P.P.*, posterior pole; *V.A.*, visual axis. ×3. (Redrawn and modified from Salzmann.)

nearby optic vesicle are totally surrounded by mesenchyme. A concomitant change now occurs in the configuration of the optic vesicle; an invagination of its distal (anterior) half, much like a depression on the side of a tennis ball, results in a conversion of the single walled optic vesicle into a double walled hemispheric *optic cup.* The invagination is particularly pronounced along the ventral surface of the lens vesicle and along the optic stalk where it produces a transient groove termed the *optic fissure* (or *choroid fissure*). Within the newly formed optic cup, the apical surfaces of the two layers are brought into contact or close proximity. The outermost layer of the optic cup will remain a simple, but highly pigmented layer, the *pigment epithelium,* whereas the inner layer undergoes proliferation and stratification not unlike that encountered in other parts of the neural tube wall. It becomes the highly complex photoreceptive *neural retina.* The mesenchyme which occupies the invagination of the optic cup will eventually occupy the *vitreous chamber* of the eye. The lens vesicle becomes partially enveloped by the free margins of the optic cup and the mesen-

chyme surrounding all of these components begins its differentiation to form nourishing, protecting and supportive tunics.

Hence, in its basic structure, the wall of the eyeball consists of two epithelial layers (derived from the neuroectodermal cup) and two mesodermally derived connective tissue tunics which taken together enclose the lens and the transparent media through which light is transmitted to a sensitive retina. The overlying surface epithelium of the head differentiates into *conjunctival* epithelium and, in conjunction with underlying mesenchyme, into the transparent *cornea.* The posterior wall of the lens vesicle thickens with the development of its highly specialized cells and the whole vesicle becomes the solid, biconvex and highly transparent *lens.*

The outermost connective tissue tunic is the *tunica fibrosa,* comprising the stroma of the *cornea* and *sclera.* The cornea forms the anterior portion of this tunic and is transparent. A fact not commonly appreciated is that most of the refraction of light takes place at the air-cornea interface rather than in the lens, the refractive power of the cornea being about 2½ times that of the lens. The remainder of the outer tunic is the sclera, a grayish-white tough protective coat, a part of which is seen through the overlying transparent conjunctiva as the "white" of the eye. The tendons of the extrinsic ocular muscles insert into the sclera.

The inner connective tissue tunic of the eye is the *tunica vasculosa,* or *uvea,* which includes the *choroid, ciliary body* and the stroma of the *iris.* All three regions of this tunic are laid down upon the outer epithelium of the optic cup. Each is characterized by extreme vascularity and considerable amounts of pigment. In addition, the ciliary body and iridial stroma contain smooth muscle. The latter muscle fibers, interestingly, have originated by differentiation of optic cup ectodermal epithelial cells. That in the ciliary body serves as the muscle of accommodation; by its contraction, the tension on the *suspensory ligament* supporting the lens is relaxed and the lens assumes a greater curvature to bring the image of near objects into correct focus on the retina. The smooth muscle in the iris acts to regulate the diameter of the pupil (Fig. 22-2).

The epithelial optic cup derivatives enclosed by those tunics include the photosensitive *neural retina* and the *pigment epithelium* layer. The forward extension of both of these epithelial layers forms the double internal lining layers of the ciliary body and iris.

As the epithelium of the neural retina differentiates, axons from ganglion cells lo-

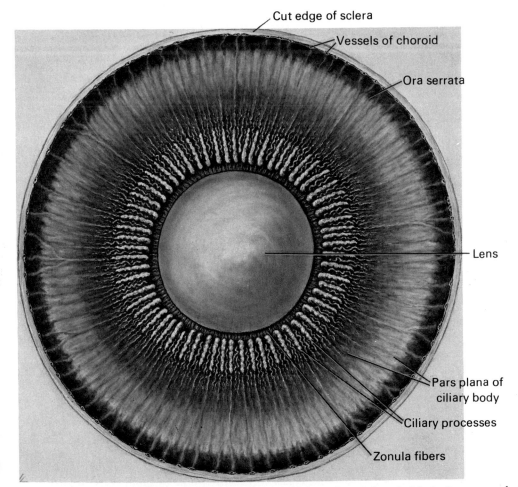

Fig. 22-2. Ora serrata, ciliary body, zonula ciliaris and lens viewed from behind after removal of the vitreous body. ×4.6. (Courtesy of Dr. S. R. Detwiler, labels added.)

cated along its basal (vitreal) surface are directed toward the optic stalk. These are the pathways for impulses generated from all parts of the retina. Eventually these axons converge at the optic stalk where, still following the basal epithelial surface, they course along the walls of the optic fissure toward the brain. As their numbers increase, the optic stalk epithelium becomes filled with nerve fibers and is then recognizable as the *optic nerve*. Closure of the optic fissure along the optic nerve and ventral surface of the optic cup normally completes enclosure of the central artery and vein which nourish the retina from its vitreal surface. In the adult eye, the retinal axons converge into the optic nerve about 3 mm medial to the posterior pole of the eye. Since this disc of convergence consists solely of nerve fibers, this area constitutes a *blind spot*. Almost at the posterior pole is a small area of the retina known as the *macula lutea*, in the center of which is a depression—the *fovea centralis*. This is the region of most acute vision.

Certain commonly used descriptive terms facilitate discussion of the histology of the eyeball. Thus, the anterior pole of the eye is coincident with the midpoint of the cornea. A point diametrically opposite is the posterior pole. A line connecting the anterior and posterior poles is the *geometric axis* of the eye. This must be distinguished from the *visual axis,* which is a line joining the fovea centralis and the nodal point of the optic system. This latter point, which is the optical center, lies in the posterior part of the lens.

A section of the eyeball passing through the anterior and posterior poles is designated a meridional section. Most instructive of the various meridional sections is that which passes through the horizontal meridian. At an angle of 90° to this plane is the vertical meridian, dividing the eyeball into a medial, or nasal, half and a lateral, or temporal, half. The equator of the eye is a circle taken equidistant from the two poles; sections parallel to this plane are called equatorial sections.

The term "outer" (or external) refers to that which is nearer the surface of the eyeball; "inner" (or internal) refers to that which is nearer the midpoint of the bulb.

Anterior and posterior refer to points which are nearer the anterior or posterior poles, whether such points be in a sagittal plane or along a meridian.

Tunica Fibrosa

The Sclera. The sclera (Figs. 22-1 and 22-10), which forms the opaque posterior five-sixths of the protective outer tunic, is composed of dense fibrous connective tissue, thickest at the posterior pole (about 1 mm) and gradually thinner until it is only 0.3 mm thick at the insertion of the recti muscles. It is pierced by three sets of apertures, or *emissaria,* through which pass nerves, blood vessels and lymphatics. At the optic nerve, the sclera is sieve-like because its fibrous components have developed in such a way as to infiltrate among the optic nerve axons which leave the retina there. This region of infiltration is termed the *lamina cribrosa*. Although the sclera and corneal stroma are structurally continuous, their line of junction is marked externally by a slight circular furrow, the *external scleral sulcus*. On the inner surface of the sclera, close to its junctions with the cornea, there is also a shallow furrow, the *internal scleral sulcus*. The posterior margin of this furrow projects slightly inward and forward to form the *scleral spur* (scleral roll), to which the ciliary body is attached (Figs. 22-1 and 22-5). The furrow itself is filled in by the *meshwork of the iris angle*. At the base of the furrow lies the *canal of Schlemm*.

For descriptive purposes, three layers of tissue may be designated in the sclera but they are in no sense sharply delimited from each other. The outermost is the *episcleral tissue,* composed of loose collagenous and elastic fibers. Superficially, it is continuous with the loose tissue of *Tenon's space*; inwardly, it merges with the sclera proper; anteriorly, it attaches the conjunctiva to the sclera. It is distinguished by its relatively large number of blood vessels.

The *sclera proper* is a dense feltwork of collagenous fiber bundles running parallel to the surface. Near the cornea and around the optic nerve the bundles of fibers are disposed chiefly in an equatorial direction; elsewhere, they cross and interlace. Numerous delicate elastic fibers are interspersed with the collagenous fibers, particularly at the periphery of the bundles. The cellular component consists chiefly of flattened fibroblasts located between the fiber bundles.

The tendons of the extrinsic ocular muscles resemble the sclera in structure except that the fiber bundles are all parallel and there are many thick elastic fibers. At their insertions, the tendons continue directly into the sclera, the tendon bundles spreading out and interweaving among those of the sclera.

The *lamina fusca,* the third zone, represents a transition between the sclera and the choroid. Here elastic fibers increase in number and thickness, the collagenous bundles become smaller and a number of branched pigment cells appear. These are also characteristics common to the adjacent outer layer of the choroid.

The Cornea. Viewed from in front, the cornea appears slightly elliptical, with a horizontal diameter of about 12 mm and a vertical diameter of about 11 mm. Viewed from behind, it is circular, the difference in the two aspects being due to the fact that the sclera overlaps the anterior surface of the cornea above and below more than it does laterally and medially. The zone of transition between the cornea and sclera, known as the *limbus,* is about 1 mm in width and has histological features differing from the remainder of the cornea.

The *corneal epithelium* (Fig. 22-3) is stratified squamous, five or six cell layers in thickness (50 to 100 μm). The deepest cells are columnar with the base of each cell resting on a basal lamina that is tenuously attached to the thick underlying Bowman's (basement) membrane. The cells of the remaining layers range from polyhedral to very flat. Although the surface cells are somewhat thickened in the regions of their nuclei, the cell thickenings are directed toward the deeper cell layers. This accounts for the smooth surface that is a characteristic feature of the cornea.

None of the corneal cells lose their nuclei or normally undergo keratinization. They are attached to each other by desmosomes.

Bowman's membrane appears homogeneous and structureless under the light mi-

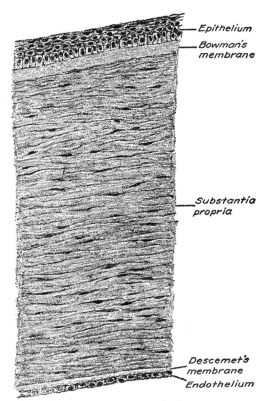

Fig. 22-3. Section through human cornea. (From a section by Dr. R. Castroviejo.)

croscope. However, electron micrographs show that it contains a network of relatively fine collagenous fibers having an irregular arrangement. The basal lamina at the anterior border of this basement membrane is sharply defined from the corneal epithelium whereas the fibers of the posterior border blend with the superficial lamellae of the corneal stroma.

The *substantia propria (corneal stroma)* forms about 90% of the thickness of the cornea and is composed of connective tissue fibers and cells. The characteristic transparency of the cornea is related, in part, to the pattern of its ultrastructural components. The predominant structural elements are collagenous fibrils arranged in layers, or lamellae, which course parallel with the surface of the cornea. Electron micrographs show that the fibrils within any one lamella are strictly parallel to one another but those of adjacent lamellae differ in direction (Fig. 22-4). Some fibrils also course from one lamella to another, thus

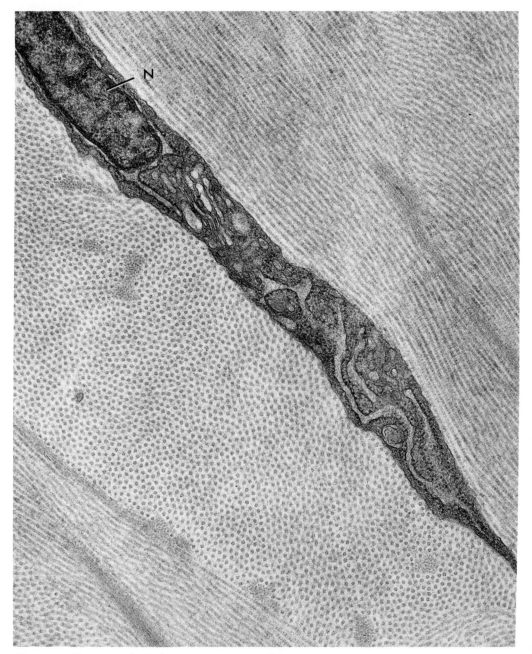

Fig. 22-4. Electron micrograph of a section through a portion of the substantia propria of the cornea. A portion of a stromal cell, with its nucleus (N), is seen between lamellae of collagenous fibrils. Note the precise alignment of collagenous fibrils at right angles to each other in adjacent lamellae. The endoplasmic reticulum of the stromal cell is not as prominent in the cornea of an adult as it is in the case illustrated, a chicken 5 days after hatching. ×34,000. (Courtesy of Drs. Elizabeth D. Hay and Jean-Paul Revel, Monographs in Developmental Biology, vol. 1, 1969.)

anchoring the lamellae together. The fibrils within each lamella, as well as the different lamellae themselves, are also held together by a mucopolysaccharide matrix rich in chondroitin sulfate A, keratosulfate and hyaluronic acid. These macromolecules apparently contribute to corneal transparency by maintaining the reversible swelling properties of the tissue. Continual loss of water from the corneal surface, which prevents turgescence of the tissue, is an additional and important factor in maintaining corneal transparency.

Most of the connective tissue cells of the corneal stroma are modified fibroblasts. They are located between and parallel to the lamellar collagenous fibers and are flat. In sections cut tangential to the corneal surface it can be seen that the fibroblasts have branching processes that often come into close apposition with neighboring cell processes.

During formative stages of the corneal stroma, the earliest collagen is actually secreted by the corneal epithelial cells. Thereafter mesenchymal cells invade the region between lens and corneal epithelium and contribute further to the building of collagenous lamellae. This sequence is significant also in that a cavitation occurs in the mesenchyme between the corneal stromal layers and the margins of the optic cup and the lens, leading to the formation of the fluid-filled *anterior ocular chamber*. This chamber is lined over its anterior (corneal) margin by simple low cuboidal epithelium which by tradition has been termed the *corneal endothelium* (more accurately a mesenchymal epithelium or mesothelium rather than a true endothelium since it is quite different morphologically from the endothelium of blood and lymphatic vessels). The endothelium is continuous at the margins of the anterior chamber with a less tightly knit epithelium that forms a network over the anterior surface of the mesenchymally derived iris stroma (Fig. 22-5).

The basement membrane of the endothelium is prominent and separates the latter from the corneal stroma. Traditionally it has been termed *Descemet's membrane*. It appears homogeneous and highly refractile under the light microscope. It has resiliency and elasticity, and while it stains, to some extent, with elastic tissue dyes (e.g., resorchin-fuchsin) it is doubtful that elastic fibers are present. It consists of a basal lamina and reticular fibers of a collagenous type lacking typical 640 Å interval cross bands.

The cornea proper is entirely devoid of blood vessels, deriving its nutrition from the anterior chamber and the superficial marginal plexus of vessels, which is discussed below under "The Limbus."

The cornea has a rich sensory nerve supply derived from the ophthalmic division of the trigeminal nerve. Small branches of this nerve enter at the periphery and branch extensively in the substantia propria as they course toward the surface and the center of the cornea. Near Bowman's membrane, this *plexus proprius* ends in a terminal net from which fibers, both individually and in bundles, pass as the corneal *rami perforantes* through pores in Bowman's membrane. There they break up into finer branches which extend forward and terminate between the epithelial cells. Other nerve endings are found in the stroma and just under the epithelium at the limbus.

The Limbus. Transitional between the cornea and the adjacent sclera and conjunctiva is a zone about 1 mm wide known as the *limbus* (Figs. 22-1 and 22-5). The corneal epithelium, as it passes over into the limbus, increases in thickness up to 10 or more cells. The surface cells retain the characteristics of those of the cornea, but the basal cells become smaller and the basal border becomes irregular in contour. These are characteristics of the conjunctival epithelium with which the epithelium of the limbus is continuous. Here also the corneal stroma loses its regular lamellar arrangement, the fiber bundles becoming irregular like those of the sclera. Some elastic fibers are also found.

The only blood vessels which nourish the cornea are found in the limbus, where they form the superficial marginal plexus in the superficial stroma and a series of meridonally directed loops which extend to the border of Bowman's membrane. These vessels are derived from the anterior ciliary artery, a derivative of the ophthalmic division of the internal carotid.

Descemet's membrane and the corneal endothelium become thinner as they approach the scleral meshwork of the iris angle. The surface over the scleral meshwork has an irregular contour and numerous spaces extending inward toward the canal of Schlemm (see "The Iris Angle").

Tunica Vasculosa (Uvea)

The tunica vasculosa comprises the *cho-*

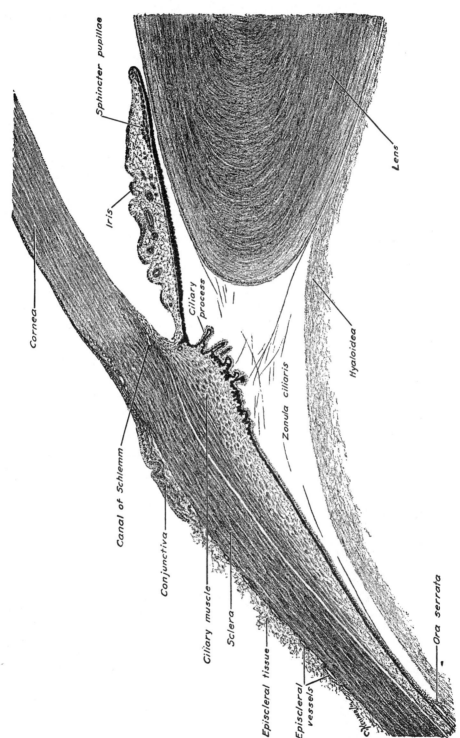

Fig. 22-5. Horizontal meridional section through anterior portion of human eye.

roid, ciliary body and iridial stroma and is characterized by the presence of numerous blood vessels and pigment cells. After removal of the overlying sclera and cornea, it greatly resembles a grape (uva); hence the synonym uvea.

The Choroid. The term choroid (chorioid) is derived from the resemblance of this layer, in vascularity, to the chorion serving the fetus. It forms the posterior part of the uvea. Superficially, it is separated from the sclera by a potential space, the perichoroidal space, across which delicate lamellae of the choroid pass obliquely to blend with the lamina fusca of the sclera. It is limited anteriorly by the insertion of the ciliary muscle into the scleral spur (Fig. 22-9), and posteriorly, it ends a short distance in front of the optic nerve. In life, this space is probably nonexistent; in the fixed specimen, it may enlarge as the result of shrinkage of tissues (Fig. 22-5).

Internally, the choroid is intimately related to the pigment epithelium layer of the retina. When the retina is detached, the pigment epithelium remains adherent to the choroid.

Histologically, the choroid may be divided into four layers. The suprachoroid (lamina suprachoroidea; epichoroid), the superficial layer of the choroid, consists of loosely arranged collagenous and elastic fibers which course obliquely backward from choroid to sclera, bridging the perichoroidal space. Within the meshwork of fibers, there are occasional fibroblasts, some histiocytes and numerous chromatophores that contain black-brown melanin granules.

The vessel layer (stratum vasculosa) is, in the thicker portions of the choroid, sometimes regarded as being subdivided into an outer layer of large vessels (Haller's layer) and an inner layer of medium-sized vessels (Sattler's layer). In the region of the fovea, only smaller vessels are present; anterior to the equator, the small vessels merge with the capillary layer, leaving as a distinct layer only the large vessels.

The veins of the vessel layer converge to form four whorl-like patterns—the vortices. In each vortex, the veins unite in an ampulla from which a single vortex vein arises. The vortex veins (venae vorticossae) leave the eye through emissaria in the sclera, two

superiorly and two inferiorly. Choroidal stroma occupies the spaces between the vessels. Its structure resembles that of the suprachoroid, but the stellate chromatophores have longer and more slender processes.

The capillary layer (lamina choriocapillaris), the only layer not continued forward into the ciliary body, contains vessels which supply nutrition for the outer layers of the retina. Its capillaries form a network in which the components are mostly in the same plane and are unique in having lumina of sufficient width to accommodate several red blood corpuscles side by side. Structurally they are irregular, but simple endothelial tubes (Fig. 22-10).

The interspaces of the capillary net are filled in by a stroma of delicate collagenous and elastic fibrils which becomes continuous with that of the vessel layer. Toward the vessel layer, pigment cells are lacking. On the inner aspect of the capillary layer, a condensation of elastic fibrils forms the outer lamella of the lamina vitrea.

The lamina vitrea (Bruch's membrane, glassy membrane) has traditionally been considered as the innermost layer of the choroid. In fact, it is mostly a prominent basement membrane of the retinal epithelium, and hence primarily of optic cup derivation (Fig. 22-10). It is about 2 to 2.5 μm thick with a thin outer lamella composed of slender collagenous fibers and a plexus of elastic fibers, likely of mesenchymal origin. Electron micrographs show that the basement membrane portion is similar to that of other regions in that it consists of a basal lamina and a reticular lamina.

The ciliary nerves course in the perichoroidal space and give off fine branches which form plexuses in the suprachoroid and the choroidal stroma. Multipolar ganglion cells associated with the plexuses are probably concerned with the sympathetic innervation of blood vessels.

In certain teleost fishes a silvery layer (argentea) is found between the suprachoroid and the vessel layer. It is formed by specialized cells containing crystals of guanine and extends into the iris, giving that membrane a characteristic silvery luster.

In most mammals, but not in man, a reflecting layer, the tapetum lucidum, is developed in the posterior region of the choroid. Lying between the choriocapillaris and the vessel layer, it consists either of several layers of flattened cells, the *cellular tapetum* (carnivores) or several layers of fine fibers, the *fibrous tapetum* (herbivores).

The Ciliary Body. The choroid extends anteriorly as far as the *ora serrata,* which is the anterior margin of the sensory portion of the retina (Figs. 22-1 and 22-2). In front of the ora serrata, the uvea is thickened to form the *ciliary body,* a ring to which the *suspensory ligament* of the lens is attached and from which the iris extends. In meridional section, the ciliary body is triangular in shape (Fig. 22-5). Its outer surface is separated from the sclera by the perichoroidal space. Its inner surface faces the vitreous body and lens, and when viewed macroscopically from behind, it displays two zones (Fig. 22-2). The posterior two-thirds appears darkly pigmented and is relatively smooth. This is the *orbiculus ciliaris* or *pars plana.* The anterior one-third bears some 70 to 80 radially arranged pale ridges, the *ciliary processes;* this region is the *corona ciliaris* (*pars plicata*).

The anterior surface of the ciliary body, from which the iris arises, faces the anterior chamber; its outer edge is attached to the scleral spur. The greater part of the anterior surface is obscured by the overlying *meshwork of the iris angle.*

The ciliary body represents a forward continuation of all the elements of the choroid except the capillary layer, plus epithelial layers continued from the retina as the *pars ciliaris retinae.*

The outermost layers constitute the *suprachoroid* and *ciliary muscle.* Reference has been made to the presence of smooth muscle fibers in the suprachoroid. In the ciliary body, this smooth muscle forms a mass of very appreciable bulk (Fig. 22-5). According to the directions in which they are disposed, three sets of fibers are distinguished in the ciliary muscle.

(a) The *meridional fibers* (longitudinal fibers, *Brücke's muscle*) are the outermost ones. They begin in the relatively sparse star-shaped groups in the suprachoroid in front of the equator and, increasing in number, form bundles which run anteriorly to insert into the scleral spur (Fig. 22-9).

(b) The *radial fibers* lie internal to the meridional fibers. They are intermingled with connective tissue elements which become continuous anteriorly with the meshwork of the iris angle.

(c) The *circular fibers* (*Müller's muscle*) are continuous with the radial fibers and lie at the inner edge of the ciliary body. These fibers course in a circular direction around the ciliary body just posterior to the root of the iris. Immediately anterior to them is the *circulus arteriosus iridis major,* source of the arterial supply to the iris, and ciliary processes.

The blood vessels of the ciliary muscle run in the interstitial tissue and are of small caliber. The arteries are branches of the long posterior ciliary and anterior ciliary arteries.

The ciliary muscle is innervated by parasympathetic fibers of the oculomotor nerve. Preganglionic fibers reach the ciliary ganglion by way of the short motor root; the postganglionic fibers are the axons of ganglion cells in the ciliary ganglion and course to the ciliary muscle through the short ciliary nerves. These postganglionic fibers are unique in that they are myelinated, an exception to the general rule that postganglionic fibers are nonmyelinated.

The collective action of the ciliary muscles is to relax the tension in the suspensory ligament of the lens, thus allowing the lens to assume a more convex form.

The *vessel layer* underlying the muscles is similar in structure to that of the choroid, except that there are fewer chromatophores and more collagenous fibers, and the vessels consist for the most part of veins. The arteries supplying this region enter through the perichoroidal space and the ciliary muscle, leaving the vessel layer as the almost exclusive avenue of the returning veins.

In the pars plana, the vessels are arranged almost in a single layer. Further forward in the pars plicata, the vessels are disposed in several layers. The ciliary processes are formed by localized thickenings of the vessel layer (Fig. 22-6).

The *lamina vitrea* of the ciliary body is a continuation of the vitreous lamina of the choroid and it contains the same structures: an outer elastic lamella and an inner lamella that is the basement membrane of the pigment epithelium. In the ciliary re-

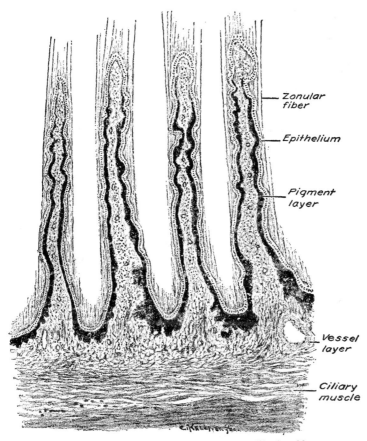

Fig. 22-6. Equatorial section through corona ciliaris of human eye.

gion, however, an added layer of connective tissue is interposed between the two lamella. The elastic lamella fades out at about the middle of the pars plicata and the intermediate zone of collagenous fibers merges with the stroma of the vascular layer. The inner lamella, or basement membrane, continues onto the iris.

The *pigment epithelium* of the ciliary body is a forward continuation of the pigment epithelium layer of the retina. Its cells are so heavily filled with round melanin granules that cell borders are difficult to distinguish by light microscopy, except on the summits of the ciliary processes, where the cells are more cuboidal and have less pigment (Fig. 22-6). This accounts for the characteristic white appearance of the ciliary processes.

The *ciliary epithelium* represents a continuation of the neural retina. Over the inner (vitreal) surface of the ciliary body, this becomes a single layer of columnar epithelial cells, unpigmented except in the region of the iris root, where they acquire increasing amounts of pigment and together with the pigment epithelium continue over the back surface of the iris. Over the summits of the ciliary processes, the ciliary epithelial cells become cuboidal in shape. Electron micrographs show cytological characteristics commonly found in epithelial cells that are active in transport, such as numerous infoldings of the basal plasma membrane and the presence of a fenestrated type of endothelium in the capillaries of the ciliary processes (chapter 12, Fig. 12-6).

The *aqueous humour* (intraocular fluid) is not only a fluid refractive medium in the eye; its circulation is also essential for the nutritive support of the retina and other refractile elements. Maintenance of proper intraocular fluid pressure ensures the physical stability of the eye and the functional interrelationship of its refractile components. Aqueous humour is constantly formed in the posterior chamber and, after circulating through that chamber as well as percolating through the interstices of the vitreous body, it is drained at a balanced rate at the angle of the anterior chamber. Formation of aqueous humour involves activity by the ciliary epithelium and its numerous ciliary processes. Although details of aqueous humour formation are not fully understood, one hypothesis is that a filtrate from the blood capillaries passes through the epithelial cells where some proteins, glucose and urea are subtracted and other substances, such as ascorbic acid, sodium chloride and bicarbonate are added.

When different substances are injected into the blood, some reach the aqueous humour in amounts approaching that in plasma whereas many others such as protein, inulin and trypan blue do not usually enter the aqueous humour. The lack of passage of certain substances from the blood to the aqueous humour is regarded as being due to a *blood-aqueous barrier.* A principal site for such a barrier against extracellular passage seems to be the occluding junctions of the ciliary epithelium. The cells of the epithelium probably determine which substances pass via an intra- or transcellular route.

The *internal limiting "membrane"* of the retina is a thin layer that is actually the basal lamina and reticular lamina of the optic cup. It continues over the inner (vitreal) side of the ciliary epithelium.

The Iris. The *iris* is a thin circular diaphragm placed directly in front of the lens. It forms a distensible aperture, the *pupil,* located slightly to the nasal side of its center. Its peripheral border (*ciliarly border, iris root*) is attached to the anterior surface of the ciliary body (Fig. 22-9); its *pupillary border* rests on the lens. The iris, therefore, inclines forward from the ciliary body; its shape is thus that of a low truncated cone. The iris divides the space between the cornea and the lens into the *anterior chamber* of the eye ahead and the *posterior chamber* behind. The two communicate through the pupil.

The anterior surface of the iris shows a division into two regions, an inner *pupillary zone* and an outer *ciliary zone,* which differ in structure and frequently also in color. The irregular circular line (about 1.5 mm from the pupillary margin) which forms the junction between these two zones is known variously as the *collarette, iris frill* or *angular line.* It marks the position of an underlying system of arteriovenous anastomoses, the *circular vasculosus iridis minor.*

The pupillary zone is radially striated and, near the collarette, shows a number of depressions, the *pupillary crypts,* which may also occur in the neighboring part of the ciliary zone. At the pupillary margin is a dark border which represents the limit of the pigmented double layered posterior epithelium, the rim of the embryonic optic cup.

The ciliary zone is marked by a series of fine radial striations formed by blood vessels. In its outer half are a number of concentric circular *contraction furrows.* Near the ciliary border, *ciliary crypts* are seen. These are smaller than the pupillary ones.

Like the ciliary body, the iris consists of structural continuations from both the tunica vasculosa and the tunica interna. Five layers can be distinguished. An *endothelium, anterior border layer* and a *vessel layer* (stroma) form the uveal portion of the iris. *Dilator pupillae* muscles and a *pigment epithelium* represent a forward continuation of the tunica interna and constitute the *pars iridica retinae.*

The endothelium of the anterior surface of the iris is continuous with the endothelium of the iris angle and, in turn, with that of the cornea (Fig. 22-5). It is a thin discontinuous and delicate layer that is difficult to demonstrate in sections prepared for light microscopy (Figs. 22-7 and 22-9).

The anterior border layer (Fig. 22-7) lies immediately under the endothelium and is the layer which determines the color of iris. It is essentially a condensation of the iris stroma but has fewer collagenous fibers and no blood vessels. It is formed principally of *chromatophores*—branched connective tissue cells containing granules of yellowish-brown pigment. The layer is lacking over the crypts and is thin on the contraction furrows.

The color of the iris depends upon the thickness of the anterior border layer and

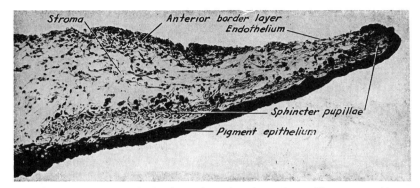

Fig. 22-7. Photomicrograph of a horizontal section through pupillary zone of human iris.

the degree of pigmentation of its cells. In the brown iris, the layer is thick and the cells heavily pigmented. In the blue iris, the layer is thin with a minimum of pigment. Light striking it, therefore, will pass through this layer and the underlying stroma and be reflected as blue from the darkly pigmented posterior epithelium. Since the pigmentation of the border layer and stroma in the white races is acquired chiefly in the first few years of life, it follows that in these races, the ultimate color of the eyes is not apparent at birth.

The vessel layer consists of a great number of blood vessels inbedded in a loose stroma of delicate collagenous fibrils, with some elastic fibers and a number of stromal cells. Most of the latter are pigmented (chromatophores).

The arteries of the iris are branches of the greater arterial circle, located at the root of the iris and derived from the anterior and posterior ciliary arteries. Within the stroma of the iris, the arteries course radially and spirally. In comparison with arteries of most other parts of the body (see chapter 12) those of the iris have a poorly developed intima, a relatively thin muscular layer and an unusually thick collagenous adventitia. The spiral patterns and firm connective tissue walls permit the vessels to straighten or coil without stretching or kinking; these structural modifications are well-suited to the changes in the radial dimensions of the iris.

In the stroma of the pupillary zone there is a circular band of smooth muscle fibers, the *sphincter pupillae* (Fig. 22-7). Their contraction reduces the diameter of the opening. This smooth muscle is of ectodermal origin, derived from the pigment epithelium layer by a transformation of epithelial cells into smooth muscle fibers, an unusual fact now firmly established by electron microscopic studies. Mesenchymal origin of the muscle cells can be ruled out because the pigment epithelial cells are clearly separated from mesenchyme by a basal lamina through all stages of differentiation.

Contraction of the *dilator pupillae* muscle (Fig. 22-9) produces dilation of the pupil. It too seems to be derived from pigment epithelial cells. The smooth muscle cells remain in close association with the ciliary epithelial cells which have become deeply pigmented over the posterior surface of the iris. The two layers can be distinguished best after bleaching (Fig. 22-8) or in tissues from albino animals. Because the smooth muscle cells retain some of the characteristics of epithelial cells they are sometimes described as "myoepithelial cells."

Together with the ciliary muscle, the sphincter and dilator pupillae comprise the *intrinsic muscles* of the eye. The sphincter is innervated by parasympathetic fibers of the oculomotor nerve. These follow the same course as those described for the ciliary muscle. The dilator pupillae is innervated by the sympathetic division of the autonomic nervous system, receiving nonmyelinated postganglionic fibers from the superior cervical ganglion. These travel in the internal carotid nerve to the carvernous plexus, thence to the Gasserian ganglion and ophthalmic division of the trigeminal nerve and finally by way of the nasociliary nerve and long ciliary nerves to reach the dilator muscle.

The ciliary epithelium, as it nears the root of the iris, acquires increasing amounts of pigment. From the ciliary body, it is continued over the posterior surface of the iris juxtaposed to and indistinguishable

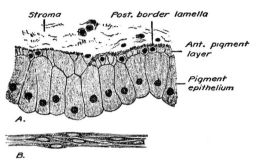

Fig. 22-8. *A*, transverse section, bleached, of the ectodermal layers of posterior surface of the iris; *B*, surface view of elements of dilator pupillae in middle of ciliary zone of the iris (teased preparation). (Redrawn from Salzmann.)

from the pigment epithelium (Figs. 22-7 and 22-9). So densely pigmented is this layer that neither cell boundaries nor nuclei can be distinguished in routine preparations for light microscopy. If the pigment is bleached out, however, the cells of both layers can be seen as columnar or prismatic elements with round nuclei (Fig. 22-8, *A*). The two layers represent remnants of the two layers of the embryonic cup. At the pupil, they become confluent, bending slightly forward around the pupillary border as the *pigment seam*. There they join the endothelium lacing over the anterior surface of the iris.

The Iris Angle. The lateral borders of the anterior chamber have, in meridional section, an angular shape. This *iris angle,* or the angle of the anterior chamber, is occupied by a triangle of loose spongy tissue, the *meshwork of the iris angle*. This

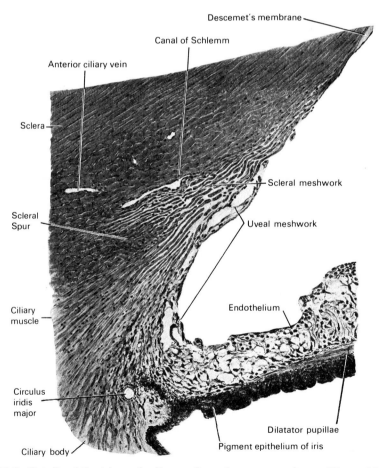

Fig. 22-9. Details of the iris angle. Drawn from the same section as Figure 22-5.

tissue fills in the scleral furrow and extends behind to the ciliary body (Fig. 22-9). The apex of the triangle is continuous with Descemet's membrane and the posterior lamellae of the cornea. Its base unites with the scleral spur and the anterior surface of the ciliary body, its outer border adjoins the tissues of the adjacent sclera and cornea, and, its inner border bounds the anterior chamber.

The major portion of the tissue is known as the *scleral meshwork*. The true nature of the meshwork is revealed by studies of tangential sections which show perforated, flattened lamellae piled on top of one another. Interposed fluid-filled channels are connected by holes through the lamellae. Each lamella consists of a central core (or plate) of collagenous tissue, a layer of elastic fibers, a homogeneous glassy basement membrane and a covering endothelium. The latter layer is continuous with the endothelium of the cornea. The spaces of the meshwork, known as the *spaces of Fontana,* are in direct communication with the anterior chamber.

Along the inner border of the scleral meshwork, there is a thin layer of trabeculae that lack elastic fibers and that are round instead of flat. In some species, the trabeculae along the inner border form a well-defined structure known as the *pectinate ligament.* This name is sometimes used for the similarly located, but poorly developed, trabeculae in the human eye.

The *canal of Schlemm* also lies in the scleral furrow, close to its bottom. In meridional sections, it appears as one or more endothelial lined oval spaces, just in front of the scleral spur and adjacent to the meshwork of the iris angle (Figs. 22-5 and 22-9). Actually, it encircles the eye as a canal which irregularly divides and recombines into two or more branches. It communicates peripherally by means of 20 to 30 small branches with the anterior ciliary veins in the neighboring scleral tissue (Fig. 22-9). The outer borders of the endothelial cells of Schlemm's canal are in contact with the lining cells of some of the spaces of Fontana.

Together with the meshwork of the angle, Schlemm's canal forms a means of exit from the eye for the intraocular fluid. The aqueous humour passes readily through the spaces of Fontana and into the canal. Particulate matter is caught by the trabeculae of the meshwork. Under normal conditions, only aqueous humour is found in Schlemm's canal. It has been suggested that the action of the ciliary muscle on the scleral spur provides a pumping mechanism for the canal.

The aqueous humour carries nutrients, substrates and metabolites. As outlined previously, it also maintains an intraocular pressure which is higher than that in the surrounding tissues and thus, together with the fibrous tunics, it plays an important role in maintaining stability of optical dimensions. A normal intraocular pressure is present when the aqueous humour is formed and drained at normal rates. An increase in intraocular pressure, known as *glaucoma,* occurs when there is defective drainage by the outflow channels at the iris angle.

The Retina

The retina forms the *pars optica retinae* of the tunica interna and is the part of the eye which transduces the stimulus of light into nerve impulses, resulting in the sensation of vision. Thus it might be considered that all other parts of the eye assist the retina in the proper performance of its highly specialized function.

The retina, having arisen from the optic cup, consists of an outer layer, the *pigment epithelium*, and an inner layer, the *neural retina*. In pathological detachment of the retina, or as often occurs in fixed specimens, the two parts of the retina separate, the pigment epithelium remaining adherent to the choroid. The pigment epithelium will be discussed after examination of the neural retina.

The neural retina is firmly attached to underlying structures at only two regions— at its scalloped anterior margin, the ora serrata (Figs. 22-2 and 22-5) and at the optic disc, where the nerve fibers pass through the wall of the bulb to form the optic nerve (Fig. 22-23). Detached from the pigment epithelium, it is a delicate layer which in life is transparent.

Except at the optic disc (optic papilla),

the fovea centralis and the extreme periphery, the neural retina consists of nine layers (Fig. 22-10), which from without inward, are arranged as follows: (1) layer of rod and cone outer and inner segments; (2) external limiting membrane (outer zone of intercellular attachments); (3) outer nuclear layer; (4) outer plexiform layer; (5) inner nuclear layer; (6) inner plexiform layer; (7) ganglion cell layer; (8) nerve fiber layer; and (9) internal limiting membrane (basal lamina).

The nature and significance of the layers of the neural retina will be better understood if it is realized that the stratification depends upon the location and interrelationships of the photoreceptor cells and the intraretinal neurons of the afferent pathway. Considering them in the order of the initiation and conduction of an impulse, we find that the photoreceptor portions of the *rod* and *cone cells* occupy the layer of that name. The *outer nuclear layer* consists of the nuclei and cell bodies of the photoreceptor cells, and the *outer plexiform layer* is where axon-like photoreceptor cell processes make synaptic junctions with dendrites of bipolar neurons and with processes of horizontal cells. The nuclei of the bipolar cells lie in the *inner nuclear layer*; their axons pass into the *inner plexiform layer*,

where they effect synapse with the dendrites of the ganglion cells. The relatively large cell bodies of the latter form the *ganglion cell layer*; their long axons course in the *nerve fiber layer* to the optic disc, where all the axons converge to form the optic nerve. These fibers are continuous to the brain, where the great majority end in the lateral geniculate body, from which another neuron system carries the nerve impulse to the visual areas in the occipital cortex.

The true photoreceptive elements, the rods and cones, lie furtherest removed and oriented *away* from the light stimulus, which to affect them must first pass through all the intervening layers and their organelles (except at the fovea). These are all maintained in a remarkably transparent state. Also, the nervous pathway at first travels directly toward the source of the stimulus before turning to course toward the brain. This seemingly *inverted* retina is characteristic of all vertebrates.

The layer of rod and cone outer and inner segments lies between the *external limiting "membrane"* and the pigment epithelium, facing the latter. The apical portions of rod and cone cells are known as outer segments and are arranged in parallel fashion, perpendicular to the surface.

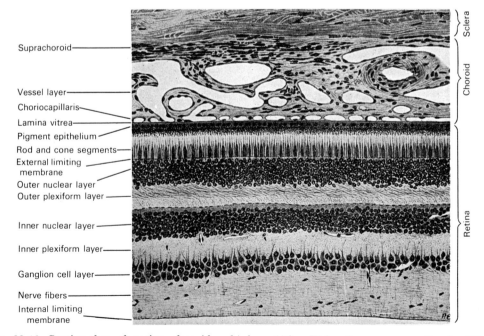

Suprachoroid

Vessel layer
Choriocapillaris
Lamina vitrea
Pigment epithelium
Rod and cone segments
External limiting membrane
Outer nuclear layer
Outer plexiform layer

Inner nuclear layer

Inner plexiform layer

Ganglion cell layer

Nerve fibers
Internal limiting membrane

Sclera
Choroid
Retina

Fig. 22-10. Section through retina, choroid and sclera. (After Eisler, from a preparation by Stieve.)

The Rod Cells. The apical protrusions of *outer* and *inner segments* of these cells, (sometimes known as the *rods proper*) are slender cylindrical elements, 40 to 60 μm in length and about 2 μm in diameter. Although the rod outer and inner segments vary in length and width in different species (Fig. 22-11), they are similarly organized in all vertebrates.

The outer segment is the most distal part and is the receptor of the cell that "traps" light which reaches the retina. Electron micrographs show that the outer segment is made up of hundreds of flattened membranous sacs piled in a stack of uniform diameter (Figs. 22-12 to 22-16). The membranes of the sacs contain molecules of visual pigment which absorb the light and undergo steric chemical conformational changes that lead to the production of a

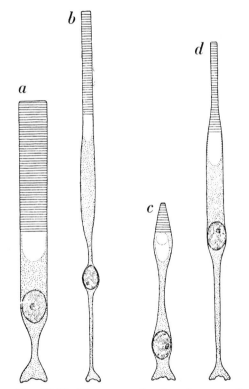

Fig. 22-11. Diagrams of rod and cone cells. Although the retinal photoreceptors differ somewhat in different species, they have a similar general organization in all vertebrates. *Left,* typical rod cells from the frog retina (*a*) and the human retina (*b*); *right,* typical cone cells from the frog (*c*) and human (*d*). (After R. W. Young, Sci. Am., vol. 223, 1970.)

generator potential by the photoreceptor cell. It is clear that the compact stacked arrangement of the flattened sacs increases enormously the membrane surface over which photic absorption and transduction can occur.

The base of the outer segment is connected with the inner segment by a slender stalk or cilium (really a flagellum) which contains nine peripheral doublet microtubules that emanate from a centriole or basal body. Striated ciliary rootlets extend from the centriole into the inner segment cytoplasm. Thus, the outer segment is revealed to be a specialized cilium that differs from the cilia of most other types of epithelium (chapter 4) mainly in the lack of a central pair of microtubules and in the unique and massive development of the surrounding cell membrane to form the flattened sacs. The outer portion of the inner segment, identified as an "ellipsoid" by light microscopists, contains mitochondria, in some species quite closely packed. The inner portion of each inner segment contains the Golgi complex and granular and smooth endoplasmic reticulum. In the retinas of some lower vertebrates, filamentous elements in the inner segment are contractile, serving to advance or retract the outer segment with reference to the pigment epithelium in response to light or dark.

Radioautographic studies of retinas from animals sacrificed at intervals after injection of radioactive amino acids show that rod cells synthesize new proteins in the inner segments and that these poteins are conducted by the ciliary stalks to the bases of the outer segments where groups of new sacs are formed by infoldings of the cell membrane. The older sacs are displaced outward as new sacs are built below, and they are eventually shed from the tips of the rods into the region of the pigment epithelium. Thus, the outer segments of the rod cells are continually renewed, and during their life spans, held in register perpendicular to the direction of incoming light rays (Fig. 22-16). (See additional disussion regarding this pattern in relation to the pigment epithelium.)

When the retina is freshly removed from the eye of an animal which has been kept in the dark, it appears purplish-red in color

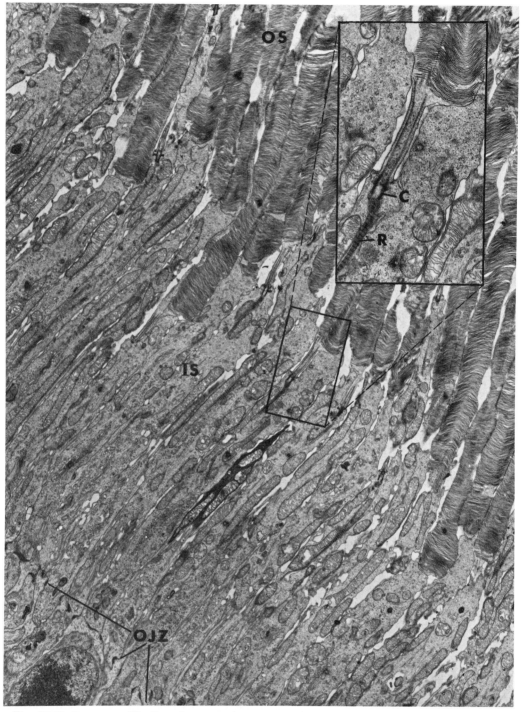

Fig. 22-12. Low magnification electron micrograph of a section through the retina of an albino rat (a pure rod retina). The region of outer segments (*OS*) and inner segments (*IS*) covers most of the field. The outer junctional zone (*OJZ*) separates the above region from the outer nuclear layer (*lower left corner*). Details of the connection between outer and inner segments of one rod cell are shown at higher magnification in the *inset*. The outer segment begins as a narrow ciliary stalk with a centriole (*C*) at its base. A ciliary rootlet (*R*) extends from the centriole into the inner segment cytoplasm. ×6000; inset ×15,000. (Courtesy of Dr. David Chase.)

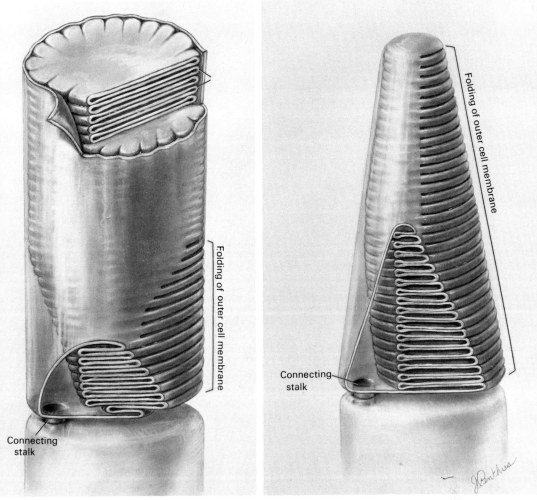

Fig. 22-13. Diagrammatic representation of the ultrastructure of rod and cone cell outer segments. In the rod, there is a continual formation of new sacs by repeated infolding of the cell membrane. As the older sacs are displaced away from the base of the outer segment, they lose their attachment to the cell membrane, and they are eventually cast off. The sacs of the cone outer segment are also continually replaced, but in a less obvious sequential fashion. (Courtesy of Dr. Richard W. Young.)

when viewed in subdued light. The color fades rapidly when the preparation is exposed to light. Chemical studies have shown that rod pigment, *visual purple,* consists of vitamin A aldehyde, now known as *retinal* (formerly called retinene) combined with a protein known as *rod opsin.* When a pigment molecule is exposed to light, there is a steric change (from *cis* to *trans*) in the form of the retinal and the relationship between retinal and its combined protein is broken. This leads to a change in electrical potential in the cell that results in the formation of a membrane generator potential (signal) which is released at the

synaptic contact of the rod basal process to the dendrites of a biopolar ganglion cell. After light stimulation, the visual purple is rapidly reconstituted.

It was noted many years ago that animals that are particularly active at night (e.g., rats and mice) have many rods and few or no cones. On the other hand, animals active only in daytime have retinas composed almost entirely of cones (e.g., diurnal lizards and turtles). The respective roles of the mixed population of rods and cones in the human eye are well-established. The rods have a low threshold of stimulation by light, are particularly important in intensity

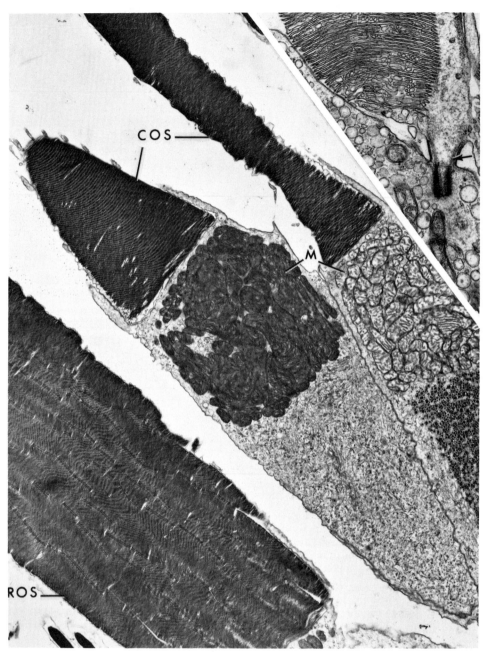

Fig. 22-14. Electron micrograph of portions of rod and cone cells. The field includes a portion of the outer segment of a rod (*ROS*) and the outer segments of a double cone (*COS*). The field also includes cone inner segments, showing closely packed mitochondria (*M*) in the outer portion of the inner segment. Endoplasmic reticulum is found chiefly in the inner portion of the inner segment. The electron-dense granules seen in the inner segment of one of the cones represent glycogen. *Inset, upper right,* junction of outer and inner segments of a photoreceptor cell at higher magnification. *Arrow,* connecting stalk. The electron-dense material subjacent to the stalk is the basal body. *Lower figure,* from a newt, *Taricha torosa,* ×7200; inset, a photoreceptor cell from the same species at higher magnification, ×16,450. (Lower figure, courtesy of Dr. Anita Hendrickson.)

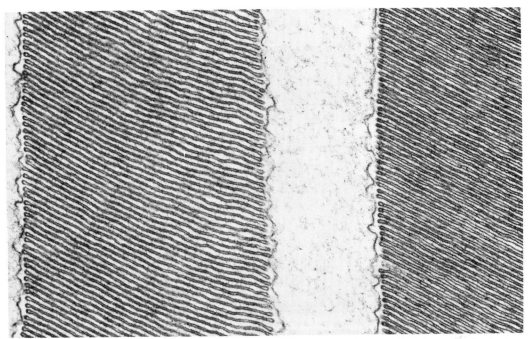

Fig. 22-15. Electron micrographs of portion of a cone segment (*left*) and a rod outer segment (*right*) from the retina of a monkey. Note that the rod disks are more closely packed than those of the cones. ×53,000. (Courtesy of Dr. Richard W. Young.)

(dark and light) discrimination and are active in night vision. The cones have a higher threshold of stimulation and are particularly important in wavelength discrimination and in visual acuity. They are most active under daylight intensity.

The Cone Cells. Except in the region of the fovea centralis and its immediate vicinity, the cones are flask-shaped, having a relatively short and conical outer segment and a relatively broad and bulbous inner segment. The region that connects the cone inner segment to the cone body is short and it is not constricted as it is in the rods (Fig. 22-11). Variations in shapes of cones from different areas of the human retina are shown in Figure 22-17.

Electron microscopic studies show that the cone outer segments are composed of sacs somewhat like those of the rods. The cone sacs differ, however, in that they remain attached to the cell plasmalemma from which they arise and are less closely packed, and they become progressively smaller in diameter along the length of the cone (Figs. 22-13 through 22-15). The cone outer segment is attached to the cone inner segment by a ciliary stalk that is similar in structure to that in the rod.

In some species, the inner segment often contains a characteristic oil droplet or accumulations of glycogen just beneath the connecting cilium. Otherwise it resembles the rod inner segment in having a region of closely packed mitochondria followed by a region containing the Golgi complex and smooth and rough endoplasmic reticulum.

Radioautographic studies of retinas taken from animals sacrificed at intervals subsequent to injection of labeled amino acids show that new proteins are also synthesized in the inner segments of the cones (i.e., in the regions of the rough endoplasmic reticulum and Golgi complex) just as in the rods. The new proteins, however, diffuse quickly into the cone outer segments by comparison to the longer sequential pattern in the rods. However, there is no doubt that the cone is renewed by the progressive formation of new sacs. When new sacs form during the continuous regeneration of a cone outer segment, each newly formed sac at the base of the stack is larger than the preceding one, and thus the cone becomes

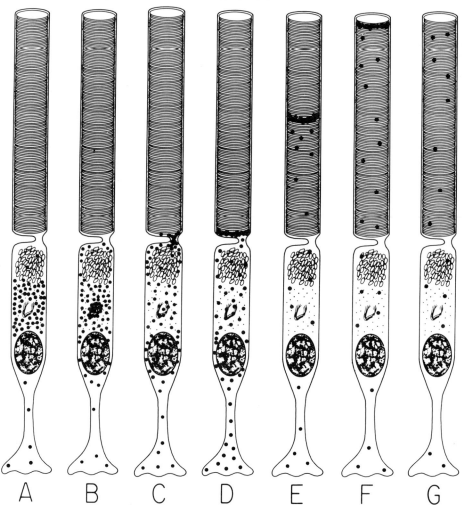

Fig. 22-16. Diagrammatic representation of the results of radioautographic studies of frog retinae fixed at different intervals of time after injection of labeled amino acids. Labeled material in newly synthesized protein (*dots*) is found in the region of the endoplasmic reticulum and the Golgi complex within 10 minutes after the injection (*A* and *B*). At later intervals, the newly formed protein passes around the mitochondria of the outer segment and reaches the connecting stalk (*C*). The synthesized protein is found in a newly formed basal disk of the outer segment in about 1 week (*D*), then moves outward (*E*) and reaches the end of the disk in about 8 weeks (*F* and *G*). (Courtesy of Dr. Richard W. Young.)

tapered or conical in shape. The functional significance of this fact and mechanism by which it is achieved remain mysteries.

The visual pigment of the cones is associated with the sacs of the outer segment, as it is in the rods. In the cones, the pigment is known as *iodopsin* and it consists of retinal (retinene) combined with a cone opsin. The basic steps in light absorption and in the generation of an impulse are similar to those described above for the rods. The cones respond to light of rela-tively high intensity, and they function for visual acuity and for color perception. Detection of different colors apparently depends upon the presence of different pigments in the cones, each apparently absorbing light most efficiently at red, blue or green wavelengths. Rods, on the other hand, apparently have only one type of pigment.

The external limiting "membrane" is really not a discrete membrane, but rather, as seen in electron micrographs, a region

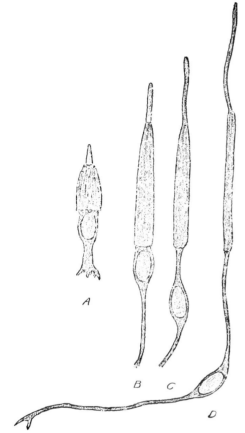

Fig. 22-17. Cones from different areas of the human retina. *A*, from near the ora serrata; *B*, from periphery of macula lutea; *C*, from the macula lutea; *D*, from the fovea centralis. (After Greeff.)

of junctional complexes between the outer ends of the supporting neuroglial (Müller) cells and the adjoining photoreceptor cells. It is more accurately termed the *outer junctional zone.*

The outer nuclear layer consists of rod and cone cell bodies containing rod cell and cone cell nuclei, respectively. The cone nuclei are located close to the outer junctional zone, and with the exception of the region of the fovea, they are limited to a single row. The rod nuclei are more numerous than cone nuclei, except in the fovea, and are distributed in several layers. Rod nuclei are rounded and they stain intensely in most routine preparations for light microscopy.

The outer plexiform layer is composed chiefly of the basally directed processes

(*spherules* or *pedicles*) of rod and cone cells, the dendrites of bipolar cells, and processes of horizontal cells. These are in synaptic relationship with the spherules or pedicles acting as presynaptic components in transferral of the photoreceptor generator potential to the bipolar cells where it is converted to a membrane potential. Synaptic contacts with the horizontal cells and between spherules and pedicles themselves integrate and modify the photoreceptor input. The spherules of rods are indented, enclosing the dendrites of one or more bipolar cells and several horizontal cells in an enclosed synaptic cleft (Figs. 22-18 and 22-19). The presynaptic (photoreceptor) element is characterized by typical hollow synaptic vesicles plus a *synaptic ribbon,* an unusual organelle common to several types of receptor cells. Synaptic ribbons are dense proteinaceous plaques oriented perpendicular to the synaptic surface and bounded by numerous vesicles (Fig. 22-20). Cone pedicles are much larger in their dimensions, contain several synaptic indentations incorporating the processes of many bipolar and horizontal cells and display multiple synaptic ribbons (Fig. 22-20).

The *inner nuclear layer* is thinner than the outer nuclear layer but resembles it in general appearance. It contains the nuclei of the *bipolar neurons,* nuclei of association neurons known as *horizontal cells* and *amacrine cells* and nuclei of the supporting *Müller's cells.* In general, the nuclei of this layer are arranged in three zones: an outer one of horizontal cell nuclei; a middle one of bipolar cell nuclei; and an inner one in which amacrine cell nuclei predominate (Fig. 22-19). The morphology and interrelationships of these cells are discussed below. Müller's cells are the most obvious glial population of the neural retina. Their distribution and relationships resemble to some degree the fibrous astrocytes of the central nervous system (CNS). The Müller's cell processes course among receptor and other cell bodies and processes, extending from the inner to outer limiting "membranes." They are probably physically supportive in function.

The *inner plexiform layer* consists of the processes of the amacrine cells, the axons of the bipolar cells and the profusely branched dendrites of the ganglion cells.

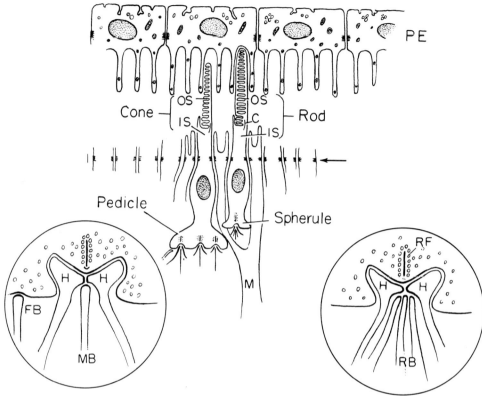

Fig. 22-18. Diagram of the utlrastructural organization of a portion of the retina showing the relationship of the rod and cone cells to the pigment epithelial cells and to the processes of Müller's cells. Desmosomes are seen at the lateral borders of apposing pigment epithelial cells (*P*). Processes of Müller's cells (*M*) project outward almost to the level of the connecting stalks (*C*) between the outer segments (*OS*) and inner segments (*IS*) of the photoreceptor cells. *Arrow,* the position of junctional complexes between the cell membranes of the processes of Müller's neuroglial cells and membranes of rod and cone cells; this region is known as the outer limiting membrane of light microscope studies. The cone cell terminates in an expansion known as a pedicle, whereas the rod cell has a knoblike ending or spherule. *Inset at lower left,* the synaptic contacts of a cone cell pedicle with processes of midget bipolar cells (*MB*), flat bipolar cells (*FB*) and horizontal cells (*H*). *Inset at lower right,* synaptic contacts of a rod cell spherule with processes of rod bipolar cells (*RB*) and horizontal cells (*H*). An electron-dense line in the presynaptic terminal is known as a synaptic ribbon (*RF*). (Courtesy of Drs. Charles R. Noback and Lois K. Laemle, The Primate Brain, vol. 1, 1970.)

An intricate array of synaptic interconnections of all these cells provides an appropriately integrated and controlled input to the ganglion cells. The axonal terminals of bipolar cells are unusual for neurons in that they contain synaptic ribbons.

The *ganglion cell layer* is composed of multipolar ganglion cells, among which are scattered neuroglial cells. Branches of the retinal blood vessels are also present. The ganglion cells are variable in size (11 to 30 μm) with clear round nuclei containing one or more prominent nucleoli.

The *nerve fiber layer* consists of the ax-ons of the ganglion cells. These nonmyelinated fibers are arranged in bundles which run parallel to the inner surface of the retina and converge at the optic disk to form the optic nerve. Between the bundles are numerous fibrous neuroglia cells (*spider cells*) and rows of Müller's cell processes. Also present in this layer are the retinal blood vessels, indented into the retinal epithelium much in the manner seen for vessels supplying the central nervous system.

The *"internal limiting membrane"* is formed by the apposition of the expanded inner ends of processes of Müller's cells and

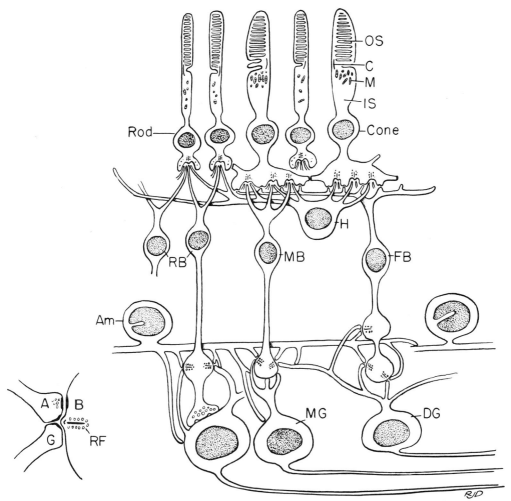

Fig. 22-19. Diagram of the ultrastructural organization of the retina showing the relationship of the photoreceptor cells and the intraretinal neurons. The rod cell terminals have synaptic contacts with rod bipolar cells (*RB*) and horizontal cells (*H*). Cone cell terminals have synaptic contacts with midget bipolar cells (*MB*), flat bipolar cells (*FB*) and horizontal cells. The amacrine cells (*Am*) have processes which have synaptic contacts with the processes of all types of bipolar cells and with the midget ganglion cells (*MG*) and diffuse ganglion cells (*DG*). *Inset at lower left,* a schematic representation of the synaptic contacts between an amacrine cell terminal (*A*), ganglion cell process (*G*) and bipolar cell process (*B*). *C,* connecting stalk; *IS,* inner segment; *M,* mitochondria; *OS,* outer segment; *RF,* synaptic ribbon. (Courtesy of Drs. Charles R. Noback and Lois K. Laemle, The Primate Retina, vol. 1, 1970; adapted from Dowling and Boycott, 1966.)

by their basal lamina. Here Müller's cells are particularly similar to astrocytes of the CNS and their relation to the basal (vitreal) surface of the retina is homologous to the glia limitans externa of the CNS. Müller's cells are the chief supporting cells of the retina although other cells of neuroglial type are also present.

Retinal Modification in the Maculae Lutea and Fovea Centralis. Near the posterior pole of the eye, the human neural retina undergoes a localized modification of its layers and shows a funnel-shaped depression. This region has a yellowish color when viewed in gross specimens; hence, it is named the *macula lutea,* or yellow spot. The inner layers of the retina spread apart and deviate from the center of the region, leaving a small pit known as the *fovea centralis* (Figs. 22-1 and 22-21).

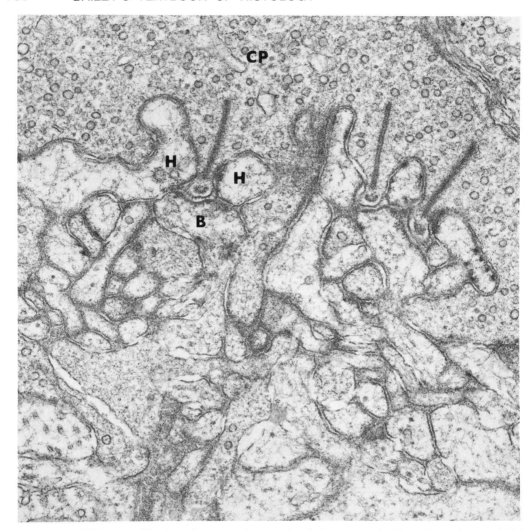

Fig. 22-20. High magnification electron micrograph of the outer plexiform layer in a goldfish retina. A cone pedicle (*CP*) is seen with numerous synaptic vesicles distributed in its cytoplasm. Three synaptic ribbons occupy positions juxtaposed to areas of synaptic contact along the basal surface of the indented pedicle. Bipolar (*B*) and horizontal (*H*) cell processes make synaptic contact with the pedicle at these points. ×48,750 (Courtesy of Dr. Dean Bok.)

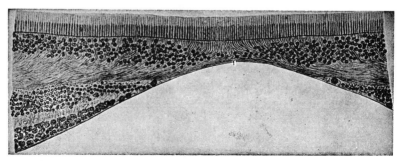

Fig. 22-21. Section through center of fovea centralis. The outer nuclear layer is represented in the fovea by only a few scattered cells. (After Eisler.)

There the photoreceptors consist only of cones. In the center of the fovea, in an area which is about 0.5 mm in diameter, the cones are extremely slender and closely packed (Fig. 22-17). This appears to explain partly the high visual acuity of the fovea.

Peripheral to the foveal region, rod receptors begin to appear among the cones and they gradually increase in numbers until three to four rods intervene between individual cones in areas peripheral to the macula. It has been estimated that there are about 7,000,000 cones in the retina; of this number, about 13,000 are said to be in the macular region and about 4,000 in the fovea centralis. Estimates of the number of rods range from 75,000,000 to 170,000,000.

Retinal Interneuronal Associations and Functions. The chief interneuronal relationships in the retina, as currently described and interpreted from electron microscopic studies, are shown schematically in Figures 22-18 and 22-19. The cone pedicles make separate synaptic contacts with dendrites of two types of bipolar cells: *midget bipolars* and *flat bipolars*. It seems functionally significant that, in the fovea of the retina at least, a single midget bipolar cell is in synaptic contact with a single cone. This appears to be correlated with the high visual acuity of the central part of the fovea. Contact of the midget bipolar cell dendrite with the cone cell terminal forms a part of a triadic synaptic complex, with the dendritic ending of the bipolar cell located between endings of two separate horizontal cells. Contacts between rod and cone cell terminals are present also, but the significance of some of these contacts is not fully understood.

Each *rod bipolar* cell synapses with several rod cells (only two are included Fig. 22-19). This correlates with the finding that rods generally function as groups. Rod cell terminals are also in contact with processes of the horizontal cells.

The cell bodies of the amacrine cells, located in the inner cell layer of the retina, have processes that extend into the inner plexiform layer where they make contact with axon terminals of all types of bipolar cells and with the dendrites of both types of ganglion cells. They also make contact with each other; i.e., amacrine to amacrine contact.

Two types of ganglion cells have been identified: *midget ganglion cells,* with each cell dendrite in contact with the axon of a single midget bipolar cell, and *diffuse ganglion cells* which make contact with all types of bipolar cells. The synapses of the bipolar cells with the diffuse ganglion cells are both axodendritic and axosomatic in type.

The above retinal interneuronal relationships are significant in relation to the arrangement of retinal visual fields. The *visual field* of a particular ganglion cell is defined as that area of the retina which, upon stimulation, affects the ganglion cell. Each visual field consists functionally of a central region and a peripheral region; in light-adapted retinas, these two concentric fields function antagonistically. For example, if a given ganglion cell is excited when light is applied to the center of its visual field it will be inhibited when light is applied to the periphery of its field. When light is applied to the periphery and center of the field of the particular ganglion cell at the same time, there is a summation of effects and the ganglion cell gives a weak response. In the case of color vision, it appears that the center of a field responds maximally to light of another wavelength. In other words, the antagonistic central and peripheral zones of a field may be color coded.

The diameters of visual fields, particularly the diameters of the central portions of the fields, differ in different parts of the retina. In visual fields of the fovea, the diameter of the center of the field may be within the magnitude of the diameter of a single cone. This is one of the explanations for the greater visual acuity of the foveal region.

The antagonistic responses to stimulation of "central" and "surround" regions of visual fields appear to correlate with the arrangement of neurons shown in Figures 22-18 and 22-19. A change in light intensity at the center of a field sets up a stimulus which is probably transmitted by direct receptor-bipolar-ganglion cell contacts. In the case of cone vision, this is by cone cell-midget bipolar cell-midget ganglion cell. On the other hand, a change in light intensity in the peripheral portion of the visual field of a ganglion cell sets up a stimulus which reaches the ganglion cell by a circuitous route that is apparently mediated by amacrine-amacrine cell contacts along the way.

The intricate circuitry of bipolar, ganglion, horizontal and amacrine cells undoubtedly underlies many more modulating, feedback and coordinating processes in this first level of visual integration. Some of these are beginning to be uncovered with newer methods. Functional understanding of the system is further complicated by recent reports of *efferent* fibers coursing from the brain to the retina, presumably performing some feedback or modulating task.

Blood Vessels or the Retina. The layer of rod and cone outer and inner segments, the outer nuclear layer, and the outer plexiform layer are devoid of blood vessels. Their nourishment comes from the choriocapillaris of the choroid. The remaining layers of the retina are supplied by a system of retinal vessels derived from the central retinal artery, which enters the eye in the optic nerve (into which it gained entrance via the embryonic optic fissure). The larger arteries lie indented into the nerve fiber layer, with finer branches looping into the ganglion cell and inner plexiform layers. Two capillary networks are formed, one in the nerve fiber layer and another which extends as far as the outer border of the inner nuclear layer. The retinal veins follow the course of the arteries.

The Ora Serrata. The scalloped anterior border of the retina is known as the ora serrata (Fig. 22-1). Here the retina ends abruptly, its margin forming a step which may be rounded, angular or even overhanging. Approaching this region, the rods and cones become shorter and thicker (Fig. 22-17, *A*), the nuclear layers become thinner and the ganglion cell and nerve fiber layers cease altogether. There is a corresponding increase in the number of glial cells (Müller's fibers).

The Pigment Epithelium. A full realization of the functional role of the pigment epithelium is only recently beginning to unfold, in part coincident with the experiments cited above concerning membrane protein turnover in photoreceptor inner and outer segments. For many years, it has been known that the thin apical processes of the pigment epithelial cells surround and interdigitate with the outer segments. Hence, it has long been suspected that they might serve a role of physical and/or metabolic support for the photoreceptors. In many lower vertebrates the processes are rich in pigment granules, and these migrate up and down each process in response to illumination, seemingly masking to a degree the outer segments in conditions of bright light and, conversely, exposing them in dim light or darkness. The processes are also present and closely associated with outer segments in the human retina, but they are not highly pigmented, so dim/bright retinal accommodation occurs chiefly through other mechanisms. However, tracer experiments with labeled vitamin A and studies of hereditary- and vitamin A deficiency-induced retinal dystrophy strongly suggest that the epithelium, via its processes, serves as a storage site in the continual cyclic supply of this vitamin to the outer segment membranes. Just as new flattened membrane sacs are continually being added in packets to the bases of rod and cone outer segments, so too are bunches of them released at the distal tips. These cast-off membranes are rapidly phagocytosed by the nearby pigment epithelial cells (Fig. 22-22) and their components are either degraded and removed or recycled to the photoreceptors by mechanisms and pathways as yet incompletely understood. Interestingly, it is now known that packets of rod sacs are shed to the pigment epithelium just after the outset of daylight, while cone sacs are shed just following the onset of darkness. This means that outer segments are replenished just following their diurnal period of maximum activity (R. W. Young, personal communication).

The Optic Nerve

The nerve fibers of the retina converge at the optic disc and turn outward to pass through the sieve-like *lamina cribrosa* of the sclera as the optic nerve (Fig. 22-23). In this intraocular portion, the nerve has a structure similar to that of the nerve fiber layer; i.e., bundles of nonmyelinated fibers surrounded by glial cell processes.

Immediately behind the lamina cribrosa,

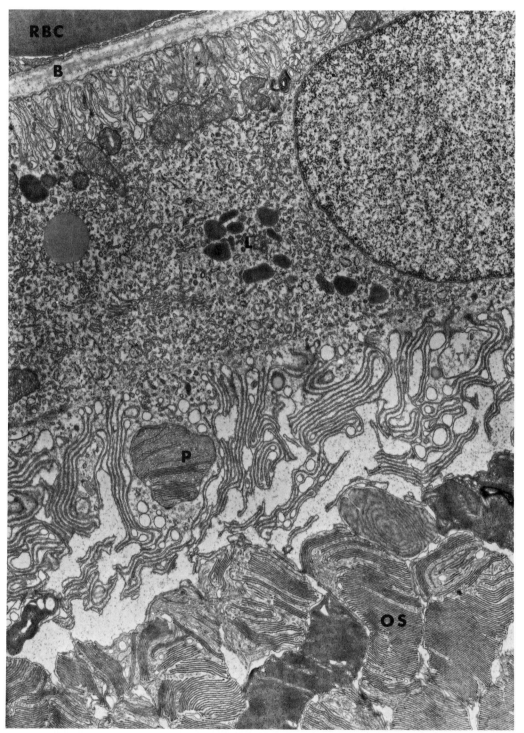

Fig. 22-22. Electron micrograph depicting the relationship between the pigment epithelium and retinal rod outer segments (*OS*) in an albino rat. A pigment epithelial cell is seen with its nucleus (*upper right*), lysosomes (*L*) and numerous apical processes extending toward the disorganized tips of the outer segments. Unlike normally pigmented animals the albino rat does not possess pigment granules in its pigment epithelial cells. A portion of one outer segment tip (*P*) has been phagocytosed by the pigment epithelial cell. Bruch's membrane (*B*) is seen to consist of the epithelial basal lamina, connective tissue and the basal lamina of a capillary in the choroid. A red blood cell (*RBC*) occupies the capillary whose endothelial wall is richly fenestrated. Note the pleated basal surface of the pigment epithelial cell. ×14,000. (Courtesy of Dr. David Chase.)

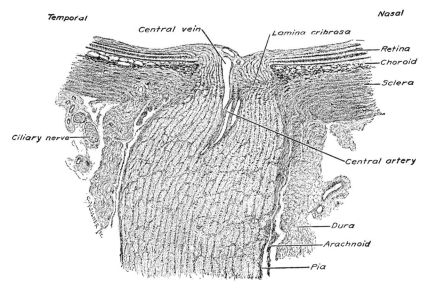

Fig. 22-23. Horizontal section of human optic nerve head.

the nerve fibers acquire myelin sheaths, with a consequent increase in diameter of the entire nerve. Since the optic nerve actually is a tract of the brain rather than a true peripheral nerve, it is not surprising that it should resemble the CNS in its coverings and its histological characteristics.

A cross section of the myelinated orbital portion of the optic nerve shows that it is surrounded by three connective tissue sheaths: an outer *dura,* an inner *pia* and an intermediate *arachnoid,* which divides the *intervaginal space* into a subdural space and a *subarachnoid space.* These sheaths are continuous with the corresponding meninges of the brain; at the bulb, the dura becomes continuous with the sclera, and the arachnoid and pia vaguely continuous with the choroid.

From the pial sheath, connective tissue trabeculae invaginate with basal laminae into the nerve and in conjunction with the arrangement of neuroglial elements form a system of septa which enclose groups of nerve fiber bundles. Between the bundles are glial cells whose processes and fibers penetrate between the individual nerve fibers.

In the anterior part of the nerve, for a distance of about 12 mm behind the eye, the septa are united to a central core of connective tissue, the *central supporting*

tissue strand (a remnant of the fused embryonic optic fissure). This carries the *central artery* and *central vein* of the retina. Small branches from these vessels course in the septal system to supply the nerve itself.

The Lens

The lens (Fig. 22-24) is a transparent and somewhat plastic biconvex epithelial body situated between the iris and the vitreous body. Its posterior surface has a greater convexity than the anterior surface (Fig. 22-1). Three structural components make up the lens, a *capsule,* an *anterior epithelium* and the *lens substance.*

The capsule consists of a basal lamina and reticular lamina ensheathing the lens. Actually, it is the basement membrane that has surrounded the lens since its emergence as an epithelial lens vesicle. It is of varied thickness in different parts of the lens but always thinnest at the posterior pole. On either surface a zone concentric with the equator serves for the insertion of the *zonular fibers* of the *suspensory ligament* (Fig. 22-25).

The anterior epithelium is a single layer of cuboidal cells on the anterior lens surface, just under the capsule (Fig. 22-25). The posterior epithelial cells have been greatly modified to form the primitive *lens*

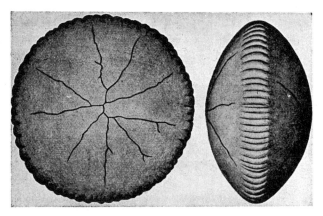

Fig. 22-24. The lens, viewed from behind and from the side. (From Eisler, after Rabl.)

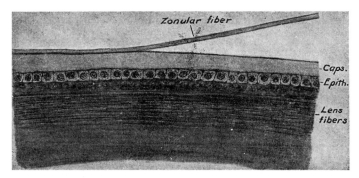

Fig. 22-25. Portion of anterior surface of equatorial zone of the lens, showing attachment of zonular fiber to the capsule. *Caps.*, anterior capsule of lens; *Epith.*, lens epithelium.

fibers during embryonic development. At the equator, or margin, the cells are elongated and arranged meridionally in rows (Fig. 22-26). This is the region where new lens fibers are constantly being formed during lens growth, and the cells themselves may be regarded as young lens fibers.

The lens substance consists of elongated prismatic lens fibers. The first lens fibers that form during embryonic development arise by elongation and differentiation of the posterior epithelial cells of the lens vesicle, and they are oriented in an anteroposterior direction. Succeeding fibers are formed superficially by mitosis, elongation and differentiation of epithelial cells at the equator of the lens. Consequently, these fibers are arranged meridionally in concentric layers. The older and deeper fibers lose their nuclei but the epithelial cells of the region of the equator continue to multiply and differentiate into new lens fibers. As a result, the concentric layers show varying

degrees of differentiation. Individual fibers can be identified more readily in the outer part of the lens, known as the *cortex*, than in the inner part, sometimes called the *nucleus* of the lens. In the inner region the fibers are condensed and appear more homogeneous. The regions of the lens where cortical fibers from opposite sectors converge and make contact are known as lens *sutures*.

Electron micrographs show that the epithelial cells of the equatorial region have numerous interdigitations and occasional desmosomes. The lens fibers also show interdigitations, particularly in the so-called sutures. The intercellular spaces of epithelial cells and of lens fibers are very narrow, being similar in this respect to intercellular spaces of other types of epithelium. It should be noted that the lens, like the cornea, is avascular and totally dependent for its nutrition upon the circulating intraocular fluid and transport by its own cells.

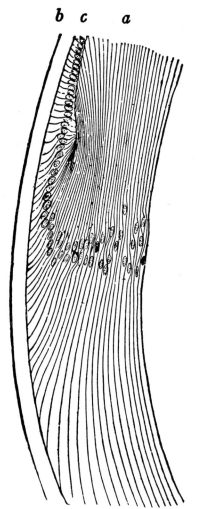

b c a

Fig. 22-26. From section through margin of lens, showing longitudinal sections of lens fibers and transition from epithelium to lens fibers. *a*, lens fibers; *b*, capsule; *c*, epithelium. (Merkel-Henle.)

The Zonula Ciliaris

The *zonula ciliaris* (*zonule of Zinn, suspensory ligament*) is a system of delicate collagenous fibers which form a fairly thick band radiating from the equatorial zone of the lens capsule to the inner surface of the ciliary body, thereby fixing the lens in place (Fig. 22-5). Many of the fibers arise from the orbiculus ciliaris and sweep forward over the surface of the ciliary body to the lens capsule. Others come from the corona ciliaris. They arise from the basement membrane in the valleys between the cili-

ary processes (Fig. 22-6) and are closely applied to the sides of the latter as they course radially inward to the lens.

The zonular fibers are inserted on the lens capsule in two main zones: in front of the equator and just behind it. Fibers which insert on the anterior capsule are thicker.

Recalling the arrangement of the smooth muscle fibers of the ciliary muscle and its attachment anteriorly to the scleral spur, it becomes evident that contraction of this muscle will cause the ciliary body and choroid to be pulled forward, while the ciliary processes will at the same time be displaced toward the equator of the lens. The result of both actions will be to relax the tension normally maintained on the zonular fibers. The highly elastic lens capsule, released from tension, is thus enabled to mould the plastic lens cortex to a more spherical form. This constitutes the process of accommodation, by which images of near objects are brought to correct focus on the retina. It should be noted that in a state of rest, the ciliary muscle is relaxed and the zonula ciliaris and lens are under tension.

The Vitreous Body

The *vitreous body* occupies the space between the lens and the retina. (This space is not the posterior chamber.) In the fresh condition, the vitreous body is a transparent, firm jelly-like body (actually a form of connective tissue). The molecular meshwork provided by its fibers and ground substance molecules provides for percolation of the intraocular fluid (aqueous humor) during its normal circulation through anterior, posterior and vitreous chambers. The vitreous body is particularly adherent to the retina in the region of the ora serrata and at the optic disc. On its anterior surface is a broad shallow depression, the *patellar fossa,* which accommodates the posterior convexity of the lens. Through its axis, from the optic disc to the patellar fossa, runs the *hyaloid canal,* which marks the site of the fetal hyaloid artery. In electron micrographs, the vitreous body appears to have a dispersed collagenous fibrillar structure. The peripheral condensation of the vitreous body seen in such sections is like a basement membrane, particularly adjacent to the lens and neural retina.

The Eyelids

The eyelids are essentially movable folds of skin which protect the eye both from injury and from excessive light. Each lid is covered by a thin skin, which on the posterior surface is modified to form a transparent mucous membrane, the *conjunctiva*. This lines the lid as the *palpebral conjunctiva* and is reflected onto the anterior surface of the eye up to the cornea as the *bulbar conjunctiva*. The reflection forms a deep recess known as the *fornix*. The form of the lid is maintained by a tough fibrous *tarsal plate*. In the connective tissue between this and the anterior surface are the palpebral fibers of the *orbicularis oculi muscle*. Associated with the free margin of the lid are the *eyelashes* and certain small glands (Fig. 22-27).

The upper and lower lid are similar in all main respects. The skin is very thin. It is provided with many fine downy hairs, with which are associated small sebaceous glands. Numerous small sweat glands and pigment cells are also present. The subcutaneous layer is a loose connective tissue, rich in elastic fibers but containing no fat. It is loosely adherent to the underlying muscle.

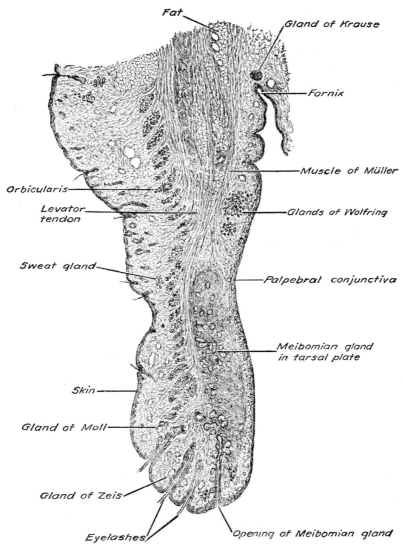

Fig. 22-27. Vertical section through human upper lid.

The *orbicularis oculi* is a thin oval sheet of skeletal muscle which covers the lids. It is innervated by the facial nerve and its action is to close the eye by bringing the lids together. The muscle bundles are disposed concentrically and are loosely united to the underlying tarsal plate by the submuscular connective tissue. Tendon fibers of the *superior levator palpebrae* muscle pass through the latter tissue either to insert on the lower anterior surface of the tarsal plate or to attach to the skin of the lid. This muscle acts to raise the lid.

The *tarsal plate,* or *tarsus,* is a curved plate of dense fibrous connective tissue with some elastic fibers. Its lower free border extends to the lid margin and its upper border serves for attachment of the involuntary *superior palpebral muscle* (muscle of Müller). Embedded in the tarsal plate are a number of simple branched alveolar glands, the *tarsal* or *Meibomian glands.* These sebaceous glands are arranged in a single row with their long axes perpendicular to the lid margin.

Each Meibomian gland consists of a long straight central duct surrounded by numerous alveoli which open into it. The ducts are lined by simple cuboidal epithelium and open onto the lid margin by a series of minute orifices. The fatty secretion of these glands lubricates the edges of the lids, preventing them from sticking together and also helping to form a water-tight seal when the lids are closed.

In the lid margin are the eyelashes, arranged in two or three irregular rows. They are short heavy curved hairs. Their follicles extend obliquely up to the tarsal plate and show the structure typical of hair follicles elsewhere in the body, with the exception that they lack arrector muscles. The large sebaceous glands associated with them are known as the *glands of Zeiss.* Between the follicles are large spiral sweat glands, the *glands of Moll.*

The conjunctiva consists of an epithelium and a connective tissue substantia propria. At the lid margin, the epithelium has the stratified squamous character of the epidermis with which it is continuous. Over the tarsal plates (palpebral conjunctiva), it becomes reduced to two layers of cells; the surface cells are tall columnar and the deeper ones, low cuboidal. In the region of the fornix a third layer of cells appears. Toward the limbus, the epithelium of the bulbar conjunctiva gradually increases in thickness, the superficial cells becoming flatter and the deep cells more cuboidal. At the limbus it is again stratified squamous. Throughout the conjunctiva, but particularly in the fornix and bulbar region, goblet cells occur in the epithelium.

The substantia propria consists of a thin layer of fine connective tissue fibers in which a profuse infiltration of lymphocytes occurs. This is especially marked in the region between the upper border of the tarsal plate and the fornix. Over the tarsal plate, the substantia propria firmly anchors the epithelium; elsewhere, it merges with the richly elastic subconjunctival connective tissue.

In the subconjunctival tissue above the upper border of the tarsal plate are several small tubuloalveolar glands, the *glands of Wolfring.* Their ducts open on the surface of the conjunctiva.

The *glands of Krause* are small accessory lacrimal glands which lie in the loose connective tissue beneath the fornix conjunctivae. Their ducts open into the margin of the fornix.

The Lacrimal Glands

The lacrimal gland lies in the superior temporal region of the orbit, just within the orbital margin. It is divided into a *superior* and an *inferior lobe,* which are continuous around the lateral horn of the aponeurosis of the levator muscle. It secretes the tears, which empty into the conjunctival sac through 10 or 12 ducts opening just in front of the superior fornix.

The lacrimal gland is a compound tubuloalveolar gland of serous type. It bears considerable resemblance to the parotid gland, differing slightly in that the secretory cells of its terminal alveoli are more columnar in form. Between them and their basal lamina, there are numerous myoepithelial cells (see chapter 16, Fig. 16-61). The smaller excretory ducts are lined by a single layer of cuboidal cells; the larger ducts have a double-layered epithelium.

The stroma consists of loose connective

tissue which blends peripherally with the surrounding structures. In the adult, considerable lymphatic tissue occurs in the stroma.

The Ear

The ear contains a series of receptors specialized for hearing and also for the perception of the position of the head and head movement. The fact that the receptors for these diverse functions are housed within the same organ is not surprising because each employs the same basic cytological mechanism—an epithelial cell surmounted by a group of projections called cell "hairs" (actually modified microvillar and ciliary projections). When these hairs are bent the hair-carrying cell signals nerve fibers contacting its base, and these convey signals to the brain. The simple hair cell may accomplish these diverse functions by three remarkable adaptations: (1) certain of the cells have minute weights positioned near the end of their projecting hairs; *gravity or linear movement* will variously bend these hairs and provide the basis for a series of nerve signals to the brain; (2) certain of the hair cells are surmounted by a gelatinous keel which is displaced by fluid flowing through a narrow channel; by placing such a device in each of three body planes the amount and direction of any *angular movement* of the head can be signaled by the subjacent nerve endings; (3) certain hair cells are mounted between two flexible membranes so that sound waves will cause their hairs to bend as one membrane vibrates; the signals sent to the brain from the nerve endings on these cells form the basis for *hearing.*

The special apparatus for each of these types of reception is mounted within fluid-filled spaces deep within the temporal bone (which forms part of the base of the skull). The complex of interconnecting channels containing these receptors is called the *inner ear.* The receptors for position and motion need no access to the external environment, but the mechanism for hearing requires a chamber, the *middle ear,* across which sound waves from the air are transmitted to the fluid spaces of the inner ear. In addition, a channel is required for the passage of sound waves from the external environment to the middle ear; this passageway is part of the *external ear.*

The sound waves collected by the external ear produce vibrations of the *tympanic membrane,* also known as the *ear drum* (Figs. 22-28 and 22-29). The latter forms the outer wall of the *tympanic cavity,* which, with the *auditory (Eustachian) tube,* comprises the middle ear. The tympanic cavity contains the *auditory ossicles* (ear bones) with which two small muscles are associated. By movement of the ossicles, vibrations produced by the sound waves reach the inner ear. The inner ear consists of a complex of fluid-filled membranous chambers and canals known as the *membranous labyrinth* (Fig. 22-30), in turn suspended within a fluid-filled cavity lined by layers of particularly hard bone, the *osseous labyrinth.* The osseous labyrinth of the inner ear is in contact with the middle ear by two small membrane-covered apertures known, respectively, as the *oval window* and the *round window* (Figs. 22-28 and 22-29). The membrane of the former houses the base of the stapes; the membrane of the latter is known as the *secondary tympanic membrane.*

Localized areas of neuroepithelium in the membranous labyrinth comprise the sensory mechanisms discussed above. These areas are supplied by the eighth cranial nerve and they are described subsequently under "Innervation of the Organ of Corti."

The membranous labyrinth is an evolutionary derivation of the anterior parts of a much simpler and superficial segmented system of vibratory sensing organs known in lower swimming vertebrates as the *lateral line system.* Concurrently, the middle ear ossicles have evolved from some of the articulating bones of more primitive jaws. This evolution is reflected in the patterns of embryonic development of the mammalian ear, a pattern which also helps to clarify the adult morphology.

The membranous labyrinth is an ectodermal, epithelial component derived embryonically as an invaginating mesenchyme-surrounded saccule from a surface placode. Through a series of outgrowths, constrictions and coilings it is shaped into its delicate *saccular* and *macular* parts plus

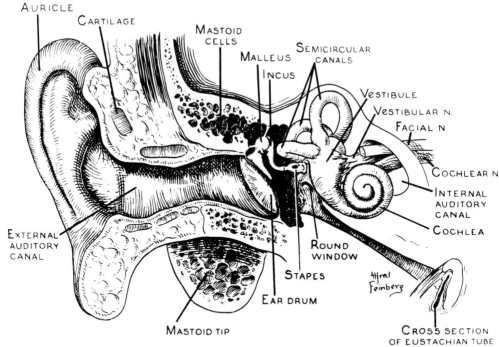

Fig. 22-28. Diagram of the external ear (extending from the auricle to the eardrum), the middle ear (containing the malleus, incus and stapes and communicating with the pharynx via the Eustachian tube) and the inner ear (formed by the three semicircular canals, the vestibule and the cochlea). The nerve signals arising from the inner ear travel to the brain via the cochlear and vestibular divisions of the eighth cranial nerve. (From Davis, H. (editor) Hearing and Deafness: A Guide for Laymen. Holt, Rinehart and Winston, Inc., New York, 1947.)

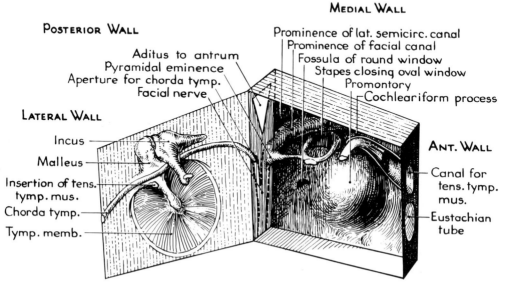

Fig. 22-29. The narrow air-filled cavity of the middle ear shown diagrammatically. The lateral wall of the middle ear is turned back to show its inner face. If the lateral wall were in its normal position, the tensor tympani muscle would attach to the middle part of the malleus and the incus would articulate with the stapes. (From Boies, L. Fundamentals of Otolaryngology, ed. 4. Saunders, Philadelphia, 1964.)

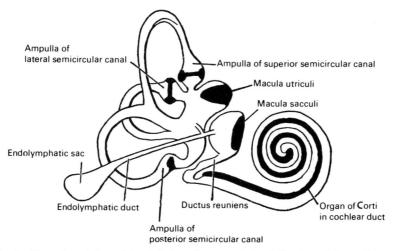

Ampulla of
lateral semicircular canal

Ampulla of superior semicircular canal

Macula utriculi

Macula sacculi

Endolymphatic sac

Endolymphatic duct

Ductus reuniens

Organ of Corti
in cochlear duct

Ampulla of
posterior semicircular canal

Fig. 22-30. Outline of cavities of the left membranous labyrinth viewed from the medial aspect. Receptor regions of the neuroepithelium are sketched in black. (Redrawn from Schaffer.)

three *semicircular canals* and the *cochlea.* Surrounding mesenchyme encases these in a fluid-filled casket of bone, while nearby the three ossicles take form by intramembranous ossification. All this development is occurring in the upper reaches of the first and second branchial arches. The first pharyngeal pouch will also be a major contributor. The rapidly expanding pouch engulfs the region of ossicle formation and extends well beyond, forming the large endodermal epithelium-lined tympanic cavity within the developing temporal bone. The ossicles remain articulated with each other, suspended across the tympanic cavity. Each is left enshrouded with a thin coat of mesenchyme and an endodermal epithelial covering that is continuous with that covering the walls of the cavity. The tympanic cavity similarly overgrows two muscles, the *stapedius* and *tensor tympani,* and a branch of the facial nerve, the *chorda tympani.* Concomitantly, the first branchial groove has deepened to form the *external auditory meatus.* Its close relationship to the pouch is maintained so that the endodermal lining of the tympanic cavity remains closely adherent to the ectoderm of the meatus (with only scant intervening mesenchyme) in the area of the future *tympanic membrane* (eardrum). After the outermost ossicle, the *malleus,* is positioned on the tympanic surface of the eardrum, and the most medial one, the *stapes,* is

similarly situated on the membrane of the oval window, the adult relationships of the ear have been established.

The External Ear

The external ear consists of the part we see, the *auricle* or *pinna,* plus the *external auditory canal* (meatus). The auricle contains an irregularly shaped plate of elastic cartilage except in the region known as the *lobule.* The skin of the auricle is of thin epidermal type (chapter 13), and it contains numerous hairs and sebaceous glands; the skin of the posterior surface also has some sweat glands.

In its final form, the *external auditory canal* (meatus) is a slightly S-shaped channel leading to the middle ear and separated from the latter by the tympanic membrane. The wall of the outer portion of the canal contains elastic cartilage while that of the inner portion is formed by a part of the temporal bone (Fig. 22-28). Both portions of the canal are lined by skin which is continuous with that of the auricle.

The skin which lines the cartilaginous portion of the auditory canal contains stiff hairs which guard against the entrance of foreign objects. It also contains sebaceous glands associated with the hairs. Simple coiled tubular glands are present and these open directly to the surface of the skin by long narrow ducts; these are known as *cer-*

uminous glands because they contribute to the ear wax, or *cerumen,* which consists of secretion from both types of glands plus desquamated epithelial cells. The cells of the ceruminous glands are columnar in shape and they contain numerous brown pigment granules and fat droplets.

The skin of the bony portion of the auditory canal is thinner than that of the cartilaginous portion and it adheres closely to the periosteum. The hairs of this portion are fine; they and the sebaceous glands are present only on the superior wall of the canal.

The Middle Ear

The middle ear consists of an extensive air-filled space in the temporal bone known as the *tympanic cavity;* this cavity is ventilated by the *auditory* (Eustachian) *tube* which, as a remnant of the first pouch, leads to the pharynx. The tympanic cavity is a laterally compressed chamber composed of the middle ear proper, the *atrium,* and an *epitympanic recess,* the *attic,* which lies above the level of the tympanic membrane. The cavity is continuous posteriorly, via the *tympanic antrum* with the *mastoid cells* which are air-filled spaces in the mastoid process of the temporal bone.

The lateral wall of the middle ear cavity is formed almost entirely by the *tympanic membrane.* The periphery of the membrane is fixed firmly by fibrocartilage in a groove (the *tympanic sulcus*) in the surrounding bony ring. Superiorly, the bony ring is notched, so that a small area of the membrane remains lax. This is the *pars flaccida;* the remaining and greater part of the membrane is the *pars tensa.*

The bone-supported inner wall of the middle ear cavity bears a rounded eminence, the *promontory,* which marks the position of the first, or basal, coil of the underlying cochlea. Somewhat above and behind this is an oval aperture, the *oval window* onto the membrane of which fits the base of the stapes. Behind and below the promontory is a funnel-shaped recess which leads to a second aperture in the bone, *the round window* which is closed by the thin *secondary tympanic membrane.*

Extending across the tympanic cavity is the chain of three small bones, the *auditory ossicles* (Fig. 22-29). These, from without inward, are the *malleus* (hammer), the *incus* (anvil) and the *stapes* (stirrup). The *manubrium* (handle) of the malleus is firmly attached to the tympanic membrane. The head of the malleus lies in the epitympanic recess, where it articulates with the head of the incus. The long process of the latter bends sharply near its end to articulate with the head of the stapes. The base of the stapes is firmly fixed to the border of the oval window by a ring of elastic fibers.

Associated with the auditory ossicles are several ligaments and two small muscles, the *tensor tympani* and *stapedius* muscles.

Lining the tympanic cavity, and investing all the structures contained within, is a mucous membrane, the *tympanic mucosa.* This consists of a thin connective tissue layer covered in part by simple squamous epithelium and in part by pseudostratified epithelium which is composed of ciliated columnar cells interspersed with secretory cells. The secretory portion of this epithelium is thought to be the source of fluid in middle ear infections; the ciliated cells may play a part in removal of this fluid. This mucosa forms the linings of the tympanic antrum and the air-filled spaces of the mastoid bone and covers the inner surface of the tympanic membrane.

The *tympanic membrane* is a thin, rather rigid, semitransparent structure in which three layers can be distinguished. The outer cutaneous layer is composed of very thin skin in which the epithelium is reduced to a thin stratum germinativum and a thin stratum corneum. The inner layer consists of a single layer of squamous epithelial cells on a sparse lamina propria. Between the two surface membranes is the substantia propria, which forms the main mass of the tympanic membrane. It consists of two layers of tendon-like collagenous fiber bundles. The fibers of the outer layer are disposed in a radial manner from the manubrium of the malleus outward to the fibrocartilaginous ring. The inner fibers course in a circular direction and are most numerous near the periphery. Both layers are lacking in the upper, pars flaccida portion of the membrane.

The auditory ossicles, malleus, incus and stapes, are composed of compact bone with interstitial lamellae interspersed with osteons. Their articular surfaces are covered by a thin layer of hyaline cartilage and the bases of the stapes, manubrium and malleus have patches of hyaline cartilage. The stapes alone contains a marrow cavity.

The *tensor tympani* and the *stapedius muscles* contain striated skeletal muscle. The tensor tympani lies in a canal just above the auditory tube and it ends in a tendon which is inserted into the upper end of the malleus. When this muscle contracts, it draws the malleus inward and thus tenses the tympanic membrane. It is innervated by the fifth cranial (trigeminal) nerve.

The stapedius muscle lies within a small conical bony projection, the *pyramidal eminence,* on the posterior wall of the tympanic cavity. Its tendon passes through a minute aperture in the summit of the eminance and is inserted into the stapes. It is innervated by the seventh cranial (facial) nerve.

The middle ear serves the important function of amplifying the weak forces of the sound waves that move the eardrum to provide larger force vibrations at the foot plate of the stapes in the oval window. This amplification necessitates no added energy, because the eardrum is about 18 times as large as the opening in the oval window. Therefore, the movements transmitted through the ossicle chain have enough force to move the stapes against the fluid of the inner ear. Thus the eardrum and the membrane covering the oval window move together, their impedance (the amount of resistance to movement) being well-matched.

In addition to allowing impedance matching, the middle ear provides (through its muscular components) an opportunity to adjust the responsiveness of the ossicle chain. It was previously thought that the primary function of the contraction of the tensor tympani and stapedius muscles was to dampen ossicle movement and thus to protect the delicate inner ear structures from excessive vibrations caused by very loud noises. Their contraction is now also thought to play an important role in setting the degree of tension in the tympanic membrane so that transmission of sounds of moderate intensity through the middle ear is facilitated, to improve hearing in a noisy environment and to prevent us from hearing our own voices too loudly.

The *auditory (Eustachian) tube* is a flattened canal leading from the anterior wall of the tympanic cavity to the nasopharynx (Fig. 22-28). In its upper extent, near the middle ear, it is surrounded by a bony wall. Below this osseous part, the reinforcing wall is formed partly by a cartilaginous plate and partly by fibrous connective tissue.

In cross section, the cartilage is shaped like a hook and forms the wall of the posterior surface, the upper margin and the superior portion of the anterior surface of the canal. The remainder of the wall is supported by the fibrous connective tissue. At its upper end, the cartilage is of the hyaline variety. In its lower portion, patches of elastic fibers occur in the matrix.

The mucosa which lines the auditory tube consists of a connective tissue lamina propria covered by ciliated columnar epithelium. In the bony part, the mucosa is thin and firmly united to the underlying bony wall. The epithelium is a low ciliated columnar type. In the cartilaginous part of the tube, the mucosa is loose and the epithelium is of the pseudostratified ciliated variety. Goblet cells occur near the pharyngeal opening, as well as tubuloacinar mucous glands.

The auditory tube serves as a means of ventilating the middle ear. Normally collapsed, the tube is opened during chewing and swallowing to allow pressure equilibration between throat and middle ear. Unfortunately, it also serves as a route for the spread of infection between these two regions.

The Internal Ear

The internal ear is contained in the petrous part of the temporal bone and consists of an interconnected series of bony-walled chambers and passages containing similarly shaped membraneous sacs and canals (Figs. 22-28 and 22-33). These are known as the *osseous labyrinth* and the *membranous labyrinth,* respectively. Intervening between the two is a space, the *perilymphatic* space (actually a highly fluid connective tissue space) which contains the fluid *peri-lymph*. Within the membranous labyrinth there is also a fuid, the *endolymph*.

The Osseous Labyrinth. Although the osseous labyrinth is not a separate entity, its bony wall is harder than that of the surrounding bone from which it can be freed by careful dissection. Seen thus, it consists of an ovoid central chamber, the *vestibule*, from which are given off the three *semicircular canals* and the *cochlea*.

The osseous vestibule of the inner ear is separated from the osseous middle ear by a plate of bone which is pierced by the *oval window* and the *round window*. A narrow canal that extends from the vestibule to the posterior surface of the petrous portion of the temporal bone is known as the *ves-tibular aqueduct*, and it houses the mem-branous endolymphatic duct (Fig. 22-30).

The three osseous semicircular canals are arranged with their respective planes per-pendicular to each other. Thus, there are two *vertical canals* and one *horizontal canal*. The two vertical ones are *superior* (anterior) and *inferior* (posterior) canals; the horizontal one is known as the *lateral*, or external canal. The lateral canals of the two sides lie in the same horizontal plane. The orientation of the vertical canals is such that the plane of the superior canal on one side is approximately parallel to the plane of the inferior canal of the opposite side. Just after leaving the vestibule, each canal has a dilation known as the *ampulla*.

The central chamber of the osseous ves-tibule of each ear is continuous anteriorly with a spiral cavity which constitutes the bony *cochlea*. The latter is a spiral chamber which houses the *organ of Corti* (Fig. 22-30). In man, the apex of the cochlear canal is directed forward, outward and downward (Fig. 22-33).

The Membranous Labyrinth. The *membranous labyrinth* consists of a con-nected series of sacs and canals whose walls are formed of a fibrous connective tissue lined internally by simple squamous epithe-lium of ectodermal origin. In general, the membranous labyrinth has the same form as the osseous labyrinth in which it is con-tained. However, that part enclosed within the osseous vestibule is divided into two

sacs (compare Figs. 22-28 and 22-30). The larger of these, the *utricle*, is an elliptical sac from which are given off the membra-nous semicircular canals. In front of the utricle is the smaller spherical *saccule* which connects by a short and narrow canal, the *ductus reuniens*, with the mem-branous cochlea, *cochlear duct*. The utricle and the saccule are connected by the *utri-culosaccular duct*, the two parts of which converge and continue backward through the vestibular aqueduct as the slender *en-dolymphatic duct*. Under the dura of the posterior surface of the temporal bone, this duct terminates in a blind enlargement, the *endolymphatic sac* (Fig. 22-30).

The membranous labyrinth only par-tially fills the space within the osseous lab-yrinth. At places, it lies close to the perios-teum of the osseous wall, with which its connective tissue layer then blends. For the most part, however, it lies suspended in the perilymph by a number of connective tissue trabeculae which pass from the periosteum to the membranous wall.

In certain definite regions, the wall of the membranous labyrinth is considerably modified to form the true sensory areas. In these areas, the epithelium takes on a spe-cial complexity and among its cells the fi-bers of the vestibulocochlear (eighth cra-nial) nerve terminate. There are six such neuroepithelial areas in each labyrinth: one in each macula, the *macula utriculi* and the *macula sacculi;* one in each ampulla, the *cristae ampullares;* and one in the cochlear duct, the *organ of Corti* (Fig. 22-30). The maculae and cristae ampullares (concerned with position and motion sense) are within the vestibule of the osseous lab-yrinth and are supplied by the vestibular portion of the eighth nerve; the organ of Corti (concerned with hearing) is located in the cochlea and is supplied by the coch-lear division of the eighth nerve.

The Vestibule. The *maculae* represent local thickenings of the membranous walls, each covering an area about 3 mm by 2 mm in extent and forming an elevation into the endolymphatic space. The epithelium is columnar in type and is composed of *supporting* (sustenacular) cells and *hair cells* (Fig. 22-31).

The supporting cells are tall columnar

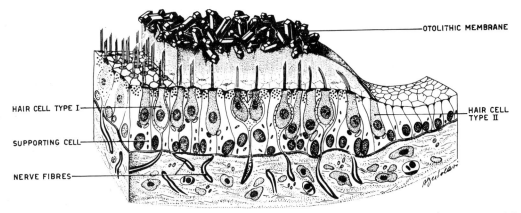

Fig. 22-31. Schematic drawing of the macula, as found either in the saccule or in the utricle of the vestibule. (From Iurato, S. Submicroscopic Structure of the Inner Ear, p. 18. Pergamon Press, New York, 1967.)

elements with their bases resting on the basal lamina and with their apical portions extending to the lumen and forming a support for the hair cells. Their lateral borders are irregular and difficult to follow in sections. The nuclei are oval in shape, and they stain rather densely (Fig. 22-31). Electron micrographs show that the cytoplasm contains the usual organelles plus numerous "secretory" granules and an abundance of microtubules. The latter join a dense terminal web (Fig. 22-32). The function of these cells, other than for physical support for the hair cells, is not well understood. At the edge of the macula, the supporting cells show a gradual transition into the simple squamous epithelium characteristic of the remainder of the membranous labyrinth.

The hair cells occupy the outer part of the epithelium. Two types have been described (Fig. 22-32). The first is a flask-shaped cell embraced over its entire inferior aspect by a single large nerve terminal. The second is a cylindrical cell contacted by a series of nerve endings only around its base. Some of these nerve endings are thought to receive signals from the hair cell while others deliver signals from the brain to the hair cell. Both the afferent and efferent nerve fibers belong to the vestibular branch of the eighth cranial nerve and both types are myelinated. They lose their myelin in the lamina propria, just prior to contacting the hair cells (Fig. 22-32).

In the apical portion of each hair cell,

there is a dense terminal web which is usually described as a *cuticular plate* (Fig. 22-32). Extending from this region, there are long tapering processes composed of bundles of nonmotile projections (called *sterocilia*) and one conventional cilium (a *kinocilium*). The latter has nine doublets of microtubules like ordinary cilia. The sterocilia are arranged in regular hexagonal patterns and they extend outward from the epithelium for 20 to 25 μm to penetrate a peculiar deposit which covers the surface of the macula.

This deposit, the *otolithic "membrane,"* consists of a gelatinous substance containing a great number of small bodies—the *otoconia* or *otoliths* (Fig. 22-31). The otoconia are minute crystals composed chiefly of calcium carbonate.

The hair cells are thought to alter their resting potential when their hairs are bent by the action of linear movement or of gravity on the overlying otolithic membrane. By an unknown mechanism this causes the generation of an action potential in the underlying nerve endings. This cytological mechanism provides the brain with information both on the position of the head in space and on linear head movements.

Each *semicircular canal* forms an arc which is slightly more than a semicircle. It does not occupy the center of the osseous canal but lies against the periosteum of the outer border to which it is attached (Fig. 22-33). Connective tissue trabeculae from

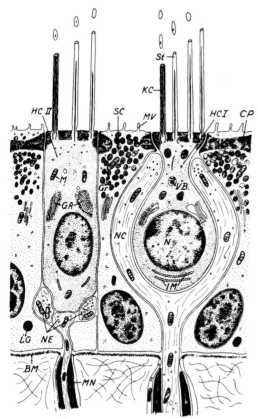

Fig. 22-32. This schematic drawing represents a section through the specialized sensory epithelium found in the maculae of the saccule and utricle and in the crista ampullaris of each semicircular canal. *HC I,* hair cell of type *I; HC II,* hair cell of type II; *SC,* supporting cell; *St,* stereocilia; *kc,* kinocilia; *N,* nucleus; *GA,* Golgi apparatus; *IM,* intracellular membranes; *VB,* multivesicular body; *NC,* nerve calyx; *CP,* cuticular plate; *M,* mitochondrion; *NE,* nerve endings both afferent and efferent; *BM,* basement membrane; *MN,* myelinated nerve fiber; *LG,* lipid granule; *MV,* microvilli. (From J. Wersall Acta Otolaryngol. (suppl. 126:1, 1956.)

the wall of the osseous canal also serve to anchor it in the perilymphatic space.

The histological structure of the canals does not vary essentially from that described for the remainder of the membranous labyrinth. Certain special features are present, however, in the structure of the cristae ampullares, the sensory areas which are found in each ampulla. Here the membranous wall is thickened to form a ridge, placed transversely to the long axis of the canal. This ridge consists of the connective

tissue tunica propria, containing many nerve fibers and blood vessels, surmounted by a specialized columnar epithelium.

The epithelium of the cristae consists of *sustenacular cells* and *hair cells* that are remarkably similar to those described above for the maculae. In fixed preparations, a rounded and longitudinally striated mass, the *cupula,* is seen over the surface of the cells (Fig. 22-34). This is a gelatinous structure which is separated from the epithelium by a narrow space containing endolymph. The long tapering hairs of the cells pass through this space and penetrate for some distance into the cupula, each hair occupying a narrow canal filled with endolymph. The hairs in the middle of the crista stand perpendicular to its surface, whereas those at the border are inclined toward the median plane of the cupula.

Fibers of the vestibular nerve terminate in the epithelium of the crista in much the same manner as they do in the maculae. The naked axons pierce the basement membrane and form contacts around each of the two types of hair cells similar to those in the maculae.

Because the cupula has a flexible attachment to the crista ampullaris, it can be swayed by the flow of endolymph within the semicircular canals. A change in the speed of rotation of the head will cause a deflection of the cupula in two or more of the semicircular canals resulting in movement of the hairs embedded in its base. The underlying nerve endings are then signaled and the brain thus receives information regarding the speed and direction of rotation of the head.

The Cochlea. The osseous cochlea consists of a conical axis of spongy bone, the *modiolus,* or hub, around which winds a spiral bony canal. This canal in man makes about two and one-half turns and ends at the rounded tip of the cochlea, which is known as the *cupula.* The base of the modiolus forms the bottom of the internal auditory meatus, through which the fibers of the cochlear nerve pass and enter the modiolus (Fig. 22-35). These fibers are processes of the bipolar ganglion cells of the spiral ganglion, which is lodged in the *spiral canal of the modiolus* (Fig. 22-36).

Projecting from the modiolus partly

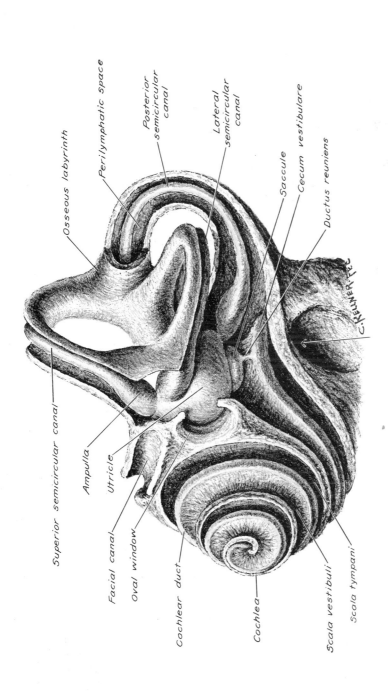

Fig. 22-33. The membranous labyrinth (in yellow) is shown within the channels of the bony labyrinth. The outer and lateral walls of the bony labyrinth have been removed in order to show the membranous labyrinth. Perilymph fills the spaces around the membranous labyrinth; endolymph is within the cavities of the membranous labyrinth. Compare with Figure 22-30. (Based on a model by Tramond but considerably modified.)

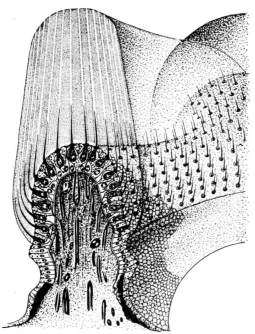

Fig. 22-34. Schematic drawing of one-half of a crista ampullaris, showing innervation of its epithelium. Thick nerve fibers form nerve calyces around type I hair cells at the summit of the crista, medium caliber fibers innervate type I hair cells on the slope of the crista, and medium caliber and fine nerve fibers from a nerve plexus which innervates hair cells of type II. The gelatinous mass surmounting the hair cells is the cupula, which is pushed to and fro by the flow of the endolymph in the semicircular canal. (From J. Wersall Acta Otolaryngol. (suppl.) 126:1, 1956.)

across the osseous canal of the cochlea is a shelf of bone, the *osseous spiral lamina,* which follows the spiral turns of the cochlea and ends at the cupula. Along the outer wall of the canal, opposite the osseous spiral lamina, is a projection of thickened periosteum, the *spiral ligament.* A connective tissue membrane, the *membranous spiral lamina,* bridges the space intervening between the spiral ligament and the osseous spiral lamina. Thus, the osseous canal of the cochlea is divided into two spirally parallel parts, an upper *scala vestibuli* and a lower *scala tympani** (Figs. 22-37 and 22-38).

---

* The terms "upper" and "lower" are here used arbitrarily as if the cochlea were oriented with its base downward and its apex upward. "Inner" and "outer" are used to designate directions with respect to the axis of the cochlea, the modiolus.

From the thickened periosteum covering the upper surface of the osseous spiral lamina, a thin membrane, the *vestibular membrane* (membrane of Reissner), extends obliquely outward to the upper part of the spiral ligament. This membrane forms the roof of a triangular-shaped canal known as the *cochlear duct (scala media).*

The scala vestibuli and scala tympani course parallel with the cochlear duct as outlined above. The scala vestibuli arises in the vestibule and is in close relation to the oval window whereas the scala tympani has its base at the round window; the two communicate directly only at the apex of the cochlea through a small canal known as the *helicotrema.*

The cochlear duct is a narrow tube in which the organ of hearing is located (Fig. 22-30). It is the cochlear portion of the membranous labyrinth. At the apex of the cochlea, its closed end is known as the *cecum cupulare.* The cochlear duct is triangular in transverse section, thus allowing a division of its walls into upper, outer and lower (Figs. 22-37 and 22-38).

The upper or vestibular wall is formed by the vestibular (Reissner's) membrane which consists of a thin central lamina of connective tissue covered on either side by simple squamous epithelium. The epithelium on the upper surface is continuous with a mesenchymal epithelium lining the scala vestibuli whereas on the lower surface, the epithelium is continuous with that of the cochlear duct and is of ectodermal origin.

The outer wall of the cochlear duct is formed by the *spiral ligament,* a thickening of the periosteum which appears triangular in cross section (Figs. 22-36 and 22-37). The outer portion of the ligament, that is, the portion that is adjacent to the osseous wall, is composed of dense fibrous connective tissue while that of the inner portion consists of more loosely arranged connective tissue. The portion of the ligament along the lateral border of the scala media is known as the *stria vascularis* due to the numerous capillaries in its subepithelial connective tissue. The cochlear duct epithelium of this region is relatively thick and is pseudostratified.

The vascular stria is thought to be active in the production of endolymph within the

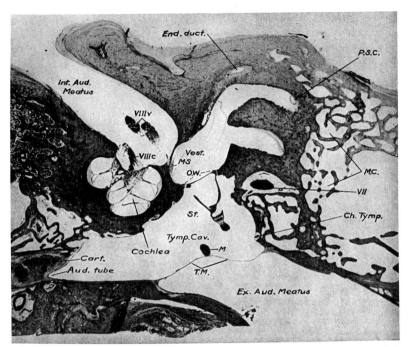

Fig. 22-35. Section through left temporal bone of a man (age 17 years). *Aud. tube,* auditory (Eustachian) tube; *Cart.,* cartilage of auditory tube; *Ch. Tymp.,* chorda tympani nerve; *End. duct,* endolymphatic duct; *Ex. Aud. Meatus,* external auditory meatus; *Int. Aud. Meatus,* internal auditory meatus; *M,* manubrium of malleus; *M.C.,* mastoid air cells; *MS,* macula sacculi; *O.W.,* oval window; *St.,* stapes; *T.M.,* tympanic membrane; *Tymp. Cav.,* tympanic cavity; *Vest.,* vestibule; *VII,* seventh cranial (facial) nerve; *VIIIc,* cochlear division of eighth cranial (auditory) nerve; *VIIIv,* vestibular division of eighth cranial nerve. (Photomicrograph of a section from the collection of Dr. E. P. Fowler, Jr.)

cochlear duct, and in the regulation of ion content. The regulation of ion content is of special interest because the endolymph, unlike extracellular fluids in any other part of the body (and unlike perilymph), has a high potassium (144 mEq/l) and a low sodium (15 mEq/l) content. It thus resembles intracellular fluid. Reabsorption of endolymph may also take place in the stria vascularis (and perhaps also in the endolymphatic sac).

The lower or tympanic wall of the cochlear duct has an extremely complex structure. It is formed by the outer part of the osseous spiral lamina and the whole of the membranous spiral lamina, together with certain special modifications of their epithelial and connective tissue layers.

A thickening of periosteal connective tissue along the upper border of the osseous spiral lamina forms an elevation known as the *limbus* (Figs. 22-35 and 22-36). The limbus has upper and lower projections

known, respectively, as the *vestibular lip* and the *tympanic lip*. They partially enclose a groove, the *internal spiral sulcus* (Figs. 22-37 and 22-38). The connective tissue of the limbus is firm and unusually cellular. Lateral to the point of attachment of the vestibular membrane to the limbus, the latter is covered by columnar epithelium the surface of which bears a cuticular formation continuous with the *tectorial membrane* (Figs. 22-36 and 22-37).

The tympanic lip projects slightly farther outward than the vestibular lip. Its upper surface forms the floor of the internal spiral sulcus and is lined by a single layer of clear flat cuboidal cells, which continue to the vestibular lip as the lining of the sulcus. The lower surface of the tympanic lip is covered by a thin layer of mesenchymal epithelium continuous with that lining the scala tympani.

Continued directly from the tympanic lip is the *basilar membrane,* which extends

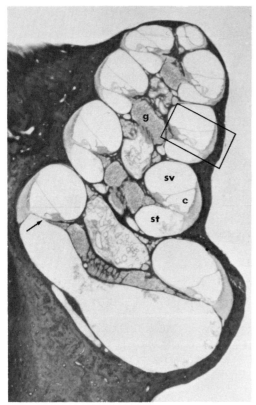

Fig. 22-36. Axial section through the cochlea of a guinea pig. In the spaces of the bony core are the ganglia (*g*), which contain sensory neurons supplying the hair cells of the organ of Corti. The cochlear duct (*c*), scala tympani (*st*) and scale vestibuli (*sv*) are marked in one turn of the cochlea. The area outlined in black is the region depicted in Figure 22-37. In this guinea pig, a portion of the hair cells in the basal turn was damaged before death by exposure to excessive sound. In this region, the hair cells are absent (*arrow*). Note the increasing length of the basilar membrane toward the apex of the cochlea. (Courtesy of Dr. W. Marovitz.)

outward to the *crista basilaris* of the spiral ligament. The basilar membrane consists of fine straight unbranched fibers, the *basilar fibers* or *auditory strings,* embedded in a sparse homogeneous ground substance.

The breadth of the basilar membrane varies in the different turns of the cochlea. It is greatest at the apex, gradually diminishing toward the base until its narrowest extent is reached in the proximal end of the basal coil.

The Organ of Corti. On the upper sur-

face of the basilar membrane, an arrangement of the cochlear duct epithelial cells forms a complex structure which is the sensory part of the organ of hearing. This structure is the spirally disposed *organ of Corti*—the cochlear receptor. The cochlear receptor has three principal components: (1) a framework which supports the receptive hair cells and provides a mechanism for the transformation of acoustic energy into the proper stimulus for the hair cells, (2) the receptor cells themselves, the hair cells, which serve as the transducer of mechanical into electrochemical energy, and (3) the nerve endings which receive signals from the hair cells and provide signals to them.

The organ of Corti extends the entire length of the cochlear duct with the exception of a short distance at either end. The specialized cells which provide the components listed above, are border cells, inner hair cells, inner phalangeal cells, inner and outer pillar cells, outer phalangeal cells (cells of Deiters), outer hair cells and cells of Hensen (Fig. 22-39). The last named are continuous with the cells of Claudius, which extend over the remainder of the basilar membrane to the spiral ligament. All except the hair cells may be considered as sustentacular or supporting cells. The hair cells are intimately related to the endings of the cochlear division of the vestibulocochlear nerve.

The *border cells* are slender columnar elements which rest on the tympanic lip and form a single row along the inner side of the inner hair cells. Their surfaces are provided with a cuticle.

The *inner hair cells* are larger than the outer hair cells, being broader and slightly longer. They form a single row occupying only the upper part of the epithelial layer. The rounded base of each cell rests on the adjacent supporting cells. The surface of this cell has a number of processes (traditionally described as hairs) which are in contact with the tectorial membrane. The processes and numerous other features of the inner hair cells resemble those of the outer hair cells described in more detail below.

The *inner phalangeal cells* are arranged in a row along the inner surface of the inner

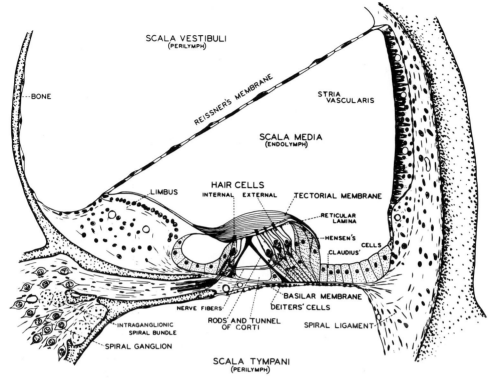

Fig. 22-37. This schematic diagram illustrates the membranous labyrinth as it is considerably modified in the region of the scale media. The drawing was prepared from a section through the lower part of the second turn of the guinea pig cochlea and illustrates the tectorial membrane in its normal position. (From Davis, H., et al. J. Acoust. Soc. Am. 25:1180, 1953.)

pillar cells. Their bases rest on the basilar membrane. The nucleus lies in the lower portion of the cell, which is continued as a slender process to the surface. Here it ends in a small cuticular plate. When viewed from above, this cuticular plate has a shape not unlike that of the phalanges, the finger bones.

The *inner and outer pillar cells* each consist of a broad curved protoplasmic base which contains the nucleus, and an elongated body or pillar which contains a stout bundle of closely packed microtubules. The thickened end of the pillar away from the base is known as the head. Its cytoplasm contains a dense "cuticular plate" into which the microtubules are attached. The head of the outer pillar presents a convexity on its inner side, which fits into a corresponding concavity on the head of the inner pillar, the heads of opposite pillars thus "articulating" with each other. From their articulation, the pillars diverge, so that

their bases, which rest on the basilar membrane, are widely separated. There are thus formed by the pillars a series of arches which enclose a triangular canal, the *inner tunnel* or Corti's tunnel (Fig. 22-39). This is crossed by delicate nerve fibers.

The *outer phalangeal cells* (*cells of Deiters*) are the supporting elements for the outer hair cells, one for each cell. Like the hair cells, therefore, their number varies in different regions of the cochlear duct. They form three rows in the basal coil, four in the middle coil and five in the apical coil. Between the innermost of the outer phalangeal cells and the outer pillar there is a space, the *space of Nuel*.

Each outer phalangeal cell is an elongated element with its basal portion resting on the basal lamina and its slender apical portion extending between the hair cells. The nucleus is rounded and is located within the basal portion of the cell (Fig. 22-39). Each phalangeal cell has a facet

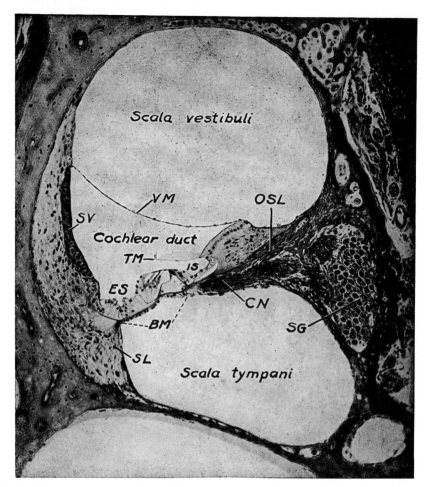

Fig. 22-38. Photomicrograph of a radial section through basal turn of cochlea of the guinea pig. *BM*, basilar membrane; *CN*, cochlear nerve; *ES*, external spiral sulcus; *IS*, internal spiral sulcus; *OSL*, osseous spiral lamina; *SG*, spiral ganglion; *SL*, spiral ligament; *SV*, stria vascularis; *TM*, tectorial membrane; *VM*, vestibular (Reissner's) membrane.

in its lateral wall which supports the base of the neighboring hair cell.

The cytoplasm of each phalangeal cell contains bundles of microtubules which divide into two groups at the level of the neighboring hair cells. One group of microtubules terminates in the cup-shaped facet which houses the hair cell and the other group continues to the surface where it spreads out into a flat "cuticular plate." Adjacent plates interdigitate and are collectively known as the *reticular lamina* (Fig. 22-39). The cuticular plates of each row of phalangeal cells interdigitate with those of the next row and also with the outer ends of the hair cells.

The *outer hair cells* are columnar in

shape and their apical surfaces bear a number of short sensory hairs which are in contact with the tectorial membrane. The base of each cell, supported by a phalangeal cell, contains the nucleus and a granular cytoplasm that stains more deeply than that of the remainder of the cell.

Electron micrographs show that the hairs are straight projecting rods surrounded by a typical plasma membrane (Fig. 22-40). Internally the hair contains longitudinally arranged filamentous material similar to that which constitutes the cuticular plate. Electron micrographs also show that the lateral border of the apical end of the hair cell is in contact with the apical end of its supporting cells by occluding junctions

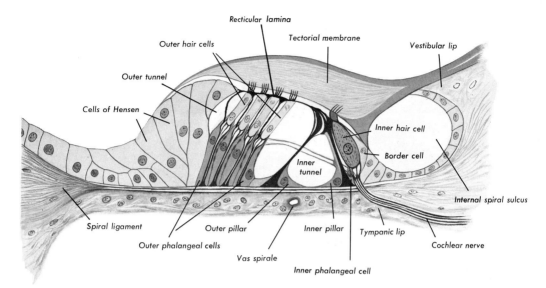

Fig. 22-39. Idealized diagram of a section through the human organ of Corti (from the upper end of the first coil). Note the position of the tectorial membrane; it is rarely preserved in this position in histological sections. (Redrawn and modified from Held, with assistance from Dr. E. P. Fowler, Jr.)

(Fig. 22-40) which separate endolymph from perilymph. In freeze-fracture images, these tight junctions resemble those seen between the apical ends of neighboring epithelial cells in a number of other locations.

Electron micrographs of freeze-fracture preparations of the cochlea show specializations of the hair cells not only at the apical and basal regions but also show special patterns of particles on the cytoplasmic faces of the nonjunctional, lateral borders of the hair cells. These findings strengthen the view that the inner and outer hair cells differ in their functions, and they also suggest that the nonjunctional portions of the membranes play an important role in transduction.

The hairs project from the surface in a regular pattern, with three rows forming a W- (or in some mammals a V-) shape facing the modiolus (Fig. 22-41). The hairs are in contact with, but apparently not firmly embedded in, the tectorial membrane. The number of outer hair cells varies; there are three rows in the basal coil of the cochlea (Fig. 22-41), four rows in the upper end of the basal coil and in the middle coil and five rows in the apical coil.

The *cells of Hensen* are tall columnar elements which form the outer border cells of the organ of Corti. They are arranged in several rows on the basilar membrane lateral to the outer phalangeal cells. The base of each cell is narrower than its upper part, which contains the nucleus. The outer cells decrease in height and pass into the cells of Claudius. The space between the outer phalangeal cells and the cells of Hensen is known as the *outer tunnel.*

The *cells of Claudius* are cuboidal in shape and have a clear cytoplasm. They line the outermost portion of the basilar membrane.

The cuticular plates of the sustentacular cells collectively form the *lamina reticularis.* It covers the organ of Corti and in surface view appears as a mosaic pierced by regularly arranged rows of holes into which the heads of the hair cells are inserted (Fig. 22-41).

The *tectorial membrane* consists of extracellular material that is continuous with the cuticle-like covering of the columnar cells of the limbus region of the cochlea (Fig. 22-37). It is apparently formed by certain connective tissue cells of the limbus region. After extending over the limbus region it becomes thickened into a striated gelatinous structure which overhangs the internal spiral sulcus and extends outward

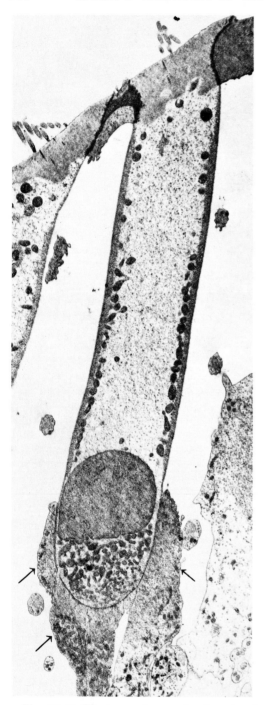

Fig. 22-40. Electron micrograph of parts of two of the outer hair cells from the organ of Corti of the chinchilla. One of the hair cells is shown in its entirety. At its base, this cell contains a nucleus and numerous mitochondria and receives several nerve endings (*lower arrows*). The middle portion is relatively empty. The apical portion is closely associated with sur-

as far as the cells of Hensen. The upper surface is more convex than the lower one.

The tectorial membrane is particularly susceptible to distortion from the action of fixing reagents. Therefore, it is usually shrunken and separated from the processes of the hair cells in fixed preparations. In the living condition it is in contact with the processes of the hair cells and the processes of these cells are stimulated by movements of the tectorial membrane which are related to vibrations in the endolymph (see below).

The organ of Corti is innervated by the cochlear division of the auditory nerve which enters the axis of the modiolus from the internal auditory meatus and divides into a number of branches. From these, numerous fibers radiate to the osseous spiral lamina, in the base of which they enter the *spiral ganglion* (Fig. 22-37).

The cells of the spiral ganglion are peculiar, in that while of the same general type as the spinal ganglion cell, they maintain their embryonic bipolar condition throughout life. Their central processes follow their course through the modiolus and thence through the internal auditory meatus to their terminal nuclei in the medulla. Their peripheral processes also become myelinated and pass outward in bundles in the osseous spiral lamina. From these are given off branches which enter the tympanic lip of the limbus, where they lose their myelin and pass through the *foramina nervosa* (minute apertures in the tympanic lip) to their terminations in the organ of Corti. In the latter, the fibers run in three bundles parallel to the inner tunnel. One bundle lies just inside the inner pillar beneath the row of inner hair cells (Fig. 22-39). A second bundle runs in the tunnel to the outer side of the inner pillar. The third bundle crosses the inner tunnel (*tunnel fibers*) and turns at right angles to course between the outer phalangeal cells. From all of these bundles of fibers, delicate terminal fibers are given off which end in branching telodendria around the bases of the hair cells.

rounding cuticular plates. Note the extensive extracellular space between hair cells and the apical portions of the outer phalangeal cells. ×3500. (From C. Smith Advan. Sci. 24:419, 1968.)

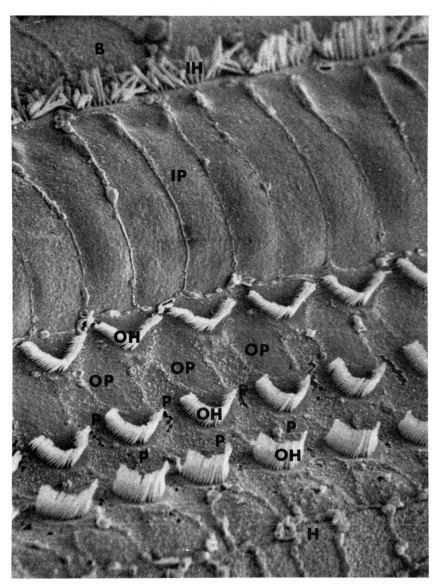

Fig. 22-41. Scanning electron micrograph showing a surface view of the reticular lamina of a cat's organ of Corti after removal of the tectorial membrane. Three rows of outer hair cells (*OH*) and one row of inner hair cells (*IH*) are visible. Border cells (*B*) and Hensen cell (*H*) apical surfaces are also seen. The interdigitating cuticular plates formed by the apices of inner pillar (*IP*), outer pillar (*OP*) and outer phalangeal (P) cells is well demonstrated in this view. ×2800. (Courtesy of Dr. Masayuki Miyoshi.)

Apparently not all of the nerve fibers serving the hair cells are afferent (transmit impulses from the hair cells). Electron microscopy of the endings around the hair cells (Figs. 22-40 and 22-42) discloses that some harbor large populations of synaptic vesicles. This strongly suggests that they are conveying some form of efferent or feedback (perhaps inhibitory) input to the hair cells, but the functional significance of this finding remains unclear.

Physiology of the Auditory Mechanism

Sound vibrations which impinge upon the tympanic membrane will cause it to vibrate at the same frequency as the incident sound waves. The movement conse-

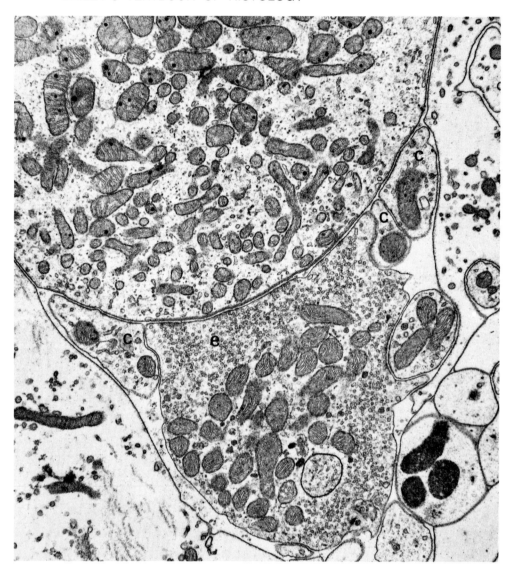

Fig. 22-42. Electron micrograph of the nerve endings on the basal part of the outer hair cell of the chinchilla organ of Corti. One large efferent (*e*) and three small afferent (cochlear) (*c*) nerve endings terminate on the hair cell. Note the large number of mitochondria in this portion of the hair cell. ×31,500. (From Smith, C., and Rasmussen, G., J. Cell Biol. 26:63, 1965.)

quently imparted to the auditory ossicles will serve to move the base of the stapes in and out of the oval window at the same frequency as that of the stimulating sound. Since the fluid perilymph on the other side of the oval window lies in a chamber with rigid bony walls and is itself incompressible, it follows that the inward movement of the stapes will produce a pressure within the perilymph which can be relieved only by a compensating outward movement of the

secondary tympanic membrane covering the round window.

Two avenues for the transfer of this change in pressure are available. It could travel the length of the scala vestibuli and pass by way of the slender helicotrema to the perilymph of the scala tympani, thence to be relieved by the outward bulging of the secondary tympanic membrane of the round window, or it could be transmitted across the vestibular membrane of Reissner to the fluid endolymph of the cochlear duct. This would cause a displacement of the basilar membrane toward the scale tympani; consequently, the pressure is transmitted to the perilymph of the scala tympani and released at the round window. Thus a sound vibration of a given frequency would cause movements of the basilar membrane of equal frequency.

Because the hair cells are held within a framework mounted on the basilar membrane and their hairs are in contact with the overlying tectorial membrane, and because these membranes are "hinged" at different points, movements of the basilar membrane will cause the hairs to bend (Fig. 22-43). This bending constitutes the effective stimulus for the hair cells, with consequent activity which is translated into nerve impulses in the associated nerve fibers.

Although the above may represent a reasonable description of the chain of events resulting in stimulation of the hair cells, it fails to account for the fact that the auditory mechanism is capable of differentiating between vibrations of different frequencies—in other words, pitch or tone. It is known that damage to structures at the base of the cochlea leads to a loss of hearing for high tones and that damage near the apex affects reception of lower tones. Because the length of the basilar membrane is shorter near the base of the cochlea and longer near the apex, it has been assumed that the basilar membrane vibrates in a specific region for different sound frequencies.

It is now known, however, that large regions of the basilar membrane vibrate for all frequencies but that the waves of vibration that travel up the cochlear spiral produce maximum displacement of the membrane at different sites depending on the tone of the incident sound. The lower the frequency of the sound waves, the farther from the oval window the maximum displacement of the basilar membrane occurs. Central nervous system mechanisms then sort out the input signals so that the site of maximum basilar membrane displacement (as well as vibratory patterns in adjacent regions) and thus the pitch and quality of a sound is discerned. The loudness of a tone is thought to be determined by the amount of basilar membrane set into maximum motion. It has also been suggested that the outer hair cells are particularly concerned with determining the intensity of sound and the inner hair cells with pitch discrimination. It should also be recalled that the nerve endings on hair cells are arranged not only for the reception of excitation but also for inhibition. This brings to the organ of Corti central nervous system mechanisms of inhibition for use in providing for pitch and loudness discrimination.

It is well to remember that the total number of hair cells in man is probably less than 20,000. These cells can be damaged or destroyed by sounds of exceptionally high intensity and are not replaced if lost. One cannot lose many cells from the extraordinarily delicate and sensitive organ of Corti without suffering significant hearing loss. The protection of the ear against excessive noise must be taken seriously.

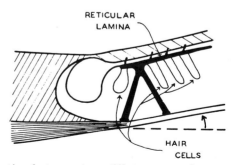

Fig. 22-43. Diagram showing how the shearing action between two stiff structures, the tectorial membrane and the reticular lamina, bends the hairs of the hair cells. (From Davis, H. *In* Physiological Triggers and Discontinuous Rate Processes (Bullock, T., editor). American Physiological Society, Washington, D.C., 1957.)

The Organ of Smell

The sense of smell is perceived in a restricted specialized portion of the mucosa in the upper part of each nasal cavity. This *olfactory mucosa* contains nerve cell bodies which provide the mechanism for olfactory reception on their exposed ends and send an axon from their basal end to the first olfactory way station in the brain—the *olfactory bulb.*

The olfactory mucosa can be distinguished with the naked eye by its brownish-yellow color which contrasts with the reddish tint of the surrounding respiratory mucosa. The epithelium is pseudostratified columnar, and is considerably thicker than that of the respiratory region. The surface cells are of two kinds: sustentacular cells and olfactory cells (Figs. 22-44 and 22-45).

The *sustentacular cells* are the more numerous. Each cell consists of: (1) a superficial portion which is shaped like a stout cylinder and contains pigment and granules arranged in longitudinal rows, (2) a middle portion which contains an oval nucleus and (3) a thin filamentous process which extends from the nuclear portion down between the cells of the deeper layers. The luminal surface of the cell is covered with microvilli. Immediately subjacent to the surface, a series of desmosomes bind the apical portion of the cell to the adjacent olfactory cells.

The *olfactory cells* lie between the sustentacular cells. Their nuclei are spherical, lie at different levels, and most of them are more deeply placed than those of the sustentacular cells. From the nuclear portion of each cell a delicate process extends to the surface, where it is expanded in a minute knob (sometimes called the olfactory vesicle). From this terminal knob several cilia arise, each from a typical basal body. Near their base these are typical cilia, but more distally their long, narrow extensions contain only two microtubules. The cilia do not project vertically but are flattened against the mucosal surface; they are thought to be the portion of the olfactory cell that reacts with odor-producing chemicals. The mucosal surface and the cilia are constantly bathed by the product of special tubular glands (the *glands of Bowman*) which underlie the olfactory mucosa and

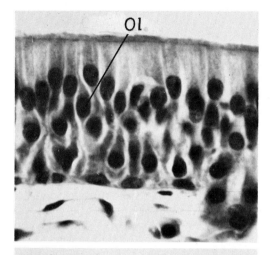

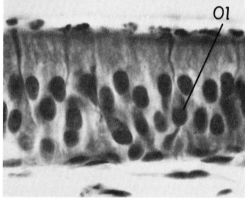

Fig. 22-44. Photomicrographs of the olfactory mucosa showing the olfactory receptor cells (*Ol*) between the sustentacular cells. The *upper figure,* stained with hematoxylin and eoxin, also shows part of a gland of Bowman (*lower right*); the *lower figure* is a silver-stained preparation which demonstrates the bipolar nature of the olfactory neurons. ×1100. (From preparations by Dr. G. Hamlett.)

deliver their products to its surface.

From the opposite pole of the olfactory cell a longer process extends centrally which, as a centripetal nerve fiber of one of the olfactory nerves, passes through the cribriform plate of the ethmoid bone to terminate in the olfactory bulb. The olfactory cell is thus seen to be of the nature of a bipolar ganglion cell with a short peripheral and a longer central process. This is the only example in man of the peripherally placed sensory ganglion cells found in certain lower animals. Between the basal portions of the olfactory cells and the basal

The basement membrane supporting this epithelium is not well-developed. The underlying *stroma* consists of loosely arranged collagenous fibers, delicate elastic fibers and connective tissue cells. Embedded in the stroma are the numberous simple branched tubular glands (mentioned above). Each gland consists of a duct, a body and a fundus. The secreting cells are large and irregular and contain a yellowish pigment which, with that of the sustentacular cells, is responsible for the peculiar color of the olfactory mucosa.

The *olfactory bulb* of man is a small structure relative to the massive cerebral hemispheres; in some lower animals it constitutes a much more substantial portion of the brain. It consists of both gray matter and white matter arranged in six distinct concentric layers. These are (from superficial to deep): (1) the layer of olfactory fibers, (2) the layer of glomeruli, (3) the plexiform layer, (4) the layer of mitral cells, (5) the granule layer and (6) the layer of longitudinal fiber bundles. Through the center of the last named layer runs a band of neuroglia which represents the obliterated lumen of the embryonal lobe.

The layer of olfactory fibers consists of a dense plexiform arrangement of the axons of the above-described olfactory cells. From this layer the axons pass into a layer containing discrete fiber nests, the olfactory glomeruli. Here the olfactory cell axons make contact with the dendritic terminals of the main relay neurons of the bulb, the *mitral cells* and the *tufted cells*. These are large neurons; their axons leave the bulb to form the olfactory tract which carries signals to the central parts of the brain.

This direct relay path is influenced by the presence of several other neurons in the bulb, especially the prominent granule cells. These have cell bodies in the granule cell layer and dendrites extending into the plexiform layer. The *granule cell* is a form of anaxonic interneuron, distinguished by having no definitive axon and both providing and receiving synapses on adjacent regions of its dendritic surfaces (reciprocal synapses). The granule cells are thought to provide inhibitory activity for the initial processing of olfactory information that occurs in the olfactory bulb.

From the above discussion, it is clear

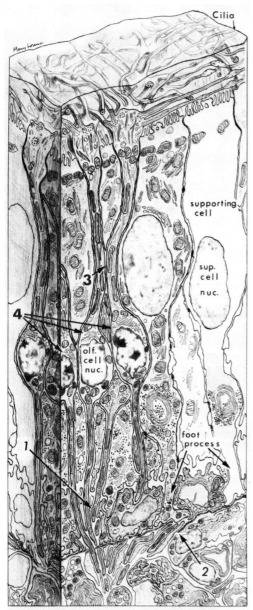

Fig. 22-45. Schematic drawing showing the olfactory mucosa with the sensory cells terminating in apical expansions from which many modified cilia arise and lie on the mucosal surface. The supporting cells are surmounted by microvilli. *1*, axons arising from olfactory neurons; *2*, basement membrane; *3*, apical portion of olfactory neuron; *4*, cell bodies of olfactory neurons. (Drawing by Mary Lorenc, from Frisch, D. Am. J. Anat. 121:87, 1967.)

processes of the sustentacular cells are small irregular cells of unknown function termed *basal cells*.

that the olfactory cells of the nasal mucosa are very much akin to sensory ganglion cells as, for example, in the dorsal root ganglion. These cells have the responsibility to receive chemical stimuli, to provide for transduction to a nervous impulse and to conduct this signal to a region of the central nervous system. The mechanism by which chemicals stimulate the olfactory cells is not known but it is known that effective stimuli must be volatile and must be at least slightly soluble in both water and lipid. Olfactory cells have extraordinary sensitivity; certain substances can be detected at concentrations much lower than those measurable by any method of chemical analysis. The sense of smell is closely related to the sense of taste, discussed below, but of the two, olfaction is by far the more sensitive.

The Organ of Taste

The organ of taste consists of specialized *taste buds* located mainly within the mucosa of the tongue but also within parts of the palate and the pharynx. Taste buds are concentrated in the tongue, especially in the side walls of the circumvallate papillae (Fig. 22-46), in some of the fungiform papillae and in folds (foliate papillae) which occur along the posterolateral margin of the tongue.

The taste bud (Figs. 16-8, 22-46 and 22-47) is an ovoid epithelial structure embedded in the epithelium and connected with the surface by means of a minute canal, called a *taste pore*. In light microscope preparations of well-fixed tissues from laboratory animals, one can distinguish three varieties of cells: (1) a few relatively small cells scattered along the basal and lateral borders of the taste bud, (2) columnar cells with fairly dark staining round or oval nuclei and (3) columnar cells with oval nuclei and light staining cytoplasm. The light cells have been described as the taste receptor elements and the dark cells as supporting (sustentacular) cells although there has been disagreement on this. Electron microscope studies indicate that there are several types of cells which are designated as types I to IV. Type IV is the basal cell of light microscopy and it apparently functions as a stem cell which divides and differentiates

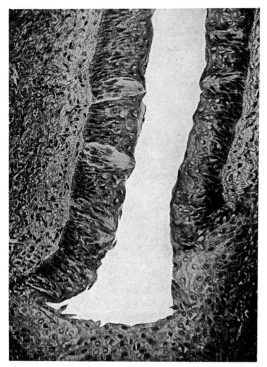

Fig. 22-46. Photomicrograph of a section through trench surrounding circumvallate papilla (human). Several taste buds are shown.

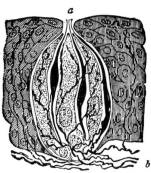

Fig. 22-47. Taste bud from side wall of circumvallate papilla. *a*, taste pore; *b*, nerve fibers, some of which enter the taste bud while others end freely in the surrounding epithelium. (Merkel-Henle.)

into the other categories. Type II is distinguished from type I by the presence of the considerable rough endoplasmic reticulum it is beginning to differentiate. Type III has less rough endoplasmic reticulum and more smooth reticulum and it has microvilli (commonly described as hairs) which project into the taste pore. These types may be merely different developmental or functional stages; the cells have a relatively short life span with a fairly rapid turnover.

In studies on degeneration and regeneration of taste buds in rabbits after transection of the nerves to the taste buds, it has been found that the first degenerative change appears in about 12 hr and that the buds disappear completely within 10 days. However, the taste buds regenerate rapidly after they become reinnervated. The type IV cell (basal cell) apparently survives and serves as a stem cell.

Sensory fibers of the 7th, 9th and 10th cranial nerves end within the taste buds. An efferent, presumably feedback or inhibitory, input to the taste buds has also been reported. Because the sensory nerve endings are found related to more than one cell type, it is not altogether certain which cell or cells may act as the taste receptor and excite the related nerve endings. It is known that different taste buds are specialized for the perception of salty, sweet, sour or bitter tastes, and that these tastes are better perceived on certain parts of the tongue than on others. Substances must be in solution to be tasted, and the amounts required to stimulate sensation are much greater than for the sense of smell. As with many of the other receptors discussed above the acuteness of the sense of taste declines with age.

References

The Eye

ASHTÜN, N., BRINI, A., AND SMITH, R. Anatomical studies of the trabecular meshwork of the normal human eye. Br. J. Ophthalmol. 40:257–282, 1956.

AURELL, G., AND HOLMGREN, H. Metachromatic substance in cornea with special reference to question of its transparency. Nord. Med. 30:1277–1279, 1946.

BOK, D., AND HALL, M. The role of the pigment epithelium in the etiology of inherited retinal dystrophy in the rat. J. Cell. Biol. 49:664–682, 1971.

BOK, D., AND HELLER, J. Transport of retinal from the blood to the retina: an autoradiographic study of the pigment epithelial cell surface receptor for plasma retinal-binding protein. Exp. Eye Res. 22:395–402, 1976.

BOK, D., AND YOUNG, R. W. The renewal of diffusely distributed protein in the outer segments of rods and cones. Vision Res. 12:161–168, 1972.

COHEN, A. I. Vertebrate retinal cells and their organization. Biol. Rev. 38:427–459, 1963.

DAVSON, H. (editor) The Eye, vols. 1–4. Academic Press, New York, 1962.

DEROBERTIS, E. Morphogenesis of the retinal rods; an electron microscope study. J. Biophys. Biochem. Cytol. (suppl.) 2:209–218, 1956.

DETWILER, S. R. Vertebrate Photoreceptors. The Macmillan Company, New York, 1943.

DOWLING, J. E., AND BOYCOTT, B. B. Organization of the primate retina: electron microscopy. Proc. Roy. Soc. London Biol. 166:80–111, 1966.

DOWLING, J. E. The site of visual adaptation. Science 155:273–279, 1967.

DOWLING, J. E. Organization of vertebrate retinas. Invest. Ophthalmal. 9:665–680, 1970.

DUKE-ELDER, S., AND GLOSTER, J. The physiology of the eye and vision. In System of Ophthalmology (Duke-Elder, S., editor), vol. 4. The C. V. Mosby Company, St. Louis, 1968.

DUKE-ELDER, S., AND WYBAR, K. C. The anatomy of the visual system. In System of Ophthalmology (Duke-Elder, S., editor), vol. 2. The C. V. Mosby Company, St. Louis, 1961.

HAY, E. D., AND MEIER, S. Stimulation of corneal differentiation by interaction between cell surface and extracellular matrix. II. Further studies on the nature of transfilter "induction." Dev. Biol. 52:141–157, 1976.

HAY, E. D., AND REVEL, J-P. Fine structure of the developing avian cornea. In Monographs in Developmental Biology, vol. 1. S. Karger, Basel, 1969.

HECHT, S. The nature of the visual process. Harvey Lect., Ser. 33, pp. 35–64, 1938.

HELLER, J., AND BOK, D. Transport of retinal from the blood of the retina: involvement of high molecular weight lipoproteins as intracellular carriers. Exp. Eye Res. 22:403–410, 1976.

JAKUS, M. A. Studies on the cornea. J. Biophys. Biochem. Cytol. (suppl.) 2:243–252, 1956.

JAKUS, M. A. The fine structure of the human cornea. In The Eye (Smelser, G. K., editor), pp. 343–366. Academic Press, New York, 1961.

KRONFELD, P. C. The gross anatomy and embryology of the eye. In The Eye (Dawson, H., editor), vol. 1, pp. 1–62. Academic Press, New York, 1962.

MANN, I. The Development of the Human Eye. Grune & Stratton, Inc., New York, 1950.

MEIER, S., AND HAY, E. D. Stimulation of corneal differentiation by interaction between cell surface and extracellular matrix. I. Morphometric analysis of transfilter "induction." J. Cell. Biol. 66:275–291, 1975.

NOBACK, C. R., AND LAEMLE, L. K. Structural and functional aspects of the visual pathway of primates. In The Primate Brain, Advances in Primatology, vol. 1, pp. 55–81, 1970.

PAPACONSTANTINOU, J. Molecular aspects of lens cell differentiation. Science 156:338–346, 1967.

PAPPAS, G. D., AND SMELSER, G. K. The fine structure of the ciliary epithelium in relation to aqueous humor secretion. In The Structure of the Eye (Smelser, G. K., editor), pp. 453–467. Academic Press, New York, 1961.

POLYAK, S. L. The Retina. University of Chicago Press, Chicago, 1941.

RASMUSSEN, K. E. A morphometric study of the Müller cell cytoplasm in the rat retina. J. Ultastruct. Res. 39:413–429, 1972.

RAVIOLA, E. Intercellular junctions in the outer plexiform layer of the retina. Invest. Ophthalmol. 15:881–895, 1976.

RAVIOLA, E., AND GILULA, N. B. Intramembrane organization of specialized contacts in the outer plexiform layer of the retina. A freeze fracture study in monkeys and rabbits. J. Cell. Biol. 65:192–222, 1975.

RAVIOLA, G. The fine structure of the ciliary zonule and ciliary epithelium. Invest. Ophthalmol. 10:851–869, 1971.

ROHEN, J. W. Das Auge und seine Hilfsorgane. Handb. mikr. Anat. Menschen. (v. Möllendorff, W., and Bargmann, W., editors), vol. 3, part 4. Springer-Verlag, Berlin, 1964.

SALZMANN, M. The Anatomy and Histology of the Human Eyeball in the Normal State. Trans. by E. V. L. Brown. Lippincott, Philadelphia, 1933.

SJOSTRAND, F. A search for the circuitry of directional selectivity and neural adaptation through three-dimensional analysis of the outer plexiform layer of the rabbit retina. J. Ultrastruct. Res. 49:60–156, 1974.

SMELSER, G. K. (editor) The Structure of the Eye. Academic Press, New York, 1961.

TONOSAKI, A., AND KELLY, D. E. Fine structural study of the origin and development of the sphincter pupillae muscle in the West Coast newt (Taricha torosa). Anat. Rec. 170:57–74, 1971.

WALD, G. The molecular organization of visual systems. In Light and Life (McElroy, W. D., and Glass, B., editors), p. 724. The Johns Hopkins Press, Baltimore, 1960.

WALD, G. The receptors of human color vision. Science 145:1007–1016, 1964.

WALLS, G. L. The Vertebrate Eye and Its Adaptive Radiation. Cranbrook Institute of Science, Bloomfield Hills, Mich., 1942.

WALSH, F. B., AND HOYT, W. F. Clinical Neuro-Ophthalmology, ed. 3, Williams & Wilkins, Baltimore, 1969.

WOLFF, E. The Anatomy of the Eye and Orbit, ed. 6, Revised by R. J. Last. Saunders, Philadelphia, 1968.

YOUNG, R. W. Visual cells. Sci. Am. 223:80–91, 1970.

YOUNG, R. W. Visual cells and the concept of renewal. Invest. Ophthalmol. 15:700–725, 1976.

YOUNG, R. W., AND BOK, D. Autoradiographic studies on the metabolism of the retinal pigment epithelium. Invest. Ophthalmol. 9:524–536, 1970.

The Ear

BAST, T. H., AND ANSON, B. J. The Temporal Bone and the Ear. Charles C Thomas, Publisher, Springfield, Ill., 1949.

DAVIS, H. Excitation of auditory receptors. In Handbook of Physiology, sect. 1, vol. 1, pp. 565–584. American Physiological Society, Washington, D.C., 1959.

DEREUCK, A., AND KNIGHT, J. (editors) Hearing Mechanisms in Vertebrates. Little, Brown and Company, Boston, 1968.

ENGSTROM, H. The innervation of the vestibular receptor cells. Acta Otolaryngol. (suppl.) 163:30–41, 1961.

FRIEDMANN, I. The cytology of the ear. Br. Med. Bull. 18:209–213, 1962.

GULLEY, R. L., AND REESE, T. S. Intercellular junctions in the reticular lamina of the organ of Corti. J. Neurocytol. 5:479–507, 1976.

GULLEY, R. L., AND REESE, T. S. Regional speciali-

zations of the hair cells in the organ of Corti. in press, 1977.

GULLEY, R. L., AND REESE, T. S. Freeze-fracture studies on the synapses in the organ of Corti. J. Comp. Neurol. 171:517–544, 1977.

HENTZER, H. Histologic studies of the normal mucosa in the middle ear, mastoid cavities and Eustachian tube. Ann. Otol. Rhin. Laryngol. 79:825–833, 1970.

IURATO, S. (editor) Submicroscopic Structure of the Inner Ear. Pergamon Press, New York, 1967.

JAHNKE, K. The fine structure of freeze-fractured intercellular junctions in the guinea pig inner ear. Acta Otolaryngol. (suppl.) 336:1–40, 1975.

NADOL, J. B., MULROY, M. J., GOODENOUGH, D. A., AND WEISS, T. F. Tight and gap junctions in the vertebrate inner ear. Am. J. Anat. 147:281–302, 1976.

RASMUSSEN, G. L., AND WINDLE, W. F. Neural Mechanisms of the Auditory and Vestibular Systems. Charles C Thomas, Publisher, Springfield, Ill., 1960.

SHAMBAUGH, G. E. Cytology of the internal ear. In Special Cytology, ed. 2 (Cowdry, E. V., editor), vol. 3, pp. 1335–1367. Paul B. Hoeber, Inc., New York, 1932.

SMITH, C. A. Electron microscopy of the inner ear. Ann. Otol. Rhin. Laryngol. 77:629–643, 1968.

V. ILBERG, C., AND VOSTEEN, K.-H. Permeability of the inner ear membranes. Acta Otolaryngol. 67:165–170, 1969.

VON BÉKÉSY, G. Experiments in Hearing. Edited and Translated by E. G. Wever. McGraw-Hill Book Company, New York, 1960.

WERSALL, J. Studies on the structure and innervation of the sensory epithelium of the cristae ampullares in the guinea pig. Acta Otolaryngol. (suppl.) 126:1–85, 1956.

WERSALL, J. Vestibular receptor cells in fish and mammals. Acta Otolaryngol. (suppl.), 163:25–29, 1961.

Organs of Smell and Taste

ARSTILA, A., AND WERSALL, J. The ultrastructure of the olfactory epithelium of the guinea pig. Acta Otolaryngol. 64:187–204, 1967.

BEIDLER, L. M., AND SMALLMAN, R. L. Renewal of cells within taste buds. J. Cell Biol. 27:263–272, 1965.

FRISCH, D. Ultastructure of the mouse olfactory mucosa. Am. J. Anat. 121:87–119, 1967.

FUJIMOTO, S., AND MURRAY, R. G. Fine structure of degeneration and regeneration in denervated rabbit vallate buds. Anat. Rec. 168:393–414, 1970.

KARE, M. R., AND HALPERN, B. P. (editors) Physiological and Behavioral Aspects of Taste. University of Chicago Press, Chicago, 1961.

LANDIS, D. M. D., REESE, T. S., AND RAVIOLA, E. Differences in membrane structure between excitatory and inhibitory components of the reciprocal synapse in the olfactory bulb. J. Comp. Neurol. 155:67–92, 1974.

MURRAY, R. D., AND MURRAY, A. Fine structure of taste buds of rabbit foliate papillae. J. Ultrastruct. Res. 19:327–353, 1967.

OAKLEY, B., AND BENJAMIN, R. M. Neural mechanism of taste. Physiol. Rev. 46:173–211, 1966.

REESE, T. S. Olfactory cilia in the frog. J. Cell Biol. 25:209–230, 1965.

ZOTTERMAN, Y. (editor) Olfaction and Taste. The Macmillan Company, New York, 1963.

Index